ADVANCES in WOUND CARE

Volume 1

2010
Yearbook
of the
WHS
Wound
Healing
Society

ADVANCES in WOUND CARE

Volume I

Translational Medicine:
From Benchtop to Bedside to Community and Back

Editor-in-Chief:
Chandan K. Sen
Director, Comprehensive Wound Center
The Ohio State University Medical Center
Columbus, Ohio

Mary Ann Liebert, Inc. publishers
www.liebertpub.com

Library of Congress Cataloging-in-Publication Data

Translational medicine : from benchtop to bedside to community and back / editor-in-chief, Chandan K. Sen.
p. ; cm. — (Advances in wound care ; v. 1)
Includes bibliographical references and index.
ISBN-13: 978-1-934854-01-3
ISBN-10: 1-934854-01-8
1. Wounds and injuries. I. Sen, Chandan K. II. Series: Advances in wound care ; v. 1.
[DNLM: 1. Wounds and Injuries—therapy. 2. Translational Research. 3. Wounds and Injuries—surgery. WO 700 T772 2010]
RD93.T665 2010
617.1—dc22

2010006903

Cover military photo courtesy of Alexander Stojadinovic.

ISBN: 978-1-934854-01-3

Mary Ann Liebert, Inc.
140 Huguenot Street
New Rochelle, NY 10801

Printed in the United States of America.

CONTENTS

Advances in Wound Care

Evangelos Van Badiavas
University of Miami Miller School of Medicine
Miami, Florida

Robert Bartlett
The Ohio State University
Columbus, Ohio

Damien Bates
Organogenesis, Inc.
Canton Massachusetts

B.M. Bates-Jensen
UCLA
Los Angeles, California

A.C. Beekley
Madigan Army Medical Center
Ft. Lewis, Washington

Adam Belley
The Medicines Company
St-Laurent, Quebec, Canada

Dustin Miguel Bermudez
University of Pennsylvania School of Medicine
Philadelphia, Pennsylvania

François Berthod
Université Laval
Quebec City,
Quebec, Canada

Sabyasachi Biswas
The Ohio State University
Columbus, Ohio

Thomas Bjarnsholt
University of Copenhagen
Copenhagen, Denmark

Adriana Blakaj
Yale University
New Haven, Connecticut

Melodie Blakely
Osceola Regional Medical Center
Kissimmee, Florida

Laura Bolton
UMDNJ
Metuchen, New Jersey

Nancy Boudreau
University of California San Francisco
San Francisco, California

Harold Brem
New York University
New York, New York

George Broughton II
Landstuhl Regional Medical Center
APO, New York

Austin H. Chhoeu
D.D. Eisenhower Army Medical Center
Fort Gordon, Georgia

Pierre-Alain Clavien
University Hospital Zurich
Zurich, Switzerland

Neeltje Coolen
ADBC, Beverwijk
Noord-Holland
The Netherlands

George Coppit
Walter Reed Army Medical Center
Washington, D.C.

Renee Cordrey
The George Washington University
Washington, DC

Ross W. Crawford
Queensland University of Technology
Brisbane, Australia

Tengjiao Cui
University of Miami
Miami, Florida

Stephen C. Davis
University of Miami Miller School of Medicine
Miami, Florida

Marcela Del Rio
CIEMAT-CIBERER
Madrid, Spain

Robert H. Demling
Natick, Massachusetts

Robert F. Diegelmann
VCU Medical Center
Richmond, Virginia

Edward J. Doolin
Children's Hospital of Philadelphia
Philadelphia, Pennsylvania

Scot E. Dowd
Research and Testing Laboratory, Pathogenius Diagnostics
Lubbock, Texas

James Robert Dunne
National Naval Medical Center
Bethesda, Maryland

Christophe Egles
Tufts University School of Dental Medicine
Boston, Massachusetts

William J. Ennis
University of Illinois
Chicago, Illinois

Elof Eriksson
Brigham and Women's Hospital
Boston, Massachusetts

Tim Eubank
The Ohio State University
Columbus, Ohio

Matteo Fabbi
Boston Medical Center
Boston, Massachusetts

Kevin Fitzpatrick
Walter Reed Army Medical Center
Washington, D.C.

Jonathan Agner Forsberg
Walter Reed National Military Medical Center
Washington, D.C.

Jenny Ellen Freeman
JEF Core, Inc.
Weston, Massachusetts

Rollin McCulloch Gallagher
Philadelphia VA Medical Center
Philadelphia, Pennsylvania

Michael Gabriel Galvez
Stanford University School of Medicine
Stanford, California

George D. Garcia
Rockville, Maryland

William V. Giannobile
University of Michigan
Ann Arbor, Michigan

Karen Ann Gibbs
Texas State University
San Marcos, Texas

Nicole S. Gibran
University of Washington
Seattle, Washington

Amos Gilhar
Appaport Faculty of Medicine
Haifa, Israel

Finn Gottrup
Copenhagen Wound Healing Center, Bispebjerg University Hospital
Copenhagen, Denmark

Mikel Gray
University of Virginia
Charlottesville, Virginia

Jianjun Guan
The Ohio State University
Columbus, Ohio

Anandev N. Gurjala
Northwestern Feinberg School of Medicine
Chicago, Illinois

Geoffrey Gurtner
Stanford University
Stanford, California

Rose Hamm
University of Southern California
Los Angeles, California

Patricia Hebda
University of Pittsburgh School of Medicine
Pittsburgh, Pennsylvania

Benjamin J. Herdrich
The University of Pennsylvania School of Medicine
Philadelphia, Pennsylvania

Cathy Thomas Hess
Wound Care Strategies, Inc.
Harrisburg, Pennsylvania

Allen Holloway
Maricopa Medical Center
Phoenix, Arizona

Harriet Hopf
University of Utah
Salt Lake City, Utah

Thomas K. Hunt
University of California
San Francisco, California

Mark Iafrati
Tufts Medical Center
Boston, Massachusetts

Lars-Peter Kamolz
Vienna Burn Centre
Vienna, Austria

Robert M. Kellman
SUNY Upstate Medical University
Syracuse, New York

Sundeep G. Keswani
Cincinnati Children's Hospital Medical Center
Cincinnati, Ohio

Mahmood Khan
The Ohio State University Medical Center
Columbus, Ohio

Sorabh Khandelwal
The Ohio State University
Columbus, Ohio

George Kontakis
University of Crete
Heraklion, Greece

Anastasios V. Korompilias
University of Ioannina Medical School
Ioannina, Greece

Anand Raj Kumar
National Naval Medical Center
Bethesda, Maryland

Periannan Kuppusamy
The Ohio State University
Columbus, Ohio

Lynn Lambert
The Ohio State University Comprehensive Wound Center
Columbus, Ohio

Gerald Lazarus
Johns Hopkins School of Medicine
Baltimore, Maryland

James B. Lutz
Lutz Consulting LLC
Buellton, California

John M. Macdonald
University of Miami
Miami, Florida

Liam C. Macleod
Stanford University
School of Medicine
Stanford, California

Arturo R. Maldonado
Cincinnati Children's Hospital
Medical Center
Cincinnati, Ohio

David J. Margolis
University of Pennsylvania
Philadelphia, Pennsylvania

Clay Marsh
The Ohio State University
Columbus, Ohio

Manuela Martins-Green
University of California
Riverside, California

Jodi McDaniel
The Ohio State University
Columbus, Ohio

W. Scott Melvin
The Ohio State University
Arthur G. James Cancer
Hospital and Research
Institute
Columbus, Ohio

Patricia Mertz
University of Miami Miller
School of Medicine
Miami, Florida

Michael Miller
The Ohio State University
Columbus, Ohio

Gregory Moeck
The Medicines Company
St. Laurent, Quebec, Canada

Nicanor Moldovan
The Ohio State University
Medical Center
Columbus, Ohio

Sean Montgomery
Walter Reed Army Medical
Center
Washington, D.C.

Zena Elizabeth Helen Moore
Royal College of Surgeons
Dublin, Ireland

Lee Mathew Morris
Cincinnati Children's Hospital
Medical Center
Cincinnati, Ohio

Thomas A. Mustoe
Northwestern University
Chicago, Illinois

Lillian Nanney
Vanderbilt School
of Medicine
Nashville, Tennessee

Sean O'Connell
Mt. Sinai School of Medicine/
Englewood Hospital
Morris Plains, New Jersey

James P. O'Gara
Dublin, Ireland

Oluyinka O. Olutoye
Baylor College of Medicine
Houston, Texas

Martin Oudega
University of Pittsburgh
Pittsburgh, Pennsylvania

Narasimham Parinandi
The Ohio State University
Columbus, Ohio

Laura K.S. Parnell
Precision Consulting
Missouri City, Texas

Maurizio Parola
University of Torino
Torino, Italy

Kyle Petersen
Naval Medical Research
Center
Silver Spring, Maryland

Anie Philip
McGill University
Montreal, Quebec, Canada

Donald G. Phinney
Tulane University
New Orleans, Louisiana

Barbara Pieper
Wayne State University
Detroit, Michigan

Michael S. Pinzur
Loyola University Medical
Center
Maywood, Illinois

Heather M. Powell
The Ohio State University
Columbus, Ohio

Glenn D. Prestwich
The University of Utah
Salt Lake City, Utah

Supparerk Prichayudh
Chulalongkorn University
Bangkok, Thailand

Katherine A. Radek
UCSD
San Diego, California

Derren Ready
Eastman Dental Hospital
UCLH NHS Foundation
Trust
London, United Kingdom

Ann Richmond
Vanderbilt University
Nashville, Tennessee

G.L. Rommers
UMC Groningen
Groningen, The Netherlands

Vincent Ronfard
Organogenesis, Inc.
Canton, Massachusetts

Karen Rose
The Ohio State University
Comprehensive Wound Center
Columbus, Ohio

Andreas Rümelin
Johannes Gutenberg–
University Mainz
Mainz, Germany

Richard Edward Schlanger
The Ohio State University
Columbus, Ohio

Susie Seaman
Sharp Rees-Stealy Medical Group
San Diego, California

Heather A. Shankowsky
University of Alberta
Edmonton, Alberta
Canada

Peter Sheehan
New York, New York

Forest R. Sheppard
Naval Medical Research Center
Silver Spring, Maryland

John Sheridan
The Ohio State University
Columbus, Ohio

Braham Shroot
Priority-Derm LLC
Princeton, New Jersey

Vijay A. Singh
Sinai Hospital of Baltimore
Baltimore, Maryland

Lars Tue Sørensen
Bispebjerg Hospital
Copenhagen, Denmark

Barbara K. Sosnowski
Tissue Repair Company
San Diego, California

Scott R. Steele
Madigan Army Medical Center
Fort Lewis, Washington

Steven Steinberg
The Ohio State University
Columbus, Ohio

Kurt S. Stenn
Aderans Research Institute, Inc.
Philadelphia, Pennsylvania

M.G. Stineman
University of Pennsylvania
Philadelphia, Pennsylvania

C. Stuehmer
Hannover Medical School
Hannover, Germany

Karl G. Sylvester
Hagey Laboratory, Stanford
University School of Medicine
Stanford, California

Douglas Tadaki
Naval Medical Research Center
Silver Spring, Maryland

Kenichi Tamama
The Ohio State University
Columbus, Ohio

Bill Tawil
UCLA, Bioengineering
Department
Los Angeles, California

Richard Peter ten Broek
Radboud Medical University
Nijmegen, Gelderland
The Netherlands

Luc Teot
Montpellier University Hospital
Montpellier, France

Stephen R. Thom
University of Pennsylvania
Philadelphia, Pennsylvania

Pankaj Tiwari
The Ohio State University
Comprehensive Wound Center
Columbus, Ohio

Nancy Tomaselli
Cherry Hill, New Jersey

Marjana Tomic-Canic
University of Miami
Miller School of Medicine
Miami, Florida

Chloé Trial
Montpellier University Hospital
Montpellier, France

Tai-Lan Tuan
The Saban Research
Institute of Children's
Hospital Los Angeles
Los Angeles, California

Paul L. Vaughn
Arizona Vascular Surgery
Consultants, P.C.
Mesa, Arizona

Amy Vertrees
Walter Reed Army Medical
Center
Washington, D.C.

Loretta Vileikyte
University of Manchester
Manchester, United Kingdom

Susan Volk
University of Pennsylvania School of Veterinary Medicine Philadelphia, Pennsylvania

Peter J. Weina
Walter Reed Army Institute of Research Silver Spring, Maryland

Alan Wells
University of Pittsburgh Pittsburgh, Pennsylvania

Traci Wilgus
The Ohio State University Columbus, Ohio

Randall Wolcott
Southwest Regional Wound Care Center Lubbock, Texas

Jacqueline Wolfrum
Genzyme Biosurgery Cambridge, Massachusetts

Daniel Wozniak
The Ohio State University Columbus, Ohio

Jacquelyn Youssef
Brown University Providence, Rhode Island

Jonathan Zenilman
Johns Hopkins University Baltimore, Maryland

Min Zhao
UC Davis Davis, California

Karen Zimmerman
New York University New York, New York

PREFACE

Strengthening the Interdisciplinary Continuum of Wound Care

Healing is a matter of time, but it is sometimes also a matter of opportunity

—Hippocrates

The opportunity we attempted to seize in committing to produce this volume was to strengthen the interdisciplinary continuum of wound care. Quantum leaps in wound care can come only from effective synchrony between the numerous disciplines the wound care community represents. Given the numerous clinical as well as basic science disciplines involved in developing the science of wound care, this is not a trivial task, and it calls for a strategic approach. Even for accomplished scientists, staying abreast of the latest developments in wound care is a daunting task. It is almost impossible for wound care professionals to closely monitor relevant scientific developments in such a diverse atmosphere. Thus, there is a fast-growing gap between the frontiers of science and the quality of education and patient care.

Wounds represent a major and escalating public health problem.[1] The Wound Healing Society, founded in 1989, is committed to fostering interaction among scientists, physicians, licensed practitioners, industry representatives, and government agencies, with the final objective of improving the care of those suffering from wounds. In 2009, the Society decided to address an unmet need by initiating its first book series aimed at publishing digest articles that would, in straightforward language and simple format, present the essence of the latest discoveries in the field to the broader wound care community. The first in an annual book series, *Advances in Wound Care* addresses the broader wound care community and serves as a forum for facilitating cross-pollination between disciplines. For the scientist, this volume presents a digest of the clinical aspects of wound care. Such understanding should help improve the translational value of investigator-initiated research. For basic scientists who advance the frontiers of the fundamental sciences of wound healing, this volume should inspire innovative directions. Wound care physicians, nurses, and staff will find the latest discoveries presented in a succinct format. The volume also addresses industry-academia partnership, a key element in motivating inventions and in effectively rolling out novel therapies.

At a time when our nation is fighting multiple wars, we are generating a wealth of information from our battleground experiences. In this opening volume, the spotlight is therefore placed on military wound care. I salute the wound care community of soldiers who contributed to the spotlight section despite their very hectic schedules in a time of war. I am particularly thankful to Dr. Alexander Stojadinovic, COL MIL USA MEDCOM WRAMC, for his help with the spotlight section and book cover.

I extend my sincere thanks to over a hundred volunteers representing different disciplines who gave their time and effort to peer-review chapters of this volume. Special efforts were made to create brief, stylistically uniform chapters that deliver key take-home messages. I hope you enjoy reading this volume as much as I have enjoyed putting the pieces together.

Chandan K. Sen, Editor-in-Chief
Director, The Ohio State University
Comprehensive Wound Center

1. Sen CK, Gordillo GM, Roy S, Kirsner R, Lambert L, Hunt TK, Gottrup F, Gurtner GC and Longaker MT. Human skin wounds: A major and snowballing threat to public health and economy. *Wound Repair & Regeneration* 2009 Nov-Dec;17(6):763–71.

Section 1

Military Wound Care

Section Editors: Alexander Stojadinovic and Eric Elster

War and Medicine: A Brief History of the Military's Contribution to Wound Care Through World War I

George Broughton II[1,*] and David Burris[2]

[1]Department of Plastic and Reconstructive Surgery, Landstuhl Regional Medical Center, Landstuhl, Germany.
[2]Norman M. Rich Department of Surgery, Uniformed Services University of the Health Sciences, Bethesda, Maryland.

As man finds better and efficient ways to kill and maim each other, he also had to learn to care for the survivors. This chapter is a brief history of the military's contribution to wound care from antiquity through World War I.

Abbreviation and Acronym

WWI = World War I

*Correspondence: Col. George Broughton, CMR 402 Box 1812, APO AE 09180 (e-mail: georgebroughton@gmail.com; george.broughton@amedd.army.mil).

"It is only the dead who have seen the end of war"
—*Plato* (428–348 BC)

WHEN MAN DECIDED to use force and violence to satisfy his greed for power and wealth, he also decided that he must find a way to treat and heal his injuries so that he could continue his campaign to possess what he desired or protect what he owned. "Notwendigkeit bringt uns alle Machen bei" (necessity teaches us all things) is a German proverb that succinctly summarizes surgery's birth and rebirth from war. The importance of the modern U.S. Army Medical Department's motto, "maintaining the fighting strength," was appreciated for hundreds of years (but maybe not always in the same spirit). Sixteenth-century French military officers would hire surgeons to work for them on their campaigns. Having a "celebrity" surgeon could be very advantageous for the fighting morale of the troops. Ambroise Paré (1510–1590) is said to be "worth the equivalent of 10,000 soldiers on the battlefield, as the men knew their chances of survival were greatest if he was present."[1]

The military is not responsible for all advancements in wound care, but it certainly has provided plenty of opportunity for many civilian-initiated innovations to be tested. L.F. Pilcher noted in his 1919 American Surgical Association Presidential Address, "The Influence of War Surgery Upon Civil Practice," that during World War I (WWI) 35,000 physicians had joined the military and 14,000 were sent overseas. The surgical experience learned during this time caused significant change in civilian practices of surgical technique and antisepsis.[2] This paper briefly touches the advancements of wound care by the military through WWI.

ANCIENT

Homer's *The Iliad* (800 BC) is considered the first written description of the treatment of a battle wound.[2] King Melelaus (former husband of Helen of Troy), survives after having an arrow removed from his side by Machaon, son of Asclepius (the Greek God of medicine and healing):

> When he [Machaon] saw the wound where the bitter arrow was driven, he

The opinions or assertions contained herein are the private views of the author and are not to be construed as official or as reflecting the views of the Department of the Army or the Department of Defense.

Printed in U.S.A.
DOI: 10.1089/awc.2009.0013

> sucked the blood and in skill laid healing medicines on it that Chiron in friendship long ago had given his father [Asclepius].

Asclepius was the son of Apollo and Coronis. His mother was killed for being unfaithful to Apollo and was laid out on a funeral pyre to be consumed. When the body of Coronis was to be burnt, Apollo, or perhaps Hermes, saves the child from the flames, and carried it to the centaur Chiron, who instructed the boy in the art of healing.[3]

Galen (130 to 200 AD) was court physician to Roman Emperor Marcus Aurelius and a gladiatorial surgeon, and is most notable for his anatomical dissections (Galen's nerve). He wrote that hemorrhage should be treated in one of four ways—applying direct pressure with a finger, twisting the cut end with a hook, grasping the cut end and tying it off, or applying styptics (an example of his mixture was made from frankincense, aloe, egg white-mix to a consistency of honey and add a "pinch" of clippings from the fur of a hare).[4] Marcus Aurelius sent a mission of merchants from Rome to China and brought back silk that Galen used to tie off bleeding vessels. Galen wrote 400 works describing trepanning of the skull and suturing penetrating intestinal and abdominal wall wounds.[4]

THE MIDDLE AGES

For over a thousand years, Galen's work was dogma. Galen had a teleological view of "purpose" to every bodily function and illness. The early Christian Church embraced it and made it the absolute authoritative word on medicine—to question it would be heresy.[1] However, he is considered to have an overall negative effect on surgical progress because of his position that suppuration is an essential component of wound healing.[5] Galen's writings and the edicts of two Ecclesiastical Councils (The Council of Clermont, 1130, and Council of Tours, 1163) put a stop to any advancement of medicine and surgery during the Middle Ages. The Council of Clermont prohibited priests and monks from practicing medicine, and the Council of Tours proclaimed *Ecclesia Abhorrent a Sanguine* ("the church abhors bloodshed") and physicians are prohibited from practicing surgery,[5,6] and so the barber surgeon was born. The reader may be interested to know that the Council of Clermont of 1095 was convened by Pope Urban II to assemble a Christian army to fight the First Crusade.

THE BATTLE OF CRÉCY—1346

The Battle of Crécy was fought during the Hundred Year's War and marks the first time cannons were deployed and strategically used in battle in Europe. The first hand cannon appeared during the 1260 Battle of Ain Jalut between the Egyptians and Mongols in the Middle East. Many historians consider the Battle of Crécy the beginning of the end of chivalry.[7]

Metal projectiles and explosions created new wounds and new challenges. A German surgeon, von Pfolspeundt, originated the belief that gunpowder was poison and must be removed.[5] Hieronymous Brunschwig, also a German surgeon, wrote the first book on the treatment of firearm wounds in 1497. He wrote

> In case a man has been shot with a gun and the bullet is still in place, he is poisoned by the powder, or part of the powder is still in the body, in the arm or leg or wherever the wound may be. Take a seton, push it through the wound, and pull it back and forth to force the powder out[8]. . .

His work established the standard treatment for extremity missile wounds for almost 300 years—cauterize the wound with a hot iron or boiling oil and plug the wound. Amputation was not done unless gangrene was present—and only through dead tissue to avoid the problem of blood loss.[8] Brunschwig is also credited with reporting the first bowel repair from a war wound.[5]

16TH AND 17TH CENTURIES

Ambroise Paré (1510–1590) became barber surgeon in the army of Francis I (1536–1538). In 1536 at the siege of Turin, Paré did not have any "seething" elder oil available to him to treat the wounded. Paré substituted egg yolk and turpentine and bandaged the wounds, and observed that the healing was better under this treatment. He resolved "never so cruelly, to burne poor men wounded with gunshot."[9] His observations, published in 1545, gave the impetus to a rational reform of the whole system of dealing with wounds, and did away with the theory of poisoned gunshot wounds. Paré was reluctant to explore gunshot wounds unless it was to remove foreign bodies, detached pieces of bone, and congealed blood. Fractures were treated by reduction, immobilization, and various concoctions to hinder development of "paine, inflammation, feaver, abscesse, gangrene, and sphacell [mortification]."[1]

Vascular ligation was revived by Paré for amputations. A surgeon during this era had about 30 seconds to amputate the limb and 3 minutes to complete the operation. Working without anesthesia and a tourniquet, this was not enough time for a surgeon (other than Paré) to complete the surgery and is why many, such as Guillemeau,

Paré's student, again abandoned this method for direct cautery. It was not until later with the reintroduction of the tourniquet in 1674 by Etienne J. Morel (1648–1710), also a French Army surgeon, during the Siège of Besançon, that ligation would have more widespread use.[9] Perhaps the most significant advance in the performance of amputation was the tourniquet of Jean Louis Petit (1674–1750). Petit modified Morel's tourniquet so that it was easier to apply, and tension could be adjusted using a screw.[1] Petit's modification allowed the surgeon to perform the surgery alone or with only one assistant (perhaps to hold the patient), whereas before several people were needed. His device was also recognized to be useful to control bleeding from massive wounds.[1] Henri François LeDran (1685–1770) recommended Petit's tourniquet to the military[1] and described the importance of fasciotomy—"incising into muscle compartments was essential to release pressure from bleeding, injury, or inflammation."[10]

William Clowes was a surgeon in the British Navy and considered the preeminent surgeon in Elizabethan England. In 1536, he published a book advocating debridement, extraction of foreign bodies, and avoidance of cautery when treating wounds. He also reignited the debate "gunpowder is poison" by announcing that the bullet could be smeared with poison before it was fired. This was eagerly accepted and is thought to have been responsible for many prisoners of war being executed when their injured captors died with infected wounds.[5]

18TH AND 19TH CENTURIES

Napoleon's surgeon, Dominique Jean Larrey (1766–1842), wrote extensively on the necessity for early amputation for any limb injured that cannot be saved. Hospital gangrene was frequently seen in untreated wounds and was almost universally fatal. Larrey reasoned that an early amputation would obviate this danger by creating a relatively clean viable wound.[4] This belief was held by most (but not all) through the American Civil War—30% of gunshot and fragment wounds to the extremities resulted in amputation.

Larrey developed *ambulance volantes* (flying hospitals)—carriages that had a spring suspension so that a cushioned ride was possible. His surgical team would race through the battlefield treating the wounded and performing amputations on the battlefield.[8] He reasoned that shock of the wound rendered it relatively insensate and the patient more cooperative. He tested his postulate in 1793 at the Battle of Metz and was so successful in saving patients and improving troop morale, that he was tasked with reorganizing the medical care of all the 14 armies of the French Republic.[5]

Carl Reyher (1846–1890), a Russian military surgeon, recommended adding a more extensive mechanical wound cleansing, which he termed *débridement.* He demonstrated a significant reduction in mortality from patients he treated during the Russo-Turkish war.[4]

In the Americas, wound care varied very little from that being done in Europe. The biggest advancements came in the way the wounded received their care. Jonathan Letterman (1824–1872) was tasked by Major General George B. McClellan to fix an inefficient medical care system of the Union Army. Letterman devised a system of forward first aid stations at the regimental level where one medical officer was tasked with performing triage. He established mobile field hospitals to be located at division and corps headquarters. In August 1862, Letterman established an efficient ambulance corps and supply system that he placed under the control of medical staff instead of the Quartermaster Department. At each hospital, one physician was responsible for keeping records on all admissions and the second was delegated to provide shelter, bedding, fuel, and nutrition services.[11] Ira Rutkow, a surgical historian, said the title "Operating Surgeon" was "one of the most momentous medical reforms to come out of the Civil War."[5] Letterman instituted a policy that only the three most experienced physicians in each division are permitted to perform surgical procedures. This was the first time professional privileging was instituted and was dependent on documentation of the physician's proficiency and experience.[5] Letterman proved the efficiency of his systems at the Battle of Fredericksburg, in which the Army of the Potomac suffered 12,000 casualties. His system was adopted by other Union armies and was eventually officially established as the medical procedure for the entirety of the United States' armies by an Act of Congress in March 1864.[11]

J.J. Chisholm, the Chairman of Surgery at the Medical College of South Carolina, received the first medical appointment for active military service for the Confederacy, and he recommended that surgeons be examined by senior surgeons before they were allowed to perform amputations.[5]

THE 20TH CENTURY

Many credit French surgeons of the 18th and early 19th centuries (particularly French surgeon Pierre Joseph Desault [1744–1795]) for the modern concept of débridement. However, full credit for the modern practice of débridement belongs to Belgian Army surgeon Colonel Antoine Depage (1862–1925). Depage was not satisfied with simple débridement, or wound exploration. In the course of his débridement of soldiers injured during World War I, he stressed the importance of removing contaminated tissue and contused, necrotic flesh in addition to foreign bodies.[10] He reasoned that necrotic tissue is fertile ground for the growth of pathogens, particularly the spore-forming anaerobes responsible for many cases of *gangrene gazeuse* (gas gangrene). Depage was enthusiastic on bacteriology and kept up to date—the discoverer of penicillin, Alexander Fleming (1881–1955), was doing many of his bacteriologic studies in the research laboratories of Depage's military hospital at La Panne.[4]

Antitetanic serum was widely used during the war and virtually eliminated tetanus in the wounds.[2] Other improvements made during WWI include

- Field blood transfusions: The A, B, and O blood groups were described in 1901. In 1917, O.H. Robertson took Harvey Cushing's Harvard Unit and traveled to France and developed a safe and efficient system to transfuse blood to combat casualties.[5]
- Fluoroscopic localization of foreign bodies: Wilhelm C. Roentgen discovered X-rays in 1895. In 1917 J.M. Flint describes using fluoroscopy with "astonishing accuracy" for removing foreign bodies—80% were done using local anesthesia only.[2]
- Crystalloid and colloid administration: E.W. Archibald and W.S. McLean stated that shock was a consequence of plasma deficiency and gave "a great deal of salt solution" intravenously. To compensate for the transient effects of salt solutions, they also gave a colloid solution consisting of 25 g of gelatin in 1 L of saline.[2]
- Specialized surgical care: Specialized treatment centers were established to deal with unique wounds. In a 1919 speech delivered at the American Surgical Association, E. Cuttler stressed the importance of transporting "head cases" to a site where specialist could carry out the necessary surgery.[2]
- Dakin's solution: Dakin's solution is known by most surgeons as an old treatment for treating contaminated wounds. Dakin's solution was originally called "Carrel-Dakin solution" named after the inventors—Alexis Carrel (1873–1944) and Henry Drysdale Dakin (1880–1952). Mr. Dakin was an English chemist and teamed up with Dr. Carrel, who was serving as a Major in the French Army. They were tasked to develop a method for treating contaminated and infected wounds—a common occurrence during trench warfare. Their method required rubber tubes to be interspersed in the dressings and the solution was irrigated through the tubes into the dressings (and into the bed necessitating frequent bed sheet changes). However, as one nurse remarked about the messy regime, "but [it] is surely is remarkable how those wounds heal."[12] Why was "Carrel" dropped from the "Carrel-Dakin solution" name? The authors could not find a specific date or an editorial calling for the removal of his name—it just started fading away in the literature before WWII. Alexis Carrel became a *persona non grata* for his controversial beliefs of fascism and eugenics. Even more titillating is the American hero he collaborated with.

Carrel won the Nobel Prize in medicine in 1912 for extracorporeal tissue perfusion and was renowned for his vascular surgery techniques. Carrel was also interested in the phenomenon of cellular senescence. In 1930, Charles A. Lindbergh (1902–1974) teamed up with Carrel after his sister-in-law developed a fatal heart condition. While living in France, Lindbergh studied extracorporeal perfusion of organs with Carrel. Lindbergh invented a glass perfusion pump, named the "Model T" pump, and with Carrel's work on membrane oxygenation, they are credited with making future heart surgeries possible.[13] In 1935, Lindbergh and Carrel summarized their work first in *Science*[14] and later in their book, *The Culture of Organs* (1938). Both Lindbergh and Carrel appeared on the cover of *Time* magazine on June 13, 1938. After WWI, Carrel was an outspoken admirer of fascism and eugenics. His writings on selective breeding and euthanasia for undesirables attracted the attention of the German National Socialist Party. In 1936, Carrel authored his eugenics book *Man, the Unknown*. Carrel and Lindbergh talked about eugenics and Lindbergh promoted the thought that the white races of Germans, French, British, and Americans should unite against the Asian hordes (led by Soviet Russia).[15] Carrel's agenda was a little more broad in its goals—he advocated the use of gas chambers to rid humanity of "inferior stock," thus endorsing the scientific racism discourse. His endorsement of this idea began in the mid-1930s, before the Nazi implementation of such practices in Germany. In 1944 he was accused of collaboration with the fascist wartime government of Vichy. Throughout the occupation, Carrel had plenty of money for research under the big Fondation Française Pour L'Etude Des Problèmes Humains, created for him by Vichy.[16] He was imprisoned and died later that year at the age of 71 while awaiting charges for war crimes.[17]

CONCLUSION

This brief synopsis of medical history attempts to whet the curiosity of the reader to learn more about the paths our surgical ancestors traveled and how often we repeatedly keep walking down these same paths. Knowing surgical history is critical to the discovery (or "re-discovery") of future advances. The contributions military medicine has made to wound care is not a finished chapter in the book of medical history; for as long as there will be conflict there will always be a necessity for military medicine to devise better ways to treat the wounded. The interested reader is encouraged to study the references used in this article for a much more detailed discussion.

AUTHOR DISCLOSURE STATEMENT

G.B. has nothing to disclose. D.B. has nothing to disclose.

REFERENCES

1. Bagwell CE: "Respectful image": revenge of the barber surgeon. Ann Surg 2005; **241:** 872.
2. Pruitt BA, Jr.: Centennial changes in surgical care and research. Ann Surg 2000; **232:** 287.
3. Atsma AJ: *Theoi Greek Mythology*, vol. 2000–2008. Auckland, New Zealand, 2008. www.theoi.com.
4. Majno G (ed): *The Healing Hand: Man and Wound in the Ancient World.* Cambridge: Harvard University Press, 1975, p. 570.
5. Pruitt BA, Jr.: Combat casualty care and surgical progress. Ann Surg 2006; **243:** 715.
6. Holzman RS: The legacy of Atropos, the fate who cut the thread of life. Anesthesiology 1998; **89:** 241.
7. Wikipedia Contributors: Battle of Crécy, 2009. www.wikipedia.org/wiki. Accessed February 3, 2009.
8. Helling TS and McNabney WK: The role of amputation in the management of battlefield casualties: a history of two millennia. J Trauma 2000; **49:** 930.
9. Hamby WB (ed): *Ambroise Paré, Surgeon of the Renaissance.* St. Louis: W.H. Green, 1967, p. 251.
10. Helling TS and Daon E: In Flanders fields: The Great War, Antoine Depage, and the resurgence of debridement. Ann Surg 1998; **228:** 173.
11. Musto R: The treatment of the wounded at Gettysburg: Jonathan Letterman: The father of modern battlefield medicine. Gettysburg Magazine 2007; **37:** 120.
12. King M: Our historical roots: Dr. Richard Drysdale Dakin, DSc, and his solution. J Wound Ostomy Continence Nurs 2008; **35:** 289.
13. Frazier OH, Shah NA, Myers TJ. Total artificial heart. In: *Cardiac Surgery in the Adult*, edited by Cohn LH and Edmunds LH Jr. New York: McGraw-Hill, 2003, pp. 1507–1514.
14. Carrel A and Lindbergh CA: The culture of whole organs. Science 1935; **81:** 621.
15. Ward GC: Lindbergh: In "The American Experience," edited by Ives S. New York: Insigna Films, 1990.
16. Science: Data from France. Time Magazine, vol. XLIV, no. 16, October 16, 1944.
17. Milestones, Nov. 13, 1944. Time Magazine vol. XLIV, no. 20, November 13, 1944.

WHS
Wound
Healing
Society

History of Bacteriology of War Wounds

Forest R. Sheppard[1–3,*] and Martin C. Robson[4]

[1]Department of Surgery, National Naval Medical Center, Bethesda, Maryland.
[2]Naval Medical Research Center, Silver Spring, Maryland.
[3]Department of Surgery, Uniformed Services University of Health Sciences, Bethesda, Maryland.
[4]Emeritus Professor of Surgery, University of South Florida, Tampa, Florida.

Abbreviations and Acronyms

WWI = World War I

WWII = World War II

*Correspondence: Naval Medical Research Center, Regenerative Medicine Department—CCCD, 503 Robert Grant Ave., Silver Spring, Maryland 20910 (e-mail: forest.sheppard@med.navy.mil).

War wounds are, as all traumatic wounds, uniformly contaminated and the contaminating organisms can be of various species. The change of the predominating species over the various armed conflicts can be due to several factors such as medical knowledge and practice of the era, munitions used, climate where and season when injury occurred, time from battlefield to medical care, initial treatment and resuscitation regimens, and antibacterial measures. The history of war wound microbiology is extensive; it is the authors' goal to present a concise treatise acknowledging these factors that may serve as both a general reference and a starting point for more in-depth study by the reader.

HISTORY PRIOR TO 1850

Infection has plagued man since his beginning and indeed predates man by nearly 5 million years.[1,2] The theory that "minute animals" invisible to the eye might in some way cause disease was postulated in the first century BC by Marcus Terentius Varro; however, another 1,600 years would pass before this theory was further elucidated.[1,2] In the first century AD, A. Cornelius Celsus enumerated the first four signs of inflammation: rubor, tumor, calor, and dolor.[2] In his *De re medicina*, he suggested that wounds should be sutured or approximated by clamps, but only after "the internal surface of the wound be cleansed, lest clotted blood be left there. For it becomes converted into pus, and by exciting inflammation impedes the agglutination of the wound."[2]

Guy de Chauliac, in 1363, listed eight conditions in which delayed closure should be employed.[1] These conditions, which remain a basis for military surgery, included the need for debridement. This concept of early debridement was emphasized in 1545 by Ambrose Pare, who used early debridement for gunshot wounds and condemned the application of boiling oil for cautery of such wounds.[2]

A return to the "germ theory" of Varro occurred in 1546 when Hieronymus Fracastorius (Gerolamo Fracastoro) published in *De Contagione et contagiosis morbis*, "Infection itself is composed of minute and insensible particles and proceeds from them."[2] These invisible organisms, which he termed "seminaria," could cause infection both by air and direct contact. In 1763 John Morgan stated in his student thesis, "The production of pus is the work of a living organism, very similar to a secretion . . . developed in accordance with the proper stage of a preceding inflammation."[3] Lazaro Spallazani discovered in 1776 that flasks of meat infusion broth, when boiled and hermetically sealed, did not allow bacterial growth.[4] These observations were not recognized for what

ADVANCES IN WOUND CARE, VOLUME 1

Printed in U.S.A.
DOI: 10.1089/awc.2009.0062

they were and it would take almost another 100 years for Pasteur to disprove the concepts of "spontaneous generation."[1] Military surgery and the understanding of war wound bacteriology would have been very different had Spallazani's observations been truly understood. Since microscopy had improved sufficiently by 1676 for Leeuwenhoek to identify bacteria, bacteriology of war wounds might have been a subject for military surgeons during the American Revolutionary War and the War of 1812.[2] Because Spallazani's observations were not understood, war wounds from those conflicts routinely became infected and were frequently not survivable. One surgeon who stood out during the turn of the 18th century was Napoleon Bonaparte's surgeon-in-chief, Dominique Jean Larrey. Larrey realized that if death following combat wound infection was to be avoided, operation must be performed as soon as possible after wounding. This led to his institution of what was known as the "flying ambulance," a mobile transportation from the battlefield to the surgeon.[5]

HISTORY OF THE LATE 19TH CENTURY

It remained until the latter half of the 19th century for discoveries and reports to substantiate the "germ theory" and place it in the realm of practicality with formalization of the science of bacteriology and the institution of antiseptic and aseptic surgical techniques.[1] By 1850 it was well established that infection in a wound or incision came from without. The chief sources appeared to be the air or direct contact with unclean objects.[1] To prevent this contact, in 1855 Auguste Nelaton placed alcohol-soaked dressings on open wounds with a decrease in infection rates.[6] Nelaton's treatment, although sound, was not based on the beliefs in vogue in 1855 which held that spontaneous generation was the source of bacteria in wounds. It took a series of experiments by Louis Pasteur in the 1860s to disprove the hypothesis of spontaneous generation.[4]

In 1867 Joseph Lister, having heard of Pasteur's work, used carbolic acid compresses on open fractures to prevent contamination from the air by invisible living organisms.[7] He based his treatment on the observation that closed fractures healed without infection, whereas open fractures routinely became infected.[1,7] Lister's belief that the air was the prime source of contamination led to his use of carbolic acid spray to purify the air of the operating room as an extension of his use of antibacterial dressings.[1]

The understanding and treatment of war wounds was much different in 1861 at the outbreak of the American Civil War than had the war commenced 10 years later.[8] The existence of microbes had not yet been accepted. At the beginning of the Civil War, combat wounds were treated by dressings, with considerable difference of opinion concerning the best dressing, and most without attempt at closure.[9] Wounds always became infected. Many formed white pus that drained and was called laudable pus. Others became red and swollen, a condition called erysipelas by the surgeons and subsequently identified as infection by streptococcus.[9] Today it would be considered cellulitis. If the infection remained localized, the patient's natural defenses might allow the patient to recover. If it became widespread and entered the bloodstream, it was fatal. Some wounds became complicated by a newly identified infection called hospital gangrene. It was probably due to two different organisms growing in the same wound in symbiosis, most likely a strain of staphylococcus and a strain of clostridia.[9]

Several complicating factors led to the outcomes of combat-related wounds during the Civil War. The munitions, specifically the minie ball, caused more tissue destructive wounds than previously seen. The minie ball flattened when it encountered human flesh and did not pass through tissues as do modern bullets with metal jackets.[9] Bones were splintered, shattered, and driven through muscle and skin. This required amputation above the level of shattered bone. Sanitation in the troop areas was dismal leading to the presence and multiplication of bacteria. At the outbreak of the war, First Battle of Bull Run, there was no method to evacuate the wounded. This was corrected when Jonathan Letterman organized an ambulance service and had control of the ambulances transferred from the Quartermaster Department to the Medical Department.[9] Finally, great strides were made with combat wound care when J.S. Billings reorganized the medical services and moved the medical facilities closer to the battlefield.[8]

Pasteur's and Joseph Lister's work of the 1860s would require decades for acceptance and implementation, and antisepsis would remain a source of skepticism, only to be slowly adopted in the decades to come following Robert Koch's confirmation of bacteria as the cause of wound infections.[10,11] Even the advent of surgical gloves was a comfort-driven development, subsequently to be shown to reduce infections.[12] At the dawn of the 20th century, the practice of asepsis, antiseptic use, sterile surgical clothing, and the use of rubber gloves and masks had begun.[1]

The Spanish American War (1898) witnessed antiseptic dressings that were applied in an occlusive manner to wounds on the battlefield. However, the ratio of disease : death due to battlefield wounds increased, a reversal of the previous trend in U.S. casualties. The reduction in death from initial wounding was attributed to the prompt delivery of field medical care, notably occlusive antiseptic dressings; however, controversy regarding the appropriate timing and indications for operations, including laparotomy, existed and would continue to World War I (WWI).[12]

HISTORY OF THE 20TH CENTURY

Following the Spanish American War, A, B, O, and AB blood groups were identified and *in vitro* blood compatibility testing developed. The ability to provide blood transfusions in combination with improved resuscitation contributed to improved laparotomy outcomes, especially if performed within 3 h of injury.[13,14] However, mortality of laparotomy remained high, reported as 60% in the British and 45–60% in the American experiences.[13]

Effective vaccination against typhoid, which had been devastating during the Spanish American War, and anti-tetanus serum virtually eliminated these infections in WWI. Improved methods to treat wounds during the initial incubation period, including continuous irrigation of dirty wounds, and radiology-guided foreign body extraction were implemented and enhanced foreign body extraction and wound debridement.[1,15,16] Carrel in collaboration with Henry Dakin advocated catheter placement deep into wounds with continuous irrigation of what we now know as Dakin's solution to prevent and treat infections with a reduction in amputations noted.[1,4,15]

By the conclusion of WWI the beginnings of the modern, mechanized, MEDEVAC system had begun, permitting relatively rapid transit from time of injury to true surgical specialists for care. Blood transfusion was a relatively safe and fieldable reality; the understanding and resuscitation of shock had improved as had the outcomes of laparotomy and the delayed primary closure of dirty wounds had been popularized and accepted as standard practice.[1]

In the decades between WWI and World War II (WWII), agents to control and eliminate microorganisms were further developed and most notably the antibiotic era was born with the development of an efficacious antibacterial, the sulfonamide prontosil.[17] Fleming discovered penicillin in 1929 and a decade later Florey was able to isolate and produce it with initial clinical trials in 1941.[18,19]

During the 1930s the existence of hospital-acquired infections was identified and nosocomial *Streptococcus pyrogenes* documented to negatively impact wound healing.[20] A change in bacterial serotype in hospitalized patients and 40% and 6–13% of the hospital staff as carriers of *Staphylococcus aureus* and *Streptococcus pyrogenes*, respectively, was reported.[20] The delayed primary closure of dirty wounds was the accepted civilian practice and would become the standard of care throughout WWII with war reports of wound infection rate of 15% when wounds were closed within 10 days versus approximately 49% when closed more than 10 days after surgery.[1]

The initial use of antibiotics in WWII was in Pearl Harbor casualties, with sulfonamides being successfully utilized. Subsequently, sulfonamide was widely utilized as a topical wound agent though penicillin largely took its place as the war progressed. Penicillin would first be used by American forces in the North African theater in 1942 and would subsequently be used in all theaters with remarkable success.[21,22] Penicillin, however, was not to replace aggressive surgical debridement of wounds and was most effective when used in conjunction with debridement.[23]

Coincident with the use of antibiotics in casualties, the U.S. Army Surgical Research Unit was established in 1943. The collection and review of clinical data and casualty outcomes would continue and expand in subsequent U.S. wars. WWII witnessed dramatic improvements in logistics and transportation. The development of an Army Medical Corps trauma system provided continuity of care from field to rehabilitation hospitals and utilized ground vehicles, trains, ships, and aircraft to do so. This expanded the availability of surgical specialists, and additionally auxiliary surgical groups were utilized and deployed as mobile teams to areas of need.

Combat casualty care of WWII was a marked improvement throughout in comparison to previous wars with abdominal wound mortality being reduced to 15–24% in American troops and 42% in British troops. The improved American survival was attributed to the closer proximity of definitive surgical care in the American forces where advanced surgical, resuscitative, and antibiotic administration were available.[13]

During the Korean War the evaluation and collection of patient and treatment outcome data continued and expanded within theater surgical research teams.[13] Microbiology revealed that at the time of presentation to medical care, wounds were contaminated with bacteria.[23] The bacterial contamination varied by season with staphylococci and streptococci being predominant in the winter months and fecal bacteria and clostridium species more commonly identified during the summer.[23] The standard of care for wounds was aggressive surgical debridement and the use of penicillin in conjunction with streptomycin. The continued use of a relatively limited number of antibiotics gained appreciation as resistance to penicillin and streptomycin was demonstrated in 48 and 49 of the 50 cases, respectively, upon evacuation of wounded to Japan.[23]

The Korean War saw the further development of forward surgical facilities into Mobile Army Surgical Hospitals. Helicopters were first used for casualty transport and advancements such as hemodialysis were available.[13] The mortality of abdominal wounds declined to 8.85% during the Korean War, and the effect of evacuation time on infectious complications and death was appreciated.[24]

In Vietnam the abundant use of helicopters reduced time from injury to surgical care to <2 h.[13,23] The impact on time from injury to surgical care was further elucidated: mortality was 10% with arrival within the first hour increasing to 75% with arrival to surgical care >8 h. Assessment of casualties documented mortality rates of 1.8–2.3% (compared with 3.3% in WWII and 2.4% in Korea) with mortality of abdominal wounds improving to 4.5–9%.[24] Hemorrhage and head injuries replaced infections as the most common causes of death in Vietnam. In Vietnam 70% of the patients received antibiotics in association with wound care. Most commonly penicillin was used, but streptomycin (51%) and chloromycetin (27%) were also commonly administered. Only 2% of the patients were treated with topical agents. A trend of initially mixed gram-positive and -negative wound isolates was observed with transition to predominantly gram negative by day 5 and high incidences of antibiotic resistance reported.[25,26] Seasonal differences in flora were observed with *Staphylococcus epidermidis* being most common in January, *Pseudomonas aeruginosa* in July, and *Escherichia coli* in June. Upon return to the United States, bacteria recovered from wounds were predominantly gram negative with a predominance of single bacterial species (92%) with *P. aeruginosa* (43%) being the most common and *S. aureus* (18%) being the second most common.[27]

HISTORY OF THE 21ST CENTURY

Present day conflicts in the Middle East and Southwest Asia benefit from an evolved military medical system developed during 20th century wars. Gram-negative bacteria remain the most commonly isolated bacteria in U.S. war wounds with acinetobacter the predominant isolate in wounds from Iraq and Afghanistan as it was during Desert Storm.[23] This gram-negative predominance may be partially influenced by the delayed timing of majority of these cultures as there is evidence of an acutely early gram-positive predominance in U.S. troops injured in Iraq.[26] Though there has been debate as to whether acinetobacter was a prominent gram negative in Vietnam, the trend of gram-negative wound infections and appearance of resistant organisms seen in wars of the latter half of the 20th century has continued.[23] It remains to be elucidated how the microbiology of present-day combat wounds is selected for/determined; however, given the history of war wound microbiology and evolution of military medicine described within this text, it seems likely that regardless of initial inocula, how we care for casualties plays a central role in the etiology of war wound infections. It seems likely that the present dilemma with resistant strains of acinetobacter in the wounds of casualties will one day be but a footnote in the history of combat wound microbiology.

DISCLAIMER

The views expressed in this article are those of the authors and do not necessarily reflect the official policy or position of the Department of the Navy, Department of Defense, nor the U.S. Government. This work was prepared as part of official duties. Title 17 U.S.C. 105 provides that "Copyright protection under this title is not available for any work of the United States Government." Title 17 U.S.C. 101 defines a U.S. Government work as a work prepared by a military service member or employee of the U.S. Government as part of that person's official duties.

AUTHOR DISCLOSURE STATEMENT

The authors (F.R.S. and M.C.R.) have no commercial associations or financial interests that might create or seem to pose a conflict of interest in connection with the submitted manuscript.

REFERENCES

1. Robson MC, Krizek TJ, and Heggers JP: Biology of surgical infection. In: *Current Problems in Surgery*, edited by Ravitch MM. Chicago: Yearbook Medical Publishers Inc., 1973.

2. Major RH: *A History of Medicine*, vol. 1. Springfield: Charles C. Thomas Publisher, 1954.

3. Meade RH: *An Introduction to the History of General Surgery*. Philadelphia: W.B. Saunders Co., 1968, Chap. 3.

4. Jamor RH: *A History of Medicine*, vol. 2. Springfield: Charles C. Thomas Publisher, 1954.

5. Larrey DJ: *Memoirs of Military Surgery*, vol. 1. Baltimore: Joseph Cushing Publisher, 1814.

6. Atler WF: *Clinical Lectures on Surgery by M. Nelaton*. Philadelphia: J.B. Lippincott Co., 1856.

7. Lister J: On a new method of treating compound fracture, abscess, etc. with observations on the conditions of suppuration. Lancet 1867; **1:** 326.

8. Denney RE: *Civil War Medicine: Care & Comfort of the Wounded*. New York: Sterling Publishing Co., 1995.

9. Freemon FR: *Gangrene and Glory: Medical Care During the American Civil War*. London: Associated University Presses, 1998.

10. Cameron HC: Lord Lister and the evolution of modern surgery. Glasgow, 1861–1869. BMJ 1902; **2:** 1844.

11. Koch R: Investigations into the etiology of traumatic infective diseases. London 1880. Roberts W. Address in Medicine. BMJ 1877; **2:** 168.

12. McBurney C: The use of rubber gloves in operative surgery. Ann Surg 1898; **28:** 108.

13. Pruitt BA: Combat casualty care and surgical progress. Ann Surg 2006; **243:** 715.

14. Adams DB: Abdominal gunshot wounds in warfare: a historical review. Mil Med 1983; **148:** 15.

15. Bennet J: Abdominal surgery in the war: the early story. J R Soc Med 1991; **84:** 554.

16. Depage A: General consideration as to the treatment of war wounds. Ann Surg 1979; **68:** 575.

17. Domagk GA: A contribution to the chemotherapy of bacterial infections. Rev Infect Dis 1986; **8:** 163.

18. Abraham E: Selective reminiscences of beta-lactam antibiotics: early research on penicillin and cephalosporins. Bioessays 1990; **12:** 601.

19. Fleming A: On the antibacterial action of cultures of a penicillium, with special reference to their use in the isolation of B influenza. Br J Exp Pathol 1929; **10:** 226.

20. Miles AA, Schwabacher H, and Cunliffe AC: Hospital infection of war wounds. BMJ 1940; **2:** 895.

21. Fraser I: Penicillin: early trials in war casualties. BMJ 1984; **289:** 1723.

22. Poole LT: Army progress with penicillin. Br J Surg 1944; **32:** 110.

23. Murray CK, Hinkle MK, and Yun HC: History of infections associated with combat-related injuries. J Trauma 2008; **64:** S221.

24. Pruitt BA: The symbiosis of combat casualty care and civilian trauma care: 1914–2007. J of Trauma 2008; **64:** S4.

25. Tong MJ: Septic complications of war wounds. JAMA 1972; **219:** 1044.

26. Kovaric JJ, Matsumoto T, Dobek AS, *et al.*: Bacterial flora of one hundred and twelve combat wounds. Mil Med 1968; **133:** 622.

27. Heggers JP, Barnes ST, Robson MC, *et al.*: Microbial flora of orthopedic war wounds. Mil Med 1969; **134:** 602.

Trauma System Approach to Complex Wounded

Mathew J. Bradley and James R. Dunne*

Department of General Surgery, National Naval Medical Center, Bethesda, Maryland.

Background: The military trauma system, throughout its history, has adapted to changes in military tactics to improve treatment and evacuation of the combat wounded. Prior U.S. military conflicts in the 20th century saw the development of the Mobile Army Surgical Hospital units and the introduction of the helicopter as an air ambulance.
The Problem: Conflicts, such as Mogadishu, Operation Iraqi, and Operation Enduring Freedom, have resulted in a new nonlinear type of warfare and have created new dilemmas for military medicine to overcome.
Basic/Clinical Science Advances: Solutions to address these challenges include advances in training of first responders (tactical combat casualty care) and more mobile, flexible surgical trauma support, in the form of the Navy and Marine Corps' Forward Resuscitative Surgical Support System and the Army's Forward Surgical Teams. In addition, the joint theater trauma system was developed to assist in coordinating and standardizing care throughout the system as well as to provide educational feedback and a process for robust and comprehensive performance improvement.
Clinical Care Relevance: The foundation of the current military trauma system remains based on five echelons of care. Treatment starts on the battlefield and advances through several echelons of care until patients reach the highest level, a major military treatment facility in the continental United States.
Conclusion: The key to continued success of the military trauma system will be its ability to effectively coordinate and maintain the continuity of care from point of injury, through rehabilitation and beyond.

Abbreviations and Acronyms

ASG = auxiliary surgical group

CONUS = continental United States

CSH = combat support hospital

FRSS = forward resuscitative surgical support system

FST = forward surgical team

JTTS = joint theater trauma system

MASH = mobile army surgical hospital

STP = shock trauma platoons

TCCC = tactical combat casualty care

*Correspondence: Department of General Surgery, National Naval Medical Center, 8901 Wisconsin Ave., Bethesda, Maryland 20889 (e-mail: james.dunne@med.navy.mil; twobdun@aol.com).

BACKGROUND

The U.S. military trauma system, throughout its history, has adapted to changes made on the battlefront in order to maximize support to combat casualties. Each war has brought new challenges to military medicine, and efforts to provide expeditious trauma support can be traced back to World War II. At the beginning of the war, casualties were taken from the site of injury to battalion aid stations; from there, they were triaged and, if necessary, sent to field hospitals for further care. The field hospitals were large, fixed buildings that were unable to advance with the troops but were equipped to provide definitive surgical care. Although they were situated near airfields to hasten transport out of the combat zone, evacuation to them depended on ground transport. This resulted in long evacuation times and increased mortality for the wounded patients. To address this problem, Colonel DeBakey and other surgical advisors recommended the development of mobile surgical units, auxiliary surgical groups (ASGs), to maneuver with the troops. Each ASG consisted of two surgeons, an anesthesiologist, a nurse, and two technicians. These smaller units provided earlier

Printed in U.S.A.
DOI: 10.1089/awc.2009.0041

surgical support, improvements in resuscitative efforts, and a reduction in mortality.[1]

The ASGs were the precursor to the mobile army surgical hospital (MASH) units popularized in the Korean War. The goal of the MASH units was to provide earlier resuscitation and stabilization prior to transport to field hospitals located farther away. Although they were capable of providing support within 24 h of assembly and could move with the combat troops, MASH units were still relatively large and situated several miles from the frontlines. In fact, the division rear area was the farthest forward the MASH could be deployed. Because of their large logistical footprint, they were not able to insert into the opening stages of a combat operation until D+4 or D+5. MASH units were initially designed to support a capacity of 60 inpatients; however, some had to expand to 200 beds to meet the larger number of casualties they received during the conflict.

The mountainous terrain of Korea, not encountered in previous wars, was a new obstacle for the transport of patients. However, the evolution of aeromedical evacuation, especially the advent of the helicopter, offered a vital solution for this treacherous landscape. The first helicopter used as an air ambulance was the Bell H-13. It allowed for rapid transport of casualties but was limited to transporting only two patients. Further aeromedical developments during the Vietnam War led to the Huey, UH-1D, helicopter capable of transporting nine patients per flight.[1] In addition to the increased carrying capacity, each Huey had trained flight medics capable of providing in-flight care.

CLINICAL PROBLEM ADDRESSED

There were many innovations to improve trauma support in the wars of the early 20th century, but modern warfare has changed drastically since those conflicts. Marines are no longer used to secure beach heads and soldiers are no longer fighting battles in open areas. The battlefront has become asymmetric and urbanized. It is often difficult to discern between enemy and civilians. The battle in Mogadishu, Somalia, in 1993, which pitted a U.S. Army special operations task force against supporters of a warlord, is early evidence of the closed-quartered, city warfare that troops now face more regularly.[2] With modern technology and lighter units, troops can cover remarkable distances at a considerable pace. For example, Marines are now traveling several hundred miles inland to secure areas that are far removed from their sea-based support. This new era of combat has created logistical challenges for military medicine with regards to rapid surgical support and expeditious evacuation.[3,4]

As the combat troops have made tactical adjustments to this new asymmetric, nonlinear warfare, military medicine has had to parallel in its adaptations and solutions to prevent delays in care. The tactical combat casualty care (TCCC) project was developed in the early 1990s by the Naval Special Warfare Command and has expanded to provide prehospital trauma training for combat Navy corpsmen, Army medics, and Air Force Pararescuemen and medics.[5,6] Through the use of didactic sessions, trauma simulators, and procedure laboratories, the course provides a set of combat trauma care guidelines and skills to bring to the combat zone. Prehospital field care, such as needle decompression, extremity tourniquet application, hemostatic dressings, and airway management, has resulted in countless lives saved on the battlefield.[7–9] To provide more mobile and flexible surgical trauma support for the troops, the Navy and Marine Corps developed the Forward Resuscitative Surgical Support System (FRSS). Similarly, the Army's Forward Surgical Teams (FSTs) were designed to move with the rapidly advancing ground troops. Together, these small units afford immediate damage control surgery in far forward areas.

DISCUSSION OF FINDINGS AND RELEVANT LITERATURE

The current military trauma system is highly integrated and is designed to triage, treat, and expedite evacuation of the wounded. Treatment starts on the battlefield and advances through several echelons of care until patients reach the highest level, a major military treatment facility in the continental United States (CONUS). There are five echelons with each one providing more advanced resources, personnel, and supplies. However, depending on the tactical situation, availability of aircraft for evacuation, and the severity of injuries, the casualty may not be sequentially evacuated through each level in order that the right patient is evacuated to the right echelon of care at the right time.[10]

Level I care begins on the battlefield with first aid and includes self-aid, buddy aid, or treatment by a combat medical technician. Simple maneuvers such as tourniquet application and dressing of open wounds can be rendered by nonmedical service members. The emergency medical technicians, medics, and corpsmen assigned to each combat unit are the first medical personnel to provide care to the wounded. Through the skills and knowledge learned in the TCCC course, they have the ability to perform needle decompression for a tension pneumothorax, endotracheal intubations, cricothyroidotomies, and initial intravenous fluid resuscitation.[6,11,12] Wound care at this level is limited to tourniquet placement and application of hemostatic dressings for injuries not amenable to tourniquets. The chitosan-based HemCon or the zeolite powder QuikClot hemostatic dressing has also been useful in austere environments when pressure dressings have been ineffective.[13,14]

Following initial stabilization, casualties are often evacuated to "Level II a" facilities. These include Army battalion aid stations and Marine Corps shock trauma platoons (STPs) where a physician or physician's assistant awaits to provide advanced trauma life support. Patient support is only limited to a few hours. Those who require surgery or are deemed unable to return to duty within 24 h are often directly evacuated to "Level II b" facilities. These facilities consist of surgical units that are small and highly mobile, often located within 3–5 km of the battlefield. Medical supplies are limited, and electricity is often from portable generators. Although there is different nomenclature, Level II b care is served in the same manner by all services. The goal is to provide life and limb-sparing, damage control surgery.[15] The FRSS is the echelon II b unit for the Navy and Marines. These units are often colocated with an STP, a mobile emergency room, which provides triage, advanced trauma life support, and resuscitation efforts. STPs are composed of 2 emergency department physicians, a physician's assistant, an emergency room nurse, 14 corpsmen, and 7 marines. In addition to emergency room care, STPs can also provide supplemental preoperative and postoperative care. An FRSS team consists of eight personnel, including two general surgeons, an anesthesiologist, a critical care nurse, two surgical technicians, an independent duty corpsman, and a basic corpsman. They are designed to be functional within 1 h time and to perform a total of 18 surgical procedures on two operating room tables over 48 h without resupply or relief.[16,17] Laboratory and radiographic capacity for FRSS teams depends on the tactical situation and location. They have the ability to carry and store type O blood but often have no access to component therapy. However, these units frequently encounter mass casualty situations resulting in the need for massive transfusions and therefore have relied heavily on the use of whole blood obtained from military personnel often referred to as the "walking blood bank." Damage control resuscitation and further hemostasis is initiated here. This strategy involves permissive hypotension, treatment of hypothermia, the use of ratios of plasma to red blood cells approaching 1:1, and the early administration of recombinant Factor VIIa in patients requiring massive transfusions.[18] Surgical care rendered at Level II facilities includes damage control celiotomies, craniectomies, thoracotomies, placement of arterial shunts, completion amputations, and fracture splinting. Wound care at this level includes aggressive debridement of necrotic tissue and copious low-pressure irrigation with normal saline of every wound. All wounds are left open and treated with wet to dry dressings prior to transport to the next echelon of care.

The Army's equivalent of the FRSS is the FST. Similar to FRSSs, these units can be assembled and disbanded within 1 h. The team is comprised of roughly 20 service members, including 3 general surgeons, an orthopedic surgeon, 2 nurse anesthetists, 1 critical care nurse, an emergency room nurse, an operating room nurse, an executive officer, and 5 emergency medical technicians or scrub technicians. They contain enough equipment and supplies to sustain 30 operations in two operating rooms for a 72-h period. Postoperative critical care can be maintained for four ventilated patients or eight nonventilated patients for up to 6 h.[19,20]

Similarly, the Air Force's Level II units consist of the mobile field surgical team and the Expeditionary Medical Support Basic team. The mobile field surgical team is a 5-member team with minimal supplies devised to supplement an aid station, and the Expeditionary Medical Support Basic is a 25-member team with one operating room table capable of providing surgical support for up to 48 h.[10]

Level I and II facilities have minimal holding capacity and therefore require rapid evacuation to higher echelons of care and this evacuation is often performed by rotary wing aircraft. The most advanced level of care within the combat zone is provided by a Level III treatment facility. More resources are offered at these facilities compared to lower echelons, but these units are larger, relatively immobile, and require up to several weeks to become fully operational. The Navy has several Level III capable units, including the land-based fleet hospital, the sea-based Hospital Ships, and the Casualty Receiving and Treatment Ships. A fleet hospital has 1,000 personnel and consists of 6 operating rooms, 80 intensive care unit beds, and 500 general purpose beds. Navy Hospital Ships, such as the USNS Comfort, have 12 operating rooms, 100 ICU beds, and 1,000 general beds. The Echelon III facility of the Army is the combat support hospital (CSH). A typical CSH is an approximately 250-bed hospital with general, orthopedic, thoracic, vascular, and urologic surgeons available. It can support up to four operating rooms and 24 critical care patients.[10] Resources for a CSH include laboratory facilities, a blood bank, a radiology department, and physical therapy. The Air Force Level III is similar to the CSH. Depending on the status of the casualty and initial care provided, care involves initial damage control surgery, amputations, and initial/repeat aggressive debridement and irrigation of all wounds. The only definitive care provided at this level is arterial and venous reconstructions. All other definitive care including fracture fixation and wound closure is delayed until transport out of theater due to the increased risk of infection. The majority of wounds are dressed with wet to dry dressings though in some cases negative pressure therapy has been used during transport out of theater.

Level IV represents the first level of care outside the combat zone. A CSH, a Navy Fleet hospital, Casualty Receiving and Treatment Ships, or a fixed medical facility can all function as Level IV centers based on the situation and evacuation route. The major Level IV center in the current war on terrorism is Landstuhl Regional Medical Center in Germany.[21] These facilities have blood banks, laboratory, and multiaxial imaging capabilities. Inpatient capacity can be up to 1,000 beds. Most surgical subspecialties are available, along with a multidisciplinary intensive care team. However, when performing more intensive modalities such as hemodialysis, a nephrology consultation must occur via teleconference due to the lack of on-site medical subspecialists.[22] Second-look abdominal operations and interval wound irrigations and debridements occur at this stage including the application of wound Vacuum-Assisted Closure devices prior to transport to CONUS.

Level V care is provided in CONUS. These military treatment facilities are major hospitals that can offer all surgical and medical subspecialties. It is here that any definitive abdominal and thoracic operation, extremity reconstruction, amputation revision, and complex soft tissue coverage procedures are performed. Given the multisystem nature of these injuries, these patients require multidisciplinary care that needs to be highly coordinated to ensure their optimal outcome. The major Level V military hospital for the Navy and Marine Corps is the National Naval Medical Center in Bethesda, MD. The Army-wounded warriors are sent to Walter Reed Army Medical Center in Washington, DC, or Brook Army Medical Center in San Antonio, TX. Wounded airmen are often evacuated to National Naval Medical Center, Walter Reed Army Medical Center, or Brook Army Medical Center depending on the nature of their injuries. In addition, the Institute of Surgical Research, the only burn center within the Department of Defense, provides all burn care for the services (Fig. 1). These Level V centers also serve as sites for initial physical rehabilitation. As the injured complete their surgeries and meet their initial rehabilitation goals, plans are made to transfer them to definitive rehabilitation centers located both in the Veterans Administration and the Department of Defense.

With the advent of the Critical Care Air Transport program enacted by the U.S. Air Force in 1996, evacuation of the injured to specialized Level IV centers can occur within 24 h and to CONUS Level V centers within 48–72 h. Critical Care Air Transport teams have allowed transport of critical-injured patients, on fixed-wing aircraft; thousands of miles away from the combat zone and back home in the United States within a few days from injury.

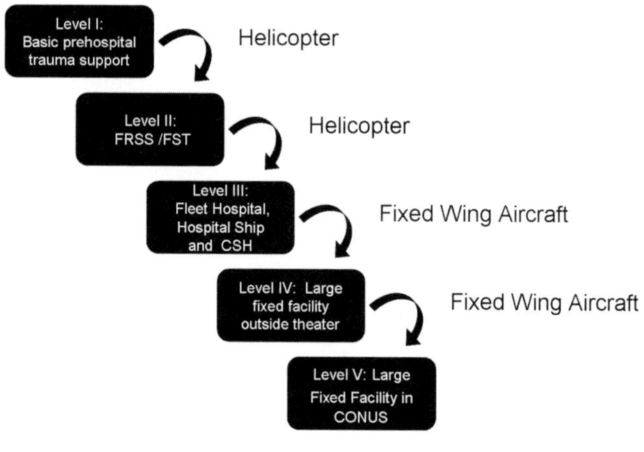

Figure 1. Military Trauma System Structure. Care begins on the battlefield with Level I care that includes Army medic and Navy corpsman Tactical Combat Casualty Care. Depending on the situation, the wounded are transported, usually by rotary winged aircraft, to Level II or Level III units where limb and life-saving, damage control surgery is performed. Further stabilization and wound management occurs at the Combat Support Hospital or Fleet Hospitals prior to transfer from the combat zone. Within 24 h the wounded can reach a large Level IV center, currently Landstuhl Regional Medical Center in Germany. Finally, casualties are evacuated to Level V facilities in continental United States where all definitive surgical management and initial rehabilitation occurs. STP = shock trauma platoon; FRSS = forward resuscitative surgical system; FST = forward surgical team.

Continued improvements to the integrated military trauma system have led to the development of the joint theater trauma system (JTTS). Its main purpose is to assist in the coordination and standardization of care throughout the entire system. At its core is the JTTS director who is stationed in theater. His main duties include collection of injury data far forward and to assist in process improvement efforts throughout the theater. He chairs a tri-service video teleconference between Iraq, Afghanistan, Landstuhl Regional Medical Center, and the Level V centers in the United States. This conference occurs once a week to discuss the troops wounded in the previous week. It is designed to provide educational feedback and process improvement for all echelons of care. The key to any combat casualty process improvement program is the collection of quality data from point of injury through rehabilitation. This fact led to the development of the joint trauma theater registry. This registry documents injury data, therapeutic interventions, and outcomes for all combat casualties injured in Operation Iraqi and Operation Enduring Freedom. Retrospective reviews of these data will assist with quality improvements now and in the future.[22-24]

CRITICAL REMARKS AND RECOMMENDATIONS

Although the current trauma system is well organized and structured, it has its limitations. First, in theater, there are often situations when wounded need to bypass a Level II facility but the distance required to reach the next echelon is beyond the evacuation range of current rotary wing aircraft. One possible solution is the V-22 Osprey. This aircraft has a significantly longer range than current rotary wing aircraft but maintains the ability to land in tight locations similar to rotary wing aircraft. Second, trauma training remains a significant challenge. During peace time, military personnel often have little consistent exposure to trauma care. The advent of courses like TCCC and Prehospital Trauma Life Support have exposed enlisted personnel to just in time trauma training as well as the potential for trauma sustainment training. Opportunities for physicians have developed as well including the Emergency War Surgery course. Emergency War Surgery trains all surgeons regardless of specialty to perform procedures frequently encountered in combat but rarely if ever performed during peace time such as cranial burr holes and placement of external fixators. To further improve combat trauma preparedness, each branch of service has teamed up with a civilian Level I trauma center to provide not only just in time trauma training but also sustainment training. In today's warfare, surgical support needs to be far forward as this is frequently the best option to provide early damage control, life-saving surgery, and every military surgeon needs access to this type of training.

FUTURE DEVELOPMENT

The military trauma system has undergone significant advances in recent years and will continue to adapt as needed to provide medical support to the war fighter. Lessons learned from the recent development of the JTTS as well as developments in specific echelons of care will need to be adapted based on the number and location of future conflicts. The key to continued success of the military trauma system will be its ability to effectively coordinate and maintain the continuity of care from point of injury, through rehabilitation and beyond.

ACKNOWLEDGMENTS

There was no NIH funding or grants used in research or writing of this manuscript.

AUTHOR DISCLOSURE STATEMENT

M.J.B., and J.R.D. have confirmed that no competing financial interests exist.

REFERENCES

1. King B and Jatoi I: The mobile Army surgical hospital (MASH): a military and surgical legacy. J Natl Med Assoc 2005; **97:** 648.

2. Mabry RL, Holcomb JB, Baker AM, Cloonan CC, Uhorchak JM, Perkins DE, Canfield AJ, and Hagmann JH: United States Army Rangers in Somalia: an analysis of combat casualties on an urban battlefield. J Trauma 2000; **49:** 515.

3. Bilski TR, Baker BC, Grove JR, Hinks RP, Harrison MJ, Sabra JP, Temerlin SM, and Rhee P: Battlefield casualties treated at Camp Rhino, Afghanistan: lessons learned. J Trauma 2003; **54:** 814.

4. Chambers LW, Green DJ, Gillingham BL, Sample K, Rhee P, Brown C, Brethauer S, Nelson T, Narine N, Baker B, and Bohman HR: The experience of the US Marine Corps' Surgical Shock Trauma Platoon with 417 operative combat casualties during a 12 month period of operation Iraqi freedom. J Trauma 2006; **60:** 1155.

5. Butler FK, Jr., Hagmann J, and Butler EG: Tactical combat casualty care in special operations. Mil Med 1996; **161 Suppl:** 3.

6. Butler FK, Jr., Holcomb JB, Giebner SD, McSwain NE, and Bagian J: Tactical combat casualty care 2007: evolving concepts and battlefield experience. Mil Med 2007; **172(11 Suppl):** 1.

7. Butler FK, Holocomb JB, Giebner SD, McSwain NE, and Bagian J: Tactical combat casualty care 2007:

evolving concepts and battlefield experience. Mil Med 2007; **172(11 Suppl):** 1.

8. Tien HC, Jung V, Rizoli SB, Acharya SV, and MacDonald J: An evaluation of tactical combat casualty care interventions in a combat environment. J Am Coll Surg 2008; **207:** 174.
9. Kragh JF, Walters TJ, Baer DG, Fox CJ, Wade CE, Salinas J, and Holcomb JB: Survival with emergency tourniquet use to stop bleeding in major limb trauma. Ann Surg 2009; **249:** 1.
10. Bagg MR, Covey DC, and Powell ET, 4th: Levels of medical care in the global war on terrorism. J Am Acad Orthop Surg 2006; **14:** S7.
11. Sohn VY, Miller JP, Koeller CA, Gibson SO, Azarow KS, Myers JB, Beekley AC, Sebesta JA, Christensen JB, and Rush RM, Jr: From the combat medic to the forward surgical team: the Madigan model for improving trauma readiness of brigade combat teams fighting the Global War on Terror. J Surg Res 2007; **138:** 25.
12. Tien HC, Jung V, Rizoli SB, Acharya SV, and MacDonald JC: An evaluation of tactical combat casualty care interventions in a combat environment. J Am Coll Surg 2008; **207:** 174.
13. Wedmore I, McManus JG, Pusateri AE, and Holcomb JB: A special report on the chitosan-based hemostatic dressing: experience in current combat operations. J Trauma 2006; **60:** 655.
14. Rhee P, Brown C, Martin M, Salim A, Plurad D, Green D, Chambers L, Demetriades D, Velmahos G, and Alam H: QuikClot use in trauma for hemorrhage control: case series of 103 documented uses. J Trauma 2008; **64:** 1093.
15. Brethauer SA, Chao A, Chambers LW, Green DJ, Brown C, Rhee P, and Bohman HR: Invasion vs insurgency: US Navy/Marine Corps forward surgical care during Operation Iraqi Freedom. Arch Surg 2008; **143:** 564.
16. Chambers LW, Rhee P, Baker BC, Perciballi J, Cubano M, Compeggie M, Nace M, and Bohman HR: Initial experience of US Marine Corps forward resuscitative surgical system during Operation Iraqi Freedom. Arch Surg 2005; **140:** 26.
17. Stevens RA, Bohman HR, Baker BC, and Chambers LW: The U.S. Navy's forward resuscitative surgery system during Operation Iraqi Freedom. Mil Med 2005; **170:** 297.
18. Beekley AC: Damage control resuscitation: a sensible approach to the exsanguinating surgical patient. Crit Care Med 2008; **36(7 suppl):** S267. Review.
19. Beekley AC and Watts DM: Combat trauma experience with the United States Army 102nd Forward Surgical Team in Afghanistan. Am J Surg 2004; **187:** 652.
20. Patel TH, Wenner KA, Price SA, Weber MA, Leveridge A, and McAtee SJ: A U.S. Army Forward Surgical Team's experience in Operation Iraqi Freedom. J Trauma 2004; **57:** 201.
21. Beekley AC: United States military surgical response to modern large-scale conflicts: the ongoing evolution of a trauma system [review]. Surg Clin North Am 2006; **86:** 689.
22. Fang R, Pruitt VM, Dorlac GR, Silvey SV, Osborn EC, Allan PF, Flaherty SF, Perello MM, Wanek SM, and Dorlac WC: Critical care at Landstuhl Regional Medical Center. Crit Care Med 2008; **36(7 Suppl):** S383.
23. Eastridge BJ, Jenkins D, Flaherty S, Schiller H, and Holcomb JB: Trauma system development in a theater of war: experiences from Operation Iraqi Freedom and Operation Enduring Freedom. J Trauma 2006; **61:** 1366.
24. Moore EE, Knudson MM, Schwab CW, Trunkey DD, Johannigman JA, and Holcomb JB: Military-civilian collaboration in trauma care and the senior visiting surgeon program. N Engl J Med 2007; **357:** 2723.

In-Theater Wound Care

Sean P. Montgomery[1,*] and Lorne Blackbourne[2]

[1]Department of Surgery, Walter Reed Army Medical Center, Washington, District of Columbia.
[2]Department of Surgery, US Army Institute of Surgical Research, San Antonio, Texas.

Background: There are many differences between combat and noncombat wounds, both in mechanisms and the initial treatment of the wounds. Additionally, the current conflicts in Iraq and Afghanistan have allowed the introduction of cutting edge products and techniques into the battlefield.
The Problem: War wounds are often dirty and high energy. This is especially true in the current conflicts, where improvised explosive devices have accounted for the majority of all combat wounds. Additionally, the initial first aid and medical care is delivered in an austere and limited resource environment.
Basic/Clinical Science Advances: The current wars have seen the widespread use of advanced hemostatic dressings for initial wound care. Tourniquets have also made a resurgence and will need to be accounted for in all future research on wound care. In the hospital setting, the concept of damage control resuscitation has been widely implemented, with the early use of fresh frozen plasma, platelets, and fresh whole blood becoming common.
Clinical Care Relevance: The advances in military combat wound care are already being transferred to the civilian setting. Specifically, the topical hemostatic agents pioneered in soldiers are becoming widespread among civilians, and increasing ratios of plasma to blood have been widely adapted in civilian trauma centers.
Conclusion: Advances in wound care in the theater of war have centered around achieving rapid local hemostasis with tourniquets and hemostatic agents.

Abbreviations and Acronyms

ATLS = advanced trauma life support

PRBCs = packed red blood cells

*Correspondence: Department of Surgery, Walter Reed Army Medical Center, 6900 Georgia Ave. NW, Washington, District of Columbia 20307 (e-mail: sean.p.montgomery@us.army.mil).

BACKGROUND

COMBAT WOUNDS FROM THE WARS in Iraq and Afghanistan differ from civilian wounds in both mechanism and the initial care provided. The current approach to wounds and the wound research performed during these wars are based on the analysis of the military's experiences in Vietnam and Somalia.

Blast or explosive injury is the leading cause of injury and death in this conflict, accounting for 56–79% of the casualties.[1] The improvised explosive device has seen widespread use in this war. In addition to the direct fragments from the bombs themselves, many soft-tissue wounds contain a great deal of dirt, rocks, and other foreign bodies resulting from the buried explosives. Additionally, this war has seen the most extensive use of body armor in a modern military conflict, resulting in patients surviving with severe blast and fragmentation injuries to multiple extremities that may have died from truncal injuries in prior conflicts.[2]

The initial care provided to wounds in this conflict is also different than that provided in civilian situations. The military divides care into different

Printed in U.S.A.
DOI: 10.1089/awc.2009.0065

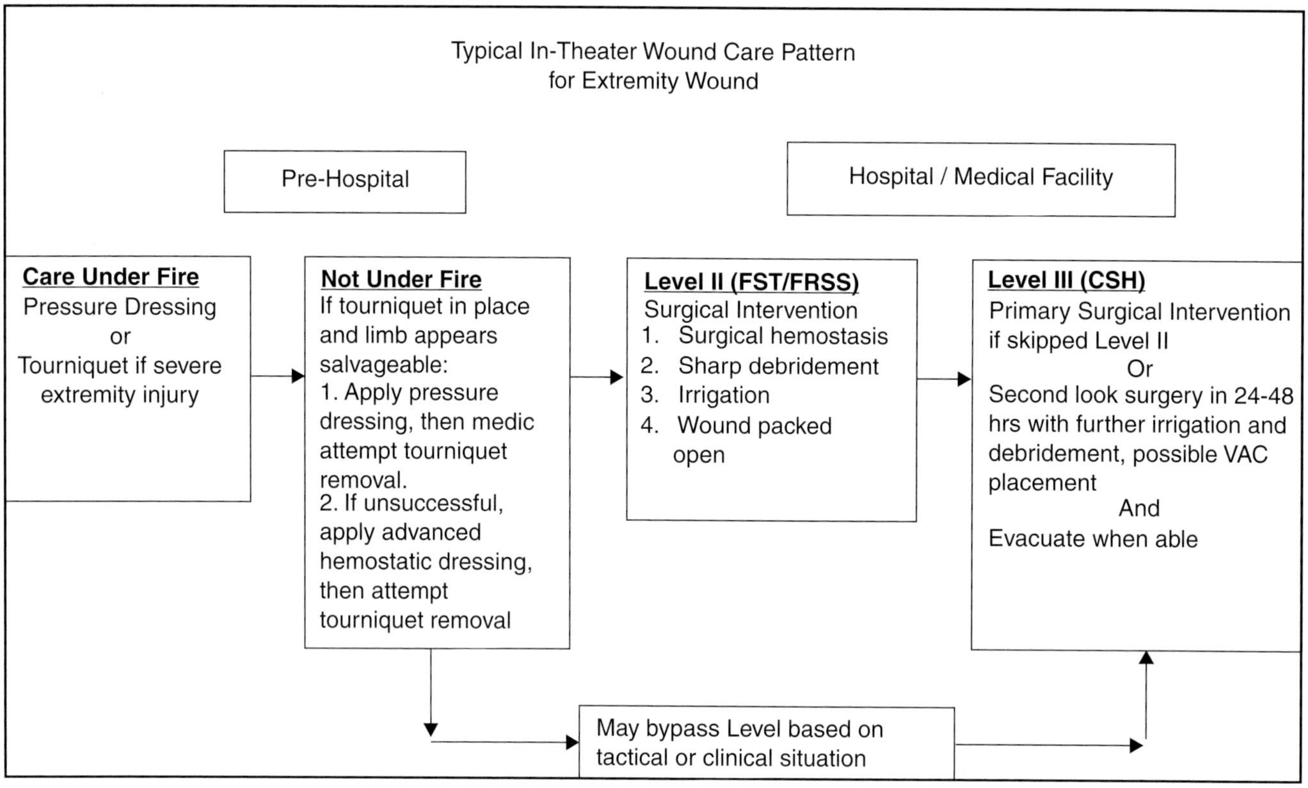

Figure 1. A typical pathway for in-theater wound care. An extremity soft-tissue wound is used as the example here since this is the common area of injury in Iraq and Afghanistan.

levels, with levels I–III occurring in theater and levels IV and V being large hospitals outside of theater, such as Landstuhl Regional Medical Center in Germany and American hospitals. A schematic overview is provided in Figure 1.

The initial care given to a wound occurs at level I, which is self-aid or buddy aid given by a combatant or medic. This frequently occurs while under fire. Medics and soldiers employ the doctrine of Tactical Combat Casualty Care. The aspects of this pertinent to wounds are the control of hemorrhage with pressure dressings, tourniquets, or hemostatic dressings.

Physicians become involved at levels II and III. Level II care consists either of a battalion aid station staffed by an advanced trauma life support (ATLS) provider without surgical capability or a Forward Surgical Team (Army) or Forward Resuscitative Surgery System (Navy/Marines). In these teams, limited surgeries are performed to control hemorrhage and minimize contamination. Level III is typically a Combat Support Hospital with multiple operating rooms, a full array of blood products, and multiple surgical teams. At a Combat Support Hospital, wounds may again undergo irrigation and debridement. They are left open and managed with dressings or negative pressure wound therapy. Definitive closure or coverage is usually deferred to a standard hospital outside of the theater of war in Europe or America, as war wounds often involve extensive devitalization of tissues and early closure is often doomed to failure.

CLINICAL PROBLEM ADDRESSED

The primary clinical problems that need to be addressed with in-theater wound care are control of hemorrhage, debridement of devitalized tissue, prevention of invasive infection, maximizing later function, and facilitating future closure or grafting. It has been well demonstrated in prior wars and again with this one that primary closure of a wound at the time of injury is fraught with peril and results in frequent infection. An additional challenge is to implement the initial wound care while under fire from the enemy.

Hemorrhage was the leading cause of death in the Vietnam War[3] and remains the leading of cause of death in Operation Iraqi Freedom.[1] An analysis of deaths from Vietnam[3] and Somalia[4] revealed many injuries that would not be treatable even by immediate surgical intervention. However, there were also a number that hemorrhaged to death from extremity wounds and other injured areas that were potentially amenable to the immediate, direct control of hemorrhage. Therefore, much of the research leading to this current conflict focused on the development of hemostatic agents that could be applied by medics and soldiers shortly after the time of injury and achieve hemostasis before evacuating the soldier to get surgical treatment.

Research on wounds also has to account for the difficulties of providing care under fire. Even in a wound where direct pressure arrests hemorrhage, it may be helpful to use a tourniquet or advanced hemostatic agent to control hemorrhage, so the soldier applying pressure will be free to return to fire or assist another casualty. The modern doctrine of Tactical Combat Casualty Care has been developed to manage this process.

However, even patients who survive surgical intervention can die from coagulopathy. Severe bleeding can result in the triad of coagulopathy, acidosis, and hypothermia. This can in turn cause life-threatening coagulopathic bleeding. The coagulopathy of trauma is another key clinical problem that has been focused on with research in this war.

BASIC SCIENCE CONTEXT

The increasing use of tourniquets has been poorly studied at the basic science level. Tourniquet use for extremity wounds in theater is creating an ischemia reperfusion scenario. Much basic science work has shown the deleterious effect of ischemia reperfusion injury in many models. However, it is unclear how much ischemia reperfusion impacts wound healing after tourniquet use.

The hemostatic mechanisms of topical hemostatics have been well investigated. However, the science on the effect of these agents on the wound-healing environment has been minimal. Some agents may have the potential to alter the microenvironment in the wound and modulate the inflammatory response.

EXPERIMENTAL MODEL OR MATERIAL

Several experimental models of lethal hemorrhagic shock have been developed. The swine groin injury is the one most applicable to cutaneous wounds.[5,6] In this model, a combined skin, muscle, and vascular injury is created by transection of the thigh muscles and the femoral artery and vein. The animal is allowed to hemorrhage for 3 to 5 minutes to simulate field response time, and then the agent to be tested is applied to the wound. The endpoint in experiments using this model has been survival, and wound healing has not been tested. The advantage of this model is that it simulates a realistic war wound of the type not amenable to tourniquet placement, such as a high groin wound. Other models have used a partial injury to the femoral artery.[7] This prevents the artery from retracting into the wound. This may yield a more standardized model as the effects of vasospasm are minimized.

The complex contaminated wounds after war injury have also been modeled in animals. Goats have been used for studies, where a reproducible complex musculoskeletal wound has been inoculated with genetically modified *Pseudomonas aeruginosa*.[8] Photon counts can then be used to determine bacterial concentrations after various interventions.

DISCUSSION OF FINDINGS AND RELEVANT LITERATURE

The predominant change in wound care in theater has been the use of hemostatic agents applied topically to wounds. Animal data have shown a significant increase in survival when granular zeolite was applied in the swine groin injury model. For this reason, it was adopted by the Marine Corps. Clinical data have been less definitive. A case series of 103 human uses of zeolite has been presented, showing control of hemorrhage in 95 of the 103 cases, but without any controls.[9] There were also no anatomic details of the injuries and no follow-up on the long-term outcome of the wounds. Another case series reported four instances of significant burns from the use of the zeolite product.[10] Since this time, the zeolite product has undergone reformulation to decrease the exothermic reaction. There has been no analysis on the effects of zeolite on wound healing and functional outcome in survivors. Although the Marine Corps has been the primary user of zeolite, the Army has used a chitosan-based dressing (HemCon; HemCon Inc., Portland, OR) for topical hemostasis. An uncontrolled series of 64 cases of the use of this dressing was reported.[11] Hemorrhage was stopped or greatly decreased in 97% of the cases. There were no reported complications.

Two new products, a kaolin-impregnated gauze (Combat Gauze; Z-Medica Corporation, Wallingford, CT) and a granular smectite (WoundStat; TraumaCare, Bethesda, MD),[7] have been tested in swine models of arterial hemorrhage and offer superior hemostasis to the QuikClot and HemCon dressings in current use, but again the impact of these products on wound healing has been untested. The Combat Gauze has been provided to some field units, while the WoundStat is not being used because of the concerns of embolism of the granules.

Tourniquet use is by no means a new technology, but it has assumed a new prominence in this conflict. Tourniquet use has been discouraged in civilian trauma and by some authors.[12,13] However, analyses during this war confirmed a survival benefit to the use of tourniquets.[14,15] This benefit was greatest when applied in the prehospital setting and before the onset of shock. In patients with indicated tourniquet use, the mortality was 11% with prehospital use and 24% when application was delayed to the emergency department.[15] This study also suggests that the application of tourniquets before the onset of shock is most helpful. When tourniquet usage is compared in studies from the beginning of the war to now, the use of tourniquets has increased from less than 50%[14] to over 90%[15] of the severely injured extremities. What is missing is any information on the long-term effects of tourniquet use on wound healing or coverage rates. Amputation rates do not appear to be affected by tourniquet use, but there are no data on later wound complications or healing rates in these extremities.

This is also the first military conflict where negative pressure wound therapy has been widely employed. The wounds of American servicemen are always left open in theater and managed with either serial dressing changes or vacuum-assisted closure devices. There are no published results of wounds managed with primary closure in theater, but in the author's personal experiences essentially all wounds closed in theater have become infected and required opening by the time of arrival in the United States. Patients who are local nationals are not evacuated out of theater and have their wounds managed at an in-theater hospital. One published cohort of 88 patients with high-energy wounds had their wounds managed entirely in theater.[16] The wounds were managed with serial operative debridement, pulse lavage, and negative pressure dressings. The patients were managed with all dressing care in the operating room. When the wounds were clean and viable, direct closure, skin graft, or closure by local skin flap was performed. This achieved a 0% infection rate.

The concept of damage control resuscitation has also become prominent during this war.[17–19] This is not a direct wound therapy, but it is important for those performing research or clinical care on wounds to be familiar with this concept. In brief, the use of crystalloid or packed red blood cells (PRBCs) to resuscitate a trauma patient can contribute to systemic coagulopathy in severely injured patients. This war has contributed to an emerging doctrine that using fresh whole blood or increasing the ratio of plasma to PRBCs to 1:1 is appropriate for hemorrhagic shock. Hard data to confirm better survival in war casualties are still pending as of this time. The impact of damage control resuscitation on wound healing or the systemic inflammatory profile has not been fully investigated.

CAUTION, CRITICAL REMARKS, AND RECOMMENDATIONS

War has frequently led to advances in wound care because of a high concentration of patient volume and clinical experience. However, modern research has evolved away from case series and experience-based research to carefully controlled prospective studies. These will never be possible in a subject as demanding as wound care in the theater or war. It will be necessary to gather as much data as possible during the remainder of the war, so that the true effects of interventions such as topical hemostatics can be evaluated.

TAKE-HOME MESSAGE

Basic science advances

- The effect of hemostatic agents on the inflammatory response in the wound and on wound healing is unknown.
- The impact of ischemia reperfusion following the use of tourniquets is unknown.

Clinical science advance

- Topical hemostatics have shown great success in swine arterial injury models.

Relevance to clinical care

- Tourniquets are proven to control hemorrhage from serious extremity wounds and should be applied in the prehospital setting.
- Following initial debridement, war wounds should be left open for closure or coverage in a delayed fashion. Negative pressure wound therapy is an acceptable choice for management of major soft-tissue injuries.
- The use of fresh whole blood and higher ratios of plasma to PRBCs is common in battle casualties.

FUTURE DEVELOPMENTS

None of the advances in wound care seen during this war has

addressed the issue of noncompressible hemorrhage. This is a daunting challenge, but to have medications or devices available to the first responder that affect internal bleeding would dramatically increase the lives saved after injury. The impact of the devices that we are using for hemostasis, such as tourniquets and topical hemostatics, on wound healing and later function needs to be better examined. If ischemia reperfusion injury can be shown after tourniquet use, the development of agents targeted at preventing this injury will be important.

AUTHOR DISCLOSURE STATEMENT

None.

REFERENCES

1. Kelly JF, *et al.*: Injury severity and causes of death from Operation Iraqi Freedom and Operation Enduring Freedom: 2003–2004 versus 2006. J Trauma 2008; **64(2 Suppl):** S21; discussion S26–S27.
2. Montgomery SP, Swiecki CW, and Shriver CD: The evaluation of casualties from Operation Iraqi Freedom on return to the continental United States from March to June 2003. J Am Coll Surg 2005; **201:** 7; discussion 12–13.
3. Bellamy RF: The causes of death in conventional land warfare: implications for combat casualty care research. Mil Med 1984; **149:** 55.
4. Mabry RL, *et al.*: United States Army Rangers in Somalia: an analysis of combat casualties on an urban battlefield. J Trauma 2000; **49:** 515; discussion 528–529.
5. Alam HB, *et al.*: Comparative analysis of hemostatic agents in a swine model of lethal groin injury. J Trauma 2003; **54:** 1077.
6. Alam HB, *et al.*: Application of a zeolite hemostatic agent achieves 100% survival in a lethal model of complex groin injury in swine. J Trauma 2004; **56:** 974.
7. Kheirabadi BS, *et al.*: Comparison of new hemostatic granules/powders with currently deployed hemostatic products in a lethal model of extremity arterial hemorrhage in swine. J Trauma 2009; **66:** 316; discussion 327–328.
8. Owens BD, White DW, and Wenke JC: Comparison of irrigation solutions and devices in a contaminated musculoskeletal wound survival model. J Bone Joint Surg Am 2009; **91:** 92.
9. Rhee P, *et al.*: QuikClot use in trauma for hemorrhage control: case series of 103 documented uses. J Trauma 2008; **64:** 1093.
10. McManus J, *et al.*: A case series describing thermal injury resulting from zeolite use for hemorrhage control in combat operations. Prehosp Emerg Care 2007; **11:** 67.
11. Wedmore I, *et al.*: A special report on the chitosan-based hemostatic dressing: experience in current combat operations. J Trauma 2006; **60:** 655.
12. Navein J, Coupland R, and Dunn R: The tourniquet controversy. J Trauma 2003; **54(5 Suppl):** S219.
13. Welling DR, *et al.*: A balanced approach to tourniquet use: lessons learned and relearned. J Am Coll Surg 2006; **203:** 106.
14. Beekley AC, *et al.*: Prehospital tourniquet use in Operation Iraqi Freedom: effect on hemorrhage control and outcomes. J Trauma 2008; **64(2 Suppl):** S28; discussion S37.
15. Kragh JF, Jr., *et al.*: Survival with emergency tourniquet use to stop bleeding in major limb trauma. Ann Surg 2009; **249:** 1.
16. Leininger BE, *et al.*: Experience with wound VAC and delayed primary closure of contaminated soft tissue injuries in Iraq. J Trauma 2006; **61:** 1207.
17. Fox CJ, *et al.*: Damage control resuscitation for vascular surgery in a combat support hospital. J Trauma 2008; **65:** 1.
18. Holcomb JB: Damage control resuscitation. J Trauma 2007; **62(6 Suppl):** S36
19. Holcomb JB, *et al.*: Damage control resuscitation: directly addressing the early coagulopathy of trauma. J Trauma 2007; **62:** 307.

WHS
Wound
Healing
Society

Update on Bioburden Control and Treatment of War Wound Infections

Kyle Petersen,[1,*] Duane Hospenthal,[2] and Glenn Wortmann[3]

[1]Undersea Medicine Division, Naval Medical Research Center, Silver Spring, Maryland.
[2]Infectious Disease Service, San Antonio Military Medical Center, Fort Sam Houston, Texas.
[3]Infectious Disease Service, Walter Reed Army Medical Center, Washington, District of Columbia.

Abbreviations and Acronyms

CFU = colony forming unit

Flt3L = FMS-like tyrosine kinase ligand

HBO = hyperbaric oxygen

MRSA = methicillin-resistant *Staphylococcus aureus*

NPWT = negative pressure wound therapy

QPCR = quantitative polymerase chain reaction

RIP = RNA-inhibiting peptide

VAC = vacuum-assisted closure

*Correspondence: Undersea Medicine Division, Naval Medical Research Center, 503 Robert Grant Ave., Silver Spring, Maryland 20910 (e-mail: kyle.petersen@med.navy.mil).

Background: Combat injury–related wounds are generally acute, and occur in young, otherwise healthy adults. The most significant sequelae of wound bioburden, sepsis, which previously affected 90% of casualties in the preantibiotic era, continues to occur in 5–10%, causing considerable morbidity and some mortality. Controlling or eradicating bioburden before the critical colonization stage of 10^5 colony forming unit/g or more than four bacterial species might decrease infectious sequelae.
The Problem: Modern combat wounds are complex, usually blast-related injuries, with extensive soft tissue damage, which is often complicated by vascular impairment and underlying bone injury. Persons developing infection may be critically ill, have received multiple transfusions, and suffer multiorgan impairment. With modern debridement and posttrauma antibiotic use, combat wound pathogens have changed from *Clostridia* and *Streptococcus* to multidrug-resistant nosocomial pathogens such as *Staphylococcus aureus*, *Pseudomonas aeruginosa*, and *Acinetobacter baumannii.* New modalities that prevent the selection of drug-resistant bacteria, and prevent wound-related sepsis and death are needed.
Basic/Clinical Science Advances: In 2008 numerous approaches to bioburden reduction were published. Several having potential for combat wound care include novel diagnostics, dressings, negative pressure devices, topical solutions, antimicrobial peptides, and innovative approaches to surgical care.
Clinical Care Relevance: Application of some of these aforementioned novel approaches might reduce multidrug-resistant bacterial colonization and wound infection, but more study is required.
Conclusion: Limited studies were done on combat-related bioburden reduction in 2008. Work focused on chronic wound infections may have potential crossover utility in combat wounds; however, more studies are needed in this unique population.

BACKGROUND

Combat wounds result from high-velocity gunshots or explosive devices. In the current wars in Iraq and Afghanistan multiorgan blast injuries predominate and wound contamination with environmental debris and device fragments is common. Advances in body armor often spare the thorax and abdomen in survivors of the initial blast. Improvised bombs and rocket attacks remain our adversaries' weapon of choice, inflicting devastating injury on the extremities, including vascular disruption, traumatic amputations, and multiple large soft tissue wounds, often with underlying open fractures.[1]

Advances in trauma care have resulted in a population of critically ill

ADVANCES IN WOUND CARE, VOLUME 1

Printed in U.S.A.
DOI: 10.1089/awc.2009.0058

patients, often with iron overload from massive transfusions, surviving with these complex wounds. Coupled with the selective pressure of perioperative and empiric antibiotic therapy, multidrug-resistant nosocomial bacteria, including methicillin-resistant *Staphylococcus aureus* (MRSA), *Acinetobacter baumannii*, *Pseudomonas aeruginosa*, and enteric bacteria such as extended-spectrum β-lactamase–producing *Klebsiella*, have emerged as the predominant agents of wound and orthopedic infection.[2] These organisms colonize wounds within days after injury; however, the usual wound bioburden stages (contamination, colonization, etc.) are uncommon because of repeated debridement every 2–3 days. Antimicrobial selection is often limited to the carbapenems with these multidrug-resistant bacteria, and carbapenem-resistance rates in military hospitals are increasing.[3] The usual challenges of distinguishing colonization from infection are amplified due to the size and complexity of many of these wounds and the coexisting multiorgan dysfunction in these injured personnel. Distinguishing inflammation from infection is difficult, resulting in the overuse of empiric broad-spectrum antibiotics. Some bacteria, such as *A. baumannii*, have developed resistance to carbapenem antibiotics, often leaving colistin sulfate (associated with significant

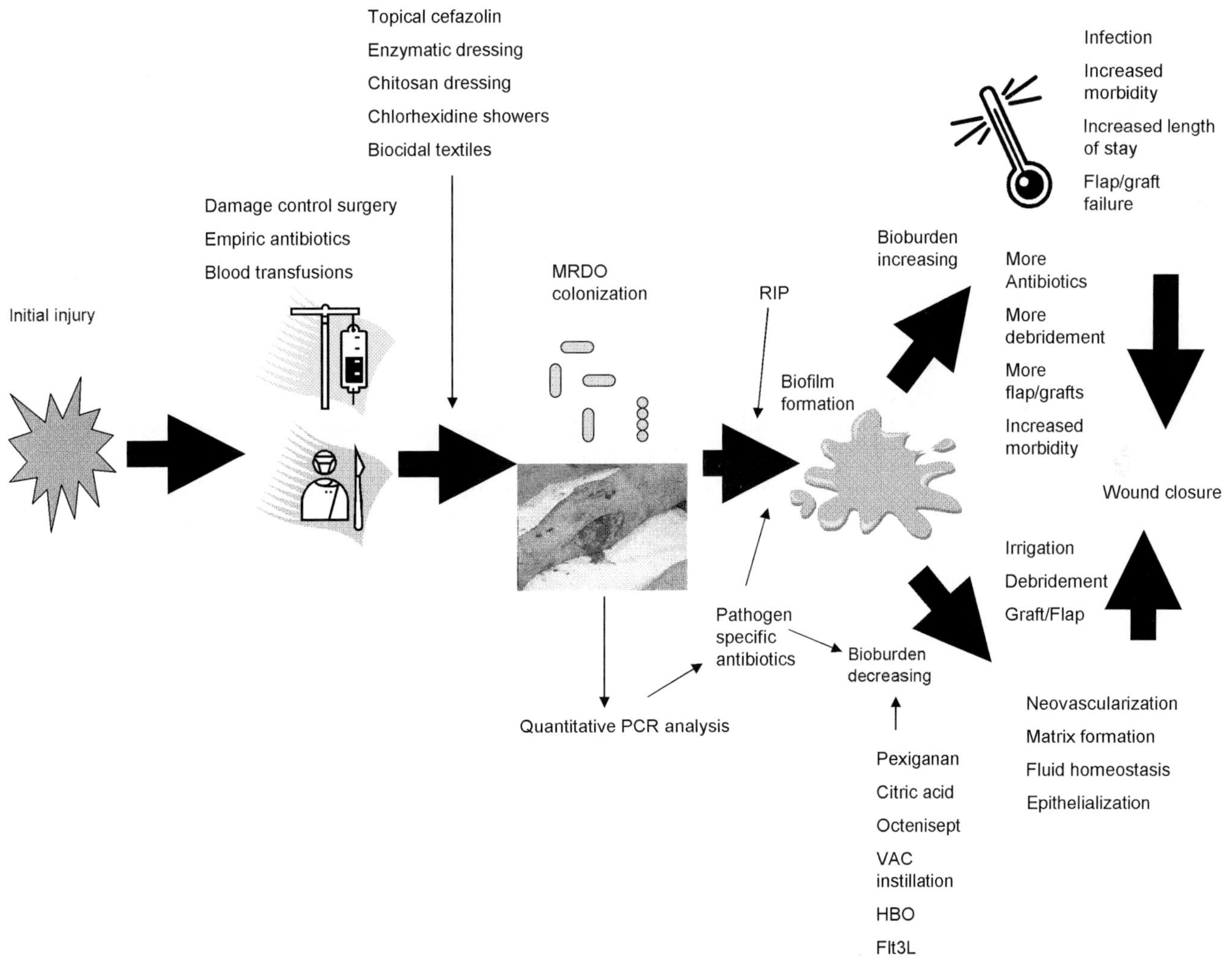

Figure 1. Typically, within 1 h after wounding, patients are transferred to a forward surgical unit, where life-saving surgery is performed. Patients may receive up to 100 U of whole blood or packed RBCs, providing an iron-rich environment for bacteria. Additionally, perioperative antibiotics such as cefazolin, administered to prevent infection, may select for subsequent multidrug-resistant colonization. The patient is then transferred to other facilities with wounds that become colonized with multidrug-resistant bacteria. The development of immunologic dysregulation secondary to massive trauma and/or the development of wound biofilms may allow bacteria to exceed a critical threshold, resulting in invasive infection. Possible sites of implementation for the technologies reviewed in the text are indicated by arrows.

nephrotoxicity) as the only therapeutic option. New or novel classes of broad-spectrum antibiotics are not on the horizon.

Approaches to decrease use of empiric broad-spectrum agents, reduce antibiotic resistance, and prevent or control initial host contamination are needed (Fig. 1).

CLINICAL PROBLEM ADDRESSED

Several studies of wound bioburden and wound infection treatment were published in 2008.[4–30] While specific combat wound studies were limited, several papers of interest relating to acute or chronic wound bioburden reduction, diagnosis, prophylaxis, and treatment had broad applicability.

Recent approaches to mitigating bioburden in combat wounds can be broadly divided into five areas. Diagnostics, particularly novel molecular ones, might better differentiate colonization from infection allowing for tailored antibiotic therapy or reducing empiric broad-spectrum usage. Novel devices including negative pressure wound therapy (NPWT), such as vacuum-assisted closure (VAC), might remove wound inflammatory exudates, including potential harmful cytokines and bacteria, via continuous suction. Impregnated dressings would mitigate bioburden via dressings that elute their relevant compound into the wound. Topically applied products act like impregnated dressings, but are applied directly into the wound bed at dressing changes. Finally modification of existing wound care techniques, such as the use of biocidal textiles incorporated into medical gowns and drapes might also mitigate bioburden.

RELEVANT BASIC SCIENCE CONTEXT

Bioburden is described in the following continuum: contamination (presence of nonreplicating bacteria); colonization (presence of replicating organisms in the wound); critical colonization (replicating organisms exceeding a threshold to cause host harm and impede wound healing); local invasion (infection of the wound or contiguous tissue structures); and disseminated infection (spread to the bloodstream or remote sites). Studies have suggested that greater than 10^5 colony forming unit (CFU)/g tissue biopsied or more than four bacteria species in a wound might predispose to invasive infection. Exceptions include β-hemolytic *Streptococcus* (lower invasive threshold) and *Pseudomonas* (impairs matrix healing via proteolysis).[31]

The role of wound biofilms is critical in the formation of bioburden. While planktonic bacteria are susceptible to antibiotics at the tested minimum inhibitory concentration, minimum inhibitory concentrations for bacteria in biofilm can be 1000-fold greater, rendering antibiotic agents useless. Biofilms can form in as little as 6–8 h and appear to have the same 10^5 CFU/g threshold.

EXPERIMENTAL MODEL OR MATERIAL—ADVANTAGES AND LIMITATIONS

Wound bioburden studies are difficult to conduct in war trauma patients. The study population is small, as opposed to that of patients with chronic wounds. It is difficult to replicate the actual scenario of blast exposure, which includes complex musculoskeletal injury, polymicrobial colonization/infection, underlying orthopedic injury, massive transfusion burden with possible iron overload, and multiorgan dysfunction in animal models. One goat model of complex musculoskeletal injuries reviewed comes closest, but it has been limited to the study of one bacterial species at a time.[4] We included reviews of multiple studies in chronic wounds for potential applicability, but caution that these are more conceptual ideas for future study rather than having immediate applicability in trauma wounds.

DISCUSSION OF FINDINGS AND RELEVANT LITERATURE

Diagnostics

An interesting case report examined the use of molecular diagnostics in optimally treating bioburden.[5] A patient suffered a chronic ulcer recalcitrant to healing with antibiotic treatment. Quantitative polymerase chain reaction (QPCR) revealed *P. aeruginosa* where standard culture was negative, resulting in a modification of therapy and subsequent improvement. While more studies are needed, tailoring antimicrobials to the individual wound ecology via QPCR might be preferred over broad-spectrum empiric therapy, particularly when organisms are present in low numbers or exhibit fastidious growth, but is limited in that it does not distinguish between planktonic and biofilm growth. 16S ribosomal RNA might also have applicability for diagnosis.[6]

Impregnated dressings

Silver has been used for decades as a wound adjunct, is bactericidal, and does not tend to select for resistance. A recent meta-analysis of silver dressings examined their effectiveness and commented on the methodological quality of the studies.[7] Of over 1,900 papers examined (1950 to present), only 14 (1,200 patients) were of sufficient quality for inclusion in their analysis, and only 4 examined silver dressings and infection. All 4 showed significant "relative infection control reduction" but were of moderate quality and lacked adequate power and size. A second study on silver and infection used a novel polymer of polyethylene glycol and gelatin.[8] This dressing's advantage is its ability to conform to large/complicated wounds (common in war trauma) and one-time application. A dressing matrix imbedded with an antimicrobial (silver sulfadiazine) and an analgesic (bupivacaine) was studied for inhibitory activity against *S. aureus* and *P. aeruginosa*. Results showed that both the silver-impregnated matrix and the dual-impregnated matrix eluted greater than 96% of their drug, without antagonism between drugs. The silver was bactericidal to both organisms.

Two studies investigated dressings with chitosan, a biopolymer that effects hemostasis, stimulates healing, provides a wound scaffold, is a vehicle for drug delivery, and has antimicrobial properties. One study examined chitosan dressings applied to a burn wound model and the effects on *Pseudomonas* and *Proteus*.[9] In *Pseudomonas* infections, chitosan had the highest survival rates. In *Proteus* infections, it was equivalent to the silver dressing. The authors reported the dressing superior to silver sulfadiazine due to its faster bactericidal activity. A study limitation, however, was the short dwell times between infection and dressing application. Another study reported efficacy of chitosan dressings in 85 patients.[10] All wounds were colonized at baseline. At 21 days polymicrobial or streptococcal infection had developed in 45% of the control wounds but in none of the chitosan-treated wounds, suggesting that chitosan has promise and merits further study.

Enzymatic debridement dressings have been considered unsafe for wounds with high bioburdens, as previous burn injury studies demonstrated a sepsis risk.[32] These agents, however, have not been well studied in nonburn, open wounds. Using a chronic wound infection model with 10^8 CFU *Escherichia coli*, treatment with collagenase or papain-urea dressings was studied.[11] A significant reduction in CFU occurred by day 4 with papain and day 7 with collagenase. While the study demonstrated safety, it was not superior to wet to dry dressings or sharp debridement.

Several therapies considered alternative to traditional medicine have been investigated, including triphala, an Indian compound of three herbs with catechin-based antibacterial properties.[12] Triphala-impregnated collagen dressing significantly reduced bioburden 4 days after wounding compared to control or collagen alone, but more study of the active agents is required.

While honey has been used for centuries, its effect in human wounds was disappointing in two recent trials. Manuka honey (the most bactericidal) was compared to hydrocolloid dressings in venous ulcers and reduced MRSA colonization, but showed no difference in infection and performed worse than hydrocolloid against *Pseudomonas*.[13] A well-controlled, randomized trial demonstrated no benefit of honey-impregnated dressings on wound healing,[14] suggesting that further investigation would be fruitless.

Topical agents of interest in 2008 included citric acid. Two case reports showed that 3% citric acid substantially reduced *S. aureus* and *E. coli* growth from foot wounds at 2 days, and completely in 6 days, with increases in angiogenesis and fibroblasts.[15] Another study reported the effect of a 4% citric acid gel containing 1% acetic acid on *Pseudomonas* infection in a rat wound model.[16] In less heavily contaminated wounds, the gel was equivalent to 5% mafenide. However, previous efforts have shown impaired healing at one-fourth of the acetic acid concentration in this product.[33] While citric acid is promising, more analysis is required.

Cefazolin is well established in preventing perioperative surgical-site infections. However, its broad-spectrum activity has been postulated as the cause of widespread *Pseudomonas* wound infection in the 1970s' Israeli wars.[34] One study compared topical cefazolin solution bulb syringe irrigation to intravenous administration and measured wound and serum drug concentrations 5 h postoperatively.[17] Serum peak drug levels were four times higher in the intravenous group than in the topical group, but both were therapeutic for the inhibition of *Staphylococcus*, and serum drug levels persisted only 1 h longer than the topical group. Wound fluid levels were 190-fold higher in the topical arm. No infections or differences in healing were noted, but the study was not powered to detect a difference. Nevertheless, this study suggests that topical cefazolin irrigation to prevent surgical-site infections is worth further study.

Peptides have been a recent therapy focus. Pexiganan is a synthetic peptide with broad antibacterial activity. In a randomized trial in diabetic foot wounds,[18] patients were treated with ofloxacin or Pexiganin for 2–4 weeks. There were no differences in eradication rates in the wound bed, but a Pexiganin advantage was an absence of induced drug resistance to *Staphylococcus*. A common criticism/concern of peptide therapy is that host proteases will degrade peptides, but that did not occur in this study.

Another peptide recently tested is an RNA-inhibiting peptide (RIP), which blocks quorum sensing, an important action in bacterial biofilm formation.[19] In a mouse model using MRSA, RIP-impregnated foam dressing (when combined with teichoplanin) was found to increase revascularization and up-regulate growth factors. When used alone, the foam dressing significantly decreased bioburden and increased wound repair. This agent might have promise in combat wounds if also effective against Gram-negative bacteria.

Octenisept, an antiseptic, was recently studied in infected malignant ulcers,[20] reducing Gram-negative and Gram-positive bacterial colonization and completely eradicating coagulase-negative *Staphylococcus* and *Enterococcus* species from the wounds. More studies are required before commenting on its applicability in war wounds.

Finally, existing topical treatments were evaluated for *A. baumannii*, a common colonizer of current combat wounds.[21] Mafenide had the most activity, followed by mupirocin, Neosporin, polysporin, and silver dressings. This study did not use a war-associated clinical isolate, but it suggests that mafenide, an established agent for burn wounds, deserves further investigation.

Novel devices

Several recent papers looked at the effect of NPWT therapy, applied either via the traditional sponge suction device or via several newer devices, including one that includes a reservoir to instill antiseptics into the wound. A recent meta-analysis of all previous VAC studies (13 trials of 573 wounds in 554 patients) reported two that examined effect on bioburden. Neither showed any reduction in bacterial growth (approximately 10^5 CFU/g organisms after VAC therapy).[22] Acute wound studies suggested no benefit and possible harm (number needed to harm = 9). A second trial comparing VAC versus alginate dressings in diabetic foot ulcers showed no significant difference in infections, suggesting a more neutral effect.[23] Theoretically, combining antiseptic irrigation with VAC could reduce bioburden, but a channel effect (where not all irrigation fluid is distributed evenly across the wound) has been observed with some devices.[24] A recent pilot study appears to have overcome this effect.[25] Fifteen patients receiving VAC with instillation of silver nitrate were compared to historical controls treated with standard wet dressings. Infection resolution, wound closure, and time to hospital discharge were significantly faster than in controls. However, the study suffered from a lack of a VAC group without silver nitrate instillation.

Modification of existing wound care technique

In 2008, only one study evaluated war wound infections. That study involved hyperbaric oxygen (HBO) treatment.[26] HBO was used as an adjunct for open fracture blast leg wounds in 99 patients and compared with 289 controls. HBO-treated patients had a decreased rate of soft tissue infection, skin graft lysis, and flap necrosis. Impact on osteomyelitis was insignificant, but time to granulation increased 25%.

Immunoaugmentation is a clever and unique approach to reducing wound bioburden that does not engender bacterial resistance. A recent paper reported the effect of a dendritic cell growth factor (FMS-like tyrosine kinase ligand [Flt3L]) on *Pseudomonas*-infected burn wounds.[27] In mice, infections were reduced to almost zero after inoculation and significant

TAKE-HOME MESSAGE

Basic science advance

- QPCR is an emerging technology that may help diagnose bacteria in biofilms and allow for targeted therapy.

Clinical science advances

- Silver dressings appear to reduce bioburden and can be incorporated into a novel polymer dressing better suited to large combat wounds.
- Of existing U.S. Food and Drug Administration–approved topical agents, mafenide demonstrated the best activity against *A. baumannii in vitro.*
- Immunoaugmentation by the dendritic cell growth factor Flt3L is very promising and needs more studies.

Relevance to clinical care

- NPWT has a negative or neutral effect on wound bioburden. Next-generation devices with drug delivery reservoirs may be more effective at bioburden reduction, especially when used with silver nitrate solution.
- Chitosan reduces bioburden and may emerge as a multipurpose combat dressing.
- From the available data, honey does not appear to be an effective therapy for bioburden control.
- Perioperative wound prophylaxis with topical cefazolin is an intriguing idea that needs further study. Peptide therapies such as Pexiganan and RIP blockade of quorum sensing are novel therapies with encouraging initial results.
- Octenisept reduces bioburden, but toxicity to healing tissue remains unknown.

reductions in bacterial burden and increased survival in Flt3L-treated animals occurred. Clearly this is an exciting technology that merits more research in war wounds.

Topical decolonization with preoperative showers with chlorhexidine recently demonstrated reduced surgical-site infections[28] and might have applicability in combat wounds, as might biocidal sheets woven with copper.[29] In burn patients, enhanced glycemic control maintained wound CFU under 10^5 CFU/g.[30]

CAUTION, CRITICAL REMARKS, AND RECOMMENDATIONS

Many of these studies were performed in animal models or in patients with chronic wounds and may not translate to the care of complex combat wounds. However, they may serve as a springboard for future combat wound care research.

FUTURE DEVELOPMENT

Evaluation of the most promising multipurpose products, such as chitosan, silver/bupivacaine composite dressings, and next-generation NPWT is needed. Efforts to reduce the spread of multidrug-resistant bacteria by the use of targeted therapies and immunoaugmentation might spare existing antibiotics for the future.

ACKNOWLEDGMENTS

The authors would like to thank Ms. Diana Temple for her assistance in editing the manuscript.

DISCLAIMER

The views expressed herein are those of the authors and do not reflect the official policy or position of the Department of the Army, Department of the Navy, Department of Defense, or the U.S. Government. The authors are employees of the U.S. Government. This work was prepared as part of their official duties and, as such, there is no copyright to be transferred.

AUTHOR DISCLOSURE STATEMENT

No competing financial interests exist.

REFERENCES

1. Ramasamy A, Harrisson SE, Clasper JC, and Stewart MP: Injuries from roadside improvised explosive devices. J Trauma 2008; **65:** 910.
2. Murray CK, Hinkle MK, and Yun HC: History of infections associated with combat-related injuries. J Trauma 2008; **64:** S221.
3. Hujer KM, Hujer AM, Hulten EA, Bajaksouzian S, Adams JM, Donskey CJ, Ecker DJ, Massire C, Eshoo MW, Sampath R, Thomson JM, Rather PN, Craft DW, Fishbain JT, Ewell AJ, Jacobs MR, Paterson DL, and Bonomo RA: Analysis of antibiotic resistance genes in multidrug-resistant *Acinetobacter* sp. isolates from military and civilian patients treated at the Walter Reed Army Medical Center. Antimicrob Agents Chemother 2006; **50:** 4114.
4. Svoboda SJ, Owens BD, Gooden HA, Melvin ML, Baer DG, and Wenke JC: Irrigation with potable water versus normal saline in a contaminated musculoskeletal wound model. J Trauma 2008; **64:** 1357.
5. Wolcott RD and Dowd SE: A rapid molecular method for characterising bacterial bioburden in chronic wounds. J Wound Care 2008; **17:** 513.
6. Janda JM and Abbott SL: 16S rRNA gene sequencing for bacterial identification in the diagnostic laboratory: pluses, perils, and pitfalls. J Clin Microbiol 2007; **45:** 2761.
7. Lo SF, Chang CJ, Hu WY, Hayter M, and Chang YT: The effectiveness of silver-releasing dressings in the management of non-healing chronic wounds: a meta-analysis. J Clin Nurs 2009; **18:** 716.
8. Kleinbeck KR, Bader RA, and Kao WJ: Concurrent *in vitro* release of silver sulfadiazine and bupivacaine from semi-interpenetrating networks for wound management. J Burn Care Res 2009; **30:** 98.
9. Dai T, Tegos GP, Burkatovskaya M, Castano AP, and Hamblin MR: Chitosan acetate bandage as a topical antimicrobial dressing for infected burns. Antimicrob Agents Chemother 2009; **53:** 393.
10. Kordestani S, Shahrezaee M, Tahmasebi MN, Hajimahmodi H, Haji Ghasemali D, and Abyaneh MS: A randomised controlled trial on the effectiveness of an advanced wound dressing used in Iran. J Wound Care 2008; **17:** 323.
11. Payne WG, Salas RE, Ko F, Naidu DK, Donate G, Wright TE, and Robson MC: Enzymatic debriding agents are safe in wounds with high bacterial bioburdens and stimulate healing. Eplasty 2008; **8:** 151.
12. Kumar MS, Kirubanandan S, Sripriya R, and Sehgal PK: Triphala incorporated collagen sponge—a smart biomaterial for infected dermal wound healing. J Surg Res 2008 Aug 15. [Epub ahead of print.]
13. Gethin G and Cowman S: Bacteriological changes in sloughy venous leg ulcers treated with manuka honey or hydrogel: an RCT. J Wound Care 2008; **17:** 241.
14. Jull A, Walker N, Parag V, Molan P, and Rodgers A: Randomized clinical trial of honey-impregnated dressings for venous leg ulcers. Br J Surg 2008; **95:** 175.
15. Nagoba BS, Gandhi RC, Wadher BJ, Potekar RM, and Kolhe SM: Microbiological, histopathological and clinical changes in chronic infected wounds after citric acid treatment. J Med Microbiol 2008; **57:** 681.
16. Martineau L and Dosch HM: Management of bioburden with a burn gel that targets nociceptors. J Wound Care 2007; **16:** 157.
17. White RR, Pitzer KD, Fader RC, Rajab MH, and Song J: Pharmacokinetics of topical and intravenous cefazolin in patients with clean surgical wounds. Plast Reconstr Surg 2008; **122:** 1773.
18. Lipsky BA, Holroyd KJ, and Zasloff M: Topical versus systemic antimicrobial therapy for treating mildly infected diabetic foot ulcers: a randomized, controlled, double-blinded, multicenter trial of pexiganan cream. Clin Infect Dis 2008; **47:** 1537.
19. Simonetti O, Cirioni O, Ghiselli R, Goteri G, Scalise A, Orlando F, Silvestri C, Riva A, Saba V, Madanahally KD, Offidani A, Balaban N, Scalise G, and Giacometti A: RNAIII-inhibiting peptide enhances healing of wounds infected with methicillin-resistant *Staphylococcus aureus.* Antimicrob Agents Chemother 2008; **52:** 2205.
20. Sopata M, Ciuplnska M, Głowacka A, Muszynski Z, and Tomaszewska E: Reducing bacterial flora in pressure ulcers of patients with advanced cancer. J Wound Care 2008; **17:** 452.

21. Davis SC, Pisanni F, and Montero RB: Effects of commonly used topical antimicrobial agents on *Acinetobacter baumannii*: an *in vitro* study. Mil Med 2008; **173:** 74.

22. Ubbink DT, Westerbos SJ, Nelson EA, and Vermeulen H: A systematic review of topical negative pressure therapy for acute and chronic wounds. Br J Surg 2008; **95:** 685.

23. Blume PA, Walters J, Payne W, Ayala J, and Lantis J: Comparison of negative pressure wound therapy using vacuum-assisted closure with advanced moist wound therapy in the treatment of diabetic foot ulcers: a multicenter randomized controlled trial. Diabetes Care 2008; **31:** 631.

24. Lee SS, Chang KP, Lai CS, and Lin SD: Does continuous negative-pressure and irrigation treatment really rinse the whole closed wound? Plast Reconstr Surg 2008; **122:** 319.

25. Gabriel A, Shores J, Heinrich C, Baqai W, Kalina S, Sogioka N, and Gupta S: Negative pressure wound therapy with instillation: a pilot study describing a new method for treating infected wounds. Int Wound J 2008; **5:** 399.

26. Roje Z, Roje Z, Eterović D, Druzijanić N, Petrićević A, Roje T, and Capkun V: Influence of adjuvant hyperbaric oxygen therapy on short-term complications during surgical reconstruction of upper and lower extremity war injuries: retrospective cohort study. Croat Med J 2008; **49:** 224.

27. Bohannon J, Cui W, Cox R, Przkora R, Sherwood E, and Toliver-Kinsky T: Prophylactic treatment with fms-like tyrosine kinase-3 ligand after burn injury enhances global immune responses to infection. J Immunol 2008; **180:** 3038.

28. Edmiston CE Jr., Krepel CJ, Seabrook GR, Lewis BD, Brown KR, and Towne JB: Preoperative shower revisited: can high topical antiseptic levels be achieved on the skin surface before surgical admission? J Am Coll Surg 2008; **207:** 233.

29. Borkow G and Gabbay J: Biocidal textiles can help fight nosocomial infections. Med Hypotheses 2008; **70:** 990.

30. Hemmila MR, Taddonio MA, Arbabi S, Maggio PM, and Wahl WL: Intensive insulin therapy is associated with reduced infectious complications in burn patients. Surgery 2008; **144:** 629.

31. Edwards R and Harding KG: Bacteria and wound healing. Curr Opin Infect Dis 2004; **17:** 91.

32. Hummel RP, Kautz PD, MacMillan BG, and Altmeier WA: The continuing problem of sepsis following enzymatic debridement of burns. J Trauma 1974; **14:** 572.

33. Cooper ML, Laxer JA, and Hansbrough JF: The cytotoxic effects of commonly used topical antimicrobial agents on human fibroblasts and keratinocytes. J Trauma 1991; **31:** 775.

34. Simchen E and Sacks T: Infection in war wounds: experience during the 1973 October War in Israel. Ann Surg 1975; **182:** 754.

Damage Control in the War Wounded

Scott R. Steele[1,*] and George E. Peoples[2]

[1]Department of Surgery, Madigan Army Medical Center, Fort Lewis, Washington.
[2]Department of Surgery, Brooke Army Medical Center, Fort Sam Houston, Texas.

Background: Present-day wartime conflicts have highlighted the controversy regarding the optimal treatment for combat casualties. One such component, damage control surgery (DCS), has made it into mainstream practice for the most severely injured patients, and brought improved survival to injuries that previously resulted in death.
The Problem: Despite system and technological improvements in combat casualty care, continued efforts are needed to reduce morbidity and mortality. DCS has emerged as a leading effort. This article describes its role on the modern-day battlefield and highlights the impact on contemporary military medicine.
Basic/Clinical Science Advances: Evidence has demonstrated the high mortality associated with the commencement of an irreversible physiological insult connected with the "lethal triad" of hypothermia, acidosis, and coagulopathy. DCS attempts to halt this process through an abbreviated initial surgery aimed at controlling hemorrhage and preventing further contamination. Subsequently, the patient is rewarmed and metabolic derangements are corrected before returning for definitive surgical care.
Clinical Care Relevance: While DCS is widely practiced in the civilian arena, its routine use in the combat wounded has been implemented during recent conflicts, and represents one of the major surgical shifts to improve outcomes and reduce mortality.
Conclusion: Caring for combat injured provides unique challenges to surgeons due to multiple influences, including austere conditions, limited resources, and worldwide evacuation requirements. Yet, the implementation of DCS principles has had a significant impact on providing state of the art care, and improved outcomes for those wounded in battle.

Abbreviation and Acronym

DCS = damage control surgery

*Correspondence: Department of Surgery, Madigan Army Medical Center, 9606 Piperhill Dr SE, Fort Lewis, Washington 98513 (e-mail: harkersteele@gmail.com).

BACKGROUND

Injuries suffered in the combat environment remain some of the most devastating and lethal. In an attempt to counterbalance this, the evolution of care for the trauma patient has seen major changes over the past few decades, including improved prehospital care, formal implementation of an in-theater trauma system, worldwide evacuation capabilities, and the incorporation of damage control surgery (DCS) principles into the combat setting.[1] DCS attempts to prevent the onset of the "lethal triad" of hypothermia, coagulopathy, and acidosis through an abbreviated initial surgery, followed by aggressive rewarming and resuscitation, before embarking on the definitive surgical care. The present day concept of DCS takes its roots in both the civilian and military sectors. The high mortality and increasing difficulty associated with controlling further hemorrhage from high-grade liver injuries found new success through the practice of hepatic packing and

Printed in U.S.A.
DOI: 10.1089/awc.2009.0015

avoiding prolonged surgical attempts at vascular control.[2] In 1983, Stone and colleagues applied similar concepts to cold and coagulapathic trauma patients with multisystem injuries, defining the modern-day three-phase practice of (i) surgery, (ii) resuscitation and correction of physiological abnormalities, and (iii) a definitive operation, while demonstrating a 64.7% survival rate in 17 patients.[3] The term "damage control" has its origins, in part, from the United States Navy surface fleets' ability to "absorb damage and maintain mission integrity."[4] Similarly, surgeons attempt to control the anatomical and physiological insults after battlefield traumatic injuries, and to keep the human vessel afloat before eventual definitive care. It is vastly different from an admission of defeat, or even a classical surgical "bailout option." Rather, DCS is a well-thought-out and deliberate attempt to avoid prolonged surgery, massive blood loss, and irreversible physiological changes at both the micro- and macrolevel. Through this deliberate strategy, surgeons continue to practice well-established techniques while improving outcomes.[5]

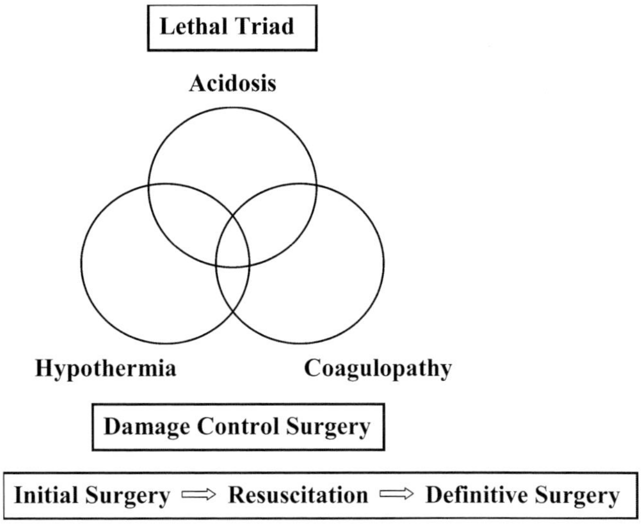

Figure 1. Avoiding the lethal triad with damage control surgery. The lethal triad consists of acidosis, coagulopathy, and hypothermia. Avoiding this severe physiological insult is imperative to improving outcomes. Damage control surgery attempts to aid in this effort by performing an initial abbreviated surgery with the goals of achieving hemostasis and preventing ongoing contamination. This is followed by resuscitation, classically in the intensive care unit, before returning to the operating room for definitive surgical reconstruction once the patient has been stabilized.

CLINICAL PROBLEM ADDRESSED

System-based and technological improvements in combat casualty care have ranged from increased use of tourniquets,[6] changes in patterns of blood product and fluid resuscitation,[7] and education and implementation of optimal prehospital care guidelines.[8] Yet, despite these improvements, continued efforts are needed to reduce morbidity and mortality. Among the most severely injured of patients in combat include those undergoing a massive transfusion protocol—often defined as requiring >10 units of packed red blood cells in 24 h—where mortality rates range from 25% to 65%.[7,9] In addition, those patients sustaining penetrating abdominal and pelvic injuries often present in extremis with severe multisystem involvement, including concomitant vascular, genitourinary, orthopedic, and bowel injuries.[10] Further, the presence of hypothermia has been shown to be an independent predictor of higher mortality in a study of almost 3,000 patients injured in combat.[11] Finally, those patients presenting with an acute coagulopathy (international normalized ratio >1.5) on arrival to the battlefield emergency department have been shown to have an almost fivefold (odds ratio, 5.38; 95% confidence interval, 1.55–11.37) increase in mortality, while acidosis at presentation was associated with a sevenfold increase in the death rate (odds ratio, 6.9; 95% confidence interval, 2.1–19.5).[12] Each of these scenarios depicts the gravity associated with the presence or development of one of the lethal triad components. Unfortunately, acidosis, coagulopathy, and hypothermia are often present simultaneously, leading to even higher rates of morbidity and mortality (Fig. 1). Thus, it is imperative that resuscitative and surgical intervention take place ideally before the development of these physiologic states, or shortly thereafter. It is also in the management of these types of injury complexes, and in these severely compromised patients, where DCS has emerged as a leading effort to counteract and attempt to reverse the accompanying physiological disturbances. It is the DCS principles that provide a deliberate and staged approach to guide both resuscitation and repair.

BASIC SCIENCE CONTEXT

Devastating combat injuries all tend to have one unifying factor—major blood loss. Exsanguinating hemorrhage leads to tissue hypoxia, acidosis, loss of coagulation factors, and hypothermia—further compounding the problems associated with the development of a trauma-induced coagulopathy. Further, although the ensuing massive transfusion attempts to correct this state, cold blood products, dilution of present clotting factors, and the occasional development of disseminated intravascular coagulation can lead to a futile cycle of uncorrectable bleeding, worsening acidosis, and death.[13] Additional evidence has supported the early use of adjuncts such as fresh warm whole blood as the initial resuscitation fluid under certain circumstances, including the austere conditions often experienced by those in the military, and where component therapy is not available.[14] In this model, termed "damage control resuscitation," the most seriously injured patients are allowed an initial degree of hypotension, while control of mechanical bleeding is pursued, along with invocation of both active and passing rewarming measures to avoid hypothermia.[1,15] Critical to this model, however, is the aggressive and immediate transfusion of clotting factors in a 1:1 ratio with packed red blood cells and up-front use of platelets. Unlike traditional resuscitation strategies, blood products play the lead role, while all efforts are geared at stopping the onset or propagation of the lethal triad. While still mostly applied in the military setting, definitive trials are needed to validate this approach across a broad clinical setting. Yet, early surgical intervention is still required to stop ongoing hemorrhage. However, prolonged efforts in the operating room, often with an open abdomen, ongoing blood loss, and further cooling of core body temperature, are associated with worse outcomes.[16] As such, DCS, along with damage control resuscitation, aims to help minimize these losses and maximize resuscitative efforts.

EXPERIMENTAL MODEL OR MATERIAL

From its roots with ongoing abdominal hemorrhage after liver injury,[2] the basic tenets of DCS have been successfully applied to a wide range of traumatic injuries ranging from the pancreas,[17] colorectal,[18] major vascular structures,[19] head and neck,[20] genitourinary,[21] hepatic,[22] spleen,[22] and orthopedic.[23] Despite these seemingly diverse injury patterns and even underlying etiologies, the goals of DCS remain the same—stabilize the organ system from further damage, correct or avoid the onset of a physiological state that will promote worsened impairment, and ultimately provide definitive repair. In each case, these precepts are simply tailored to the organ system(s) involved.

Unlike many efforts where bench-top research attempts to translate to the clinical realm, the focus with DCS-related research has been on developing models of exsanguinating hemorrhage, the role that DCS plays in improving outcomes, and how resuscitation in both pre- and posthospital settings can support this strategy. In one such model, Ding and colleagues have developed a trauma-shock-hypothermia model using pigs by creating a superior mesenteric artery injury, and allowing loss of nearly 50% of total blood volume. The authors have demonstrated the importance of not only aggressive resuscitation but also the need for early surgical intervention using DCS within the first 60 min.[24] However, in the combat environment, injuries often occur to soldiers in remote locations where prolonged evacuation times are unfortunately unavoidable. Thus, further research is ongoing evaluating interventions such as widespread combat lifesaver classes, hemostatic dressings, and tourniquet use to help stabilize the patient after initial injury and during transport to medical facilities where DCS can be performed. Exciting advances in medical resuscitation include the use of histone deacetylase inhibitors such as antiseizure medication valproic acid that promote transcription of genes that provide cell protective effects and improved survival in animal models of hemorrhagic shock.[25] Although not ready for clinical use on the battlefield, these promising endeavors, combined with DCS strategies, can hopefully one day be of regular use on the battlefield and provide lower morbidity and improved survival to those injured in combat.

Highlighting this DCS concept, a 27-year-old man sustained a blast injury with multiple shrapnel wounds to the abdomen and chest during Operation Iraqi Freedom. Initial DCS techniques involved left chest tube thoracostomy, discontinuity stapled-off resection of multiple small bowel and left colon injuries, left nephrectomy, pancreatic drain placement, and temporary closure. After air-evacuation to a higher-level echelon of care, resuscitation, stabilization, and correction of physiological derangements were performed. The next day, abdominal exploration revealed no contamination and healthy viable tissues, along with a pancreatic tail duct injury. After distal pancreatectomy, the small bowel continuity was restored, end colostomy performed, along with primary fascial closure. The patient ultimately underwent a successful colostomy takedown before resuming full function.

DISCUSSION OF FINDINGS AND RELEVANT LITERATURE

At first glance, it may seem hard for nontrauma surgeons to comprehend the concept of leaving the

TAKE-HOME MESSAGE

Basic science advances

- Severely injured patients with traumatic injuries involving multiple organ systems may experience the lethal triad of hypothermia, coagulopathy, and acidosis.
- Onset of the lethal triad is associated with a high mortality.
- Massive transfusion, while necessary, has additional drawbacks that can exacerbate each of the components of the lethal triad.
- Experimental models have demonstrated that early surgical intervention is critical to minimizing morbidity and mortality.
- Although emerging medical therapies such as histone deacetylase inhibitors work to stabilize damage on a cellular level and provide additional promise, surgical intervention is still the primary method of treatment for these patients.

Clinical science advances

- Prolonged initial attempts at definitive operative intervention may lead to a worsening of one or more component(s) of the lethal triad, which will directly affect the other components, leading to worse outcomes.
- DCS attempts to interrupt the onset of this process through an abbreviated surgery, followed by aggressive resuscitation in the intensive care unit, before returning to the operating room for a definitive surgery.
- Major principles in DCS include controlling further contamination through use of resection or diversion of bowel injuries, achieving hemostasis of ongoing bleeding, and packing and draining other damaged organs (*i.e.*, liver and pancreas).
- During the intervening resuscitation, abdominal wounds are kept open through the use of temporary closures to facilitate return to the operating room.
- Once the coagulopathy, acidosis, and electrolyte abnormalities have been corrected, definitive surgery is performed with attempted restoration of gastrointestinal continuity (with or without diversion), formal repair of injured organs, and closure of the abdomen.

Relevance to clinical care

- DCS allows for stabilization and resuscitation of even the most severely injured patients.
- Initially described in the civilian sector, these principles are being properly and effectively applied to various organ systems in the combat arena as well.
- Although often hampered by austere conditions and limited resources, deployed military surgeons faced with these difficult injury patterns have an effective strategy to help stabilize patients before worldwide evacuation for more definitive care.
- Continued care including resuscitation is required through all levels of evacuation from the site of injury with topical hemostatic dressings and tourniquets, to the closest military surgical facility, and ultimately during helicopter or fixed-wing transport to higher levels of care, including those both within and outside of the combat theater. Depending on stability, this can include transatlantic flights to fixed military medical facilities in the United States all within days of the inciting event.
- DCS principles may be needed at one or more levels during this process.[30]

operating room without "finishing" what needs to be done. From the time most surgeons begin training, the maxim of completing all steps of an elective operation from initial incision to final closure, analogous to an airplane pilot's checklist, has been instilled and followed. Thus, the concept of leaving the operating room in the middle, or even shortly after arriving, is one initially foreign to many surgeons. Yet, prolonged attempts at stopping all bleeding and leakage, performing detailed and vast reconstructions for what are often colossal injury patterns, and further worsening coagulopathy in the face of massive transfusions have led to poor outcomes.[1] As such, DCS does not only involve the operation itself, as it represents both the technical and the organizational approach to the most severely injured. Therefore, when encountering an exsanguinating and multisystem injured patient, a decision-tree algorithm starting with early recognition of the severity, urgent intervention, and defined therapeutic response is crucial. Therefore, prior planning, with each team member recognizing and understanding his role, is vital. Typical triggers for invocation of DCS include hypothermia (temperature $< 35°C$), acidosis ($pH < 7.30$), and coagulopathy (nonsurgical bleeding with elevated coagulation parameters).[26] To avoid the onset or further propagation of the lethal triad, surgeons have readily adopted the practice of DCS.

DCS has bridged the gap across all fields of trauma. Adapted from major hepatic trauma,[2,3] DCS has demonstrated decreased morbidity (12–62%) and mortality (23–70%) in pancreatic injuries—previously not felt to be amenable to this type of approach.[17] Orthopedic DCS includes splinting and external fixation to maintain stabilization of bony and extremity injuries during transport or vascular repair.[23] For vascular injuries, use of temporary shunts can rapidly provide necessary distal blood flow without prolonged bypass or reconstructive efforts until more stable or reaching a higher echelon of care.[19] Temporary abdominal closures with open abdomen techniques such as vacuum assistance or packing with suction drains are widely used before definitive closure to protect abdominal wall fascia, decrease operating time, and avoid abdominal compartment syndrome.[27] Thus, despite the various organ systems, the critical concepts encompassing DCS remain the same—concomitant resuscitation and stabilization with contamination and hemorrhage control, followed by subsequent restoration of the physiological milieu and definitive surgery. In patients with colon and rectal pathology, for example, DCS has been shown effective in both the elective setting and after trauma. Miller and colleagues evaluated delayed primary anastomosis after an initial damage control procedure, finding similar anastomotic leak rate (0% vs. 5%), abscess rate (36% vs. 24%), and colon-related death rate (9% vs. 0%; all $p > 0.05$) as those undergoing immediate primary repair.[18] Since DCS stabilization can be performed initially, reevaluation in the next 24–36 h can then help dictate the appropriate surgical procedure; thus, potentially making this once emotionally charged debate of diversion versus primary repair a moot point. DCS, for both civilian and combat injuries, may hopefully then lead to not only decreased mortality and morbidity rates, but also less need for diversion.

Proper education on damage control procedures is integral to success. Currently, combining DCS with more standard procedures, such as packing off of pelvic injuries, has been incorporated into training programs, such that trauma surgeons feel comfortable and competent implementing these concepts into their daily care of trauma patients.[28] Additionally, while widely practiced at many busy civilian trauma centers, DCS skills have similarly been taught to active duty and reservist personnel before deployment, by an integration program at select trauma centers before heading to the combat theatre.[29] Thus, the opportunity exists to become more familiar or reacquainted with DCS under the guidance of those who practice it regularly before exposure on the battlefield. This is especially critical as, unique to military trauma, continued care including both resuscitation and even DCS is often required through all levels of evacuation from the site of injury, to the closest military surgical facility, and ultimately during transport to higher levels of care, including those both within and outside of the combat theater.[30] Depending on stability, this may include transatlantic flights to fixed military medical facilities in the United States all within days of the inciting event.

DCS also has an important impact on wound management. Most commonly, after the initial or subsequent operations, the abdomen is closed temporarily with the use of protective layers for the underlying viscera and drains or negative pressure for fluid evacuation to avoid abdominal compartment syndrome. After the definitive operation, the goal is to close the abdominal fascia primarily. Yet in ~25–50% of cases primary closure is not possible, as fascial retraction and adherence of the viscera to the abdominal wall prevents this objective.[31] The resultant open abdominal wound requires a well-thought-out approach to successful management. Options include planned ventral hernia with delayed closure, controlled fascial tensioning devices, vacuum-assisted closure, mesh repair, split-thickness skin grafting, and component separation with rates of success ranging from 22% to 91%.[31–34] Regardless of the method chosen, the surgeon should be cognizant of the wound implications that result from DCS techniques, and be well-versed in the multiple options to deal with them.

CAUTION, CRITICAL REMARKS, AND RECOMMENDATIONS

Despite our improvements in the care of the critically wounded, and even with proper invocation of the damage control surgical principles, these patients remain critically ill, and morbidity and mortality remain significant. Because we are also in the infancy in terms of some of the other medical and resuscitative measures, we hope to continue to see improved outcomes in the future. Although focus on this chapter has been on the surgical principles, further knowledge of methods and endpoints of proper resuscitation—the middle aspect of DCS—will also play an intricate part in achieving this goal. Similarly, expanding that golden hour of time from injury to intervention through methods and technology brought to the patient may allow more patients to reach battlefield surgical facilities where DCS can be performed.

FUTURE DEVELOPMENTS

Although the practice of DCS in the combat wounded highlights improvements in the care of those injured on the battlefield, it remains only one aspect of the continued attempts to minimize morbidity and mortality. Further efforts at both the site of injury and preinjury care are needed to allow more patients to reach surgeons to invoke these damage control principles. Additionally, the evolving strategy of "damage control resuscitation," characterized by early and aggressive use of all components of blood, highlights an important shift away from crystalloid and more traditional manners of fluid resuscitation in the most severely injured. Similarly, experience in both recognizing patients at need for DCS and proper execution of DCS tactics, along with improvements in resuscitation, is needed to improve outcomes. Only then can we accomplish our mission goal of leaving no soldier behind on the battlefield.

ACKNOWLEDGMENTS

We have no acknowledgments for this article.

AUTHOR DISCLOSURE STATEMENT

Financial Disclosure: No outside financial support or provision of supplies was solicited or received in connection with this work and no conflict of interest disclosed.

Disclosure and Proprietary Statement: This is an original work by the above authors. The opinions expressed are the authors' and authors' alone. They do not necessarily reflect the opinion of the United States Government, the U.S. Department of Defense, Madigan Army Medical Center, or Brooke Army Medical Center.

REFERENCES

1. Beekley AC: Damage control resuscitation: a sensible approach to the exsanguinating surgical patient. Crit Care Med 2008; **36(7 Suppl):** S267.
2. Walt AJ: The surgical management of hepatic trauma and its complications. Ann R Coll Surg Engl 1969; **45:** 319.
3. Stone HH, Strom PR, and Mullins RJ: Management of the major coagulopathy with onset during laparotomy. Ann Surg 1983; **197:** 532.
4. US Navy: Surface ship survivability. Navy War Publications 3–20.31. Department of Defense, Washington, DC, 1996.
5. Rotondo MF, Schwab CW, McGonigal MD, Phillips GR, III, Fruchterman TM, and Kauder DR: "Damage control": an approach for improved survival in exsanguination penetrating abdominal injury. J Trauma 1993; **35:** 375.
6. Kragh JF, Jr., Walters TJ, Baer DG, Fox CJ, Wade CE, Salinas J, and Holcomb JB: Survival with emergency tourniquet use to stop bleeding in major limb trauma. Ann Surg 2009; **249:** 1.
7. Spinella PC, Perkins JG, Grathwohl KW, Beekley AC, Niles SE, McLaughlin DF, Wade CE, and Holcomb JB: Effect of plasma and red blood cell transfusions on survival in patients with combat related traumatic injuries. J Trauma 2008; **64(2 Suppl):** S69.
8. Tien HC, Jung V, Rizoli SB, Acharya SV, and MacDonald JC: An evaluation of tactical combat casualty care interventions in a combat environment. J Am Coll Surg 2008; **207:** 174.
9. Borgman MA, Spinella PC, Perkins JG, Grathwohl KW, Repine T, Beekley AC, Sebesta J, Jenkins D, Wade CE, and Holcomb JB: The ratio of blood products transfused affects mortality in patients receiving massive transfusions at a combat support hospital. J Trauma 2007; **63:** 805.
10. Arthurs Z, Kjorstad R, Mullenix P, Rush RM, Jr., Sebesta J, and Beekley A: The use of damage-control principles for penetrating pelvic battlefield trauma. Am J Surg 2006; **191:** 604.
11. Arthurs Z, Cuadrado D, Beekley A, Grathwohl K, Perkins J, Rush R, and Sebesta J: The impact of hypothermia on trauma care at the 31st combat support hospital. Am J Surg 2006; **191:** 610.
12. Niles SE, McLaughlin DF, Perkins JG, Wade CE, Li Y, Spinella PC, and Holcomb JB: Increased mortality associated with the early coagulopathy of trauma in combat casualties. J Trauma 2008; **64:** 1459.
13. Hess JR and Lawson JH: The coagulopathy of trauma versus disseminated intravascular coagulation. J Trauma 2006; **60(6 Suppl):** S12.
14. Repine TB, Perkins JG, Kauvar DS, and Blackborne L: The use of fresh whole blood in massive transfusion. J Trauma 2006; **60(6 Suppl):** S59.
15. Holcomb JB, Jenkins D, Rhee P, Johannigman J, Mahoney P, Mehta S, Cox ED, Gehrke MJ, Beilman GJ, Schreiber M, Flaherty SF, Grathwohl KW, Spinella PC, Perkins JG, Beekley AC, McMullin NR, Park MS, Gonzalez EA, Wade CE, Dubick MA, Schwab CW, Moore FA, Champion HR, Hoyt DB, and Hess JR: Damage control resuscitation: directly assessing the early coagulopathy of trauma. J Trauma 2007; **62:** 307.
16. Lee JC and Peitzman AB: Damage-control laparotomy. Curr Opin Crit Care 2006; **12:** 346.
17. Seamon MJ, Kim PK, Stawicki SP, Dabrowski GP, Goldberg AJ, Reilly PM, and Schwab CW: Pancreatic injury in damage control laparotomies: is pancreatic resection safe during the initial laparotomy? Injury 2009; **40:** 61.
18. Miller PR, Chang MC, Hoth JJ, Holmes JH, 4th, and Meredith JW: Colonic resection in the setting of damage control laparotomy: is delayed anastomosis safe? Am Surg 2007; **73:** 606.
19. Fox CJ, Gillespie DL, Cox ED, Kragh JF, Jr., Mehta SG, Salinas J, and Holcomb JB: Damage control resuscitation for vascular surgery in a combat support hospital. J Trauma 2008; **65:** 1.
20. Rezende-Neto J, Marques AC, Guedes LJ, and Teixeira LC: Damage control principles applied to penetrating neck and mandibular injury. J Trauma 2008; **64:** 1142.
21. Ball CG, Hameed SM, Navsaria P, Edu S, Kirkpatrick AW, and Nicol AJ: Successful damage control of complex vascular and urological gunshot injuries. Can J Surg 2006; **49:** 437.
22. Sutton E, Bochicchio GV, Bochicchio K, Rodriguez ED, Henry S, Joshi M, and Scalea TM: Long term impact of damage control surgery: a preliminary prospective study. J Trauma 2006; **61:** 831.
23. Pape HC, Hildebrand F, Pertschy S, Zelle B, Garapati R, Grimme K, Krettek C, and Reed RL, 2nd: Changes in the management of femoral shaft fractures in polytrauma patients: from early total care to damage control orthopedic surgery. J Trauma 2002; **53:** 452.
24. Ding W, Wu X, Gong G, Meng Q, Ni L, and Li J: Establishment of an acute superior mesenteric artery injury model for damage control surgery. J Surg Res. 2009 Apr; **152**:249. Epub 2008 Mar 26.
25. Gonzales ER, Chen H, Munuve RM, Mehrani T, Nadel A, and Koustova E: Hepatoprotection and lethality rescue by histone deacetylase inhibitor valproic acid in fatal hemorrhagic shock. J Trauma 2008; **65:** 554.
26. Rotondo MF and Zonies DH: The damage control sequence and underlying logic. Surg Clin N Am 1997; **77:** 761.
27. Fabian TC: Damage control in trauma: laparotomy wound management acute to chronic. Surg Clin N Am 2007; **87:** 73.
28. Bach A, Bendix J, Hougaard K, and Christensen EF: Retroperitoneal packing as part of damage control surgery in a Danish trauma centre–fast, effective, and cost-effective. Scand J Trauma Resusc Emerg Med 2008; **16:** 4.
29. Koehler RH, Smith RS, and Bacaner T: Triage of American combat casualties: the need for change. Mil Med 1994; **159:** 541.

30. Blackbourne LH: Combat damage control surgery. Crit Care Med 2008; **36(7Suppl):** S304.

31. Miller PR, Meredith JW, Johnson JC, and Chang MC: Prospective evaluation of vacuum-assisted fascial closure after open abdomen: planned ventral hernia rate is substantially reduced. Ann Surg 2004; **239:** 608.

32. Fantus RJ, Mellett MM, and Kirby JP: Use of controlled fascial tension and an adhesion preventing barrier to achieve delayed primary fascial closure in patients managed with an open abdomen. Am J Surg 2006; **192:** 243.

33. Cothren CC, Moore EE, Johnson JL, Moore JB, and Burch JM: One hundred percent fascial approximation with sequential abdominal closure of the open abdomen. Am J Surg 2006; **192:** 238.

34. Jernigan TW, Fabian TC, Croce MA, Moore N, Pritchard FE, Minard G, and Bee TK: Staged management of giant abdominal wall defects: acute and long-term results. Ann Surg 2003; **238:** 349.

WHS
Wound
Healing
Society

Management of the Open Abdominal Wound

Amy Vertrees* and Craig Shriver

General Surgery Service, Walter Reed Army Medical Center, Washington, District of Columbia.

Abbreviation and Acronym

PVH = planned ventral hernia

*Correspondence: General Surgery Service, Walter Reed Army Medical Center, Building 2, 5th floor, 6900 Georgia Ave. NW, Washington, District of Columbia 20307 (e-mail: amy.vertrees@us.army.mil).

Background: Loss of abdominal domain is common in trauma and sepsis due to generalized edema. Leaving the abdominal fascia open prevents abdominal compartment syndrome, but it creates another problem with associated morbidity and mortality.

The Problem: Intraabdominal contents are contained within a myofascial sleeve. After laparotomy, intraabdominal contents may not be able to be replaced into the abdomen resulting in an open abdomen. Management of the open abdomen must address potential for evaporative losses, contamination, and reversal of causative factors. Retraction of fascial edges and granulation tissue forming a "visceral block" may preclude eventual closure. Avoiding complications including enterocutaneous fistula, prolonged, or recurrent hospitalizations, and recurrence of hernia are other important aspects of open abdominal management.

Basic/Clinical Science Advances: Open abdomen management has progressed from simple and inexpensive containment of abdominal contents with Bogotá bag closure to more costly negative pressure closure systems and use of mesh. Numerous methods of closure have been described with eventual fascial closure ranging from 25% to 100%.

Clinical Care Relevance: Ideal management of the open abdomen must consider several aspects of patient care. Minimizing or reversing factors causing intraabdominal hypertension include judicious fluid administration, optimization of ventilator settings, adequate hemostasis, and control of sepsis. Providing tension to fascial edges prevents retraction, although excessive tension may devitalize fascial edges. Recurrence of hernia occurs with closing under suboptimal circumstances or using a material that would fail long term.

Conclusion: Open abdomen management continues to evolve. Primary fascial closure with minimal complications is ideal. Temporary closures allow time for reversal of causative factors and increase the probability of primary fascial closure. Techniques providing tension to fascia increase the probability of closure. Supplemental closure devices vary in cost, effectiveness, and complications. There is currently no consensus regarding the ideal method that would allow a high rate of closure and minimize complications.

BACKGROUND

Abdominal compartment syndrome resulting from intraabdominal hypertension is a well-described clinical problem.[1] The abdomen is a finite compartment, and generalized edema decreases the available space resulting in the compression of susceptible structures. Renal vein compression leads to acute renal failure, and upward pressure on the diaphragm results in pulmonary compromise.[1] Generalized edema can occur in trauma patients requiring massive resuscitation and in septic patients with disruption of vascular integrity and

ADVANCES IN WOUND CARE, VOLUME 1

Printed in U.S.A.
DOI: 10.1089/awc.2009.0027

increased fluid requirements.[2] Damage control surgery and open abdomen management is an important life-saving strategy to avoid the morbidity of abdominal compartment syndrome and provide a method for abbreviated initial operations to avoid the lethal triad of acidosis, coagulopathy, and hypothermia.[2] Second look operations are also facilitated with temporary closure.[2] The resulting open abdomen can be difficult to manage, specifically finalizing closure efficiently with minimal complications.

CLINICAL PROBLEM ADDRESSED

Management of the open abdomen must consider protection of intraabdominal contents, attention to reversal of causative factors of the loss of abdominal domain, and methods of final closure with primary fascial closure as the ideal. Intraabdominal contents must be protected from desiccation and from insensible losses, and temporary closures have been used to achieve this goal. Many different strategies for temporary closure have been described. Most recent studies describe variations of Bogotá bag closure.[3] The most common method of contemporary closure involves using any type of plastic occlusive barrier such as large sterile irrigation bags or Steri-Drape® (3M®, St. Paul, MN) plastic sheeting with small slits cut in the plastic to allow egress of fluid. This sheeting is then tucked under the fascia down to the pericolic gutters (Fig. 1).[2–7] Gauze dressings or operative towels are placed over the plastic barrier then covered with occlusive dressings like Ioban® (3M). Fluid egress is achieved with large tubes (often nasogastric tubes with the air vent portion of the sump drain tied into a knot) placed on top of the towels or gauze and underneath the occlusive dressing with attachment to continuous wall suction. Commercially available temporary abdominal closure kits are available (V.A.C.® dressing; Kinetic Concepts, San Antonio, TX) that provide polyurethane foam dressing sandwiched in between perforated plastic sheeting and adhesive drapes. A T.R.A.C. pad® (Kinetic Concepts) is attached over a hole placed in the adhesive dressing with attached tubing delivering fluid into a canister attached to a self-contained vacuum machine. Any method of temporary closure is acceptable if viscera are contained, desiccation is avoided, and damage to underlying bowel is prevented.

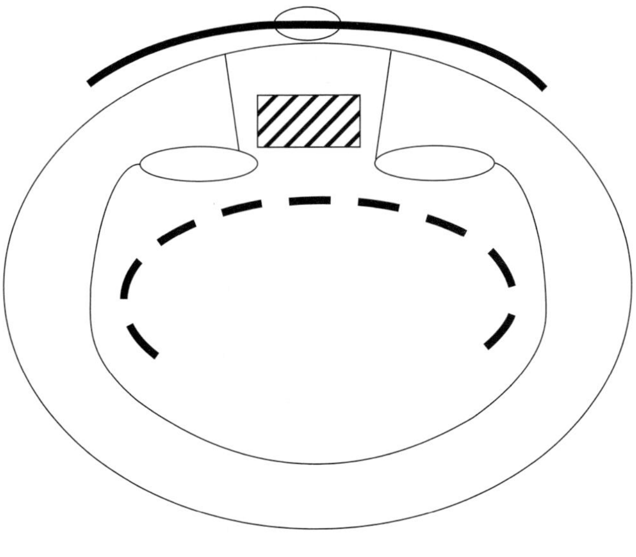

Figure 1. Transverse section of abdomen demonstrating temporary closure. Dashed line, plastic sheeting; striped box, vacuum sponge or operative towels; solid line, occlusive dressing with vacuum device either under or through the dressing.

Temporary closure allows time for reclaiming the abdominal domain. When the abdomen is amenable to closure, primary fascial closure is ideal. If this is not possible, the surgical standard of care for open abdomen used to be planned ventral hernia (PVH). PVH involves initial placement of absorbable mesh sewn to the retracted fascial edges, granulation tissue ingrowth into the mesh over time, and subsequent delayed split-thickness skin graft placement. The resultant large ventral hernia requires another surgery several months to a year later with its own morbidity and mortality including high rates of enterocutaneous fistula formation (9–25%).[8,9] Significant morbidity associated with PVH led to a search for better methods of closure.

Temporary closures can increase the ability to primarily close the abdominal fascia. Closures utilizing negative pressure systems (V.A.C. dressing; Kinetic Concepts) have become prominent to assist with fluid control with the added benefit of stimulating granulation tissue formation and speeding wound healing.[4,10] The negative pressure has been postulated to increase the window of opportunity for fascial closure and provide traction on the fascial edges and the abdominal wall.[4] V.A.C.-assisted closure has improved the rate of closure, but enterocutaneous fistula is still a common complication.[11]

Modification of temporary closure to include traction of fascial edges has the highest closure success rates.[5,12] This modification limits the retraction of fascial edges with retention sutures or mesh that is shortened over time with Velcro-like dressing (Wittmann patch) or mesh revision as the abdominal domain is reclaimed.[5,13]

Biological meshes including acellular human dermis or acellular porcine submucosa were enthusiastically embraced for their ability to be in contaminated wound, in proximity to bowel.[3,14–16] Previous reports of laxity of repair were initially attributed to failure to adequately stretch the mesh before use or reclaiming abdominal domain after mesh was placed.[3] Enthusiasm for biological mesh has waned as many recent studies have noted significant laxity of the mesh over time.[15,16]

BASIC SCIENCE CONTEXT

There is a narrow window of opportunity for successful closure of the open abdomen. Although the abdominal domain may be reclaimed over time, the fascial edges retract, and creation of a "visceral block" or "frozen hostile abdomen" makes safe dissection of the fascial edges impossible. Successful management of the open abdomen patient requires an understanding of the timeline of wound healing. Generalized edema will decrease 3–5 days from surgery unless there are continued physiologic insults (sepsis and multiorgan dysfunction) causing continued fluid accumulation. This continued insult may explain a recent study noting less success with sepsis-related abdominal closure compared to trauma-related closure.[17] Temporary closures will allow time for the causative factors to lessen. The dressings are changed every 2–4 days with continued reassessment of the possibility of primary fascial closure.

If primary fascial closure is not possible within a week of creating the open abdomen, consideration must be given to ensuring continued access to the fascial edges and providing traction to those edges to prevent significant retraction. Formation of granulation tissue creates adherence of bowel loops together and to the edges of the fascia creating a visceral block. Adherence to the abdominal wall prevents access to the abdominal contents and fascial edges. This process is usually seen after a week of the abdomen being open. Placement of plastic barriers tucked under the fascia down to the pericolic gutters assists with continued separation of the visceral block from the abdominal wall. Conscientious and careful disruption of adhesions at each open abdominal dressing change (usually twice a week) allow longer access to the fascial edges, extending the window of closure to at least a month from the opening of the abdomen.[5,13,11]

Retraction of fascia over time has also been described, often evident within a week of opening the abdomen.[5,13,18] The reasons for this retraction are unknown. Techniques that provide traction to the fascial edges have shown improved rates of closure.[5,12,13,19,20] Strategies range from inexpensive retention sutures to more expensive interposition mesh allowing distributed tension on the fascial edges. Care must be taken to avoid damage to the fascial edges to further compromise the ability to primarily close the abdominal fascia.

Understanding and correcting causative factors involved with the loss of abdominal domain may lead to better success of closure. Variations in intensive care management are likely to influence closure rates but have not yet been elucidated. Aggressive use of positive pressure ventilation decreases venous return resulting in increased congestion of liver and bowel that would logically affect reclaiming the abdominal domain. Achieving a negative fluid balance would also logically influence the closure rate with its decrease in generalized edema and has gained interest over time as a modifiable factor.[13,18] Most studies involve a single-institution study, and successful abdominal closure may not translate to other hospitals if perioperative management is significantly different.

EXPERIMENTAL MODEL OR MATERIAL

Studies of open abdominal closure have focused on the surgical strategies used for closure. The previous standard of care of PVH has been replaced with a wide variety of different meshes, retention suture, and vacuum-assisted systems. Vacuum-assisted closure devices include a commercially available system from KCI®[4,6,13] Addition of retention sutures in addition to vacuum dressing is thought to improve the closure rate by preventing retraction of fascia.[18] Attachment of the mesh to the fascial edges provides equal tension to improve closure.[5,13,19,20]

DISCUSSION OF FINDINGS AND RELEVANT LITERATURE

Damage control surgery has become a valuable tool for managing complex surgical patients. Open abdomen management was required in nearly 25% of the trauma laparotomy patients returning to Walter Reed from the current conflicts in Iraq and Afghanistan.[13] Establishing an algorithm for treatment is helpful in open abdomen management to ensure successful fascial closure and avoidance of PVH (Fig. 2).

After initial laparotomy, temporary closure is required. Attention to reversal of causative factors (judicious fluid management, improved ventilator settings, and control of sepsis) is most important in this time frame. At each dressing change, the

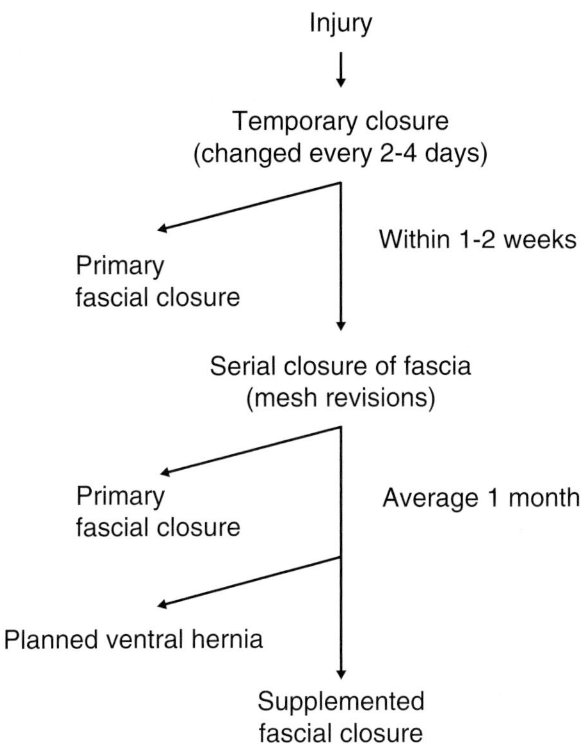

Figure 2. Algorithm for open abdominal closure.

extent of fascial separation is noted, and closure should be attempted if the closure would not be under tension. If closure is not possible, then the dressing is replaced and the process is repeated in 2–4 days.

The choice of temporary closure may improve closure rates. Improved results have been shown with V.A.C.-assisted closures, compared to previous closures not utilizing this system. The negative pressure from the vacuum dressing is thought to indirectly decrease fascial retraction by providing constant tension to the subcutaneous tissue attached to the fascia. Recent series have noted primary closure ranging from 68% to 100%.[4,6,18] Failures of closure in these series undergo PVH.

After a week of failing to close the open abdomen, consideration should be given to supplementation of temporary closure to increase the possibility of primary fascial closure. Although fascial closure has been obtained beyond a week with temporary closure alone, the visceral block and fascial retraction decrease the likelihood of primary closure.[4,5,13,18] Plastic sheeting used in temporary closures should be placed under the fascial edges extending to the pericolic gutter to facilitate later isolation of the fascial edges from the visceral block. Attachment of interposition mesh or retention sutures are examples of supplementation, and a recent Cochrane review noted improved closure with these techniques.[5,12,13,18–20] Excessive tension on the fascia must be avoided with these methods to prevent damage to the fascial edges.

Serial closure allows constant and even traction on the fascia to prevent retraction by sewing mesh to the fascial edges. As the causative factors lessen, and the fascial edges are closely approximated, the prosthetic mesh can be removed and permanent fascial closure achieved. We have favored serial closure with Gore-Tex® mesh (Dualmesh®; WL Gore & Associates) to provide equal tension on the fascial edges. Serial gathering of the mesh as abdominal domain is reclaimed allows the fascial edges to remain undisturbed while enclosing and protecting the intraabdominal contents. Gore-Tex is an ideal mesh as it does not adhere to the viscera and avoids the inflammatory reaction associated with polypropylene mesh that would increase the risk of enterocutaneous fistula.[5,13] It is important to note that the Gore-Tex mesh should be used as a temporary prosthetic and must be removed once the abdominal domain has been reclaimed and the rectus muscles are as close

TAKE-HOME MESSAGE

Basic science advances

- Understand wound-healing evolution and time-sensitive considerations for successful closure.
- Understand how overall management may influence outcomes of closure, specifically fluid and ventilator management. Judicious use of fluids without over-resuscitation and ventilator management that allows adequate oxygenation without using pressures affecting bowel and liver edema are important considerations that require further study.

Clinical science advances

- Understand the underlying cause of loss of abdominal domain.
- Treat the underlying cause.
- Apply knowledge of wound evolution to optimize successful fascial closure.

Relevance to clinical care

- Provide traction on fascia to prevent retraction.
- Protect underlying viscera from desiccation and to prevent fistulas.
- Avoid PVH by providing adequate final closure to avoid morbidity of second operation.
- Cost analysis must consider all consequences of closure including associated complications and long-term hernia.

together as possible (usually 4–6 cm apart in the midline). Although decreases in PVH have been achieved with vacuum-assisted and serial closures, supplemental material is still often required.[5,13,18]

Final closure after serial closure often involves use of supplemental material or component separation of fascia.[5,13,18] Prosthetic mesh is not advisable with exposed bowel as resulting inflammation may create adhesions and enterocutaneous fistulas.[3,13] Component separation alters the anatomy of the abdominal wall to gain extra movement of the otherwise unyielding abdominal myofascial layer. Component separation involves incision of the external oblique aponeurosis to increase the circumference of the abdominal wall and allow greater space for intraabdominal contents.[21] The most common technique involves creating skin flaps over the fascial layer and identifying the external oblique aponeurosis just lateral to the rectus abdominal muscle. This layer is incised, but also included the perforating arteries that supply the abdominal wall. Rosen *et al.* (2007)[22] described a small series of patients where they performed the procedure laparoscopically and decreased the complications associated with open component separation. This technique involves making an incision laterally on the abdominal wall to allow a 10-mm port to be placed. The external oblique aponeurosis is incised, and the space below is entered. A laparoscopic port with balloon used for hernia repair is placed in this space to allow blunt dissection of the space between the external and internal oblique muscles. Insufflation is achieved, and a 5-mm port is placed to allow an instrument to bluntly take down the avascular attachments between these layers. Another 5-mm port is used to incise the external oblique from the underside of the external oblique, avoiding the extensive skin flaps used in open component separation. Although component separation increases the ability to close the fascia primarily, there is a high failure rate (32% in one series).[23] Biological mesh has been enthusiastically supported despite its significant cost for its ability to succeed initially in these complex wounds, but long-term results have been very disappointing with up to 80% failure rates reported often within the first year after closure.[15,16] In our experience, our approach avoids the extensive long-term morbidity of PVH or placement of large pieces of biological mesh, which have been shown to result in unacceptably high ventral hernia rates after 6–12 months. It also avoids the need for an extensive component separation that can result in weakening of the core musculature and additional abdominal wall hernia formation at separation sites, even with mesh underlay.

CAUTION, CRITICAL REMARKS, AND RECOMMENDATIONS

Management of the open abdomen has evolved significantly over the last few decades. Analysis of literature must consider all aspects of the described closure, specifically the cause of the loss of abdominal domain, length of time to closure, the method of final closure, the costs of materials used, and need for reoperation. There has not been a study to directly compare all these factors. Initial enthusiasm with methods of closure should be tempered with need for adequate comparison to other closures, include an adequate number of patients, and long-term follow-up data to identify complications.

FUTURE DEVELOPMENTS

Better understanding and treatment of the factors causing loss of abdominal domain will lead to improvement in abdominal closure. Advances in surgical management should focus on the use of affordable materials that are readily available. Primary fascial closure or use of a material that resists infection and expansion should provide closure in less than a month. Identifying ways to avoid complications, especially enterocutaneous fistula, are important considerations.

AUTHOR DISCLOSURE STATEMENT

No conflict of interest disclosed

REFERENCES

1. Schein M, Wittmann DH, Aprahamian CC, *et al.*: The abdominal compartment syndrome. The physiological and clinical consequences of elevated intra-abdominal pressure. JACS 1995; **180:** 745.
2. Rotondo MF, Schwab CW, McGonigal MD, Phillips GR 3rd, Fruchterman TM, Kauder DR, Latenser BA, and Angood PA: "Damage control": an approach for improved survival in exsanguinating penetrating abdominal injury. J Trauma 1993; **35:** 375.
3. Rutherford EJ, Skeete DA, and Brasel KJ: Management of the patient with an open abdomen: techniques in temporary and definitive closure. Curr Probl Surg 2004; **41:** 815.
4. Barker DE, Green JM, Maxwell RA, *et al.*: Experience with vacuum pack temporary abdominal wound closure in 258 trauma and general and vascular surgical patients. JACS 2007; **204:** 782.
5. Vertrees A, Greer L, Pickett C, *et al.*: Modern management of complex open abdominal wounds of war: a 5-year experience. JACS 2008; **207:** 801.
6. Garner GB, Ware DN, Cocanour CS, *et al.*: Vacuum-assisted wound closure provides early

fascial reapproximation in trauma patients with open abdomen. Am J Surg 2001; **182:** 630.

7. Tremblay LN, Feliciano DV, Schmidt J, *et al.*: Skin only or silo closure in the critically ill patient with an open abdomen. Am J Surg 2001; **182:** 670.

8. Fabian TC, Croce MA, Pritchard E, *et al.*: Planned ventral hernia: staged management for acute abdominal wall defects. Ann Surg 1994; **219:**643.

9. Sutton E, Bochicchio GV, Bochicchio K, *et al.*: Long term impact of damage control surgery: a preliminary prospective study. J Trauma 2006; **61:** 831.

10. Cothren CC, Moore EE, Johnson JL, *et al.*: One hundred percent fascial approximation with sequential abdominal closure of the open abdomen. Am J Surg 2006; **192:** 238.

11. Miller PR, Meredith JW, Johnson JC, *et al.*: Prospective evaluation of vacuum-assisted fascial closure after open abdomen. Ann Surg 2004; **239:** 608.

12. van Hensbroek PB, Wind J, Dijkgraaf MGW, *et al.*: Temporary closure of the open abdomen: a systematic review on delayed primary fascial closure in patients with an open abdomen. World J Surg 2009; **33:** 199.

13. Vertrees A, Kellicut D, Ottman S, *et al.*: Early definitive abdominal closure using serial closure technique on injured soldiers returning from Afghanistan and Iraq. JACS 2006; **202:** 762.

14. Franklin ME Jr., Treviño JM, Portillo G, *et al.*: The use of porcine small intestinal submucosa as a prosthetic material for laparoscopic hernia repair in infected and potentially contaminated fields: long-term follow-up. Surg Endosc 2008; **22:** 1941.

15. Bluebond-Langner R, Keifa ES, Mithani S, *et al.*: Recurrent abdominal laxity following interpositional human acellular dermal matrix. Ann Plast Surg 2008; **60:** 76.

16. Jin J, Rosen MJ, Blatnik J, *et al.*: Use of acellular dermal matrix for complicated ventral hernia repair: does technique affect outcomes? JACS 2007; **205:** 654.

17. Wondberg D, Larusson HJ, Metzger U, *et al.*: Treatment of the open abdomen with the commercially available vacuum-assisted closure system in patients with abdominal sepsis. World J Surg 2008; **32:** 2724.

18. Scott BG, Feanny MA, and Hirshberg A: Early definitive closure of the open abdomen: a quiet revolution. Scand J Surg 2008; **94:** 9.

19. Wittmann DH, Aprahamian C, Bergstein JM, *et al.*: Etappenlavage: advanced diffuse peritonitis managed by planned multiple laparotomies utilizing sippers, slide fasteners, and Velcro analogue for temporary abdominal closure. World J Surg 1990; **14:** 218.

20. Weinberg JA, George RL, Griffin RL, *et al.*: Closing the open abdomen: improved success with Wittmann Patch staged abdominal closure. J Trauma 2008; **65:** 345.

21. Kaplan M, Banwell P, Orgill D, *et al.*: Guidelines for the Management of the Open Abdomen, Supplement to Wounds: A Compendium of Clinical Research and Practice, October 2005 http://www.ovm.com/files/doc/KCI_AbdomenSuppl_Oct05.pdf (accessed Dec 2009).

22. Rosen MJ, Jin J, McGee MF, *et al.*: Laparoscopic component separation in the single-stage treatment of infected abdominal wall prosthetic removal. Hernia 2007; **11:** 435.

23. de Vries Reilingh TS, van Goor H, Rosman C, *et al.*: "Components separation technique" for the repair of large abdominal wall hernias. JACS 2003; **196:** 32.

Heterotopic Ossification in High-Energy War Wounds

Jonathan Agner Forsberg* and Benjamin Kyle Potter

Orthopaedic Surgery Service, Integrated Department of Orthopaedics and Rehabilitation, Walter Reed National Military Medical Center, Bethesda, Maryland/Washington, District of Columbia.

Abbreviations and Acronyms

BMP = bone morphogenic protein

FDA = food and drug administration

HO = heterotopic ossification

ISS = injury severity score

*Correspondence: Orthopaedic Surgery Service, Integrated Department of Orthopaedics and Rehabilitation, Walter Reed National Military Medical Center, 8901 Wisconsin Ave., Bethesda, Maryland 20889 (e-mail: jaforsberg@mac.com).

Background: Heterotopic ossification (HO) refers to the formation of mature bone in nonosseous tissue. In moderate to severe cases, this disorder can lead to ankylosis of joints, neuropathy, limb pain, and subsequent disability.
The Problem: The development of heterotopic bone has been observed to be more common than previously reported in patients sustaining high-energy wartime extremity wounds. This is especially problematic in the periarticular setting and in the residual limbs of amputees.
Basic/Clinical Science Advances: Animal models and human histology samples suggest that HO formation follows a predictable sequence of events culminating in endochondral ossification. Additionally, progenitor cells of endothelial, neural, and muscular origin have been implicated various stages of HO development.
Clinical Care Relevance: Most cases of HO are asymptomatic. Conservative management is recommended as first-line treatment and includes rest, local and systemic medications, activity modification, and prosthetic socket/suspension modifications. Surgical excision is reserved for pain, ulceration, or joint stiffness attributable to HO that remains refractory to exhaustive conservative measures. Before surgical excision, other sources of limb pain such as painful bursae, myodesis failure, and neuromata must be ruled out.
Conclusion: HO is a complex disorder with numerous proven and putative risk factors and varied initiating external stimuli, ultimately resulting from both local and systemic internal biologic factors. Lesions are often asymptomatic but can result in profound patient disability due to pain and joint stiffness. When practicable, primary prophylaxis via radiation therapy or nonsteroidal antiinflammatory drugs is effective in a majority of patients at risk. After an appropriate trial of conservative measures, operative excision of symptomatic heterotopic bone provides generally good results with low recurrence rates in appropriately selected patients treated with secondary prophylaxis. Future research regarding biomarker-based prognostication and identification of initiating chemokines, genes, and cellular origin of ectopic bone may permit expanded early prophylaxis and development of novel targeted therapies for prophylaxis.

BACKGROUND

Heterotopic ossification (HO) refers to the formation of mature bone in nonosseous tissue. In moderate to severe cases, this disorder can lead to ankylosis of joints, neuropathy, limb pain, and subsequent disability. Development of HO has traditionally been associated with severe systemic insults including spinal cord injury, traumatic brain injury, and neoplasm.[1–9] HO also forms as sequelae of hip arthroplasty and fractures of the acetabulum or elbow, particularly

ADVANCES IN WOUND CARE, VOLUME 1

Printed in U.S.A.
DOI: 10.1089/awc.2009.0081

those requiring operative fixation. These associations imply a relationship between HO and muscle traumatized due to injury and/or surgical dissection.[10–25] Less common causes of heterotopic bone formation include the genetic disorders fibrodysplasia ossificans progressiva and progressive osseous heteroplasia.[26–28] Although both proven risk factors and genetic predispositions exist, the underlying cause(s) of HO is largely unknown.

CLINICAL PROBLEM ADDRESSED

Recently, the development of heterotopic bone has been observed to be more common than previously reported in patients sustaining high-energy wartime extremity wounds.[29,30] Explosive blasts inflict a high percentage of modern war wounds and predominately affect the extremities.[31–42] This results in a unique injury pattern, comprised of severely traumatized limbs, open fractures, and extensive zones of injury with frequent bone and soft tissue loss, often in association with both gross foreign body and bacterial contamination. Despite the severity of these injury patterns, patient survival, due in part to improved body armor, the judicious use of tourniquets, and a robust casualty evacuation system approaches 90%.[43]

The incidence of HO in combat-wounded servicemembers has consistently been reported as 63–64.6%, far greater than that described in civilian trauma centers. Formation of HO in this patient population is significantly associated with patients who have sustained a blast injury, a combat-related amputation within the zone of injury, and those with injury severity scores (ISSs) greater than 16.[30,44] In contrast, the largest civilian series examining fracture care and HO found that the disorder complicated the extremities in 11% of the severe traumatic brain-injured patients and 20% of the spinal cord injuries.[45] Earlier work reported rates of ectopic bone growth in various long-bone fractures including forearm fractures (20%),[17] femoral shaft fractures (52%),[46] and tibial shaft fractures (0%),[47] all in the setting of significant head injury.

BASIC SCIENCE CONTEXT

As mentioned above, literature focusing on risk factors in a susceptible patient population identifies the ISS and traumatic amputees as risk factors. Though the formation of HO in these patients is theorized to stem from a prolonged inflammatory response, the cause of HO is largely unknown. Considerable efforts are underway to define the mechanistic pathways responsible for this unique phenomenon. Animal models have been developed to evaluate pathways associated with the expression of bone morphogenic protein (BMP), a member of the transforming growth factor superfamily. Despite this seemingly appropriate approach, the cell(s) that ultimately differentiate into bone-forming cells need also be identified and characterized.

EXPERIMENTAL MODEL OR MATERIAL

Recent HO research by Gannon *et al.*[48] has successfully identified genetic mutations that localize to chromosome 4q 27-31. Though the *BMP4* gene itself does not harbor a genetic mutation, overexpression of *BMP4* and its receptor BMPRIA coupled with underexpression of its antagonists is thought to be required for HO formation.[48–51] This phenomenon, first identified in patients with fibrodysplasia ossificans progressiva, firmly establishes a link between some forms of HO and traditional osteoblastic signaling. Davis, in association with Gannon, further defined the microenvironment by identifying the presence of brown (hypoxic) adipocytes in the early stages of HO development. The hypoxic environment induces both chondrogenesis and neovascularization. The result is an increase in oxygen tension enabling endochondral ossification to occur. Nesti *et al.*[52] isolated a population of mesenchymal progenitor cells present in traumatized muscle. The authors concluded, based on their ability to demonstrate pluripotency, that these cells may play a central role in the pathologic osteogenic response. However, in a more recent study, Lounev *et al.*[53] implicate progenitor cells of a vascular lineage.

Ongoing studies from our own institutions examine sera, tissue, and wound effluent from high-energy wartime extremity wounds. We are developing predictive biomarker and gene-based profiles for HO formation in these patients. These profiles will permit the early identification of patients most at risk for HO via computer-based algorithms, potentially allowing aggressive primary prophylaxis. Additionally, we have successfully induced stem-cell production of bone *in vitro* utilizing patient sera, with the composite goal of identifying molecular triggers of HO production, evaluating therapeutic targets and developing and testing novel preventative treatments.

DISCUSSION OF FINDINGS AND RELEVANT LITERATURE

Few case series evaluating both head-injured and nonhead-injured patients with fractures contain a control group for comparison. Spencer[54] compared the healing times and radiographic callus appearance in 82 fractures in 53 patients with head injuries to 30 patients with extremity fractures and no head injury. Based on the graphical representation of his data, an exuberant healing response was present in 52.6% of the tibia fractures, 60.0% of the femur fractures, and 36.4% of the humerus fractures in patients with head injuries compared to an average of 10.0% across the three fracture sites in patients without head injury. He also demonstrated a decreased time to union in the head-injured group and concluded that the term HO may be more appropriate in describing exuberant fracture callus. Giannoudis *et al.*[55] reported similar findings in patients with femur fractures, noting a shorter time to union and a higher callus-to-diaphyseal bone diameter ratio in patients with a head injury when compared to nonhead-injured controls. More recent literature corroborates these findings, reporting a twofold shorter time to union but, more importantly, a linear relationship between the amount of radiographically apparent (exuberant) callus and the *in vitro* proliferation rates of a human osteoblastic cell line in response to sera from study participants.[56] We are aware of no consensus regarding the rate of HO in civilian long-bone extremity trauma without head injury. Nevertheless, the incidence of clinically relevant or symptomatic HO in this setting is generally considered to be low.[8,54,55,57]

Other estimates of injury severity and subsequent systemic inflammation can be used to predict HO. The occurrence of autonomic dysfunction or evidence of systemic infection correlates with an increased risk of HO formation. The ISS has also been shown to predict the development of HO.[44,58] Critics of ISS utility as a prognostic factor for HO growth argue that head-injured patients score higher and therefore are inherently more likely to develop heterotopic bone. However, Steinberg *et al.*[57] reported that the ISS, independent of a head injury, remained an important predictor of the development of HO after intramedullary nailing of femoral fractures. These findings add to the growing body of evidence suggesting that systemic factors, arguably related to the degree of systemic inflammation, initiate or contribute to an exaggerated osteogenic response that may ultimately be responsible for the development of heterotopic bone.

Other associations

The relationship between age and the development of HO remains unclear. Recent studies have demonstrated a statistical increase in HO formation in younger adults.[44,57,59] Conversely, there is also evidence of increased risk of HO with advancing age[60–62]; however, the bulk of the available literature supports no association between patient age and ectopic bone growth.[8,30,45,63–69] The apparent increased risk observed in younger adults may be related to a more severe injury pattern and the resultant systemic insult,[44] but the exact mechanism initiating HO formation and the systemic influence remain unknown.

Likewise, the available literature reports contradictory results regarding a predisposition based on gender. The bulk of the available literature reports higher rates of more severe grades of HO in males undergoing arthroplasty, as well as operative fixation of acetabular fractures, presumably due to increased muscle mass.[11,22,23,57,64,69–72] Nevertheless, a small number of large series report higher rates of development in females, but provide no explanation for this finding other than postulating that systemic or hormonal factors may play a role in HO formation.[24,59,62,65] Independent of age, smoking has been identified in one retrospective study as an independent risk factor for HO formation in patients undergoing operative fixation of acetabular fractures.[13]

The association between heterotopic bone growth and the number and method of surgical debridement procedures, including the use of intermediate-pressure pulsatile lavage irrigation devices and negative pressure wound therapy, is not well understood. Two recent studies reported trends toward an association between HO formation and the number of debridement procedures as well as the duration of negative pressure dressing therapy.[30,44] However, these results should be interpreted with caution because the increases in both the number of debridement procedures and the duration of negative pressure dressing therapy are ostensibly also indicators of greater local injury severity; therefore, establishment of a causal linkage between local ectopic bone and these wound care modalities is difficult and fraught with confounding factors.

The type of definitive fracture treatment (internal fixation, external fixation, or amputation) appears unrelated to the formation of HO in extremity trauma, despite an historic association with certain surgical approaches to the hip and acetabulum.[15,20,24,71,73–77] This theoretical concern has not been borne out in clinical studies of extremity trauma.[44]

Amputees

The predilection of heterotopic bone for growth within the residual limbs of amputees is an important recent observation.[30,44] In combat-wounded servicemembers, serial debridement procedures are performed every 24–72 h before definitive wound closure or coverage in an effort to remove devitalized tissue and gross contamination. Antibiotic-impregnated polymethylmethacrylate beads are routinely used to reduce the bacterial bioburden, as are negative pressure wound dressings. Definitive amputations are often performed within or near the zone of injury (which is extensive in blast injuries) in an effort to preserve residual limb length, joint levels, and subsequent function. As a result, there exists a strong association between these injuries and the subsequent development of both radiographic and symptomatic HO.[30]

Several grading classification systems exist to classify its formation about the hip, knee, and elbow.[6,20,24,62,64,65,69] These were later extrapolated to other joints, but none is directly applicable or adaptable to the residual limbs of amputees. For these patients, a classification system, originally described by one of us (B.K.P.), has been adopted. The severity of HO is graded using a single radiographic projection (anteroposterior, lateral, or oblique) that maximizes the extent of the ectopic bone within the soft tissues of the residual limb. For example, ectopic bone formation is considered to be mild if it occupies less than 25%, moderate if it occupies 25–50%, and severe if it occupies >50% of the soft tissues on a single radiographic projection (Fig. 1).

Primary and secondary prophylaxis

Numerous randomized studies have documented the efficacy of primary prophylaxis to prevent HO in patients at risk. This type of prophylaxis is given following high-risk index procedures, such as total hip arthroplasty or operative fixation of acetabular fractures.[70,78–87] Typically, 5–10 Gy of local radiation therapy is dosed in a single fraction, with or without nonsteroidal anti-inflammatory medication. Nonsteroidal anti-inflammatory medications alone can be expected to provide a cost-effective, dose-related decrease in heterotopic bone formation, though the risk of complications, gastrointestinal and otherwise, appears higher.[72,79] Though some randomized series have demonstrated no difference in ectopic bone formation between nonsteroidal treatment and radiation therapy,[78,83,86] the bulk of the existing literature, including two meta-analyses, modestly favors radiation therapy, arguably related to compliance issues with medical treatment.[70,87–89] Two randomized series found no difference between preoperative and postoperative radiation when dosing single fraction of 7–10 Gy, provided it is given less than 4 h before or 48 h after surgery.[80,85]

Evidence supporting secondary prophylaxis following excision of symptomatic HO is lacking. To our knowledge, there exist no randomized trials of any secondary prevention modality. Nevertheless, the rate of recurrence in the appropriate surgical candidate is generally accepted to be low, and the theoretical benefit of secondary prophylaxis outweighs the risks of symptomatic recurrence for most patients.

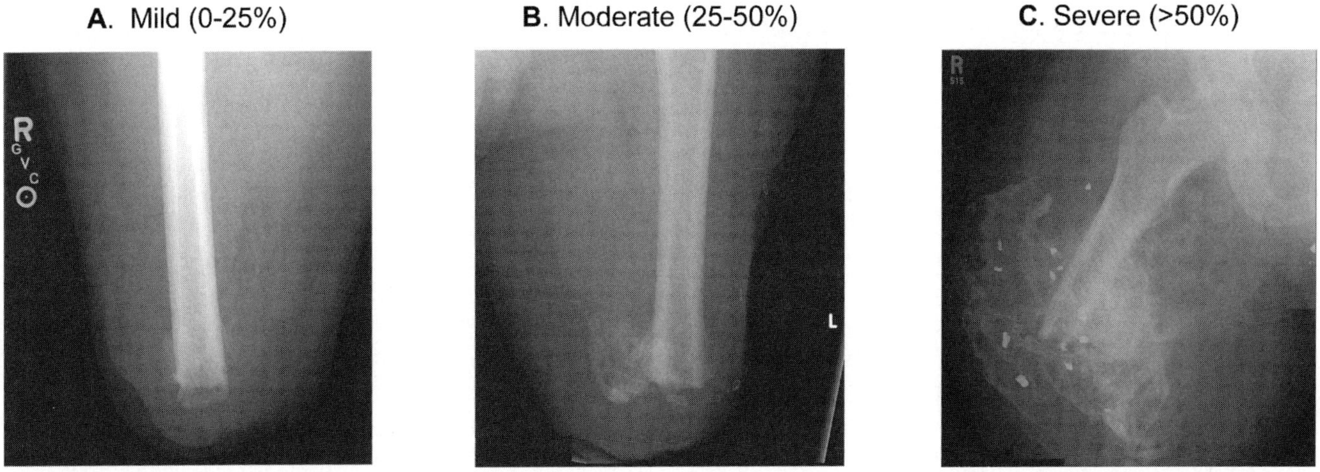

Figure 1. The Walter Reed classification for heterotopic ossification in the residual limbs of amputees. **A.** Mild, if the ectopic bone occupies < 25% of the residual limb; **B.** Moderate, if the ectopic bone occupies 25–50% of the residual limb; **C.** Severe, if the ectopic bone occupies > 50% of the residual limb.

Pitfalls of prophylaxis

Unfortunately, the use of HO prophylaxis is not without consequence. Following radiation, therapy, wound-, and implant-related complications have been reported.[74,87] For this reason, close consultation with a radiation oncologist will help ensure that the skin incision is protected and any press-fit implants are properly shielded. Patients with high-energy penetrating extremity wounds exhibit a relatively high baseline incidence of wound and fracture-related complications. The use of radiation therapy on these complex wounds is highly controversial and is theorized to result in an unacceptably high wound complication rate. Considering this, radiation as primary prophylaxis for HO is not currently used in this patient population.

Nonsteroidal anti-inflammatory medications (NSAIDS) may also be problematic in certain patient populations. Cyclooxygenase-2 is required for endochondral bone formation, a mechanism critical to the development of HO, as well as early fracture healing.[90] Concerns about NSAIDS in an orthopaedic population stem from this blunting of "helpful" inflammation necessary for endochondral ossification,[91–95] leading to increased time to union and increase in the number of delayed unions in several studies.[91,92,94–97] The potential benefit of NSAIDS for HO prophylaxis must be weighed heavily against potential fracture-related complications.

Etidronate is the only drug U.S. Food and Drug Administration (FDA) approved for the primary prophylaxis of HO and thus deserves consideration as well as a complete discussion. The FDA label states that etidronate is indicated following total hip replacement or spinal cord injury, though the drug has been evaluated off-label in other settings such as civilian trauma and in burns. Etidronate blocks the aggregation, growth, and mineralization of hydroxyapatite crystals, necessary for the formation of heterotopic bone. Early randomized and pseudorandomized trials demonstrated efficacy,[98–103] but only as long as the drug was administered. "Rebound" formation of HO following cessation of therapy was common,[98–101,103] and follow on studies failed to corroborate the earlier results.[104–106] In fact a recent Cochrane database review did not demonstrate pharmacologic efficacy and could not recommend etidronate treatment for the primary prophylaxis of HO.[107]

Treatment

The treatment of HO is individualized. Most cases are mild, minimally or asymptomatic, and result in little or no functional impairment.[13–16,18,20,22,58,62,64–72,76,77,81,82,84,85,108–110] Moderate to severe cases can be highly debilitating, particularly in periarticular locations or in the residual limbs of amputees.[16,30,111] Once HO has been identified radiographically, an assessment should be made as to the impact on the patient's level of function and activities of daily living. In amputees, it is important to identify and treat other sources of residual limb pain such as painful bursae, myodesis failure, and neuromata.[112,113] Conservative management including rest, local and systemic medications, activity modification, and prosthetic socket/suspension modifications requires close consultation with skilled prosthetists, physical therapists, and physiatrists. Likewise, in nonamputees, alternative causes of pain and functional limitations including infection, fracture nonunion, and neuropathic pain syndromes should be evaluated and treated. Surgical excision is reserved for pain, ulceration, or joint stiffness attributable to HO that remains refractory to exhaustive conservative measures.

Timing and results of excision

The timing of excision HO is controversial. Historically, excision was advocated only after prolonged observation ensuring that the ectopic bone was "mature," as evidenced by quiescent three-phase bone scans and normalization of the serum alkaline phosphatase.[114–116] This practice has recently been called into question, as these measures do not accurately predict recurrence.[6] Numerous studies support earlier excision based on the roentgenographic appearance of the lesion.[30,117–127] This approach allows earlier range of motion and return of functional mobility and a recurrence rate similar to late excision.[118] Garland[6] identified other prognostic factors for HO excision in patients with head injuries, using a classification system based on the patient's cognitive and physical disability (Table 1). In his series, motion-related outcomes and recurrence rates were excellent in classes I and II and uniformly poor, with a 100% recurrence rate, in class V. He theorized that the latter group of patients possessed a systemic oste-

Table 1. *Garland classification, prognostic factors of heterotopic ossification excision*

Class I	Minimum cognitive and physical disability
Class II	Minimum cognitive, but moderate physical disability
Class III	Minimum cognitive with severe physical disability
Class IV	Moderate to severe cognitive deficits with minimal physical deficits
Class V	Moderate to severe cognitive deficits with severe physical disability

ogenic stimulus that may persist for years after the initial injury. Knowledge of this can help set patient and family expectations, particularly in cases involving severe traumatic brain injury. After appropriate patient selection and preoperative counseling, we advocate surgical excision as soon as symptoms warrant following appropriate efforts at conservative management. Regarding the amputee with variable cognitive and minimal other physical disability, excellent results of excision can be achieved. In one series of 25 combat-related amputations, an 8% recurrence rate of mild, asymptomatic ectopic bone has been reported with secondary prophylaxis treatment in 84% of the cases.[30]

TAKE-HOME MESSAGE

Basic science advances

- Animal models and human histology samples suggest that HO formation follows a predictable sequence of events. Aberrant BMPs in soft tissues stimulate differentiation of progenitor cells into brown adipocytes. The resultant hypoxic environment, in turn, stimulates chondrogenesis and neovascularization. Then, as the oxygen tension increases, endochondral ossification occurs.
- Endothelial precursor cells are thought to contribute to every stage of HO development.

Clinical science advances

- The incidence of HO in combat-wounded servicemembers has consistently been reported as 63–64.6%, far greater than that described in civilian trauma centers.
- Important risk factors include
  - blast injury
  - combat-related amputations within the zone of injury
  - ISSs greater than 16

Relevance to clinical care

- Most cases of HO are asymptomatic
- Conservative management is recommended and includes rest, local and systemic medications, activity modification, and prosthetic socket/suspension modifications
- Surgical excision is reserved for pain, ulceration, or joint stiffness attributable to HO that remains refractory to exhaustive conservative measures.

CONCLUSION

HO is a complex disorder with numerous proven and putative risk factors and varied initiating external stimuli, ultimately resulting from both local and systemic internal biologic factors. Lesions are often asymptomatic but can result in profound patient disability due to pain and joint stiffness. When practicable, primary prophylaxis via radiation therapy or nonsteroidal anti-inflammatory drugs is effective in a majority of patients at risk. After an appropriate trial of conservative measures, operative excision of symptomatic heterotopic bone provides generally good results with low recurrence rates in appropriately selected patients treated with secondary prophylaxis. Future research regarding biomarker-based prognostication and identification of initiating chemokines, genes, and cellular origin of ectopic bone may permit expanded early prophylaxis and development of novel targeted therapies to prevent or limit HO.

ACKNOWLEDGMENT

HO research in the author's laboratory is funded by a grant from the Department of the Navy, Bureau of Medicine Advance Development Program.

CAUTION, CRITICAL REMARKS, AND RECOMMENDATIONS

Before surgical excision, other sources of limb pain such as painful bursae, myodesis failure, and neuromata must be ruled out.

FUTURE DEVELOPMENTS

- It is important, and perhaps essential to better identify the molecular pathway(s) responsible for HO production. Novel prophylactic therapies may then be developed.
- Prediction and risk stratification methods, using biomarker analysis and modeling, are also necessary.

AUTHOR DISCLOSURE STATEMENT

No competing financial interests exist.

REFERENCES

1. Mansoor A and Beals RK: Enchondral ossification of muscles of the calf: a case report on a new form of heterotopic ossification. J Pediatr Orthop B 2008.
2. Kypson AP, Morphew E, Jones R, Gottfried MR, and Seigler HF: Heterotopic ossification in rectal cancer: rare finding with a novel proposed mechanism. J Surg Oncol 2003; **82:** 132; discussion 137.
3. Kaplan FS, Glaser DL, Hebela N, and Shore EM: Heterotopic ossification. J Am Acad Orthop Surg 2004; **12:** 116.
4. Hoffer MM, Garrett A, Brink J, Perry J, Hale W, and Nickel VL: The orthopaedic management of brain-injured children. J Bone Joint Surg Am 1971; **53:** 567.
5. Garland DE, Razza BE, and Waters RL: Forceful joint manipulation in head-injured adults with heterotopic ossification. Clin Orthop Relat Res 1982; **169:** 133.
6. Garland DE, Hanscom DA, Keenan MA, Smith C, and Moore T: Resection of heterotopic ossification in the adult with head trauma. J Bone Joint Surg Am 1985; **67:** 1261.
7. Garland DE and Keenan MA: Orthopedic strategies in the management of the adult head-injured patient. Phys Ther 1983; **63:** 2004.
8. Garland DE. A clinical perspective on common forms of acquired heterotopic ossification. Clin Orthop Relat Res 1991; **263:** 13.
9. Como JJ, Yowler CJ, and Malangoni MA: Extensive heterotopic mesenteric ossification after penetrating abdominal trauma. J Trauma 2008; **65:** 1567.
10. Sanchez-Sotelo J, Torchia ME, and O'Driscoll SW: Complex distal humeral fractures: internal fixation with a principle-based parallel-plate technique. J Bone Joint Surg Am 2007; **89:** 961.
11. Rama KR, Vendittoli PA, Ganapathi M, Borgmann R, Roy A, and Lavigne M: Heterotopic ossification after surface replacement arthroplasty and total hip arthroplasty: a randomized study. J Arthroplasty 2009; **24:** 256–262.
12. Mikic ZD and Vukadinovic SM: Late results in fractures of the radial head treated by excision. Clin Orthop Relat Res 1983; **181:** 220.
13. Kreder HJ, Rozen N, Borkhoff CM, *et al.*: Determinants of functional outcome after simple and complex acetabular fractures involving the posterior wall. J Bone Joint Surg Br 2006; **88:** 776.
14. Kamineni S, and Morrey BF: Distal humeral fractures treated with noncustom total elbow replacement. J Bone Joint Surg Am 2004; **86A:** 940.
15. Giannoudis PV, Grotz MR, Papakostidis C, and Dinopoulos H: Operative treatment of displaced fractures of the acetabulum. A meta-analysis. J Bone Joint Surg Br 2005; **87:** 2.
16. Garland DE, Blum CE, and Waters RL: Periarticular heterotopic ossification in head-injured adults. Incidence and location. J Bone Joint Surg Am 1980; **62:** 1143.
17. Garland DE and Dowling V: Forearm fractures in the head-injured adult. Clin Orthop Relat Res 1983; **176:** 190.
18. Garland DE and O'Hollaren RM: Fractures and dislocations about the elbow in the head-injured adult. Clin Orthop Relat Res 1982; **168:** 38.
19. Dias DA: Heterotopic para-articular ossification of the elbow with soft tissue contracture in burns. Burns Incl Therm Inj 1982; **9:** 128.
20. Brooker AF, Bowerman JW, Robinson RA, and Riley LHJ: Ectopic ossification following total hip replacement. Incidence and a method of classification. J Bone Joint Surg Am 1973; **55:** 1629.
21. Broberg MA and Morrey BF: Results of treatment of fracture-dislocations of the elbow. Clin Orthop Relat Res 1987; **216:** 109.
22. Back DL, Smith JD, Dalziel RE, Young DA, and Shimmin A: Incidence of heterotopic ossification after hip resurfacing. ANZ J Surg 2007; **77:** 642.
23. Ahrengart L: Periarticular heterotopic ossification after total hip arthroplasty. Risk factors and consequences. Clin Orthop Relat Res 1991; **263:** 49.
24. Morrey BF, Adams RA, and Cabanela ME: Comparison of heterotopic bone after anterolateral, transtrochanteric, and posterior approaches for total hip arthroplasty. Clin Orthop Relat Res 1984; **188:** 160.
25. Ozer H, Solak S, Turanli S, Baltaci G, Colakoglu T, and Bolukbasi S: Intercondylar fractures of the distal humerus treated with the triceps-reflecting anconeus pedicle approach. Arch Orthop Trauma Surg 2005; **125:** 469.
26. Kaplan FS, Hahn GV, and Zasloff MA: Heterotopic ossification: two rare forms and what they can teach us. J Am Acad Orthop Surg 1994; **2:** 288.
27. Kaplan FS, McCluskey W, Hahn G, Tabas JA, Muenke M, and Zasloff MA: Genetic transmission of fibrodysplasia ossificans progressiva. Report of a family. J Bone Joint Surg Am 1993; **75:** 1214.
28. Kaplan FS and Shore EM: Progressive osseous heteroplasia. J Bone Miner Res 2000; **15:** 2084.
29. Potter BK, Burns TC, Lacap AP, Granville RR, and Gajewski D: Heterotopic ossification in the residual limbs of traumatic and combat-related amputees. J Am Acad Orthop Surg 2006; **14:** S191.
30. Potter BK, Burns TC, Lacap AP, Granville RR, and Gajewski DA: Heterotopic ossification following traumatic and combat-related amputations. Prevalence, risk factors, and preliminary results of excision. J Bone Joint Surg Am 2007; **89:** 476.
31. London PS: Medical lessons from the Falkland Islands' campaign. Report of a meeting of the united services section of the royal society of medicine held at the Royal College of Surgeons on February 17 and 18, 1983. J Bone Joint Surg Br 1983; **65:** 507.
32. Gofrit ON, Leibovici D, Shapira SC, Shemer J, Stein M, and Michaelson M: The trimodal death distribution of trauma victims: military experience from the Lebanon war. Mil Med 1997; **162:** 24.
33. Mabry RL, Holcomb JB, Baker AM, *et al.*: United states army rangers in Somalia: an analysis of combat casualties on an urban battlefield. J Trauma 2000; **49:** 515; discussion 528.
34. Islinger RB, Kuklo TR, and McHale KA: A review of orthopedic injuries in three recent U.S. military conflicts. Mil Med 2000; **165:** 463.
35. Covey DC: Blast and fragment injuries of the musculoskeletal system. J Bone Joint Surg Am 2002; **84A:** 1221.
36. Champion HR, Bellamy RF, Roberts CP, and Leppaniemi A: A profile of combat injury. J Trauma 2003; **54:** S13.
37. Lin DL, Kirk KL, Murphy KP, McHale KA, and Doukas WC: Evaluation of orthopaedic injuries in operation enduring freedom. J Orthop Trauma 2004; **18:** S48.
38. Patel TH, Wenner KA, Price SA, Weber MA, Leveridge A, and McAtee SJ: A U.S. Army forward surgical team's experience in operation Iraqi freedom. J Trauma 2004; **57:** 201.
39. Covey DC: Combat orthopaedics: a view from the trenches. J Am Acad Orthop Surg 2006; **14:** S10.
40. Hofmeister EP, Mazurek M, and Ingari J: Injuries sustained to the upper extremity due to modern warfare and the evolution of care. J Hand Surg [Am] 2007; **32:** 1141.
41. Fox CJ, Gillespie DL, Cox ED, *et al.*: Damage control resuscitation for vascular surgery in a combat support hospital. J Trauma 2008; **65:** 1.
42. Hayda RA, Mazurek MT, Powell Iv ET, *et al.*: From Iraq back to Iraq: modern combat orthopaedic care. Instr Course Lect 2008; **57:** 87.
43. Kragh JFJ, Walters TJ, Baer DG, *et al.*: Survival with emergency tourniquet use to stop bleeding in major limb trauma. Ann Surg 2009; **249:** 1.
44. Forsberg JA, Pepek JM, Wagner S, *et al.*: Heterotopic ossification in high-energy wartime extremity injuries: prevalence and risk factors. J Bone Joint Surg Am 2009; **91:** 1084.
45. Garland DE: Clinical observations on fractures and heterotopic ossification in the spinal cord and traumatic brain injured populations. Clin Orthop Relat Res 1988; **233:** 86.
46. Garland DE, Rothi B, and Waters RL: Femoral fractures in head-injuries in adults. Clin Orthop Relat Res 1982; **166:** 219.
47. Garland DE and Toder L: Fractures of the tibial diaphysis in adults with head injuries. Clin Orthop Relat Res 1980; 198.

48. Shafritz AB, Shore EM, Gannon FH, *et al.*: Overexpression of an osteogenic morphogen in fibrodysplasia ossificans progressiva. N Engl J Med 1996; **335:** 555.

49. de la Pena LS, Billings PC, Fiori JL, Ahn J, Kaplan FS, and Shore EM: Fibrodysplasia ossificans progressiva (fop), a disorder of ectopic osteogenesis, misregulates cell surface expression and trafficking of bmpria. J Bone Miner Res 2005; **20:** 1168.

50. Roush W: Protein builds second skeleton. Science 1996; **273:** 1170.

51. Feldman G, Li M, Martin S, *et al.*: Fibrodysplasia ossificans progressiva, a heritable disorder of severe heterotopic ossification, maps to human chromosome 4q27-31. Am J Hum Genet 2000; **66:** 128.

52. Nesti LJ, Jackson WM, Shanti RM, *et al.*: Differentiation potential of multipotent progenitor cells derived from war-traumatized muscle tissue. J Bone Joint Surg Am 2008; **90:** 2390.

53. Lounev VY, Ramachandran R, Wosczyna MN, *et al.*: Identification of progenitor cells that contribute to heterotopic skeletogenesis. J Bone Joint Surg Am 2009; **91:** 652.

54. Spencer RF: The effect of head injury on fracture healing. A quantitative assessment. J Bone Joint Surg Br 1987; **69:** 525.

55. Giannoudis PV, Mushtaq S, Harwood P, *et al.*: Accelerated bone healing and excessive callus formation in patients with femoral fracture and head injury. Injury 2006; **37(Suppl 3):** S18.

56. Cadosch D, Gautschi OP, Thyer M, *et al.*: Humoral factors enhance fracture-healing and callus formation in patients with traumatic brain injury. J Bone Joint Surg Am 2009; **91:** 282.

57. Steinberg GG and Hubbard C: Heterotopic ossification after femoral intramedullary rodding. J Orthop Trauma 1993; **7:** 536.

58. Brumback RJ, Wells JD, Lakatos R, Poka A, Bathon GH, and Burgess AR: Heterotopic ossification about the hip after intramedullary nailing for fractures of the femur. J Bone Joint Surg Am 1990; **72:** 1067.

59. Simonsen LL, Sonne-Holm S, Krasheninnikoff M, and Engberg AW: Symptomatic heterotopic ossification after very severe traumatic brain injury in 114 patients: incidence and risk factors. Injury 2007; **38:** 1146.

60. Eastell R, Delmas PD, Hodgson SF, Eriksen EF, Mann KG, and Riggs BL: Bone formation rate in older normal women: concurrent assessment with bone histomorphometry, calcium kinetics, and biochemical markers. J Clin Endocrinol Metab 1988; **67:** 741.

61. Hierton C, Blomgren G, and Lindgren U: Factors associated with heterotopic bone formation in cemented total hip prostheses. Acta Orthop Scand 1983; **54:** 698.

62. Lazansky MG: Complications revisited. The debit side of total hip replacement. Clin Orthop Relat Res 1973; **95:** 96.

63. Sneath RJ, Bindi FD, Davies J, and Parnell EJ: The effect of pulsed irrigation on the incidence of heterotopic ossification after total hip arthroplasty. J Arthroplasty 2001; **16:** 547.

64. Ritter MA and Vaughan RB: Ectopic ossification after total hip arthroplasty. Predisposing factors, frequency, and effect on results. J Bone Joint Surg Am 1977; **59:** 345.

65. Riegler HF and Harris CM: Heterotopic bone formation after total hip arthroplasty. Clin Orthop Relat Res 1976; **117:** 209.

66. Kasetti RJ, Shetty AA, and Rand C: Heterotopic ossification after uncemented hydroxyapatite-coated primary total hip arthroplasty. J Arthroplasty 2001; **16:** 1038.

67. Higo T, Mawatari M, Shigematsu M, and Hotokebuchi T: The incidence of heterotopic ossification after cementless total hip arthroplasty. J Arthroplasty 2006; **21:** 852.

68. Ebraheim NA, Patil V, Liu J, and Haman SP: Sliding trochanteric osteotomy in acetabular fractures: a review of 30 cases. Injury 2007; **38:** 1177.

69. Dalury DF and Jiranek WA: The incidence of heterotopic ossification after total knee arthroplasty. J Arthroplasty 2004; **19:** 447.

70. Kolbl O, Knelles D, Barthel T, Kraus U, Flentje M, and Eulert J: Randomized trial comparing early postoperative irradiation vs. the use of nonsteroidal antiinflammatory drugs for prevention of heterotopic ossification following prosthetic total hip replacement. Int J Radiat Oncol Biol Phys 1997; **39:** 961.

71. Griffin DB, Beaule PE, and Matta JM: Safety and efficacy of the extended iliofemoral approach in the treatment of complex fractures of the acetabulum. J Bone Joint Surg Br 2005; **87:** 1391.

72. Matta JM and Siebenrock KA: Does indomethacin reduce heterotopic bone formation after operations for acetabular fractures? A prospective randomised study. J Bone Joint Surg Br 1997; **79:** 959.

73. Oh CW, Kim PT, Park BC, *et al.*: Results after operative treatment of transverse acetabular fractures. J Orthop Sci 2006; **11:** 478.

74. Petsatodis G, Antonarakos P, Chalidis B, Papadopoulos P, Christoforidis J, and Pournaras J: Surgically treated acetabular fractures via a single posterior approach with a follow-up of 2–10 years. Injury 2007; **38:** 334.

75. Rath EM, Russell GVJ, Washington WJ, and Routt MLJ: Gluteus minimus necrotic muscle debridement diminishes heterotopic ossification after acetabular fracture fixation. Injury 2002; **33:** 751.

76. Schara K and Herman S: Heterotopic bone formation in total hip arthroplasty: predisposing factors, classification and the significance for clinical outcome. Acta Chir Orthop Traumatol Cech 2001; **68:** 105.

77. Triantaphillopoulos PG, Panagiotopoulos EC, Mousafiris C, Tyllianakis M, Dimakopoulos P, and Lambiris EE: Long-term results in surgically treated acetabular fractures through the posterior approaches. J Trauma 2007; **62:** 378.

78. Burd TA, Lowry KJ, and Anglen JO: Indomethacin compared with localized irradiation for the prevention of heterotopic ossification following surgical treatment of acetabular fractures. J Bone Joint Surg Am 2001; **83A:** 1783.

79. Fransen M and Neal B: Non-steroidal anti-inflammatory drugs for preventing heterotopic bone formation after hip arthroplasty. Cochrane Database Syst Rev 2004; 3: CD001160.

80. Gregoritch SJ, Chadha M, Pelligrini VD, Rubin P, and Kantorowitz DA: Randomized trial comparing preoperative versus postoperative irradiation for prevention of heterotopic ossification following prosthetic total hip replacement: preliminary results. Int J Radiat Oncol Biol Phys 1994; **30:** 55.

81. Knelles D, Barthel T, Karrer A, Kraus U, Eulert J, and Kolbl O: Prevention of heterotopic ossification after total hip replacement. A prospective, randomised study using acetylsalicylic acid, indomethacin and fractional or single-dose irradiation. J Bone Joint Surg Br 1997; **79:** 596.

82. Kolbl O, Knelles D, Barthel T, Raunecker F, Flentje M, and Eulert J: Preoperative irradiation versus the use of nonsteroidal anti-inflammatory drugs for prevention of heterotopic ossification following total hip replacement: the results of a randomized trial. Int J Radiat Oncol Biol Phys 1998; **42:** 397.

83. Moore KD, Goss K, and Anglen JO: Indomethacin versus radiation therapy for prophylaxis against heterotopic ossification in acetabular fractures: a randomised, prospective study. J Bone Joint Surg Br 1998; **80:** 259.

84. Pakos EE, Pitouli EJ, Tsekeris PG, Papathanasopoulou V, Stafilas K, and Xenakis TH: Prevention of heterotopic ossification in high-risk patients with total hip arthroplasty: the experience of a combined therapeutic protocol. Int Orthop 2006; **30:** 79.

85. Pellegrini VDJ, Konski AA, Gastel JA, Rubin P, and Evarts CM: Prevention of heterotopic ossification with irradiation after total hip arthroplasty. Radiation therapy with a single dose of eight hundred centigray administered to a limited field. J Bone Joint Surg Am 1992; **74:** 186.

86. Seegenschmiedt MH, Keilholz L, Martus P, *et al.*: Prevention of heterotopic ossification about the hip: final results of two randomized trials in 410 patients using either preoperative or postoperative radiation therapy. Int J Radiat Oncol Biol Phys 1997; **39:** 161.

87. Sell S, Willms R, Jany R, *et al.*: The suppression of heterotopic ossifications: radiation versus nsaid therapy—a prospective study. J Arthroplasty 1998; **13:** 854.

88. Blokhuis TJ and Frolke JP: Is radiation superior to indomethacin to prevent heterotopic ossification in acetabular fractures? A systematic review. Clin Orthop Relat Res 2009; **467:** 526.

89. Pakos EE and Ioannidis JP: Radiotherapy vs. nonsteroidal anti-inflammatory drugs for the prevention of heterotopic ossification after major hip procedures: a meta-analysis of randomized trials. Int J Radiat Oncol Biol Phys 2004; **60:** 888.

90. Olmsted-Davis E, Gannon FH, Ozen M, *et al.*: Hypoxic adipocytes pattern early heterotopic bone formation. Am J Pathol 2007; **170:** 620.

91. Bergenstock M, Min W, Simon AM, Sabatino C, and O'Connor JP: A comparison between the effects of acetaminophen and celecoxib on bone fracture healing in rats. J Orthop Trauma 2005; **19:** 717.

92. Herbenick MA, Sprott D, Stills H, and Lawless M: Effects of a cyclooxygenase 2 inhibitor on fracture healing in a rat model. Am J Orthop 2008; **37:** E133.

93. Mullis BH, Copland ST, Weinhold PS, Miclau T, Lester GE, and Bos GD: Effect of cox-2 inhibitors and non-steroidal anti-inflammatory drugs on a mouse fracture model. Injury 2006; **37:** 827.

94. Simon AM, Manigrasso MB, and O'Connor JP: Cyclo-oxygenase 2 function is essential for bone fracture healing. J Bone Miner Res 2002; **17:** 963.

95. Simon AM, and O'Connor JP: Dose and time-dependent effects of cyclooxygenase-2 inhibition on fracture-healing. J Bone Joint Surg Am 2007; **89:** 500.

96. Macfarlane RJ, Ng BH, Gamie Z, *et al.*: Pharmacological treatment of heterotopic ossification following hip and acetabular surgery. Expert Opin Pharmacother 2008; **9:** 767.

97. O'Connor JP and Lysz T: Celecoxib, nsaids and the skeleton. Drugs Today (Barc) 2008; **44:** 693.

98. Banovac K: The effect of etidronate on late development of heterotopic ossification after spinal cord injury. J Spinal Cord Med 2000; **23:** 40.

99. Banovac K, Gonzalez F, and Renfree KJ: Treatment of heterotopic ossification after spinal cord injury. J Spinal Cord Med 1997; **20:** 60.

100. Banovac K, Gonzalez F, Wade N, and Bowker JJ: Intravenous disodium etidronate therapy in spinal cord injury patients with heterotopic ossification. Paraplegia 1993; **31:** 660.

101. Spielman G, Gennarelli TA, and Rogers CR: Disodium etidronate: its role in preventing heterotopic ossification in severe head injury. Arch Phys Med Rehabil 1983; **64:** 539.

102. Finerman GA and Stover SL: Heterotopic ossification following hip replacement or spinal cord injury. Two clinical studies with ehdp. Metab Bone Dis Relat Res 1981; **3:** 337.

103. Stover SL, Niemann KM, and Miller JMr: Disodium etidronate in the prevention of postoperative recurrence of heterotopic ossification in spinal-cord injury patients. J Bone Joint Surg Am 1976; **58:** 683.

104. Garland DE, Alday B, Venos KG, and Vogt JC: Diphosphonate treatment for heterotopic ossification in spinal cord injury patients. Clin Orthop Relat Res 1983; **176:** 197.

105. Hu HP, Kuijpers W, Slooff TJ, van Horn JR, and Versleyen DH: The effect of biphosphonate on induced heterotopic bone. Clin Orthop Relat Res 1991; **272:** 259.

106. Thomas BJ and Amstutz HC: Results of the administration of diphosphonate for the prevention of heterotopic ossification after total hip arthroplasty. J Bone Joint Surg Am 1985; **67:** 400.

107. Haran M, Bhuta T, and Lee B: Pharmacological interventions for treating acute heterotopic ossification. Cochrane Database Syst Rev 2004; 4: CD003321.

108. Grohs JG, Schmidt M, and Wanivenhaus A: Selective cox-2 inhibitor versus indomethacin for the prevention of heterotopic ossification after hip replacement: a double-blind randomized trial of 100 patients with 1-year follow-up. Acta Orthop 2007; **78:** 95.

109. Saudan M, Saudan P, Perneger T, Riand N, Keller A, and Hoffmeyer P: Celecoxib versus ibuprofen in the prevention of heterotopic ossification following total hip replacement: a prospective randomised trial. J Bone Joint Surg Br 2007; **89:** 155.

110. van der Heide HJ, Rijnberg WJ, Van Sorge A, Van Kampen A, and Schreurs BW: Similar effects of rofecoxib and indomethacin on the incidence of heterotopic ossification after hip arthroplasty. Acta Orthop 2007; **78:** 90.

111. Hendricks HT, Geurts AC, van Ginneken BC, Heeren AJ, and Vos PE: Brain injury severity and autonomic dysregulation accurately predict heterotopic ossification in patients with traumatic brain injury. Clin Rehabil 2007; **21:** 545.

112. BK P, RR G, MR B, *et al.*: Special surgical considerations for the combat casualty with limb loss. In: *Rehabilitation of Combat Casualties with Limb Loss*, edited by Pasquina PCR. Washington, DC: Borden Institute, 2008. (in press)

113. Ehde DM and Smith DG: Chronic pain management. In: *Atlas of Amputations and Limb Deficiencies: Surgical, Prosthetic, and Rehabilitation Principles* (edition 3), edited by Smith DG, Michael JW, and Bowker JH, 2004, pp. 711–726.

114. Furman R, Nicholas JJ, and Jivoff L: Elevation of the serum alkaline phosphatase coincident with ectopic-bone formation in paraplegic patients. J Bone Joint Surg Am 1970; **52:** 1131.

115. Hsu JD, Sakimura I, and Stauffer ES: Heterotopic ossification around the hip joint in spinal cord injured patients. Clin Orthop Relat Res 1975; **112:** 165.

116. Pittenger DE: Heterotopic ossification. Orthop Rev 1991; **20:** 33.

117. Beingessner DM, Patterson SD, and King GJ: Early excision of heterotopic bone in the forearm. J Hand Surg [Am] 2000; **25:** 483.

118. Chalidis B, Stengel D, and Giannoudis PV: Early excision and late excision of heterotopic ossification after traumatic brain injury are equivalent: a systematic review of the literature. J Neurotrauma 2007; **24:** 1675.

119. Ellerin BE, Helfet D, Parikh S, *et al.*: Current therapy in the management of heterotopic ossification of the elbow: a review with case studies. Am J Phys Med Rehabil 1999; **78:** 259.

120. Freebourn TM, Barber DB, and Able AC: The treatment of immature heterotopic ossification in spinal cord injury with combination surgery, radiation therapy and nsaid. Spinal Cord 1999; **37:** 50.

121. Garland DE and Orwin JF: Resection of heterotopic ossification in patients with spinal cord injuries. Clin Orthop Relat Res 1989; **242:** 169.

122. McAuliffe JA and Wolfson AH: Early excision of heterotopic ossification about the elbow followed by radiation therapy. J Bone Joint Surg Am 1997; **79:** 749.

123. Mitsionis GI, Lykissas MG, Kalos N, *et al.*: Functional outcome after excision of heterotopic ossification about the knee in icu patients. Int Orthop 2008 .

124. Moritomo H, Tada K, and Yoshida T: Early, wide excision of heterotopic ossification in the medial elbow. J Shoulder Elbow Surg 2001; **10:** 164.

125. Tsionos I, Leclercq C, and Rochet JM: Heterotopic ossification of the elbow in patients with burns. Results after early excision. J Bone Joint Surg Br 2004; **86:** 396.

126. Viola RW and Hanel DP: Early "simple" release of posttraumatic elbow contracture associated with heterotopic ossification. J Hand Surg [Am] 1999; **24:** 370.

127. Wysocki RW and Cohen MS: Radioulnar heterotopic ossification after distal biceps tendon repair: results following surgical resection. J Hand Surg [Am] 2007; **32:** 1230.

WHS
Wound
Healing
Society

The Mangled Extremity

Romney C. Andersen,[1–4,*] Scott B. Shawen,[1,2,4] John J. Keeling,[1,2,4] and Robert V. O'Toole[3]

[1]Orthopaedic Surgery Service, Integrated Department of Orthopaedics & Rehabilitation, Walter Reed Army Medical Center, Washington, District of Columbia.
[2]Orthopaedic Surgery Service, Integrated Department of Orthopaedics & Rehabilitation, National Naval Medical Center, Bethesda, Maryland.
[3]Division of Orthopaedic Traumatology, R Adams Cowley Shock Trauma Center, University of Maryland Medical Systems, Baltimore, Maryland.
[4]Department of Surgery, Uniformed Services University of the Health Sciences, Bethesda, Maryland.

Background: The global war on terror has produced devastating mangled extremities. Choosing whether or not to salvage the limb is a difficult decision for the surgeon and the patient.
The Problem: There are no definitive studies that demonstrate which limbs would benefit from limb salvage and which ones would be best treated with an early amputation. Attempts at reconstruction involve replacing lost skin, bone, muscle, nerve tissue, and vasculature. Reconstructed extremities often are complicated by limited function and chronic pain, while amputation requires life-long prosthetic care.
Basic/Clinical Science Advances: Stem cell research affords the potential to regenerate some of the lost tissues. Clinical studies like the Military Extremity Trauma and Amputation/Limb Salvage (METALS) study will potentially help better define which patients would benefit from limb salvage and which would benefit from early amputation.
Clinical Care Relevance: If the Military Extremity Trauma and Amputation/Limb Salvage study is able to demonstrate groups of patients who would benefit with one type of treatment over another it would afford the surgeon the ability to better counsel their patients on whether they recommend limb salvage or amputation. However, the study is retrospective in nature, and there will be difficulties in stratifying injuries.
Conclusion: Currently, there are no clear indicators as to which patients would benefit from limb salvage or amputation. Surgeons must rely on their clinical judgment, taking into account the patients' desired goals to make recommendations on the advantages and disadvantages of different surgical treatments.

Abbreviations and Acronyms

BMPs = bone morphogenetic proteins

LEAP = Lower Extremity Assessment Project

METALS = Military Extremity Trauma and Amputation/Limb Salvage

MSCs = mesenchymal stem cells

SIP = sickness impact profile

*Correspondence: Orthopaedic Surgery Service, Integrated Department of Orthopaedics & Rehabilitation, Walter Reed Army Medical Center, 6900 Georgia Ave., Washington, District of Columbia 20307 (e-mail: romney.andersen@us.army.mil).

BACKGROUND

THE GLOBAL WAR ON TERRORISM has produced some of the worst injuries seen by the current generation of military surgeons.[1,2] The advent of improved body armor has increased the severity of extremity wounds in patients who survive. Protection of the extremities has not advanced as quickly as that of the head and torso resulting in patients with extremity injuries that would not likely have survived in previous conflicts. The injuries sustained have significant damage to all of the tissue groups in the extremity including skin, muscle, nerve, blood vessel, and bone. Reconstructed extremities often have significantly reduced function, and the patient is often faced with chronic pain. Amputation is often considered for these devastating injuries, and some patients benefit from amputation over salvage of their limb. Often, patients initially undertake limb salvage only to decide on amputation

Printed in U.S.A.
DOI: 10.1089/awc.2009.0026

later, thus expending large amounts or resources both in dollars and patient emotional costs.[3] Limb salvage is associated with high complication rates and even in the best care can fail. Protracted attempts to optimize a salvaged but dysfunctional limb are associated with some psychological problems.[4] The age-old question is which extremities would benefit most from limb salvage over early amputation. Generally, it is felt that the only absolute indications for an acute amputation are amputation to save the life of the patient, and a traumatic amputation with a skin bridge only remaining. Relative indications for an acute amputation are warm ischemia time greater than 6 h, severe ipslilateral foot trauma, polytrauma, and poor physiologic status. The decision as to what treatment course to take should be a shared responsibility between the surgeon and an informed patient with realistic expectations of likely outcomes.

CLINICAL PROBLEM ADDRESSED

When considering which limbs can even be salvaged there are several factors to consider. First and foremost is saving life over limb. With the technology available today many extremities can be salvaged and one should never focus on saving the extremity at the cost of the patient's life.[5] The extremity is comprised of several different types of tissues all of which have varying capability to reconstruct or replace. The extremity is covered with skin and frequently the mangled extremity has a significant amount of skin loss, or skin that will be removed during the debridement process. This is generally felt to be the easiest tissue to replace in a mangled extremity. Bone is the structural portion of the extremity, and relative success can be achieved in managing bone that is lost or destroyed.[6,7] For bone to heal, it needs well-vascularized muscle surrounding it. Muscles can relatively easily be moved around the body to achieve this coverage; however, the muscle transferred usually loses its function, and the muscle that was lost never has its function reproduced. Similarly, vasculature that is injured can be repaired or reconstructed fairly reproducibly. Nerve tissue can also be repaired or reconstructed; however, normal function is rarely achieved. When the injury includes the loss of a significant portion of an articular joint, one must recognize that there are very few good options at replacing the joint. Other important factors in deciding whether or not to salvage a mangled extremity are the patient's access to medical care, personality traits, medical comorbidities, socioeconomic status, substance abuse, and education level.[8] These issues are of less concern in the U.S. military population, as all patients have access to care and have been screened or treated for many of the items that portend poor results after limb salvage.

RELEVANT BASIC SCIENCE CONTEXT

Basic science research has shown much potential in recent years in the area of stem cell research. Optimum healing of wounds requires a well-orchestrated integration of the complex biological and molecular events of cell migration and proliferation, and of extracellular matrix deposition and remodeling. Studies suggest that mesenchymal stem cells (MSCs) may be involved in these processes, contributing to skin cells or releasing regulatory cytokines. Direct injection of bone marrow–derived MSCs into injured tissues shows improved repair through mechanisms of differentiation and/or release of paracrine factors.[9,10] Recent basic science studies have shown that MSCs can be derived from traumatized tissue. Histological lineage-specific markers demonstrated the potential of these cells to produce different mesenchymal tissue lineages.[11,12] If this technology can be developed to a point where MSCs can be extracted from traumatized tissue that would normally be discarded and can be used to grow new genetically similar tissues to the patient, it could obviate autograft or allograft tissue in reconstruction.

EXPERIMENTAL MODEL OR MATERIAL—ADVANTAGES AND LIMITATIONS

The long-term consequences of major limb trauma and the optimal treatment algorithms of major limb trauma in the military setting are presently not known. To address this knowledge void, the Military Extremity Trauma and Amputation/Limb Salvage (METALS) retrospective study has been undertaken to identify outcome differences between limb salvage and amputation. The study will be conducted at the four facilities receiving the most severely injured casualties from the global war on terror: the Walter Reed Military Medical Center, the National Naval Medical Center, Brooke Army Medical Center, and the San Diego Naval Medical Center. The study will be conducted by reviewing casualty databases and then abstracting their medical records looking for extremity injuries that meet the criteria of a severely injured limb that might be a candidate for amputation. Interested subjects are then surveyed for a number of outcome measures. Outcome measures include

(1) Pain: Chronic Pain Grade scale
(2) Depression: Center for Epidemiologic Studies Depression Scale
(3) Posttraumatic Stress Disorder: Posttraumatic Stress Disorder Checklist
(4) Self-Efficacy: Modified Arthritis Self-Efficacy Scale
(5) Social Support: Multidimensional Perceived Social Support
(6) Quality of Life: Satisfaction of Life Scale
(7) Restriction in Activities and Participation: Short Form Musculoskeletal Function Assessment and the Paffenberger Physical Activity Questioner
(8) Return to Usual Activity: Standard questions
(9) Use and Satisfaction with Prosthesis/Prosthetist: Prosthetic Profile of the Amputee

This study will be the first of its kind to analyze this difficult problem in a purely military setting; however, the study will be limited by its retrospective nature (Fig. 1).

DISCUSSION OF FINDINGS AND RELEVANT LITERATURE

Recent studies have been performed and are in progress to look at the results of treatment with regard to treatment of severe extremity wounds with either limb salvage or amputation. Clinical advances have also been made in fixation modes, bone morphogenetic proteins (BMPs), dermal substitutes, amputation techniques, and prosthetics.

The first of the treatment comparison studies was the Lower Extremity Assessment Project (LEAP). In this study at both 2 and 7 years there was little difference between amputation or limb salvage with regard to the Sickness Impact Profile (SIP) or return to work rates; however, both groups had significant disability.[13] However, there were significant differences in the total cost to the health care system.[14]

The METALS study will be attempting to assess the same question in the military population in both the upper and lower extremities. The overall objectives of the study are to

(1) describe the long-term consequences of major limb trauma sustained by U.S. service

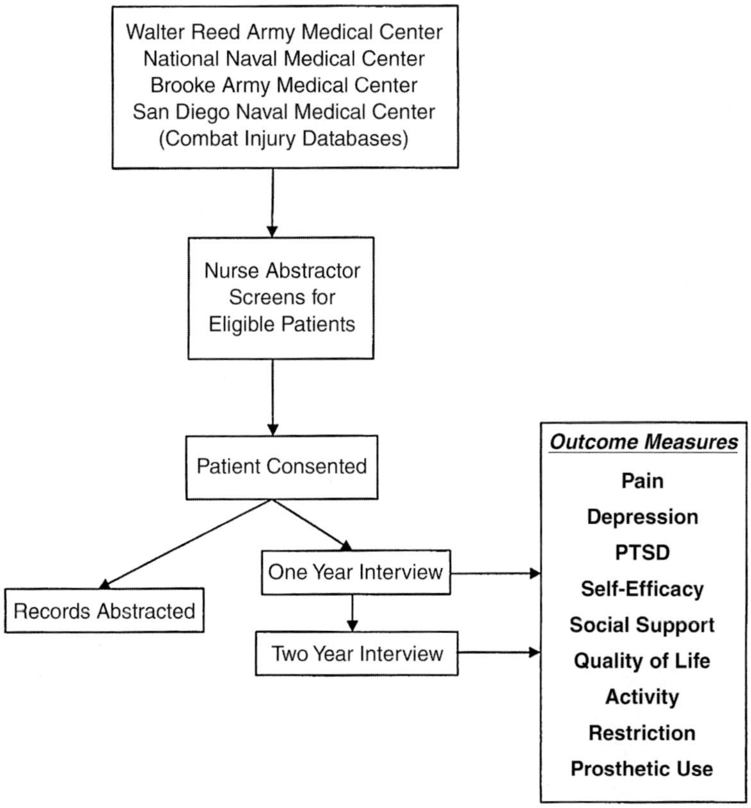

Figure 1. Military Extremity Trauma and Amputation/Limb Salvage (METALS).

members during the Global War on Terrorism;

(2) identify significant clinical, environmental, and patient characteristics that explain variations in secondary conditions, physical and psychosocial outcomes, and quality of life;

(3) determine differences in long-term outcomes for amputation versus limb salvage;

(4) identify unmet needs; and

(5) make recommendations for treatment adjustments.

Open explosion–related extremity trauma continues to present numerous challenges in management. The outside–in mechanism of tissue damage and contamination present unique obstacles not encountered in similar grade civilian extremity injuries. Several surgeons worldwide have adopted similar methods of treatment for these unique injuries.[1,15,16] Recently, circular external fixation has grown popular in treating combat-related fractures in mangled extremities. A study of 38 blast-related grade III tibial shaft fractures treated with a protocol-based approach to wound management followed by conversion of temporary monolateral external fixation to ring external fixation was recently published, and it showed good outcomes with this type of fixation.[17] Several benefits of this form of treatment for high-energy blast injuries were outlined, including minimal soft tissue handling, possible treatment of deep infection without implant removal, and immediate weight-bearing without hardware retention after fracture healing.

Another advancement in the treatment of severely injured extremities is in the use of BMPs. These proteins have shown to be effective in treating small bone defects as well as reducing the number of reoperations in tibia fractures and decreasing infection rates.[18] Military studies, however, have not shown the same promise.[17]

The treatment of complex soft tissue wounds with exposed structures is a difficult problem. The Integra dermal regeneration template (Integra Lifesciences, Plainsboro, NJ), initially developed in the late 1970s for the treatment of burn wounds,[19] has been utilized to cover these structures in preparation for skin grafting. Application of the material requires a wound bed that is free of devitalized tissue and infection. It requires

TAKE-HOME MESSAGE

Basic science advances

- Advances in stem cell research, BMPs, and dermal substitutes have markedly increased the tools available to the surgeon to use in the reconstruction of severely damaged limbs.
- Stem cells afford the potential of regeneration of several types of tissues within the body, particularly muscle, which currently is not able to be regenerated.
- BMPs are already in clinical use and greatly affect the bone's ability to heal.
- Dermal substitutes offer promise in the regeneration of skin tissue, providing a more durable and robust skin surface as compared to split-thickness skin grafting.

Clinical science advances

- The LEAP study gave us much important information as to the nature of these devastating injuries and the difficult nature of trying to predict which injury would benefit from limb salvage over amputation.
- The METALS study should be able to provide similar data in a military-specific population. By looking at many outcomes based measures, the potential exists to know which injuries are best served with limb salvage over amputation. This will afford the surgeon and patient the best information as to which course of treatment to choose. It will also potentially identify what more can be done for these devastating injuries.
- Advances in BMP use in the healing of fractures have shown to be associated with decreased infections and increased healing potential. Circular external fixation in the military blast injury has shown excellent healing rates with low infection rates.
- Dermal substitutes have clinically been used to provide a thicker skin tissue than split-thickness skin grafting alone.
- Amputation and prosthetic care advances in the areas of new surgical techniques and understanding of maintaining amputation length improve the patient care if the limb cannot be salvaged.

Relevance to clinical care

- The METALS study has the potential to lend insight to when limb salvage is optimal to amputation. If a relative set of injuries or a constellation of patient parameters can be identified that show which patients benefit from limb salvage over amputation, it will be much easier to educate and counsel patients with regard to which option would be best for them. Although this is the goal of the study, results are still pending and it may follow the same fate as the LEAP study, which was not able to demonstrate a statistical difference for limb salvage versus reconstruction with regard to SIPS or return to work rates. However, the LEAP study was able to identify some characteristics of those patients with higher sickness impact profiles scores and that the outcomes of both the amputee and limb salvage groups deteriorated over time. It also confirmed that there were more complications with the reconstruction group, as well as showing that patient satisfaction was driven by the final resultant function, pain, and depression.[26]

fenestration of the silicone covering of the bilayer material, placement, attachment of the edges, and coverage with a negative pressure dressing. After 7 to 21 days, changing the dressing every 3 to 5 days, a split-thickness skin graft is applied.[20]

In the event that extremity salvage fails, or the patient does not want to undergo a protracted salvage course, amputation should be considered. This can occur at any time in the treatment process either acutely or after a course of attempted salvage. Amputation surgery should be viewed by patient and surgeon as the next step toward reconstructive recovery. Surgically removing diseased and nonfunctional distal extremity tissues and fashioning a competent and painless residual limb for ambulation is the ultimate goal, although this goal is not uniformly obtained.[21] Transtibial and transfemoral amputation have become the most commonly performed amputation levels for trauma above and below the knee, respectively, at the U.S. military treatment centers. Blast-related traumatic amputation presents several challenges and competing priorities. Maintenance of length and joint function is critical. However, amputation closure within the zone of injury approaches a 67% wound complication rate.[22] Additionally, approximately 63% of blast-related amputations are complicated by the formation of heterotopic ossification, which is most closely correlated with closure through the zone of injury.[23] In addition to obtaining uncomplicated wound closure, optimizing functional outcome is paramount. For transtibial amputation, bone bridge synostosis seems to offer several benefits to optimize functional prosthetic use.[24] Similarly, transfemoral amputation length should be maximized and an adequate adductor myodesis performed to maximize functional outcome.[25]

CAUTION, CRITICAL REMARKS, AND RECOMMENDATIONS

Although the METALS study will potentially identify patients who will benefit from specific treatment alternatives, it is important to remember that it is a retrospective study and nonrandomized. At this point there are no clear recommendations for amputation over limb salvage. Stratifying injuries is also very difficult; for example, not all type III B tibia fractures (open fracture with need for soft tissue coverage) are the same. The amount of skin loss, muscle loss, neurovascular function, and bone loss all play an important role in determining the likely resultant function in a reconstructed extremity. It is also important to recognize that every patient is different and that appropriate treatment for identical injuries in two different patients may not be the same. A patient with goals of high function and activity may choose an amputation, whereas a patient with low functional demands may prefer to keep his extremity and avoid some of the complications of prosthetic wear. At this point it is strongly recommended that every patient be treated individually and counseled about their injury giving the best information available on the benefits and downsides to each treatment option.

FUTURE DEVELOPMENT

Many offshoots of the METALS study are being investigated. One such funded study looking at the results of open tibia fractures is already underway and will attempt to look at the same parameters that are being investigated in the METALS study. The goal of this study is to look at the individual parameters of the leg and see if any are associated with worse outcomes both in patient satisfaction and ability to heal the fractures. Other studies are also being planned to look at other significant extremity injuries to see if specific factors contribute to outcome. The knowledge of these specific factors will better allow military surgeons to more fully educate their patients. Another exciting area is the potential for stem cells basic science research to translate into clinical practice where normally discarded tissue can be utilized to harvest stem cells from and regenerate tissue that can be utilized in difficult reconstructions.

AUTHOR DISCLOSURE STATEMENT

R.C.A.: TRUE Research Foundation—Travel Support
Orthopaedic Trauma Research Program: Funded Grant
Military Amputee Research Program: Funded Grant
S.B.S.: TRUE Research Foundation—Travel Support
J.J.K.: TRUE Research Foundation—Travel Support
Orthopaedic Trauma Research Program: Funded Grant
Military Amputee Research Program: Funded Grant
R.V.O.: DePuy, KCI, Synthes, Stryker, Smith & Nephew—Research Support Synthes—Consultant

REFERENCES

1. Andersen RC, Frisch HM, Farber GL, and Hayda RA: Definitive treatment of combat casualties at military medical centers. J Am Acad Orthop Surg 2006; **14:** S24.

2. McGuigan FX, Forsberg JA, and Andersen RC: Foot and ankle reconstruction after blast injuries. Foot Ankle Clin 2006; **11:** 165.

3. Hansen ST Jr.: The type-IIIC tibial fracture. Salvage or amputation. J Bone Joint Surg Am 1987; **69:** 799.

4. Rödl R, Pohlmann U, Gosheger G, Hoffmann C, Leidinger B, Lindner N, and Winkelmann W: Ablative and extremity salvage tumor surgery of the lower extremity—a 10 year comparison. Z Orthop Ihre Grenzgeb 2001; **139:** 183.

5. War Surgery in Afghanistan and Iraq, A Series of Cases 2003–2007: Office of the Surgeon General, Borden Institute, Washington, DC, 2008, pp. 31–32.

6. Jones AL, Bucholz RW, Bosse MJ, Mirza SK, Lyon TR, Webb LX, Pollak AN, Golden JD, and Valentin-Opran A; BMP-2 Evaluation in Surgery for Tibial Trauma-Allograft (BESTT-ALL) Study Group: Recombinant human BMP-2 and allograft compared with autogenous bone graft for reconstruction of diaphyseal tibial fractures with cortical defects. A randomized, controlled trial. J Bone Joint Surg Am 2006; **88:** 1431.

7. El-Gammal TA, Shiha AE, El-Deen MA, El-Sayed A, Kotb MM, Addosooki AI, Ragheb YF, and Saleh WR: Management of traumatic tibial defects using free vascularized fibula or Ilizarov bone transport: a comparative study. Microsurgery 2008; **28:** 339.

8. MacKenzie EJ, Bosse MJ, Kellam JF, Burgess AR, Webb LX, Swiontkowski MF, Sanders RW, Jones AL, McAndrew MP, Patterson TM, and McCarthy ML: Characterization of patients with high-energy lower extremity trauma. J Orthop Trauma 2000; **14:** 455.

9. Slater BJ, Kwan MD, Gupta DM, Panetta NJ, and Longaker MT: Mesenchymal cells for skeletal tissue engineering. Expert Opin Biol Ther 2008; **8:** 885.

10. Fu X and Li H: Mesenchymal stem cells and skin wound repair and regeneration: possibilities and questions. Cell Tissue Res 2009; **335:** 317.

11. Nesti LJ, Jackson WM, Shanti RM, Koehler SM, Aragon AB, Bailey JR, Sracic MK, Freedman BA, Giuliani JR, and Tuan RS: Differentiation potential of multipotent progenitor cells derived from war-traumatized muscle tissue. J Bone Joint Surg Am 2008; **90:** 2390.

12. Jackson WM, Aragon AB, Djouad F, Song Y, Koehler SM, Nesti LJ, and Tuan RS: Mesenchymal progenitor cells derived from traumatized human muscle. J Tissue Eng Regen Med 2009; **3:** 129.

13. Bosse MJ, MacKenzie EJ, Kellam JF, Burgess AR, Webb LX, Swiontkowski MF, Sanders RW, Jones AL, McAndrew MP, Patterson BM, McCarthy ML, Travison TG, and Castillo RC: An analysis of outcomes of reconstruction or amputation after leg-threatening injuries. N Engl J Med 2002; **347:** 1924.

14. MacKenzie EJ, Jones AS, Bosse MJ, Castillo RC, Pollak AN, Webb LX, Swiontkowski MF, Kellam JF, Smith DG, Sanders RW, Jones AL, Starr AJ, McAndrew MP, Patterson BM, and Burgess AR: Health-care costs associated with amputation or reconstruction of a limb-threatening injury. J Bone Joint Surg Am 2007; **89:** 1685.

15. Johnson EN, Burns TC, Hayda RA, Hospenthal DR, and Murray CK: Infectious complications of open type III tibial fractures among combat casualties. Clin Infect Dis 2007; **45:** 409.

16. Zeljko B, Lovrc Z, Amc E, Busic V, Lovrc L, and Markovc I: War injuries of the extremities: twelve-year follow-up data. Mil Med 2006; **171:** 55.

17. Keeling JJ, Gwinn DE, Tintle SM, Andersen RC, and McGuigan FX: Short-term outcomes of severe open wartime tibial fractures treated with ring external fixation. J Bone Joint Surg Am 2008; **90:** 2643.

18. Govender S, Csimma C, Genant HK, Valentin-Opran A, Amit Y, Arbel R, Aro H, Atar D, Bishay M, Börner MG, Chiron P, Choong P, Cinats J, Courtenay B, Feibel R, Geulette B, Gravel C, Haas N, Raschke M, Hammacher E, van der Velde D, Hardy P, Holt M, Josten C, Ketterl RL, Lindeque B, Lob G, Mathevon H, McCoy G, Marsh D, Miller R, Munting E, Oevre S, Nordsletten L, Patel A, Pohl A, Rennie W, Reynders P, Rommens PM, Rondia J, Rossouw WC, Daneel PJ, Ruff S, Rüter A, Santavirta S, Schildhauer TA, Gekle C, Schnettler R, Segal D, Seiler H, Snowdowne RB, Stapert J, Taglang G, Verdonk R, Vogels L, Weckbach A, Wentzensen A, and Wisniewski T; BMP-2 Evaluation in Surgery for Tibial Trauma (BESTT) Study Group: Recombinant human bone morphogenetic protein-2 for treatment of open tibial fractures: a prospective, controlled, randomized study of four hundred and fifty patients. J Bone Joint Surg Am 2002; **84-A:** 2123.

19. Burke JF, Yannas IV, Quinby WC Jr., Bondoc CC, and Jung WK: Successful use of a physiologically acceptable artificial skin in the treatment of extensive burn injury. Ann Surg 1981; **194:** 413.

20. Helgeson MD, Potter BK, Evans KN, and Shawen SB: Bioartificial dermal substitute: a preliminary report on its use for the management of complex combat-related soft tissue wounds. J Orthop Trauma 2007; **21:** 394.

21. MacKenzie EJ, Bosse MJ, Pollak AN, Webb LX, Swiontkowski MF, Kellam JF, Smith DG, Sanders RW, Jones AL, Starr AJ, McAndrew MP, Patterson BM, Burgess AR, and Castillo RC: Long-term persistence of disability following severe lower-limb trauma. Results of a seven-year follow-up. J Bone Joint Surg Am 2005; **87:** 1801.

22. Gwinn DE, Keeling JJ, Froehner JA, McGuigan FX, and Andersen RC: Perioperative Differences Between Bone Bridging and Non-bone Bridging Transtibial Amputations for Wartime Lower Extremity Trauma. Foot Ankle Int 2008; **29:** 787.

23. Potter BK, Burns TC, Lacap AP, Granville RR, and Gajewski DA: Heterotopic ossification following traumatic and combat-related amputations. Prevalence, risk factors, and preliminary results of excision. J Bone Joint Surg Am 2007; **89:** 476.

24. Keeling JJ and Schon LC: Tibiofibular bridge synostosis in below knee amputation. Tech Foot Ankle Surg 2007; **6:** 156.

25. Pickard-Gabriel CJ, Ledford CL, Gajewski DA, Granville RR, and Andersen RC: Traumatic transfemoral amputation with concomitant ipsilateral proximal femoral fracture. A report of two cases. J Bone Joint Surg Am 2007; **89:** 2764.

26. O'Toole RV, Castillo RC, Pollak AN, MacKenzie EJ, and Bosse MJ; LEAP Study Group. Determinants of patient satisfaction after severe lower-extremity injuries. J Bone Joint Surg Am 2008; **90:** 1206.

WHS Wound Healing Society

Advances in Amputee Care

Kevin F. Fitzpatrick,[1,*] Paul F. Pasquina,[2,3] and Charles Scoville[4]

[1]*Physical Medicine and Rehabilitation, Walter Reed Army Medical Center, Washington, District of Columbia.*
[2]*Integrated Department of Orthopaedics and Rehabilitation, Walter Reed Army Medical Center, Washington, District of Columbia.*
[3]*National Naval Medical Center, Bethesda, Maryland.*
[4]*Amputee Care Program, Walter Reed Army Medical Center, Washington, District of Columbia.*

Background: Recent military conflicts have resulted in a relatively high number of young, previously healthy traumatic amputees. This has provided the setting to explore recent advances in the field of amputee care.
The Problem: Major limb amputation results in a significant loss of functional abilities. It is the responsibility of the rehabilitation team to maximize the postamputation function of these patients by providing a comprehensive approach to rehabilitation. This requires the integration of a multidisciplinary team.
Basic/Clinical Science Advances: Recent advances in several fields have the potential to change functional outcomes in traumatic amputees. The development of interdisciplinary centers in which comprehensive amputee care can be performed provides an efficient model for the delivery of care. The utilization of a sports medicine model of physical therapy is a recent development that may improve the method in which rehabilitation is performed. Finally, surgical advances include targeted reinnervation to improve the control of an upper limb prosthesis and osseointegration to improve the limb/prosthesis interface. Advances in the design of prostheses, such as microprocessor-controlled knees and externally powered knees, have shown promise in improving the functional abilities of amputees.
Clinical Care Relevance: These advances may prove to be beneficial and improve functional outcome in the full spectrum of amputee patients.
Conclusion: Ongoing developments in amputee care provide continuing improvement to the rehabilitation and functional outcomes of amputees.

Abbreviations and Acronyms

EMG = electromyography
HO = heterotopic ossification
TBI = traumatic brain injury

*Correspondence: Physical Medicine and Rehabilitation, Walter Reed Army Medical Center, 6900 Georgia Ave., Washington, District of Columbia 20307; e-mail: kevin.f.fitzpatrick@us.army.mil

BACKGROUND

As of January 2009, military operations in support of the global war on terrorism have resulted in the loss of life of more than 4,000 U.S. service members. Additionally, over 30,000 soldiers, sailors, airmen, and marines have been injured, including over 850 service members whose injuries resulted in major limb loss.

Advances in body armor, improved medical evacuation techniques, and state-of-the-art surgical resuscitation have contributed greatly to the increased survival rates of catastrophic injuries sustained in Iraq and Afghanistan.[1,2] Despite these improvements, however, the overall rates of amputations observed in the current conflicts have not significantly changed from that reported in previous wars. While the exact reasons for this have not been fully elucidated, it is theorized that surgical advances in treating catastrophic limb injuries have led to the ability to preserve limbs that in prior conflicts would have required amputation.

Printed in U.S.A.
DOI: 10.1089/awc.2009.0023

CLINICAL PROBLEM ADDRESSED

Military amputees represent a much different patient population than those seen in the civilian community. Most civilian amputations occur as the result of disease (diabetes and vascular disease), compared to the type and magnitude of trauma sustained by military service members. Additionally, more than 85% of the amputations from the current conflicts have occurred in patients under 35 years, in contrast to the civilian population, where 81% of the amputations are in patients older than 44 years.[3] These factors contribute to unique challenges encountered in the rehabilitation of the combat amputee. Issues such as complex soft-tissue wounds, associated comorbid injuries (traumatic brain injury [TBI], infection, nerve injury), complicated pain syndromes, and psychosocial stressors, including posttraumatic stress disorder, all require individualized attention in a unified rehabilitation plan. In addition, the premorbid high activity level of this patient population contributes greatly to their expectation to return to the highest level of functioning. For many, this means returning to full military operations.

Maximizing functional outcomes in this unique patient population requires the integration of management strategies for myriad medical and surgical complications; unique psychosocial factors; and expectations of the patient, family, government, and society. Because of the relatively high numbers of young, previously healthy amputees that have been treated in the military healthcare system in recent years, we have been afforded the opportunity to explore recent advances in amputee care.

RELEVANT BASIC SCIENCE CONTEXT

Despite the fact that major limb loss has been prevalent with every major military conflict in the history of our nation, relatively few advances have been made in the basic science principles underlying amputate care. One notable exception is in the treatment of heterotopic ossification (HO) following limb loss. Early studies on the prevalence of HO in traumatic amputations from the current conflicts have revealed high rates in our patient population.[4] Further research is necessary to examine the pathophysiology and etiology of HO formation, prophylactic regimens, and appropriate timing of surgical excision.

Additionally, there have been significant advances made in material designs of prosthetic components. Lighter weight carbon fiber materials, aluminum, and titanium alloys have allowed the fabrication of much more dynamic and responsive prostheses. The invention of silicon has contributed to more comfortable limb–prosthetic interfaces and microprocessor technology allows more intelligent prostheses that better approximate normal gait.

EXPERIMENTAL MODEL OR MATERIAL—ADVANTAGES AND LIMITATIONS

Many technological advances related to amputee care have recently been developed, including novel surgical techniques, creative rehabilitation strategies, and high-tech prosthetic components. Despite this, there is a paucity of clinical studies demonstrating the effectiveness of these advances in terms of improving overall functional outcomes. Moreover, there are very few studies comparing one prosthetic component with another on the same patient. Complicating this problem are the inherent problems with conducting research related to rehabilitation, given the numerous variables that influence outcomes that are nearly impossible to control for. Additionally, as prosthetic companies continue to fabricate and market new devices, it is hard to conduct a study that will not be outdated by the time it is published. Despite these challenges, professionals involved in the care of individuals with amputation are obligated to track and critically examine functional outcomes. With advances in technology, this will hopefully become more standard practice within the field.

DISCUSSION OF FINDINGS AND RELEVANT LITERATURE

Interdisciplinary centers of excellence

In the military healthcare system, Amputee Centers of Excellence have been developed at military treatment facilities throughout the continental United States. The development of these centers has allowed a wide range of specialists and subspecialists with expertise in treating patients with traumatic amputations to share experiences and collaborate to form more integrated care plans for even the most complex of patients. Specialists in physical and occupational therapy, prosthetics, orthopedic surgery, physical medicine and rehabilitation, nursing, pain management, mental health, and social work, have all been critical to the expert care of combat amputees within these centers. The development of these centers has been vital to successful rehabilitation and reintegration of injured military service members after a traumatic amputation. In addition to providing experience and developing clinical skills among providers, these centers have also improved access of patients to a full range of specialists, advanced equipment, and a therapeutic milieu of fellow soldiers, sailors, airmen, and marines confronting similar challenges together.

Advances in therapy strategies

The recent adoption of a Sports Medicine Model for guiding the physical and occupational therapy of military amputees has changed the paradigm in approach to amputee rehabilitation. In this model, the "team physician" is represented by the physiatrist who has oversight of the entire medical treatment plan, while the "coach" is represented by physical and occupational therapists who provide immediate assessment, correction, and progression through daily activities. To take the model even further, the multidisciplinary center represents the team training facility, and each patient is a member of the team, experiencing similar wins and losses, but functioning better united with those around them rather than isolated as an individual. This model also emphasizes preventing the effects of deconditioning, maintaining ideal body weight, improving fitness, and vigilant monitoring of medical complications and psychosocial factors that may be detrimental to full recovery. Specific to amputee rehabilitation, the Sports Medicine Model includes the early use of closed-kinetic chain exercises, emphasizing co-contraction of muscle groups that have been found to resemble the functional use of a prosthesis, as well as a focus on ergonomics, proper biomechanics, strengthening and stretching of remaining limbs, and core stabilization exercises. This approach strives for "maximal" functional recovery and is not satisfied with basic mobility, but challenging patients to achieve their best. At the core of this program is goal setting and creating a therapeutic environment to support and help motivate each individual's recovery and reintegration.

Advances in surgical techniques

The surgical management of complex extremity war wounds often involves the participation of multiple subspecialists over a protracted time course. Advanced techniques in the application of external fixation devices, muscle and soft-tissue flaps and grafts, along with vascular and nerve reconstructive techniques have contributed to the ability to preserve limbs and vital length that would not have been possible during earlier wars. Because of the "dirty" nature of these wounds and the extensive soft-tissue damage caused by blast injuries, definitive amputation and wound closure is often not performed until weeks after the injury. This allows for the rehabilitation team, including the surgeon, prosthetist, patient, and family to participate in the decision for optimizing residual limb length.

Despite the advances that have occurred in surgical reconstructive techniques, the basic elements of myodesis, myoplasty, and muscle balancing within the residual limb remain largely dependent on the empirical experience of the operating surgeon. There is evidence, however, that specific surgical techniques that focus on the primary use of myodesis for the attachment of the adductors magnus to the femur to promote preservation of muscle balance between thigh abductors and adductors may improve limb control and stability and increase ambulatory functioning in transfemoral amputees.[5] Clearly more research is needed in this area.

While not necessarily a recent innovation, the Ertl procedure warrants discussion as a surgical technique that is frequently considered and may be gaining popularity. Originally described in 1949, this technique includes, among other specifications, the surgical placement of a bony bridge between the distal ends of the tibia and fibula and the construction of a bony cap that is placed over the distal amputated ends of the tibia and fibula.[6] The theoretical benefits of the procedure include the ability for weight bearing on the distal end of the residual limb, decreased "scissoring" or relative movement of the tibia and fibula, and the prevention of terminal overgrowth of the tibia and fibula. Potential drawbacks of the procedure include an increased amount of time between surgical amputation and weight bearing to allow for healing and maturation of the bony bridge. Anecdotal reports suggest that the Ertl procedure is effective in reducing pain and providing increased function in transtibial amputees. While we have not observed any significant differences in our military population, controlled trials involving the comparison of functional outcomes of the Ertl procedure with traditional surgical techniques are warranted. In general, however, most practitioners consider the Ertl procedure to be reserved for stabilization of the tibia and fibula in the face of instability and pain. It is not often utilized during the primary amputation procedure and potentially contraindicated in the event of extensive trauma in the zone of injury and if significant risk exists for HO formation.

A more recent advancement in the surgical management of upper limb amputees, currently being explored, is "targeted muscle reinnervation." Targeted reinnervation involves the transfer of amputated nerves to intact motor nerves that supply muscles that are no longer functional. The result of this surgical procedure is that the reinnervated muscles will contract in response to voluntary activation of the nerves that have been amputated to create a more "natural" control. For example, in a transhumeral amputation, the amputated median nerve may be transferred to a portion of the biceps muscle, so when the patient thinks to "close hand," the median nerve signal will be transferred to the biceps and the surface electromyography (EMG) recording can be translated to terminal device hand closure. Similarly, the musculocutaneous nerve may be transferred to the pectoralis muscle in a patient with a shoulder disarticulation to activate pectoralis contraction to signal prosthetic elbow flexion. The result is that native neurological pathways that previously controlled a particular movement can now be utilized to control the same movement in a prosthetic limb. This would be expected to result in a control system for the prosthetic device that is extremely intuitive and may provide function that is superior to systems currently available today.[7–9] At present, targeted reinnervation has been used only in a very small number of carefully selected patients in controlled settings. Additionally, prosthetic devices that are capable of utilizing these control strategies are currently not commercially available. Early case reports, however, seem to indicate promising results.[8] The technique involves relatively little risk to the transhumeral amputee—no intact function is lost, no implanted devices are necessary, and the procedure does not preclude the use of traditional prosthetic devices. For these reasons, we feel that targeted reinnervation may have a dramatic impact on the design of upper limb prosthetic devices in the future.

Another surgical technique that has recently received greater attention is "osseointegration"—the direct skeletal attachment of a prosthesis to the residual limb bone. Advancement in this area would likely revolutionize prosthetic fitting and eliminate the inherent challenges encountered with today's socket designs. While many advances have been made in socket design and fabrication (computer-aided design, lighter and more flexible materials, and novel suction and silicone sleeve suspension systems), one of the most important and challenging aspects of amputee rehabilitation is the effectiveness of the prosthesis–limb interface. The shape and size of a residual limb are dynamic variables. Due to fluid shifts, changes in muscle mass, and changes in body habitus, these variables are constantly changing. This makes designing a socket-suspension system that is perfectly fitted to a residual limb extremely challenging. A poor socket fit can have a dramatic negative impact, leading to increased pain, skin breakdown, and decreased acceptance of the prosthesis. Osseointegration attempts to solve these problems by attaching a prosthesis directly to bone through a bone-implanted abutment that penetrates the patient's skin. While osseointegration seems to have significant potential, it is currently limited by the risk of contamination and infection. Because the device is exposed to the environment and also attached to the bone, the risk of bacteria or other contaminants being transferred to bone is significant. Until an improved method for sealing the skin to the device that reliably prevents infection is developed, osseointegration will not be practical for routine use.[10] However, if the seal can be perfected, this technique may dramatically change the way that prosthetic systems are designed and constructed. Another significant limitation in the current approaches to osseointegration is the protracted time course with this phased surgery over months and nearly 1 year rehabilitation period.

TAKE-HOME MESSAGE

Clinical science advances

- An interdisciplinary center of excellence design has been found to be an efficient and effective method of delivering care to combat-related traumatic amputees.
- A Sports Medicine Model of amputee rehabilitation may improve the quality of care and short- and long-term outcomes.
- Advances in surgical management have the potential to improve functional outcomes, prevent complications, and improve quality of life.
- Technological advances in prosthetic design will likely have a revolutionary impact on future amputee care.

Relevance to clinical care

- These new advances provide important new strategies for caring for amputees and have the potential to change the way the amputee rehabilitation is accomplished.

Advances in prosthetic design

Recent technological developments applied to the design of prosthetic devices have resulted in a vast array of options for the amputee. Perhaps the most significant advances have occurred in the design of knee components for transfemoral amputees and control systems for upper limb amputees. The development of microprocessor-controlled knees allows for a more responsive variable cadence gait, reduced energy consumptions, and improved stability. Our experience has also shown that microprocessor-controlled knees are an excellent option for early ambulation training following a transfemoral amputation and may be beneficial for elderly amputees with limited options for prosthetic knees. Even more recently, prototypes of externally powered knee and ankle components have been developed. These components provide active knee and ankle motion through an externally powered motor. Currently, externally powered prosthetic joints add a significant amount of weight to a prosthetic device that may result in skin breakdown and increased energy expenditure associated with ambulation. If these issues can be addressed with technological advancements, the introduction of "powered" prostheses will likely dramatically reduce the energy consumption needed for amputee ambulation and significantly improve outcomes. Because these advanced technologies are not appropriate for every amputee, a team approach to the development of prosthetic prescriptions must be implemented to ensure that amputees are carefully selected to receive appropriate prescriptions and components.

Myoelectric-controlled upper limb prostheses continue to improve and have gained increased acceptance in the rehabilitation of upper limb amputees. Myoelectric prostheses are controlled by surface EMG recordings over intact muscles. This input is used to control the movement of externally powered prosthetic components. Newer components allow better response times, more robust mechanics, and the ability to simultaneously control elbow and terminal devices. While myoelectric prostheses offer the advantage of reducing the need for straps and cables, their increased weight and mechanical vulnerability still limit their universal acceptance. For combat amputees with complex upper limb residual wounds, we have found that myoelectric prosthetic training can commence earlier than body-powered prosthetic fitting, and therefore may promote long-term acceptance and improved bimanual activities.

SUMMARY

A summary of recent advances in the field of amputee care.

Administrative advances

- Development of Interdisciplinary Centers of Excellence

Surgical advances

- Ertl procedure
- Targeted reinnervation
- Osseointegration

Advances in therapy techniques

- Development of the Sports Medicine Model of Rehabilitation

Advances in prosthetic design

- Microprocessor-controlled knees
- Externally powered knees and ankles
- Myoelectric upper limb prostheses

CAUTION, CRITICAL REMARKS, AND RECOMMENDATIONS

As noted above, a variety of advances in multiple fields relating to the treatment and rehabilitation of amputees have the potential to change the way the amputee rehabilitation is accomplished. Further clinical studies are necessary to determine the efficacy of each of these treatment methods, compare different treatment options, and determine their impact on functional outcomes.

FUTURE DEVELOPMENT

Amputee rehabilitation is an evolving field of medicine involving numerous healthcare subspecialists, scientists, and engineers. As technology improves, new surgical techniques are explored, and novel treatment paradigms are developed; they will need to be transitioned into clinical practice and integrated into the holistic care of individuals with limb loss. It is important that each new development be critically examined, compared to similar options, and evaluated based on their contribution to functional outcomes in this patient population. Further, it is clear that the Department of Defense should take the lead in addressing the unique challenges faced by service members with amputation.

AUTHOR DISCLOSURE STATEMENT

No competing financial interests exist.

REFERENCES

1. Holcomb JB, Stansbury LG, Champion HR, Wade C, and Bellamy RF: Understanding combat casualty care statistics. J Trauma Inj Infect Crit Care 2006; **60:** 397.
2. Gawande A: Casualties of war: military care for the wounded from Iraq and Afghanistan. N Engl J Med 2004; **351:** 2471.
3. Ziegler-Graham K, MacKenzie EJ, Ephraim PL, Travison TG, and Brookmeyer R: Estimating the prevalence of limb loss in the United States: 2005 to 2050. Arch Phys Med Rehabil 2008; **89:** 422.
4. Potter BK, *et al.*: Heterotopic ossification in the residual limbs of traumatic and combat-related amputees. J Am Acad Orthop Surg 2006; **14:** S191.
5. Pinzur MS, *et al.*: Controversies in lower-extremity amputation. J Bone Joint Surg Am 2007; **89A:** 1118.
6. Drvaric DM, and Kruger LM: Modified Ertl osteomyoplasty for terminal overgrowth in childhood limb deficiencies. J Pediatr Orthop 2001; **21:** 392.
7. Miller LA, *et al.*: Control of a six degree of freedom prosthetic arm after targeted muscle reinnervation surgery. Arch Phys Med Rehabil 2008; **89:** 2057.
8. O'Shaughnesy KD, *et al.*: Targeted reinnervation to improve prosthesis control in transhumeral amputees. J Bone Joint Surg Am 2008; **90:** 393.
9. Hijjawi JB, *et al.*: Improved myoelectric prosthesis control accomplished using multiple nerve transfers. Plast Reconstr Surg 2006; **118:** 1573.
10. Aaron RK, *et al.*: Horizons in prosthesis development for the restoration of limb function. J Acad Orthop Surg 2006; **14:** S198.

Plastic Surgery Challenges in War Wounded

Anand R. Kumar,[1,2,*] Raymond Harshbarger,[1,3] and Barry Martin[1,3]

[1]Department of Surgery (Plastic Surgery), Uniformed Services University of the Health Sciences (USUHS), Bethesda, Maryland.
[2]Department of Plastic and Reconstructive Surgery, National Naval Medical Center (NNMC), Bethesda, Maryland.
[3]Department of Plastic and Reconstructive Surgery, Walter Reed Army Medical Center (WRAMC), Washington, District of Columbia.

Background: Military treatment facilities continue to treat injured personnel supporting the Global War on Terrorism. Optimal reconstruction of massive soft tissue and bone defects of the extremities and craniofacial skeleton secondary to high-energy wounding mechanisms remain poorly characterized.
The Problem: The ideal method to care for these injuries has continued to evolve and has yet to be completely defined. Effects of high-energy blast trauma on tissues, and the unusual bacteria (*Acinetobacter baumanii*) existing within the wounds, characterize these unique military wounds. Despite the relatively quick triage time, definitive care is delayed, and multiple concomitant injuries exist per patient.
Basic/Clinical Science Advances: In addition to practicing established concepts from prior military conflicts, new technology for the advancement of trauma care has been applied. Treatment with novel flap reconstructions, distraction osteogenesis, bone grafting, and bone-engineering techniques including use of bone morphogenetic protein-2 has led to improved outcomes.
Clinical Care Relevance: Modern battlefield care in conjunction with treatment protocols at continental United States Military Treatment Facilities has resulted in improved limb and craniofacial reconstruction.
Conclusion: Successful limb salvage and craniofacial reconstruction can be accomplished in the subacute period using treatment protocols, which incorporate the use of novel flaps, fixation devices, and bone-engineering techniques.

Abbreviation and Acronym

IED = improvised explosive device

*Correspondence: Department of Plastic and Reconstructive Surgery, National Naval Medical Center, 8901 Wisconsin Ave., Bethesda, Maryland 20889-5000 (e-mail: arkumar@mac.com).

BACKGROUND

Military treatment facilities continue to treat injured personnel supporting the Global War on Terrorism. Optimal reconstruction of massive soft tissue and bone defects of the extremities and craniofacial skeleton secondary to high-energy wounding mechanisms remain poorly described. The optimal care of these injuries has yet to be defined. Wounds from modern high-energy blast trauma mechanisms are unique. Blast trauma wounds are characterized by severe composite tissue damage, large zones of injury, extensive devitalization, significant foreign body loading, and nearly ubiquitous bacterial colonization with *Acinetobacter Baumanii* (a significant pathogen from Iraq). Despite advances in triage, and access to critical care far forward in the battlefield, definitive care can be delayed. Once stateside, delivery of reconstructive care is often complicated by the multiple concomitant injuries that exist per patient, and prolonged ICU stays. Major civilian principles of early radical debridement, fixation of fractures with bone grafting, and wound coverage with vascularized tissue are followed

Printed in U.S.A.
DOI: 10.1089/awc.2009.0087

when possible. Given the complexity and multiplicity of these blast wounds, along with extensive concomitant injuries, early closure of wounds and fracture fixation can be difficult to achieve. In many cases the subacute (3 weeks after injury) period has been the most appropriate time for definitive wound treatment. The application of traditional wound and fracture treatment techniques along with introduction of novel approaches has met with early success in these difficult military wounds.

CLINICAL PROBLEM ADDRESSED

Evidence in the civilian trauma literature indicates that early wound coverage provides better outcomes and that subacute reconstruction is plagued with high complication rates.[1–12] Conversely, war extremity wounds have been reconstructed in the subacute time period.[13–15] This variation in the treatment algorithm is necessary due to temporal evacuation factors, large zones of injury, complex desert microflora in battlefield wounds, and multiple concurrent injuries.[13–15]

BASIC SCIENCE CONTEXT

Injured soldiers are treated using evolving protocols developed over the course of the Iraq/Afghanistan conflicts. Extremity-injured patients are initially treated with serial debridement until the wounds appear clinically clean with viable tissue. Between operative wound evaluations, negative pressure dressing therapy was applied to the wounded extremity. Uni-planar external fixation for extremity fractures is placed far forward in the theatre of operation and modified as necessary at the Level V (definitive stateside) military treatment facility.[16] Wounds are then accessed for primary closure, skin grafting, and/or flap reconstruction as indicated. At the time of flap inset, bone defects are filled with OSTEOSET® (Wright Medical Technology, Arlington, TN), antibiotic beads, and INFUSE® Bone Graft (Medtronic, Minneapolis, MN) as indicated in extremity reconstruction. After extremity flap reconstruction, patients are converted within 2 weeks to multiplanar weight-bearing external frames (Taylor Spatial Frame).

Cranial defects are reconstructed in a delayed fashion when necessary, allowing for cerebral edema to resolve. Facial fractures are treated with internal fixation and supplemental bone grafting as indicated and as early as possible. Subsequently, all patients underwent early rehabilitation regaining ambulatory status with functional ability expected for their injuries and preexisting conditions. Intensive traumatic brain injury rehabilitation remains a critical adjunct to the patients' overall physical and mental restoration.

EXPERIMENTAL MODEL OR MATERIAL

Craniofacial reconstruction

Blast trauma with high-energy transfer to the cranial vault has necessitated decompressive craniectomy, a life-saving maneuver performed far forward in the theater of war. Patients once considered expectant have now been aggressively treated and have survived devastating neurologic trauma. Patients surviving a decompressive craniectomy after military blast trauma represent a diverse and unique population that has been poorly studied[17] (Fig. 1). This group of patients ultimately requires reconstruction of the cranial defect not only for brain protection and cosmetic restoration of the calvarium but also for correction of the syndrome of the trephined (dizziness, fatigability, vague discomfort at the site of the defect, mental depression, apprehension and insecurity, and intolerance to vibration). Currently, there are gaps in the literature detailing the incidence, natural history, and appropriate treatment of this unique population of patients.[18–20]

Operation Iraqi/Enduring Freedom has resulted in the largest concentration of penetrating head trauma since the Vietnam War. Due to severe impairment of tissue perfusion and heavy wound contamination at the time of initial injury, reconstruction is often delayed for 6 to 12 months. In the presence of soft-tissue deficiencies, either acute or chronic, calvarial reconstruction is delayed. Soft-tissue reconstruction using tissue expansion or free

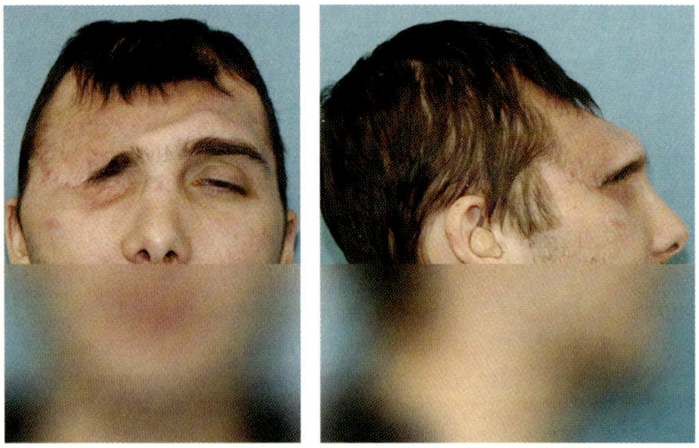

Figure 1. Soldier 5 months post-IED (improvised explosive device) blast injury with loss of right frontal, temporal, and supra orbital bone.

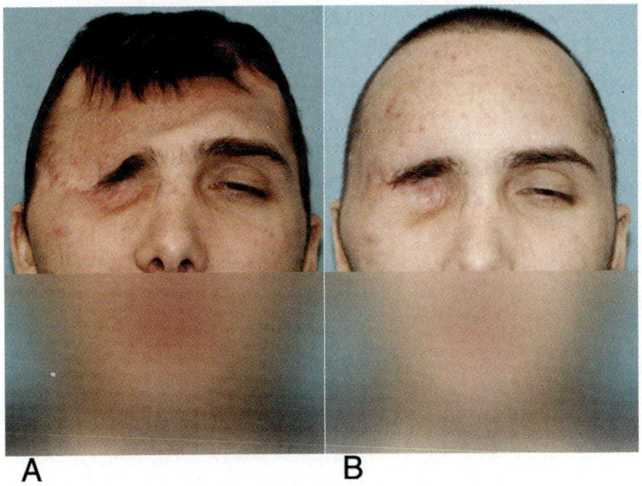

Figure 2. Postoperatively, brain protection and more natural contours have been restored. (**A**) Preoperative anterior view. (**B**) Postoperative anterior view.

tissue transfer has been the main treatment used to augment deficient tissue in the region of the planned cranioplasty. The cranial defect can be safely addressed once adequate soft tissue is available. Hemi-craniectomy defects represent the majority of defects. Due to their large size, the desire to avoid further intracranial surgery on the contralateral hemisphere and concerns with banked cranial bone, implant-based reconstruction has been the first choice of replacement.[19–22] Banked craniectomy bone autograft was utilized for reconstruction during the early phase of the Iraq War. This practice was largely abandoned due to evidence of bone resorbtion and concerns with bacterial colonization/infection. With the advent of rapid prototyping technologies, patient-specific, computed tomography–guided, three-dimensional prefabricated poly methyl methacrylate and Ti Mesh (woven titanium mesh) reconstructive implants are the most common choices (Fig. 2). Although implants have been used to reconstruct the upper orbits (bandeau region), our preference has been cranial or iliac crest bone grafts and cranialization of the frontal sinus as indicated.[19] This strategy separates the alloplastic cranial implants from the facial skeleton and adjacent frontal/ethmoid sinus, lessening potential infectious complications.

Facial fractures in isolation or more commonly in conjunction with major cranial injury are repaired when clinically appropriate. Classic timeframes to reduce and fixate facial fractures are within 7 days of injury. This allows for reconstitution of the skeletal framework before soft-tissue contracture. Military blast trauma craniofacial injury patients typically have severe prolonged swelling (due to mechanism and transport times 3–7 days to definitive care) and multiple concurrent injuries including severe closed head injury with vasospasm. Fixation within 1 week of injury is rarely accomplished. Most of these severely injured soldiers have undergone facial fracture fixation and grafting between 2 and 4 weeks after injury. Combined craniofacial approaches used in civilian practice are often not possible due to severe brain edema.[20,21] Internal fixation with bone grafts is used as indicated. In the critically injured patient, bone grafting may be delayed, and distraction osteogenesis or free tissue transfer is used when indicated.

Torso/extremity reconstruction

For these unique extremity and torso injuries no standard protocol exists. The major principle of early radical debridement and wound coverage with vascularized tissue is followed (Figs. 3 and 4). Modern civilian wound reconstruction principles may be used; however, the timing and type of flap reconstruction for these lower extremity battlefield injuries are generally based on evolving experience and surgeon judgment. Evidence in the civilian literature indicates that early wound coverage provides better outcomes and that subacute

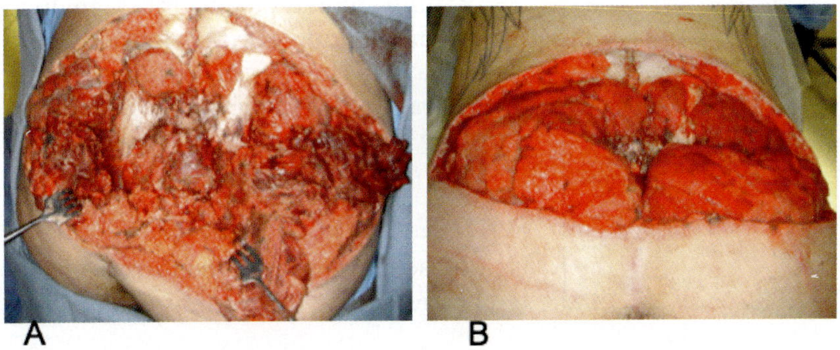

Figure 3. Marine after high-energy torso wound. Massive sacral wound with exposed bone. (**A**) Initial injury with exposed sacral bone. (**B**) Sacral wound after bilateral gluteus maximus advancement flaps.

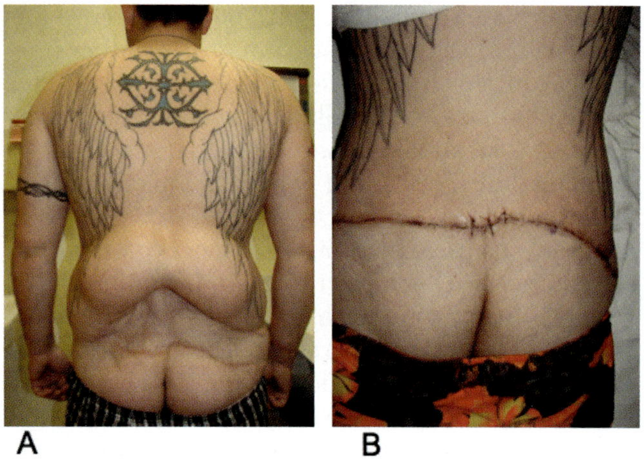

Figure 4. (A) Secondary reconstruction with lumbar tissue expanders in place. (B) Expanders removed and flaps advanced for complete coverage.

reconstruction is plagued with high complication rates.[6–12] Due to multiple factors including transport times, war extremity wounds are routinely reconstructed in the subacute time period.[13]

TAKE-HOME MESSAGE

Basic science advances

- Bone morphogenetic protein-2 is a potent osteoinductive agent when placed in bone defects at the time of wound reconstruction.
- Hydroxyapatite bone cement with antibiotic impregnation is a useful osteoconductive agent when placed in bone defects at the time of wound reconstruction.

Clinical science advances

- Multiplanar weight-bearing frames used in conjunction with lower extremity reconstruction allow early weight bearing without endosteal blood supply associated with intramedullary nails.
- Transport distraction osteogenesis is a useful technique for bone regeneration even in the setting of adjacent soft-tissue injury.

Relevance to clinical care

- Multidisciplinary care incorporating novel bone regeneration techniques along with wound reconstruction with vascularized tissue (flaps) has increased limb and craniofacial salvage.
- Delay in reconstruction has not been associated with increased complications.
- Microsurgical free flap reconstruction has been uniformly successful in craniofacial and extremity wounds using longer pedicled (*e.g.*, anterior lateral thigh flap vs. lateral arm flap) flaps with anastomosis in the relative lesser zone of injury.
- Operating out of the zone of injury is nearly impossible due to the wide blast trauma zone of injury.
- Soft tissue and bone reconstruction can be safely performed in the subacute period when the comorbid patient conditions are controlled.

DISCUSSION OF FINDINGS AND RELEVANT LITERATURE

Subtle variations in care are necessary with the uniquely large zones of injury, complex desert microflora in battlefield extremity wounds, and multiple concurrent injuries.[1–5,23] Unique in military medicine are highly motivated patients who reap benefits from surgeon's constant exposure to complex battle injuries (Fig. 1). In addition to practicing established concepts from prior military conflicts, new technology for the advancement of trauma care has been applied. Treatment with novel flap reconstructions, bone grafting, and bone-engineering techniques including use of bone morphogenetic protein-2 has lead to improved outcomes.[24] Also, early involvement of a wide array of professionals and intense rehabilitation facilities is a critical component of comprehensive care.

We have demonstrated that this delay in reconstruction does not unfavorably affect outcomes.[24] If surgeons adhere to the established principles of creating a clean wound bed and using healthy vascularized coverage, infection and flap failure can be minimized. Compared to the body of orthopedic and plastic surgical literature, our experience demonstrated low flap failure rates and reasonably low infection rates without the need for amputation.[3–5,8] This represents a significant improvement in the management of devastating open lower extremity fractures in the subacute period, also corroborated by the experience at Balboa Naval Hospital.[25]

CAUTION, CRITICAL REMARKS, AND RECOMMENDATIONS

- Soft tissue and bone reconstruction can be safely performed in the subacute period only when the comorbid patient conditions are controlled.
- Wound management must include prompt and serial debridements along with negative pressure dressing therapy during the interval to definitive war wound reconstruction.

FUTURE DEVELOPMENTS

Use of soft tissue and bone regenerate templates in the future may obviate the need for donor site flap and associated morbidity. Further integration of sophisticated biocompatible synthetic constructs with tissue engineering will improve both form and function in the reconstruction of composite tissue defects. More sophisticated distraction devices will allow for greater soft tissue and bone regeneration.

ACKNOWLEDGMENTS

Wound healing research in the author's institution is not financed by external sources.

AUTHOR DISCLOSURE STATEMENT

No conflict of interest disclosed.

REFERENCES

1. Bermudez LE: Abstract: Microsurgery in war wounds. Presented at the 69th Scientific Meeting of the American Society of Plastic Surgeons (ASPS). Los Angeles, CA: October 14–18, 2000.
2. Stalekar H, Fuckar Z, Ekl D, *et al.*: Primary vs. secondary wound reconstruction in Gustilo type III open tibial shaft fractures: follow up study of 35 cases. Croat Med J 2003; **44:** 746.
3. Byrd HS, Cierny G, III, and Tebbetts JB: The management of open tibial fractures with associated soft tissue loss: external pin fixation with early flap coverage. Plast Reconstr Surg 1981; **68:** 73.
4. Godina M: Early microsurgical reconstruction of complex trauma of the extremities. Plast Reconstr Surg 1986; **78:** 285.
5. Heller L and Levin LS: Lower extremity microsurgical reconstruction. Plast Reconstr Surg 2001; **108:** 1029.
6. Francel TJ, Vander Kolk CA, Hoopes JE, *et al.*: Microvascular soft-tissue transplantation for reconstruction of acute open tibial fractures: timing of coverage and long-term functional results. Plast Reconstr Surg 1992; **89:** 478.
7. Hertel R, Lambert SM, Muller S, *et al.*: On the timing of soft-tissue reconstruction for open fractures of the lower leg. Arch Orthop Trauma Surg 1999; **119:** 7.
8. Khouri RK and Shaw WW: Reconstruction of the lower extremity with microvascular free flaps: a 10-year experience with 304 consecutive cases. J Trauma 1989; **29:** 1086.
9. Hallock GG: Utility of both muscle and fascia flaps in severe lower extremity trauma. J Trauma 2000; **48:** 913.
10. Hallock GG: Lower extremity muscle perforator flaps for lower extremity reconstruction. Plast Reconstr Surg 2004; **114:** 1123.
11. Yildirim S, Gideroglu K, and Akoz T: Anterolateral thigh flap: ideal free flap choice for lower extremity soft-tissue reconstruction. J Reconstr Microsurg 2003; **19:** 225.
12. Yazar S, Lin CH, Lin YT, *et al.*: Outcome comparison between free muscle and free fasciocutaneous flaps for reconstruction of distal third and ankle traumatic open tibial fractures. Plast Reconstr Surg 2006; **117:** 2468.
13. Kumar A: Standard wound coverage techniques for extremity war injury. J Am Acad Orthop Surg 2006; **14(10 Suppl):** S62.
14. Gustilo RB, Mendoza RM, and Williams DN: Problems in the management of type III open fractures. A new classification of type III open fractures. J Trauma 1984; **24:** 742.
15. Caudle RJ and Stern PJ: Severe open fractures of the tibia. J Bone Joint Surg 1987; **69A:** 801.
16. Bagg MR, Covey DC, and Powell ET: Levels of medical care in the global war on terrorism. J Am Acad Orthop Surg 2006; **14(10 Spec No.):** S7.
17. Lee C, Antonyshyn OM, and Forrest CR: Cranioplasty: indications, technique, and early results of autogenous split skull cranial vault reconstruction. J Craniomaxillofac Surg 1995; **23:** 133.
18. Rish BL, Dillon JD, Meirowsky AM, *et al.*: Cranioplasty: a review of 1030 cases of penetrating head injury. Neurosurgery 1979; **4:** 381.
19. Manson PN, Crawley WA, and Hoopes JE: Frontal cranioplasty: risk factors and choice of cranial vault reconstructive material. Plast Reconstr Surg 1986; **77:** 888.
20. Isago T, Nozaki M, Kikuchi Y, Honda T, and Nakazawa H: Sinking skin flap syndrome: a case of improved cerebral blood flow after cranioplasty. Ann Plast Surg 2004; **53:** 288.
21. Schiffer J, Gur R, Nisim U, and Pollak L: Symptomatic patients after craniectomy. Surg Neurol 1997; **47:** 231.
22. Segal DH, Oppenheim JS, and Murovic JA: Neurological recovery after cranioplasty. Neurosurgery 1994; **34:** 729.
23. Pollack AN and Ficke JR: Exremity war Injuries III, session moderators. J Am Acad Orthop Surg 2008; **16:** 628.
24. Kumar AR, Navanjun S, Grewal M, Chung TL, and Bradley JP: Lessons from Operation Iraqi Freedom: successful subacute reconstruction of complex lower extremity battle injuries. Plast Reconstr Surg 2009; **23:** 218.
25. Geiger S, McCormick F, Chou R, and Wandel AG: War wounds: lessons learned from Operation Iraqi Freedom. Plast Reconstr Surg 2008; **122:** 146.

WHS
Wound
Healing
Society

The Use of Three-Dimensional Models in the Treatment of Craniomaxillofacial Injuries

Phillip Littlefield, Christopher Cote, and George Coppit*

Department of Otolaryngology/Head & Neck Surgery, Walter Reed Army Medical Center, Washington, District of Columbia.

Abbreviations and Acronyms

3D = three-dimensional

CT = computed tomography

PMMA = polymethylmethacrylate

*Correspondence: Department of Otolaryngology/Head & Neck Surgery, Walter Reed Army Medical Center, 6900 Georgia Ave. NW, Washington, District of Columbia 20307 (e-mail: george.coppit@us.army.mil).

Background: The use of explosive weaponry and high-powered ordnance in modern combat has resulted in increasingly complex patterns of craniomaxillofacial injures. These injuries include high-velocity penetrating injuries, relatively low-velocity penetrating injuries, burns, and over pressurization blast effect injuries. These injuries typically involve extensive loss of and injury to soft tissue, dentition, ocular, bony, and neurovascular structures. Reestablishment of proper function and cosmesis in these patients presents special challenges to the reconstructive surgeon. We have found that scale three-dimensional (3D) models generated from fine-cut computed tomography scans of the defect are useful in preoperative counseling, planning and rehearsing the operative procedure, reducing operative times, and improving outcomes.

The Problem: Massive traumatic head and neck injuries present special challenges to the reconstructive surgeon. Significant functional (speech, swallowing, and visual) and cosmetic defects can occur, making rehabilitation of these patients difficult. The balance between form and function in the reconstruction of these patients is facilitated by the use of preoperative 3D scanning.

Basic/Clinical Science Advances: Advances in imaging techniques (3D modeling) allow for more precise interpretation of the traumatic defect. The extent of soft tissue and bony injury can be accurately assessed, and the operative plan tailored to each individual patient. This aspect can also be utilized to create patient- and defect-specific implants (polymethylmethacrylate or titanium) to aid in reconstruction. Further, stereolithic models can be created, allowing for model surgery to be performed in a test run before the actual procedure. This allows for preoperative modification of the treatment plan and more accurate determination of the reconstructive needs of the case, as well as allowing for prebending of reconstruction plates.

Clinical Care Relevance: Improved preoperative imaging techniques allow for better and more individualized surgical planning, shortened operative times, and improved outcomes. The ability to perform model surgery results in shortened operative times and improved outcomes.

Conclusion: The widespread use of high-velocity weapons and explosive devices in modern combat has resulted in devastating complex craniomaxillofacial injuries. The ability to restore form and function to these patients is extremely challenging. Three-dimensional stereolithic models generated from fine-cut computed tomography scans have been employed to enhance preoperative counseling and preoperative planning, to reduce operative times and to improve functional and cosmetic outcomes.

The opinions and views expressed here do not represent the position of the US Army Medical Corps, Department of the Army, or the Federal Government.

ADVANCES IN WOUND CARE, VOLUME 1

Printed in U.S.A.
DOI: 10.1089/awc.2009.0025

BACKGROUND

MODERN WEAPONRY PRODUCES a spectrum of injury different from what is commonly seen in most civilian trauma. The most common mechanism of injury tends to be penetrating wounds caused by gunshot wounds or fragmentary devices,[1] whereas in civilian trauma blunt force injury is more common. Combat-related wounds tend to be larger in both number and size, and have a significant amount of associated soft tissue trauma.

In modern combat, up to 31% of patients have significant head and neck injuries.[1–3] These injuries typically involve extensive loss of and injury to soft tissue and bony structures, dentition, ocular structures, and neurovascular structures. The treatment and rehabilitation of these patients is particularly challenging. Massive swelling and concomitant injuries often preclude treatment outside of the traditional 14–21-day window for bony injuries.

Combat-related trauma has characteristics unique from civilian trauma. A large explosion frequently results in a mix of traumatic injuries, including blast injury, penetrating injuries, and thermal injuries. The mechanism of blast injury can be divided into primary blast effect and secondary blast effect. The primary blast effect is caused by the initial shock wave, traveling up to 1,600 feet/s. This high-pressure wave results in high-velocity propulsion of fragments resulting in craniofacial fractures and soft tissue injuries. Secondary blast effect is caused by high-pressure air, up to 1,000 times that of normal atmospheric pressure, rushing in to fill the vacuum created by the primary blast wave. This phenomenon causes concussions, loss of consciousness, tympanic membrane rupture/hearing loss, and traumatic brain injury.[1–3]

The complex anatomical relationships in the head and neck are important for proper function (speech, swallowing, and vision), and important in what is considered to be normal in terms of cosmesis. The balance between reestablishing proper form and function is especially difficult in the head and neck region, and is compounded when significant bony and soft tissue loss occurs, as in combat-related injuries.

At our institution we sought to improve the outcomes for these patients and maximize the balance between form and function in our reconstructions. In our experience, the use of three-dimensional (3D) stereolithographic models allows for improved preoperative evaluation of the defect, improved preoperative counseling of patient and family, improved quality of reconstruction, creation of patient- and defect-specific implants, reduced operative time, and improved outcomes in our patient population.

CLINICAL PROBLEM ADDRESSED

Combat-related injuries in the head and neck represent a special challenge to the reconstructive surgeon. The combination of bony and soft tissue injuries, with associated ocular and neurovascular injuries, is complex anywhere in the body; when coupled with the delicate function and important cosmetic considerations in the head and neck, the complexity is greater than perhaps anywhere else in the body. The use of stereolithography and 3D modeling in head and neck reconstruction has been described in the literature since 1988.[4,5] Advances in the preoperative evaluation and treatment of these injuries provide for marked improvement in the treatment and outcome for these patients. Using 3D models based on data from standard-format computed tomography (CT) scans, accurate models of comminuted injuries and defects are created. These models allow for preoperative assessment and planning in a manner not available using conventional techniques. Additionally, in cases of extensive bony loss 3D models enable the creation of implantable models of the defect to help guide the use of autologous grafts or the creation of biocompatible implants (polymethylmethacrylate [PMMA] or titanium) to aid in reconstruction. The overall goals of reconstruction using these new techniques are to (i) restore function, (ii) restore cosmesis, (iii) reduce morbidity, (iv) reduce the need for follow-on surgeries for the same issues, and (v) improve outcomes.

BASIC SCIENCE CONTEXT

The faster processing speed of today's computers, coupled with advances in CT scanning and imaging software, provides the ability to produce scale 3D models of traumatic defects at an affordable cost. In-house capability to produce these stereolithographic models further reduces overall cost and improves turn-around time in the creation of these models. Additionally, 3D models provide the potential for the creation of defect-specific implants (PMMA or titanium) in cases of significant bony loss.

Preoperatively, patients undergo thin-cut CT scans (1–1.25 mm) in the axial and coronal planes of the traumatic defects. Using stereolithographic technology (3D Systems, Rock Hill, SC), data from the CT scans are utilized to create scale 3D light-activated epoxy resin models. After evaluation of the 3D models, in cases of significant bone loss where autologous tissue transfer may be utilized, planned donor sites are scanned in a similar fashion. This creates a 3D model not only of the defect, but of the donor bone as well. The overall result is a highly accurate, detailed model of the traumatic defect, improved preoperative planning, shortened surgical times, and improved outcomes.

EXPERIMENTAL MODEL OR MATERIAL

No applicable experimental model exists that is comparable to the techniques described in this article.

DISCUSSION OF FINDINGS AND RELEVANT LITERATURE

There has been an increase in the frequency and severity of head and neck injuries in modern combat operations. In our experience, these injuries are typically severe and involve extensive soft tissue and bony injury, as well as extensively comminuted fractures of the midface and mandible. Concomitant ocular and neurovascular injuries further complicate the clinical picture. Massive swelling and other injuries (*e.g.*, orthopedic and thoracic) that take precedence may preclude timely treatment of the craniomaxillofacial injuries, making successful treatment, and rehabilitation of these patients even more difficult.

We sought to improve the quality of our reconstruction through all phases of treatment: preoperative assessment and planning, preoperative counseling of patients and family, and improved surgical outcomes.

The use of stereolithography and 3D modeling in head and neck reconstruction has previously been described. Most of these reports involve the use of 3D CT scanning only.[4–8] Today's faster computing speeds, combined with advances in CT scanning (helical CT) and imaging software, have given us the ability to produce scale 3D models based on standard 1 mm format CT scans at an affordable cost. The result is a highly accurate and detailed model of the defect. The creation of stereolithographic 3D models represents an evolution in the assessment and treatment of complex craniomaxillofacial injuries.

Our approach to the treatment of these injuries involves multidisciplinary care of the patient: neurology, neurosurgery, ophthalmology, oromaxillofacial surgery, otolaryngology, speech pathology, occupational and physical therapy, as well as general surgery and intensive care specialists as necessary. This multifaceted care ensures that all aspects of the patients care, both acute and long-term, are addressed, helping to maximize functional outcomes.

In cases of severely comminuted fractures, intraoperative reduction and stabilization is a challenging process. Utilizing the 3D models, the location and rotation of individual fragments can be accurately assessed preoperatively. Fragments can then be manipulated and reduced using the model—what we term "model surgery." Reconstruction plates can be prebent based on this model surgery. This is typically done the day or evening before the actual procedure. We have found this to be a highly accurate technique, reducing operative times by 2 to 4 h (data maturing) and improving reduction of fracture segments.

When significant bony loss is present, traditional planning, harvesting, and molding of autologous grafts to the defect site can be extremely challenging and time consuming. In cases requiring microvascular free flap reconstruction, minimizing ischemic time is paramount to the success of the procedure. Utilizing the 3D methods described above, it is possible to premeasure and precut the bone grafts on highly accurate anatomic models, perform simulated osteotomies, and rehearse the reconstruction preoperatively. Additionally, these preplanned osteotomies can then be applied *in situ* before graft harvest, reducing ischemic time in microvascular cases. In cases involving complex 3D reconstructions (such as massive midface defects), this has saved many hours of operative time, reduced ischemic times, and helped to improve surgical outcomes in our hands.

In some cases, the extent of bony loss precludes the use of autologous free bone grafts or vascularized bone grafts. This may be due to the absolute size and/or shape of the defect, or due to the loss of donor sites secondary to concomitant injuries. The 3D modeling technology allows for the creation of biocompatible 3D implants that precisely match the defect and mirror the uninjured side. Both PMMA and titanium implants have been used successfully to reconstruct massive, complex craniomaxillofacial defects with excellent cosmetic and functional results. Each type of implant has unique characteristics; however, both are widely accepted to be extremely biocompatible. PMMA implants can be fashioned in-house, in a process that can take up to 14 days. It is necessary to use secondary titanium fixation plates to anchor the PMMA implant to surrounding uninjured bony structures. One advantage of the PMMA implant is the ability to modify the implant intraoperatively if the need arises. PMMA implants do not allow for native tissue ingrowth, and are not visible on radiographs. Titanium implants currently are designed in-house, and fabricated at a separate facility (Medical Modeling, Golden, CO), but can be fabricated within 24 h of receipt of the design. The titanium implants have built in fixation points, allow for native tissue ingrowth, and are clearly visible on radiographs. However, titanium implants cannot be modified intraoperatively (we have several broken drills and instruments that can attest to this fact).

To date, we have treated over 275 complex craniomaxillofacial injuries utilizing the 3D modeling technique. While any one of these cases could have been treated without the use of 3D modeling, we believe that this technology has significantly improved our ability to accurately assess the extent of injury preoperatively, allowing for better counseling of patients and families as to the nature of the injury and proposed reconstruction. Further, we have been able to better plan for the surgical reconstruction and perform model surgery. We feel that this has dramatically reduced operative times, improved resource utilization, reduced the need for revision surgery, and improved outcomes (Figs. 1–8).

CAUTION, CRITICAL REMARKS, AND RECOMMENDATIONS

It is important to remember that a multidisciplinary approach to the treatment of trauma patients maximizes the long-term functional outcome. Often, while maybe the most visually startling, craniomaxillofacial injuries are not the most life threatening. It is possible to achieve excellent functional and cosmetic outcomes with delayed reconstruction, especially utilizing the 3D imaging techniques described in this article.

While 3D imaging and stereolithography help to maximize surgical outcomes, it is still often difficult to achieve true one-stage reconstruction of massive craniomaxillofacial injuries. More complex injuries are likely to require revisions, most commonly involving adjustments of ocular structures (eyelid repositioning), placement of ocular prostheses (in cases of enucleation), and thinning or repositioning of soft tissues (more common in cases of microvascular free flap reconstruction). However, the overall trend is to a reduced number of procedures and revisions when using stereolithography in the treatment of these injuries.

Restoration of the anatomic defect is only one part of the treatment of complex craniomaxillofacial injuries. These patients face long-term rehabilitation to maximize functional outcomes. Early involvement of speech therapists and occupational and physical therapists helps aid the

TAKE-HOME MESSAGE

Basic science advances

- Advances in computer processing and CT scanning have enabled the creation of highly accurate 3D models at an affordable cost.
- PMMA and titanium represent highly versatile biocompatible materials that can be used to create accurate, individualized implants for the repair of complex craniomaxillofacial injuries.

Clinical science advances

- Three-dimensional stereolithic modeling allows for unparalleled preoperative assessment of traumatic defects.
- Three-dimensional stereolithic modeling allows for individualized treatment of complex craniomaxillofacial injuries by providing an accurate assessment of the defect.
- Three-dimensional stereolithic modeling provides the reconstructive surgeon with the ability to assess the injury in real-time 3D preoperatively, which aids in surgical planning and treatment.
- Model surgery can be performed utilizing 3D stereolithic models. This essentially allows a dry run of the surgery using an anatomically accurate model. Further, reconstruction plates can be accurately preformed according to the model surgery, thus reducing operative times. Similarly, stereolithic models of donor sites can be created, allowing for the creation and adjustment of osteotomies before the actual surgery. In cases of microvascular free tissue transfer, this significantly shortens ischemic times.

Relevance to clinical care

- The overall goals of the reconstruction of complex craniomaxillofacial injuries are to (i) restore function, (ii) restore cosmesis, (iii) reduce morbidity, (iv) reduce the need for revision surgery, and (v) improve outcomes. The use of 3D CT scanning and stereolithography allows for enhanced preoperative assessment of injury, and provides for better preoperative counseling of the patient and family. Scale models created using this technology have allowed for precise preoperative reduction of severely comminuted fractures, as well as prebending of reconstruction plates. Additionally, simulated bone grafts can be created and osteotomies performed during model surgery, providing an opportunity to assess and modify the reconstructive plan without compromising patient care. Customized, precise implants of either PMMA or titanium can be created using this same technology, providing highly individualized and specific treatment of complex craniomaxillofacial injuries. All of this translates into improved preoperative assessment, reduced operative times, a reduction in revision surgery, and improved patient outcomes.

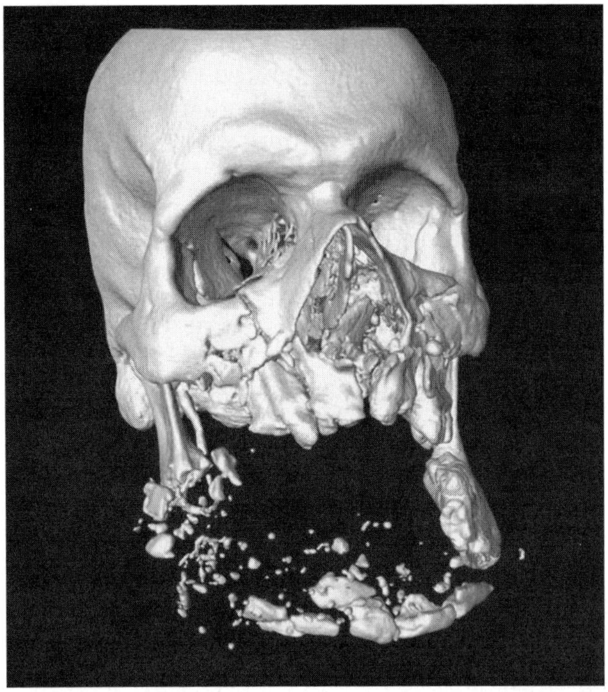

Figure 1. Three-dimensional model representing a severely comminuted mandible fracture.

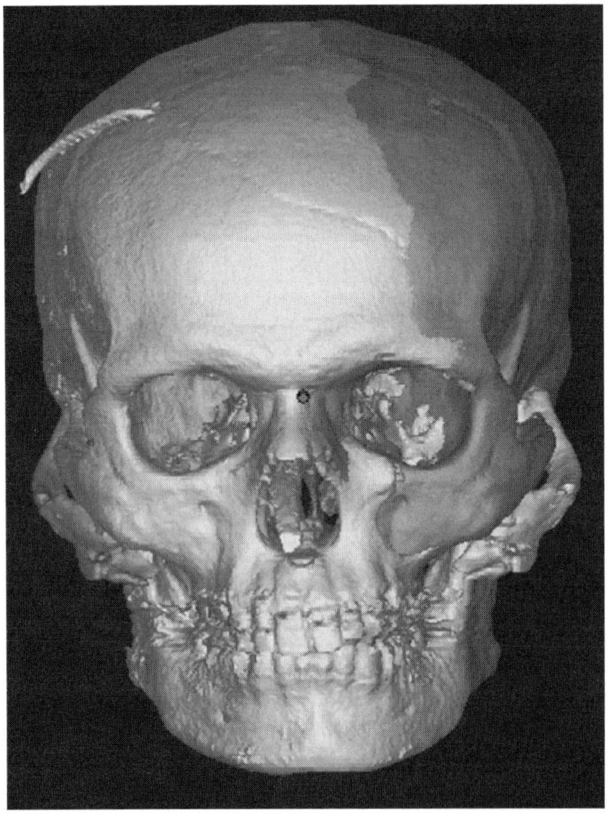

Figure 2. Application of three-dimensional imaging technology to create a mirror image of the uninjured side and project into the defect.

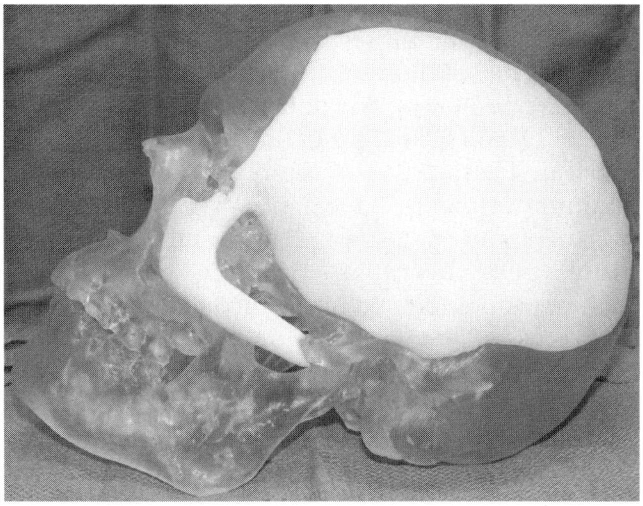

Figure 3. Three-dimensional model based on mirror image of uninjured side onto defect.

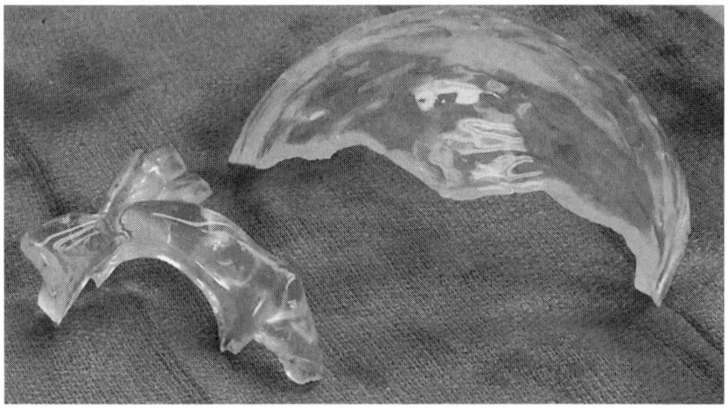

Figure 4. Example of cranial and orbital polymethylmethacrylate implants.

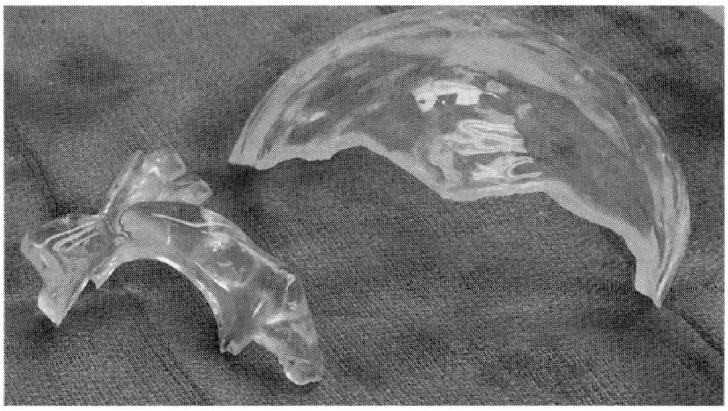

Figure 5. Representative patient reconstructed with polymethylmethacrylate implants (Fig. 4).

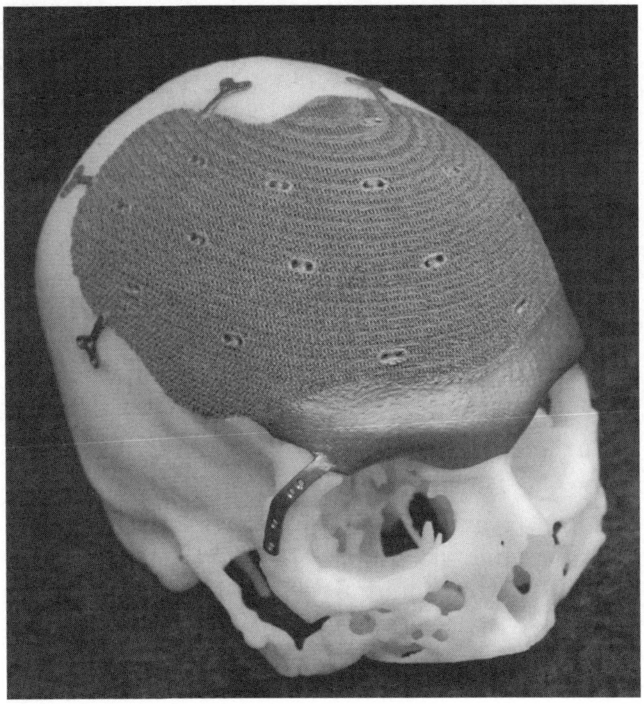

Figure 6. Example of titanium cranial implant.

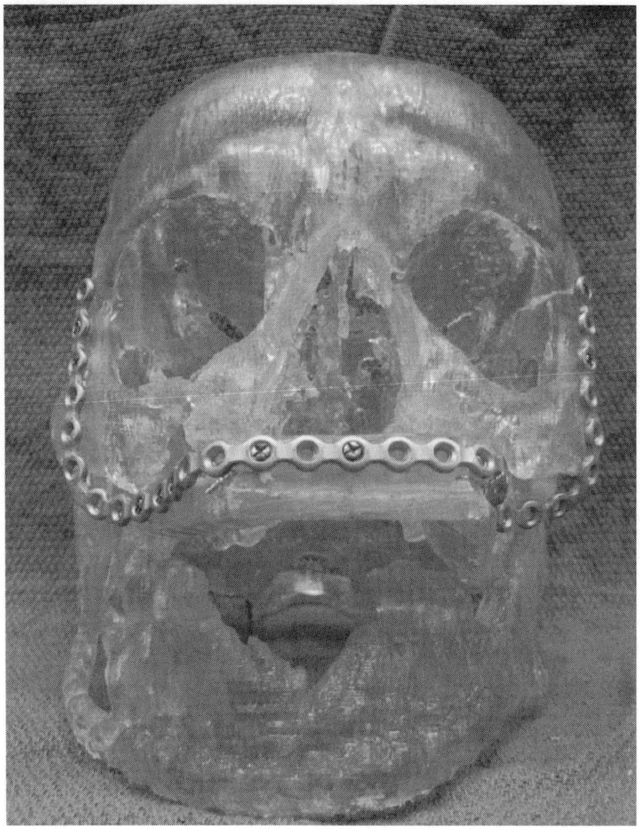

Figure 8. Example of three-dimensional model after model surgery.

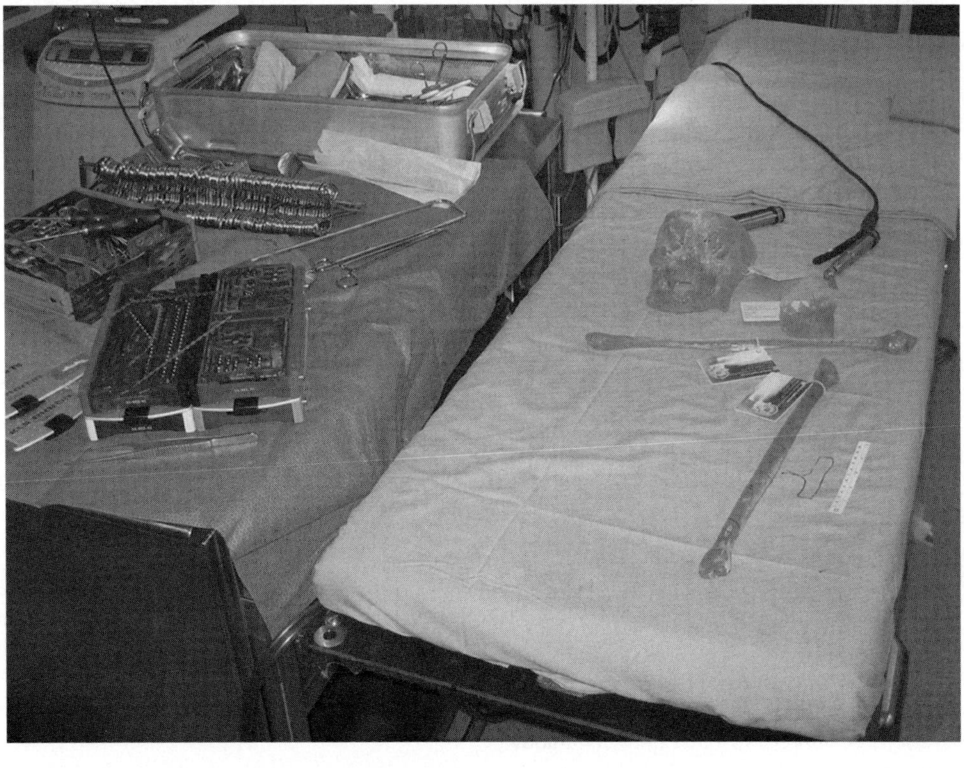

Figure 7. Operating room setup for model surgery.

patient in maximizing the long-term goal of full rehabilitation.

FUTURE DEVELOPMENT

The use of 3D stereolithography has been shown to be an effective tool in the treatment of complex craniomaxillofacial injuries. This technology could be applied even more effectively if a preinjury scan existed. This would allow even more accurate assessment of the dimensions of the injury. While this may not be practical in the civilian setting, in the military a database of preinjury CT scans could be completed upon entry to active duty, similar to what is today accomplished with panorex dental imaging. Comparison of preinjury models to post-injury models would provide an even more accurate assessment of the injury, and avoid using mirror images of the uninjured site to create a model of the defect.

Optical 3D surface scanning has been shown to provide a superior means of objectively quantifying facial soft tissues.[9] It is possible to correlate the data obtained from 3D surface scanning with the data obtained using 3D CT scanning. This provides an accurate anatomic assessment not only of bony anatomy, but of the overlying soft tissue envelope as well. The relationship and relative thickness of soft tissue at varying points on the facial skeleton can be accurately assessed, and this information utilized in reconstructive planning. We have recently started to employ this technology with our own patients; however, it is too early to asses its impact.

AUTHOR DISCLOSURE STATEMENT

P.L., C.C., and G.C. disclose that they have no commercial associations that might create or seem to pose a conflict of interest in connection with the submitted article.

REFERENCES

1. Peoples GE, Gerlinger T, Craig R, and Burlingame B: Combat casualties in Afghanistan cared for by a single Forward Surgical Team during the initial phases of Operation Enduring Freedom. Mil Med 2005; **170:** 462.
2. Xydakis MS, Fravell MD, Nasser KE, and Casler JD: Analysis of battlefield head and neck injuries in Iraq and Afghanistan. Otolaryngol Head Neck Surg 2005; **133:** 497.
3. Montgomery SP, Swiecki CW, and Shriver, CD: The evaluation of casualties from operation Iraqi freedom on return to the continental United States from March to June 2003. J Am Coll Surg 2005; **201:** 7.
4. Toth BA, Ellis DS, and Stewart WB: Computer-designed prosthesis for orbitocranial reconstruction. Plast Reconstr Surg 1998; **81:** 315.
5. Powers DB, Edgin WA, and Tabatchnick L: Stereolithography: a historical review and indications for use in the management of trauma. J Craniomaxillofac Trauma 1998; **4:** 16.
6. DeRosa V, Ionna F, Mozzillo N, Parascandolo S, and Ziviello M: 3D spiral computerized tomography in the reconstructive treatment of malignant maxillofacial tumors. Radiol Med 2000; **100:** 424.
7. Franca C, Levin-Plotnik D, Sehgal V, Chen GT, and Ramsey RG: Use of three-dimensional spiral computed tomography imaging for staging and surgical planning of head and neck cancer. J Digit Imaging 2000; **13(2 Suppl 1):** 24.
8. Saigal K, Winokur RS, Finden S, Taub D, and Pribitkin E: Use of three-dimensional computerized tomography reconstruction in complex facial trauma. Facial Plast Surg 2005; **21:** 214.
9. Lin SJ, Patel N, O'Shaughnessy K, and Fine N: A new three-dimensional imaging device in facial aesthetic and reconstructive surgery. Otolaryngol Head Neck Surg 2008; **139:** 313.

Section 2

ACUTE WOUNDS

Section Editors: Adrian Barbul and David Leaper

ACUTE WOUNDS

WHS
Wound
Healing
Society

Surgical Site Infections

David Leaper[1] and Adrian Barbul[2,*]

[1]Department of Wound Healing, Cardiff University, Cardiff, United Kingdom.
[2]Department of Surgery, Sinai Hospital and Johns Hopkins Medical Institutions, Baltimore, Maryland.

Surgical wound infections continue to represent a significant clinical and economic problem. Herein, we review several contributions to the world's literature on epidemiology, clinical aspects, and guidelines aimed at reducing the incidence of surgical site infection.

INTRODUCTION

Surgical site infection (SSI) continues to be an important topic with two guidelines being published last year from different sides of the Atlantic (the United States of America and the United Kingdom). Both have been compiled by appropriate and expert groups after extensive searches of the evidence base. Although the reviews are systematic, they have not been limited to the constraints of the Cochrane Collaboration methodology so that when further research has been perceived as being needed, the authors have used best available evidence to formulate guidelines for clinical practice. Most of the recommendations are designed on level I evidence-based medicine, but where it is lacking consensus opinion has been given with highlighting of the fields where more research could be usefully and realistically undertaken. The third manuscript, which has been appraised in this acute wound section, is a large retrospective review of 10,253 general surgical and vascular operations that has analyzed data, using bivariate and regression analysis, for predictive factors for SSIs.

Definitions of SSI and the method of surveillance, postdischarge in particular, continue to pose difficulties and may be the cause of guidelines and predictive factors not working equally well on an international basis. For example, the National Nosocomial Infection Surveillance study data used for SSI prediction do not work in all countries as well as its parent country of origin. The North American Centers for Disease Control (CDC) definition is the most widely used for reviews and studies in this field but is also open to interpretation; for example, the recording of an SSI can depend on the attending physician's opinion. Surgeons do tend to under-report their SSI rates. In addition, and more importantly, the CDC definition does not differentiate the severity of SSIs particularly well. Infections can be relatively trivial or life threatening and need a more discriminant scoring system, such as the well-established ASEPSIS score, to allow these important distinctions to be made. Continuous or interval data, rather than categorical data, are also more useful in statistical analysis and the calculation of power for randomized controlled trials. Increasing numbers of operations, particularly in elective surgery, are undertaken on a day case basis. If the incidence or prevalence of SSI is to be accurately computed, postdischarge surveillance (PDS) must extend beyond the hospital or secondary care period. SSIs take several days to be apparent and

Abbreviations and Acronyms

ASA = American Society of Anesthesiologists

ASEPSIS = Additional treatment, Serious discharge, Erythema, Purulent exudate, Separation of deep tissue, Isolation of bacteria, Stay in hospital

BMI = body mass index

CDC = Centers for Disease Control

NICE = National Institute of Health and Clinical Excellence

PDS = postdischarge surveillance

SSI = surgical site infection

*Correspondence: Department of Surgery, Sinai Hospital and Johns Hopkins Medical Institutions, 2435 W. Belvedere Ave., Baltimore, Maryland 21215 (e-mail: abarbul@jhmi.edu).

Printed in U.S.A.
DOI: 10.1089/awc.2009.0157

surveillance must closely follow patients into primary care. Optimally, PDS should involve a trained, validated, unbiased observer and is an expensive option when undertaken adequately. After orthopedic surgery, PDS should continue for a year, but infection, after hip and knee replacement, for example, can be missed in the early postoperative period when patients are allowed home within 4–5 days.

BACKGROUND

SSIs cause significant morbidity and mortality in the postoperative period and are the second most common nosocomial infection in the United States. Overall, approximately 25% of all nosocomial infections in hospitalized patients are SSIs. However, among surgical patients SSIs are the most common nosocomial infection and complicate 2.6% of all surgical procedures performed. Patients with SSIs are more likely to need admission to an intensive care unit, have a longer length of stay, and are more likely to die than their counterparts without SSIs. However, rather than treating all operative patients with broad-spectrum antibiotics in an effort to decrease the prevalence of SSIs, the emergence of widespread antibiotic resistance has required a more judicious use of antimicrobial prophylaxis.

SSIs have a dramatic impact on the morbidity and mortality of affected individuals. While the mortality attributable to SSIs is less than 5%, when surgical patients with nosocomial SSI die, a majority of deaths are attributable to the infection. Most deaths occur after organ/space infections.

The morbidity associated with SSI is more difficult to quantify. While superficial incisional infections may only increase the length of hospitalization by a few days, organ/space infections may result in a prolonged hospitalization and the need for additional procedures. In 2004, SSIs increased hospital length of stay an average of 6.5 days. Finally, individuals with substantial wounds after debridement may require discharge to a nursing facility or daily home visits by a skilled wound care nurse.

The authors of this review trawled the indexed publications of 2008/2009, and in the field of SSI felt that these were the outstanding communications worthy of presentation and review for the *Year Book of Wound Healing Society*.

1. Predictive factors for surgical site infections in general surgery

Haridas H, Malangoni MA
Surgery 2008; 144: 496–501

This is an interesting retrospective survey of over 10,000 general surgical and vascular operations, at a single institution, for a 6-year period looking for SSIs using ICD-9 and CDC definitions. It has concentrated on the identification of predictive factors with particular relevance to the complications of deep or organ/space infections.

Their hypothesis was based on the fact that the widely reported numbers of SSIs (2–7%) were associated with increased morbidity and mortality and increased duration of stay and healthcare costs, and that better recognition of additional predictive factors might help to reduce them further. The widely quoted National Nosocomial Infection Surveillance risk factors of American Society of Anesthesiologists (ASA) grade, wound classification, and length of operation do not work equally well on an international basis, so further predictive factors for deep and organ/space SSIs, provided they could be acted on preoperatively, would be particularly welcome. However, the deep and organ/space infections are relatively uncommon, but they represent a huge drain on resources when they occur.

Retrospective reviews always suffer from not having a complete dataset (which the authors admit is a limitation), and therefore they had no data on the adequacy of antibiotic prophylaxis, hair removal, bowel and skin preparation, presence of a high body mass index (BMI), avoidance of hypothermia or perioperative management of blood sugar, supplemented oxygen, or blood transfusion. All of these have been implicated in SSI risk, some with a level I evidence base. Nevertheless, they identified 50 discrete variables. No reference is made to the extent of PDS, which is so important in these days of increasing short-stay surgery; nor was there any comment on who decided on the presence of an SSI, which should ideally be a trained, validated, independent practitioner on a prospective basis. Their low incidence of SSI was surely influenced by this. The CDC definition also only gives a categorical result, and scoring systems, such as the well-validated ASEPSIS system, give interval data that are more amenable to inferential statistical analysis.

The actual number of patients reviewed who had a deep/organ space infection was small (also admitted by the authors), a convenient 300 or 16.3% of the total who had SSIs. Compared with a comparable reference group, they undertook bivariate and multivariate analysis, and the factors coming up with a significant risk of SSI were low albumin, low hemoglobin, excess alcohol intake, previous surgery, a history of chronic obstructive pulmonary disease, and long operation. These factors were also controlled for the effects of ASA grade, wound type, and type of procedure. The latter factor clearly relates to a complex combination of factors such as difficult operations taking longer with more blood loss. The authors do speculate briefly on the predictive factors they have identified, but it would have been useful to have had more advice on how their institution attempts to counteract or minimize the effect of these.

Comments

Such retrospective studies of large patient populations, while having limitations, do afford the opportunity for examining risk factors and clinical factors that impact on the occurrence of SSI. Given the enormous economic and clinical cost of these events, such efforts are welcome, although limited. Given the difficulty in conducting randomized studies on SSIs, since it is such a multifactorial event, such retrospective studies fill a valuable niche that can influence clinical practice in a positive way. The only randomized studies usually examine a single factor such as antibiotic therapy or are limited to examining single aspects of care (preoperative washing, shaving, dressing types, etc.). The full story of SSI is still untold and the bacteria are getting smarter by the minute.

2. Guidelines to aid healing of acute wounds by decreasing impediments of healing

Franz MG, Robson MC, Steed DL, Barbul A, Brem H, Cooper DM, Leaper D, Milner SM, Payne WG, Wachtel TL, Wiersema-Bryant L

Wound Repair and Regeneration 2008; 16: 723–748

This paper is very different as it does not confine itself to SSIs but includes the whole picture of aids to optimal healing of acute wounds. The authors are a panel of general, vascular, plastic, trauma, burn, and cancer surgeons, with nurse clinicians and researchers, drawn from academic, government and private practice, and industrial backgrounds. They are certainly representative in the field and all active. Although the review was not commissioned or led by the Wound Healing Society, the document was sent for appraisal through their Web site. The panel's remit was to identify detriments or deterrents to acute wound healing (healing in bone, cartilage, neural tissue, or viscera was not addressed) that could be used practically to eliminate or reduce complications of healing.

The panel undertook reviews in 11 areas of impediments to wound healing using PubMed, MEDLINE, EMBASE, and Cochrane databases, and published reviews and guidelines. Three levels of modified, strength of evidence base were used (I [best] to III [worst]). Somewhat unconventionally, they also included experimental, nonclinical studies where there was proof of principle. The decision to place guidelines in each category of evidence was undertaken using DELPHI consensus where there had to be a minimum of 10 out of 11 reviewer agreements to be included. Areas where further research is indicated, categories II and II, were made clear. The 11 categories for guidelines were as follows: five local (wound perfusion, tissue viability, hematoma or seroma, infection, and mechanical factors) and six systemic (immunology, oncology, miscellaneous systemic factors, thermal injury, external agents, and excessive scarring). The guidelines are presented with strength of evidence in Table 1.

The huge amount of work presented in this guideline does not come with any authority to be

Table 1. *Impediments to acute wound healing that should be ruled out*

Level I strength of evidence
Arterial insufficiency (recognize and correct)
Hypotension and skin hypoperfusion (correct and consider local or systemic warming)
Presence of necrotic tissue, foreign material, and bioburden (debride using sharp, enzymatic, biological, or autolytic methods)
Hematoma or seroma (correct coagulopathy, ensure meticulous hemostasis, recognize prosthetic risk, avoid dead space, undertake early evacuation or drainage)
Contaminated wounds (consider avoidance of wound closure and encourage healing by secondary intention, but in clean wounds ensure primary closure, use of prosthetic material in hernia repair and suture technique must be optimal)
Inadequate antibiotic prophylaxis (needs rationalization and appropriate administration)
Inappropriate skin preparation (avoid inappropriate scrubbing or hair removal)
Systemic immune disease (needs maximal medical support)
Immunosuppressant therapy (needs minimization whenever possible)
Blood transfusion (keep to a minimum around the time of wounding)
Chemotherapy (maximize time between neoadjuvant therapy and wounding)
Radiotherapy (avoid irradiated tissue)
Cancer cachexia and malnutrition (recognize and give enteral supplementation)
Burn injury (excise eschar early and use advanced wound care dressings)
Burn injury (use skin substitutes appropriately)
Burn injury (cytokine and growth factors can accelerate epithelialization)
External agents (stop smoking)
Excessive scar formation (use silicone sheets, intralesional steroids)
Level II strength of evidence
Hyperbaric oxygen
Negative pressure therapy
Leucopenia (correction with GM-CSF or blood transfusion)
Optimization of blood glucose
Older patients
Obesity (consideration for elective surgery)
Burn injury (early excision and grafting at extremes of age or specific conditions)
Burn injury (use of topical antimicrobials)
Chronic corticosteroid use (minimize before surgery)
Exogenous vitamin use
Excessive scar formation (use of TGFβ, laser therapy, or postoperative radiotherapy)
Level III strength of evidence
Zinc deficiency (zinc supplements)
Excessive scar formation (attacking the collagen deposition–lysis equilibrium, *e.g.*, with vitamin E and lathrogens)

included as a mandatory exercise in clinical practice. It will be interesting to see if the Colleges of Surgeons and Nurses, Hospital Boards and Universities will do so. Some of the guidelines will be contentious.

3. Surgical site infection: prevention and treatment of surgical site infection
Clinical Guideline no.74. October 2008
National Institute of Health and Clinical Evidence (www.nice.org.uk)

This set of guidelines has been promulgated by a large group of societies and individuals from the United Kingdom. The National Institute of Health and Clinical Excellence in Great Britain commissioned the current document. It is an outstanding document that is available as a download. Several factors stand out in this document:

1. The comprehensiveness of the membership of the working group that included a wide variety of health care providers, state organizations, and specialists all involved in various aspects of health care, epidemiology, bacteriology, and surgical specialties.
2. The document is exhaustive in examining every aspect of the surgical continuum of care, from admission to perioperative holding area, from the intraoperative phase to the postoperative period. No aspect was considered too minute or trivial to examine and to provide evidence that would support interventions that could possibly affect societal developments.
3. Although clinical data are paramount, there is strong consideration given to economic factors, particularly when several factors are found to be of equal efficacy. This is novel and very helpful as most guidelines tend to not tackle such considerations.
4. Recommendations are made based on best available evidence, which is thoroughly reviewed and analyzed.

The document should be required reading for most health practitioners involved in surgical care.

Comments

Both sets of guidelines are state of the art and present cogent arguments for various effective interventions in the aim of reducing the incidence of SSI. There are differences between the UK and U.S. sets, but these differences are minor and should not detract from the main message, which is that all should be done to prevent SSI rather than have to treat. It would perhaps be desired for most busy clinicians if the full sets of guidelines were available as an abbreviated pocket document that would highlight in bullet point fashion the main recommendations, without providing the in-depth background materials. With efforts like this on both sides of the Atlantic, this is going to lead to improvements in health care and eradicating or minimizing the affects of SSI. It would be outstanding to see further international debate and comment, encouraged by respective governments, academic and professional bodies, and relevant societies, to enable definitions, surveillance, and guidelines to be optimized and universally agreed.

AUTHOR DISCLOSURE STATEMENT

Professor Leaper chaired the National Institute of Health and Clinical Excellence-UK (NICE) guideline and was a coauthor of the guideline published in *Wound Repair and Regeneration*. Professor Barbul led the review of these papers with agreement and deference to Professor Leaper.

Smoking and Postsurgical Wound Healing—An Update on Mechanisms and Biological Factors

Lars Tue Sørensen[1] and Finn Gottrup[2,*]

[1]Department of Surgery K, Bispebjerg University Hospital, Copenhagen, Denmark.
[2]Department of Dermatology S42, Copenhagen Wound Healing Center, Bispebjerg University Hospital, Copenhagen, Denmark.

Background: Delayed postsurgical healing and postoperative wound complications like tissue and wound dehiscence and surgical-site infection represent a major problem in surgery. A wide range of factors seem to affect the outcome of healing: (1) the patient's lifestyle and comorbidity, (2) disease characteristics, (3) the surgical procedure, and (4) the organizational setting.
The Problem: It is unclear why some patients develop postoperative wound infections and others do not after identical surgical procedures. Growth factors, metalloproteinases, and cytokines are probably involved, but because of the complexity of the healing processes, it is unresolved which biological factors may predict adverse wound events, monitor postoperative healing, and serve as targets for therapeutical intervention.
Basic/Clinical Science Advances: Smoking is now recognized as one of the most significant lifestyle factors for adverse wound events across the range of surgical specialties. Smoking has a temporary detrimental vasoactive effect on blood flow and tissue oxygen and a prolonged negative effect on collagen deposition and neutrophil oxidative killing mechanisms. Also, growth factors and metalloproteinases are affected. Recent evidence has demonstrated that nicotine has little or no effect on any of these mechanisms.
Clinical Care Relevance: Smoking cessation for a minimum of 4 weeks before surgery reduces postoperative wound infections, but is not enough to reverse the negative effect of smoking on tissue and wound dehiscence.
Conclusion: Considering smoking as a pathophysiologic model that delays healing and increases wound infection rate, biological markers of acute wound healing affected by smoking may appear to be valuable predictors for adverse wound events after surgery.

Abbreviations and Acronyms

ePTFE = expanded polytetrafluoroethylene

MMP = matrix metalloproteinase

*Correspondence: Department of Dermatology S42, Copenhagen Wound Healing Center, Bispebjerg University Hospital, Copenhagen, Denmark 2400 (e-mail: fgottrup@post4.tele.dk).

BACKGROUND

Surgical-site infections and delayed healing followed by tissue and wound dehiscence constitute a major problem in surgery resulting in reoperations, prolonged wound care, and hospitalization. As for other complications after surgery patient lifestyle appears to play a significant role. In the last decades increasing evidence has documented that smoking is a significant risk factor for the poor outcome of postsurgical wound healing. Accordingly, smokers have a higher incidence of surgical-site infections, wound disruption, anastomotic leakage, dental implant failure, and loss of tissue flaps.[1–4] The effects may also be seen months to years after surgery with incisional hernia and recurrence of inguinal hernia occurring more frequently in smokers.[5,6] However, not all studies find that smoking is associated with adverse wound events after surgery.[7] This is most often due to methodological flaws

Printed in U.S.A.
DOI: 10.1089/awc.2009.0134

and lack of adjustment for other risk factors for poor outcome of wound healing.

Many surgeons and health care professionals have until now believed that nicotine released from tobacco smoke is the primary mechanism for impaired healing in smokers. Due to the adreno-mediated stimulatory effect on the sympathetic nervous system, nicotine has been suggested as causative for smoking-induced reductions in blood flow and tissue oxygen resulting in reduced cellular functions and impaired wound healing.[8] However, recent evidence has changed this perception, suggesting that the impaired wound-healing mechanisms in smokers are more complex and that altered metabolic pathways and cellular functions seem to be involved.

CLINICAL PROBLEM ADDRESSED

The smoking prevalence in the Western world has decreased significantly for the past decades. However, still almost 20% of the adult population continue to smoke despite ongoing health campaigns and bans on smoking. In many developing countries, like China, the smoking prevalence increases and currently over 300 million people are smokers.[9] For this reason surgeons will continue to face patients who smoke and deal with smoking-related diseases and complications. From clinical studies of the association between smoking and postoperative wound complications, it has become obvious that the lifestyle and comorbidity of the patient also must be taken into consideration. Several studies indicate that smoking cessation 4 weeks before surgery reduces the incidence of wound infections, but seems not to be enough to decrease wound ruptures and dehiscence of sutured tissue.[10] Change of lifestyle is difficult and more evidence is needed before it is possible to say to which extent it may improve healing outcome for the individual patient.

Like other risk factors resulting in adverse wound events after surgery, it is not clear why some smokers develop postoperative wound complications and some don't after identical surgical procedures. Tools to monitor wound healing and predict the outcome are therefore needed to provide the optimal treatment for smokers and other patients for that matter. Biological factors like growth hormones, cytokines, proteinases, and adhesion molecules involved in acute wound healing may in theory be valuable to monitor wound healing and serve as indicators for healing outcome. However, due to the complexity of the wound-healing processes and the limitations of wound-healing models it remains unclear which biological markers are useful in the clinical setting.

BASIC SCIENCE CONTEXT

Various *in vitro* and animal wound-healing models have been used to describe the mechanisms for postoperative acute wound healing.[11] These include biological factors like growth hormones and cytokines and their specific effects and interactions on mobilization, proliferation, and activation of cell populations. In humans, the study of these complex processes has been made difficult due to ethical problems, but the use of human models is critical because of methodological problems when animal data have to be extrapolated to human reality. For this reason human models are increasingly used,[11] ranging from postsurgical epithelialization of skin donor sites, wound biopsies, postoperative accumulation of wound fluid, tissue deposition in implanted material (*e.g.*, expanded polytetrafluoroethylene [ePTFE], polypropylene) to studies of dynamic physiologic outcome measures (*e.g.*, blood flow, tissue oxygen tension, and metabolites).

Beyond doubt, the physiologic environment in which the cellular mechanisms take place plays an immense role for the wound-healing processes.[12] Adequate blood supply, tissue oxygen tension, temperature and hydration, and nutritional status constitute the basic fundament for normal wound healing. The importance of many of these factors has been clarified in studies of animals and healthy individuals, and most of the surgical and anesthetic procedures aim to optimize these factors for successful outcome. Yet, in patients who suffer from chronic diseases or have an unhealthy lifestyle the fundament for normal wound healing may be significantly altered.

EXPERIMENTAL MODEL OR MATERIAL—ADVANTAGES AND LIMITATIONS

In a recent study, an experimental human model was applied to examine the immediate physiologic response to nicotine infusion and cigarette smoking. Blood flow of the skin and subcutis, tissue oxygen, and metabolic markers were recorded to clarify the role of nicotine in the pathophysiologic mechanisms of smoking-induced impaired wound healing.[13] Nicotine infused intravenously had a temporary effect by increasing skin blood flow marginally and decreasing subcutaneous blood flow. Surprisingly, tissue oxygen tension increased and no effect on metabolic markers was found. In contrast, smoking of one cigarette decreased blood flow, tissue oxygen, and aerobe metabolism for a

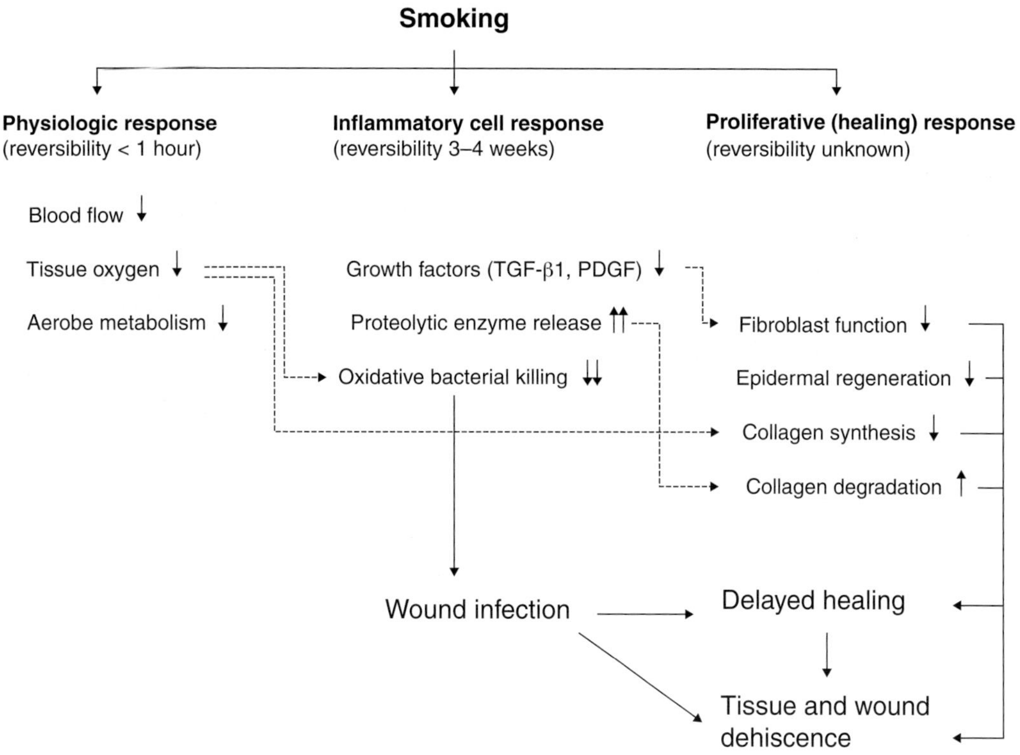

Figure 1. Overview of the major mechanisms involved in the detrimental effect of smoking on wound healing. An immediate physiologic response (reversible after less than 1 h) reduces blood flow, tissue oxygen, and aerobe metabolism. An inflammatory cell response (reversible after 3–4 weeks) reduces oxidative killing mechanisms and growth factors, and increases proteolytic enzymes release. A proliferative healing response (reversibility unknown) reduces fibroblast function, epidermal regeneration, and collagen synthesis, and increases collagen degradation. These mechanisms may exclusively or combined lead to wound infection, delayed healing, and tissue and wound dehiscence.

period of 45 min, thus confirming previous reports.[8] No difference was found between smokers and ex-smokers, suggesting that the vasoactive effect of smoking is temporary and reversible and that no prolonged detrimental effects of smoking on blood flow, tissue oxygen, and metabolism of the skin and subcutis exists (Fig. 1).

These findings have made it clear that previous reports of experimental studies of the acute effect of smoking have been limited. Only a few have studied nicotine *per se*, whereas some have extrapolated from pharmacologic nicotine studies to suggest that nicotine was the primary mediator of the vasoactive effect of smoking.[8] Besides a few studies of nicotine applied to fibroblast cultures showing a detrimental effect on cell proliferation, nicotine applied in human and some animal wound-healing models have not been found to impair wound healing. In contrast, recent studies have found that nicotine appears to stimulate collagen synthesis and other wound-healing parameters.[14,15] Further, clinical studies have found that nicotine replacement drugs used by abstinent smokers do not impose a higher risk of adverse wound events after surgery.[9]

DISCUSSION OF FINDINGS AND RELEVANT LITERATURE

Clinical observations of postoperative wound healing and adverse wound events in relation to the surgical procedure and the patient's disease characteristics, lifestyle, and comorbidity are necessary to make the understanding of human wound healing comprehensive and guide the basic research performance. However, biological factors involved in the underlying wound-healing processes may also be used to monitor healing and eventually predict outcome.

In a recent study of postmastectomy wound fluid a number of biological markers of early postoperative healing were assessed.[16] The quantitative and temporal profiles of growth factors, cytokines, and metalloproteinases during the first postoperative days showed a complex picture of the inflammatory phase of wound healing. Interestingly, platelet-derived growth factor level in wound fluid on the first postoperative day was a significant predictor of wound infection, whereas other growth factors studied were not associated with outcome. The proinflammatory cytokines interleukin-6 and tumor necrosis factor alpha and matrix metalloproteinases (MMP)-2, (MMP)-8, and (MMP)-9 have in other studies been shown to play an important role in the early inflammatory phase of wound healing and predict outcome.[17] As an intermediate indicator for the outcome of healing, we previously found that collagen deposition in an ePTFE wound-healing model was inversely correlated with MMP-9 levels in postherniotomy wound fluid.[18]

In a recent study, we studied suction blister fluid retrieved from never smokers, smokers, and abstinent smokers.[19] Neutrophil collagenase (MMP-8) was significantly associated with smoking, showing a twofold higher level in smokers compared to never smokers. Four weeks of abstinence from smoking normalized MMP-8 levels. Interestingly, MMP-8 was linearly correlated with neutrophil blood count, suggesting that the effect of smoking on MMP-8 has an immunomodulatory origin. This finding implies that not only local factors like tissue perfusion and oxygen levels but also general pathophysiologic mechanisms are affected by smoking. This is in line with other studies that have found that the systemic neutrophil and mononuclear cell function is significantly altered by smoking.[20] Smoking enhances the chemotactic responsiveness by many-fold and attenuates the oxidative killing mechanisms (Fig. 1). These mechanisms may generate smokers' higher postoperative wound infection rate and the apparent higher connective tissue turnover, which may explain the higher incidence of abdominal aorta aneurisms, paradontosis, face wrinkling, and pulmonary emphysema as found in smokers.[21–24]

Not only inflammation but also the proliferative mechanisms of wound healing appear to be affected by smoking. Deposition of collagen in a subcutaneously implanted ePTFE wound-healing model has been found to be impaired in smokers.[25] Also, epidermal healing appears to be impaired.[19] In a model of epidermal wounds, transepidermal water loss, which is inversely correlated with the stratum corneum barrier function, was studied in never smokers, smokers, and abstinent smokers. The epidermal wounds of smokers healed significantly slower than the wound of never smokers. Up to 3 months of abstinence from smoking did not affect healing, as the wounds of abstinent smoker showed the same course of healing as the smokers' wounds (Fig. 1).

CAUTION, CRITICAL REMARKS, AND RECOMMENDATIONS

Studies of basic wound-healing mechanisms using *in vitro* and animal models are essential but cannot stand alone since the complex processes of healing in humans make it difficult to assess the significance of these biological factors in relation to patient outcome.

The study of wound-healing mechanisms and research in pathophysiologic mechanisms underlying the higher wound complication rate associated with smoking, lifestyle, and comorbidities must embrace various human wound-healing models to clarify the relevant aspects of healing for outcome. As exemplified by studies of nicotine and smoking not one model can stand-alone. Biological factors related to the inflammatory and proliferative phases of healing have been identified as being affected by smoking. Wound fluid appears to provide a good model for the study of biological factors involved in postoperative wound healing, although the significance of the underlying disease, that is, cancer, is unknown.[16]

TAKE-HOME MESSAGE

Basic science advances

- Smoking decreases blood flow, tissue oxygen, and aerobe metabolism in the skin and subcutis.
- Nicotine increases tissue oxygen and cannot explain the detrimental effect of smoking on wound healing.
- Smoking impairs inflammatory processes by altering the function of neutrophils and mononuclear cells.
- Smoking decreases collagen production and increases connective tissue turnover.

Clinical science advances

- Smokers have more postsurgical wound infections than never smokers.
- Smokers have more disruptions of sutured tissue and wounds than never smokers.
- Abstinence from smoking for 4 weeks reduces wound infections, but is not enough to reduce wound and tissue dehiscence.

Relevance to clinical care

- Smokers are more likely to have adverse wound events after surgery and the patient's lifestyle has to be taken into consideration. Smoking cessation reduces wound infections, but it is unclear if other aspects of healing are improved. Biological markers of the wound-healing processes may in the future be valuable to monitor healing and predict outcome. For example, platelet-derived growth factor in postmastectomy wound fluid was significantly associated with wound infection. Markers of tissue physiology or collagen turnover like procollagens and MMPs may prove to be valuable as well, but the feasibility in the postoperative observation of wound healing needs still to be established.

FUTURE DEVELOPMENT

Human studies that aim to assess the association of biologic markers like growth hormones, cytokines, and proteinases with the clinical outcome of wound healing are essential. Considering smoking as a pathophysiologic model that delays healing and increases wound infection rate, biological markers of acute wound healing that are affected by smoking may appear to be valuable predictors for adverse wound events in patients with other types of hazardous lifestyle and comorbidities.

More, well-designed, good-quality human studies relevant to the clinician that combine the study of biologic markers of healing and clinical outcome are needed. Such studies may clarify which biologic factors may serve as useful indicators of successful healing to provide knowledge for prevention of adverse wound-healing events and to move the science of wound care forward.

AUTHOR DISCLOSURE STATEMENT

No conflict of interest disclosed.

REFERENCES

1. Klokkevold PR and Han TJ: How do smoking, diabetes, and periodontitis affect outcomes of implant treatment? Int J Oral Maxillofac Implants 2007; **22 Suppl:** 173.
2. Sorensen LT, Hemmingsen U, Kallehave F, Wille-Jorgensen P, Kjaergaard J, Moller LN, *et al.*: Risk factors for tissue and wound complications in gastrointestinal surgery. Ann Surg 2005; **241:** 654.
3. Nickelsen TN, Jorgensen T, and Kronborg O: Lifestyle and 30-day complications to surgery for colorectal cancer. Acta Oncol 2005; **44:** 218.
4. Spear SL, Ducic I, Cuoco F, and Hannan C: The effect of smoking on flap and donor-site complications in pedicled TRAM breast reconstruction. Plast Reconstr Surg 2005; **116:** 1873.
5. Sorensen LT, Hemmingsen UB, Kirkeby LT, Kallehave F, and Jorgensen LN: Smoking is a risk factor for incisional hernia. Arch Surg 2005; **140:** 119.
6. Sorensen LT, Friis E, Jorgensen T, Vennits B, Andersen BR, Rasmussen GI, *et al.*: Smoking is a risk factor for recurrence of groin hernia. World J Surg 2002; **26:** 397.
7. Dixon AJ, Dixon MP, Dixon JB, and Del Mar CB: Prospective study of skin surgery in smokers vs. nonsmokers. Br J Dermatol 2009; **160:** 365.
8. Jensen JA, Goodson WH, Hpf HW, and Hunt TK: Cigarette smoking decreases tissue oxygen. Arch Surg 1991; **126:** 1131.
9. Mackay J, Eriksen M, and Shafey O: *The Tobacco Atlas* (2nd edition). Atlanta: American Cancer Society, 2006.
10. Sørensen LT, Karlsmark T, and Gottrup F: Abstinence from smoking reduces incisional wound infection: a randomized controlled trial. Ann Surg 2003; **238:** 1.
11. Gottrup F, Agren MS, and Karlsmark T: Models for use in wound healing research: a survey focusing on *in vitro* and *in vivo* adult soft tissue. Wound Repair Regen 2000; **8:** 83.
12. Hunt TK, Hopf HW, and Hussain Z: Physiology of wound healing. Adv Skin Wound Care 2000; **13(2 Suppl):** 6.
13. Sørensen LT, Jørgensen S, Petersen LJ, Hemmingsen U, Bülow J, Loft S, and Gottrup F: Acute effects of nicotine and smoking on blood flow, tissue oxygen, and aerobe metabolism of the skin and subcutis. J Surg Res 2009; **152:** 224.
14. Sørensen LT, Jorgensen LN, Zillmer R, Vange J, Hemmingsen U, and Gottrup F: Transdermal nicotine patch enhances type I collagen synthesis in abstinent smokers. Wound Repair Regen 2006; **14:** 247.
15. Jacobi J, Jang JJ, Sundram U, Dayoub H, Fajardo LF, and Cooke JP: Nicotine accelerates angiogenesis and wound healing in genetically diabetic mice. Am J Pathol 2002; **161:** 97.
16. Baker EA, Kumar S, Melling AC, Wetter D, and Leaper DJ: Temporal and quantitative profiles of growth factors and metalloproteinases in acute wound fluid after mastectomy. Wound Repair Regen 2008; **16:** 95.
17. Loo WTY, Sasano H, and Chow LWC: Pro-inflammatory cytokine, matrix metalloproteinases and TIMP-1 are involved in wound healing after mastectomy in invasive breast cancer patients. Biomed Pharmacol 2007; **61:** 548.
18. Agren MS, Jorgensen LN, Andersen M, Viljanto J, and Gottrup F: Matrix metalloproteinase 9 level predicts optimal collagen deposition during early wound repair in humans. Br J Surg 1998; **85:** 68.
19. Sørensen LT, Zillmer R, Ågren M, Ladelund S, Karlsmark T, and Gottrup F: Effect of smoking, abstention and nicotine patch on epidermal healing and collagenase in skin transudate. Wound Rep Reg 2009; **17:** 347.
20. Sørensen LT, Nielsen HB, Kharazmi A, and Gottrup F: Effect of smoking and abstention on oxidative burst and reactivity of neutrophils and monocytes. Surgery 2004; **136:** 1047.
21. Abboud RT and Vimalanathan S: Pathogenesis of COPD. Part I. The role of protease-antiprotease imbalance in emphysema. Int J Tuberc Lung Dis 2008; **12:** 361.
22. Derubertis BG, Trocciola SM, Ryer EJ, Pieracci FM, McKinsey JF, Faries PL, *et al.*: Abdominal aortic aneurysm in women: prevalence, risk factors, and implications for screening. J Vasc Surg 2007; **46:** 630.
23. Taybos G: Oral changes associated with tobacco use. Am J Med Sci 2003; **326:** 179.
24. Freiman A, Bird G, Metelitsa AI, Barankin B, and Lauzon GJ: Cutaneous effects of smoking. J Cutan Med Surg 2004; **8:** 415.
25. Jorgensen LN, Kallehave F, Christensen E, Siana JE, and Gottrup F: Less collagen production in smokers. Surgery 1998; **123:** 450.

WHS Wound Healing Society

Pilonidal Sinus: Healing by Primary Closure Versus Open Healing Surgery

Luc Téot* and Pascal Granier

Burns and Plastic Surgery Unit, Montpellier University Hospital, Montpellier, France.

Abbreviation and Acronym

NR = not reported

*Correspondence: Burns and Plastic Surgery Unit, Hôpital Lapeyronie, 371 Avenue Doyen Giraud 34295 Montpellier cedex 5, France (e-mail: lteot@aol.com).

Background: Twenty-six out of 10,000 young adults were found to have pilonidal sinus. Pain, chronic abcess, and psychological disorders are more pronounced when the rate of recurrence is higher. Open healing versus midline and off-midline technique has been proposed. In this review, a comparison of two techniques is proposed.

The Problem: Open healing technique after extensive debridement of the inverted hair and the surrounding abcess in the fold offers a better guarantee concerning recurrence, but time to closure is higher than when using midline or off-midline immediate surgical closure.

Basic/Clinical Science Advances: A systematic review and a meta-analysis of trials was developed on healing by primary closure versus open healing after surgery of pilonidal sinus.

Clinical Care Relevance: The pilonidal sinus surgical cure needs to remove as completely as possible the inverted hair subcutaneous pouch, and to heal the wound as fast as possible, and to prevent recurrence. In a recent article published in the British Medical Journal, McCallum *et al.* presented a systematic review and meta-analysis of articles comparing healing by primary closure versus open healing after surgery of pilonidal sinus, following the Cochrane register of controlled trials. Included trials compared two or more surgical techniques on patients aged 14 years or more.

Conclusion: The authors concluded that wounds heal more quickly after primary closure than after open healing but at the expense of increased risk of recurrence. Off-midline closure should become the standard management for pilonidal sinus when closure is the desired surgical option.

BACKGROUND

Pilonidal sinus is a disease that may concern emergency physicians, general surgeons, plastic surgeons, nurses, and wound care specialists. The incidence rate is 26 per 100,000 and it touches deeply the young males and females from 14 years of age. This painful disease is a source of chronic pain for young adults.[1]

The most common etiology is referring to an inverted folliculitis of the natal cleft of the sacrococcygeal zone, issuing to a chronic purulent wound that includes a hair follicle. Pilonidal sinuses may appear as asymptomatic, or as an acute abcess. Recurrent purulent formation is a usual characteritics of the disease, issuing to a difficult management, often source of the problems.

The aim of the treatment is ideally to remove the inverted hair to heal the wound without ongoing complications. The morphology of the buttocks, the skin biomechanic around this fold-like shearing forces, and grinding makes this area more problematic in terms of mechanical stress, an obstacle to healing.

Printed in U.S.A.
DOI: 10.1089/awc.2009.0181

The usual surgical strategy is to largely excise an inflamed area around the abcess, and to leave it open and progressively closing by spontaneous healing, or to close it directly using a midline or an off-midline incision by means of rotation flap.[2–5] Other procedures include curettage of tracts and phenol injections.

In a recent article published in the British Medical Journal, McCallum *et al.*[6] developed a systematic review and a meta-analysis of trials on healing by primary closure versus open healing after surgery of pilonidal sinus.

EXPERIMENTAL MODEL OR MATERIAL

Pilonidal sinus poses the problem of a chronic purulent disease occuring in an adolescent or a young adult, and localized on a very sensitive area, the sacrococcygeal fold. This disease is psychologically devastating, because of repetitive surgical complications leading to chronicity at an age when relationship to others and intimacy are real issues. The permanent purulent discharge is the source of chronic pain, aggravating the poor self-esteem; surgery is seen by the patient as a saving technique, but unfortunately many complications will render the final closure dificult to obtain.

Several opposite solutions have been proposed and extensively used, like debriding abcess and the inverted hair area, the wound being left opened, others advocating the use of closing procedures, either leaving a scar longitudinally located in the fold or realizing a rotation flap with an off-side incision.

Open technique

The surgical excision with a wound left opened to spontaneous healing was advocated some decades ago, when poor hygienic conditions were still observed in some communities. Arguments in favor of this technique are that no tension is exerted over the wound edges, with a lower recurrence rate.

Primary closure technique

Primary closure techniques using midline incision were also popularized, with a consistent rate of postoperative complications. The midline technique removes in the same procedure the pits, the abcess, and the hair follicle entrapped in it.

Primary closure using the off-midline incisions was recently developed, like the rhomboid or limberg flaps. These techniques are more demanding in terms of training in reconstructive surgery. The rotation flap was initially designed for recurrent sinuses. It is a large well-vascularized flap. The technique avoids a midline incision. The midline pits and the small epithelial tissue annexed to it are removed. The procedure can be applied either under local or general anesthesia.

CLINICAL PROBLEM ADDRESSED

The pilonidal sinus poses two different problems for the surgeon, one of them being the need to remove as completely as possible the inverted hair subcutaneous pouch, the other, more difficult to get, is to heal the wound as fast as possible, keeping in mind to prevent recurrence.

Strategy should be determined with a perfect knowledge of the main surgical procedures, their respective advantages and complications, to excise the whole sinus tract, obtain a complete healing, and prevent recurrence.

In a recent article published in the British Medical Journal, McCallum *et al.* presented a systematic review and meta-analysis of articles comparing healing by primary closure versus open healing after surgery of pilonidal sinus, following the Cochrane register of controlled trials.

The aim of this article was to determine the relative effects of open healing compared with the primary closure and optimal closure method, using randomized control trials already published withdrawn from the Cochrane register of controlled trials, Cochrane Wounds Group specialized trials register (2006), Medline (1950–2007) Embase (1980–2006), and CINAHL (1982–2006) databases, without language restrictions. Included trials compared two or more surgical techniques on patients aged 14 years or more.

The authors concluded that wounds heal more quickly after primary closure than after open healing but at the expense of increased risk of recurrence. Benefits were clearly shown with off-midline closure compared with midline closure. Off-midline closure should become the standard management of pilonidal sinus when closure is the desired surgical option.

BASIC SCIENCE CONTEXT

Pilonidal sinus can be considered difficult to heal surgical situation where several obstacles exist, which impair closure of the wound, like the nature of the skin fold, submitted to an intense mechanical stress related to the movements of the powerful buttock muscles. Tendency to enlarge is the usual way of any wound observed in this area (also observed in sacral pressure ulcer). This pressure is majored on the midline, and any surgical incision parallel to the fold will lead to disunion.

Table 1. *Time to wound healing using open healing compared with midline closure techniques*

	Sample Size		Time (days) to Wound Healing			
Study	Open Healing	Midline Closure	Open Healing	Midline Closure	*p*-Value	Result Format
Gencosmanoglu	73	69	79 (21–112)	14 (14–63)	<0.001	Median
Kronborg	33	32	64 (17–157)	13 (7–203)	NR	Median
Rao	30	29	61 (34–132)	27 (24–68)	<0.001	Median
Khawaja	23	23	41NR	14NR	NR	Median
Al-Hassan	40	42	91 (28–546)	10 (10–15)	NR	Mean
Sondenaa	59	60	70 (28–266)	14 (14-11)	<0.001	Median
Hameeed	20	23	70 (59–91)	15 (12–21)	<0.05	Mean

NR = not reported.

During pilonidal sinus excision, a subsequent amount of tissue should be resected to completely remove the inverted hair and the surrounding fibrotic "capsule." This relatively long, deep to the fascia and large loss of tissue contributes to increase the rate of postoperative complications. The tendency for recurrence is mainly due to an insufficient packing with well-vascularized tissue of the surgically induced wound.

TAKE-HOME MESSAGE

Clinical science advance

Pilonidal sinus heals more quickly after off-midline closure than with any other method, but the rate of recurrence is higher. Available data suggest that off-midline closure should become the standard of care for pilonidal sinus (Fig. 1).

Basic science advances

Evidence is still lacking as to whether open healing or primary closure methods should be used.

Since the last decade deep cavity wounds are treated using many different techniques. The need to transpose some of them to the pilonidal sinus, located in a problematic perineal zone, has to be experimented.

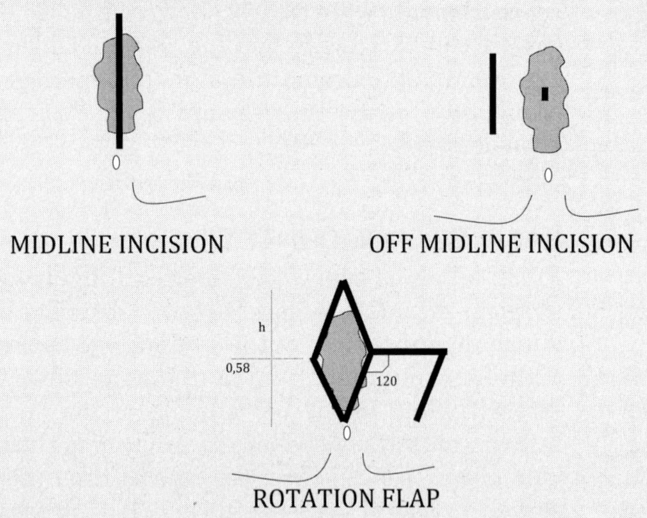

Figure 1. Possible techniques used in pilonidal sinus surgery.

DISCUSSION OF FINDINGS AND RELEVANT LITERATURE

The objectives of McCallum *et al.*[6] were to determine the relative effects of open healing compared with the primary closure for pilonidal sinus and optimal closure methods.

In the 18 selected trials, primary outcomes were time to healing, infection of the surgical site, and recurrence rate.

Data were extracted independently by two reviewers. Eighteen randomized control trials were included ($n = 1573$).

Closed intervention was defined as midline closure (inside the natal cleft) or off-midline if located outside the natal cleft. Marsupialization or open wound healing were realized if wound edges were not closed at the end of the intervention.

Of the 1367 potentially relevant trials, 45 were reviewed for full critical appraisal. Eighteen were included in the review; 12 trials compared open healing with primary closure (Table 1). Time to healing was quicker after primary closure, but the recurrence rate was more pronounced in this group. In six trials, surgical closure and midline versus off-midline methods were compared. The postoperative period for midline closure was longer in midline incisions, than in off-midline incisions.

Time to wound healing was compared, even if in the trials describing open technique, some inconsistencies in reporting the data were noted. Four trials reported significant statistical differences when practising primary closure.

When comparing midline closure versus off-midline closure, it was noted that midline wounds took significantly longer to heal than off-midline rhomboid flaps.

When comparing the rate of surgical site infection, no statistical differences could be found between open healing and primary closure.

When comparing midline versus off-midline techniques, rate of post-operative infections were higher (statistically significant) when using midline techniques, and a trial comparing modified rhomboid flap versus classic one was in favor of the modified rhomboid flap (less infection).

Recurrence rate was commonly reported. Meta-analysis indicated that the open healing of pilonidal sinus is the source of lower risk of recurrence than primary closure (58% less).

Midline versus off-midline closure recurrence rate was higher after midline closure.

When analyzing time to return to work, patients undergoing open procedures took longer time to return to work than with midline closure, whatever be the method of closure.

Other items like patient satisfaction and length of hospital stay were analyzed and compared.

Pain was less after techniques closing primarily the skin in three studies, but in two others, pain was not statistically different when open versus closed surgery was practiced.

Wound healing rate was comparable in all the studies.

The authors concluded that after surgery wounds healed more quickly when primary closure was used, but the risk of recurrence is higher than with open healing. Recurrence of pilonidal sinus was noted more common with midline closure (11.7%).

Open wounds took longer to heal than closed wounds, and this reflects the other outcomes such as the length of hospital stay and time taken to return to work.

It is generally accepted that open healing leads to a lower rate of infection at surgical sites, but this review does not conclude in this direction. When surgeons opt for excision and primary closure, a significant benefit was found when the incision was off-midline. The rates of infection (10.4% vs. 6.3%) and recurrence (1.4% vs. 10.3%) were lower when using this technique.

Due to the existence of possible bias, the conclusions should be cautiously analyzed. Important outcomes like the rate of infection and recurrence are not reported systematically in the analyzed trials. Standardization was lacking, and late recurrence was not reported (after 4 years).

AUTHOR DISCLOSURE STATEMENT

No competing financial interests exist.

REFERENCES

1. Sondenaa K, Andersen E, Nesvik I, and Soreide JA: Patient characteristics and symptoms in chronic pilonidal sinus disease. Int J Colorectal Dis 1995; **10:** 39.
2. Petersen S, Koch R, Stelzner S, Wendlandt T, and Ludwig K: Primary closure techniques in chronic pilonidal sinus: a survey of results of different surgical approaches. Dis Colon Rectum 2002; **45:** 1458.
3. Acartürk TO, Parsak CK, Sakman G, and Demircan O: Superior gluteal artery perforator flap in the reconstruction of pilonidal sinus. J Plast Reconstr Aesthet Surg 2008. Int J Colorectal Dis 1995; **10:** 39–42.
4. Başterzi Y, Canbaz H, Aksoy A, Sar A, Türkmenoğlu MO, and Cağlkülekçi M: Reconstruction of extensive pilonidal sinus defects with the use of S-GAP flaps. Ann Plast Surg 2008; **61:** 197.
5. Darwish AM, and Hassanin A: Reconstruction following excision of sacrococcygeal pilonidal sinus with a perforator-based fasciocutaneous limberg flap. J Plast Reconstr Aesthet Surg 2009. J Plast Reconstr Aesthet Surg 2008; Nov 13.
6. McCallum I, King PM, and Bruce J: Healing by primary versus secondary intention after surgical treatment for pilonidal sinus. Cochrane Database Syst Rev 2007; **4:** CD006213. Doi: 10.1002/14651858.CDoo6213.pub 2.
7. Higgins JPT, and Green S (eds): Cochrane Handbook for Systematic Reviews of Interventions Version 4.2.5 [updated May 2005]. The Cochrane Collaboration, 2005. www.cochrane-handbook.org

WHS
Wound
Healing
Society

Honey as a Topical Treatment for Wounds

Zena Elizabeth Helen Moore*

Faculty of Nursing and Midwifery, Royal College of Surgeons in Ireland, Dublin, Ireland.

Abbreviations and Acronyms

CI = confidence interval

RCT = randomized controlled trial

*Correspondence: Faculty of Nursing and Midwifery, Royal College of Surgeons in Ireland, 123 St. Stephens Green, Dublin, Ireland D2 (e-mail: zmoore@rcsi.ie).

Background: The interest in the use of honey as a topical wound treatment has received a great deal of attention over the past 10 years. However, as yet the exact role of honey in wound healing has to be clarified.
The Problem: The optimal method of covering acute and chronic wounds remains an elusive goal. The aim of the review was to determine the effects of honey on wound healing in both acute and chronic wounds.
Basic/Clinical Science Advances: Honey is a viscous, supersaturated sugar solution derived from nectar gathered and modified by the honeybee, *Apis mellifera*. Evidence from animal studies and human studies suggested that honey may accelerate wound healing. A previous systematic review had been undertaken; however, since then, further evidence had emerged. The authors of the original review had no plans to conduct an update. Therefore, Jull *et al.*[1] argue that an updated review of the evidence was necessary.
Clinical Care Relevance: Honey may improve healing times in mild to moderate superficial and partial thickness burns compared with some conventional dressings. Honey significantly improved healing and debridement outcomes in larger, longer duration, sloughy venous ulcers compared with a hydrogel, whereas little effect seems evident on small, short duration venous ulcers that would likely heal with adequate compression independent of dressing.
Conclusion: Outside the management of burn injuries and longer duration, sloughy venous ulcers, there is currently insufficient evidence to guide practice regarding the use of honey. However, randomized controlled trials are not the only form of evidence, and the selection of the most appropriate methodology for a study will depend on the question being asked.

BACKGROUND

THE INTEREST IN the use of honey as a topical wound treatment has received a great deal of attention over the past 10 years. Indeed, Jull *et al.*[1] argue that there are over 40 case reports or series in 875 patients published in December 2006. However, the exact role of honey in wound healing has yet to be clarified. Therefore, Jull *et al.*[1] describe a systematic review undertaken to explore whether honey increases the rate of healing in acute wounds (burns, lacerations, and other traumatic wounds) and chronic wounds (venous ulcers, arterial ulcers, diabetic ulcers, pressure ulcers, and infected surgical wounds). This article provides a review and critique of the systematic review.

CLINICAL PROBLEM ADDRESSED

Wounding can occur for a multiplicity of different reasons, for example, physical, mechanical, or thermal damage, or indeed due to some underlying physiological or medical disorder.[2] Wounds also affect a wide variety of people, all with their own unique set of circumstances, including both physical and psychosocial dimensions.[3] The

ADVANCES IN WOUND CARE, VOLUME 1

Printed in U.S.A.
DOI: 10.1089/awc.2009.0172

variety of wounds seen in any clinical setting is enormous. For the purpose of clarity these wounds may be broadly divided into acute and chronic wounds. Acute wounds are those which generally progress through the wound-healing process unhindered. Chronic wounds include pressure ulcers, leg ulcers, and diabetic foot ulcers. These wounds may be described as those which fail to progress through the wound-healing process at a rate that would be expected from a wound of similar depth and tissue loss.[4]

The optimal method of covering acute and chronic wounds remains an elusive goal. Although methods of wound coverage have been described since biblical times, the evolution of technology and biological understanding has been slow. The current paradigm of maintaining a moist wound environment to maximally enhance reepithelialization represents just a beginning. The ideal wound coverage should conform to the wound shape, provide pain and odor control, be nonallergenic and nonirritating, be permeable to gas (oxygen primarily), be safe, nontraumatic, convenient and lastly, but not least, cost effective. Clearly technology that meets all these desired endpoints is lacking.

The aim of this review was to determine the effects of honey on wound healing in both acute and chronic wounds. The primary outcomes of interest were the time to complete wound healing and the proportion of participants with completely healed wounds. The secondary outcomes of interest were the incidence of adverse events, length of hospital stay, change in wound size, incidence of infection, cost, and quality of life.

RELEVANT BASIC SCIENCE CONTEXT

Honey is a viscous, supersaturated sugar solution derived from nectar gathered and modified by the honeybee, *Apis mellifera*.[1] Honey is composed of glucose, fructose, sucrose, and water.[1] Honey also contains other substances, such as amino acids, vitamins, minerals, and enzymes.[1] Honey is not a modern treatment for the management of wounds; there is documented evidence of the use of honey since ancient Egyptian times.[1] Over the past decade there has been a growth in the interest in the use of honey as a topical wound treatment. Evidence from animal studies and human studies suggested that honey may accelerate wound healing. A previous systematic review had been undertaken;[5] however, since then, further evidence had emerged. The authors of the original review had no plans to conduct an update. Therefore, Jull *et al.*[1] argue that an updated review of the evidence was necessary.

EXPERIMENTAL MODEL OR MATERIAL—ADVANTAGES AND LIMITATIONS

Randomized controlled trials (RCTs) and quasi-RCTs involving participants of any age, with an acute wound healing by primary or secondary intention, or chronic wound healing by secondary intention, were included. The primary intervention was any honey topically applied by any means, alone or in combination with other dressing components, to the wound. Comparison interventions were dressings or other topical agents applied to the wound.

Nineteen trials met the inclusion criteria. Twelve of the trials recruited participants with acute wounds, nine with burns, two with minor surgical excisions, and one with minor trauma. Six of the trials recruited participants with chronic wounds, one with infected surgical wounds, one with pressure ulcers, one with Fournier's gangrene, and two with leg ulcers. Two trials recruited participants with mixed groups of chronic or acute wounds.

In acute wounds, honey may reduce time to healing compared with some conventional dressings in partial thickness burns (weighted mean difference 4.68 days; 95% confidence interval [CI] 4.28–5.09 days). In chronic wounds, honey in addition to compression bandaging did not significantly increase healing in venous leg ulcers (relative risk 1.15; 95% CI 0.96–1.38). There was insufficient evidence to determine the effect of honey compared with other treatments for burns or in other acute or chronic wound types.

The authors[1] therefore conclude that honey may improve healing times in mild to moderate superficial and partial thickness burns compared with some conventional dressings. Honey dressings as an adjuvant to compression did not significantly increase leg ulcer healing at 12 weeks. While there is insufficient evidence for a significant increase in venous ulcer healing at 12 weeks, a modest effect of honey on larger, longer duration, sloughy venous ulcers merits further research. There was insufficient evidence to guide clinical practice in other areas.

DISCUSSION OF FINDINGS AND RELEVANT LITERATURE

The use of objective outcome measures such as the time to complete wound healing or the proportion of participants with completely healed wounds is considered an important quality marker. The rationale for this is that there is a wide margin of error in the use of subjective outcome measures such as ease of use, comfort, or improvement in wound bed condition. However, wound-healing rates may not always be expected to differ between groups. For example, Jull *et al.*[1] identified that honey dressings used alongside compression therapy did not significantly increase leg ulcer healing at 12 weeks. This is unsurprising, as compression therapy is the mainstay of treatment for individuals with venous leg ulceration.[6] There is no evidence that dressings influence the rate of ulcer healing,[7] and recommendations from The Royal College of Nursing (United Kingdom) are that in combination with compression therapy, simple low-adherent dressings should be used.[8] One of the studies included by Jull *et al.*[1] was that of Gethin and Cowman[9] whose primary aim was to compare the desloughing efficacy of honey versus gel in individuals with venous ulcers. This aim appears more clinically applicable, because, although compression therapy is the mainstay of treatment, one must still manage the local wound condition to move toward wound healing. In wounds with slough present, the objective would be to remove the slough to promote the production of granulation tissue as demonstrated by Gethin and Cowman.[9]

The Cochrane review derives a conclusion of "no significant effect of honey on ulcer healing at 12 weeks" by combining two studies that should not have been combined due to *a priori* heterogeneity based on: (1) The Cochrane review combines previous own study Jull *et al.*[1] on small, short duration venous ulcers with that of Gethin and Cowman[9] on larger, longer duration, sloughy venous ulcers. (2) The analyzed Jull *et al.*[1] study had a control of usual practice more variable than the more rigorous gel control study by Gethin and Cowman.[9] (3) The treatment duration differed for the two studies.

TAKE-HOME MESSAGE

Basic science advances

- Honey is a viscous, supersaturated sugar solution derived from nectar gathered and modified by the honeybee, *A. mellifera.*
- Honey is composed of glucose, fructose, sucrose, and water. Honey also contains other substances, such as amino acids, vitamins, minerals, and enzymes.
- Honey is not a modern treatment for the management of wounds; there is documented evidence of the use of honey since ancient Egyptian times.
- Evidence from animal studies and human studies suggested that honey may accelerate wound healing.

Clinical science advances

- In acute wounds, honey may reduce time to healing compared with some conventional dressings in partial thickness burns (weighted mean difference 4.68 days; 95% CI 4.28–5.09 days).
- In chronic wounds, honey in addition to compression bandaging did not significantly increase healing in venous leg ulcers (relative risk 1.15; 95% CI 0.96–1.38). While there is insufficient evidence for a significant increase in venous ulcer healing at 12 weeks, a modest effect of honey on larger, longer duration, sloughy venous ulcers merits further research.
- There is insufficient evidence to determine the effect of honey compared with other treatments for burns or in other acute or chronic wound types.

Relevance to clinical care

- Honey may improve healing times in mild to moderate superficial and partial thickness burns compared with some conventional dressings.
- In the management of uncomplicated venous leg ulceration, compression therapy is the mainstay of treatment; however, one must still manage the local wound condition to move toward wound healing.
- RCTs are not the only form of evidence, and the selection of the most appropriate methodology for a study will depend on the question being asked.

CAUTION, CRITICAL REMARKS, AND RECOMMENDATIONS

Jull *et al.*[1] have completed a systematic review exploring the effect of honey on the healing rate of acute and chronic wounds. They conclude that honey may improve healing times in mild to moderate superficial and partial thickness burns compared with some conventional dressings. Further, honey dressings as an adjuvant to compression did not significantly increase leg ulcer healing at 12 weeks. However, honey significantly improved healing and debridement outcomes in larger, longer duration, sloughy venous ulcers compared with a hydrogel. Thus, their overall conclusion is that there is insufficient evidence to guide clinical practice for the use of honey in other areas.

It is important to consider the findings from this review in terms of the studies included. Fundamentally, this review has only included RCT evidence and as such there may be other evidence available, such as controlled clinical trials, cohort studies, and case studies, but are not referred to. Thus, the review provides a summary of only one component of the potential evidence relating to the use of honey in wound healing. Further, the review focused on wound healing as the primary outcome of interest, it is contended that other endpoints, such as wound debridement, are also clinically important. This should be borne in mind in interpreting the findings of the review. It is evident that from an RCT point of view there is insufficient evidence to clearly support or refute the use of honey in wounds other than in moderate superficial and partial thickness burns and longer duration, sloughy venous ulcers.

FUTURE DEVELOPMENTS

As the interest in the use of honey as a topical wound management product grows, there will need to be a corresponding increase in the clinical evaluation of this product to place in context its use within the clinical arena. Future studies should be designed to answer clinical applicable problems. It is contended that other endpoints, such as wound debridement, are also clinically important. While there is insufficient evidence for a significant increase in venous ulcer healing at 12 weeks, a modest effect of honey on larger, longer duration, sloughy venous ulcers merits further research.

AUTHOR DISCLOSURE STATEMENT

No competing financial interests exist.

REFERENCES

1. Jull AB, Rodgers A, and Walker N: Honey as a topical treatment for wounds. Cochrane Database Syst Rev 2008; Issue 4, (CD005083).
2. Harding KG and Boyce DE: Wounds: the extent of the burden. In: *Wounds Biology and Management*, edited by Leaper D and Harding KG. Oxford: Oxford University Press, 1998, pp. 1–4.
3. Cole-King A and Harding KG: Psychological factors and delayed healing in chronic wounds. Psychosom Med 2001; **63:** 216.
4. Schultz GS, Sibbald G, Falanga V, Ayello EA, Dowcett C, Harding K, Romanelli M, Stacey MC, Teot L, and Vanscheidt W: Wound bed preparation: a systematic approach to wound management. Wound Repair Regen 2003; **11 (Suppl 1):** S1.
5. Moore OA, Smith LA, Campbell F, Seers K, McQuay HJ, and Moore RA: Systematic review of the use of honey as a wound care dressing. BMC Complement Altern Med 2001; 1(2).
6. Cullum N, Nelson EA, Flemming K, and Sheldon T: Systematic reviews of wound care management: (5) beds; (6) compression; (7) laser therapy, therapeutic ultrasound, electrotherapy and electromagnetic therapy. Health Technol Assess 2001; **5:** 1.
7. Palfreyman S, Nelson EA, and Michaels JA.: Dressings for venous leg ulcers: systematic review and meta-analysis. BMJ 2007; **335:** 244.
8. The Royal College of Nursing (United Kingdom): The nursing management of patients with venous ulcers. In: *Clinical Practice Guidelines*. London, 2006.
9. Gethin G and Cowman S: Manuka honey vs hydrogel—a prospective, open label, multicentre, randomised controlled trial to compare desloughing efficacy and healing outcomes in venous ulcers. J Clin Nurs 2009; **18:** 466.

WHS Wound Healing Society

Prolene Hernia System, Lichtenstein Mesh, and Plug and Patch for Primary Inguinal Hernia: A 3-Year Randomized Controlled Trial

Vijay A. Singh,* Sandra L. Kavalukas, and Adrian Barbul

Department of General Surgery, Sinai Hospital of Baltimore, Baltimore, Maryland.

Abbreviations and Acronyms

L = Lichtenstein mesh

P = PerFix plug

PHS = Prolene Hernia System

*Correspondence: Department of General Surgery, Sinai Hospital of Baltimore, 2401 West Belvedere Avenue, Baltimore, Maryland 21215 (e-mail: sghva@hotmail.com).

Background: Herniorrhaphy is one of the most common procedures performed around the world. Open, tension-free repairs involve the placement of a synthetic mesh to strengthen the inguinal region; some popular techniques include the Lichtenstein repair, plug and patch, Kugel, and Prolene Hernia System (PHS).

Clinical Problem Addressed: There are only a few randomized controlled trials that compare the various types of open, tension-free techniques. Although these techniques share the same principles of repair without tension, the operative dissections and the repair techniques do differ. Thus, it is important to know if any one technique is inferior in terms of recovery time, length of hospitalization, and recurrence rates.

Experimental Model or Material: A prospective study using 472 men between the ages of 30 and 75 years with primary inguinal hernias who were randomized to one of three types of open, mesh-based repair: the PHS, PerFix plug, or Lichtenstein mesh.[1] All patients were seen postoperatively at 2 weeks, 3 months, 1 year, and 3 years.

Discussion of Findings and Relevant Literature: The only significant difference found was the length of operative time. Specifically, the PHS and PerFix plug repair required less operative time than the Lichtenstein mesh repair did. The current literature shows that a surgeon who is experienced with a certain type of open, tension-free repair, regardless of type, has the best chance of limiting recurrence as well as allowing for the most favorable outcome.

BACKGROUND

Herniorrhaphy is a very common procedure performed in the United States and around the world. Almost 1,000,000 are performed each year in the United States. There are a number of ways to repair a hernia. Described in the 1880s, the traditional Bassini technique was a repair under tension, in which the edges of the defect were sewn back together without any reinforcement or prosthesis. Because of the high recurrence rate of the hernia (8–15%), long recovery period, and postoperative pain, few tension repairs are still in use today.[2,3]

Many repairs currently performed are open, tension-free repairs that involve the placement of a synthetic mesh to bridge and strengthen the inguinal floor; some popular techniques include the Lichtenstein repair (flat mesh patch placed on top of the defect), plug and patch (mesh plug placed in the defect and covered by a Lichtenstein-type patch), Kugel (mesh device placed behind the defect), and Prolene Hernia System (PHS) (a two-layer mesh device placed over

ADVANCES IN WOUND CARE, VOLUME 1

Printed in U.S.A.
DOI: 10.1089/awc.2009.0153

and behind the defect). The rate of recurrence is considerably lower with the tension-free repair versus the tension repair.[3,4]

Recently, laparoscopic repair has become another alternative method of repair. It is also tension free; however, the mesh is placed in the preperitoneal space posterior to the defect as opposed to plugging the defect or covering it anteriorly.

CLINICAL PROBLEM ADDRESSED

There has been recent literature comparing various aspects of laparoscopic versus open techniques of hernia repair.[5] However, there are still only a few randomized controlled trials that compare the various types of open, tension-free techniques.

The goal is to assess what factor, if any, has a significant impact on the outcome of a patient who undergoes an inguinal herniorrhaphy. Is the extent of dissection the determining factor? Is it type of mesh used? Is it the surgeon's experience that is the most important factor? Answering these questions may help define the ideal method to repair an inguinal hernia.

RELEVANT BASIC SCIENCE CONTEXT

All meshes discussed in this paper are made of synthetic polypropylene. This material is not absorbed by the body. Instead, it provides a matrix for ingrowth of inflammatory and scar tissue. Because it is a foreign body, there is a vigorous patient response resulting in scarring.

EXPERIMENTAL MODEL OR MATERIAL

Four hundred seventy-two men between ages of 30 and 75 years with primary inguinal hernias were randomized to one of three types of open, mesh-based repair: the PHS, PerFix plug (P), or Lichtenstein mesh (L).[1] All the patients were seen postoperatively at 2 weeks, 3 months, 1 year, and 3 years. The goal was to assess if the different extents of dissection required by the three types of repair resulted in different operative times, return of functionality, and wound healing (*i.e.*, wound infections).

This was a randomized, single-blind, multicenter study with patients randomly allocated to one of three types of different surgical techniques (PHS, P, or L) for repair of an inguinal hernia. The main hypothesis tested in this study was that the extent of dissection impacts on overall cost, length of stay, and recovery time. The three repair systems (*i.e.*, PHS, P, and L) are among the more common types of mesh-based repairs used in the United States and Sweden. The patients were stratified by demographics, type of anesthesia administered, and application of the main steps of the respective procedure that were strictly followed according to preset criteria developed by all the operating surgeons.

DISCUSSION OF FINDINGS AND RELEVANT LITERATURE

The only significant finding was the length of operative time. Specifically, the PHS and P repair required less operative time than the L repair did. Despite this finding, no other aspect of comparison, namely, time of full recovery, length of stay, or wound complications, showed any significant difference between the three types of repair. This would give an indication that the extent of dissection may not affect the healing or the overall progression of the hernia wound, or have any impact on postoperative pain. Despite different operative techniques and time involved in the three types of hernia repairs described (PHS, P, and L), none have significant advantages in outcomes such as return to functional activity, pain scores, or recurrence rates (Table 1). Therefore, one can deduce that the driving force in a surgeon's decision to select a type of primary hernia repair should be based mainly upon comfort and experience with the specific procedure. The literature does support that performing even the more extensive dissection, as required by the Lichtenstein repair, had no major bearing on the overall outcome of the patient.

There are other factors besides the type of repair that play a role in the outcome of patient who

Table 1. *Results by time frame of outcome measures*

	L (3 Months)	P (3 Months)	PHS (3 Months)	L (1 Year)	P (1 Year)	PHS (1 Year)	L (3 Years)	P (3 Years)	PHS (3 Years)
Pain	2.5%	4.4%	2.6%	3.2%	3.9%	5.2%	2.0%	2.6%	2.7%
Recurrence	0	1	0	1	1	2	1	1	0
Function	98%	97%	96%	97%	99%	99%	100%	100%	97%

L = Lichtenstein mesh; P = PerFix plug; PHS = Prolene Hernia System.

> **TAKE-HOME MESSAGE**
>
> **Clinical care**
>
> - Tension-free herniorrhaphy has a drastically smaller recurrence rate than tension repairs have.
> - Operative time is slightly less for plug repairs compared with the Lichtenstein repair.
> - Regardless of patient demographics, size of defect, extent of dissection, and repair type used, there is no difference in patient outcomes for pain, recurrence, or functional return.

undergoes a herniorrhaphy. These include type of approach (anterior or posterior), type of mesh used,[6] experience of the surgeon,[7] and type of anesthesia administered.[8] Each of these factors by itself and when combined with the other factors has a significant impact on patient outcome.

There is evidence that surgeon experience[7] as reflected in outcome is the principal determinant of recurrence and complication rates. A hernia repair can be arduous, for many reasons, such as distorted anatomy and extensive scar tissue in recurrent hernias. Long-term numbness, pain, and sometimes even impotence caused by nerve damage are some of the more distressing complications related to an inguinal herniorrhaphy. Although the incidence of complications of low-volume hernia surgeons is significantly higher compared with high-volume hernia surgeons, these complications can occur to anyone.

In summary, it is clear that a surgeon who is experienced with a certain type of open, tension-free repair, regardless of type, has the best chance of limiting recurrence as well as assuring a successful outcome.

CAUTION, CRITICAL REMARKS, AND RECOMMENDATIONS

Mesh is a nonabsorbable foreign body that can pose real problems in the face of infection. There are two instances in which Prolene mesh systems should not be placed in a patient. The mesh should never be placed into the hernia defect if the peritoneum has been violated. This can result in migration of the mesh into the abdominal cavity causing bowel adherence and potential obstruction or fistula formation.

The second contraindication to mesh placement is in the face of enterotomy or infection. If entrance has been made into the bowel, a contaminated field has been created. Even if the bowel is repaired and the peritoneal defect is closed, it is still not advised to continue with Prolene mesh placement. If the mesh does get infected, antibiotics may be attempted, but many times removal of mesh is necessary.

FUTURE DEVELOPMENT

This operation has seen many evolutions since Bassini's time. The open technique discussed above has very little morbidity and mortality. It would seem perhaps that only future advances will address the mesh material's properties and function.

AUTHOR DISCLOSURE STATEMENT

No competing financial interests exist.

REFERENCES

1. Dalenback C, Andersson B, Anesten S, Bjorck S, Eklund S, Magnusson O, Rimback G, Stenquist B, and Wedel N: Prolene Hernia System, Lichtenstein mesh and plug-and-patch for primary hernia repair: 3-year outcome of a prospective randomized controlled trial. Hernia 2009; **113:** 121.
2. Elsebae MM, Nasr M, and Said M: Tension-free repair versus Bassini technique for strangulated inguinal hernia: a controlled randomized study. Int J Surg 2008; **6:** 302.
3. Zsolt B and Csíky M: Recurrence rate in Bassini operation after five years. Magy Seb 2001; **54:** 307.
4. Miyazaki K, Nakamura F, Narita Y, Dohke M, Kashimura N, Matsunami O, and Katoh H: Comparison of Bassini repair and mesh-plug repair for primary inguinal hernia: a retrospective study. Surg Today 2001; **31:** 610.
5. Pokorny H, Klingler A, Schmid T, Fortelny R, Hollinsky C, Kawji R, Steiner E, Pernthaler H, Függer R, and Scheyer M: Recurrence and complications after laparoscopic versus open inguinal hernia repair: results of a prospective randomized multicenter trial. Hernia 2008; **12:** 385.
6. Campanelli G, Catena F, and Ansaloni L: Prosthetic abdominal wall hernia repair in emergency surgery: from polypropylene to biological meshes. World J Emerg Surg 2008; **3:** 33. http://www.wjes.org/content/3/1/33.
7. Nordin P and Van der Linden W: Volume of procedures and risk of recurrence after repair of groin hernia: national register study. BMJ 2008; **336:** 934. http://www.bmj.com/cgi/content/full/336/7650/934?view=long&pmid=18426843.
8. Nordin P, Haapaniemi S, Van Der Linden W, and Nilsson E: Choice of anesthesia and risk of reoperation for recurrence in groin hernia repair. Ann Surg 2004; **240:** 187.

Use of Human Acellular Dermal Matrix for Hernia Repair: Friend or Foe?

Vijay Singh,* Sandra L. Kavalukas, and Adrian Barbul

Department of General Surgery, Sinai Hospital of Baltimore, Baltimore, Maryland.

Background: A hernia develops when the outer layers of the abdominal wall weaken, bulge, or actually rip. Hernias range from being asymptomatic to causing operative emergencies. It is one of the most common operative procedures performed in the United States.
Clinical Problem Addressed: Although a herniorrhaphy is a common procedure, there remain a lot of questions that are not clearly answered: the issue of recurrence with primary repairs, managing loss of domain for complex hernias, and repair in areas of active infection. The idea is that human acellular dermal matrix (HADM), a cadaveric dermal graft in which all epidermis and cellular elements of dermis have been separated, is used in a hostile or complex wound to avoid tissue rejection and graft failure. HADM can effectively close contaminated abdominal wall defects in a single-staged, tension-free manner.
Experimental Model or Material: A retrospective review of a single institution's experience with use of HADM was analyzed to assess the overall effectiveness in using a cadaveric dermal graft as the prosthetic material of choice. Between May 2004 and October 2007, HADM was implanted in 46 patients undergoing ventral hernia repair. The patients' age range was 26–77 years with similar comorbidities. HADM was used as fascial reinforcement and, in some instances, as fascial replacement.
Discussions of Findings and Relevant Literature: HADM is instrumental in the idea of giving surgeons a viable option for treating infected hernia wounds in a single-staged, tension-free fashion. When used as a bridging component for large fascial defects, there was a tendency for eventration. The literature shows a distinct benefit in using these materials in an infected or hostile environment.

Abbreviation and Acronym

HADM = human acellular dermal matrix

*Correspondence: Department of General Surgery, Sinai Hospital of Baltimore, 2401 West Belvedere Avenue, Baltimore, Maryland 21215 (e-mail: sghva@hotmail.com).

BACKGROUND

A HERNIA IS THE PROTRUSION OF A TISSUE through the wall that normally contains it. An incisional hernia usually occurs in the abdomen in an area of a previous surgical scar. This protuberance can cause a bulge in the abdominal area. This type of hernia is often reducible and painless. However, when the bulge cannot be pushed back into the abdomen, it means a segment of bowel or a surrounding structure has become entrapped or incarcerated. This can eventually lead to an intestinal obstruction. If a hernia is incarcerated for a considerable period of time, there is a possibility of compromise to intestinal blood supply to that region, which can lead to ischemia or strangulation. In general, an incisional hernia has an incidence rate of up to 11–20% following all major abdominal surgeries.[1–3] Considering

Printed in U.S.A.
DOI: 10.1089/awc.2009.0154

there are ~2.5 million abdominal surgeries per year, the actual number of incisional hernias can be quite daunting.

This is a dilemma that has plagued the field of general surgery for many years. Previously, the options of repair would be restricted to either attempting a primary closure or using an alloplastic material to buttress and reinforce the repair.

CLINICAL PROBLEM ADDRESSED

Incisional hernias present a surgeon with three distinct problems: high recurrence with primary repairs, how to manage loss of domain for complex hernias, and repair in cases of infection. The use of prosthetic mesh can alleviate some of these concerns. It has been especially useful in significantly reducing the rate of recurrence with primary repairs. In some instances, the incidence of recurrence has been reported as high as 54%, but with mesh repair this incidence drops to 34%.[4] The ideal nonabsorbable mesh for use in complex or hostile incisional hernias has not been described. Initially, surgeons either implanted an absorbable synthetic mesh or allowed the wound to granulate and heal by secondary intention with or without an overlying skin graft. Each of these scenarios predisposed patients to a staged repair and also added morbidity to an already challenging procedure. It was found that absorbable synthetic prostheses could indeed be applied into hostile wounds without the fear of exacerbating the infection. Conversely, the use of absorbable prostheses exposed the patient to predictable hernia recurrence. These materials, once implanted, lead to a vigorous inflammatory reaction that, through a hydrolytic reaction, removes and digests the implanted prosthetic material completely. Therefore, there remains a high risk of hernia recurrence due to the complete dissolution of the absorbable prosthetic support.

RELEVANT BASIC SCIENCE CONTEXT

Biological substitutes were found to be an adequate replacement for synthetic mesh. In particular, human acellular dermal matrix (HADM) was studied in complex and/or infected hernias. HADM is a cadaveric dermal graft in which all epidermal and cellular elements of dermis have been removed to avoid rejection and graft failure. The biologic material can then act as a scaffold that allows for ingrowth of cellular elements and revascularization. Eventually, the material is replaced by host scar tissue.

Initially used in burn wounds as a prelude to skin grafts, HADM is increasingly used to repair contaminated abdominal wall defects. HADM can effectively close contaminated abdominal wall defects in a single-staged, tension-free manner. Its recurrence rate, when used as a reinforcement tool in hernia repair, is comparable, if not superior to results seen with use of other prostheses.[5] However, when used as a bridge to close large noninfected fascial defects, the recurrence rate of a hernia is high. A high rate of eventration is observed when used as a method of bridging fascial defects together. Therefore, using HADM for bridging purposes provides only a temporary solution.

EXPERIMENTAL MODEL OR MATERIAL

A retrospective review of a single institution's experience with use of HADM was analyzed to assess its overall effectiveness. Between May 2004 and October 2007, HADM was implanted in 46 patients undergoing ventral hernia repair. The patients' age range was 26–77 years with similar comorbidities.[5]

An infected wound was considered to be any wound which at the time of HADM placement had a history of feculent peritonitis, an iatrogenic enterotomy, incarcerated hernia with bowel necrosis, bowel resection at the time of hernia repair, or fascial dehiscence with evisceration. A complex wound was defined as a recurrent incisional/ventral hernia with or without removal of preexisting mesh.

HADM was used as fascial reinforcement and, in some instances, as fascial replacement. In the bridged group, HADM was placed in the intraperitoneal position, with a variable degree of underlay (1–4 cm), which then acted as the conduit between the separated fascial edges. For a reinforced repair, HADM was placed as an underlay or onlay (extraperitoneal), or in a sandwich technique (intra- and extraperitoneal) before and/or after primary reapproximation.

DISCUSSION OF FINDINGS AND RELEVANT LITERATURE

Candage *et al.*[5] were able to demonstrate the benefits of HADM in infected hernia wounds. This may afford surgeons a viable option for treating infected hernia wounds in a single-staged, tension-free fashion, with results showing a 28% recurrence rate. When used as a bridging component for large fascial defects, the results are less impressive because of high eventration rate resulting in recurrence rates as high as 60%. This high rate of recurrence leads one to conclude that large fascial defects will most likely need a multistaged procedure in order to be closed, irrespective of the type of prosthesis applied.

There are many types of biological prosthetic material that have been developed and proposed for clinical use in hostile and complex fields. These materials all have the same characteristic of adapting into the environment for the way by which they are replaced after their implantation within the patient.

The eventual incorporation of these types of prostheses into the tissue leads to a reproduction of tissue similar to the original host. This matrix can be composed of porcine small intestine submucosa, cadaveric human dermis, and others. As stated earlier, there are many types of these "new" biological prostheses available in the market today. The main indication of use is for repair of hernias in hostile environments and for soft tissue reconstruction. There remains a lack of good data to clearly define the use of these materials. Examples of materials discussed in current literature include acellular cadaveric dermis,[6,7] the porcine small intestine submucosa,[8,9] porcine dermal collagen,[10] and the acellular extracellular matrix.[11]

Clearly there is evidence that HADM and the other biological prostheses play a role in addressing the problems associated with incisional hernias. These materials show a distinct benefit in infected or hostile environment. Recurrence rates (when these materials are used as reinforcement for primary repairs) are comparable to their synthetic counterparts. These materials show an absence of significant effect on reduction of recurrence when used as a bridge for complex wounds. Although this is a good start for advocating use of biological materials in incisional hernia, more studies are needed to further define its role.

CAUTION, CRITICAL REMARKS, AND RECOMMENDATIONS

HADM is gaining arenas' acceptance as an alloplastic material for complex hernia repair; however, it is important to understand the limitations of this application. Often the tensile strength is less than desirable (resulting in eventration in larger repairs) and should be reserved for smaller hernia repairs with good fascial edges. There are new matrices that have been used to improve this aspect of the repair, although at this time there is insufficient research to attest to outcomes of recurrences.

It is important to keep in mind that many of these substances have specific polarity—one side which promotes granulation and not safe against bowel, and the other which is nonadherent. Care should be taken to implant these substances correctly so that the surfaces are facing the elements for which they are intended.

FUTURE DEVELOPMENT

Although new meshes and matrices are available in the market everyday, as yet there is no product with the combined strength of prolene or gortex and with the biologic adaptability of HADM. It will be to the patient's advantage when a combination substance comes out which will allow use in fistula formation, enterotomy, and infected wounds as well as provide definitive management of hernia that will result in low recurrence rates.

AUTHOR DISCLOSURE STATEMENT

No competing financial interests exist.

TAKE-HOME MESSAGE

Basic science advances

- Development of dermal matrix, stripped of cells, allows for migration over a scaffold native to the patient's body and, at the same time, avoids rejection issues.
- Once implemented, a series of enzymatic reactions hydrolyze the mesh, allowing for complete resorption of the matrix.
- Eventually, the body revascularizes this graft and repopulates the area with the patient's own cellular elements.

Clinical science advances

- HADM is indicated and particularly useful in the case of infection or contamination without ensuing morbidity which occurs with prosthetic meshes.
- Because it is made of nonreactive material (in contrast to prosthetic mesh), it can be used against bowel without fistula formation or ingrowth of bowel contents.

Relevance to clinical care

- May be safely used in hernia repair when entrance into the peritoneal cavity has occurred; frequently used in both the inlay and onlay techniques.
- Has shown success with smaller hernias and primary closure, as well as infected wounds.
- However, may be of limited use when a bridging technique is employed for large defects and result in eventration, leading to further operative management.

REFERENCES

1. Mudge M and Hughes LE: Incisional hernia: a 10 year prospective study of incidence and attitudes. Br J Surg 1985; **72:** 70.
2. Lewis RT and Wiegand FM: Natural history of vertical abdominal parietal closure: Prolene versus Dexon. Can J Surg 1989; **32:** 196.
3. Sugerman HJ, Kellum JM, Reines HD, DeMaria EJ, Newsome HH, and Lowry JW: Greater risk of incisional hernia with morbidly obese than steroid-dependent patients and low recurrence with prefascial polypropylene mesh. Am J Surg 1996; **171:** 80.
4. Luijendijk RW, Hop WC, van den Tol MP, de Lange DC, Braaksma MM, Ijzermans JN, Boelhouwer RU, de Vries BC, Salu MK, Wereldsma JC, Bruijninckx CM, and Jeekel J: A combination of suture repair vs mesh repair for incisional hernia. N Engl J Med 2000; **343:** 392.
5. Candage R, Jone K, Luchette F, Sinacore J, Vandevender D, and Reed R: Use of human acellular dermal matrix for hernia repair: friend or foe? Surgery 2008; **144:** 703.
6. Buinewicz B and Rosen B: Acellular cadaveric dermis [Alloderm]; a new alternative for abdominal hernia repair. Ann Plast Surg 2004; **52:** 188.
7. Espinosa-de-los-Monteros A, de la Torre JI, Marrero I, Andrades P, Davis MR, and Vasconez LO: Utilization of human cadaveric acellular dermis for abdominal hernia reconstruction. Ann Plast Surg 2007; **58:** 264.
8. Edelman DS and Selesnick H: Sports hernia: treatment with biologic mesh [Surgisis]; a preliminary study. Surg Endosc 2006; **20:** 971.
9. Edelman DA and Hodde JP: Bioactive prosthetic material for treatment of hernias. Surg Tech Int 2006; **15:** 104.
10. Hiles M and Hodde J: Tissue engineering a clinically useful extracellular matrix biomaterial. Int Urogynecol J 2006; **17:** S39.
11. Ma SZ, Li XH, and Hu J: Acellular extracellular matrix for inguinal hernia repair. Hernia 2006; **10:** 229.

Section 3

DRESSINGS

Section Editors: Dot Weir and Harriett Loehne

DRESSINGS

Introduction to Dressings

Patricia Mann Mertz*

Department of Dermatology and Cutaneous Surgery, Miller School of Medicine, University of Miami, Miami, Florida.

Abbreviations and Acronyms

MMP = matrix metalloproteinase

MRSA = methicillin-resistant *staphylococcus aureus*

SSC = silver sulfadiazine creme

TOE = topical oxygen emulsion

UCFS = University of California, San Francisco

*Correspondence: Patricia M. Mertz, 5950 SW 129 Ter, Miami, Florida 33156 (e-mail: pmertz@bellsouth.net).

INTRODUCTION

In preparation to write this introductory chapter, I reread the thesis of George D. Winter, Ph.D.[1] His early observation of the role of moisture in the wound healing process was ahead of time and not supported by the general public. He discussed the role of the hair follicles and other skin appendages as a source for migrating epidermal cells and the possibility of the presence of collagenase to aid epithelial cells in their migration. Collagenase was first described in the amphibian skin by J. Gross and C.M. Lapiere and was not described in human skin until 1967.[2,3]

To develop a reliability model for wound healing, we used as sources of information the publications of George Winter, Ph.D., David Rovee, Ph.D., and that of C. Hinman and Howard Maibach, M.D.[4–6] They had all published on moist wound healing: George Winter in the domestic pig, David Rovee in the guinea pig paw, and C. Hinman, and Howard Maibach in a human model. I sought to learn more about Dr. Winter from his colleagues and contacted David Rovee Ph.D., Warren Rottman Ph.D., and Howard Maibach, M.D. who shared some anecdotal information with me which is detailed below.

Warren Rottman, Ph.D., wrote:

"George Winter's contribution to the art and science of wound management is testimony to how the intersection of circumstances and history often leads to discovery . . . or rediscovery. The management of wounds has a very long history . . . at times throughout history, so-called 'moist wound healing' was actively practiced, but often abandoned . . . not for clinical reasons, but for reasons of 'tradition' . . . the tradition can be dated as far back as Hippocrates who reasoned (but may not have had data) that 'it (the wound) should not be moistened nor should it be bandaged; after cleaning the wound, one should dry the wound . . . for what is soonest dried up . . . thereby separates from the rest of the tissues which is full of blood and life.'"

It is interesting that one year before his landmark article in 1962, George Winter coauthored an article that ended by stating, "Our explanation of the better results obtained with cotton lint and stockinette are that they allow the wound to dry most rapidly.[7,8] Thus he agreed with Hippocrates, "one should dry the wound, for what is soonest dried up, thereby most rapidly separates." What changed between 1961 and 1962?

To make a guess, one must recall certain points of confusion at that time (which are relevant today also):

1. Not all wounds are alike either in either biology or best management. (especially, depth, extent, localization, microbial colonization/infection, origin, or underlying pathology).

Printed in U.S.A.
DOI: 10.1089/awc.2009.0183

2. A breach of the skin allows for microbial colonization or infection, and there has always existed an *a priori* argument on how to manage the problem. The chief reason why it took many years between the report on moist wound healing and the introduction of dressings designed to promote the practice was the fear of promoting infection.
3. The lessons learned in managing one class of wounds, for example, burns, often failed to translate to the management of other types of wounds.

For example, it was learned through the pioneering efforts of treating horrific battle wounds during World War II by Archibald McIndoe that the best way to manage burns initially included (as well as other procedures) moist saline dressings. (*i.e.*, tulle gras moistened every 2 h, to prevent further desiccation of the eschar). Despite this practice, it failed to become a standard global practice in burn therapy or in the management of other types of wounds.

4. The standard dressings in 1961 were fiber (mostly cotton) based, and the chief clinical concern was with the adherence of the dressing to the wound surface, leaving fibers in the wound bed and causing patient discomfort. Many clinicians argued that adhesion was good because it served to clean the wound. In light of these controversies, the article by Scales and Winter suggested that drying the wound was the best treatment, which was based on the work that was funded by Courtaulds Limited (who were one of the largest producers of fibrous materials in the United Kingdom).[7] It is understandable that they could make such an interpretation, especially since they never had a "Control" which would be the fiber dressing that was not allowed to desiccate. It is tough to go against the Standard of Practice of the day, and it is interesting to note that this landmark article was very conservative in the authors' discussion and interpretation.

George Winter's landmark research resulted from several circumstances:

1. He started medical studies at South Hampton University but was drafted into the military in 1945. After his discharge in 1948, he embarked on his academic career as a research assistant at the Royal National Orthopaedics Hospital at Stanmore, United Kingdom, working under J.T. Scales. This situation was unique because their institute was capable of large animal experimentation and Scales had a biomechanical interest in pressure-relieving mechanisms for bed-ridden patients, including the management of patients with bed sores.
2. *Opportunity #1*: George worked in his spare time toward his degrees (The motive). But in his work environment he had the opportunity to pioneer research on the histological analysis of how wounds heal in an animal species (domestic pigs) that have skin quite similar to that of humans. It is with the biology of wound repair that his discovery was made.
3. *The interest:* R&D on the potential use of new fiber-based materials was of business interest to a major U.K. manufacturer, Messrs. Courtaulds Limited, London, UK. They provided research funding for the laboratory to test some of their materials, which in turn sponsored George's basic research.
4. *Opportunity #2*: As noted above, the key observation that desiccation has its consequences was somewhat counter-culture at the time.
5. *The discovery:* For some years after, the basic observation was interpreted as "Moist wound environments accelerate wound healing" (The misinterpretation). We now recognize that what George actually observed was that "Moist wound healing eliminates the adverse effects of desiccation."

The legacy: David Rovee, Ph.D., wrote of fond recollection of George Winter:

"As a graduate student I became aware of George Winter's work during my research into epidermal wound healing. His findings that simple films could dramatically alter the healing process was intriguing. The polyethylene film he studied prevented tissue dehydration necrosis, eschar formation and consequently, enhanced epithelial migration in pig excisions. His ideas affected my work in the area of wound treatment. His paper published in *Nature* (1962) and subsequent studies by others formed the basis for the now-accepted concepts of 'moist wound healing.' I had the opportunity to visit with George in his laboratory in England in the mid-to-late 1960s when he invited me to see the procedures he developed for studying excisions in pig skin. Our friendship from that meeting extended for many years until his death. In 1971, I was pleased to include George in a conference on wound healing held in California and hosted by Howard Maibach and me. It was a pleasure to follow him to the podium and present work showing the application and relevance of his preclinical findings to human wounds. His contribution to the published work of this conference presented a thorough and complete record of his pioneering studies in healing, a paper to which I still refer for information. George visited my laboratories in the U.S. many times, made many friends there, and always inspired my colleagues with his ideas. Our last visit occurred in his laboratories in Minnesota."

Howard Maibach, M.D. dictated this recollection of George Winter's article in *Nature*.

"I read George Winters' paper in *Nature* with interest and thought how unlikely this finding of occlusion speeding epithelization was. I discussed this with the chief of surgery at the University of California, San Francisco (UCFS) and he had lots of doubt regarding the similarities of pig skin to human skin and also that a film covering wounds could change the healing outcome. Because each freshman medical student had to complete a two week research program, I summoned Carmon Hindmen, then a second year medical student, to complete his research requirement by helping read the slides of a human wound healing model of partial thickness wounds as his project. We both read the slides in a blinded fashion and found George's findings in pigs were the same in humans. I felt this was a very important finding and even considered patenting the idea but decided not to follow that road. I became very friendly with George and suggested he interview at 3M, where he later worked until his untimely death."

George Winter, with his legacy of using biomaterials for moist wound healing, has inspired the search for new materials that can be used for maintaining a moist wound environment and will interact with the cells responsible for healing. We look to the past to introduce the so-called "new materials." This chapter will outline some materials that are now being investigated for their effects on wound healing and may soon enter the wound care marketplace.

THE FOLLOWING "NEW" HAVE "OLD" HISTORY

Spider silk

The silk from spider webs was used in ancient times with some anecdotal success for wound coverings. The silk spider web was obtained from the spiders. More recently spider silk has been reported to be antimicrobial, hemostatic, and nonimmunogenic, all perfect properties for a wound covering.[9,10] Panilaitis *et al.* studied the *in vitro* direct inflammatory potential of silk fibers and macrophage cells. They found that the proteins extracted from native silk fibers did not induce a significant macrophage reaction.[11] An international patent to use spider silk as a wound dressing was filed by three scientists in 2006[12]; the title of their patent is *Implant of Cross-linked Spider Silk Threads*. They describe the treatment of venous and decubitus ulcers treated with a dressing made of spider silk obtained from *Nephilia clavipes*.

To obtain the silk, the spider is sedated with CO_2 and cooled to a temperature of 4°C. The silk is then molded into a mixture comprised of spider silk and a cross-linking agent.

The patentees presented clinical studies that supported their application. However, the studies were not well controlled. Their findings were that spider silk dressings enhance healing of chronic wounds such as venous and decubitus ulcers. No conclusive studies have been performed on this natural material.

Spiders themselves generally are not used to obtain silk because they attack and kill one another and are difficult to handle. The molecular makeup of spider silk was described by Randolph V. Lewis in 2006.[9] Scheibel has developed a method of growing spider silk in *Escherichia coli* and plans on developing wound coverings.[13]

Honey

Stone Age wall painting dating back to 6000 BC depicts honey collecting. Its use for medicinal purposes was recorded in ancient scrolls, tablets, and books. The Egyptians describe using honey with lint and fat for a dressing for chronic wounds. Honey had been used in Europe and other countries shortly after World War I. However, the first honey-containing dressing approved by the Food and Drug Administration was cleared in April 2008. It is manufactured and marketed by Derma Science (Derma Science, Inc., Princeton, NJ). It contains 95% Manuka honey and calcium alginate. It has a wide spectrum of antimicrobial activity even including antifungal activity.[14] Honey has also been shown to have a strong osmotic effect that helps draw moisture to the wounded tissue and promotes debridement. As in ancient times, this modern-day dressing honey has been teamed with calcium alginate. It seems as though our ancient ancestors had an idea for moist wound healing.

Oak bark extract

The extract of oak bark has a long history for use in wound healing by Native American warriors. They used the preparation to stop bleeding and also as an astringent.[15] In 1992 a patent was granted to

Thomas Stanley for the treatment of skin ulcers with an aqueous extract of oak bark ash.[16] The ointment he developed contained 3% oak bark extract, 6% benzoic acid, 6% salicylic acid in polyethylene glycol-8, and polyethylene glycol-75. Our laboratory at the Miller School of Medicine, University of Miami, studied this ointment in pig models of burn wounds and wounds with bacterial biofilms. We evaluated burn wound healing using a salt split technique and found that 33% were healed on day 8, and 88% were healed when treated with the oak bark extract ointment. By contrast, only 5% and 43% were healed in the control-treated burns. In a Methicillin-resistant *Staphylococcus aureus* (MRSA) biofilm assay, the active treatment had a significant reduction in the numbers of MRSA in 24 h as compared with the vehicle and air-exposed control ($p < 0.005$).[17] Other investigators have studied the production of matrix metalloproteinase (MMPs) in nonhealing wounds that were treated with oak bark extract. They found that the MMP-2 expression paralleled the healing of the wounds that were treated with oak bark extract.[18] Jacobs and Tomczak described a clinical trial of the oak bark extract ointment on diabetic foot ulcers. Forty subjects were randomized to be treated with the Bensal Hp (oak bark extract) versus silver sulfadiazine cream (SSC). The results showed that in the Bensal Hp group, ulcers decreased in size 72% compared with 54.7% in the SSC treatment group. Although the subject numbers were small, this study suggests that the oak bark ointment is effective.[19] This material is now licensed to 3M, where it is distributed in Asia, Europe, and Canada. Perhaps it will be available soon in the United States.

Zinc and iron solution

Oken published a work showing that topical zinc application enhanced collagen biosynthesis and epithelization.[20] Iron is essential for wound healing because wound DNA synthesis requires iron as a cofactor so that cells can divide. Iron is also required for hydrolization of proline and for collagen biosynthesis.

In 2003 we studied a zinc iron solution in our epithelization model in domestic pigs. We found that the zinc iron solution enhanced epithelization in partial-thickness and burn wounds.[21,22] Feiner evaluated the effects of the zinc iron solution in an *in vitro* wound model on the migration of fibroblasts. The results suggested that the zinc iron solution enhanced fibroblast migration over either control zinc or iron alone.[23] BioDerm Science (Bioderm, Oxford, MS) now markets a zinc iron solution and a dressing with the zinc iron solution for wound healing. The preparations are approved by the Food and Drug Administration.

Topical oxygen

Wound repair requires oxygen for some aspects of healing. Topically applied gaseous oxygen has been tested to improve oxygenation of superficial wound tissue[24] and improve clinical outcomes.[25] Recently, a new technology of perfluorcarbon droplets made into an emulsion that contains supersaturated oxygen has been developed. This emulsion can carry oxygen at a higher capacity into the skin. The perfluorcarbon oxygen emulsion has been studied in our laboratory at the Miller School of Medicine, University of Miami.[26] Assays were performed *ex vivo* to determine the pO_2 levels over time. Viable tissue treated with topical oxygen emulsion (TOE) had increased pO_2 levels when compared with the controls of vehicle or phosphate-buffered saline. *In vivo*, eight pigs received partial-thickness wounds, and eight pigs received second-degree burn wounds. Topical application of TOE daily stimulated epithelization as well as vascularization of partial-thickness wounds and also stimulated epithelization in ischemic second-degree burn wounds. Using the same pig model we evaluated some possible mechanisms of topical oxygen treatment. The studies found the upregulation of vascular endothelial growth factor, collagen I and III, and matrix metalloproteinase levels in TOE-treated wounds when compared with the vehicle control.[27]

Other investigators studied topical oxygen as delivered from a device into chronic wounds and found a reduction in wound size and that topical oxygen was associated with higher gene expression of vascular endothelial growth factor as compared with the hyperbaric oxygen therapy.[25]

This device described in the pig protocols was not studied in humans. A very similar technology is now being developed for wound healing and other medical uses. The name of the company is Oxygen Biotherapeutics, and they have developed a therapeutic oxygen carrier based on perfluorcarbon.

CONCLUSION

The search for new materials to cover wounds is continuing, and some unusual materials are being added to the list of active wound dressings. George Winter, Ph.D., set us on the path to look at materials in a new light and now the list includes spider silk, honey, oak bark extract, zinc iron solution, and perfluorcarbon oxygen. All these natural agents have the possibilities to be used as a dressing or in some cases as an antimicrobial agent for wound treatment.

ACKNOWLEDGMENTS

My thanks to Howard Maibach, M.D., David Rovee, Ph.D., and Warren Rottman, Ph.D., for their contributions.

AUTHOR DISCLOSURE STATEMENT

There are no commercial associations that might create or seem to pose a conflict of interest.

REFERENCES

1. Winter G: A study of wound healing in the domestic pig [Ph.D. thesis]. Department of Biomechanics and Surgical Materials, Institute of Orthopaedics, University of London Stanmore, Middlesex, United Kingdom. Thesis submitted for the Degree of Ph.D. Birkbeck College, 1966.
2. Gross J and Lampiere CM: Collagenolytic activity in amphibian tissues: a tissue culture assay. Proc Natl Acad Sci USA 1962; **48:** 1014.
3. Riley WB and Peacock EE: Identification, distribution and significance of a collagenolytic enzyme in human tissues. Proc Soc Exp Biol Med 1967; **124:** 207.
4. Winter GD: Formation of the scab and the rate of epithelization of superficial wounds in the skin of the young domestic pig. Nature 1962; **193:** 293.
5. Rovee DT and Miller CA: Epidermal role in the breaking strength of wounds. Arch Surg 1968; **86:** 43.
6. Hinman C and Maibach H: Effect of air exposure and occlusion on experimental human skin wounds. Nature 1963; **200:** 377.
7. Scales JT and Winter GD: The adhesion of wound dressings. An experimental study. In: *Wound Healing*. Oxford: Pergamon Press, 1961.
8. Scales JT: Wound healing and the dressing. Brit Jr Industr Md 1963; **20:** 82.
9. Lewis RV: Spider silk: ancient ideas for new biomaterials. Chem Rev 2006; **106:** 3762.
10. Altman GH, Diaz F, Jakuba C, Calabro T, Horan RL, Chen J, Lu H, Pichmond J, and Kaplan DL: Silk based biomaterials. Biomaterials 2003; **24:** 201.
11. Panilaitis B, Altman GH, Chen J, Jin JH, Karageorgiou V, and Kaplan DL: Macrophage response to silk. Biomaterials 2003; **24:** 3079.
12. Vogt P, Allmeling C, and Reimers K: International Intellectual Property Organization 19 June 2008. International Publication Number: WO 2008/071226 A1.
13. Scheibel T: Spider silks: recombinant synthesis, assembly, spinning and engineering of synthetic proteins. Microb Cell Fact 2004; **3:** 14.
14. Koc AN, Silici S, Ercal BD, Kasap F, Hormet-Oz HT, and Mavus-Buldu H: Antifungal activity of Turkish honey against *Candida* spp. and *Trichosporon* spp: an *in vitro* evaluation. Med Mycol 2008; **2:** 1.
15. Behrman CH: *The Indian Wars: Chronicle of American Wars*. Twenty First Century Book, 2005; Lerner Publications.
16. United States Patent 5080900. Issued to Stanley, Thomas R.
17. Davis SC and Mertz PM: Determining the effect of an oak bark formulation on methicillin-resistant *Staphylococcus aureus* and wound healing in porcine wound models. Ostomy Wound Manage 542008;54 (10).
18. Karim RB, Brito BL, Dutrieux RP, Lassance FP, and Hage JJ: MMP-2 assessment as an indicator of wound healing: a feasibility study. Adv Skin Wound Care 2006; **19:** 324.
19. Jacobs AM and Tomczak R: Evaluation of Bensal Hp for the treatment of diabetic foot ulcers [Departments: APWCA Clinical Rounds]. Adv Skin Wound Care 2008; **21:** 461.
20. Oken E: Update on micronutrients: iron and zinc. Curr Opin Pediatr 2002; **14:** 350.
21. Cazzaniga AL, Davis SC, Drosou A, and Mertz PM: The effect of a zinc/iron solution as compared to a topical growth factor on epithelization of partial thickness wounds. J Invest Dermatol 119 (1), 2002. Abstract no. 842.
22. Davis SC, Cazzaniga AL, Drosou A, and Mertz PM: A zinc/iron solution stimulates epithelization of second-degree burn wounds. J Invest Dermatol 119 (1), 2002. Abstract no. 847.
23. Feiner A, Cazzaniga A, Davis SC, Berman D, and Mertz PM: Evaluation of the effects of a zinc/iron solution on the migration of fibroblasts in an *in vitro* incisional wound healing model. J Invest Dermatol 121 (1), 2003. Abstract no. 0692.
24. Fries RB, Wallace WA, Roy S, Kuppusamy P, Bergdall V, Gordillo GM, Melvin WS, and Sen CK: Dermal excisional wound healing in pigs following treatment with topically applied pure oxygen. Mutat Res 2005; **579:** 172.
25. Gordillo GM, Roy S, Khanna S, Schlanger R, Khandelwal S, Phillips G, and Sen CK: Topical oxygen therapy induces vascular endothelial growth factor expression and improves closure of clinically presented chronic wounds. Clin Exp Pharmacol Physiol 2008; **35:** 957.
26. Davis S, Cazzaniga AL, Ricotti C, Zalesky P, Hus L-C, Creech J, Eaglstein WH, Mertz PM, Hsu L-C, Creech J, Eaglstein WH, and Mertz PM: Topical oxygen emulsion: a novel wound therapy. Arch Dermatol 2007; **143:** 1252.
27. Li J, Zhang YP, Zhu L, Mertz PM, Cazzaniga AL, Ricotti C, Zalesky PJ, Hus LC, Creech J, Eaglstein WH, and Davis SC: The effect of an oxygen emulsion on collagen deposition in second degree burn wound repair. Wound Rep Regen 12 (2), 2004. Abstract no. A-16.

WHS Wound Healing Society

Hydrocolloids: Healing by Occlusion

Cathy Thomas Hess*

Wound Care Strategies, Inc., Harrisburg, Pennsylvania.

*Correspondence: Wound Care Strategies, Inc., 4080 Deer Run Court, Suite 1114, Harrisburg, Pennsylvania 17112 (e-mail: cthess@woundcare strategies .com).

Decades of research has demonstrated that in a moist wound environment, scabbing or crusting of the wound was inhibited, growth factors were available for new cell and vessel formation, proteolytic enzymes deterred the wound of necrotic tissue, white blood cells were used to protect against infection, and epidermal cells were allowed to freely migrate over the moist dermal surface. Modern research continues to build upon documented findings. Hydrocolloid dressings were introduced to practitioners in the 1980s specifically as an occlusive choice to manage the healing of acute and chronic wounds and continue to be used in clinical practice today. Studies have shown that hydrocolloids improved healing rate, increased epithelialization, reduced infection, and enhanced collagen synthesis compared with the traditional gauze dressings. Hydrocolloid dressings continue to provide a key role for the wound care practitioner when caring for wounds.

BACKGROUND

THE USE OF OCCLUSIVE DRESSINGS and their ability to influence moist wound healing was brought to the forefront by George Winter in 1962.[1] Winter's work revealed many important aspects of wound healing that would began to build the foundation for the arsenal of dressings used in clinical practice today.[1–5]

Occlusive dressings, specifically hydrocolloids, were first developed as adhesive flanges used to protect the skin around a stoma. Because of its adhesive properties and ability to protect the skin from bodily fluids, the hydrocolloid dressing technology was developed to manage acute and chronic wounds.

Hydrocolloid dressings were introduced to practitioners in the 1980s specifically as an occlusive choice to manage the healing of acute and chronic wounds. By virtue of its occlusive properties, clinicians feared that these dressings would lead to wound infection by increased proliferation of microorganisms occurring on the skin.[6] Research has shown that chronic wounds managed only with an occlusive dressing demonstrated a rare infection despite massive bacterial overgrowth.[7] Much of the research citing wound infection under occlusive dressings was referring to the use of films. Buchan *et al.* demonstrated that the wound fluid beneath Opsite® (Smith and Nephew, London, UK) showed viable neutrophils able to phagotocize and destroy pathogenic bacteria.[8] It was also demonstrated that the wound's fluid had antibacterial activity.[8] In addition to maintaining a moist wound environment, some of the occlusive dressings serve as highly effective protective barriers against external contamination. *In vivo* studies of the hydrocolloid dressings (specifically DuoDERM® [ConvaTec, Skillman, NJ]) demonstrated that the dressings serve as a barrier against *Pseu-*

ADVANCES IN WOUND CARE, VOLUME 1

Printed in U.S.A.
DOI: 10.1089/awc.2009.0159

domonas, *Staphylococcus aureus*, human immunodeficiency virus, and Hepatitis B.[9,10] Additionally, clinical studies focusing on chronic wounds, such as pressure ulcers and lower leg ulcers, had shown that the gel-like properties of the hydrocolloid dressing healed superficial wounds faster than with the use of gauze or wounds left open to air.[11]

CLINICAL PROBLEM ADDRESSED

Topical wound management varies according to the wound's characteristics, including amount of exudate, size of the wound, presence or absence of infection, and the characteristics of the surrounding skin. Moisture-retentive dressings, such as hydrocolloids, should be selected for wounds with light to moderate drainage and based on the manufacturer's indications. Table 1 provides an overview of the actions, indications, and contraindications of hydrocolloids.

Table 1. *Actions, indications, contraindications, advantages, and disadvantages of hydrocolloid dressings*

Action:

Hydrocolloids are occlusive or semiocclusive dressings composed of materials such as gelatin, pectin, and carboxymethylcellulose. The composition of the wound contact layer may differ considerably among dressings. These dressings provide a moist healing environment that allows clean wounds to granulate and necrotic wounds to debride autolytically. Some hydrocolloids may leave a residue in the wound, and others may adhere to the skin around the wound. Hydrocolloids are manufactured in various shapes and sizes, with different adhesive properties, and in various forms, including wafers, pastes, and powders. To date, the formulation of hydrocolloids includes alginates, silver, and honey.

Indications:

Hydrocolloid dressings may be used as primary or secondary dressings to manage select pressure ulcers, partial- and full-thickness wounds, wounds with necrosis or slough, and wounds with light to moderate exudate.

Advantages:

- Are impermeable to bacteria and other contaminants.
- Facilitate autolytic debridement.
- Are self-adherent and mold well.
- Provide light to moderate absorption.
- Minimize skin trauma and disruption of healing.
- Allow observation of the healing process, if transparent.
- May be used under compression products (compression stockings, wraps, pumps, and Unna's boot).

Disadvantages:

- Are not recommended for wounds with heavy exudate, sinus tracts, or infections; wounds surrounded by fragile skin; or wounds with exposed tendon or bone.
- Can make wound assessment difficult, if opaque.
- May be dislodged if the wound produces heavy exudate.
- Provide an occlusive property that limits gas exchange between the wound and the environment.
- May curl at edges.
- May injure fragile skin upon removal.
- May be difficult because of body contours, incontinence, patient mobility, and wound exudate.

Hydrocolloid dressings consist of absorptive ingredients (typically carboxymethylcellulose, pectin, or gelatin).[12] The formulation of hydrocolloid's inner layer, primarily carboxymethylcellulose, provides a place for the wound's fluid to be absorbed. This absorptive swelling action is what allows this dressing to control light to moderate amounts of exudate. This mechanism of action is maintained until the swelling of the inner layer extends to the edge of the dressing. Once the exudate has reached the dressing's inner layer surface capability or saturation point, the dressing must be changed.

Hydrocolloid dressings interact with wound drainage and swell or melt out leaving a residue in the wound. When the dressing is removed, a gel residue may be left in the wound bed. To remove this residue, the wound has to be gently cleansed with a wound cleanser before assessing the wound. A distinctive foul odor may also be present. This may be from product breakdown, not infection.

Hydrocolloids adhere best at body temperature. To promote adherence, the clinician should place his or her hand over the dressing after applying it to the wound. The heat from the clinician's hand will assist in molding the dressing to the wound and facilitating adherence. In literature, it has been documented that the adhesion of the hydrocolloid is higher than select surgical tapes.[13] It is further documented that with the use of a hydrocolloid, "after application the absorption of transepidermal water vapor modifies the adhesive flow to maintain a high-tack performance throughout the period of use."[13] Additionally, research has demonstrated that a very low oxygen gradient helps stimulate the formation of granulation tissue and new blood vessels.[14]

By virtue of the hydrocolloid's dressing profile, those hydrocolloids with thick edges may roll up and adhere to the patient's clothing or bed linens, decreasing the dressing's wear time. Dressings with a thinner profile and tapered edges generally adhere better to the periwound skin without rolling up.

Hydrocolloid sheet dressings are available in various thicknesses and in precut shapes for body areas such as the sacrum, elbows, and heels. Highly conformable to the patient's body, these dressings adhere well to high-friction areas such as the sacrum and heels. All sheet hydrocolloid dressings have a film covering to make the product waterproof. Some sheet hydrocolloids are opaque, making wound assessment difficult; others are translucent or transparent.

Because sheet hydrocolloids are adhesive, the patient's skin may be vulnerable to tearing when the dressing is removed. The clinician should evaluate the integrity of the periwound skin to determine if a hydrocolloid can be used.

CLINICAL SCIENCE ADVANCES

Since 1980s, many different types, forms, and shapes of hydrocolloids have been introduced to the clinical market. For clinical use, hydrocolloids are indicated for partial- or full-thickness acute and chronic wounds. These dressings are occlusive hydroactive wafers, pastes, or granules that promote granulation tissue formation and wound healing within a moist environment. Hydrocolloid dressings protect fragile skin and areas of the body affected by both urinary and fecal incontinence and frictional forces. Most hydrocolloid wafers react with wound exudate to form a gel-like covering to protect the wound and maintain a moist wound healing environment. Because of the hydrocolloid's occlusive nature, hydrocolloid dressings do not allow water, oxygen, or bacteria into the wound. This aids in facilitating angiogenesis and granulation tissue. Hydrocolloids also cause the pH of the wound surface to drop; the acidic environment can inhibit bacterial growth. They can help a clean wound to granulate or epithelialize and encourage autolytic debridement in wounds with necrotic tissue. However, because of their occlusive nature, hydrocolloids cannot be used if the wound or surrounding skin is infected.

Further research has documented that occlusive dressings keep the wound bed moist, reduce the formation of crust in the wound, and decrease pain and inflammation in acute and chronic wounds.[9,10] Madden *et al.*[15] demonstrated that the use of occlusive hydrocolloid dressings and polyurethane films healed donor sites significantly faster and with less pain than those covered with fine mesh gauze or silver sulfadiazine. There were no clinical infections with the wounds that were occluded.

To date, additional components have been added to hydrocolloids which in turn have changed the hydrocolloid's mechanism of action. These components include alginates, honey, and silver. As the product evolves, the clinician must understand how the components work together as a dressing. For example, honey has been found to have anti-inflammatory and antibacterial effects, promoting moist wound healing and facilitating debridement.[16] The ingredient of honey combined with the delivery system of a hydrocolloid allows the antibacterial activity of the honey to stay within the wound's site longer when in the presence of wound fluid.

Silver is another product that has been integrated into the hydrocolloid's delivery system. Silver provides an antimicrobial or antibacterial action and is activated from the dressing to the wound's surface based on the amount of exudate and bacteria in the wound.[17] Hydrocolloid dressing with silver may be employed to decrease the bacterial load, contain exudate, and optimize the appearance of the wound's granulation tissue.

RELEVANT LITERATURE

Animal and human studies focusing on the use of hydrocolloids have been well documented. In 2008, Heyneman *et al.* performed a systematic literature review methodically detailing current evidence in the field of pressure ulcer treatment with hydrocolloids.[18] They reviewed 29 publications (targeting 28 different studies) that met the inclusion criteria and included in the review. In this review, hydrocolloids were most frequently used to manage stage 2–3 pressure ulcers. It was found that hydrocolloids are more effective than gauze dressings for the reduction of the wound dimensions, absorption capacity, time needed for dressing changes, pain during dressing changes, and side effects. This review demonstrated that hydrocolloids are preferred to gauze dressings in the treatment of pressure ulcers. Last, the study compared hydrocolloids to the use of collagen-, saline- and povidine-soaked gauze. It was found that hydrocolloids were a less expensive alternative but more expensive compared to hydrogel, polyurethane foam and collagenase dressings. The study provides recommendations for clinical practice and further research.

A recent review of the literature by Thomas suggests that hydrocolloid dressings serve an important role in wound management.[19] The author found that hydrocolloids have an expanded role in acute wounds, provide a barrier to decrease pain at the wound's site, increase healing time, and provide cost savings in wound care. Additionally, Thomas found that hydrocolloids' natural covering protects wounds from the environmental elements, thereby decreasing the spread of bacteria.

Research continues to illustrate the use of hydrocolloids in acute and chronic wounds. Additional research is needed to evaluate the new technologies integrated in the hydrocolloid as a complete delivery system.

SUMMARY ILLUSTRATION

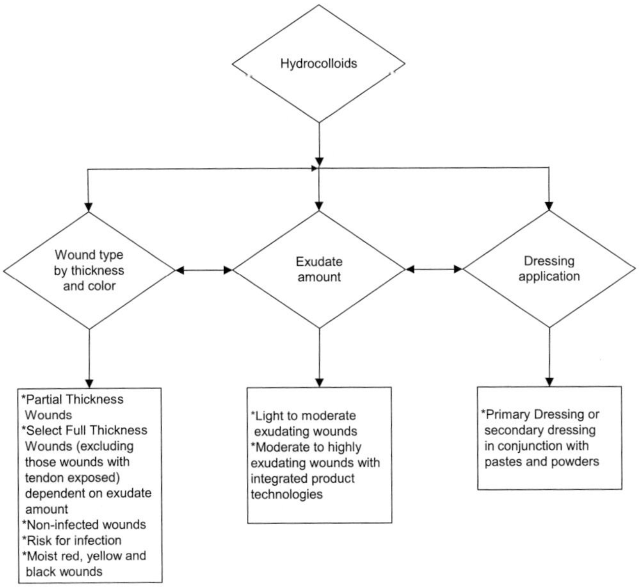

CONCLUSION

Decades of research has demonstrated that in a moist wound environment, scabbing or crusting of the wound was inhibited, growth factors were available for new cell and vessel formation, proteolytic enzymes deterred the wound of necrotic tissue, white blood cells were used to protect against infection, and epidermal cells were allowed to freely migrate over the moist dermal surface. Modern research continues to build upon documented findings. Hydrocolloids, in particular, have been shown to be safe and effective in managing acute and chronic wounds. Recent literature has confirmed that hydrocolloid dressings indeed serve as a functional wound management choice when caring for acute and chronic wounds. The studies and literature concluded that the application of hydrocolloids improve patient's satisfaction through pain management, provide a cost-effective treatment alternative, and increase wound healing outcomes. Differences in the hydrocolloid delivery systems may have advantages regarding patient's preference, bacterial killing, and exudate management. As always, it remains the clinician's responsibility to understand the hydrocolloid's action, indication, and contraindication prior to use.[20] With careful wound oversight, clinicians will continue to provide optimal wound caring.

AUTHOR DISCLOSURE STATEMENT

No competing financial interests exist.

REFERENCES

1. Winter GD: Formation of scab and the rate of epithelialization on superficial wounds in the skin of the domestic pig. Nature 1962; **193:** 293.
2. Odland G: The fine structure of the interrelationship of cells in the human epidermis. J Biophys Biochem Cytol 1958; **4:** 529.
3. Hinman CC, Maibach H, and Winter GD: Effect of air exposure and occlusion on experimental human skin wounds. Nature 1963; **200:** 377.
4. Alvarez OH, Mertz PM, and Eaglstein WH: The effect of occlusive dressing on collagen synthesis and epithelialization in superficial wounds. J Surg Res 1983; **35:** 142.
5. Eaglstein WH: The effect of occlusive dressing on wound healing. In: *Wound Healing*, edited by Eaglestein EH. Philadelphia, PA: Lippincott, 1894, pp. 107–111.
6. Leydon JL, Steward R, and Klingman AM: Update *in vivo* methods for evaluating topical antimicrobial agents on human skin. J Invest Dermatol 1979; **72:** 165.
7. Alper JC, Welch EA, Ginsberg M, Bogaars H, and Maguire P: Moist wound healing under a vapor permeable membrane. J Am Acad Dermatol 1983; **8:** 347.
8. Buchan IA, Andrews JK, and Lang SM: Clinical and laboratory investigation of the composition and properties of human skin wound exudate under semi-permeable dressing. Burns 1981; **7:** 326.
9. Mertz PM, Marshall DA, and Eaglstein WH: Occlusive wound dressing to prevent bacterial invasion and wound infection. J Am Acad Dermatol 1985; **12:** 662.
10. Bowler PG, Delargy H, Prince D, and Fondberg L: The viral barrier properties of some occlusive dressings and their role in infection control. Wounds 1993; **5:** 1.
11. Hutchinson JJ and McGuckin M: Occlusive dressings: a microbiologic and clinical review. Am J Infect Control 1990; **18:** 257.
12. Hess CT: When to use hydrocolloid dressings. In: *Advances in Skin & Wound Care*, March/April 2000, pp. 63–64.
13. Turner TD: The development of wound management products. In: *Chronic Wound Care: A Clinical Source Book for Healthcare Professionals*, 3rd edition, edited by Krasner DL, Rodeheaver, GT, and Sibbald RG. Wayne, PA: HMP Communications, 2001, pp. 293–310.
14. Knighton D, Hunt TK, Scheunstuhl H, Halliday BJ, Web Z, and Banda MJ: Oxygen tension regulates the expression of angiogenesis factor by macrophages. Science 1983; **221:** 1283.
15. Madden MR, Nolan E, Finkelstein JL, Yurt RW, Smeland J, Goodwin CW, Hefton J, and Staiano-Coico L: Comparison of an occlusive and a semi-occlusive dressing and the effect of the wound exudate upon keratinocyte proliferation. J Trauma 1989; **29:** 924.
16. Pieper B: Honey-based dressings and wound care: an option for care in the United States. J Wound Ostomy Continence Nurs 2009; **36:** 60.
17. Hess CT and Kirsner RS: Orchestrating wound healing: assessing and preparing the wound bed. Adv Skin Wound Care 2003; **15:** 246.
18. Heyneman A, Beele H, Vanderwee K, and Defloor T: A systematic review of the use of hydrocolloids in the treatment of pressure ulcers. J Clin Nurs 2008; **17:** 1164.
19. Thomas S: Hydrocolloid dressings in the management of acute wounds: a review of the literature. Int Wound J 2008; **5:** 602.
20. Hess CT: *Clinical Guide to Skin and Wound Care*, 6th edition. Springhouse, PA: Lippincott Williams & Wilkins, 2008.

Skin Protectants in the Treatment of Irritant Dermatitis Associated with Exposure to the Body's Effluents

Mikel Gray*

Department of Urology and School of Nursing, University of Virginia, Charlottesville, Virginia.

Abbreviations and Acronyms

IAD = incontinence-associated dermatitis

MASD = moisture-associated skin damage

TEWL = transepidermal water loss

*Correspondence: Department of Urology and School of Nursing, University of Virginia, PO Box 800422, Charlottesville, Virginia 22908 (e-mail: mg5k@virginia.edu).

Background: Skin protectants, also called moisture barriers, are used by wound care clinicians to prevent or treat irritant dermatitis when the natural moisture barrier of the skin is compromised.

The Problem: Exposure to urine, stool, or both results in a condition called incontinence-associated dermatitis. Exposure to exudate from a wound may lead to periwound maceration. Other clinical manifestations include intertrigo, characterized by inflammation in skin folds exposed to excessive perspiration, and peristomal irritant dermatitis, characterized by excessive exposure to effluent from the stoma. Collectively, these conditions may be referred to as moisture associated skin damage (MASD).

Basic/Clinical Science Advances: Ointments or cream-based products are typically preparations of petrolatum, dimethicone, and/or zinc oxide. Petrolatum products contain a mixture of mineral oil and petroleum wax. Dimethicone is a silicone-based organic polymer. Zinc oxide is a white powder incorporated with an ointment or cream base. A liquid polymer acrylate is also used as a skin protectant; it is applied to the skin and allowed to dry.

Clinical Care Relevance: A modest but growing body of evidence exists that supports the use of skin protectants for the prevention and treatment of two forms of MASD, periwound maceration and incontinence-associated dermatitis. In each of these clinical scenarios, a skin protectant is applied as part of a structured skin care regimen.

Conclusion: Clinical evidence supports the use of skin protectants for the treatment of MASD with cream or ointment-based formulations containing petrolatum, dimethicone, or zinc oxide or a liquid polymer acrylate. Evidence suggests that both categories of products are useful for preventing or treating irritant dermatitis associated with exposure to urine, stool, wound exudate, or excessive perspiration.

BACKGROUND

Skin protectants, also called moisture barriers, are frequently used by wound care clinicians to prevent or treat irritant dermatitis. A skin protectant is defined by the U.S. Food and Drug Administration as a prescriptive or cosmetic product that is applied to the skin or a mucus membrane to protect the underlying tissue from harmful irritants.[1,2] Dermatologists classify skin protectants as a moisturizer.[3] They label these products occlusives, based on their ability to physically block transepidermal water loss while protecting the skin from irritating substances.

Skin protectants are indicated when the moisture barrier of the skin is compromised. In addition to its other functions, the skin acts as a barrier against toxins and irritants from the external environment, while preventing excessive loss of fluids and

ADVANCES IN WOUND CARE, VOLUME 1

Printed in U.S.A.
DOI: 10.1089/awc.2009.0175

electrolytes from the internal environment. This mechanism, referred to as the skin's moisture barrier, is analogous to a brick and mortar arrangement. The bricks within this conceptual framework are hygroscopic molecules within the corneocytes, collectively referred to as the natural moisturizing factor.[4] They act as endogenous humectants, maintaining a 20% concentration of water within the stratum corneum. Keratin filaments and amino acids created by the enzymatic action of filaggrin comprise the bulk of these molecules. They are surrounded by a cross-linked protein shell called the corenodesmosome.

The mortar within this conceptual framework is the intracellular lipids, primarily ceramides, cholesterol, and free fatty acids. They are formed by lamellar granules found in the keratinocytes and exist in fine alternating layers with water, creating an endogenous emollient. Lipid production within the stratum corneum is pH dependent; it thrives in a mildly acidic environment and is impaired in an alkaline environment.[5] Aquaglyceroporin-3 is a membrane protein that facilitates the transport of water and closely associated solutes such as urea and glycerol. It provides a local circuit for water between the epidermal base and stratum corneum, enabling the skin to maintain needed water within the stratum corneum.[6]

CLINICAL PROBLEM ADDRESSED

In healthy community-dwelling adults, skin protectants and other forms of moisturizers are commonly used to treat seasonal or age-related xerosis, or as a sun screen. In contrast, wound care clinicians usually apply a skin protectant to prevent or treat irritant dermatitis associated with exposure to a bodily effluent. Exposure to urine, stool, or both results in a condition called incontinence-associated dermatitis (IAD).[7] Exposure to exudate from a wound may lead to periwound maceration.[8] Other clinical manifestations include intertrigo, characterized by inflammation in skin folds exposed to excessive perspiration, and peristomal irritant dermatitis, characterized by excessive exposure to effluent from the stoma. Collectively, these conditions may be referred to as moisture-associated skin damage (MASD).[9] Application of a skin protectant is one component of a structured skin care regimen that includes regular cleansing and application of a protectant/moisturizing agent.

RELEVANT BASIC SCIENCE CONTEXT

Ointments or cream-based products are the most common form of skin protectant. Petrolatum products contain a mixture of mineral oil and petroleum wax; available formulations comprise 30–100% white or yellow petrolatum.[10] Dimethicone, a silicone-based organic polymer, is incorporated into ointments or creams containing 1–30% dimethicone. Zinc oxide is a white powder that is incorporated into multiple cream or ointment-based formulations containing 1–25% zinc oxide per gram of vehicle. Liquid polymer acrylates are applied to the skin and allowed to dry, forming a solid film that acts as a barrier to irritating substances.[8]

A number of studies have examined the use of skin protectants (occlusives) on skin hydration and barrier function, but most focus on irritant contact dermatitis associated with xerosis or exposure to environmental irritants.[11] Only one study was identified that compared the performance of ointment-based skin protectants designed for use in patients with MASD. Hoggarth *et al.*[12] compared skin protectant and moisturization properties of products containing dimethicone, zinc oxide, and petrolatum. Phase 1 of the study evaluated the barrier properties of the skin protectants using patch testing after exposure to sodium laurel sulfate, phase 2 measured transepidermal water loss (TEWL) and skin hydration using a chromometer after repeated washing with soap and water, and phase 3 evaluated the barrier properties of the various ointments. Petrolatum-based protectants provided a potent barrier to a standardized irritant while maintaining skin hydration. Dimethicone-based products provided variable protection against the irritants, but it preserved skin hydration and avoided maceration better than petrolatum or zinc oxide–based products. Zinc oxide products provided the greatest protection against the irritant, but its ability to prevent maceration and maintain skin hydration was less than dimethicone- or petrolatum-based ointments.

EXPERIMENTAL MODEL OR MATERIAL—ADVANTAGES AND LIMITATIONS

The most common experimental model for testing skin protectants is the volar surface of the forearm of healthy volunteers. The most common main outcome measure in these studies is TEWL, defined as a measurement of the movement of water across the stratum corneum via diffusion and evaporation over time and expressed as $g/m^2/h$. Secondary outcomes included electrical capacitance, colorimetry (chromometry), and various visual scores based on the clinical assessment.

Only one study was identified that compared the performance of various ointment-based skin protectants designed for use in patients with MASD. Hoggarth *et al.*[12] used the volar surface of the arm and completed patch testing after exposure to sodium laurel sulfate, followed by repeat washing with soap and water to measure TEWL and skin hydration, and dye testing to measure their barrier properties. Alternative models should be explored. Specifically, even though the volar surface of the arm is convenient for testing, its stratum corneum differs from the perineal and perigenital skin. In addition, current models are restricted to younger volunteers, and testing should be conducted on healthy elders to better model their response to skin protectants when challenged by experimentally induced moisture barrier damage. Finally, researchers need to develop a scale for measuring product efficacy, so novel and existing formulations can be measured against new or existing skin protectants.

DISCUSSION OF FINDINGS AND RELEVANT LITERATURE

A modest but growing body of evidence exists that supports the use of skin protectants for the prevention and treatment of two forms of MASD, periwound maceration and IAD (Table 1). In each of these clinical scenarios, a skin protectant is applied as part of a structured skin care regimen. The regimen begins with gentle cleansing to remove irritants, followed by application of a skin protectant to both shield the skin from additional exposure to the irritant and preserve its moisture barrier.

Periwound maceration

Two systematic reviews have been published that focus on the management of periwound maceration. Gray and Weir[13] reviewed literature related to the prevention of periwound maceration and identified varying levels of evidence supporting several interventions for prevention and treatment of periwound maceration including: (1) selection of a dressing capable of absorbing moderate to heavy volume exudate; (2) incorporation of an antimicrobial substance into the dressing, such as ionic silver; (3) use of manuka honey or honey-soaked gauze; (4) application of negative pressure wound therapy to reduce edema and exudate, compression therapy to counteract venous hypertension, edema, and exudate; and (5) application of a skin protectant to the periwound skin.

Schuren *et al.*[8] pooled results from eight published studies identified via systematic review and data on file from 3M Corporation (Minneapolis, MN) in a meta-analysis to determine whether a liquid acrylate is effective for prevention of periwound maceration. The studies compared the liquid polymer acrylate to other treatments including ointment-based skin protectants (zinc oxide- or petrolatum-based skin protectants), a placebo, or protective dressing.[14–22] Variability in reported outcomes, small sample sizes, limited data collection periods, and independent treatment of multiple lesions of the periwound skin limit the ability to generate meaningful data using meta-analytic techniques. Nevertheless, when compared with placebo, the liquid acrylate polymer film proved more effective in preventing ($Z = 5.66$, $p < 0.0001$) and treating periwound skin maceration ($Z = 10.49$, $p < 0.00001$). However, no statistical differences were found when the film barrier was compared with two ointment-based skin protectants (petrolatum or zinc oxide).

IAD

No systematic review was identified that evaluated the efficacy of the various skin protectants for the treatment of IAD. Bliss *et al.*[23] compared the effectiveness of four skin care regimens, all of which included application of an ointment, cream, or liquid polymer acrylate as a skin protectant in a multisite, open-label, quasiexperimental study involving 16 nursing homes across the United States and 11,918 residents. The skin protectants used were 43% petrolatum-based ointment, 98% petrolatum-based ointment, 12% zinc oxide plus 1% dimethicone cream, or a liquid polymer acrylate. The study was powered to detect differences in cost, and results demonstrated that the skin regimen using the liquid polymer acrylate was less expensive than regimens that included application of a cream- or ointment-based protectant because the liquid polymer acrylate was applied less often than the other protectants. However, analysis of efficacy revealed no significant differences in the effectiveness of any of the skin care regimens for prevention of IAD in this high-risk population.

Zehrer *et al.*[24] reported results of a 6-month, multisite descriptive study that reported cost and effectiveness of four skin care regimens for prevention of IAD in 250 residents in four nursing homes based in the midwestern United States. The skin protectants used in the study were 43% petrolatum-based ointment, 99% petrolatum ointment, 12% zinc oxide, 1% dimethicone cream, and a liquid polymer acrylate. The ointments and creams were applied with routine cleansing and following incontinence episodes, and the liquid polymer acrylate was applied either once daily or three times weekly. Similar to Bliss *et al.*,[23] no differences were

Table 1. *Principal findings and supporting studies*

Conclusion	Supporting studies	Description
Application of a liquid polymer acrylate is more effective than placebo or no treatment for preventing periwound maceration, erythema, and promotion of healing of periwound skin damage	Schuren *et al.*[8,a]	Pooled data from eight studies and data on file from manufacturer for meta-analysis
	Rolstad *et al.*[21,b]	Compared alcohol-based liquid polymer acrylate to standard treatment in periwound skin of 30 subjects with ostomies, wounds, perifistular skin
	Hampton[19,b]	RCT[b], nonalcohol-based liquid polymer acrylate applied to skin, while other half subjected to standard treatment in 62 subjects
	Garcia *et al.*[17,c,e]	Case–control study compared nonalcohol-based liquid polymer acrylate to traditional treatment for periwound skin in 26 subjects with pressure ulcers
	Neander and Hesse[20,b]	RCT compared nonalcohol-based liquid polymer crylate to placebo in 227 subjects with venous leg ulcers
Use of an ointment-based liquid polymer acrylate is as effective as use of a liquid polymer acrylate in preventing periwound maceration and erythema and promoting healing of periwound skin damage	Coutts *et al.*[16,c,e]	Case–control study compared nonalcohol-based liquid polymer acrylate to zinc oxide- or petrolatum-based ointments in periwound skin of 15 patients with pressure ulcers, venous leg ulcers, and diabetic foot ulcers
	Bar and Vanscheidt[14,b,e]	RCT compared nonalcohol-based liquid polymer acrylate to zinc oxide ointment in periwound skin of 20 subjects (wound etiology not specified in available abstract)
	Cameron *et al.* [15,b]	RCT compared nonalcohol-based liquid polymer acrylate to zinc oxide–based ointment in 35 patients with venous leg ulcers
	Bliss *et al.*[23,c]	Comparison cohort study compared four skin regimens, one using a nonalcohol-based liquid polymer acrylate, one used 43% petrolatum-based ointment, one used 98% petrolatum-based ointment, and one used 12% zinc oxide/1% dimethicone-based cream in 1,918 patients
Application of an ointment- or cream-based skin protectant or a liquid polymer acrylate are equally effective for prevention of incontinence-associated dermatitis	Zehrer *et al.*[24,c]	Multisite study compared four preventive regimens that included use of skin protectants; one used 99% petrolatum-based ointment, one used 43% petrolatum-based ointment, one used 12% zinc oxide/1% dimethicone-based cream, and one used nonalcohol-based liquid polymer acrylate in 250 patients

[a] Meta-analysis of multiple studies.
[b] Randomized clinical trial.
[c] Quasiexperimental study (comparison of groups without randomization).
[d] Descriptive, nonexperimental study.

found in the effectiveness of the skin protectants for prevention of IAD.

Baatenburg de Jong and Admiraal[25] compared cost and effectiveness of a liquid polymer acrylate versus a zinc oxide oil skin protectant in 39 residents in a nonblinded, randomized clinical trial set in a single nursing home in Zaandam, Holland. Data measurement was limited to 14 days. The liquid polymer acrylate was applied every 2–3 days for patients deemed to have less severe skin damage and every 1–2 days for those judged to have more severe damage. The zinc oxide oil was applied twice daily and after every incontinent episode. Skin condition was reported to be improved in both groups, but subjects randomized to the liquid polymer acrylate were reported to have achieved better results, specifically less erythema and denudation based on visual assessment.

CAUTION, CRITICAL REMARKS, AND RECOMMENDATIONS

Consideration of the clinical evidence for use of skin protectants for prevention and treatment of IAD or periwound maceration reveals that ointment-based products, cream-based products, and a liquid polymer acrylate are effective for preventing and treating MASD. Given this equivalency in efficacy, other factors should be considered when determining the best skin protectant to use in an individual patient. For example, multiple studies reveal reduced costs associated with use of a liquid polymer acrylate, based on fewer applications when compared with an ointment- or cream-based product. However, interpretation of these findings must be considered carefully since none of the studies evaluated the effect of application of any ointment- or cream-based product using a comparable schedule. Another consideration is how the product interacts with dressings or the faceplate of a pouching system. After drying, a liquid acrylate produces a slightly tacky surface that is not anticipated to impede an adhesive seal, whereas an ointment- or cream-based product is more likely to impede an adhesive border. Applied in a thin layer, clinical experience strongly suggests that an ointment- or cream-based skin protectant does not negatively influence the absorbency of absorptive pads or briefs, but the results of one study suggest that application of a thick layer of ointment will interfere with absorbency, paradoxically increasing exposure of the skin to urine or stool.[26]

Dimethicone- and petrolatum-based ointments or creams and liquid polymer acrylates tend to be clear, enabling the clinician to observe and assess the underlying skin. However, the addition of zinc oxide to cream or especially an ointment creates an opaque white paste that obscures the underlying skin and may delay assessment of progress toward healing or deterioration of the underlying skin. Zinc oxide ointments are usually applied in a thicker layer, resulting in a greater risk for impedance of the absorptive properties of incontinence pads of briefs.

FUTURE DEVELOPMENTS

The evidence supporting the use of skin protectants for the prevention and treatment of irritant dermatitis remains limited, and research focusing on their performance in the treatment of various forms of MASD is especially sparse. A standardized outcome measure to determine efficacy or a benchmark to measure the magnitude of the barrier properties of skin protectants, such as that used to determine UV protection among sunscreens,[27] is urgently needed.

Additional research should be performed to determine the optimal frequency of application for skin protectants. Manufacturers and clinicians tend to recommend application of a "thin coat," but it is difficult to standardize this direction for professional care providers, and even more difficult for lay caregivers. The optimal frequency of application for skin protectants is also not clearly understood. For patients with IAD, clinical tradition suggests that ointment- or cream-based skin protectants should be applied during routine bathing and after each incontinent episode. Liquid polymer acrylates are typically applied every 3–4 days. However, both ointment-based and liquid polymer acrylates are known to be resistant to removal during cleansing, so it remains possible that ointment- or cream-based products might have emerged as more expensive in some studies based on the presumption that they require more frequent application when this is not, indeed, the case.

TAKE-HOME MESSAGE

Basic science advance

- Sparse evidence reveals that petrolatum- or zinc oxide–based protectants offer superior protection against irritants compared with the dimethicone-based formulations, but dimethicone-based formulations provide superior protection against skin maceration while maintaining hydration.

Clinical science advances

- Two forms of skin protectants are effective for preventing and treating IAD and periwound maceration.
- Both product categories are effective in preventing or treating MASD.

Relevance to clinical care

- Two categories of products may be applied as a skin protectant, cream- or ointment-based formulations containing petrolatum, dimethicone or zinc oxide, or a liquid polymer acrylate.
- Clinical judgment, based on the type of skin damage, severity of dermatitis, and use of adhesive-based dressings or ostomy pouching system should influence skin protectant choice.
- Further research is needed to determine product efficacy for skin protectants, including a benchmark for efficacy that novel and existing formulations can be measured against similar to the sun protection factor used to determine the protective nature of sun blockers.

AUTHOR DISCLOSURE STATEMENT

Dr. Gray is a member of a speaker's bureau for SAGE Products, Cary, IL.

REFERENCES

1. Intota Guideline Expert Services. Available at http://www.intota.com/experts.asp?strSearchType=all&strQuery=skin+protectant+product (accessed July 1, 2009).
2. Skin Protectant Drug Products for Over-the-Counter Human Use; Final Monograph. Federal Register 2003; **68:** 35290.
3. Lynde CW: Moisturizers: what they are and how they work. Skin Ther Lett 2001; **6:** 3.
4. Verdier-Sévrain SM and Bonté F: Skin hydration: a review on its molecular mechanisms. J Cosmet Dermatol 2007; **6:** 75–82.
5. Hachem JP, Man MQ, Crumrine D, Uchida Y, Brown BE, Rogiers V, Roseeuw D, Feingold KR, and Elias PM: Sustained serine proteases activity by prolonged increase in pH leads to degradation of lipid processing enzymes and profound alterations of barrier function and stratum corneum integrity. J Investig Dermatol 2005; **125:** 510.
6. Sougrat R, Morand M, Gondran C, Barre P, Gobin R, Bonte F, Dumas M, and Verbavatz JM: Functional expression of AQP3 in human skin epidermis and reconstructed epidermis. J Investig Dermatol 2002; **118:** 678.
7. Gray M, Bliss DZ, Doughty DB, Ermer-Seltun J, Kennedy-Evans KL, and Palmer MH: Incontinence-associated dermatitis: a review. J Wound Ostomy Continence Nurs 2007; **34:** 45.
8. Schuren J, Becker A, and Sibbald RG: A liquid film-forming acrylate for peri-wound protection: a systematic review and meta-analysis (3M Cavilon no-sting barrier film). Int Wound J 2005; **2:** 230.
9. Gray M, Bohacek L, Weir D, and Zdanuk J: Moisture vs pressure: making sense out of perineal wounds. J Wound Ostomy Continence Nurs 2007; **34:** 134.
10. Faust HR and Casserly AW: Petrolatum and regulatory requirements. Available at http://www.penreco.com/newsevents/tradearticles/NPRA2003_Pet_Regulations.pdf (accessed July 1, 2009).
11. Yokota M and Maibach HI: Moisturizer effect on irritant dermatitis: an overview. Contact Dermatitis 2006; **55:** 65.
12. Hoggarth A, Waring M, Alexander J, Greenwood A, and Callaghan T: A controlled, three-part trial to investigate the barrier function and skin hydration properties of six skin protectants. Ostomy Wound Manage 2005; **51:** 30.
13. Gray M and Weir D: Prevention and treatment of moisture-associated skin damage (maceration) in the periwound skin. J Wound Ostomy Continence Nurs 2007; **34:** 153.
14. Bar M and Vanscheidt W: Ulcer edge protection with a polymer protective film. Z Wundheiling 2001; **22:** 16.
15. Cameron J, Hoffman D, Wilson J, and Cherry G: Comparison of two peri-wound skin protectants in venous leg ulcers: a randomized controlled trial. J Wound Care 2005; **14:** 233.
16. Coutts F, Sibbald GR, and Queen D: Peri-wound skin protection: a comparison of a new skin barrier vs traditional therapy in wound management. Presented at the *Canadian Association of Wound Care Conference*, London, ON, Canada, November 2001.
17. Garcia RF, Gago M, Adame S, Romero J, Jimenez A, and Vega J: 3M Cavalon No Sting Barrier Film: an evaluation of peri-wounds prone to maceration. Presented at the *European Pressure Ulcer Advisory Panel Conference*, Pisa, Italy, September 2000.
18. Garcia Gonzalez RF, Verdu Soriano J, Gago Fornelis M, Rueda Lopez J, Segovia Gomez T, and Peters Guiterrez JS: The use of a no sting barrier film to prevent maceration in pressure ulcers treated with an adhesive hydrocolloid dressing. Presented at the *European Woundcare Management Association*, Granada, Spain, May 2002.
19. Hampton S: Film subjects win the day. Nurs Times 1998; **94:** 80.
20. Neander KD and Hesse F: Wound edge protection in chronic wounds. J Wound Care 2003; **12:** 369.
21. Rolstad BS, Borchert K, Magnag S, and Scheel N: A comparison of an alcohol based siloxane-based peri-wound skin protectant. J Wound Care 1994; **3:** 376.
22. Vin F and Bonnetblanc JM: Peri-wound protection with Cavalon NSBF for patients with chronic venous leg ulcers: a randomized multicenter trial, data on file, 3M Healthcare, 2003.
23. Bliss DZ, Zehrer C, Savik K, Smith G, and Hedblom E: An economic evaluation of four skin damage prevention regimens in nursing home residents with incontinence: economics of skin damage prevention. J Wound Ostomy Continence Nurs 2007; **34:** 143.
24. Zehrer CL, Lutz JB, Hedblom EC, and Ding L: A comparison of cost and efficacy of three incontinence skin barrier products. Ostomy Wound Manage 2004; **50:** 51.
25. Baatenburg de Jong H and Admiraal H: Comparing cost per use of 3M Cavilon No Sting Barrier Film with zinc oxide oil in incontinent patients. J Wound Care 2004; **13:** 398.
26. Zehrer CL, Newman DK, Grove GL, and Lutz JB: Assessment of diaper-clogging potential of petrolatum moisture barriers. Ostomy Wound Manage 2005; **51:** 54.
27. Pinnell SR, Fairhurst D, Gillies R, Mitchnick MA, and Kollias N: Microfine zinc oxide is a superior sunscreen ingredient to microfine titanium dioxide. Dermatol Surg 2000; **26:** 309.

WHS Wound Healing Society

Gauze, Impregnated Gauzes, and Contact Layers

Renee Cordrey*

Program in Physical Therapy, The George Washington University, Washington, District of Columbia.

Abbreviations and Acronyms

BIPP = bismuth, iodoform, and paraffin paste

CL = contact layer

CMS = Centers for Medicare and Medicaid Services

MRSA = methicillin-resistant *staphylococcus aureus*

MWH = moist wound healing

NPWT = negative pressure wound therapy

PHMB = polyhexamethylene biguanide

WTDD = wet-to-dry dressing

*Correspondence: Program in Physical Therapy, The George Washington University, 900 23rd St. NW, 6th Floor, Washington, DC, 20037 (e-mail: hsprxc@gwumc.edu).

Background: Gauze has long been used as a primary and secondary dressing. It is frequently impregnated with substances for bactericidal, moisture-balance, hemostatic, or debridement purposes. Contact layers (CLs) provide a nonadherent protective layer over the wound when needed.
The Problem: Though commonly used, gauze is potentially recognized to harm wound tissue through desiccation and adhesion. Contemporary research on gauze is largely limited to being the control group of a product trial. Impregnated gauzes vary widely in the materials used. Iodoform, commonly impregnated on gauze, is weakly antimicrobial and can be toxic when absorbed.
Basic/Clinical Science Advances: Wet-to-dry dressings (WTDDs) are not supported in modern wound care, as they slow healing and destroy viable tissue. Gauze dressing orders should be written "moist-to-damp." The composition of a CL can affect cell viability and interface pressure through negative pressure therapy. Gauze dressing changes release more bacteria into the air than other types of dressings. Gauze has long been impregnated with various substances. The most recently used materials have antimicrobial and hemostatic properties.
Clinical Care Relevance: WTDDs are more expensive over the course of care despite its inexpensive supply cost. Iodoform and bismuth dressings may result in allergic reactions, toxicity with cognitive changes, and multisystem problems. CLs can reduce tissue trauma with dressing changes, with different types preferred for different wounds. Gauze may be impregnated with a large number of substances to achieve different goals, both during manufacturing or at the point of care.
Conclusion: Despite evidence against the use of WTDDs, they are still used. There is limited evidence on impregnated gauzes (other than iodoform) and CLs, but they are commonly used. More research should be done on gauzes, impregnated gauzes, and CLs.

BACKGROUND

Gauze has been used to support wound healing throughout recorded history. Healers have impregnated gauze or other materials such as papyrus, lint, sponges, or wool with honey, wine, vinegar, poultices, salves, and other compounds thought to aid healing.[1,2]

Gauze is a versatile product. It is commonly used to absorb blood and exudate. It is applied with pressure to achieve hemostasis, placed as a wound filler or cover, made wet or kept dry, and used as a secondary dressing to secure a primary product. Sterile cotton gauze was first mass-produced[1] in 1891. Since then, gauze has evolved into a wider variety of products and sizes, including rolls for wrapping extremities or ribbons for packing into tracts/tunnels, and a choice of woven cotton or nonwoven synthetic gauze.

Heavily used since the early 20th century are contact layers (CLs).

ADVANCES IN WOUND CARE, VOLUME 1

Printed in U.S.A.
DOI: 10.1089/awc.2009.0155

Early CLs included tulle gras,[3] a wide-mesh net material coated with a blend of paraffin, oil, and Balsam of Peru. Later, CLs included a synthetic net or mesh, uncoated or coated. CLs serve several functions. They may be used directly on the wound to reduce trauma from dressing changes while allowing exudate and topical agents to pass through it to and from the wound. CLs also prevent adhesion to dressings, especially with negative pressure wound therapy (NPWT) or over skin grafts.

Gauze products are frequently impregnated with a number of substances (Table 1). In the quest to provide wound care for minimal cost, the pennies-per-use cost of gauze has been appealing, as well as its wide availability and general ease of use. However, there are several areas of concern with some gauze applications, and the previously popular gauze "wet-to-dry dressings" (WTDDs) has fallen out of favor because of the tissue trauma and wound desiccation associated with its use.

Table 1. *Common uses of impregnated gauzes*

Impregnated Ingredient	Non-adherent	Debridement	Moisture-retentive	Moisture-additive	Absorbent	Wound drying/ desiccation	Anti-microbial	Hemostasis	Primary Dressing	Contact Layer	Manufactured impregnated	Impregnated at point of use
Sodium Chloride (saline)		Primary	Secondary	Secondary	Primary	Secondary			Primary		Primary	Primary
Hypertonic Sodium Chloride (dry)		Primary			Primary				Primary		Primary	
Iodoform					Primary	Primary	Primary		Primary		Primary	
Petrolatum	Primary		Primary						Primary	Primary	Primary	Secondary
Paraffin	Primary		Primary						Primary	Primary	Primary	
Bismuth and Petrolatum	Primary		Primary			Secondary	Secondary		Primary	Primary	Primary	
BIPP	Primary		Primary					Primary	Primary		Primary	
Oil Emulsion	Primary		Primary						Primary	Primary	Primary	
Hydrogel	Primary			Primary					Primary		Primary	Primary
Honey	Primary	Primary	Primary		Secondary		Primary		Primary		Primary	Primary
PHMB					Primary	Primary	Primary		Primary		Primary	
Cellulose								Primary	Primary		Primary	
Chitosan								Primary	Primary		Primary	
Kaolin								Primary			Primary	
Zeolite								Primary			Primary	
Polymer	Primary		Primary	Primary	Primary				Primary		Primary	

Legend: Primary effects; Secondary effects

This table represents the most commonly used impregnation substances. Clinicians often manually impregnate gauze with other desired substances. This technique may be especially valuable in resource-poor nations where preimpregnated dressings may be unavailable or prohibitively expensive. The properties of saline gauze vary depending on use—whether placed wet, moist or dry, and whether removed wet, damp, or dry. Hemostatic dressings vary in use across manufacturers. Some are designed to be left in place as a primary dressing, whereas others are designed to be temporary until clotting occurs, at which point they are removed and a different primary dressing is applied. Dark gray shades: primary effects; light gray shades: secondary effects.

BIPP = bismuth, iodoform, and paraffin paste; PHMB = polyhexamethylene biguanide.

BASIC SCIENCE CONTEXT

In 1962, Winter published his seminal paper supporting moist wound healing (MWH) as superior to dry wounds.[4] Wounds that are kept moist heal faster, with less scarring, a better cosmetic outcome, and fewer infections.

Critical colonization and infection are well understood to impair wound healing through the production of inflammatory cytokines and bacterial toxins, which lead to a prolonged inflammatory phase of wound healing.

The choice of dressing can influence the wound bed's moisture and bacterial loads, thus influencing wound viability and progression. Depending on its use, gauze may dry or hydrate the wound and is typically very permeable to bacteria.

EXPERIMENTAL MODEL OR MATERIAL—ADVANTAGES AND LIMITATIONS

Because it has long been the "standard of care," there has been little research on gauze, especially recently. Most research has been on the treatment for the control group, with the test product usually proving superior to gauze for wound healing. These trials are often sponsored by the manufacturer of the product. As gauze and impregnated gauzes are inexpensive, there is little financial incentive to invest in studies. Published papers on these materials may be based on clinical experience or professional opinion. Studies rarely compare CLs. Those that do include few types and these studies often are not replicated or expanded.

Iodoform has proven to be more bacteriostatic than bactericidal *in vitro*.[5] However, it is thought that it may react with body fluids and become more bactericidal *in vivo*. However, the research on this question is limited, and it has not been examined for decades in the context of current knowledge. Other antimicrobial substances, such as cadexomer iodine and Dakins solution, have been studied as stand-alone products, not necessarily impregnated on gauze. (See Section 3, Antibacterial Dressings for more information on antimicrobial substances.)

The contemporary research cited in this chapter was produced in western nations with access to advanced wound care. Resource-poor nations may not have access to these more expensive products, and so more of traditional materials may be encompassed in the primary approach. Therefore, older research may prove valuable when these products are the only available ones. Research on outcomes in these settings is important.

DISCUSSION OF FINDINGS AND RELEVANT LITERATURE

Gauze has been used since ancient times, because of its availability, ease of use, inexpensive cost, familiarity, and longevity in practice, as well as clinicians' lack of knowledge about the variety of alternatives available.[6]

Plain gauze is commonly used in several manners. Dry gauze is often used on closed surgical sites to absorb any exudate and provide a mild barrier from the environment. With moistened gauze or a wet-to-moist dressing, gauze is wet with normal saline, or other liquid solution, and changed several times daily to prevent the wound from drying. For WTDDs, saline-moistened gauze is applied to the wound and allowed to dry before removal to facilitate debridement. Fifty years post-Winter, WTDDs continue to be prevalent.[6–8]

Though gauze dressings appear inexpensive, it has been demonstrated that these dressings are actually much more expensive than advanced dressings because of the labor involved multiple times per day, longer time to healing, greater need for pain medications, and a higher infection risk.[6–12] As the moisture evaporates the wound bed cools, slowing healing through vasoconstriction, reducing oxygen release by hemoglobin, and reducing the mobility and activity of leukocytes.[6] The gauze also becomes hypertonic, drawing fluid from the wound bed, causing dessication.[6,7] In addition to inhibiting MWH, WTDDs tightly adhere to slough and granulation tissue. As a result, dressing changes cause significant trauma to the newly growing tissue through nonselective debridement[6,8] and a prolonged inflammatory state. Of particular concern for patients lacking coagulation, WTDDs also increase the risk of bleeding upon dressing removal.[3] For these reasons, Centers for Medicare and Medicaid Services (CMS) regulations for long-term care indicate that this approach should be used only for mechanical debridement when the wound has no significant viable tissue.[13] Clinicians often re-wet the gauze before removal to reduce the adherence and associated pain, thus preventing mechanical debridement while maintaining the disadvantages of a dry wound bed.[8] There is a commercially available hypertonic salt-impregnated dry gauze designed to debride slough.

Iodoform gauze has been used to prevent or treat infection since 1837.[14] In the 1880s there was a debate over the toxicity of iodoform because of the complications from its use, including several deaths.[14] Iodoform and bismuth are common sensitizers,[15–17] with an allergic reaction rate for bismuth, iodoform, and paraffin paste (BIPP) dressings up to 11% after a second exposure.[18] Despite these risks, and a weak antimicrobial effect,[14,15,19–22] it is still in use.

TAKE-HOME MESSAGE

Basic science advances

There is little research on gauze, impregnated gauze, and CLs. Most modern research is on a control group's standard of care while another product is being studied. The studies focused on these products are older.

- Iodoform is incompatible with silver nitrite, metallic salts, strong oxidizers, and strong bases.[23]
- WTDDs are not supported in modern wound care.
- Iodoform is more bacteriostatic than bacteriocidal.[5]
- Iodoform and other substances may respond differently in *in vivo* and *in vitro* environments.
- CL composition affects cell viability.

Clinical science advances

- Gauze and impregnated substances have been used since ancient times.
- There is a wide variety of CLs and impregnated gauzes (which may serve as CLs or primary dressings). They serve several purposes, including the following:
  - Protection of the wound bed through nonadherence, leading to reduced pain, bleeding, and trauma,
  - Bacteriostatic or bacteriocidal environment,
  - Hemostasis,
  - Management of moisture balance.
- Gauze and impregnated gauzes may promote or hinder MWH, depending on the product and its use.
- Gauze is not an adequate bacterial barrier, especially when wet. Greasy, oily, or gel-based substances on the gauze may provide better occlusion.
- Iodoform and bismuth are strong allergic sensitizers.
- With a WTDD, evaporative cooling delays wound healing through vasoconstriction, reduced leukocyte activity, and increased oxygen binding.
- As the moisture evaporates from a WTDD, it becomes more hypertonic, desiccating the wound as it pulls fluid osmotically.
- Polyhexamethylene biguanide-impregnated gauze may be helpful in reducing the risk of Methicillin-resistant *Staphylococcus aureus* (MRSA) and other infections.
- The removal of gauze dressings releases significant amounts of bacteria into the air.

Relevance to clinical care

- Despite inexpensive supply costs, gauze dressings have a higher total cost of care.
- The clinician can impregnate gauze with nearly any solution, gel, or paste at the point of care.
- Wound-care professionals must be aware of the risks and benefits of each product being used.
- Sudden changes in behavior, mental status, neurological status, renal function, or overall medical condition should trigger assessment of iodine or bismuth levels if dressings containing them have been used. If toxicity is suspected or confirmed, the type of dressing must be changed and supportive measures implemented. Hemodialysis or chelation may be necessary in severe cases.
- With systemic absorption, iodoform can transmit to a fetus through the placenta or to an infant via breastmilk, causing hypothyroidism.[37]
- CLs are used to reduce tissue trauma and pain at dressing changes with NPWT,[35] over skin grafts, and with fragile tissue.
- Each type of CL has advantages and disadvantages, and the clinician should consider which option best serves a particular patient.

Iodoform may be absorbed systemically, especially if the wound is large or if it is used for a prolonged time. The Material Safety Data Sheet for iodoform[23] labels it a severe health risk with multiple problems, such as inhalation, ingestion, or transdermal absorption, including dermatitis, irritation, and effects on the cardiovascular system, nervous system, liver, and kidneys. Other reported symptoms of iodoform toxicity include acid/base disturbance, thyroid disorders, abnormal liver function, and neutropenia.[24]

There are many reported cases of iodoform toxicity causing reversible cognitive impairment,[5,15,25–29] with both iodopor gauze and BIPP-impregnated gauze. Bismuth can result in systemic toxicity.[24] Iodoform may affect peripheral nerves. Gauze impregnated with an iodophor paint placed adjacent to a nerve blocked conduction.[30] The same effect was not found with iodoform gauze, but facial paralysis has been noted with BIPP use.[31]

Gauze may be impregnated with antimicrobial agents. Antiseptics such as Dakin's solution have broad cytotoxicity, but may be used in limited situations. (See Section 3, Antibacterial Dressings.) One study[32] found a 24% reduction in surgical site infections and a 48% reduction in MRSA surgical site infections with an antimicrobial gauze impregnated with polyhexamethylene biguanide.

Gauze is often used as a secondary dressing to secure primary dressings and provide a bacterial barrier. However, 64 layers of dry gauze are required to block bacteria.[33] Moist gauze is even more permeable to bacteria.[6] The risk of aerosolization and cross-contamination is also higher with gauze. Compared with a hydrocolloid, gauze dressing changes resulted in five times the amount of bacteria released into the air.[33,34]

Woven cotton gauze adheres to tissue more strongly than nonwoven synthetic gauze and may shed fibers, especially if cut. These tiny foreign bodies prolong inflammation and may form granulomas in the tissue.

There has been little research on CLs; however, their value is clinically recognized. They are most commonly a synthetic mesh, either raw or coated with a nonadherent material such as petrolatum, oil, or silicone. CLs may dry and stick if left in place too long or the exudate is sanguinous.[3] The composition and permeability of a CL used under NPWT will affect the force at the surface, and so this should be considered in planning care.[35] Petrolatum-impregnated gauze resulted in lower local pressure than the foam alone or with silicone or mylar-polyester CLs. (See Section 11, Topical Negative Pressure Therapy for Acute and Chronic Wounds.)

The composition of the CL affects cell viability. *In vitro* tulle gras with chlorhexadine produced a significant reduction in fibroblasts and keratinocytes, whereas a silicone-coated viscose CL showed an increase in the number of fibroblasts after 3 days of treatment, but not 7.[36]

CAUTION, CRITICAL REMARKS, AND RECOMMENDATIONS

At this time there is little independent research on impregnated gauzes and CLs. Most product trials compare their efficacy to plain gauze, which usually is not conducive to wound healing, making the alternatives appear superior. Comparative trials of products within or across categories are rare. Many published articles are commentary or informational pieces based on opinion or experience.

There are some reports that silicone-coated CLs may be more difficult to apply and are more time consuming than other CLs.[38] They also have been reported to adhere less to the wound base, however, and may be a better choice in some cases, despite a higher cost.[39]

Despite the wide array of advanced wound products available, and the knowledge base that has accumulated about the harm WTDDs and iodoform-impregnated gauze may cause to wounds, they are still in common use by nonwound specialists. Efforts must be taken by the wound-healing community to bring the practice of wound care by all health professionals up to current standards.

Despite being highly toxic, iodoform is still used in open wounds. The Material Safety Data Sheet advises wearing protective garments to prevent skin contact when working with iodoform. It is not, however, a carcinogen.[23]

FUTURE DEVELOPMENT

There is a need for further work in this area, with new products being developed, and the efficacy of new and existing products being explored.

The older dressings, such as gauze, petrolatum gauze, BIPP, and iodoform gauze, have some evidence available about their use, both favorable and unfavorable, albeit mostly decades old. The newer products have limited independent research. As there is much variability in the composition and properties of CLs and impregnated substances, comparative research should be conducted so that wound-care professionals will be able to select the optimum product for a given wound.

New impregnations are sure to be developed, with multiple aims. Recently, several gauze impregnations previously reserved for emergency settings have become available for achieving hemostasis. Another new product impregnated with a polymer designed to maintain moisture balance by moving fluid between the dressing and the wound as needed has been developed. Real-world outcomes for these products should be studied.

ACKNOWLEDGMENT

None.

AUTHOR DISCLOSURE STATEMENT

No competing financial interests exist.

REFERENCES

1. Broughton G, 2nd, Janis JE, and Attinger CE: A brief history of wound care. Plast Reconstr Surg 2006; **117(7 Suppl):** 6S.
2. Baxter H: How a discipline came of age: a history of wound care. J Wound Care 2002; **11:** 383–386, 388, 390 passim.
3. Malone WD: Wound dressing adherence: a clinical comparative study. Arch Emerg Med 1987; **4:** 101.
4. Winter GD: Formation of the scab and the rate of epithelization of superficial wounds in the skin of the young domestic pig. Nature 1962; **193:** 293.
5. O'Connor AF, Freeland AP, Heal DJ, and Rossouw DS: Iodoform toxicity following the use of B.I.P.P.: a potential hazard. J Laryngol Otol 1977; **91:** 903.
6. Ovington LG: Hanging wet-to-dry dressings out to dry. Home Healthc Nurse 2001; **19:** 477–483; quiz 84.
7. Spear M: Wet-to-dry dressings—evaluating the evidence. Plast Surg Nurs 2008; **28:** 92.
8. Armstrong M and Price PE: Wet-to-dry gauze dressings: fact and fiction. Wounds 2004; **16:** 56.
9. Capasso VA and Munro BH: The cost and efficacy of two wound treatments. AORN J 2003; **77:** 984–992, 95–97, 1000–1004.
10. Harding K, Cutting K, and Price P: The cost-effectiveness of wound management protocols of care. Br J Nurs 2000; **9(19 Suppl):** S6, S8, S10 passim.
11. Colwell JC, Foreman MD, and Trotter JP: A comparison of the efficacy and cost-effectiveness of two methods of managing pressure ulcers. Decubitus 1993; **6:** 28.
12. Xakellis GC and Chrischilles EA: Hydrocolloid versus saline-gauze dressings in treating pressure ulcers: a cost-effectiveness analysis. Arch Phys Med Rehabil 1992; **73:** 463.
13. State operations manual: Appendix PP—guidance to surveyors for long term care facilities, 2004. http://www.cms.hhs.gov/manuals/downloads/som107ap_pp_guidelines_ltcf.pdf.
14. Van Arsdale WW: The present status of the iodoform question. Ann Surg 1889; **9:** 202.
15. Flook EP, Uddin FJ, and Johnston MN: The need to include BIPP reactions in routine consent. Clin Otolaryngol 2006; **31:** 165.
16. Roest MA, Shaw S, and Orton DI: Allergic contact otitis externa due to iodoform in BIPP cavity dressings. Contact Dermat 2002; **46:** 360.
17. Goh CL, and Ng SK: Contact allergy to iodoform and bismuth subnitrate. Contact Dermat 1987; **16:** 109.
18. Lim PV, Hughes RG, and Oates J: Hypersensitive allergic reactions to bismuth-iodoform-paraffin paste following ear surgery. J Laryngol Otol 1998; **112:** 335.
19. Wilson AP: The dangers of BIPP. Lancet 1994; **344:** 1313.
20. Estrela C, Estrela CR, Hollanda AC, Decurcio Dde A, and Pecora JD: Influence of iodoform on antimicrobial potential of calcium hydroxide. J Appl Oral Sci 2006; **14:** 33.
21. Maylard AE: An experimental investigation into the antiseptic value of iodoform. Ann Surg 1890; **11:** 17.
22. Nigam A and Allwood MC: BIPP—how does it work? Clin Otolaryngol Allied Sci 1990; **15:** 173.
23. *MSDS for Iodoform.* Phillipsburg, NJ: Mallinckrodt Baker, Inc., 2008. http://www.jtbaker.com/msds/englishhtml/i3480.htm.
24. Ovaska H, Wood DM, House I, Dargan PI, Jones AL, and Murray S: Severe iatrogenic bismuth poisoning with bismuth iodoform paraffin paste treated with DMPS chelation. Clin Toxicol 2008; **46:** 855.
25. Numata S, Murayama Y, Makino M, and Nakamura A: Temporary stupor in a patient treated with iodoform gauze for mediastinitis after coronary artery bypass grafting. Interact Cardiovasc Thorac Surg 2004; **3:** 309.
26. Matsumura Y, Tsuji A, Izawa J, Kumakura A, Hiramatsu M, Kogo K, Takahashi K, Inoue Y, Harada H, and Tonozuka N: Suspected toxicity from an iodoform preparation in a diabetic patient with multiple foot ulcers. Diabet Med 2005; **22:** 1121.
27. Youngman L and Harris S: BIPP madness; an iatrogenic cause of acute confusion. Age Ageing 2004; **33:** 406.
28. Harris RA and Poole A: Beware of bismuth: post maxillectomy delirium. ANZ J Surg 2002; **72:** 846.
29. Araki K, Hirakawa N, Kosugi T, Higashimoto I, Kakiuchi Y, and Nakashima M: Iodoform intoxication; a case report of prolonged consciousness disturbance in a patient with a high plasma iodine level. Fukuoka Igaku Zasshi 2007; **98:** 397.
30. Loescher AR and Robinson PP: The effect of surgical medicaments on peripheral nerve function. Br J Oral Maxillofac Surg 1998; **36:** 327.

31. Jones PH: BIPP allergy causing facial paralysis. J Laryngol Otol 1985; **99:** 389.

32. Mueller SW and Krebsbach LE: Impact of an antimicrobial-impregnated gauze dressing on surgical site infections including methicillin-resistant *Staphylococcus aureus* infections. Am J Infect Control 2008; **36:** 651.

33. Lawrence JC: Dressings and wound infection. Am J Surg 1994; **167:** 21S.

34. Lawrence JC, Lilly HA, and Kidson A: Wound dressings and airborne dispersal of bacteria. Lancet 1992; **339:** 807.

35. Jones SM, Banwell PE, and Shakespeare PG: Interface dressings influence the delivery of topical negative-pressure therapy. Plast Reconstr Surg 2005; **116:** 1023.

36. Dover R, Otto WR, Nanchahal J, and Riches DJ: Toxicity testing of wound dressing materials *in vitro*. Br J Plast Surg 1995; **48:** 230.

37. L'Italien A, Starceski PJ, and Dixit NM: Transient hypothyroidism in a breastfed infant after maternal use of iodoform gauze. J Pediatr Endocrinol Metab 2004; **17:** 665.

38. Briggs SL, Taylor A, and Lansdown AB: Clinical perspective on silicone dressings and wound management. J Wound Care 2008; **17:** 364–365; author reply 5–6.

39. Williams C: Mepitel. Br J Nurs 1995; **4:** 51–52, 4–5.

Transparent Film Dressings

Susie Seaman*

Wound Clinic, Sharp Rees-Stealy Medical Group, San Diego, California.

Abbreviations and Acronyms

MVTR = moisture vapor transmission rate

TEWL = transepidermal water loss

*Correspondence: Sharp Rees-Stealy Wound Clinic, 2020 Genesee Ave., San Diego, California 92123 (e-mail: susie.seaman@sharp.com).

Background: Before 1960, wound healing was believed to be optimized in a dry environment, which resulted in the formation of a dry crust or scab. The primary dressings used were made from cotton and/or wool and their function was mainly to cover and conceal the wound. It is now well accepted among wound management experts that a moist environment is advantageous to wound healing. The benefits include enhanced keratinocyte and fibroblast proliferation, keratinocyte migration, collagen synthesis, angiogenesis, wound contraction, autolytic debridement, and wound closure.

The Problem: The clinical problems addressed with transparent films are wound desiccation, wound trauma, and bacterial contamination, all of which are frequently observed with the use of gauze dressings.

Basic/Clinical Science Advances: Moisture vapor transmission rate can be measured and is a good indicator of a dressing's moisture retentiveness. Transparent film dressings have been demonstrated to speedup reepithelialization and improve pain scores without increasing the risk of infection in partial-thickness wounds.

Clinical Care Relevance: Transparent films should be considered for use in patients with superficial, low-exudating wounds, including abrasions, skin tears, stripping injuries, and split-thickness skin graft donor sites. Gauze dressings should be avoided in these wounds as they may cause significant pain and trauma upon removal.

Conclusion: Because of their ability to maintain a moist wound healing environment and provide a barrier against exogenous bacterial contamination, transparent films will continue to have a role in treating superficial wounds.

BACKGROUND

Before 1960, wound healing was believed to be optimized in a dry environment, which resulted in the formation of a dry crust or scab.[1] The primary dressings used were made from cotton and/or wool and their function was mainly to cover and conceal the wound.[2–4] It was generally believed that dressings were unimportant to the healing process. This viewpoint was challenged by Winter's landmark research which demonstrated that reepithelialization in partial-thickness porcine wounds kept covered with polyethane film occurred two times faster when compared with similar wounds left open to air.[5] This finding was substantiated by Hinman and Maibach, who found that reepithelialization rates in human partial-thickness wounds covered with polyethane film healed twice as fast as similar wounds left open to air.[6] These studies led to the concept that dressings, rather than being passive coverings, had the potential to alter the wound environment and affect healing.

It is now well accepted among wound management experts that a moist environment is advantageous

ADVANCES IN WOUND CARE, VOLUME 1

Printed in U.S.A.
DOI: 10.1089/awc.2009.0152

to wound healing. The benefits include enhanced keratinocyte and fibroblast proliferation, keratinocyte migration, collagen synthesis, angiogenesis, wound contraction, autolytic debridement, and wound closure.[7,8] However, despite evidence supporting moist wound healing, there has been concern that the same environment that promotes healing may also support bacterial growth and infection.[9] A secondary analysis of over 100 studies comparing infection rates in over 4,000 wounds treated with either moisture-retentive dressings (films, hydrocolloids, foams, and hydrogels) or dry dressings (predominantly gauze) found that the overall infection rate was 2.6% with moisture-retentive dressings versus 7.1% with dry dressings ($p < 0.001$).[10] Thus, there is evidence supporting a moist wound environment as beneficial to healing with a decreased risk of infection.

In the last four decades, hundreds of dressings have been developed to provide this moist wound environment. Transparent films were one of the first dressings of this type.

CLINICAL PROBLEMS ADDRESSED

The clinical problems to be addressed with transparent films are wound desiccation, wound trauma, and bacterial contamination. These issues are frequently observed with gauze dressings, which remain the most commonly used dressings in wound care and which perform in an opposite manner from transparent films.[11] When a wound dries out, gauze dressings may adhere to the wound, causing significant pain, bleeding, and tissue trauma.[4] Wet-to-dry gauze dressings, in which saline-moistened gauze is applied to a wound, allowed to dry out, and then is pulled out of the wound, provide nonselective debridement, in that when the gauze dries out, it adheres to both viable and nonviable tissue, stripping both upon dressing removal.[11] Delayed wound healing may result from repetitive tissue trauma. This type of dressing change is usually performed two to three times a day, which may significantly increase the cost of care from the standpoint of staff productivity. Use of gauze dressings may also result in exogenous bacterial contamination when exudate strikes through to the outer dressing, facilitating movement of bacteria into the wound. It has been shown *in vitro* that bacteria can rapidly migrate through multiple layers of wet gauze and that a layer of cellophane can block this movement.[12,13] It has also been demonstrated *in vitro* and *in vivo* that aerosolization of bacteria is greater when removing dry gauze dressings versus hydrocolloid dressings, which are occlusive and moisture retentive, from both a wound model and from small burn wounds in humans.[14] This can result in contamination of the patient care setting and lead to transmission of pathogenic bacteria among staff and other patients. Use of transparent films prevents wound desiccation, tissue trauma, and bacterial contamination of the wound, and may decrease aerosolization of bacteria with dressing changes.

RELEVANT BASIC SCIENCE CONTEXT

The degree of moisture retentiveness of dressings is measured by moisture vapor transmission rate (MVTR).[7,15] MVTR, often reported as $g/m^2/24\,h$, refers to the passage of water vapor from the wound bed, through a dressing, to the outside environment. Moisture-retentive dressings have MVTRs of less than $840\,g/m^2/24\,h$.[16] MVTR varies widely, with highly occlusive dressings having MVTRs less than $300\,g/m^2/24\,h$ and more permeable dressings such as gauze having MVTRs over $1{,}600\,g/m^2/24\,h$.[7] As a comparison, it has been shown that transepidermal water loss (TEWL) is $4–9\,mg/m^2/h$ ($96–216\,g/m^2/24\,h$) in intact skin, and $80–90\,mg/m^2/h$ ($1{,}920–2{,}160\,g/m^2/24\,h$) in partial- and full-thickness wounds.[17,18]

EXPERIMENTAL MODELS OR MATERIALS—ADVANTAGES AND LIMITATIONS

Studies examining the role of transparent films have been performed in animals and humans. Many different animals have been utilized in wound healing studies; however, the pig has emerged as one of the best animal models to use.[19] Porcine skin is comparable to human skin in multiple advantageous ways. Although most animals have thin epidermal and dermal layers and thick body hair, porcine skin resembles human skin in epidermal thickness, dermal–epidermal thickness ratio, amount of body hair, presence of rete ridges and plentiful subcutaneous fat, anatomy of dermal blood vessels, dermal collagen structure, and many other characteristics. Both in pigs and humans, partial-thickness wounds heal primarily via reepithelialization, whereas in most other animals, similar wounds heal mainly by wound contraction. Sullivan *et al.*[19] reviewed multiple studies of the use of transparent films in the porcine model of wound healing, in which the results were later replicated in humans, demonstrating that pigs make an excellent model for studying wound healing which can be applied to humans. Just as

Hinman and Maibach[6] replicated Winter's[5] early work in pigs, demonstrating enhanced epithelialization in humans, other studies on the effects of transparent films have shown an enhanced proliferation response in keratinocytes, faster reepithelialization rates, and increased rate of healing in full-thickness wounds in both pig models and humans. These studies justify the use of the porcine model to examine dressing effects on wound healing. Potential disadvantages in the use of the porcine model include anatomic differences in the skin such as a lesser developed dermal plexus in the pig, absence of eccrine glands, and wide distribution of apocrine glands in the pig, and the inability to collect subjective responses regarding dressing effects on wound pain from the pig. Thus, transparent films are also studied on humans in both experimentally induced wounds and surgically created wounds.

DISCUSSION OF FINDINGS AND RELEVANT LITERATURE

Transparent films are thin, semipermeable, clear polyurethane dressings with an adhesive layer that adheres to intact skin, but not to a moist wound bed.[20] They do not have absorptive capacity, but do transmit moisture vapor. Transparent films used in wound care have MVTRs from 300 to 800 $g/m^2/24\,h$ and will maintain a moist wound environment.[7,16,21] In contrast, transparent films used over intravenous line sites require a higher MVTR to prevent moisture accumulation under the dressing and subsequent poor adherence. These films, whose main goal is to protect the intravenous site from bacterial contamination, have MVTRs up to 3,700 $g/m^2/24\,h$,[21] and they should not be used on open wounds, as they can lead to wound desiccation. Although films are moisture vapor and gas permeable, they are impermeable to exogenous bacteria and liquids. With their nonadherence to a moist wound bed, moisture retentiveness, and barrier qualities, transparent films address the clinical problems of wound desiccation, wound trauma, and bacterial contamination observed with the use of gauze dressings.

The use of transparent films has been studied on a variety of wounds. Visscher *et al.*[22] examined the role of semipermeable films, completely occlusive films, or no occlusion on the restoration of skin barrier function in 240 partial-thickness wounds created by tape stripping in 40 healthy volunteers. The rate of skin barrier repair was measured by TEWL, skin hydration, rate of moisture accumulation, and erythema. Skin barrier restoration occurred most rapidly in wounds treated with semipermeable films versus wounds treated with total occlusion or no occlusion. Beam[23] studied the healing rates of 40 standardized partial-thickness abrasions created on 10 healthy volunteers treated with an occlusive hydrocolloid, a semipermeable transparent film, a hydrogel sheet, or no dressing. The wounds treated with the hydrocolloid and film dressings had the greatest statistically significant decreases in wound size at 7 and 10 days, and at 14 days the hydrocolloid, film, and hydrogel dressings all demonstrated significantly improved healing compared with no dressing. A prospective, randomized trial showed that the use of transparent film dressings versus fine mesh gauze in 24 patients with 60 split-thickness skin graft donor sites resulted in significantly faster reepithelialization in the donor sites treated with the film dressings.[24] When 80 patients with split-thickness skin graft donor sites were randomized to treatment with transparent polyurethane film, paraffin gauze, polyurethane foam, or polyethane film, healing rates in all groups were similar; however, the group treated with the transparent polyurethane film noted significantly less pain with dressing removal.[25] It was also noted that the polyurethane film was the easiest and fastest to remove, taking less than 5 min, whereas the paraffin gauze took the longest, in some cases requiring saline soaks for over 20 min prior to dressing removal. In a study of split-thickness skin graft donor site healing and pain management, 40 patients had their donor sites dressed with paraffin gauze covered by dry gauze, alginate covered by dry gauze, alginate covered by transparent film, or transparent film alone.[26] The healing rates were highest and pain scores were lowest in the group treated with alginate plus transparent film; the transparent film alone had the second best results. Statistical testing was not reported. Rubio[27] reported on the use of transparent film dressings, applied in the operating room and left on for 10 days, in 3,637 postoperative incisions over an 8-year period. He objectively noted no infections, better hygiene, and greater mobility in all of the patients treated. Wiechula[28] performed a systematic review of 58 studies to examine whether healing rates, infection, and pain differed in split-thickness skin graft donor sites treated with either moisture-retentive dressings (hydrocolloids, transparent films, or alginates) or dry dressings (gauze or petrolatum gauze with 3% bismuth tribromphenate). The healing rates and pain scores were found to be improved with moisture-retentive dressings versus dry dressings, and there was no increased risk of infection noted with moist dressings.

SUMMARY

- Transparent films are thin, clear, semipermeable, adhesive dressings that are moisture retentive.
- Transparent films have been found to enhance healing of partial-thickness wounds compared with dry dressings.
- Transparent films have demonstrated decreased pain in comparison to dry dressings.
- There is no evidence to support that transparent films may increase infection rates.

CAUTION, CRITICAL REMARKS, AND RECOMMENDATIONS

Transparent films are indicated primarily for superficial wounds with minimal exudate.[29] Because of their moisture retentiveness, they may be utilized to soften dry eschar via autolytic debridement. Transparent films may be used over absorptive fillers, such as alginates or starch copolymers, for wounds with higher exudate levels. Alternatively, a composite/island dressing may be used, in which an absorptive layer is bonded to and surrounded by an outer transparent film. Transparent films can be placed over any dressing to provide a bacterial barrier.

Transparent films should not be used on clinically infected wounds in which the goal is to wick infectious exudate away. They should be avoided on patients with fragile skin because removal can result in significant trauma to intact skin.

Advantages of using transparent films include protection of the wound and skin from friction and bacterial contamination, provision of a moist environment for reepithelialization and autolytic debridement, and pain reduction. They allow ongoing visual assessment of the wound, are waterproof, flexible, and may stay in place up to 7 days. However, they are not absorptive, so that excess drainage can lead to periwound skin maceration and further skin breakdown, and they may be difficult to handle, apply, and remove.

When using transparent films, it is suggested to utilize a size that covers 2 cm of the periwound skin to enhance dressing adherence. To avoid maceration and further skin breakdown, films should be

TAKE-HOME MESSAGE

Basic science advances

- MVTR can be measured and is a good indicator of a dressing's moisture retentiveness. Occlusive dressings such as hydrocolloids have MVTRs less than 300 $g/m^2/24\,h$. Semipermeable dressings, such as transparent films, have MVTRs of 300–800 $g/m^2/24\,h$. As MVTR increases, wounds may become desiccated, and healing rates are decreased.
- Porcine skin provides an excellent model to assess skin repair in response to moist versus dry dressings. Many of these studies can be later replicated in humans.

Clinical science advances

- Transparent films restore skin barrier function as measured by TEWL, skin hydration, rate of moisture accumulation, and erythema more rapidly than completely occlusive films or no dressings in partial-thickness wounds caused by tape stripping.
- Transparent film dressings have been demonstrated to speedup reepithelialization in partial-thickness wounds, including abrasions and split-thickness skin graft donor sites, in comparison to dry dressings or no dressings.
- Transparent film dressings, either with or without an alginate dressing, have been shown to decrease pain scores in patients with split-thickness skin graft donor sites in comparison to dry dressings.
- Transparent polyurethane film dressings may be removed from split-thickness skin graft donor sites with significantly less pain and at a faster rate, in less than 5 min, than paraffin gauze dressings, which require saline soaks for over 20 min prior to removal.
- Transparent films can be applied over surgical incisions and left in place for up to 10 days, resulting in no infections and in greater hygiene and mobility.
- There is no evidence to support the concern that wounds kept covered with moisture-retentive dressings are at greater risk for infection than wounds covered with dry dressings.

Relevance to clinical care

- Transparent films should be considered for use in patients with superficial wounds, including abrasions, skin tears, stripping injuries, and split-thickness skin graft donor sites. They provide a protected, moist environment for rapid reepithelialization without an increased risk of infection.
- Because superficial wounds may be quite painful with exposed dermal nerve endings, the use of transparent films should be considered to decrease pain in this type of wound.
- As they are not absorptive and have a low MVTR, transparent films cannot be expected to handle high amounts of wound drainage and hence should be avoided on wounds with heavy exudate.
- Gauze dressings should be avoided in partial-thickness wounds where they may cause significant pain and trauma upon removal. The use of gauze dressings in clinical practice may take more time because if they adhere to wounds, they require saline soaks for removal.

changed when exudate leaks onto intact skin, or at least every 7 days.

FUTURE DEVELOPMENT

Transparent film dressings have been used for over 30 years. Over that period of time, they have been improved to provide different levels of MVTR, have had antibacterials such as silver added to them, and have been bonded to exudate absorbers to create island dressings. Because they are used mainly for partial-thickness wounds, which are usually the simplest type of wound to heal, there is not much need for future development, especially as wound care is moving toward the use of active products such as growth factors, bioengineered tissues, and other constructs. Transparent films will most likely continue to have a role in protecting and healing superficial wounds.

AUTHOR DISCLOSURE STATEMENT

The author of this manuscript has no competing financial interests.

REFERENCES

1. Cho CY and Lo JS: Dressing the part. Dermatol Clin 1998; **16:** 25.
2. Cockbill SME and Turner TD: The development of wound-management products. In: *Chronic Wound Care: A Clinical Source Book for Healthcare Professionals*, 4th edition, edited by Krasner DL, Rodeheaver GT, and Sibbald RG. Malvern, PA: HMP Communications, 2007, pp. 233–248.
3. Ovington LG: The evolution of wound management: ancient origins and advances of the past 20 years. Home Healthc Nurse 2002; **20:** 652.
4. Jones VJ: The use of gauze: will it ever change? Int Wound J 2006; **3:** 79.
5. Winter GD: Formation of the scab and the rate of epithelialization of superficial wounds in the skin of young domestic pigs. Nature 1962; **193:** 293.
6. Hinman CD and Maibach HI: Effect of air exposure and occlusion on experimental human skin wounds. Nature 1963; **200:** 377.
7. Bolton LL, Monte K, and Pirone LA: Moisture and healing: beyond the jargon. Ostomy Wound Manage 2000; **46(Suppl 1A):** 51S.
8. Eaglstein WH: Moist wound healing with occlusive dressings: a clinical focus. Dermatol Surg 2001; **27:** 175.
9. Fonder MA, Lazarus GS, Cowan DA, Aronson-Cook B, Kohli AR, and Mamelak AJ: Treating the chronic wound: a practical approach to the care of nonhealing wounds and wound care dressings. J Am Acad Dermatol 2008; **58:** 185.
10. Hutchinson JJ and McGuckin M: Occlusive dressings: a microbiologic and clinical review. Am J Infect Control 1990; **18:** 257.
11. Ovington LG: Hanging wet-to-dry dressings out to dry. Home Healthc Nurse 2001; **19:** 477.
12. Owens N: Use of pressure dressings in the treatment of burns and other wounds. Surg Clin North Am 1943; **23:** 1354.
13. Colebrook L: Infection through soaked dressings. Lancet 1948; **2:** 682.
14. Lawrence JC, Lilly HA, and Kidson A: Wound dressings and airborne dispersal of bacteria. Lancet 1992; **339:** 807.
15. Palamand S, Reed, AM, and Weimann LJ: Testing intelligent wound dressings. J Biomater Appl 1992; **6:** 198.
16. Bolton LL, Johnson CL, and van Rijswijk L: Occlusive dressings: therapeutic agents and effects on drug delivery. Clin Dermatol 1992; **9:** 573.
17. Wu P, Nelson EA, Reid WH, Ruckley CV, and Gaylor JDS: Water vapour transmission rates in burns and chronic leg ulcers: influence of wound dressings and comparison with *in vitro* evaluation. Biomaterials 1996; **17:** 1373.
18. Silverman RA, Lender J, and Elmets CA: Effects of occlusive and semiocclusive dressings on the return of barrier function to transepidermal water loss in standardized human wounds. J Am Acad Dermatol 1989; **20:** 755.
19. Sullivan TP, Eaglstein WH, Davis SC, and Mertz P: The pig as a model for human wound healing. Wound Repair Regen 2001; **9:** 66.
20. Merkle Leiby D and Lott G: Topical wound product ingredient guide. Ostomy Wound Manage 1997; **43:** 42.
21. Wu P, Fisher AC, Foo PP, Queen D, and Gaylor JDS: *In vitro* assessment of water vapour transmission of synthetic wound dressings. Biomaterials 1995; **16:** 171.
22. Visscher M, Hoath SB, Conroy E, and Wickett ER: Effects of semipermeable membranes on skin barrier repair following tape stripping. Arch Dermatol Res 2001; **293:** 491.
23. Beam JW: Occlusive dressings and the healing of standardized abrasions. J Athl Train 2008; **43:** 600.
24. Barnett A, Berkowitz RL, Mills R, and Vistnes LM: Comparison of synthetic adhesive moisture vapor permeable and fine mesh gauze dressings for split-thickness skin graft donor sites. Am J Surg 1983; **145:** 379.
25. Persson K and Salemark L: How to dress donor sites of split thickness skin grafts: a prospective, randomized study of four dressings. Scand J Plast Reconstr Surg Hand Surg 2000; **34:** 55.
26. Beldon P: Comparison of four different dressings on donor site wounds. Br J Nurs 2004; **13(6 suppl):** S38.
27. Rubio PA: Use of semiocclusive, transparent film dressings for surgical wound protection: experience in 3637 cases. Int Surg 1991; **76:** 253.
28. Wiechula R: The use of moist wound-healing dressings in the management of spilt-thickness skin graft donor sites: a systematic review. Int J Nurs Pract 2003; **9:** S9.
29. Seaman S: Dressing selection in chronic wound management. J Am Podiatr Med Assoc 2002; **92:** 24.

DRESSINGS

Hydrogel Dressings

Karen Lou Kennedy-Evans[1,*] and James B. Lutz[2]

[1]K.L. Kennedy, LLC, Tucson, Arizona.
[2]Lutz Consulting LLCs, Medical Writing Services, Buellton, California.

Background: Hydrogel dressings are available as sheets or amorphous gels. They contain hydrophilic polymers in a solution containing mostly water (usually >80%). There are currently at least 66 brands and 33 manufacturers of hydrogel dressings.
The Problem: Hydrogel dressings are used for dry to moderately draining wounds. They are most often used in situations where moist wound healing is desired, and the control of drainage is of secondary concern. Hydrogels can absorb or donate moisture to the wound, depending on the relative state of hydration of the tissue and the dressing. Hydrogels are often used to facilitate autolytic debridement in necrotic wounds, but are also used to help maintain a moist wound healing environment in clean, granulating wounds.
Basic/Clinical Science Advances: Modern hydrogel products are customized by varying the numbers and types of monomers contained within the linear structure of their polymers, by controlling the degree and types of cross linking between polymer strands and by the addition of ingredients that augment certain performance features of the dressing. Functional ingredients can also be added that interact with and alter the local wound environment.
Clinical Care Relevance: As hydrogel polymer chemistry advances, so too does the body of available clinical research information and the need for additional evidence-based medicine.
Conclusion: Hydrogel dressings are a unique and versatile category of advanced wound care dressings. Numerous forms and brands are currently available. This review seeks to summarize the current body of evidence supporting the clinical use of this dressing product category.

Abbreviation and Acronym

MGD = moist gauze dressings

*Correspondence: K.L. Kennedy, LLC, 5090 N. Corte de Catalonia, Tucson, Arizona 85718 (e-mail: ktulcer@aol.com).

BACKGROUND

HYDROGELS ARE A VERSATILE CLASS of materials that are used in numerous medical applications including dental and ophthalmic materials, monitoring electrodes, diagnostic electrodes, nerve stimulation electrodes, biosensors, skin-friendly adhesives, ultrasound transducer materials, drug delivery systems, and wound dressings.[1,2] They were originally developed in the 1950s,[2] but did not find their way into wound care applications until the 1980s.[3] The first hydrogel wound dressing consisted of a cross-linked polymer of polyacrylamide and agarose.[4]

Hydrogel dressings are available as sheets or amorphous (shapeless) gels. Hydrogel sheets are generally packaged individually and may or may not have a liner or backing material. Some hydrogel sheets have adhesive borders, whereas others must be secure with secondary dressings. The amorphous varieties are usually packaged in tubes, specialty applicators, or impregnated into gauze pads or similar material. Though a comprehensive survey of the market

Printed in U.S.A.
DOI: 10.1089/awc.2009.0184

is beyond the scope of this text, the authors are aware of at least 66 brands and 33 manufacturers of hydrogel wound dressings (Table 1).

Amorphous and sheet hydrogels are chemically similar in composition. Both contain one or more hydrophilic (water loving) polymers in a solution containing mostly water (usually >80%).[2,4–6] Polymers are long chains of repeating units called monomers. Some of the monomers used extensively in wound hydrogels are ethylene oxide, various acrylamides, polyvinylpyrrolidone, prolylene glycol, carboxymethylcellulose, and various acrylates.

Even though amorphous and sheet hydrogels are chemically similar in composition, physically they are differentiated by the degree of cross linking between the polymer chains.[2,4,5,7] Cross linking results in a three-dimensional structure that can affect swelling and the rigidity of the composition[2,4,5,7]; the greater the degree of cross linking, the more solid the structure.

Performance characteristics of hydrogel products can be customized by combining different monomers in different ratios into the hydrogel polymers. Various types of monomers contain different functional side groups, which can influence the behavior characteristics of the polymer such as swelling, viscosity, and the ability of the product to absorb or donate water. Small quantities of additional ingredients, such as collagen, alginate, various ions (*e.g.*, silver, zinc, calcium, and copper), peptides, or complex carbohydrates, may be added to further augment certain performance characteristics, or for the donation of purported active ingredients into the wound environment.[5,6,8,9]

CLINICAL PROBLEM ADDRESSED

Hydrogel dressings are used for dry to minimally to moderately draining wounds with or without a clean granular wound base.[6,7,10,11] They are most often used in situations where moist wound healing is desired, and the control of drainage is of secondary concern. Hydrogels can absorb or donate moisture to the wound environment depending on the relative state of hydration of the tissue and the dressing.[2] However, the clinician should note that hydrogel products differ significantly in this regard.[12–14]

Because of their unique ability to donate moisture to the wound, hydrogels are often used to facilitate autolytic debridement in necrotic wounds and are also used to help maintain a moist wound healing environment in clean, granulating wounds.[5,7–11,15] The donated moisture helps to soften the necrotic tissue so that it can be more easily removed by sharp debridement.[15] Although Williams argues that surgical or mechanical debridement is probably a better initial choice, particularly when there is a large quantity of material to be debrided, or if it extends deep into the wound.[16]

Hydrogel sheets are often used for flat shallow wounds, skin tears, second-degree burns, and many partial- and full-thickness wounds.[1,4,6,7,9,10] They may also be used to treat chronically damaged epithelium[4,9] and radiation-induced dermatitis.[6,9] If the dressing liners can be fully removed, sheet hydrogels can also be used as a wound filler,[1] although amorphous hydrogels impregnated onto a gauze sponge may be a better choice.[5,7]

Hydrogels have been used successfully on infected wounds[7,17] and can help control odor when combined with certain antibiotics.[17] However, the clinician is advised to read and follow the manufacturer guidelines and precautions before such use.

Numerous authors have observed that the use of hydrogel dressings frequently results in a reduction of wound pain. It has been suggested that the moist wound environment created by the hydrogel protects the exposed neurons from dehydration and produces acceptable changes in pH.[4,11] Also, it has been noted that sheet hydrogels have the unique ability to immediately cool the wound surface by up to 5°C for up to 6 h,[9] which may provide a soothing effect.[1,2,4,7,8] It has been further postulated that this lowering of the wound temperature could result in the reduction of the inflammatory response.[4]

RELEVANT BASIC SCIENCE CONTEXT

Modern hydrogel products are differentiated by both their physical and chemical structures, as well as by the addition of ingredients that augment certain performance features of the dressing. Functional ingredients are also added for the purpose of interacting with or altering the local wound environment. Hydrogel dressings have come a long way since their simple formulations introduced in the 1980s; as hydrogel polymer chemistry advances, so too does the body of available clinical research to support their use and the need for additional evidence-based medicine.

EXPERIMENTAL MODEL OR MATERIAL—ADVANTAGES AND LIMITATIONS

Thomas and Hay reported an experimental *in vitro* model that compared the ability of several hydrogel dressings to absorb or donate water from agar gels of varying concentrations.[12,13] These gels were

Manufacturer	Brand Name(s)
3M™ Health Care	Tegaderm™ Gel
Acrymed™	AcryDerm™
Activa®	ActiFormCool®
Afassco	2nd Skin Burn and Wound Pads
Anacapa Technologies, Inc.	MaxGel™, Anasept®
Amerx Health Care Corp.	AmeriGel®
Braun	Askina® THINSite®, Askina® Transorbent Border®
CR Bard, Inc.	Vigilon®, Biolex™
Carrington Laboratories, Inc.	CarraSmart™, Carrasyn®, DiaB™, RadiGel™, Ultrex Gel™, CarraGauze®, CaraDres™, RadiDres™
Coloplast Corp.	Purilon™, Woun'Dres®
Conmed®	Clearsite®
ConvaTec	DuoDERM® Hydroactive Sterile Gel, SAF-Gel®
Derma Sciences, Inc.	Dermagran®, Aquasite®
DermaRite Industries LLC	DermaSyn™, DermaGauze™
DeRoyal	Aquasorb®, Aquagauze™
Dow Hickam	Flexderm®
Gentell	Gentell®
Hartmann-Conco Inc.	AquaClear®, AquaFil™, Hydrosorb®
Healthpoint	Curasol®
Hollister Incorporated	Restore®
Hyperion Medical, Inc.	Hyperion®
Johnson & Johnson Wound Management	NU-GEL™
Medline Industries, Inc.	Skintegrity™, Dermagel™, TenderWet™, XCell®, SilvaSorb®
Medi Tech International Corp	Spand-Gel®
Mölnlycke Health Care	Hypergel®, Normlgel®
MPM Medical, Inc.	Regenicare®
Noble Biomaterials, Inc.	SILVERSEAL®
ProCyte, A PhotoMedx Company	Iamin®
Sage Laboratories	Panogauze, Panoplex
Smith & Nephew Inc.	Intrasite®, Solosite®, Transgel®, Flexigel™
Southwest Technologies	Gold Dust™, Elasto-Gel™, Toe-Aid™, Comfort-Aid®
Swiss-American Products, Inc.	Elta®
Tyco Health Care/Kendall	Curafil®, Aquaflo, Curagel®

Table 1. *A compiled listing of manufacturers and brands of hydrogel wound dressings.*

intended to simulate a wound bed or necrotic tissue in varying states of hydration. The authors found significant differences among the products they tested, indicating that hydrogels that may be similar in appearance can have markedly different fluid-handling properties. Likewise, in 1998, Sprung *et al.* found similar differences using aspirated wound fluid, normal saline, and water.[14] This model further demonstrated that hydrogel dressings can differ markedly in their response to different types of fluids, and it is important to compare the products using actual wound fluid or in an actual clinical setting.

DISCUSSION OF FINDINGS AND RELEVANT LITERATURE

Though hydrogel technology has been available since the 1950s,[2] the first reported use in wound care did not occur until 1982, when Geronemus and Robins reported on the experimental use of a polyethylene oxide hydrogel dressing and a copolymer starch hydrogel dressing in pigs.[18] The first reported clinical application occurred 2 years later.[3] Since then, hydrogel dressings have been studied for numerous types of acute and chronic wounds. These include pressure ulcers, diabetic foot ulcers, leg ulcers, burns, surgical wounds, and various types of skin defects.

Arguably, the single most important advancement in wound care brought about by hydrogels was in speeding and simplifying the debridement of sloughy necrotic wounds. Several studies have compared the effectiveness of debridement with hydrogels and various other modalities. Mulder and Trudgian found that wounds debrided with a hydrogel dressing healed faster than the wet to dry mechanical debridement.[19,20] A review of the literature for randomized, controlled trials of hydrogels for the debridement of diabetic foot ulcers found five such studies.[21] A meta-analysis of these five studies indicated that debridement using a hydrogel was more effective than the standard wound care for healing of the ulcers and was associated with fewer complications. In a randomized clinical trial of 267 patients, Soares *et al.* found that a hydrogel dressing produced similar healing and costs outcomes as maggot therapy for debriding sloughy leg ulcer wounds.[22] In a randomized, comparative clinical trial of 50 pressure ulcers comparing two hydrogel products, Bale *et al.* found both products equally effective, indicating that for debridement, the clinician has flexibility in choosing a product.[23]

Due to their hydrophilic nature, hydrogel dressings resist drying out, making them the ideal replacements for moist gauze dressings (MGD). Numerous studies have demonstrated that hydrogel dressings are easier to use, produce equivalent or better outcomes, and are more cost-effective at maintaining a moist wound healing environment than MGD.[24–28] Probably the most significant benefit to hydrogels over MGD is that hydrogels generally require only once per day dressing changes, whereas MGD need to be changed every 3–4 h to maintain an adequate moist wound healing environment. Therefore, there is a strong

TAKE-HOME MESSAGE

Basic science advances

Significant advancements have been made in hydrogel chemistry since their initial introduction in the early 1980s. Modern hydrogel products are customized by varying the numbers and types of monomers contained within the linear structure of their polymers, by controlling the degree and types of cross linking that occurs between polymer strands and by the addition of ingredients that augment certain performance features such as viscosity and absorptive capacity. In recent years, functional ingredients have been added that are designed to interact with and alter the microbiology or biochemistry of the wound environment. Future developments will likely continue down this functional ingredient path.

Clinical science advances

The clinical use of hydrogels has advanced alongside with the technological improvements that have been made in their formulation. Initially, hydrogels were primarily reserved for autolytic debridement of dry eschar and as a cost-effective alternative to MGD for maintaining a moist wound environment. Since then they have proven utility with a variety of acute and chronic wounds where maintaining a moist wound environment is of primary importance, and absorption of drainage is of secondary concern. This includes some types of pressure ulcers, diabetic foot ulcers, leg ulcers, burns, surgical wounds, and various types of skin defects. Areas requiring additional clinical research include burn applications and radiation-induced moist desquamation.

Relevance to clinical care

With the addition of new purported functional ingredients to hydrogel products comes the need for additional clinical research. The clinician should be mindful that the regulatory agencies of most countries require minimal efficacy data for hydrogel dressings before market introduction. Generally, safety is not an issue with hydrogel products, as their tissue-like structure makes them highly biocompatible with wounds. However, as the fiduciary for the patient, requesting manufacturers for substantiation of product efficacy claims is the duty of the clinician.

labor cost savings associated with the use of hydrogel dressings. Unlike MGD, or any other advanced wound dressing, hydrogels have the unique ability to read the moisture environment within the wound. In dry wounds, they can donate moisture to help maintain a moist wound environment, and in draining wounds, they can also absorb a small to moderate amount of excess fluid.[12–14]

Hydrogel dressings are often recommended for use on burn wounds and radiation treatment-induced dermatitis because their soothing and cooling nature provides an analgesic effect and the belief that they may also limit the extent of thermal injury in burn patients.[2] However, there is very little clinical evidence supporting these indications. Only three fairly recent clinical studies could be found. Two of the studies support the use of hydrogels in a variety of burn patient applications,[29,30] and one study with radiation-induced moist desquamation and found that the routine use of a hydrogel actually prolonged healing times and provided no improvement in patient comfort.[31]

SUMMARY ILLUSTRATION

A compiled listing of manufacturers and brands of hydrogel wound dressings is provided in Table 1. This information was derived from various published sources and from internet searches for hydrogel dressings.

CAUTION, CRITICAL REMARKS, AND RECOMMENDATIONS

- Hydrogels are not indicated for heavily draining wounds.[7,8,10]
- Hydrogel dressings may be contraindicated for third-degree burns; the wound care clinician should consult with and follow the manufacturer's instructions for use.[7,10]
- Hydrogels may be difficult for some patients to self-apply.[7,8]
- Monitoring for overhydration of the wound, periwound skin maceration, and candidiasis is necessary.[7–9,11]
- Hydrogel sheets should be cut to the size of the wound with care taken not to overlap onto the periwound skin, as this may cause maceration of the wound edges.[2,7] A skin barrier ointment or skin sealant may help prevent periwound maceration.[7,8]
- It is not recommended that amorphous hydrogels be used as a filler material in deep wounds or in wounds with tunneling or significant undermining.[5,10] Instead, it is recommended that the wound be lined with a layer of the gel and filled loosely with gauze.[5,8] Alternatively, the gel can be impregnated into a gauze sponge and used to fill the dead space.[5,8] A preimpregnated hydrogel gauze is particularly useful in these situations.[2]
- Secondary dressings that are absorptive in nature (*e.g.*, foams or hydrocolloids) should not be used in conjunction with hydrogels.[7]
- Hydrogel sheets can be changed daily or left in place for up to 3 days.[7] Amorphous hydrogels are usually changed daily.[7] If the drainage requires twice (or more) daily dressing changes, an alternative (more absorbent) dressing should be considered.[10]
- During autolysis, close monitoring of the wound is necessary, because the wound may increase in size as debridement progresses, revealing sinuses, undermining, or other previously unobservable characteristics of the wound that should be addressed.[8]

FUTURE DEVELOPMENT

It is likely that hydrogel dressings will continue to improve and evolve in aesthetics, ease of use, and the functional capacity to absorb fluids and donate moisture to the wound environment. However, as monomer chemistry progresses, so too will the functional capability of the polymers that comprise hydrogel products. The introduction of new monomers with new functional side groups will allow polymer chemists to customize hydrogel dressings to contain and control the delivery of active ingredients to the wound. Recent years have seen advancements such as the addition of antimicrobials (*e.g.*, silver) to hydrogel products, as well as ingredients that may deliver oxygen therapy to the wound. It is likely that the additional active ingredients intend to modulate the local wound environment and/or the expression of genes controlling wound healing will find their way into hydrogel dressings.

AUTHOR DISCLOSURE STATEMENT

K.L.K.E. is a family nurse practitioner working in the area of skin and wound care in Tucson, AZ. She has worked in long-term care facilities for over 30 years, where she has conducted research for a number of skin care products including hydrogels. She has also lectured on speaker bureaus for a number of manufacturers.

J.B.L. is a medical writing consultant and does paid work for a number of medical product manufacturers. Previous to this he was a Clinical Research Associate with 3M Healthcare, where he conducted research in the areas of patient skin care and advanced wound dressings. J.B.L. has not previously conducted clinical research or writing work specifically in the area of hydrogel dressings.

REFERENCES

1. Ovington LG: Treating a thermal burn? Sheet hydrogels can help. In: *Wound Care Sourcebook: The Complete Wound Care Resource*, edited by Falcon M. Atlanta, GA: American Health Consultants, 1997, pp. 199–200.
2. Eisenbud D, Hunter H, Kessler L, and Zulkowski K: Hydrogel wound dressings: where do we stand in 2003? Ostomy Wound Manage 2003; **49:** 52.
3. Yates DW and Hadfield JM: Clinical experience with a new hydrogel wound dressing. Injury 1984; **16:** 23.
4. Turner TD: The development of wound management products. In: *Chronic Wound Care: A Clinical Source Book for Healthcare Professionals*, edited by Krasner DL, Rodeheaver GT, and Sibbald RG. Wayne, PA: HMP Communications, 2001, pp. 293–310.
5. Ovington LG: Amorphous gels can help dry escharic wounds. In: *Wound Care Sourcebook: The Complete Wound Care Resource*, edited by Falcon M. Atlanta, GA: American Health Consultants, 1997, pp. 203–204.
6. *Woundsource: The Kestrel Wound Product Sourcebook*, Krasner D, clinical editor. Twelfth edition. Hinesburg, VT: Kestrel Health Information, 2009/2010.
7. Rolstad BS and Ovington LG: Principles of wound management. In: *Acute & Chronic Wounds: Current Management Concepts*, edited by Bryant R and Nix D. Philadelphia, PA: Mosby Elsevier, 2007, pp. 391–426.
8. Rolstad BS, Ovington LG, and Harris A: Wound care product formulary. In: *Acute & Chronic Wounds: Nursing Management*, edited by Bryant R. St. Louis, MO: Mosby, 2000, pp. 113–124.
9. Maklebust J and Sieggreen MY: *Pressure Ulcers: Guidelines for Prevention and Management*, third edition. Springhouse, PA: Springhouse Corporation, 2001.
10. Milne CT and Corbett LQ: *Wound, Ostomy and Continence Nursing Secrets*. Philadelphia, PA: Hanley & Belfus, 2003.
11. Zoellner P, Kapp H, and Smola H: Clinical performance of a hydrogel dressing in chronic wounds: a prospective observational study. J Wound Care 2007; **16:** 133.
12. Thomas S and Hay NP: *In vitro* investigations of a new hydrogel dressing. J Wound Care 1996; **5:** 130.
13. Thomas S and Hay P: Fluid handling properties of hydrogel dressings. Ostomy Wound Manage 1995; **41:** 54–56, 8–9.
14. Sprung P, Hou Z, and Ladin DA: Hydrogels and hydrocolloids: an objective product comparison. Ostomy Wound Manage 1998; **44:** 36–42, 4, 6 passim.
15. Vernon T: Intrasite gel and intrasite conformable: the hydrogel range. Br J Nurs 2000; **9:** 1083.
16. Williams C: The role of Sterigel hydrogel wound dressing in wound debridement. Br J Nurs 1997; **6:** 494.
17. Thomas S and Hay NP: The antimicrobial properties of two metronidazole medicated dressings used to treat malodorous wounds. Pharm J 1991; **246:** 264.
18. Geronemus RG and Robins P: The effect of two new dressings on epidermal wound healing. J Dermatol Surg Oncol 1982; **8:** 850.
19. Mulder GD: Cost-effective managed care: gel versus wet-to-dry for debridement. Ostomy Wound Manage 1995; **41:** 68–70, 2, 4 passim.
20. Trudgian J: Investigating the use of aquaform hydrogel in wound management. Br J Nurs 2000; **9:** 943.
21. Scanlon L: Review: debridement using hydrogel appears to be more effective than standard wound care for healing diabetic foot ulcers. Evid Based Nurs 2003; **6:** 83.
22. Soares MO, Iglesias CP, Bland JM, Cullum N, Dumville JC, Nelson EA, Torgerson DJ, and Worthy G: Cost effectiveness analysis of larval therapy for leg ulcers. BMJ 2009; **338:** b825.
23. Bale S, Banks V, Haglestein S, and Harding KG: A comparison of two amorphous hydrogels in the debridement of pressure sores. J Wound Care 1998; **7:** 65.
24. Jensen JL, Seeley J, and Gillin B: Diabetic foot ulcerations. A controlled, randomized comparison of two moist wound healing protocols: Carrasyn hydrogel wound dressing and wet-to-moist saline gauze. Adv Wound Care 1998; **11(7 Suppl):** 1.
25. Thomas DR, Goode PS, LaMaster K, and Tennyson T: Acemannan hydrogel dressing versus saline dressing for pressure ulcers. A randomized, controlled trial. Adv Wound Care 1998; **11:** 273.
26. Gates JL and Holloway GA: A comparison of wound environments. Ostomy Wound Manage 1992; **38:** 34.
27. Matzen S, Peschardt A, and Alsbjorn B: A new amorphous hydrocolloid for the treatment of pressure sores: a randomised controlled study. Scand J Plast Reconstr Surg Hand Surg 1999; **33:** 13.
28. Capasso VA and Munro BH: The cost and efficacy of two wound treatments. AORN J 2003; **77:** 984–992, 995–997, 1000–1004.
29. Osti E: Cutaneous burns treated with hydrogel (Burnshield) and a semipermeable adhesive film. Arch Surg 2006; **141:** 39.
30. Burd A: Evaluating the use of hydrogel sheet dressings in comprehensive burn wound care. Ostomy Wound Manage 2007; **53:** 52.
31. Macmillan MS, Wells M, MacBride S, Raab GM, Munro A, and MacDougall H: Randomized comparison of dry dressings versus hydrogel in management of radiation-induced moist desquamation. Int J Radiat Oncol Biol Phys 2007; **68:** 864.

Foam Dressings

Melodie Blakely*

The Wound Healing Center of Osceola Regional Medical Center, Kissimmee, Florida.

Background: In 1962 with the publishing of the well-known Winter study, more thought began to be given to the idea of wound microenvironment. Polymeric dressings began to be developed in the 1960s and 1970s in an effort to better facilitate conditions favorable for healing. Foam dressings are made of foamed polymer solutions, often combined with polymeric film backings, impregnated with antimicrobial agents or coated with surfactant. They are available with adhesive borders and as cavity dressings consisting of encapsulated, absorbent foam pieces.
The Problem: Clinical problems addressed include wound bed and periwound moisture balance, local edema, wound debris, bacterial contamination, and wound trauma.
Basic/Clinical Science Advances: Foam dressings meet many of the characteristics of an ideal dressing and can be used for minimally to heavily exudating wounds. Fluid handling capacity varies according to the composition of the foam as well as the combination of foam with other components such as film backings.
Clinical Care Relevance: Foam dressings have been shown to absorb wound exudate while maintaining a moist wound bed and preventing periwound maceration, cause less pain with dressing removal, and reduce time to healing compared with the traditional dressings. They allow for less frequent dressing change, decreased nursing time, and improved patient tolerance. Foam dressings are useful for venous or edema-related wounds under compression, work well to bolster skin grafts in place, and may be helpful in the prevention of pressure ulcers in at-risk populations.
Conclusion: Given the versatility of foams and their unique characteristics, it is likely that they will continue to be used even as wound therapies become more active in nature.

Abbreviations and Acronyms

FHC = fluid handling capacity

MVTR = moisture vapor transmission rate

*Correspondence: The Wound Healing Center of Osceola Regional Medical Center, 720 W. Oak St., Suite 170, Kissimmee, Florida 34741 (e-mail: melodie.blakely@hcahealthcare.com).

BACKGROUND

THE MODERN-DAY FIELD of wound care could be argued to have had its beginnings in 1962 with the publishing of the well-known Winter study.[1] It is certain that around this time more thought began to be given to the idea of wound microenvironment. Polymeric dressings began to be developed in the 1960s and 1970s in an effort to better facilitate conditions favorable for healing.[2] One of the first references to foam dressings was from The Symposium on Wound Healing in Helsinki in 1979.[2] Dr. Lock presented a partially expanded, modified polyurethane foam dressing. It consisted of an absorbent, hydrophilic wound contact layer that expanded when moist, conforming to the contours of the wound, and a hydrophobic outer layer that reduced the loss of water vapor and prevented strike through of absorbed fluid.[2] That same year Turner proposed criteria of an ideal wound dressing.[2]

Printed in U.S.A.
DOI: 10.1089/awc.2009.0174

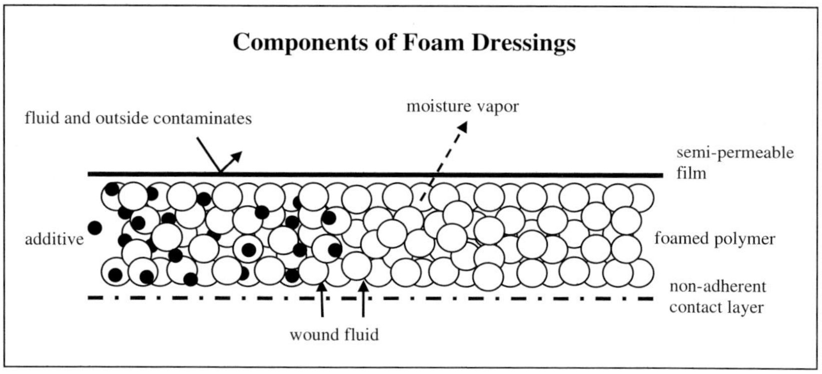

Figure 1. Anatomy of a foam dressing.

He described an ideal wound dressing as one which removes excess exudate and toxic components, maintains a moist wound environment, allows gaseous exchange, provides thermal insulation, protects from secondary infection, is free from particulate or toxic contamination, and allows removal without trauma at dressing change.[2] Foam dressings have evolved to meet many of these criteria. Foam dressings are made of foamed polymer solutions (usually polyurethane) that provide cushioning and are open celled to allow for fluid absorption.[3,4] Foam sheets are often combined with polymeric film backings that reduce the loss of water vapor and provide a bacterial barrier. They may be impregnated with antimicrobial agents (such as silver) or coated with surfactant. They are available with adhesive borders and as cavity dressings consisting of encapsulated, absorbent foam pieces (Fig. 1).

CLINICAL PROBLEM ADDRESSED

Clinical problems addressed include wound bed and periwound moisture balance, local edema, wound debris, bacterial contamination, and wound trauma. Foam dressings meet many of the characteristics of an ideal dressing. They provide a moist wound environment and thermal insulation, are absorptive and conformable, provide cushioning and protection against pressure and sheer forces, allow for moisture vapor transmission, are nonadherent to the wound bed, and can be used as either primary or secondary dressings.[4,5] Semi-permeable film backings allow for moisture vapor transmission but are impermeable to fluids, therefore providing a bacterial barrier.[6] Foam dressing moisture balance characteristics are related to the controlled absorption of wound exudate. Wound fluid is pulled away from the wound bed and captured in the open cells of the foam. Because evaporation of exudate occurs, the dressing provides a moist environment for healing to occur, in most cases without maceration to periwound tissue.[5] The absorbent and occlusive nature of foams also aids in the removal of wound debris.[2,4] Foam's physical structure provides mechanical and thermal insulation. The cells of the foam provide a cushioning effect as they conform with mechanical forces, and trapped air or fluid in the cells resist fluctuations in temperature. This is why foams are used to pad our chairs and keep our houses warm. Cell size can be manipulated to alter conformability, absorbency, and, at the dressing contact surface, wound adherence (smaller cell size prevents the ingrowth of granulation tissue and subsequent wound bed adherence). Foams can be combined with other types of nonadherent material to further prevent wound trauma at dressing removal.

RELEVANT BASIC SCIENCE

Moisture vapor transmission rate (MVTR) and fluid absorption are characteristics, helpful in differentiating between foam dressings as well as in differentiating between foams and other dressing types. Indeed, these characteristics vary widely within the category of foam dressings and are influenced by the composition of the foam as well as the combination of foam with other components such as film backings. Intact human skin has a MVTR of approximately $300\,g/m^2/24\,h$.[6] Fluid handling capacity (FHC) is a function of fluid absorption together with MVTR. In other words, the amount of fluid a dressing is able to absorb at a given time plus the amount it is able to dispel through evaporation over time. Comparison of different brands of foam dressings by one product company cite ranges from about 50 to $260\,g/m^2/24\,h$.[7] Other product information cited a range of $\sim 50–140\,g/m^2/72\,h$.[8] In comparison, a widely used hydrocolloid dressing was shown to have a FHC of approximately $40\,g/m^2/72\,h$ (the bulk of this being fluid absorption, with very little MVTR, owing to the more occlusive nature of hydrocolloid dressings).[8] Therefore, a more absorbent foam dressing without a film backing or with a very permeable outer layer could have a similar FHC to a less absorbent or thinner dressing with a more occlusive outer layer, over a given amount of time.

MATERIAL ADVANTAGES AND LIMITATIONS

Much of the science regarding foam dressings has been extrapolated from studies that have examined the effect of moist wound healing using other types of wound dressings. Winter's study used film dressings on superficial wounds in young pigs. Since that time many studies have been published, investigating the ability of various dressings to regulate moisture balance, as well as achieve other criteria of an ideal dressing. Many studies specific to foam dressings are small and are of limited scope. Published reviews of the literature often site a lack of evidential strength supporting foam. This being said, it is widely accepted that dressings that maintain moisture balance allow gaseous exchange, provide thermal insulation and a bacterial barrier, and allow removal without trauma at dressing change are supportive to healing.[2,6,9,10] It is reasonable to assume that, to the extent that foam dressings can achieve these qualities, the findings regarding their benefits to wound healing are relevant.

DISCUSSION OF FINDINGS AND RELEVANT LITERATURE

Foams are likely the most diverse and versatile category of dressings. They vary in thickness, density, conformability, texture, permeability, absorbency, and adherence, according to the polymers and processes used to create them. In a sense, there is a foam dressing for any wound. Some foam dressings employ the use of a soft silicone contact layer that is adherent to intact skin and nonadherent to a moist wound bed. An added benefit of this material is that although it adheres to intact skin, it does not cause epidermal stripping upon removal.[11] This minimizes periwound trauma and allows the dressing to be repositioned without losing its adherence. Surfactants are sometimes added to the wound contact area to decrease fluid surface tension and aid in absorption. Moisture retention can be varied according to foam cell size and presence and permeability of a film backing. Film backings provide a hydrophobic outer layer that prevents strikethrough of wound fluid and protects the wound from outside contaminates.[2,6] Some film backings have been modified to become more permeable to moisture vapor when they become moist, thereby increasing the FHC of the dressing.[5,8] One type of dressing uses a vertically wicking hydrofiber as the wound contact layer, allowing for decreased lateral seepage and periwound maceration, and relies on a foam backing to help regulate wound bed moisture balance and, together with the gel-like consistency of the hydrofiber when moist, provide protection against sheer and pressure forces.[12] Although most foam dressings are polyurethane, there is one widely available dressing made with polyvinyl alcohol. It is relatively rigid when dry and must be moistened with saline or sterile water before use. Care must be taken to keep the dressing moist, either by covering it with a more occlusive secondary dressing or through frequency of dressing change. Though there is little published data to support this, personal clinical use seems to show a reduction of hypergranulation tissue and improved edge effect with the use of this type of dressing in certain cases. Thicker foams are particularly useful for management of exudate under compression in venous ulcers.[4,13] Foams have also been shown in the literature to be an effective dressing for split-thickness skin grafts when compared with the traditional dressings.[14,15] This may be in part due to an increased area of local compression related to foam's elastic properties, causing edema reduction in the case of venous ulcers and a gentle bolstering effect in the case of skin grafts. In addition to this, foam dressings have been shown to be helpful for the prevention of pressure ulcers among at-risk patients. A study done by Brindle of surgical trauma intensive care unit patients reported a 0% incidence of pressure ulcers during the study period with the prophylactic use of soft silicone foam dressings.[16] Several negative pressure wound therapy devices use foam as the wound dressing portion of the system. Though there has been much research and discussion on this topic, negative pressure wound therapy will be discussed at length elsewhere and so will not be presented here.

Several published reviews of the literature specific to foam dressings are available. A Cochrane Database Systematic Review published in 2004 found that though only small poor-quality trials existed, foam was best studied as an alternative to gauze and appeared to be preferable in terms of pain reduction, patient satisfaction, and nursing time.[17] Another review concluded that there was a strong evidence for the use of foam dressings in surgical wound healing by secondary intention.[18] A systematic review of the use of hydrocolloids in the treatment of pressure ulcers found that hydrocolloids were more effective than gauze dressings for the reduction of wound dimensions, absorption capacity, time required for dressing changes, and pain during dressing changes, but were less effective than foam.[19] A systematic review published in the Archives of Dermatology in 2007 stated that hydrofiber and foam dressings, when compared with other traditional dressings or a silver coated dressing, respectively, reduced time to healing of acute wounds.[20] Consensus panel recommendations published concurrently stated that a strong consensus was reached for the use of foam and low-adherence dressings in the granulation stage of wound healing.[21] More recently a randomized, controlled, multicenter study of 36 patients with stage II pressure ulcers reported no difference in time to wound closure between saline gauze dressings and foam dressings, but a significantly lower cost of treatment with the use of foam.[22] Several recent studies explore the use of an ibuprofen-containing foam dressing. Romanelli *et al.* compared an ibuprofen-releasing foam with local best practice in 185 patients over a 7-day period. Patients treated with the ibuprofen-releasing foam reported less pain regardless of wound etiology.[23] A randomized, controlled, double-blind clinical investigation of 122 patients with painful venous leg ulcers compared an ibuprofen-releasing foam dressing with a foam not containing ibuprofen. Wound healing was similar in both groups but patients reported lower pain levels in the ibuprofen group.[24] One might wonder whether a nonsteroidal antiinflammatory drug used topically had any antiangiogenic effects on the wound bed. A study published in 2008 examining the effects of ibuprofen-releasing polyurethane foam implants in mice showed no decrease in new blood vessel growth over a 12-day period.[24]

TAKE-HOME MESSAGE

Basic science advances

- MVTR and fluid absorption are helpful in describing the characteristics of foam dressings. These together determine the FHC of a dressing. FHC varies according to the composition of the foam as well as the combination of foam with other components such as film backings. Foam dressings generally range from about 50 to 260 $g/m^2/24\,h$ or from ~50 to 140 $g/m^2/72\,h$ in the amount of fluid they can accommodate.
- Although there is a lack of evidential strength in the literature specific to foam dressings, the benefits of an "ideal dressing" are well documented and relevant in the support of foams.

Clinical science advances

- Foam dressings have been shown to absorb wound exudate while maintaining a moist wound bed and preventing periwound maceration.
- Foam dressings have been shown to cause less pain with dressing removal in comparison to dry dressings.
- Foam dressings have been shown to reduce time to healing compared with the traditional dressings.
- Foam dressings have been shown to have a prophylactic effect in the prevention of pressure ulcers in at-risk populations.

Relevance to clinical care

- Foams are effective in the treatment of a wide variety of wounds, from partial to full thickness as well as cavity wounds and for those with minimal to heavy exudate.
- Foam dressings allow for less frequent dressing change, decreased nursing time, and improved patient tolerance.
- Foams are useful for venous and edema-related wounds under compression.
- Foam dressings work well to bolster skin grafts in place.
- Foam dressings can be helpful in the prevention of pressure ulcers.

CAUTION, CRITICAL REMARKS, AND RECOMMENDATIONS

It is evident in reviewing the literature regarding wound dressings that much of the research available is sponsored by product companies. The main disadvantage of this is the tendency of these studies to be narrow in scope and less comparative, but the same critical thought is applied to the analysis of these as any nonindustry-sponsored study. Because of the wide variety of foam dressings available, it is important to match the dressing with the characteristics of the wound and the needs of the patient. Because foams are changed less frequently and, therefore, not observed as closely, they should be used with caution in wounds with suspected infection or deep tissue injury. Care must be taken to place foams with hydrophilic and hydrophobic sides right side up. Polyvinyl alcohol foams must be kept moist by covering them with a more occlusive secondary dressing or through frequency of dressing change. Thicker foams and polyvinyl alcohol foams can sometimes cause superficial blistering along the edge of the dressing. To avoid this simply bevel the edge of the dressing with scissors to create a sloped edge instead of a vertical one. Foams with adhesive borders should not be used in the presence of fragile periwound skin; however, those using soft silicone borders may be appropriate.

FUTURE DEVELOPMENT

Possible future development may involve the use of foams as a delivery system for drugs. The use of foam in the delivery of ibuprofen has shown promise in terms of wound pain reduction. Foams may provide a useful vehicle for other drugs or therapies useful in wound treatment. Given the versatility of foams and their unique characteristics, it is likely that they will continue to be used even as wound therapies become more active in nature.

AUTHOR DISCLOSURE STATEMENT

The author has received past poster support from Mölnlycke and ConvaTec and speaker honoraria from Mölnlycke and Healthpoint.

REFERENCES

1. Winter GD: Formation of the scab and the rate of epithelialization of superficial wounds in the skin of young domestic pigs. Nature 1962; **193:** 293.
2. Cockbill SM, and Turner TD: The development of wound management products. In: *Chronic Wound Care: A Clinical Sourcebook for Healthcare Professionals*, fourth edition, edited by Krasner DL, Rodeheaver GT, and Sibbald RG. Malvern, PA: HMP Communications, 2007, pp. 233–248.
3. Rolstad BS, Ovington LG, and Harris A: Wound care product formulary. In: *Acute & Chronic Wounds: Nursing Management*, second edition, edited by Bryant R. St. Louis, MO: Mosby, 2000, pp. 113–124.
4. Sussman G: Management of the wound environment with dressings and topical agents. In: *Wound Care: A Collaborative Practice Manual for Physical Therapists and Nurses*, second edition, edited by Sussman C and Bates-Jensen BM. Gaithersburg, MD: Aspen Publishers Inc., 2001, pp. 257–294.
5. Feedar JA: Clinical management of chronic wounds. In: *Wound healing: Alternatives in Management*, second edition, edited by McCulloch JM, Kloth LC, and Feedar JA. Philadelphia, PA: FA Davis Company, 1995, pp. 137–185.
6. Wiseman DM, Cohen IK, Rovee DT, and Alvarez OM: Wound dressings: design and use. In: *Wound Healing Biochemical and Clinical Aspects*, edited by Digelman RF and Lindbald WJ. Philadelphia, PA: WB Saunders, 1992, pp. 562–580.
7. Fluid handling capacities of a range of non-adhesive dressings over a 24 hour period. Smith & Nephew clinical evidence. Available at http://wound.smith-nephew.com/AU/node.asp?NodeId=4379. Accessed June 27, 2009.
8. Fluid handling comparative study. Today's wound care treatments from Medline. Available at http://www.medline.com/wound-skin-care/lit/AWC%20Brochure.pdf. Accessed June 27, 2009.
9. Bolton LL, Monte K, and Pirone LA: Moisture and healing: beyond the jargon. Ostomy Wound Manage 2000; **46(Suppl 1A):** 51S.
10. Okan D, Woo K, Ayello EA, and Sibbald RG: The role of moisture balance in wound healing. Adv Skin Wound Care 2007; **20:** 39.
11. Meaume S, *et al.*: Study to compare a new self adherent soft silicone dressing with a self adherent polymer dressing in stage II pressure ulcers. Ostomy Wound Manage 2003; **49:** 44.
12. Bishop SM, *et al.*: Gelling foam: the patient care advantages. White paper. ConvaTec, March, 2007.
13. Andriessen A, Polignano R, and Abel M: Monitoring the microcirculation to evaluate dressing performance in patients with venous leg ulcers. J Wound Care 2009; **8:** 145.
14. Weber RS, *et al.*: Split-thickness skin graft donor site management. A randomized prospective trial comparing a hydrophilic polyurethane absorbent foam dressing with a petrolatum gauze dressing. Arch Otolaryngol Head Neck Surg 1995; **121:** 1145.
15. Atherton D, *et al.*: A randomised controlled trial of a double layer of Allevyn compared to Jellonet and proflavin as a tie-over dressing for small skin grafts. J Plast Reconstr Aesthet Surg 2008; **61:** 535.
16. Brindle CT: Identifying high-risk ICU patients: use of an absorbent soft silicone self-adherent bordered foam dressing to decrease pressure ulcers in the surgical trauma ICU patient. J WOCN 2009; **36(3S):** Supplement S27.
17. Vermeulen H, Ubbink D, goossens A, de Vos R, and Legemate D: Dressings and topical agents for surgical wounds healing by secondary intention. Cochrane Database Syst Rev 2004; (2):CD003554.
18. Ubbink DT, Vermueulen H, and Lubers MJ: [Local wound care: evidence-based treatments and dressings] [Article in Dutch]. Ned Tijdshcr Geneeskd 2006; **150:** 1165.
19. Heneman A, Beele H, Vanderwee K, and Defloor T: A systematic review of the use of hydrocoloids in the treatment of pressure ulcers. J Clin Nurs 2008; **17:** 1164.
20. Chaby G, *et al.*: Dressing for acute and chronic wounds: a systematic review. Arch Dermatol 2007; **143:** 1297.
21. Vaneau M, *et al.*: Concensus panel recommendations for chronic and acute wound dressings. Arch Dermatol 2007; **143:** 1291.
22. Payne WG, *et al.*: A prospective, randomized clinical trial to assess the cost-effectiveness of a modern foam dressing versus a traditional saline gauze dressing in the treatment of stage II pressure ulcers. Ostomy Wound Manage 2009; **55:** 50.
23. Romanelli M, *et al.*: Ibuprofen slow-release foam dressing reduces wound pain in painful exuding wounds: preliminary findings from an international real-life study. J Dermatol Treat 2009; **20:** 19.
24. Ring A, *et al.*: *In vivo* microvascular response of murine cutaneous muscle to ibuprofen-releasing polyurethane foam. Int Wound J 2008; **5:** 464.

WHS Wound Healing Society

Absorptive Dressings: Alginates and Hydrofibers

Karen A. Gibbs*

Department of Physical Therapy, Texas State University–San Marcos, San Marcos, Texas.

Abbreviations and Acronyms

CMC = carboxymethylcellulose

DFUs = diabetic foot ulcers

PEG = percutaneous endoscopic gastrostomy

SSD = silver sulfadiazine

*Correspondence: Department of Physical Therapy, Texas State University–San Marcos, 601 University Drive, San Marcos, Texas 78666 (e-mail: kgibbs@txstate.edu).

Background: Alginate and hydrofiber dressings are popular absorptive dressings indicated for wounds with moderate to high levels of exudate. While they are similar, there are some important differences between them. Alginate dressings are biodegradable, absorb up to 20 times their weight in wound fluid, and serve as hemostatic agents. Hydrofiber dressings absorb up to 30 times their weight and provide less risk of maceration because of their vertical fluid absorption properties. Provided adequate drainage, both dressings gel with absorption promoting a moist wound-healing environment, autolytic debridement, and atraumatic removal.

The Problem: When making clinical decisions regarding dressing utilization, clinicians should refer to chemical makeup and specific dressing use guidelines because of variations between brands of dressings.

Basic/Clinical Science Advances: Alginate and hydrofiber dressings may help with infection control by holding bacteria in absorbed wound fluid, thereby reducing overall bacterial load within the wound and minimizing airborne bacteria during dressing changes.

Clinical Care Relevance: Alginate and hydrofiber combination dressings offer extended benefits, including increased absorption and antimicrobial factors, antiinflammatory and odor reduction properties, increased wear times, and reduced auxiliary supplies.

Conclusion: With high variability between patients, dressings, and research designs, clinicians should carefully consider all aspects of published research and manufacturer's recommendations regarding specific dressings before applying evidence in the literature to actual clinical practice.

BACKGROUND

Alginate and hydrofiber dressings are popular absorptive dressings indicated for wounds with moderate to high levels of exudate. While they are similar in performance and appearance, there are some important differences between them. Alginate, or alginic acid, was initially used in the pharmaceutical and food industries as a thickening and stabilizing agent.[1] Research regarding the use of alginate in wound management was first documented in the 1940s,[2] but it was not commercially available as a wound dressing until 1983.[1] Today most wound care product companies offer alginate dressings in sheet and rope form as well as in various combination dressings. Derived from seaweed, alginate dressings are biodegradeable[3] and absorb up to 20 times their weight in wound fluid.[1] Alginate dressings also serve as hemostatic agents. In the wound bed, calcium ions in the alginate exchange with sodium ions in blood stimulating coagulation and promoting hemostasis.[1] Hydrofiber dressings are relatively new in wound management,

ADVANCES IN WOUND CARE, VOLUME 1

Printed in U.S.A.
DOI: 10.1089/awc.2009.0151

Table 1. *Dressing characteristics*

Characteristic	Alginate	Hydrofiber
Moderate to high absorption	√	*
Hemostatic properties	√	X
Atraumatic removal	√	*
Bacterial sequestration	√	*
Promotes autolytic debridement	√	√
Degradable	√	X
Extended wear	√	*
Ease of application and removal	√	*
Forms a protective gel with fluid absorption	√	√
Combination dressing options	*	√

√ = yes; X = no; * = superior over the other dressing.

Table 2. *Common brand names and dressing forms*

	Alginate	Hydrofiber
Common brand names	Algicell, Carrasorb, Kalginate, Kaltostat, Melgisorb, SeaSorb, Tegaderm HI, Tegadrem HG, Sorbsan, Restore, Silvercell, and CarboFlex	Aquacel, Versiva, Melgisorb, and CarboFlex
Available dressing forms	Sheet, rope, and various combinations including silver, hydrofiber, charcoal, honey, hydrocolloid, and hydrogel	Sheet, rope, and various combinations including silver, alginate, and charcoal

becoming commercially available in 1996. Composed primarily of carboxymethylcellulose (CMC), hydrofiber dressings provide higher absorption than alginates, absorbing up to 30 times their weight in wound fluid,[1] and are available in sheet, rope, and combination dressings. (Table 1) By absorbing drainage vertically into the dressing, hydrofibers provide a decreased risk of periwound maceration compared with alginates that absorb laterally.[1] Also different from alginates, hydrofibers do not offer ion exchange hemostatic properties.[4] Depending on chemical composition,[5] some alginate dressings degrade more than others during gelling and may require irrigation for removal,[1] whereas hydrofibers typically maintain their structure after gelling and can be removed as one unit.[1] Provided adequate drainage, both alginate and hydrofiber dressings gel as they absorb, promoting a moist wound-healing environment, autolytic debridement,[6] and atraumatic dressing removal.[1]

CLINICAL PROBLEM ADDRESSED

When making clinical decisions regarding which alginate to use, clinicians should refer to the specific chemical makeup of available brands (Table 2). Alginate contains both mannuronic and guluronic acids.[3] Dressings with higher mannuronic acid form more flexible, weaker gels as they absorb fluid. These dressings may break down somewhat with absorption and gelling and may require gentle irrigation for removal from the wound bed. Alginates higher in guluronic acid tend to gel more slowly[7] and form somewhat stronger, less elastic gels promoting single-unit removal with forceps.[3] Alginate sheet dressings are available in various sizes and can be layered into deeper wounds, while rope dressings are appropriate for filling narrow tracts and tunnels. Wounds should be loosely filled with alginate since it expands with absorption and gel formation.[1] In general, alginates may remain in place for up to 7 days, depending on the amount of drainage, and may therefore facilitate less frequent dressing changes. For infected wounds, alginate should be changed daily[4]; however, utilization of a silver–alginate combination dressing can extend wear time when infection is present.

Owing to its CMC chemical makeup, hydrofiber dressings are technically classed as hydrocolloids.[1,8] The carboxy component furnishes the high absorption quality, while the methylcellulose component provides the dressing's strength and structure, allowing it to be removed as one unit even when saturated.[5] Some hydrofibers incorporate lyocel for additional structural strength making them exceptionally well designed for filling sinus tracts and undermined areas.[5] This is important since hydrofibers are not absorbable like alginates. In general and depending on the amount of drainage, hydrofiber dressings may be left in place for up to 7 days. Extended wear over 7 days is appropriate when used as a primary dressing for split thickness donor-site wounds where after initial adherence the hydrofiber is left in place until re-epithelialization causes the dressing to release and peel off.[9] Silver–hydrofiber combination dressings can further extend wear time with a 14-day slow release of silver, which can be especially beneficial when dealing with partial-thickness burn injuries.[10]

RELEVANT BASIC SCIENCE CONTEXT

While the primary role of alginate and hydrofiber dressings is absorption, as previously discussed, these dressings have many secondary benefits, including promoting moist wound healing and atraumatic removal. They also may play a role in infection control even when not combined with antibacterial components.[11] *In vitro*[12,13] and animal studies[14] demonstrate that bacteria in simulated and actual wound fluid can be captured in these absorptive dressings, thereby reducing overall bacterial load within the wound and minimizing airborne bacteria during dressing changes.[12] Hydrofiber dressings have been found superior to alginate dressings in sequestering bacteria.[12–14] Alginates suspend fluid around dressing fibers[15] versus drawing fluid into the fibers and therefore form comparatively weaker, less unified gels.[13,16] Researchers believe that the combination of individual fiber swelling and absorption with cohesive gel formation enhances the bacteria-trapping properties of hydrofiber dressings.[12,13]

EXPERIMENTAL MODEL OR MATERIAL—ADVANTAGES AND LIMITATIONS

Combining different complementary components into one dressing offers extended benefits with typically less cumbersome application and frequently less overall cost. Multiple alginate combination dressings exist pairing alginate with foam, film, hydrocolloid, gel, and charcoal. A bit newer to the market is the combination of alginate and active leptospermum honey. The primary benefits of honey (antimicrobial, antiinflammatory, debridement, moist wound healing, and odor reduction)[17] and alginate complement each other well. One such example, Medihoney™, can be used on a wide variety of wounds, including traumatic, surgical, pressure, neuropathic, venous, grafts, and burn injuries.[17]

Silver is a broad-spectrum antimicrobial component[18] available in many combination dressings. Silver–alginate and silver–hydrofiber combinations offer the antimicrobial properties of silver along with absorptive components designed for managing increased drainage frequently associated with wound infection. These combination dressings can extend wear times resulting in fewer overall dressing changes. Evidence supports effective silver delivery for up to 7 days with silver–alginate dressings[18] and up to 14 days with silver–hydrofiber dressings.[10] Researchers postulate that the combination of silver with the superior absorption and microorganism-trapping qualities of hydrofibers may work in tandem with systemic antibiotics in improving treatment for infected wounds, especially in difficult-to-treat diabetic foot ulcers (DFUs).[11]

Some dressings offer the combined benefits of alginate, hydrofiber, and silver. Melgisorb (Molnlycke Health Care, Norcross, GA), an alginate–hydrofiber combination dressing[19] has recently been updated with the addition of silver. Another dressing, Silvercel (Johnson & Johnson, Langhorne, PA), a "hydroalginate"[20] dressing, combines CMC fibers with alginate high in guluronic acid producing a highly absorbent, cohesive dressing with the advantages of silver.[20,21]

DISCUSSION OF FINDINGS AND RELEVANT LITERATURE

Literature supports the use of alginate and hydrofiber dressings in the treatment of moderately to highly exudative acute and chronic wounds of various etiologies. A randomized controlled trial including 10 clinical sites compared alginate to paraffin gauze in 66 pediatric patients with split-thickness scalp donor-site wounds.[22] Results demonstrated that subjects receiving alginate experienced overall less pain and bleeding with quality tissue regrowth allowing significantly quicker reharvesting than subjects who were treated with paraffin gauze.[22] A similar study compared 23 thigh donor sites treated with paraffin gauze and hydrofiber dressings.[9] Half of each donor site was treated with hydrofiber, and the other half with paraffin gauze. The hydrofiber areas demonstrated significantly less pain, faster reepithelialization, and produced significantly less scarring compared with the paraffin gauze. Results were attributed to the hydrofiber's gelling ability and maintenance of a moist wound environment.[9]

Another study compared a silver–hydrofiber combination dressing to silver sulfadiazine (SSD) in partial-thickness burn injuries.[10] The hydrofiber group experienced significantly less anxiety and pain with dressing changes and required fewer dressing changes overall compared with the SSD group.[10] Also, the SSD application was more labor intensive and required more supplies resulting in the hydrofiber being more cost effective.[10] Illustrating the versatility of this dressing, Owada[23] utilized a hydrofiber in conjunction with percutaneous endoscopic gastrostomy (PEG) site care. The hydrofiber outperformed the standard gauze dressings typically used for PEG site care in all eight subjects. By reducing friction, irritation, and pressure, the study demonstrated that the dressing was effective in healing or preventing PEG-site ulceration.[23]

Alginate and hydrofiber dressings are also appropriate for use with DFUs. A 2001 study documented alginate's potential in the treatment of DFUs finding the dressing to support wound healing and provide for easy dressing removal.[24] Although this study's noncomparative design results in an overall weak level of evidence, data supports that alginate can be a safe dressing to use with this population. A stronger 8-week randomized controlled study in 2007 compared alginate to a silver–hydrofiber combination dressing.[11] All subjects experienced similar healing speed and reepithelialization, but the silver–hydrofiber group demonstrated significantly quicker reduction in ulcer depth and fewer instances of wound deterioration.[11] Researchers attributed similar healing speed between groups to the bacterial sequestration properties of both dressings but linked the test group's quicker depth reduction and less wound deterioration to the combination dressing's local silver delivery.[11]

Bacterial sequestration may have contributed to positive results in a different DFU study comparing hydrofiber without silver to saline moistened gauze. After 8 weeks, the hydrofiber group demonstrated faster granulation, lower infection rates, fewer dressing changes, and significantly faster healing compared with the saline gauze group.[25] Considering these two studies, follow-up comparisons between more similar dressings (two silver dressings or hydrofiber with and without silver) could provide additional information toward the true efficacy of these dressings.

Additional studies document the usefulness of alginate and hydrofiber dressings in the treatment of other acute and chronic wounds. One study compared alginate and hydrofiber dressings in 100 acute surgical wounds healing by secondary intention.[26] Data regarding pain at dressing change and ease of application and removal were collected. While no significant differences were found between groups, results demonstrated an overall tendency for the hydrofiber dressing to outperform the alginate.[26] Similar results were found in a study comparing both dressings on 131 chronic wounds associated with lower extremity venous insufficiency.[8] Once again, both dressings performed well without significant differences in overall wound healing rates. The hydrofiber dressing, however, repeated the trend toward being more comfortable and easier to apply and, with longer wear times, was shown to be more cost effective.[8] On the other hand, these trends should not imply that alginate dressings are necessarily uncomfortable.[24] A randomized controlled trial comparing alginate to foam reported that all alginate recipients found the dressing "comfortable" or "very comfortable."[27]

TAKE-HOME MESSAGE

Basic science advances

- Alginate and hydrofiber dressings are absorptive dressings indicated for most wounds with moderate to high amounts of drainage. Since both dressings gel as they absorb, they can provide a moist wound-healing environment and atraumatic removal. They may be used as either primary or secondary dressings.
- As alginate dressings absorb, calcium ions from the dressing are exchanged with sodium ions in blood triggering the clotting cascade and aiding in wound hemostasis.
- Alginate and hydrofiber dressings possess bacterial sequestration properties that may assist in the management of local wound bioburden.

Clinical science advances

- Alginate and hydrofiber dressings are available in both sheet and rope forms, making them appropriate for wounds of various sizes and depth, with or without sinus tracts and undermining.
- Alginates with high mannuronic acid concentrations form weak gels as they absorb wound fluid, which can result in dressing degradation. These dressings may require gentle irrigation for removal. Dressings with high guluronic acid tend to form stronger gels and can typically be removed with forceps. Hydrofibers, especially those with lyocel, hold their structure after gelling, allowing for easy single-unit removal.
- Alginate and hydrofiber combination dressings greatly increase their scope of utilization and ease of application. Alginate–hydrofiber combination dressings greatly increase fluid management capabilities over single-component dressings. Honey–alginate combinations provide the benefits of exudate absorption, antimicrobial and antiinflammatory action, autolytic debridement, maintenance of a moist wound environment, and odor reduction. Silver–alginate and silver–hydrofiber dressings provide extended release of silver for highly colonized or infected wounds combined with moderate to high exudate management properties. Triple combination dressings offering alginate, hydrofiber, and silver are more recent additions to the market.

Relevance to clinical care

- Alginate and hydrofiber dressings provide for easy application and removal resulting in less wound disruption, decreased pain, and reduced patient anxiety.
- Alginate and hydrofiber dressings can provide atraumatic removal and extended wear time in infected and noninfected wounds resulting in decreased dressing changes and use of fewer auxiliary dressing supplies—all leading to potentially decreased costs associated with wound care.
- Variability among patients combined with historically small research studies with different techniques and dressing brands make comparisons in published research challenging. Clinicians should consider carefully all aspects of research studies and dressing manufacturer's recommendations before applying evidence in the literature to actual clinical practice.

A 2007 systemic review documented "weak levels of evidence on clinical efficacy" regarding the value of various modern dressings.[28] A critical examination of current research identifies low-level case study research, varying methodologies and dressings, small sample size, or a combination of these factors in making clinical comparisons of dressing performance extremely challenging.[7,15,25] More consistent, scientifically based research is required to clearly show the clinical efficacy of available dressings. Practitioners must consider carefully all aspects of individual studies when attempting to apply available evidence to practice.

CAUTION, CRITICAL REMARKS, AND RECOMMENDATIONS

Other than allergies to specific components, there are no known contraindications for the use of alginate and hydrofiber dressings.[4] However, since these are highly absorptive dressings, they should not be used on exposed bone or tendon or on lower exudating wounds due to the high risk of tissue desiccation.[4,7,19] Premoistening these dressings with saline for use on low exudating or dry wounds is not recommended,[4] and the use of a moisture-donating dressing should be explored.

Regarding dressing removal, dry, hardened alginate residue around wound edges should be removed to lower the risk of wound infection.[29] In deep wounds or tracts, alginate should not be allowed to form a dry plug preventing drainage of exudate, as this increases the risk of wound infection. Since alginate is degradable, small amounts of gelled alginate unable to be fully removed or irrigated from wound tracts should degrade without incident. However, efforts should be made to remove as much of the dressing as possible to reduce the risk of inflammation or other adverse reactions.[3] Alginate dressings also normally appear slimy, brown, and green[30] after gelling, and this should not in isolation be taken as a sign of infection.

Alginates and hydrofibers should not be tightly packed in wound spaces, as both dressings expand with absorption[7] and could place pressure on surrounding tissues. As hydrofibers are not biodegradable, they must be completely removed from the wound bed with each dressing change.[5]

FUTURE DEVELOPMENT

There have been many advances in absorptive dressings since the 1940s. Alginate dressings are now commonplace, and newer hydrofiber dressings with advanced absorption and construction qualities are becoming more popular. Combination dressings greatly extend the benefits of single-dressing components. Alginate combination dressings currently outnumber hydrofiber combinations, but new and updated dressing options are quickly becoming available. Wound journals are full of press releases advertising new and improved absorptive dressings based on alginate and hydrofiber technology. Two recent examples are Melgisorb Ag (Molnlycke Health Care), an alginate–hydrofiber–silver combination, and Restore Ag (Hollister, Libertyville, IL), an alginate–silver dressing. As older products are revitalized and new ones formulated, we should expect more alginate and hydrofiber combination dressing options in the future.

ACKNOWLEDGMENTS

The author thanks Dr. Harriett Loehne and Dr. Barbara Sanders for their mentoring and support.

AUTHOR DISCLOSURE STATEMENT

No competing financial interests exist.

REFERENCES

1. Timmons J: Alginates and hydrofibre dressings. Prof Nurse 1999; **14:** 496.
2. Blaine G: Experimental observations on absorbable alginate products in surgery. Ann Surg 1947; **125:** 102–114.
3. Pendry, E: The use of alginate dressings in the treatment of diabetic foot ulcers. Dibetic Foot 2006; **9:** 76.
4. Sussman G: Management of the wound environment with dressings and topical agents. In: *Wound Care: A Collaborative Practice Manual for Health Professionals.* 3rd edition, edited by Sussman C and Bates-Jensen B. Baltimore: Lippincott Williams and Wilkins, 2007, pp. 250–267.
5. Sibbald RG, Woo KY, and Ayello EA: M-moisture balance. Ostomy Wound Manage 2009; **5(Suppl):** 19.
6. Moues CM, Heule F, Legerstee R, and Hovius SER: Five millennia of wound care products—what is new? A literature review. Ostomy Wound Manage 2009; **55:** 16.
7. Thomas S and Loveless P: Observations on the fluid handling properties of alginate dressings. Pharm J 1992; **248:** 850.
8. Harding KG, Price P, Robinson B, Thomas S, and Hofman D: Cost and dressing evaluation of hydrofiber and alginate dressings in the management of community-based patients with chronic leg ulceration. Wounds 2001; **13:** 229.
9. Barnea Y, Amir A, Leshem D, Zaretski A, Weiss J, Shafir R, and Gur E: Clinical comparative study of Aquacel and paraffin gauze dressing for split-skin donor site treatement. Ann Plast Surg 2004; **53:** 132.
10. Caruso DM, Foster KN, Blome-Eberwein SA, Twomey JA, Herndon DN, Luterman A, Silverstein P, Antimarino JR, and Bauer GJ: Randomized clinical study of hydrofiber dressing with silver or

silver sulfadiazine in the management of partial-thickness burns. J Burn Care Res 2006; **27:** 298.

11. Jude EB, Apelqvist J, Sprault M, and Martini J: Prospective randomized controlled study of hydrofiber® dressing containing ionic silver or calcium alginate dressings in non-ischaemic diabetic foot ulcers. Diabet Med 2007; **24:** 280.

12. Bowler PG, Jones SA, Davies BJ, and Coyle E: Infection control properties of some wound dressings. J Wound Care 1999; **8:** 499.

13. Walker M, Hobot JA, Newman GR, and Bowler PG: Scanning electron microscopic examination of bacterial immobilization in a carboxymethyl cellulose (AQUACEL) and alginate dressings. Biomaterials 2003; **24:** 883.

14. Tachi M, Hirabayashi S, Yonehara Y, Suzuki Y, and Bowler P: Comparison of bacteria-retaining ability of absorbent wound dressings. Int Wound J 2004; **1:** 177.

15. Terrill P, Sussman G, and Bailey M: Absorption of blood by moist wound healing dressings. Prim Intention 2003; **11:** 7–17.

16. Castellano JJ, Shafii SM, Ko F, Donate G, Wright TE, and Mannari RJ: Comparative evaluation of silver-containing antimicrobial dressings and drugs. Int Wound J 2007; **4:** 114.

17. Acton C and Dunwoody G: The use of medical grade honey in clinical practice. Br J Nurs 2008; **17:** S38.

18. Qin Y: Silver-containing alginate fibres and dressings. Int Wound J 2005; **2:** 172.

19. Williams C: Melgisorb: A highly absorbent calcium/socium alginate dressing. Br J Nurs 1998; **7:** 975.

20. Teot L, Maggio G, and Barrett S: The management of wounds using Silvercel hydroalginate. Wounds UK 2005; **December:** 3.

21. Meaume S, Vallet D, Morere MN, and Teot L: Evaluation of a silver-releasing hydroalginate dressing in chronic wounds with signs of local infection. J Wound Care 2005; **14:** 411.

22. Rives JM, Pannier M, Castede JC, Martinot V, Le Touze A, Romana MC, Guitard J, Bohbot S, and Ebel C: Calcium alginate versus paraffin gauze in the treatment of scalp graft donor sites. Wounds 1997; **9:** 199.

23. Owada K: Use of a hydrofiber dressing to manage PEG sites. Adv Skin Wound Care 2005; **18:** 183.

24. Bale S, Baker N, Crook H, Rayman A, Rayman G, and Hardin KG: Exploring the use of an alginate dressing for diabetic foot ulcers. J Wound Care 2001; **10:** 81.

25. Piaggessi A, Baccetti F, Rizzo L, Romanelli M, Navalesi R, and Benzi L: Diabet Med 2001; **18:** 320.

26. Foster L, Moore P, and Clark S: A comparison of hydrofibre and alginate dressings on open acute surgical wounds. J Wound Care 2000; **9:** 442.

27. Dmochowska M, Prokop J, Bielecka S, Urasinska K, Krolicki A, Nagaj E, and Petkov L: A randomized, controlled, parallel group clinical trial of a polyurethane foam dressing versus a calcium alginate dressing in the treatment of moderately to heavily exudating venous leg ulcers. Wounds 1999; **11:** 21.

28. Chaby G, Senet P, Vaneau M, Martel P, Guillaume JC, Meaume S, Teot L, Debure C, Dompmartin A, Bachelet H, Carsin H, Matz V, Richard JL, Rochert JM, Sales-Aussias N, Zagnoli A, Denis C, Guillot B, and Chosidow O: Dressings for acute and chronic wounds: a systematic review. Arch Dermatol 2007; **143:** 1297.

29. Thomas S: Use of a calcium alginate dressing. Pharm J 1985; **235:** 188.

30. Marghoob AA, and Artman NN: Siegel DM. Calcium alginate dressings with second intention healing of surgical wounds: our experience. Wounds 1997; **9:** 50.

WHS
Wound
Healing
Society

Antibacterial Dressings

Rose L. Hamm*

Division of Biokinesiology and Physical Therapy, University of Southern California, Los Angeles, California.

Abbreviations and Acronyms

MRSA = methycillin-resistant Staphylococcus aureus

PHMB = polyhexamethylene biguanide

PVP-I = polyvinyl-pyrrolidine-iodine, povidone iodine

*Correspondence: Division of Biokinesiology and Physical Therapy, University of Southern California, 1540 Alcazar Street, Suite 155, Los Angeles, California 90033 (e-mail: rhammpt@msn.com).

Background: Bioburden in the wound bed impedes wound healing especially if the number of bacteria exceeds the host immune capacity to manage the load.
The Problem: There are a plethora of antibacterial dressings currently marketed, and selection of the most efficacious product for any specific wound is a challenging task for any clinician.
Basic/Clinical Science Advances: Historically topical dressings used to decrease the bacterial load were antiseptics that may be cytotoxic in concentrations traditionally used to manage infected wounds. Current best-practice antibacterial dressings contain agents that are released over a longer period of time in concentrations that (1) are not cytotoxic and (2) are delivered in an assortment of bases that also manage exudates, thereby reducing the frequency of dressing changes and improving healing outcomes.
Clinical Care Relevance: Understanding the different antibacterial agents, their bactericidal mechanisms, and their interactions with wound tissue is imperative in making wise clinical decisions.
Conclusion: Wound healing phase, exudates, wound size and shape, as well as bacterial type and count, are factors to consider when selecting the appropriate antibacterial dressing.

BACKGROUND

The presence of microbes in the acute or chronic wound bed is known to impede wound healing, especially if the number of organisms is greater than the host immune system can manage.[1] However, given the number of dressings that are considered antibacterial, selection of the most effective and efficacious dressing for any specific wound can be problematic. The purpose of this chapter is to discuss the current antibacterial topical agents that are incorporated into various dressing categories, their mechanism of action in decreasing the wound bacterial burden, indications and contraindications for their use, and any special considerations for application.

Clarification of terminology used in describing topical agents may be helpful in understanding the differences in products. Microbes are minute one-cell microorganisms (*e.g.*, bacteria, viruses, and protozoa), and agents used to destroy these organisms are termed antimicrobial.[2] Antibiotic drugs, used to treat bacterial infections, were initially defined as "a substance produced by one microorganism that selectively inhibits the growth of another microorganism"; however, they now include synthetic antibiotics that accomplish the same purpose.[3] Antibacterial agents are specifically designated to kill or retard the growth of bacteria.

Antibacterial dressings can be further classified as disinfectants (bactericidal on any surface and usually harmful to human tissue) or antiseptics (bacteriostatic on living tissue; may or may not be cytotoxic), as well

Printed in U.S.A.
DOI: 10.1089/awc.2009.0144

as antibiotic (topical or systemic medicines that inhibit microbial growth with little or no cytotoxicity).[4,5] Antiseptics are broad spectrum (effective against gram-positive, gram-negative, and some antibiotic-resistant microbes) and unlikely to cause microbial resistance. Antibiotics are selectively cytotoxic to the bacteria but can cause resistance with long-term use. Given that disinfectants are not appropriate for wound care and that antibiotics are usually reserved for systemic use for specific bacteria, only antiseptic agents used for topical treatment are discussed in this chapter.

CLINICAL PROBLEM ADDRESSED

All chronic wounds have some level of bacterial presence, termed *contamination*, which is adequately managed by the host immune system and does not interfere with wound healing. If the bacteria begin to reproduce without invading the wound tissue, the wound is *colonized*. If the bacteria continue to replicate unchecked, the condition may advance to *critical colonization*, at which point the host immune system is unable to prevent the bacterial load from interfering with wound healing processes. *Infection* occurs when the bacteria penetrate deeper tissue compartments with detrimental effects on the wound and periwound tissues with the potential for systemic complications, termed *sepsis*.[1,6]

RELEVANT BASIC SCIENCE CONTEXT

Tissue infection and sepsis require systemic antibiotics; however, wounds that are colonized or critically colonized can be treated with topical antibacterial agents. Topical applications are also beneficial for infected wounds to augment the effects of systemic antibiotics that may not reach sufficient levels in the wound tissue, especially if there is arterial insufficiency.[3] Topical antibiotics have the disadvantages of being pathogen-specific, of contributing to bacterial resistance, and of being ineffective in managing exudates. Antiseptics are broad spectrum, do not cause bacterial resistance, and can be incorporated into a variety of dressings that effectively hydrate the wound or absorb the exudates.[3] Silver, iodine, and polyhexamethylene biguanide (PHMB) have been introduced in noncytotoxic dressings during the last 10 years, and a methylene blue/gentian violet dressing was approved in 2008. Medicinal-grade honey, used for years in Australia, New Zealand, and some European countries, was approved by the Federal Drug Administration for use in the United States about 2 years ago.

MATERIALS—ACTIONS, ADVANTAGES, AND LIMITATIONS

Silver

Silver is incorporated into antimicrobial topical dressings as either the element Ag or the ion Ag^+; however, it is the ability of Ag^+ ions to bind to the bacterial wall at multiple sites, resulting in membrane damage and cytoplasm leakage that causes it to be bactericidal.[3,7] Additionally, Ag^+ binds to the cell proteins, thereby causing cell death, and to the cell DNA, thereby interfering with cell replication.[3] Silver is incorporated into a variety of dressings by complexes of silver salts or by nanocrystalline silver metal.

Silver gained popularity in the early 1970s for the treatment of burns using either 0.5% silver nitrate (a solution used in a wet gauze dressing which has to be resaturated every 2 h) or silver sulfadiazine (a cream containing both ionic silver and sulfate which has to be removed and reapplied twice daily).[8] Both dressings were labor intensive and had clinical disadvantages. Adding either elemental or ionic silver to advanced dressings that maintain moisture balance, either by hydrating or by absorbing exudates, provides the antimicrobial component, reduces frequency of dressing changes, and decreases cost. In addition, silver sulfadiazine, which contains a fast-release silver that is absorbed by the tissue, is contraindicated for infants under 2 months (may cause kernicterus) and is listed as precautionary for lactating mothers, late-term pregnant mothers, or patients with anemia, liver disease, leukopenia, renal disease, superinfection, or thrombocytopenic disorder.[9]

Studies on the efficacy of silver have been primarily carried out *in vitro* and do not reflect the changes that may occur in the wound bed when exposed to the components of exudates. Sibbald *et al.* compared total bacterial count via biopsies, number of lymphocytes, wound healing, and pain levels in patients with chronic venous wounds. Patients were treated first with multilayer compression without healing, followed by the same compression with a nanocrystalline silver primary dressing. The results were statistically significant reduced bacteria counts, elevated lymphocytes, and improved healing rates. There were slight increases in blood silver concentrations; however, they were within the normal range, indicating that nanocrystalline silver dressings are not systemically toxic, one concern that has been discussed with the use of silver sulfadiazine.[10]

In an *in vitro* study by Percival *et al.*, it was found that more than 95% of 112 bacterial strains isolated from diabetic foot ulcers were killed after 48 h of exposure to silver. Prevalence of silver resistance genes was low and confined to an enteric bacterium, *Enterobacter cloacae*, which is not a common wound pathogen.[11] Gago *et al.* compared healing of venous ulcers with dressings containing high, moderate, or low levels of silver and found that those treated with the high-concentration dressings had faster resolution of clinical signs of infection and healed faster, suggesting that the concentration of silver in the dressings is an important consideration when making dressing selections.[12]

Castellano *et al.* compared eight silver-containing dressings and reported that 100% of the bacteria were susceptible after 72 h with all of the dressings studied. Greatest susceptibility was shown to nanocrystalline products with highest concentrations and lowest susceptibility was shown to dressings with the lowest silver concentrations. They also reported that creams and gels containing silver had better bactericidal properties than other dressings with silver. The authors stated that the dressings with higher concentrations may be more appropriate for wounds that contain bacterial loads of $> 1 \times 10^5$ colony-forming units.[13]

Selection of the appropriate silver dressing is based on size, depth, shape, and tissue characteristics of the wound, as well as the amount of exudates, that is, using hydrating dressings on dry wounds and absorbent dressings on wet wounds. Based on the aforementioned studies, dressings with higher concentrations of silver are advised for wounds that are clinically infected, whereas dressings with lower concentrations may be effective on wounds that are not healing and suspected of being colonized or critically colonized, or for patients who are immunosuppressed and would benefit from prophylactic treatment. No specific recommendations were found for the length of time to use silver dressings; however, it would seem fiscally prudent to use dressings without silver whenever possible.

Iodine

Iodine reduces bacterial count by both bactericidal and bacteriostatic mechanisms. It denatures proteins and inactivates enzymes, phospholipids, and membrane structures causing immediate cell death.[10] Iodine is effective against a broad spectrum of microbes, including *Pseudomonas aeruginosa,* methycillin-resistant *Staphylococcus aureus* (MRSA), and methycillin-sensitive *S. aureus*, and may inhibit some biofilms.[4] No reports of iodine resistance have been published.

Three forms of iodine in aqueous solutions are bactericidal, with molecular iodine (I_2) having the highest antimicrobial potential.[14] The most common forms of I_2 available for wound management are polyvinyl–pyrrilidone iodophores (also known as polyvinyl–pyrrolidine–iodine, povidone iodine or PVP-I) and cadexomer iodine. PVP-I contains iodine chemically bound as triodid to the surfactant povidone; it is available in concentrations ranging from 9% to 12% (w/v).[10]

Iodine is dose dependent and numerous studies have found PVP-I to be cytotoxic in concentrations necessary for antimicrobial efficacy. These studies are discussed extensively in the studies by Leaper, Cooper, Drosou *et al.*, and Burke.[6,14,15,16] Le Duc *et al.* studied the effects of different antiseptics on skin substitutes and autografts. They concluded that PVP-I was less cytotoxic in the presence of large amounts of exudates, suggesting that it is safe to use when a wound is necrotic and infected, but should be discontinued once the wound is clean and granulating.[17] Traditionally used as an additive for whirlpool treatments or as a diluted wet-to-dry dressing, povidone iodine is currently recommended only for surgical scrubs and disinfecting intact skin, but not for direct contact with the wound surface.[15]

Cadexomer iodine consists of macrospherical, hydrophilic, biodegradable beads of cadexomer–starch with 0.9% iodine (w/w) in paste or ointment form.[4] As the base absorbs wound fluids, the iodine is slowly released at concentrations that are both noncytotoxic and effective in killing bacteria; therefore, it may be used on wounds that are in the proliferative phase of healing without destroying new cells.[15] Cadexomer iodine is available in paste, gel, ointment, and powder forms, all of which are highly absorbent. Effective in releasing safe iodine concentrations up to 48 h, the dressing is changed when it changes from brown paste or ointment to a yellowish gel. Cadexomer iodine requires a secondary dressing sufficient to contain the base as it absorbs the exudates and becomes a more fluid gel.

Any iodine product is contraindicated in patients with iodine sensitivity; caution is recommended for patients with thyroid dysfunction or full-thickness burns, children, pregnant women, or lactating mothers.[4]

Polyhexamethylene biguanide

PHMB is a polymeric biguanide that contains positive cationic biguanide groups interspersed between hydrophobic hexamethylene groups.[18] The positively charged PHMB attaches to the negatively charged bacterial cell wall, thereby displacing the metallic cations essential for the integrity of the cell outer membrane.[19] If the cell wall membrane is disrupted, the protein function is lost and the membrane becomes permeable, allowing the rapid release of K^+ and macromolecular contents and causing death of the bacteria.[20] PHMB is bactericidal to a broad spectrum of gram-positive and gram-negative bacteria, including MRSA, vancomycin-resistant *Enterococcus* (VRE), mold (*Aspergillus niger*), and yeasts.

Werthen *et al.* found that PHMB did not affect endogenous matrix metalloprotease activity in the wound fluid and did not affect dermal connective tissue components such as collagen and elastin.[18]

PHMB is available in cotton-blend gauze, biosynthesized cellulose, and nonwoven drain sponge. Unlike other antiseptic dressings that depend upon wound fluid to deliver the agent to the tissue, the biosynthesized cellulose delivers the PHMB with the sterile water contained in the dressing. The water content of the dressing allows it to either hydrate dry tissue or absorb exudates. Maintenance of the wound bed moisture balance facilitates autolytic debridement and progression of wound healing.[21]

Methylene blue/gentian violet

Hydrofera Blue wound dressings (Healthpoint, Fort Worth, TX) contain the light-activated antimicrobial agent methylene blue and gentian violet in a polyvinyl alcohol hydrophilic sponge. The sponge pulls bacteria-laden exudates away from the wound bed where the methylene blue generates singlet oxygen and free radicals that directly attack the plasma membrane, resulting in bacteriolysis.[22] Methylene blue is a bacteriostatic agent effective against a broad spectrum of bacteria including *S. aureus*, *Escherichia coli*, MRSA, and vancomycin-resistant *Enterococcus*; however, one study showed that it was less effective in killing bacteria during *in vivo* experiments than during *in vitro* experiments.[16] Dinc *et al.* also found that methylene blue may inhibit wound healing during the early phases by its effect on the nitric oxide pathway.[23]

Hydrofera Blue is applied by moistening the foam with sterile saline or sterile water, squeezing out the excess, filling or covering the wound, and applying a secondary dressing which will maintain the moisture content and prevent sponge displacement. The sponge should be kept moist and removed when it turns light or after 72 h.

Honey

Medicinal-grade honey is produced from *Leptospermum* species in New Zealand. Commonly referred to in the vernacular name, manuka honey,[24] it is marketed in the United States as Medihoney (Medihoney, Richlands, Australia). The glucose oxidase enzyme inhibine in honey breaks down into hydrogen peroxide (a mild disinfectant) and gluconolactone (a mild antibacterial)[24]. In addition, the honey creates an acidic environment (pH 3.2–4.5) that inhibits bacterial growth.[25] Medicinal honey (available in viscous form in a tube, in alginate-permeated pads, or in hydrocolloid sheets) is recommended for wounds that have been resistant to other antiseptic dressings and for malodorous wounds.

Other antiseptic agents

Other antiseptics (*e.g.*, Dakins solution, hydrogen peroxide, acetic acid, and chlorhexidine) are somewhat controversial because of potential cytotoxicity, particularly to fibroblasts, when used in concentrations necessary to be effective in killing bacteria. Recommendations for each of these agents are as follows:

Dakin's solution. A concentration of 0.025% is bactericidal, not cytotoxic, and is considered safe for infected, necrotic tissue.[26] However, Anasept (Anacapa Technologies, San Dimas, CA) is an isotonic viscous hydrogel with 0.057% sodium hypochlorite which has been tested and approved by the Federal Drug Administration as being

TAKE-HOME MESSAGE

Basic science advances

- Antiseptic agents attack bacteria by interrupting the cell wall, resulting in cytoplasmic leakage and bacterial death.
- Use of antiseptics has not led to bacterial resistance.
- Antiseptics are effective against a broad spectrum of microbes, including multidrug-resistant bacteria.

Clinical science advance

- Antiseptics in noncytotoxic concentrations are available in a variety of dressing compositions that can optimize moisture balance while reducing the bacterial load.

Relevance to clinical care

- Antimicrobial dressings can be selected based on wound characteristics, for example, healing phase, tissue type, and exudates.
- Antimicrobial dressings are recommended if the wound is known to be infected, if there are signs of critical colonization, or if the wound is at high risk for infection.

noncytotoxic. Anasept is not recommended to use with silver dressings because it contains sodium chloride which will inactivate the silver.[27]

Hydrogen peroxide. Hydrogen peroxide is effective in dissolving blood clots but has little bactericidal effect.[6]

Acetic acid. A concentration of 0.25–5% acetic acid may be effective in treating *Pseudomonas* spp. which is sensitive to low-pH acidic environments.[6,28] The recommended application is 10–15-min washes, not as dressing soaks.[29]

Chlorhexidine. Primarily used as a disinfectant, 0.02% solutions may be used for wound irrigation. Higher concentrations (0.05%) may cause tissue toxicity.[20]

DISCUSSION OF FINDINGS AND RELEVANT LITERATURE

(Included in the discussion of each antibacterial agent.)

SUMMARY ILLUSTRATION

A summary of dressings available is presented in Table 1.

CAUTION, CRITICAL REMARKS, AND RECOMMENDATIONS

Literature supports the fact that decreasing the bacterial load, especially in chronic wounds, facilitates the wound healing process and that using antimicrobial dressings decreases the bacterial load.

Given the number of vehicles available for the antibacterial agents discussed, selection of the appropriate primary dressing focuses on exudate management, cavity filling, moisture balance maintenance, and reepithelialization. The secondary dressing is based on the patient activity level, edema management (of the extremities), and contamination prevention (Table 1).

FUTURE DEVELOPMENT

Antimicrobial peptides such as pexaganan, magainin, beta-peptides, and aurien are being studied for their efficacy against a variety of bacteria and in a variety of tissues.[30,31] The only study on dermal wound healing was by Lipsky *et al.*, who compared the investigational topical antimicrobial peptide, pexiganan acetate cream, with systemic therapy for patients with diabetic foot wounds with

Table 1. *Antibacterial products*

Product	Manufacturer	Composition	Concentration
Silver:			
Acticoat 3 and 7	Smith & Nephew, Inc., Largo, FL	Polyurethane with nanocrystalline silver	107 or 120 mg/100 cm^2
Acticoat Absorbent	Smith & Nephew, Inc.	Polyethylene and calcium alginate	144 mg/100 cm^2
Actisorb	Johnson & Johnson, New Brunswick, NJ	Activated charcoal cloth	2.43–2.95 mg/100 cm^2; 220 mg/100 g cloth
Algicell	Derma Sciences, Inc., Princeton, NJ	Calcium alginate	1.4%, w/w
Aquacel Ag	ConvaTec, Skillman, NJ	Hydrofiber, sodium carboxymethylcellulose	8.3 mg/100 cm^2
Arglaes	Medline Industries, Inc., Mundelein, IL	Impregnated film or powder	100 μg/100 cm^2; 6.87 mg/g
Contreet	Coloplast Corp., Minneapolis, MN	Foam or hydrocolloid	47–85 mg/100 cm^2; 32 mg/100 cm^2
Maxorb Extra Ag$^+$	Medline Industries, Inc.	Alginate and carboxymethylcellulose	0.51%
Mepilex Ag	Molnlycke Health Care, Norcross, GA	Foam	1.73 mg/cm^2
Optifoam Ag	Medline Industries, Inc.	Foam	
Polymem Silver	Ferris Manufacturing, Inc., BurrRidge, IL	Foam	12.4 mg/100 cm^2
Restore	Hollister Wound Care LLC, Libertyville, IL	Alginate and carboxymethylcellulose; foam	(See footnote)
SilvaSorb	Medline Industries, Inc.	Polyacrylate strands or sheets	5.3 mg/100 cm^2
SILVERCEL	Systagenix Wound Management, Warren, NJ	Alginate with guluronic acid, carboxymethylcellulose, and nylon fibers	8% Elemental silver
SilverDerm 7	DermaRite Industries, Inc., Paterson, NJ	Contact layer	25% silver-coated polyamide threads
Silverlon	Argentum Medical, LLC, Geneva, IL	Contact layer with nanocrystalline silver	546 mg/100 cm^2
Iodine:			
Iodoflex pad	Smith & Nephew, Inc.	Cadexomer–starch paste	0.9%, w/w
Iodosorb gel	Smith & Nephew, Inc.	Cadexomer–starch gel	0.9%, w/w
PHMB:			
AMD dressings	Covidien, Mansfield, MA	Gauze, packing strips, discs	2%, w/w
X-Cell Antimicrobial	Xylos; Medline Industries, Inc., Langhorne, PA	Biosynthesized cellulose	3%, w/w
Methylene blue/gentian violet:			
Hydrofera Blue	Healthpoint, Fort Worth, TX	Polyvinyl alcohol sponge	

Composition and concentration information was obtained from the manufacturers' websites and from *Wound Care: A Collaborative Manual for Health Care Professionals* by Sussman and Bates-Jensen.[35] Information not reported was unavailable from either source.

favorable results.[32] These studies have not as yet resulted in an antibacterial wound dressing available for clinical use.

Antimicrobial beads, commonly used for orthopedic infections, have been used for postsurgical debridement of neuropathic wounds.[33] Prevention and treatment of biofilms is another area of research, especially in the dental field, and may result in novel approaches to wound dressings.

As dressings become more bioactive, the role of antimicrobial agents and their effects on living cells need to be investigated. Many of the currently cited studies involve *in vitro* experiments on the bacteria. More *in vivo* studies are recommended to look at the effect of the agents on living cells and to determine the optimum concentrations with the ultimate goal of creating an ideal environment for each wound that allows the natural healing processes to occur.[34]

ACKNOWLEDGMENT

The author thanks Geoffrey Cariker for his assistance in the literature search for this article.

AUTHOR DISCLOSURE STATEMENT

The author is a consultant for Davol, Inc., and is on the Speaker's Bureau for KCI. No competing financial interests exist, as these company products are not discussed in this chapter.

REFERENCES

1. Sibbald RG, Woo K, and Ayello EA: Increased bacterial burden and infection: the story of NERDS and STONES. Adv Skin Wound Care 2006; **19:** 447.
2. Ciccone CD: Treatment of infections. I. Antibacterial drugs. In: *Pharmacology in Rehabilitation*, 2nd edition, edited by Ciccone CD. Philadelphia, PA: FA Davis, 1996, pp. 501–527.
3. Definition of agent, antibiotic MedicineNet.com: 2009. Available at www.medterms.com/script/main/art.asp?articlekey=10210, (accessed June 28, 2009).
4. Landis SJ: Chronic wound infection and antimicrobial use. Adv Skin Wound Care 2008; **21:** 531.
5. Ovington LG: The truth about silver. Ostomy Wound Manag 2004; **50:** 1S.
6. Leaper DJ and Durani P: Topical antimicrobial therapy of chronic wounds healing by secondary intention using iodine products. Int Wound J 2008; **5:** 361.
7. Percival SL, Bowler PG, and Russell D: Bacterial resistance to silver in wound care. J Hosp Infect 2005; **60:** 1.
8. Rodeheaver GT and Ratliff CR: Wound cleansing, wound irrigation, wound disinfection. In: *Chronic Wound Care: A Clinical Source Book for Healthcare Professionals*, 4th edition, edited by Krasner DL, Rodeheaver GT, and Sibbald RG. Malvern, PA: HMP Communications, 2007, pp. 331–342.
9. Medscape: Silver sulfadiazine top. Available at www.medscape.com/druginfo/dosage?cid=med&drugid=13530&drugname=Silver+S, accessed July 1, 2009.
10. Sibbald RG, Contreras-Ruiz J, Coutts P, Fierheller M, Rothman A, and Woo K: Bacteriology, inflammation, and healing: a study of nanocrystalline silver dressings in chronic venous leg ulcers. Adv Skin Wound Care 2007; **20:** 549.
11. Percival SL, Woods E, Nutekpor M, Bowler P, Radford A, and Cochrane C: Prevalence of silver resistance in bacteria isolated from diabetic foot ulcers and efficacy of silver-containing wound dressings. Ostomy/Wound Manag 2008; **54:** 30.
12. Gago M, Garcia F, Gaztelu V, Verdu J, Lopez P, and Nolasco A: A comparison of three silver-containing dressings in the treatment of infected, chronic wounds. Wounds 2008; **20:** 273.
13. Castellano JJ, Shafii SM, Ko F, Donate G, Wright TE, Mannari RJ, Payne WG, Smith DJ, and Robson MC: Comparative evaluation of silver-containing antimicrobial dressings and drugs. Int Wound J 2007; **4:** 114.
14. Cooper RA: Iodine revisited. Int Wound J 2007; **4:** 124.
15. Drosou A, Falabella A, and Kirsner RS: Antiseptics on wounds: an area of controversy. Wounds 2003; **5**. Available at www.medscapte.com/viewarticle/456300, accessed August 14, 2009.
16. Burks RI: Povidone-iodine solution in wound treatment. Phys Ther 1998; **78:** 212.
17. Le Duc Q, Breetveld M, Middelkoop E, Scheper RJ, Ulrich MMW, and Gibbs S: A cytotoxic analysis of antiseptic medication on skin substitutes and autograft. Br J Dermatol 2007; **157:** 33.
18. Werthen M, Davoudi M, Sonesson A, Nitsche DP, Morgelin M, Blom K, and Schmidtchen A: *Pseudomonas aeruginosa*-induced infection and degradation of human wound fluid and skin proteins *ex vivo* are eradicated by a synthetic cationic polymer. J Antimicrob Chemother 2004; **54:** 772.
19. Xylos Corporation: *X-Cell Cellulose Wound Dressing Antimicrobial*, technical dossier. Xylos Corporation, Langhorne, PA 2004.
20. Rosin M, Welk A, Kocher T, Majic-Todt A, Kramer A, and Pitten FA: The effect of a polyhexamethylene biguanide mouthrinse compared to an essential oil rinse and a chlorhexidine rinse on bacterial counts and 4-day plaque regrowth. J Clin Periodontol 2002; **98:** 392.
21. Mulder GD, Cavorsi JP, and Lee DK: Polyhexamethylene biguanide (PHMB): an addendum to current topical antimicrobials. Wounds 2007; **19:** 173.
22. Zolfaghari PS, Packer S, Singer M, Nair SP, Bennett J, Street C, and Wilson M: *In vivo* killing of *Staphylococcus aureus* using a light-activated antimicrobial agent. BMC Microbiol 2009; **9:** 27. Available at www.biomedcentral.com/1471-2180/9/27.
23. Dinc S, Ozaslan C, Kuru B, Karaca S, Ustun H, Alagol H, Renda N, and Oz M: Methylene blue prevents surgery-induced peritoneal adhesions but impairs the early phase of anastomotic wound healing. Can J Surg 2006; **49:** 321.
24. Rund C and Sussman G: Nontraditional or alternative topical therapies for wound care. In: *Chronic Wound Care: A Clinical Source Book for Healthcare Professionals*, 4th edition, edited by Drasner DL, Rodeheaver GT, and Sibbald RG. Malvern, PA: HMP Communications, 2007, pp. 287–295.
25. George NM and Cutting KF: Antibacterial honey (Medihoney): *in-vitro* activity against clinical isolates of MRSA, VRE, and other multiresistant gram-negative organisms including *Pseudomonas aeruginosa*. Wounds 2007; **19:** 231.
26. Barillo DJ: Topical antimicrobials in burn wound care: a recent history. Wounds 2008; **20:** 192.
27. Anacapa Technologies. Available at www.anacapa-tech.net, accessed June 22, 2009.
28. Drosou A, Falabella A, and Kirsner RS: Antiseptics on wounds: an area of controversy. Wounds 2003; **15:** 149.
29. Landis S, Ryan S, Woo K, and Sibbald G: Infections in chronic wounds. In: *Chronic Wound Care: A Clinical Source Book for Healthcare Professionals*. 4th edition, edited by Drasner DL, Rodeheaver GT, and Sibbald RG. Malvern, PA: HMP Communications, 2007, pp. 299–321.
30. Savjani JK, Gajjar AK, and Savjani KT: Mechanisms of resistance: useful too to design antibacterial agents for drug-resistant bacteria. Mini Rev Med Chem 2009; **9:** 194.

31. Tamba Y and Yamazaki M: Magainin 2-induced pore formation in the lipid membranes depends on its concentration in the membrane interface. J Phys Chem B 2009; **113:** 4846.

32. Lipsky BA, Holroyd KJ, and Zasloff M: Topical versus systemic antimicrobial therapy for treating mildly infected diabetic foot ulcers: a randomized, controlled, double-blinded, multi-center trial of pexiganan cream. Clin Infect Dis 2008; **47:** 1537.

33. Myers BA: Neuropathic ulcers. In: *Wound Management*, edited by Myers BA. Upper Saddle River, NJ: Pearson, Prentice Hall, 2008, pp. 324–351.

34. Davis SC, Perez R, and Andreopoulos F: Wound environment: implications from research studies for healing and infection. In: *Chronic Wound Care: A Clinical Source Book for Healthcare Professionals*, 4th edition, edited by Drasner DL, Rodeheaver GT, and Sibbald RG. Malvern, PA: HMP Communications, 2007, pp. 205–213.

35. Sussman G: Management of the wound environment with dressings and topical agents. In: *Wound Care: A Collaborative Practice Manual for Health Professionals*, 3rd edition, edited by Sussman C, and Bales-Jensen B. Baltimore, MD: Lippincott, Williams, and Wilkins 2007, pp. 250–267.

DRESSINGS

Occlusive Versus Gauze Dressings for Local Wound Care in Surgical Patients

Zena Elizabeth Helen Moore*

Faculty of Nursing and Midwifery, Royal College of Surgeons in Ireland, Dublin, Ireland.

Background: There has been an emergence of an abundance of wound management products based on the principle of "occlusion." However, there has not been a corresponding explosion of high-quality evidence to support the use of these "occlusive" products.
The Problem: Although systematic reviews have been conducted in this area, there is relatively little evidence to support or refute the use of modern wound management products in the clinical setting.
Basic/Clinical Science Advances: A randomized controlled trial (RCT) was conducted by a group of authors to explore the relative efficacy of occlusive dressings versus gauze dressings. This article provides a review of this RCT and the author of this article was not one of the authors of the RCT.
Clinical Care Relevance: The purchase price of a dressing is not indicative of the cost effectiveness of a given method of surgical wound care, and it is more realistic to focus on key cost drivers such as nurse time taken up with frequent dressing changes and incidence of wound complications and infection. Modern wound dressings may demonstrate more benefits than gauze in the overall wound management process.
Conclusion: The performance indicators of dressings should be evaluated independent of wound-healing rates, to develop a clear evidence base. The appraisal of scientific evidence in wound care is challenging. Clinicians should be keenly aware of this and should develop and use critical appraisal skills when reviewing the existing literature. This is important to determine the clinical implications of what has been read.

Abbreviations and Acronyms

IQR = interquartile range

RCT = randomized controlled trial

RYB = Red–Yellow–Black

SSI = surgical site infection

*Correspondence: Faculty of Nursing and Midwifery, Royal College of Surgeons in Ireland, 123 St. Stephens Green, Dublin, Ireland (e-mail: zmoore@rcsi.ie).

BACKGROUND

Gauze has been the traditional choice of wound management product because of its ability to keep the wound relatively clean and dry. Since the publication of the work of Winter in 1962,[1] there has been an emergence of an abundance of wound management products based on the principle of occlusion (to block the passage of microorganisms, fluid, and dressing particles). However, there has not been a corresponding explosion of high-quality evidence to support the use of these occlusive products (occlusive dressings maintain a moist wound/dressing interface and do not allow the passage of bacteria from the wound into the environment and vice versa).[2] Further, although systematic reviews have been conducted in this area, Ubbink *et al.*[2] argued that there is relatively little evidence to support or refute the use of modern wound management products in the clinical setting. It is for this reason that the authors[2] conducted a randomized controlled trial (RCT) to explore the relative efficacy of occlusive dressings versus gauze dressings. This article provides an appraisal of the study of Ubbink *et al.*[2] The

Printed in U.S.A.
DOI: 10.1089/awc.2009.0171

author of this current manuscript was not one of the authors of the RCT.

CLINICAL PROBLEM ADDRESSED

The study was undertaken at the Department of Surgery (general, trauma, plastic surgery, and vascular surgery) of an Academic Medical Centre in Amsterdam, The Netherlands. Exclusion criteria were burn wounds, ulcerated malignancies, surgically closed wounds, wounds treated with topical negative wound therapy, ostomies, or drain openings, pin holes for external fracture fixation materials, or patients' receiving chemotherapy or local irradiation therapy or with a life expectancy of less than 6 months. The aim of the study[2] was to determine the effectiveness regarding healing time, pain during dressing change, and costs of nursing time and dressing materials of the occlusive principle versus the conventional approach using gauze. The primary outcome of interest was the time to complete reepithelialization, but how this was assessed was not alluded to in the article. Secondary outcomes were pain during dressing change (assessed using a visual analogue scale) and cost per day for nurse time and dressings used.

RELEVANT BASIC SCIENCE CONTEXT

Fifty million surgical procedures are carried out annually in the United States, with surgical site infection (SSI) estimated to be one of the leading causes of hospital-acquired infection.[3] It is argued that SSIs account for 17% of all nosocomial infections.[3] With the increasing use of ambulatory care, up to 84% of infections are diagnosed after patients are discharged from hospital, increasing the burden on community services. The direct and indirect medical costs associated with SSIs in the United States range from $1–10 billion.[3] European figures suggest that the mean length of extended hospital stay attributable to SSIs is 9.8 days, at an average cost per day of €325.[4]

Arising from the historical work of Winter,[1] the interest in the development of wound management treatment modalities has grown enormously. Winter[1] showed that when wounds were kept moist they healed more rapidly with a faster rate of epithelialization than when they were left to dry out. Interestingly, this seminal work was conducted on healthy pigs and as such there is argument regarding the relevance of these findings in the human setting. However, despite this, the principle of moist wound healing was born and adopted by most practicing clinicians.

Working on the moist wound healing concept the number and range of products available are increasing daily. Principally these products, for example, hydrogel, hydrocolloids, foams, alginates, hydrofiber, or hydropolymers, either donate fluid to the wound or absorb excess exudate from the wound, thereby maintaining a moist wound–dressing interface.[5] In a recent systematic review by Vermeulen *et al.*,[6] it was found that there is not enough evidence available, as yet, to indicate which specific dressing, or if the choice of dressing or topical agent, affects the healing of surgical wounds by secondary intention. However, gauze may be associated with greater pain or discomfort for the patient. The importance of this finding was further investigated in a study looking at which attributes of a wound dressing the doctors, nurses, and patients consider the most important.[7] From a patient's point of view, less-painful dressing changes are an important consideration. Indeed, the authors[7] found that patients would be willing to spend their own money on a dressing that would achieve this aim.

EXPERIMENTAL MODEL OR MATERIAL—ADVANTAGES AND LIMITATIONS

This was a single blind, randomized controlled clinical trial. *A priori* sample size calculation was undertaken; allocation to each arm of the study was done by computer-generated randomization, with minimization to stratify for age, sex, wound size, and underlying disease status. The methods used to implement the randomization allocation sequence are not alluded to.

Following randomization, the control group was treated with gauze (a thin, loosely woven surgical dressing usually made of cotton) or paraffin dressings (a leno-weave fabric of cotton or cotton and viscose, which has been impregnated with white soft paraffin) and the experimental group was treated with occlusive dressings. Dressing choice was based on the Red–Yellow–Black (RYB) classification.[8] The precise selection criteria are not reported in this article but in another publication.[9] The authors[2] reported that dressing frequency was determined by the manufacturer's recommendations for each dressing type. The type of dressing used was altered according to the condition of the wound. Additional treatments such as debridement, use of antiseptics, protection of the wound and periwound skin, and treatment of systemic disorders were permitted in each group. The precise nature of this additional treatment was not alluded to in the analysis.

The treatment commenced within the hospital setting and was continued following discharge. In the community setting, the patient may have been attended to by a district nurse, or may have been a patient in a nursing home or rehabilitation clinic, meaning that a diverse number of personnel would have been involved in dressing changes. The patients were monitored until wound-healing time (complete re-epithelialization) or for 6 months. The patients were followed up in the outpatient clinic and by telephonic communication to determine wound healing status, dressing use, and adverse effects. It is not clear how the telephonic communication findings were validated.

The authors[2] suggested that the analysis was by intention to treat; however, 285 patients were randomized, but the analysis was conducted in 277 patients with 417 wounds. The majority of wounds (64%) were postoperative, occurring mainly because of surgical dehiscence or infection, and the remainder were chronic or traumatic wounds. No statistical difference in pain scores were identified between the occlusive (0.90; interquartile range [IQR]: 0.29–2.34) and gauze groups (0.64; IQR: 0.22–1.95) ($p = 0.32$). Seventy-six percent of the wounds healed within the 6-month follow-up period. No statistical difference in healing rate between gauze or occlusive dressings was noted for the chronic or traumatic wounds. However, for the surgical wounds, healing rate was significantly longer in the occlusive group (median, 72 days; IQR: 36–132 days) than in the gauze group (median, 45 days; IQR: 22–92 days) ($p = 0.02$).

The median number of dressing changes in the occlusive group was significantly lower than in the gauze group (0.66; IQR: 0.43–1.00 *vs.* 1.67; IQR: 1–1.93, respectively; $p < 0.001$). No statistical difference in median time to undertake the dressing changes was noted between the groups (4.8; IQR: 3.0–8.1 *vs.* 5.0; IQR: 3.0–7.8, respectively; $p > 0.05$). Daily costs for occlusive dressings were significantly higher for the occlusive group ($p < 0.001$); however, daily nursing costs were significantly higher for the gauze group ($p < 0.001$). The overall wound care costs during hospital stay were significantly higher in the occlusive group (€7.48 [$11.74]) compared with the gauze group (€3.98 [$6.25]) ($p = 0.002$). Median duration of hospitalization was significantly longer in the occlusive group than in the gauze group (18 days; IQR: 8–36 days *vs.* 13 days; IQR: 6–27 days, respectively; $p < 0.02$).

In the occlusive group, 15.6% patients crossed over to the gauze group mainly because of excessive exudate levels which were reported by the authors[2] to exceed the capacity of the occlusive dressings. Only 3.7% of those in the gauze group crossed over to the occlusive group. No dressing-related adverse effects were noted in the gauze group, whereas four patients in the occlusive group developed dressing-related skin problems (one rash, two blisters, and one folliculitis).

DISCUSSION OF FINDINGS AND RELEVANT LITERATURE

The authors[2] have endeavored to adhere to most of the quality-reporting criteria as laid down by the Consort statement,[10] for example, *a priori* sample size calculation, allocation concealment, flow of participants through the study, and blinded outcome assessment. However, there are a number of key issues that warrant discussion pertaining to the study. These relate to the outcome measure, the dressing selection process, the cost analysis, and consideration of previous evidence from systematic reviews.

Outcome measure

Traditionally, wound healing has been used as the primary outcome measure in clinical trials of wound management products.[11] Of course it would seem logical that such an approach be taken if wound healing is the most appropriate outcome measure to be addressed. However, it was Hippocrates who first stressed the importance of observation, diagnosis, and treatment.[12] He noted the importance of a good diet, exercise, and fresh air, to allow the body to heal itself.[12] In essence, these principles are still valid today, and as such it is the body that heals itself and in the main the dressing functions to support the wound-healing process.[13] Further, most acute wounds heal uneventfully.[14] Therefore, objective measures of dressing performance are fundamental in terms of understanding the role and function of different dressings in wound management.[11] Thomas[13] reminds us that there are many different characteristics that are important in a dressing, a number of which are significant in surgical wounds, for example, to prevent or combat infection, to contain exudate, to cause minimum distress or disturbance to the patient, and to reduce pain.

Thus it is contended that it may have been more appropriate for the authors[2] to use other clinically applicable outcome measures, such as the dressing's ability to absorb and control exudate, to conform to the size and shape of the wound, to act as a barrier to the transmission of bacteria from the dressing into the environment, and *vice versa*, and also the reduced frequency of dressing changes and the role of dressings in the transmission of hospital-acquired infections.[15] It is further contended that these characteristics are considered paramount in the selection of dressings for use in surgical wound management.[16] Indeed, Chaby *et al.*[16] argued that it is these performance indicators which should be evaluated independent of wound-healing rates.

Dressing selection process

The authors[2] used the RYB classification as the basis by which the "occlusive" dressings were selected. In a previous study by the same researchers[17] the inter- and intrarater reliability of the RYB classification and the assessment of exudate was determined. Agreement among nurses was good ($k = 0.61$) for the RYB classification. This was similar for doctors ($k = 0.61$). Even with this level of agreement, there remain almost 40% of cases where nurses cannot agree on the assessment of the condition of the wound bed. Further, Stremitzer *et al.*[18] have shown that the assessment of wounds remains really challenging in clinical practice, with clinicians consistently demonstrating an inability to recognize and classify wound tissue types correctly. However, despite this inconsistency, it is this assessment that determines the choice of dressing.[18] Education was provided to the nurses within the hospital setting, pertaining to the use of the dressings. However, wound care continued postdischarge from hospital and no data are given on how training was provided to nurses working outside the hospital setting. It is likely that a large number of staff were involved in the clinical trial from hospital, community, nursing home, and rehabilitation settings. Earlier work by Lait and Smith[19] suggested that nurses often chose dressings that they are most familiar with, indicating a margin for bias in dressing choice. Therefore, both the internal and external validity of the study could be affected if the approach to dressing selection was not consistent.

For the assessment of exudate there was only moderate agreement ($k = 0.49$ for nurses; $k = °0.48$ for doctors), meaning that in over half of cases, individuals were not assessing the level of exudate in a consistent manner.[17] These findings have implications for the current study[2] where the assessment by the nurse determined the choice of dressing. The dressings in the "occlusive" group consisted of hydrogel or hydrocolloid, whose primary function is to donate fluid to the wound, or foam, alginate, and hydrofiber, whose primary function is to absorb fluid from the wound. As such, the ability to correctly assess the level of exudate was central to the appropriate selection of the dressing. In the RCT, the authors[2] identified that 15.6% patients crossed over to the gauze group mainly because of excessive exudate levels. It is reasonable to suggest that this may not have been related to the function of the "occlusive" dressings, rather may relate to the selection of an inappropriate dressing to deal with the level of exudate. Further, the fluid handling ability of the dressing is influenced by specific fluid-handling mechanisms, which are absorption, gelling, retention, and moisture vapor transmission.[20] It is argued that dressings such as foams, alginate, and hydrofiber have far greater fluid-handling mechanisms than gauze, and as such, changing to gauze, because of excessive exudate levels, does not make empirical sense.[20]

Cost

Ubbink *et al.*[2] suggested that the overall wound care costs during hospital stay were significantly higher in the occlusive group compared with the gauze group. Only a small proportion of individuals with surgical wounds are hospitalized indeed, and the majority of individuals with wounds are not managed within the hospital setting.[21] Therefore, the burden of wound management rests mainly on the community setting[21] with at least 41% of nursing time being spent on wound management.[22] Economic analysis of wound care suggests that costs of dressings and other materials associated with wound management play a relatively small overall role in the cost of wound care.[15,22] Indeed, it is nursing time and hospitalization for wound-related complications that contribute to the most important determination of costs in wound management. Thus, to focus on reducing costs of dressings alone, it is unlikely to capture the essence of the problem and will result in limited impact in terms of cost savings.[22] Indeed, the purchase price of a dressing is not indicative of the cost effectiveness of a given method of surgical wound care.[23] Therefore, it is more realistic to focus on key cost drivers such as nurse time taken up with frequent dressing changes and incidence of wound complications and infection.[22]

Previous evidence

The findings of the current study[2] are incongruent with those of the previous literature.[6,23–26] Vermeulen *et al.*[6,24] conducted a systematic review of dressings and topical agents for surgical wound healing by secondary intention. With respect to pain, four trials were identified which demonstrated that gauze was associated with significantly more pain for patients than other dressings.

Three trials found that patients treated with gauze were less satisfied compared with those receiving alternative dressings. Finally, two trials found that gauze was inexpensive but its use was associated with the use of significantly more nursing time than foam. Thus the authors[6,24] concluded that foam was best studied as an alternative to gauze and appears preferable in terms of pain reduction, patient satisfaction, and nursing time. The findings of this systematic review are further supported by work of others,[23,25,26] suggesting that modern wound dressings demonstrate more benefits than gauze in the overall wound management process.

The cornerstone of evidence-based wound management practice is the integration of high-quality research evidence into clinical decision making.[27] This evidence should be used in combination with clinical judgment and experience to plan the most appropriate patient treatment.[28] The applicability of research for clinical practice will depend on its quality.[28] Poorly conducted research will yield only poor results that have no place within the clinical arena.[29] In wound care, the challenge of achieving the standards of those expected of the Cochrane Collaboration has been well debated in the literature.[30] Indeed, the argument prevails that the way in which evidence is generated in wound care remains challenging because of difficulties in achieving all of the quality markers of the RCT.[30] As a result of issues such as inadequate sample sizes, nonblinded outcome assessment, inadequate follow-up, and lack of clear descriptions of interventions, wound care research often falls short of expectations.[31] Therefore, Gottrup[30] argued that the foundation of the problem lies in the lack of agreement regarding the conduct of research in wound management. Further, Gottrup[30] argued that the time has arrived for the development of consensus on what parameters are the most important to explore, to have acceptable evidence.

TAKE-HOME MESSAGE

Basic science advances

- Fifty million surgical procedures are carried out annually in the United States, with SSI estimated to be one of the leading causes of hospital-acquired infection.
- Working on the moist wound healing concept the number and range of products available are increasing daily.
- There is not enough evidence available, as yet, to indicate which specific dressing, or if the choice of dressing or topical agent, affects the healing of surgical wounds by secondary intention.
- Gauze may be associated with greater pain or discomfort for the patient.
- From a patient's point of view, less-painful dressing changes are an important consideration.

Clinical science advances

- No statistical difference in pain scores were identified between the occlusive (0.90; IQR: 0.29–2.34) and gauze groups (0.64; IQR: 0.22–1.95) ($p = 0.32$).
- No statistical difference in healing rate between gauze or occlusive dressings was noted for the chronic or traumatic wounds. However, for surgical wounds, healing rate was significantly longer in the occlusive group (median, 72 days; IQR: 36–132 days) than in the gauze group (median, 45 days; IQR: 22–92 days) ($p = 0.02$).
- The median number of dressing changes in the occlusive group was significantly lower than in the gauze group (0.66; IQR: 0.43–1.00 *vs.* 1.67; IQR: 1–1.93, respectively; $p < 0.001$).
- No statistical difference in median time to undertake the dressing changes was noted between the groups (4.8; IQR: 3.0–8.1 *vs.* 5.0; IQR: 3.0–7.8, respectively; $p > 0.05$).
- Daily costs for occlusive dressings were significantly higher for the occlusive group ($p < 0.001$); however, daily nursing costs were significantly higher for the gauze group ($p < 0.001$).
- There are many different characteristics that are important in a dressing, a number of which are significant in surgical wounds, for example, to prevent or combat infection, to contain exudate, to cause minimum distress or disturbance to the patient, and to reduce pain.

Relevance to clinical care

- The purchase price of a dressing is not indicative of the cost effectiveness of a given method of surgical wound care.
- It is more realistic to focus on key cost drivers such as nurse time taken up with frequent dressing changes and incidence of wound complications and infection.
- It is argued that dressings such as foams, alginate, and hydrofiber have far greater fluid-handling mechanisms than gauze, and as such, changing to gauze, because of excessive exudate levels, does not make empirical sense.
- Modern wound dressings may demonstrate more benefits than gauze in the overall wound management process.

CAUTION, CRITICAL REMARKS, AND RECOMMENDATIONS

The underlying feature of evidence-based practice is that as iterated by Sackett *et al.*[32] "The conscientious explicit and judicious use of current best evidence in making decisions about the care of individual patients . . ." (p. 71). This suggests that clinical decision making should, on the one hand, have cognizance of the specific evidence to support practice, but conversely should also bear in mind the uniqueness of each patient and their individual responses to particular treatments. It is evident in the use of wound dressings that such considerations are very important to those primarily affected by the problem of wounds.[6,24]

Ubbink *et al.*[2] have provided much food for thought; however, the review of this study has demonstrated that the choice of the most effective product is influenced by many different parameters. In the management of surgical wounds, consideration should be given to the ability of the product to address the specific wound needs, for example, exudate, infrequent dressing changes, pain, wound bed condition, infection, and the size and shape of the wound. The unit cost of the dressing is only one parameter that needs to be considered, as the purchase price of a dressing is not indicative of the overall cost effectiveness. The performance indicators of the dressing, as mentioned previously, should also be evaluated independent of wound-healing rates, to develop a clear evidence base. It is apparent that the appraisal of scientific evidence in wound care is challenging. Clinicians should be keenly aware of this and should develop and use critical appraisal skills when reviewing the existing literature to determine the clinical implications of what has been read.

FUTURE DEVELOPMENT

Changing demographics and the projected rise in the number of elderly in our society means that the number of wound problems is also set to increase correspondingly. Thus the management of such wounds will place an increasing burden on already overstretched health-care budgets. It will remain important, therefore, to target resources widely and the appropriate use of topical wound management products will be central in achieving good outcomes of care delivery. Future studies conducted in this arena should focus on clinical outcomes that are most applicable to those directly involved in wound management. The performance indicators of the dressing should be evaluated independent of wound-healing rates, to develop a clear evidence base.

AUTHOR DISCLOSURE STATEMENT

No competing financial interests exist.

REFERENCES

1. Winter GD: Formation of a scab and the rate of epithelialisation of superficial wounds in the skin of the young domestic pig. Nature 1962; **193:** 293.
2. Ubbink DT, *et al.*: Occlusive vs gauze dressings for local wound care in surgical patients: a randomized clinical trial. Arch Surg 2008; **143:** 950.
3. Perencevich EN, *et al.*: Health and economic impact of surgical site infections diagnosed after hospital discharge. Emerg Infect Dis 2003; **9:** 196.
4. Leaper DJ, *et al.*: Surgical site infection: a European perspective of incidence and economical burden. Int Wound J 2004; **1:** 247.
5. Flanagan M: Wound dressings. In: *Access to Clinical Education; Wound Management.* London: Churchill Livingstone, 1998, pp. 67–91.
6. Vermeulen H, *et al.*: Systematic review of dressings and topical agents for surgical wounds healing by secondary intention. Br J Surg 2005; **92:** 665.
7. Vermeulen H, *et al.*: Preferences of patients, doctors, and nurses regarding wound dressing characteristics: a conjoint analysis. Wound Repair Regen 2007; **15:** 302.
8. Cuzzell JZ: The new RYB colour code. Am J Nurs 1988; **88:** 1342.
9. Ubbink DT, Vermeulen H, and Van Hattem JM: Comparison of homecare costs of local wound care in surgical patients randomized between occlusive and gauze dressings. J Clin Nurs 2008; **17:** 593.
10. Begg C, *et al.*: Improving the quality of reporting of randomized controlled trials. The CONSORT statement. JAMA 1996; **276:** 637.
11. Bradley M, *et al.*: Systematic reviews of wound care management: (2) dressings and topical agents used in the healing of chronic wounds. Health Technol Assess 1999; **3(17, Part 2):** 1.
12. Majno G: The Iatros. In: *The Healing Hand: Man and Wound in the Ancient World.* London: Harvard University Press, 1975, pp. 141–206.
13. Thomas S: *A Structured Approach to the Selection of Dressings* (World Wide Wounds, Vol. 1), Surgical Materials Testing Laboratory, 1997.
14. Franz MG, *et al.*: Guidelines to aid healing of acute wounds by decreasing impediments of healing. Wound Repair Regen 2008; **16:** 723.
15. Posnett J and Franks PJ: The burden of chronic wounds in the UK. Nurs Times 2008; **104:** 44.
16. Chaby G, *et al.*: Dressings for acute and chronic wounds: a systematic review. Arch Dermatol 2007; **143:** 1297.
17. Vermeulen H, *et al.*: Inter- and intra-observer (dis)agreement among nurses and doctors to classify colour and exudation of open surgical wounds according to the Red–Yellow–Black scheme. J Clin Nurs 2007; **16:** 1270.
18. Stremitzer S, Wild T, and Hoelzenbein T: How precise is the evaluation of chronic wounds by health care professionals? Int Wound J 2007; **4:** 156.
19. Lait ME and Smith LN: Wound management: a literature review. J Clin Nurs 1998; **7:** 11.
20. White R and Cutting KF: *Modern Exudate Management: A Review of Wound Treatments* (World Wide Wounds, Vol. 1), Surgical Materials Testing Laboratory, 2006.
21. Moore Z and S. Cowman: The need for EU standards in wound care: an Irish survey. Wounds UK 2005; **1:** 20.

22. Drew P, Posnett J, and Rusling L: The cost of wound care for a local population in England. Int Wound J 2007; **4:** 149.

23. Guest JF and Ruiz FJ: Modelling the cost implications of using carboxymethylcellulose dressing compared with gauze in the management of surgical wounds healing by secondary intention in the US and UK. Curr Med Res Opin 2005; **21:** 281.

24. Vermeulen H, *et al.*: Dressings and topical agents for surgical wounds healing by secondary intention. In: *Cochrane Database of Systematic Reviews.* Wiley, 2004.

25. Beam JW: Management of superficial to partial-thickness wounds. J Athl Train 2007; **42:** 422.

26. Shinohara T, *et al.*: Prospective evaluation of occlusive hydrocolloid dressing versus conventional gauze dressing regarding the healing effect after abdominal operations: randomized controlled trial. Asian J Surg 2008; **31:** 1.

27. Moore Z and Cowman S: The Cochrane Collaboration, systematic reviews and meta analysis. In: *Nursing Research: Designs and Methods*, edited by Watson R, *et al.* London: Churchill Livingstone, 2008, pp. 101–111.

28. Sackett DL, *et al.*: Evidence-based medicine: what it is and what it isn't. BMJ 1996; **312:** 71.

29. Higgins JPT and Altman DG: Assessing risk of bias in included studies. In: *Cochrane Handbook for Systematic Reviews of Interventions*, Version 5.0.0, edited by Higgins JPT and Green S. Oxford: The Cochrane Collaboration, 2008. Available at www.cochrane handbook.org, accessed February 2008.

30. Gottrup F: Evidence is a challenge in wound care. Int J Lower Extrem Wounds 2006; **5:** 74.

31. Clark M and Price P: Evidence-based practice: sound in theory, weaker in practice? ETRS Bull 2005; **12:** 5.

32. Sackett DL, *et al.*: *Evidence-Based Medicine: How to Practice and Teach EBM.* New York: Churchill Livingstone, 1997.

Section 4

Chronic Wounds

Section Editors: Robert S. Kirsner and Robert D. Galiano

Cellular and Molecular Mechanism of Chronic Wounds

Karen Zimmerman,[1] Olivera Stojadinovic,[2] Elizabeth Lebrun,[2] Marjana Tomic-Canic,[2] and Harold Brem[1,*]

[1]Helen and Martin Kimmel Wound Center, Division of Wound Healing and Regenerative Medicine, Department of Surgery, New York University School of Medicine, New York, New York.
[2]Wound Healing and Regenerative Medicine Research Program, Department of Dermatology and Cutaneous Surgery, University of Miami Miller School of Medicine, Miami, Florida.

Background: Chronic wounds (CWs), such as diabetic foot ulcers, venous ulcers, and pressure ulcers, constitute a widespread, serious clinical problem with high morbidity and mortality. They are characterized by a distinct subpopulation of cells with different capacity to heal and physiological impairments manifested by delays in healing.
The Problem: Lack of understanding of molecular mechanisms and pathogenesis of impaired healing contributes to unnecessary debridements, biologic therapy failure, infection, amputations, and death. A major obstacle to healing of CWs is the inability to assess surgical preparation of the wound site. Objective biological/molecular markers to guide the extent of debridement and develop effective growth factor and biologic therapies are not well defined.
Basic/Clinical Science Advances: Recent advances in molecular biology of CWs include morphology pattern, pathogenic molecular markers, growth factors, and gene expression profiles used to identify genes contributing to nonhealing.
Clinical Care Relevance: Understanding the biology of CWs at the molecular and cellular level allows for better treatment and healing of all wounds. In the future, molecular markers may be used to distinguish impaired from nonimpaired tissue, thereby making treatment developments more accurate and efficacious.
Conclusion: Many of the limitations in treatment of CWs are based on the lack of knowledge of the molecular mechanism(s) of healing. Further, diagnostic tools in wound healing are still primarily macroscopic, visual, and histologic. Thus, by understanding mechanisms of wound healing at a molecular level, new treatments can be designed, prevention programs developed, and a better understanding of current treatments provided.

Abbreviations and Acronyms

ADAM12 = a disintegrin and metalloprotease 12
CW = chronic wound
DFU = diabetic foot ulcer
EGF = epidermal growth factor
EPC = endothelial progenitor cell
eNOS = endothelial nitric oxide synthase
FDA = Food and Drug Administration
GM-CSF = granulocyte macrophage colony-stimulating factor
IGF-1 = insulin-like growth factor-1
PDGF = platelet-derived growth factor
PU = pressure ulcer
VEGF = vascular endothelial growth factor
VU = venous ulcer

BACKGROUND

Chronic wounds (CWs), such as venous ulcers (VUs), diabetic foot ulcers (DFUs), and pressure ulcers (PUs), are reaching epidemic proportions. The total prevalence of all three types of ulcers in the United States is approximately 3 to 6 million. Complications from PUs result in the deaths of nearly 7% to 8% of persons with spinal cord injury.[1] An estimated 1200 amputations are performed each week, 84% of which are preceded by a DFU.[2] The United States spends over $25 billion annually on treatment of CWs.[3] The true cost, however, is the mortality and morbidity associated with CWs. Accumulation of devitalized tissue, decreased angiogenesis, increased proteases, hyperkeratotic tissue,[4] cellular exudates, and infection at the

*Correspondence: Division of Wound Healing and Regenerative Medicine, Department of Surgery, Helen and Martin Kimmel Wound Center, New York University School of Medicine, 530 First Ave., New York, New York 10016 (e-mail: harold.brem@nyumc.org).

Printed in U.S.A.
DOI: 10.1089/awc.2009.0160

outer surface of the wound are characteristics of CWs, which prevent adequate cellular response to wound-healing stimuli. Even in the absence of systemic inflammation, a CW may be associated with pain, cellulitis, drainage, or invasive soft-tissue infection, often involving bone. Wound bed preparation facilitates restoration and regeneration of damaged tissue and provides enhanced function of therapies. The standard of care in CW treatment, debridement, removes devitalized tissue, decreases bacterial contamination, and enables the stimulation of contraction and epithelialization.[5]

On the molecular level, recent studies analyzing the histology and genetics of nonhealing wounds have shown that the nonhealing edges of CWs contain distinct subpopulations of cells with a reproducible genetic expression profile that have a different capacity to heal and respond to growth factors.[6,7] Along with the gene expression profiles utilizing microarrays, identified markers of nonhealing include *β*-catenin, *c-myc*, and a disintegrin and metalloprotease 12 (ADAM12) as well as gene expression profiles utilizing microarrays.[4,6,8] These markers consistently identify impaired tissue and might be used in the future to guide surgical therapy of CWs, thereby making debridement and growth factor therapy more efficacious.

CLINICAL PROBLEM ADDRESSED

Despite development of evidence-based protocols, CWs have an enormous burden worldwide. The management of patients with CWs requires longitudinal, coordinated patient care. Patients with nonhealing wounds may present with acute complications, contributing to the alarmingly high number of 4 million patients with skin and subcutaneous tissue diseases visiting emergency departments annually. Attempts to use growth factors/ cytokines in wound therapy have had limited clinical results, and only two therapeutic modalities have been approved by the Food and Drug Administration (FDA) as efficacious in treating chronic ulcers.[9–11] These examples point to the complexity of the molecular mechanisms coordinating the cellular behavior of wound healing.

RELEVANT BASIC SCIENCE CONTEXT

Cutaneous wound healing is a multistep process that requires the collaborative effort and precise coordination of many different tissues including epidermis, dermis, local vascular structures, and the immune system. On a cellular level, wound healing depends on synchronized, multiple-signaling mechanisms involving keratinocyte proliferation and migration, matrix deposition, vascular permeability, angiogenesis, and immune responses. These signals include growth factors (*e.g.*, granulocyte/ macrophage colony-stimulating factor [GMCSF], epidermal growth factor [EGF], vascular endothelial growth factor [VEGF], basic fibroblast growth factor, platelet-derived growth factor [PDGF], and keratinocyte growth factor), cytokines (*e.g.*, interleukins IL-1 and IL-8 and interferon gamma, hormones (*e.g.*, corticosteroids), and vitamins (*e.g.*, retinoids).[12]

CWs fail to progress through the normal stages of healing and therefore enter a state of pathologic inflammation. Consequently, the healing process is delayed, incomplete, and does not proceed in a coordinated manner, subsequently resulting in poor anatomic and functional outcome.[13] There is evidence that the accumulation and remodeling of DFUs and VUs are impaired with respect to certain matrix proteins, including fibronectin.[14] Accumulation of hyperglycemia-dependent factors, including advanced glycation end products, has also been implicated in failure to heal.[15]

Resident cells of CWs have undergone phenotypic changes that impair their capacity to proliferate, migrate, and respond to growth factors. Preliminary studies demonstrate that fibroblasts cultured from DFU wound sites maintain their pathogenic phenotype and fail to respond to VEGF or GM-CSF. Fibroblasts from VUs show decreased response to PDGF and GM-CSF, correlating with diminished ability to migrate, proliferate, and close wounds. [10,16–18].

Bone marrow–derived endothelial progenitor cells (EPCs) are important in ischemic wounds. They home to sites of hypoxia by endothelial nitric oxide synthase activation (endothelial nitric oxide synthase; a signaling molecule important for the regulation of mobilization and function of EPCs) where they participate in formation of new blood vessels—a process that is impaired in diabetics and would suggest the use of supplemental oxygen for such wounds.[19–21]

EXPERIMENTAL MODEL

Studies on biologics and growth factor therapies have used animal models, skin cell cultures derived from normal cells, and clinical trials. Failure of potential therapies in clinical trial successful in animal models and *in vitro* skin model points to limitations of these models. In animal model, testing human disease cannot be precisely mimicked.

Skin cell cultures are often derived from normal cells, which do not exhibit CW pathology. In DFUs, for example, although diabetic healing deficits have been studied in animal models such as the db/db type 2 diabetic mouse, nonobese diabetic type 1 diabetic mouse, and streptozocin-induced diabetic rats, rabbits, and pigs,[22–24] therapeutic approaches evaluated in these models have not correlated well with clinical outcomes. For example, topical application of EGF accelerates healing of db/db mouse wounds[17] but shows low efficacy in clinical trials. This is likely because cells at the nonhealing edges of human CWs exhibit dysregulated expression of EGF receptor, a phenomenon not replicated in mouse models.[25,26] Therefore, more studies need to be performed on human tissue. Elucidation of molecular mechanisms of wound healing in humans has come from studies of biopsies taken from the nonhealing edge and the adjacent nonulcerated skin of human nonhealing wounds. These two areas were assessed before and after debridement for histologic examination, biological response to healing (migration using fibroblast cultures from the two distinct CW locations on each patient), and gene expression profile.[4,6,7] By comparing the wound edge before and after debridement, such methods allow for investigation of the role for surgical debridement and its effect on the molecular profile of the CW. These studies have been largely successful in identifying molecular markers of nonhealing by allowing for comparison of various parameters of the nonhealing versus the healing skin because they were performed on actual patients with nonhealing ulcers rather than on animal models; they are advantageous and should be validated in a prospective clinical trial.

DISCUSSION OF FINDINGS AND RELEVANT LITERATURE

In human CWs, keratinocytes at the nonhealing edge of the wound multiply at a higher rate than usual (hyperproliferation). Instead of migrating into the wound to close it as would be expected from normally activated keratinocytes,[7] they form thickened layers around the edge, much like a callus. Histologically, biopsies from the nonhealing VU edges show thick, hyperkeratotic (hypertrophy of the cornified layer of the skin) and parakeratotic (presence of nuclei in cornified layer) epidermis. Normally, as keratinocytes move upward, they lose their nuclei, forming sturdy layers of cross-linked proteins and creating a protective layer over the wound. However, the skin cells of CWs remain enucleated, unable to progress to this stage of differentiation. Thus, the keratinocytes of the CW seem to be trapped in the middle of these two normal processes without completing either of them.

Lack of keratinocyte migration and epithelialization, sometimes in the presence of adequate granulation tissue and stalling of the healing process, is caused by the overabundance of *c-myc*, a product of the *myc* gene. The *myc* gene is implicated in human cancers known to suppress cell migration and cause the skin to thicken, obstructing reparative cells from reaching the wound edge. β-catenin, a critical regulator of cell behavior one step up the molecular pathway, activates *c-myc* overproduction and other pathways affecting skin cell migration, growth, and regulation. Both *c-myc* and β-catenin were found to be overexpressed in the nonhealing edges of CWs in biopsies from humans.[4]

The cells that contribute to misaligned healing are regulated by specific genes that we are now beginning to identify. Gene array data and immunohistochemistry from human VUs demonstrated that ADAM12 can be used as a marker of nonhealing. There is at least fivefold greater expression in the nonhealing edge of chronic skin ulcers than in healthy skin. Additionally, studies with skin explants from ADAM-12-deficient mice revealed a significant increase in keratinocyte migration and/or proliferation compared with wild-type littermates.[8] Microarray analysis of patient biopsies confirmed the clinical findings by showing that gene transcription profiles of epithelial cells from the nonhealing edge and adjacent nonulcerated skin are distinct and recognizable. Analysis has identified a distinct subset of genes (10 induced and 10 repressed) with the most differential expression between the two locations.[7] Gene trees using these data suggested that gene expression changes may signify pathogenic progress within the wound. Specific and identifiable gene expression in nonhealing wound edges can be used to make surgical debridement more accurate in the future. The edge of surgical debridement is distinct from the nonhealing edge and is responsive to wounding. In the future, microarray profiling can be used to determine the margin of debridement within the chronic ulcer. This method is similar to Mohs microscopic surgery, where conventional hematoxylin and eosin staining is used to determine the presence of residual tumor cells in tissue around the clinical margins of the lesion. Others have observed that the cutaneous wound-healing process involves changes in the expression of specific MicroRNAs at specific phases of wound healing. Dysregulation of specific MicroRNAs is critical in derailing the healing sequence in chronic problem wounds.[27]

Clinical failure of growth factor therapy suggests that combinations of growth factors or a new delivery system may be more effective. Various dermal equivalent products would allow for sustained and timed release of growth factors in response to *in vivo* signals. The FDA approved bilayered human skin equivalent, which consists of cultured keratinocytes residing on the surface of a fibroblast-populated collagen lattice. Its potential in producing and sustaining growth factor release to enhance angiogenesis, fibroblast proliferation, matrix deposition, migration, and growth of keratinocytes has been shown *in vitro*.[28] In mice it was noted to express 15 distinct growth factors and cytokines associated with wound healing in a time-dependent distribution.[29] This would enhance angiogenesis, fibroblast proliferation, matrix deposition, migration, and growth of keratinocytes.

Viral vectors containing a growth factor gene are a recent development in gene therapy.[30] Recombinant human vascular endothelial growth factor (VEGF165 or rhVEGF; Telbermin) applied topically to chronic diabetic neuropathic foot ulcers and adenoviral vector PDGF β for VUs[31]are now in clinical trial.[32] About $72\,\mu g/cm^2$ of Telbermin applied topically three times a week for up to 6 weeks was well tolerated, but studies are required to further characterize the safety/efficacy of Telbermin.

Several studies suggest that bone marrow–derived stem cells such as mesenchymal stem cells, progenitor cells such as EPCs, and fibrocytes may be involved in wound healing by contributing to skin cells or releasing regulatory cytokines. Stem/progenitor cells may be mobilized to leave the bone marrow, home to injured tissues, and participate in their repair and regeneration. Direct injection of these cells into injured tissues shows improved repair. Enhanced understanding of these cells may help to develop cutaneous substitutes and novel therapies for CWs and hypertrophic scars.[33]

The pathologic processes found in the skin of CWs are likely to occur at many levels. Nonhealing skin has phenotypic abnormalities that include hyper and para-keratosis. Similarly, deep tissue, tendon and muscle necrosis, osteomyelitis, and fibrosis are pathologic manifestations of what is occurring at the molecular level. This suggests that pathologic processes not only in the skin but also at all levels of the CW contribute to nonhealing[34] (Table 1).

TAKE-HOME MESSAGE

Basic science advances

- In CW skin, cells multiply at a higher rate than usual and, therefore, form thickened layers around the wound edge.
- Keratinocytes at the nonhealing edges of CWs do not successfully complete either of the two possible pathways in a proper manner: proliferation or differentiation. They constantly try, without success, to achieve either of the two processes.
- The nonhealing edge keratinocytes are marked by induction of *c-myc*, nuclear presence of β-catenin, and ADAM12 overexpression leading to increased proliferation and inhibition of migration.
- Using microarrays, each location within a wound was found to have a specific gene expression profile indicating that they can be used to determine the subpopulation of cells within the wound from which a biopsy was taken.

Clinical science advances

- Surgical debridement or wound bed preparation is standard of care for removal of necrotic, infected, and unresponsive tissue.
- PDGF is the only FDA-approved growth factor for PUs and DFUs. Many growth factor therapies that were successful in animal models have failed clinical trial.
- Study of growth factor molecules and novel delivery similar to VEGF testing will increase therapeutic possibilities.
- Bilayered living skin substitutes have been successful for use in CWs, adding cells and growth factors to a deficient wound-healing environment.
- Stem cells hold a promising future for wound healing.

Relevance to clinical care

- The clinical field is missing critical information about what is occurring at the molecular level in CWs. Thus, optimal prevention and treatment strategies are not being developed.
- Based on the prevalence of amputations in DFU and sepsis and mortality in all CW, current treatment has a huge failure rate despite advances of FDA-approved therapies.
- While surgical debridement is the current standard of care, one of the major obstacles to prompt and complete CW healing is the inability to identify the nonhealing tissue that would guide the extent of surgery or gauge its success.
- Successful development of a definitive and reliable set of markers of nonhealing would lead to the development of "biomolecular debridement surgery" that will use rapid intraoperative marker analysis to guide the selective and complete removal of healing-impaired tissue.

Table 1. *Summary of chronic wound parameters with respect to the wound localization are shown*

Chronic Wound Parameter	Wound Location Nonhealing Wound Edge	Healing Wound Edge
Histopathology	• Hyperproliferative epidermis	• Normalized
• Hyperkeratosis (hypertrophy of cornified layer)	• Well-defined cornified layer	
• Parakeratosis (presence of nuclei in cornified layer)	• Less hyperproliferation than nonhealing edge	
		• Thicker epidermis than healthy skin
Keratinocytes	Inhibition of migration and/or proliferation	Proper migration and proliferation
Fibroblasts	• Misshaped	• Normalized morphology
• Larger in size	• Slightly slower than control	
• Clumped together		
• Slow migration rate		
c-myc	Overexpressed	Not overexpressed
β-catenin	Robust nuclear localization	Decreased nuclear localization
ADAM12	Upregulated at least fivefold	Normal levels
Gene expression profiles	Distinct genetic pattern compared with healing edge that correlates with wound location	Distinct genetic pattern compared with nonhealing edge that correlates with wound location
Bone marrow activity	eNOS phosphorylation is impaired, limiting EPC mobilization from the bone marrow to the circulation	VEGF induced eNOS phosphorylation and activation of eNOS increases NO levels and triggers mobilization of EPCs to the circulation

CAUTION, CRITICAL REMARKS, AND RECOMMENDATIONS

Due to the complex, multifactorial processes involved in wound healing, many therapeutic options have and will continue to be available to those who manage CWs. It is important to emphasize, however, that the best treatment is early treatment. Early intervention of VU, DFU, and PU will halt their progression. Approved evidence-based protocols based on adequate off-loading coupled with FDA-approved biological therapies should be utilized.[9] Since at present there is no definitive way to identify early on patients who are likely to heal versus those who will go on to develop CWs, all patients with impaired healing should be managed early and treated using standardized protocols.

FUTURE DEVELOPMENTS

Understanding the molecular and cellular biology of CWs lays the foundation for future treatment options. Technologies for various molecular analyses (*e.g.*, genomics, proteomics, and transgenic mice) will allow a greater fund of knowledge and ability to study wound-healing pathogenesis and treatment. Systems for sustained topical delivery (*e.g.*, polymers and adenovirus vectors) combined with major advances in tissue engineering (*e.g.*, human skin engineering, cellular matrices, and bone marrow–derived cell therapy) are a promising approach to treatment with growth factors and biologics. Developments in molecular targeting (*e.g.*, antisense oligonucleotides, siRNA, antibodies, and small molecules) may elucidate wound healing at the level of posttranslational gene regulation. Novel discoveries of disease molecular pathogenesis from studies of patient biopsies and animal models, coupled with breakthroughs in stem cell research, are powerful technologies starting at the molecular and cellular levels that hold promise of a bright future for use in CW patients.

ACKNOWLEDGMENT

Wound healing research in the author's laboratory is funded by NIH awards.

AUTHOR DISCLOSURE STATEMENT

Authors K.Z., E.L., and O.S. have no disclosures. The authors H.B. and M.T.C wish to disclose the following patent: Biological Markers of Chronic Wound Tissue and Methods of Using for Criteria in Surgical Debridement. Inventors: Brem, Harold and Tomic-Canic, Marjana. Application#PCT/US2007/010577.

REFERENCES

1. Wysocki AB: Wound fluids and the pathogenesis of chronic wounds. J Wound Ostomy Continence Nurs 1996; **23:** 283.
2. Pecoraro RE, Reiber GE, and Burgess EM: Pathways to diabetic limb amputation. Basis for prevention. Diabetes Care 1990; **13:** 513.
3. Services UDoHaH. Guidance to Surveyors for Long Term Care facilities on the World Wide Web. http://www.cms.hhs.gov//. Access date: June 19, 2009.
4. Stojadinovic O, Brem H, Vouthounis C, Lee B, Fallon J, Stallcup M, Merchant A, Galiano RD, and Tomic-Canic M: Molecular pathogenesis of chronic wounds: the role of beta-catenin and c-myc in the inhibition of epithelialization and wound healing. Am J Pathol 2005; **167:** 59.
5. Panuncialman J, and Falanga V: The science of wound bed preparation. Clin Plast Surg 2007; **34:** 621.
6. Brem H, Stojadinovic O, Diegelmann RF, Entero H, Lee B, Pastar I, Golinko M, Rosenberg H, and Tomic-Canic M: Molecular markers in patients with chronic wounds to guide surgical debridement. Mol Med 2007; **13:** 30.
7. Stojadinovic O, Pastar I, Vukelic S, Mohoney MG, Brennan D, Krzyzanowska A, Golinko M, Brem H, and Tomic-Canic M: Deregulation of keratinocyte differentiation and activation: a hallmark of venous ulcers. J Cell Mol Med 2008; **12:** 2675.
8. Harsha A, Stojadinovic O, Brem H, Sehara-Fujisawa A, Wewer U, Loomis CA, Blobel CP, and Tomic-Canic M: ADAM12: a potential target for the treatment of chronic wounds. J Mol Med 2008; **86:** 961.
9. Boulton AJ, Kirsner RS, and Vileikyte L: Clinical practice. Neuropathic diabetic foot ulcers. N Engl J Med 2004; **351:** 48.
10. Hasan A, Murata H, Falabella A, Ochoa S, Zhou L, Badiavas E, and Falanga V: Dermal fibroblasts from venous ulcers are unresponsive to the action of transforming growth factor-beta 1. J Dermatol Sci 1997; **16:** 59.
11. Steed DL: Clinical evaluation of recombinant human platelet-derived growth factor for the treatment of lower extremity ulcers. Plast Reconstr Surg 2006; **117(7 Suppl):** 143S; discussion 150S.
12. Mansbridge JN, Liu K, Pinney RE, Patch R, Ratcliffe A, and Naughton GK: Growth factors secreted by fibroblasts: role in healing diabetic foot ulcers. Diabetes Obes Metab 1999; **1:** 265.
13. Lazarus GS, Cooper DM, Knighton DR, Percoraro RE, Rodeheaver G, and Robson MC: Definitions and guidelines for assessment of wounds and evaluation of healing. Wound Repair Regen 1994; **2:** 165.
14. Loots MA, Lamme EN, Zeegelaar J, Mekkes JR, Bos JD, and Middelkoop E: Differences in cellular infiltrate and extracellular matrix of chronic diabetic and venous ulcers versus acute wounds. J Invest Dermatol 1998; **111:** 850.
15. Peppa M, Stavroulakis P, and Raptis SA: Advanced glycoxidation products and impaired diabetic wound healing. Wound Repair Regen 2009; **17:** 461.
16. Agren MS, Steenfos HH, Dabelsteen S, Hansen JB, and Dabelsteen E: Proliferation and mitogenic response to PDGF-BB of fibroblasts isolated from chronic venous leg ulcers is ulcer-age dependent. J Invest Dermatol 1999; **112:** 463.
17. Greenhalgh DG, Sprugel KH, Murray MJ, and Ross R: PDGF and FGF stimulate wound healing in the genetically diabetic mouse. Am J Pathol 1990; **136:** 1235.
18. Loot MA, Kenter SB, Au FL, Van Galen WJ, Middelkoop E, Bos JD, and Mekkes JR: Fibroblasts derived from chronic diabetic ulcers differ in their response to stimulation with EGF, IGF-I, bFGF and PDGF-AB compared to controls. Eur J Cell Biol 2002; **81:** 153.
19. Liu ZJ and Velazquez OC: Hyperoxia, endothelial progenitor cell mobilization, and diabetic wound healing. Antioxid Redox Signal 2008; **10:** 1869.
20. Sen CK: Wound healing essentials: let there be oxygen. Wound Repair Regen 2009; **17:** 1.
21. Gordillo GM, Roy S, Khanna S, Schlanger R, Khandelwal S, Phillips G, and Sen CK: Topical oxygen therapy induces vascular endothelial growth factor expression and improves closure of clinically presented chronic wounds. Clin Exp Pharmacol Physiol 2008; **35:** 957.
22. Allen TJ, Cooper ME, and Lan HY: Use of genetic mouse models in the study of diabetic nephropathy. Curr Diab Rep 2004; **4:** 435.
23. Michaels Jt, Churgin SS, Blechman KM, Greives MR, Aarabi S, Galiano RD, and Gurtner GC: db/db mice exhibit severe wound-healing impairments compared with other murine diabetic strains in a silicone-splinted excisional wound model. Wound Repair Regen 2007; **15:** 665.
24. Velander P, Theopold C, Hirsch T, Bleiziffer O, Zuhaili B, Fossum M, Hoeller D, Gheerardyn R, Chen M, Visovatti S, Svensson H, Yao F, and Eriksson E: Impaired wound healing in an acute diabetic pig model and the effects of local hyperglycemia. Wound Repair Regen 2008; **16:** 288.
25. Brem H, Golinko MS, Stojadinovic O, Kodra A, Diegelmann RF, Vukelic S, Entero H, Coppock DL, and Tomic-Canic M: Primary cultured fibroblasts derived from patients with chronic wounds: a methodology to produce human cell lines and test putative growth factor therapy such as GMCSF. J Transl Med 2008; **6:** 75.
26. Falanga V, Eaglstein WH, Bucalo B, Katz MH, Harris B, and Carson P: Topical use of human recombinant epidermal growth factor (h-EGF) in venous ulcers. J Dermatol Surg Oncol 1992; **18:** 604.
27. Shilo S, Roy S, Khanna S, and Sen CK: MicroRNA in cutaneous wound healing: a new paradigm. DNA Cell Biol 2007; **26:** 227.
28. Mazlyzam AL, Aminuddin BS, Saim L, and Ruszymah BH: Living bilayered human skin equivalent: promising potentials for wound healing. Med J Malaysia 2008; **63 Suppl A:** 32.
29. Brem H, Young J, Tomic-Canic M, Isaacs C, and Ehrlich HP: Clinical efficacy and mechanism of bilayered living human skin equivalent (HSE) in treatment of diabetic foot ulcers. Surg Technol Int 2003; **11:** 23.
30. Brem H, Kodra A, Golinko MS, Entero H, Stejadinovic O, Wang VM, Sheahan CM, Weinberg AD, Woo SL, Ehrlich HP, and Tomic-Canic M: Mechanism of sustained release of vascular endothelial growth factor in accelerating experimental diabetic healing. J Invest Dermatol 2009; **129:** 2275.
31. Margolis DJ, Morris LM, Papadopoulos M, Weinberg L, Filip JC, Lang SA, Vaikunth SS, and Crombleholme TM: Phase I study of H5.020CMV. PDGF-beta to treat venous leg ulcer disease. Mol Ther 2009; **17:** 1822.
32. Hanft JR, Pollak RA, Barbul A, Van Gils C, Kwon PS, Gray SM, Lynch CI, Semba CP, and Breen TJ: Phase I trial on the safety of topical rhVEGF on chronic neuropathic diabetic foot ulcers. J Wound Care 2008; **17:** 30–2, 34–7.
33. Wu Y, Wang J, Scott PG, and Tredget EE. Bone marrow-derived stem cells in wound healing: a review. Wound Repair Regen 2007; **15 Suppl 1:** S18.
34. Golinko MS, Joffe R, de Vinck D, Chandrasekaran E, Stojadinovic O, Barrientos S, Vukelic S, Tomic-Canic M, and Brem H: Surgical pathology to describe the clinical margin of debridement of chronic wounds using a wound electronic medical record. J Am Coll Surg 2009; **209:** 254; e251.

WHS
Wound
Healing
Society

Healing Competence of the Keratinocytes and the Chronic Wound Edge

Olivera Stojadinovic, Marilyn Zabielinski, and Marjana Tomic-Canic*

Wound Healing and Regenerative Medicine Research Program, Department of Dermatology and Cutaneous Surgery, University of Miami Miller School of Medicine, Miami, Florida.

Background: Epithelialization is an important component of successful wound healing. During acute wound healing, epidermal keratinocytes migrate, proliferate, and differentiate to cover the wound bed and reconstruct a protective barrier that prevents infection and dehydration.
The Problem: In chronic wounds, the epithelialization process is impaired. Previous studies focused primarily on a wound base, defining fibroblasts in chronic wounds. However, little is known about the biology of keratinocytes at the non-healing edge.
Basic/Clinical Science Advances: Keratinocytes at the nonhealing edges of chronic wounds are unable to migrate. They continuously proliferate, forming a thick, hyperkeratotic layer that defines the chronic wound edge. To stimulate wound healing, these healing-incompetent cells need to be identified and removed to allow healing-competent keratinocytes to epithelialize the wound. Recently, the first epidermal molecular markers of impaired wound healing were defined. Knowledge from genomics studies of human chronic wound specimens revealed that non-migratory keratinocytes are not senescent, but rather are caught in a perpetual cycle of incomplete activation and differentiation.
Clinical Care Relevance: The healing-incompetent keratinocytes contain inhibitors of healing that may be utilized as objective markers to make a clinical diagnosis, to establish a prognosis, and to determine the margin of debridement for removal of healing-incompetent cells. Moreover, defining pathological molecular markers in the non-healing edges can help in developing assays to predict healing outcomes for chronic wounds.
Conclusion: Keratinocytes at the non-healing wound edge contribute to the pathogenesis of chronic wounds. Identification of molecules participating in the non-healing phenotype may serve as a biotool for successful diagnostics and outcome measures.

Abbreviations and Acronyms

ADAM12 = a disintegrin and metalloprotease
ADV = adenoviral vectors
DFU = diabetic foot ulcer
EGF = epidermal growth factor
EGFR = epidermal growth factor receptor
ESCs = epidermal stem cells
K1 = keratin 1
K2 = keratin 2
K6 = keratin 6
K10 = keratin 10
K16 = keratin 16
K17 = keratin 17
VU = venous ulcer

*Correspondence: Wound Healing and Regenerative Medicine Research Program, Department of Dermatology and Cutaneous Surgery, University of Miami Miller School of Medicine, 1600 N.W. 10th Ave., RMSB, Room 2023-A Miami, Florida 33136 (e-mail: mtcanic@med.miami.edu).

BACKGROUND

THE INCIDENCE OF CHRONIC wounds is reaching epidemic proportions,[1] having over $25 billion expenditure annually on their treatment in the United States alone.[2] Healthy epidermis provides a protective barrier that undergoes constant renewal. Epidermal stem cells (ESCs) located in the basal layer of epidermis give rise to keratinocytes, which, as they leave the basal compartment, begin differentiation.[3] Differentiation process results in a formation of enucleated corneocytes, cross-linked insoluble proteins, and lipids forming a barrier at the surface of the skin. Upon wounding, keratinocytes at the wound edges become activated: they migrate and proliferate to seal the gap.[4] Additionally, ESCs from the bulge area of the hair follicle[5,6] and circulating

Printed in U.S.A.
DOI: 10.1089/awc.2009.0114

progenitors[7,8] migrate into the wound site to aid the process.

Epithelialization is impaired in chronic wounds. Keratinocytes at the non-healing wound edge are hyperproliferative and mitotically active in the suprabasal layers. The cornified layer is much thicker than in normal skin (hyperkeratosis) with the cell nuclei present as well (parakeratosis).[9] Moreover, studies of hard-to-heal chronic wounds demonstrated that there are two intrinsically different types of tissue: (a) the non-healing wound edge unresponsive to growth factors *in vivo* or *in vitro* that does not reepithelialize and (b) adjacent non-ulcerated skin, responsive to stimuli and healing competent.[10] These findings support the notion that healing-incompetent cells should be removed (debrided). Still, many chronic wounds heal without debridement. Additional studies are needed to determine the role of debridement in clinical outcomes. Thus, biomolecular markers that can identify healing-incompetent keratinocytes may provide a new guiding tool that would have a significant impact in the future treatment protocols.

CLINICAL PROBLEM ADDRESSED

Identification of molecules uniquely present in healing-incompetent keratinocytes at the chronic wound edge may provide a set of objective biological markers that can be used to identify wounds that are not responding to standard therapy and require aggressive early intervention to heal. Such biomarkers will allow for development of novel clinical protocols, as they may be used to guide surgical debridement, provide endpoints for future clinical trials, and predict outcomes of healing.

BASIC SCIENCE CONTEXT

In the past, the edges of non-healing chronic wounds were not considered an important tissue component in the pathology of chronic wounds. However, its epidermis has distinct biological features that make a significant contribution to the overall clinical outcome in the patient.

Keratinocytes at the chronic wound edge are hyperproliferative, hyperkeratotic, and parakeratotic. Mitotically active cells are present in the suprabasal layers and nucleated corneocytes in the cornified layer.[9] Thus, keratinocytes are not senescent, but rather deregulated. These histopathological changes have been observed in all types of chronic wounds. Therefore, they may reflect a basic non-healing mechanism of epidermal keratinocytes in chronic wounds.[9–11]

Although nonhealing edge keratinocytes resemble the activated phenotype, they express keratin 6 (*K6*), *K16*, and/or *K17*, they are different from the healing edge keratinocytes because they are overly proliferative, but not migratory. Therefore, they do not execute the complete activation cycle.[11–13] Studies on relatively small patient size revealed that these healing-incompetent keratinocytes are marked by the presence of nuclear β-catenin throughout the epidermis (Fig. 1).[9] *In vitro* studies show that presence of nuclear β-catenin inhibits keratinocyte migration and wound healing through induction of expression of its downstream target gene *c-myc*. Expression of c-myc leads to a blockade of the epidermal growth factor (*EGF*) response and represses the expression of cytoskeletal components that support migration, K6 and/or *K16*.[9] Although *K6* and *K16* were induced in non-healing wounds, indicating that the keratinocytes are in an activated state, they were downregulated in comparison to either healing chronic wounds[13] or acute wounds.[9]

Healing-incompetent keratinocytes at the venous ulcer (VU) wound edge also demonstrate deregulation in the differentiation process. Various differentiation and proliferation markers and their regulators were found deregulated in non-healing wound edges when compared to healthy skin.[11] Differentiation markers *K1*, *K10*, fillagrin, and a subset of small proline-rich proteins were suppressed, whereas involucrin, transglutaminase 1, and another subset of small proline-rich proteins were induced in keratinocytes of the VU non-healing edge,[11,12] suggesting deregulation of differentiation, which is consistent with morphological findings of hyper/parakeratosis.

EXPERIMENTAL MODEL OR MATERIAL

Experimental animal models are widely used to study wound healing. However, these models do not fully resemble the multifactorial diversity of human disease (NIH website www.niams.nih.gov/News_and_Events/Meetings_and_Events/Roundtables/2007/roundtable_wound.asp). Data generated from analyses of patient specimens yielded new information about keratinocytes derived from chronic wounds. Recently, several pilot studies emerging from a novel field of skinomics[14] contributed to the understanding of healing-incompetent keratinocytes at the non-healing chronic wounds edges. The mRNA extracted from skin specimens were analyzed using genomic approaches. These skin specimens included non-healing and healing VUs, the adjacent non-healing

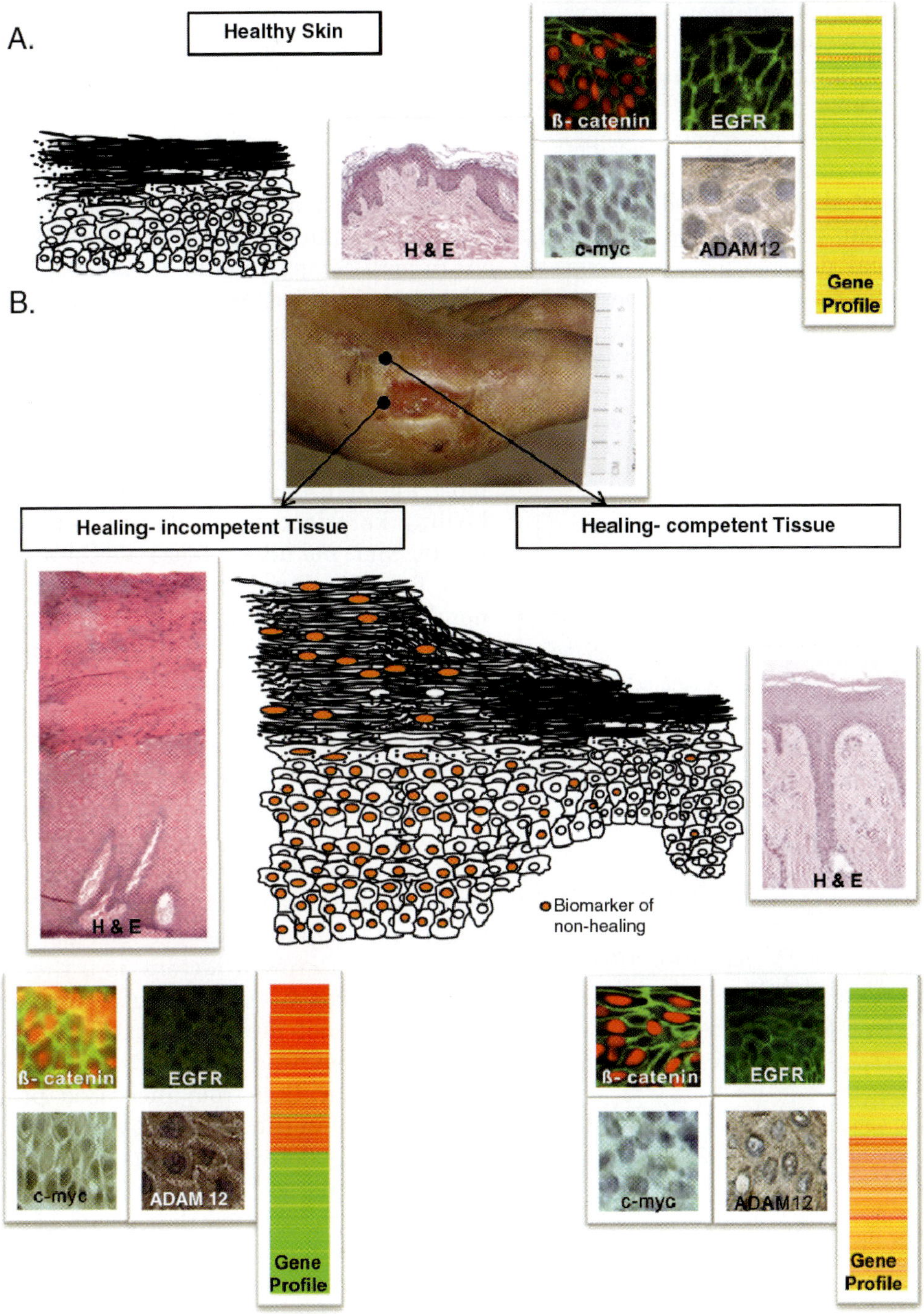

Figure 1. Healing-incompetent keratinocytes contain characteristic biomarkers. In contrast to healthy skin (**A**) edge of hard to heal wounds (**B**) consists of two distinct keratinocyte populations. Healing-incompetent keratinocytes of the nonhealing edge are hyperproliferative. They form thick cornified layer with the nuclei present throughout. These keratinocytes are marked by nuclear presence of β-catenin and c-myc, and increased cytoplasmic and membranous expression of *ADAM12* and cytoplasmic *EGFR*. However, morphology of adjacent, nonulcerated skin consists of healing-competent keratinocytes. Expression of biomarkers is similar to that of healthy skin marked by membranous presence of β-catenin and *EGFR*, absence of nuclear c-myc, and significantly lower membranous and cytoplasmic expression of *ADAM12*. *ADAM12* = a disintegrin and metalloprotease; *EGFR* = epidermal growth factor receptor.

ulcerated skin, non-healing edges of VUs, and healthy skin. Evaluation of transcriptional profiles led to characterization of biological features of healing-incompetent keratinocytes and pointed to different gene expression profiles between different wound locations,[10,11,13,15] whereas genetic analyses identified single-nucleotide polymorphisms in estrogen receptor beta as an associated factor of susceptibility to venous ulceration in elderly.[16] However, human tissue analyses are complexed by variability in collecting the specimens that may lead to diverse data. Thus, reliable tissue markers and characterization of histopathology may prove very useful in standardization of sampling.

DISCUSSION OF FINDINGS AND RELEVANT LITERATURE

Keratinocytes are important participants of the wound-healing process and are currently used as therapeutic agents in treatment of chronic wounds.[17–20] However, knowledge about the biology of keratinocytes at the non-healing edge of the chronic wounds is limited.[17]

The histopathological abnormalities and induction of *c-myc* described in chronic wounds[9] (Fig. 1) are consistent with previous findings of *c-myc* overexpression in transgenic mouse models.[21–24] Mice over expressing *c-myc* in the basal epidermal layer develop a chronic wound phenotype. Keratinocytes derived from these mice show impaired migration capacity. In addition, *c-myc* overexpression in mice leads to local deprivation of ESCs.[22] Similarly, it has been observed that there is a lack of ESCs in nonhealing VUs due to frequent cycling and loss of signals that control ESC niche.[25]

Diminished growth factor action is considered one of the hallmarks of chronic wounds.[26,27] Microarray analysis of patients' biopsies from VUs revealed that the EGF receptor (*EGFR*), localized at the cell membrane of the keratinocytes in healthy skin, is markedly reduced and present primarily in the cytoplasm of the healing-incompetent keratinocytes, resulting in the inability of the keratinocyte to respond to EGF. On the other hand, in adjacent, nonulcerated skin, the *EGFR* was present in both compartments, predominantly on the cell membrane, resuming the expression pattern of healthy epidermis (Fig. 1).[10] Also, transforming growth factor $\beta 3$ expression but not transforming growth factor $\beta 1$ or $\beta 2$ was found increased in the epithelium at the edge of VUs and diabetic foot ulcers (DFUs).[28,29] Further, a novel molecule that may contribute to the nonhealing keratinocyte phenotype, a disintegrin and metalloprotease (*ADAM12*), was found induced in keratinocytes of non-healing wound edges of VU, but not in acute wounds (Fig. 1).[30] Conversely, keratinocytes from *ADAM12(−/−)* knockout mice exhibited increased migration, indicating the possible role of *ADAM12* in the inhibition of keratinocyte migration in chronic wounds. In addition, decreased chemokines in keratinocytes, such as stromal cell–derived factor-1α, leads to decreased homing of progenitor cells to the wound site in diabetic mouse models.[31]

The use of growth factors as a therapeutic approach in treating chronic wounds did not meet expectations. The lack of efficacy was mostly attributed to rapid degeneration from increased protease activity in the wound environment, thus multiple delivery options are being currently explored.[27,32,33] For example, it has been demonstrated that electrospun silk nanofibers or self-assembling peptides are effective in slow releasing EGF. Use of such bioactive dressings for short time periods on wounded human skin equivalents leads to acceleration of wound closure.[34] Although these new experimental data are promising, further studies are necessary to validate efficacy *in vivo* and further in healing of chronic wounds in patients. Adenoviral vectors (ADVs) may also be utilized for local sustained delivery of growth factors. Recent *in vivo* studies have shown that either ADV–platelet-derived growth factor or ADV–vascular endothelial growth factor accelerates wound healing.[33,35–37]

TAKE-HOME MESSAGE

Basic science advances

- The epidermis of the chronic wound edge has distinctive morphology. It is hyperproliferative, with nuclei present in a thick cornified layer.
- Keratinocytes at the non-healing edges of VU and DFU stain for cell cycle regulators and express *K6*, *K16*, and/or *K17*, markers characteristic for their activated, non-migratory phenotype.
- Keratinocytes at the non-healing edges of chronic wounds proliferate and differentiate, but they are unable to complete either of the two processes.
- Non-healing wound edge keratinocytes are marked by nuclear presence of β-catenin and *c-myc*.
- Induction of *ADAM12* in keratinocytes at the wound edge of VU is one of the contributing factors involved in inhibition of their migration.
- EGFR is suppressed in keratinocytes of the VU edge and is localized in the cytoplasm rather than in the cell membrane.
- The gene expression profile of keratinocytes from non-healing edge and adjacent, nonulcerated skin is distinctive and many genes encoding different processes are deregulated.
- Further investigation is needed to determine molecular mechanisms that lead to the non-healing phenotype of the keratinocytes at the chronic wound edge.

Clinical science advances

- The non-healing epidermis contains inhibitors of healing, contributing to an overall negative clinical outcome.
- It might be possible to utilize the molecules that inhibit healing as objective quantitative markers of healing-incompetent tissue as an indicator for the need of a more aggressive clinical treatment.

Relevance to clinical care

- There is a critical unmet need for molecular characterization of wound healing in chronic wounds that can be used to develop effective treatment strategies. The ability to distinguish keratinocytes that are capable of responding to wound-healing stimuli, "good cells," from keratinocytes that are not capable of responding, "bad cells," as markers of a healing impaired wound edge would lead to new therapeutic targets and better outcome measures for testing novel treatment protocols. Using molecular markers could result in more effective treatment, ultimately better clinical outcome, and a decrease in health care costs.

In addition, ongoing clinical trial of ADV–platelet-derived growth factor for treatment of DFU has shown good safety profile (ClinicalTrials.gov Identifier: NCT00493051). All these developing technologies are promising and may provide new therapeutic avenues in near future. However, understanding of molecular mechanisms that lead to diminished activity of growth factors in chronic wounds in patients will allow for more advanced treatments in the future.

Understanding loss of keratinocyte migration in chronic wounds is clinically important. *K6*, *K16*, and *K17* are considered one of the first markers of keratinocyte activation that support keratinocyte migration, and thus, the wound-healing process. Interestingly, loss of *K17* in mouse model causes significant delay in embryonic healing,[38] whereas loss of *K6* does not impair migration, but does contribute to fragility of keratinocytes.[39] Keratinocytes from chronic wounds demonstrate similar complexity in keratin expression, expressing *K6* and *K16*, but at lower levels when compared to acute wounds.[9,10,12] Keratinocytes DFU wound edge are also found to express *K16*, as well, and are highly proliferative (Ki67 positive).[40] Comparison of non-healing VU to healing VU revealed greatest downregulation of *K6*, *K16*, and *K17*,[13] suggesting that a complete loss of these proteins may be a prognostic indicator of non-healing wounds.

Incomplete keratinocyte activation is coupled with incomplete differentiation.[11] Although keratinocytes from the non-healing edge initiate differentiation, they are unable to complete the process, resulting in presence of nuclei throughout cornified layer. These cells are characterized by loss of *K10* and *K2*, keratins involved in epidermal differentiation, and demonstrate a reduced expression of the uncleaved precursor of the alpha 3 chain of laminin 5, which is one of the key molecules present in migrating epithelium.[40] At the edges of VU and DFU, keratinocytes are shown to express cell cycle regulators p63+, CD29+, PCNA+, and p53.[12] In addition, expression of human β defensin 2, an endogenous antimicrobial peptide, is markedly increased in the keratinocytes of chronic VU.[41]

Taken together, keratinocytes at the chronic wound edges are not functioning properly. Unable to migrate, they are trapped in vicious cycle in which perpetuate activation, proliferation, and differentiation processes take place in unorganized fashion, without spatiotemporal control.

CAUTION, CRITICAL REMARKS, AND RECOMMENDATIONS

The epidermal edge of the non-healing wounds may contain important clinical information that can assist in predicting the clinical outcome of chronic wounds and aid in guiding the extent of debridement. Until biomarkers are validated, we suggest routine histopathological analysis to determine the presence of a hyperkeratotic and hyperproliferative edge, which would indicate the existence of healing-incompetent keratinocytes.

FUTURE DEVELOPMENTS

Identification and validation of objective quantitative markers of healing-incompetent keratinocytes will be an effective clinical tool in the future. Once established, these markers may serve as predictors of outcome and lead to development of diagnostic assays to be utilized in clinical settings and allow for the demarcation between healing and nonhealing tissue, guiding future therapeutic protocols.

ACKNOWLEDGMENT

Wound-healing research in the author's laboratory is funded by NIH awards.

AUTHOR DISCLOSURE STATEMENT

No conflict of interest disclosed.

REFERENCES

1. Brem H, Tomic-Canic M, Taranovskaya A, Ehlich HP, Baskin-Bay E, Gill K, Carasa G, Weinberger S, Entero H, and Vladeck B: Healing of elderly patients with diabetic foot ulcers, venous stasis ulcers, and pressure ulcers. Surg Technol Int 2003; **11:** 161.

2. Services UDoHaH: *Guidance to Surveyors for Long Term Care Facilities*, 2004. www.cms.hhs.gov.

3. Blanpain C and Fuchs E: Epidermal stem cells of the skin. Annu Rev Cell Dev Biol 2006; **22:** 339.

4. Tomic-Canic M, Komine M, Freedberg IM, and Blumenberg M: Epidermal signal transduction and transcription factor activation in activated keratinocytes. J Dermatol Sci 1998; **17:** 167.

5. Ito M and Cotsarelis G: Is the hair follicle necessary for normal wound healing? J Investig Dermatol 2008; **128:** 1059.

6. Ito M, Liu Y, Yang Z, Nguyen J, Liang F, Morris RJ, *et al.*: Stem cells in the hair follicle bulge contribute to wound repair but not to homeostasis of the epidermis. Nat Med 2005; **11:** 1351.

7. Sivan-Loukianova E, Awad OA, Stepanovic V, Bickenbach J, and Schatteman GC: CD34+ blood cells accelerate vascularization and healing of diabetic mouse skin wounds. J Vasc Res 2003; **40:** 368.

8. Liu ZJ and Velazquez OC: Hyperoxia, endothelial progenitor cell mobilization, and diabetic wound healing. Antioxid Redox Signal 2008; **10:** 1869.

9. Stojadinovic O, Brem H, Vouthounis C, Lee B, Fallon J, Stallcup M, *et al.*: Molecular Pathogenesis of Chronic Wounds: the role of beta-catenin and

c-myc in the inhibition of epithelialization and wound healing. Am J Pathol 2005; **167:** 59.

10. Brem H, Stojadinovic O, Diegelmann RF, Entero H, Lee B, Pastar I, *et al.*: Molecular markers in patients with chronic wounds to guide surgical debridement. Mol Med 2007; **13:** 30.

11. Stojadinovic O, Pastar I, Vukelic S, Mahoney MG, Brennan D, Krzyzanowska A, *et al.*: Deregulation of keratinocyte differentiation and activation: a hallmark of venous ulcers. J Cell Mol Med 2008; **12:** 2675.

12. Galkowska H, Olszewsk WL, Wojewodzka U, Mijal J, and Filipiuk E: Expression of apoptosis- and cell cycle-related proteins in epidermis of venous leg and diabetic foot ulcers. Surgery 2003; **134:** 213.

13. Charles CA, Tomic-Canic M, Vincek V, Nassiri M, Stojadinovic O, Eaglstein WH, *et al.*: A gene signature of nonhealing venous ulcers: potential diagnostic markers. J Am Acad Dermatol 2008; **59:** 758.

14. Blumenberg M: Skinomics. J Investig Dermatol 2005; **124:** viii.

15. Tomic-Canic M, Ayello EA, Stojadinovic O, Golinko MS, and Brem H: Using gene transcription patterns (bar coding scans) to guide wound debridement and healing. Adv Skin Wound Care 2008; **21:** 487.

16. Ashworth JJ, Smyth JV, Pendleton N, Horan M, Payton A, Worthington J, *et al.*: Polymorphisms spanning the 0N exon and promoter of the estrogen receptor-beta (ERbeta) gene ESR2 are associated with venous ulceration. Clin Genet 2008; **73:** 55.

17. Pastar I, Stojadinovic O, and Tomic-Canic M: Role of Keratinocytes in Healing of Chronic Wounds. Surg Technol Int XVII, 2008; **17:** 105.

18. Beele H, de la Brassine M, Lambert J, Suys E, De Cuyper C, Decroix J, *et al.*: A prospective multicenter study of the efficacy and tolerability of cryopreserved allogenic human keratinocytes to treat venous leg ulcers. Int J Low Extrem Wounds 2005; **4:** 225.

19. Vanscheidt W, Ukat A, Horak V, Bruning H, Hunyadi J, Pavlicek R, *et al.*: Treatment of recalcitrant venous leg ulcers with autologous keratinocytes in fibrin sealant: a multinational randomized controlled clinical trial. Wound Repair Regen 2007; **15:** 308.

20. Hartmann A, Quist J, Hamm H, Brocker EB, and Friedl P: Transplantation of autologous keratinocyte suspension in fibrin matrix to chronic venous leg ulcers: improved long-term healing after removal of the fibrin carrier. Dermatol Surg 2008; **34:** 922.

21. Waikel RL, Kawachi Y, Waikel PA, Wang XJ, and Roop DR: Deregulated expression of c-Myc depletes epidermal stem cells. Nat Genet 2001; **28:** 165.

22. Arnold I and Watt FM: c-Myc activation in transgenic mouse epidermis results in mobilization of stem cells and differentiation of their progeny. Curr Biol 2001; **11:** 558.

23. Frye M, Gardner C, Li ER, Arnold I, and Watt FM: Evidence that Myc activation depletes the epidermal stem cell compartment by modulating adhesive interactions with the local microenvironment. Development 2003; **130:** 2793.

24. Waikel RL, Wang XJ, and Roop DR: Targeted expression of c-Myc in the epidermis alters normal proliferation, differentiation and UV-B induced apoptosis. Oncogene 1999; **18:** 4870.

25. Stojadinovic O, Pastar I, Krzyzanowska A, Zimmerman K, Brem H, and Tomic-Canic M: Change of fate of epidermal stem cells contributes to pathogenesis of chronic wounds. J Investig Dermatol 2009; **129:** s5.

26. Raja, Sivamani K, Garcia MS, and Isseroff RR: Wound re-epithelialization: modulating keratinocyte migration in wound healing. Front Biosci 2007; **12:** 2849.

27. Barrientos S, Stojadinovic O, Golinko MS, Brem H, and Tomic-Canic M: Growth factors and cytokines in wound healing. Wound Repair Regen 2008; **16:** 585.

28. Jude EB, Blakytny R, Bulmer J, Boulton AJ, and Ferguson MW: Transforming growth factor-beta 1, 2, 3 and receptor type I and II in diabetic foot ulcers. Diabet Med 2002; **19:** 440.

29. Cowin AJ, Hatzirodos N, Holding CA, Dunaiski V, Harries RH, Rayner TE, *et al.*: Effect of healing on the expression of transforming growth factor beta(s) and their receptors in chronic venous leg ulcers. J Investig Dermatol 2001; **117:** 1282.

30. Harsha A, Stojadinovic O, Brem H, Sehara-Fujisawa A, Wewer U, Loomis CA, *et al.*: ADAM12: a potential target for the treatment of chronic wounds. J Mol Med 2008; **86:** 961.

31. Gallagher KA, Liu ZJ, Xiao M, Chen H, Goldstein LJ, Buerk DG, *et al.*: Diabetic impairments in NO-mediated endothelial progenitor cell mobilization and homing are reversed by hyperoxia and SDF-1alpha. J Clin Investig 2007; **117:** 1249.

32. Hardwicke J, Ferguson EL, Moseley R, Stephens P, Thomas DW, and Duncan R: Dextrin-rhEGF conjugates as bioresponsive nanomedicines for wound repair. J Control Release 2008; **130:** 275.

33. Brem H, Kodra A, Golinko MS, Entero H, Stojadinovic O, Wang VM, *et al.*: Mechanism of Sustained Release of Vascular Endothelial Growth Factor in Accelerating Experimental Diabetic Healing. J Investig Dermatol 2009; **129:** 2275.

34. Schneider A, Wang XY, Kaplan DL, Garlick JA, and Egles C: Biofunctionalized electrospun silk mats as a topical bioactive dressing for accelerated wound healing. Acta Biomater 2008; **5:** 2570.

35. Gu DL, Nguyen T, Gonzalez AM, Printz MA, Pierce GF, Sosnowski BA, *et al.*: Adenovirus encoding human platelet-derived growth factor-B delivered in collagen exhibits safety, biodistribution, and immunogenicity profiles favorable for clinical use. Mol Ther 2004; **9:** 699.

36. Keswani SG, Katz AB, Lim FY, Zoltick P, Radu A, Alaee D, *et al.*: Adenoviral mediated gene transfer of PDGF-B enhances wound healing in type I and type II diabetic wounds. Wound Repair Regen 2004; **12:** 497.

37. Margolis DJ, Crombleholme T, and Herlyn M: Clinical protocol: phase I trial to evaluate the safety of H5.020CMV.PDGF-B for the treatment of a diabetic insensate foot ulcer. Wound Repair Regen 2000; **8:** 480.

38. Mazzalupo S, Wong P, Martin P, and Coulombe PA: Role for keratins 6 and 17 during wound closure in embryonic mouse skin. Dev Dyn 2003; **226:** 356.

39. Wong P and Coulombe PA: Loss of keratin 6 (K6) proteins reveals a function for intermediate filaments during wound repair. J Cell Biol 2003; **163:** 327.

40. Usui ML, Mansbridge JN, Carter WG, Fujita M, and Olerud JE: Keratinocyte migration, proliferation, and differentiation in chronic ulcers from patients with diabetes and normal wounds. J Histochem Cytochem 2008; **56:** 687.

41. Butmarc J, Yufit T, Carson P, and Falanga V: Human beta-defensin-2 expression is increased in chronic wounds. Wound Repair Regen 2004; **12:** 439.

Age and Impaired Healing Potential

Jason Maggi,[1] Madhu Ragupathi,[1] Marjana Tomic-Canic,[2] and Harold Brem[1,*]

[1]Helen and Martin Kimmel Wound Center, Division of Wound Healing and Regenerative Medicine, Department of Surgery, NYU Langone Medical Center, New York, New York.
[2]Department of Dermatology and Cutaneous Surgery, University of Miami Miller School of Medicine, Miami, Florida.

Background: Aging patients have multiple physiological impairments to wound healing. However, aging by itself does not stop the healing process and is not a source of a chronic wound. Despite these impairments, the expectation should be maintained that elderly patients can completely heal with the same frequency of those in a younger population.
The Problem: Elderly persons tend to have a greater number of concurrent comorbidities. Increased incidence of peripheral arterial disease and venous reflux contributes to a significant local impairment to healing. Systemically, a high prevalence of type 2 diabetes further delays healing in this population. This represents a major problem not only clinically, but also economically, as the presence, and subsequently the healing, of these wounds is often used as a benchmark for quality of care.
Basic/Clinical Science Advances: Mechanisms detailing the synergy between aging, diabetes, and delayed healing are now well understood. Altered macrophage and fibroblast function, resulting in decreased collagen production and proliferative capacity, are targets of intense study. Early identification and treatment of ischemia and infection, which greatly impair healing, have become extremely important. In addition, the role of early surgical debridement, growth factor, and cellular therapy are now becoming well established and accepted as highly effective means of treatment.
Clinical Care Relevance: Care of elderly patients with wounds requires early recognition of factors that will disrupt the healing process. Immediate identification of this status should result in successful, albeit delayed healing. Adherence to established guidelines and protocol-driven care will ensure the best possible care for these patients.
Conclusion: Although healing of wounds in the elderly is delayed, increased understanding and use of current wound care advances may counter the physiologic impairments found in these patients. It should be an expectation that all persons in this population will heal, thereby decreasing the morbidity associated with these wounds.

Abbreviation and Acronym

VEGF = vascular endothelial growth factor

*Correspondence: Helen and Martin Kimmel Wound Center, Division of Wound Healing and Regenerative Medicine, Department of Surgery, New York University School of Medicine, 301 E. 17th Street, Room 1026, New York, New York 10003 (e-mail: harold.brem@nyumc.org).

BACKGROUND

As the fastest growing segment of the population, elderly patients comprise a rapidly increasing portion of patients with acute and chronic wounds. Currently, 12.6% (38 million) of the total United States population is 65 years or older, with an estimate that this group will comprise up to 20% of the population by the year 2030.[1] In addition, 1.8% of the population is 85 years or greater, and this group will also continue to grow. Given the advances in health care and increase in life expectancy of the population over the last several

Printed in U.S.A.
DOI: 10.1089/awc.2009.0161

Table 1. *Systemic and local factors affecting healing in elderly patients*

Factors Affecting Healing in the Elderly
Systemic factors:
Diabetes mellitus
Current glucocorticoid administration
Chronic immobilization
Current chemotherapy
Nutritional deficiencies
Concurrent malignancy
Hypoxemia/hypoperfusion
Lack of exercise
Decreased endogenous estrogen levels
Prolonged hospitalization
Adverse medication effects
Dehydration
Local factors:
Microbacterial contamination
Peripheral arterial disease
Venous insufficiency
Radiation
Smoking
Reduced growth factor concentration
Mechanical
Lymphedema
Neoplastic transformation

decades, it should be anticipated that this trend will continue. However, these improvements in medical care and living standards lead to an ever increasing conundrum. As the population ages, these older individuals become much more susceptible to age-related comorbid conditions. More than 80% of elderly individuals have at least one chronic condition, and 50% have at least two.[2] One specific outcome of the accretion of these conditions is a delay in the ability to heal wounds.

Aging patients have multiple physiological impairments to wound healing (Table 1). In a recent 5-year epidemiological study of 1,158 chronic wounds, it was found that the overall frequency of closed wounds within the observation period was 61.4% in the patients aged <70 years compared with 47.4% in the patients aged ≥ 70 years.[3] Although aging itself does not stop the healing process, elderly patients do show a delay in healing. Moreover, elderly persons have a higher incidence of venous reflux, type 2 diabetes, ischemic arterial disease, and being bed bound. Therefore, they will have a higher incidence of venous ulcers, diabetic foot ulcers, and pressure ulcers. Despite these medical impediments, the hypothesis should remain that their wounds can heal completely with the same frequency of those in a younger population.

CLINICAL PROBLEM ADDRESSED

Impaired wound healing in the elderly population continues to develop into a major clinical and economic problem. Concurrently, the cost of treating chronic wounds in this population continues to grow, with pressure ulcers alone easily exceeding several billion dollars per year.[4] The total cost related to diabetic foot ulcers was calculated in 2004 to be $13,179 per episode, and the cost increases as ulcers increase in severity.[5] Aside from the financial costs, it is imperative to note the role of these wounds in their effect on the quality of life of those affected. This is observed in terms of decreased physical mobility, chronic pain, and emotional stress, often resulting in depression and decreased quality of life.[6]

Elderly patients are more likely to succumb to the complications of wounds—*e.g.*, amputations or sepsis.[7] The incidence of severe sepsis was found to be increased 100-fold with age (0.2/1,000 in children to 26.2/1,000 in those aged >85 years). Further, mortality from sepsis was also significantly age dependent; it increased from 10% in children to 38.4% in those older than 85 years.[8] Patients with acute respiratory distress syndrome, often a complication from wound-induced sepsis, have significantly higher mortality rates when their age is greater than 55 years (64% mortality) when compared with patients 55 years and younger (45% mortality).[9]

Indeed, the complexity in understanding this impaired healing potential is due to the fact that changes in aged skin and resulting chronic wounds are due to a combination of intrinsic and extrinsic factors.[10] Such an intricate interaction of factors, ranging from the cellular level to variations in clinical management, culminates in progressive loss of function, loss of protection from environmental stresses, and inability to maintain homeostasis.

RELEVANT BASIC SCIENCE CONTEXT

Alterations in the normal homeostatic mechanisms in each phase of wound healing are evident in the elderly patient, especially the inflammation response and capacity for appropriate proliferation.

Macrophages, key cells in the inflammatory response, display an age-related alteration in function. In addition, changes in endothelial factors, proteinases, and growth factor concentrations all have been documented in the aged patient. Further, elderly patients show reduced proliferative response of fibroblasts and epithelial cells, and reduced overall number of cells in response to growth factors, cytokines, and angiogenic stimulation.[11,12] Uncertainty remains in determining to what extent it is the cells themselves or the local environment, which is exposed to ischemia, infection, and multiple stressors, cause the delay in healing. However, the end result of the synergy of these multiple impairments is a reduced rate of healing.

EXPERIMENTAL MODEL OR MATERIAL—ADVANTAGES AND LIMITATIONS

Despite common acceptance that aging results in delayed healing, studies focusing in this area have often been criticized for inadequate control of confounding factors. There are several comorbidities other than age, such as diabetes, ischemia, and cardiovascular disease, which make it extremely difficult to assess the exact amount these conditions affect wound healing. As such, optimal medical management of these conditions is essential to allow any study to be as focused as possible on the wound itself.

The elderly population as a whole tends to be underrepresented in most clinical trials, and as a result, information on the effects of optimal medical treatment may not be readily available. This has left possible age-related differences in diseases and responses to therapy to be inferred, and exposes elderly patients to risk from inaccurate assumptions.

As it is impossible to conduct prospective trials studying chronic wounds in the elderly, animal models have long served as the substitute. However, chronic wounds do not naturally occur in animals, leaving a large gap in our current understanding of this process.

Studies of outcomes of operative debridement in the elderly have also been limited because of the fact that these patients are often felt to be unsuitable for anesthesia or surgical intervention. There is little evidence to prove the safety of providing local anesthesia only, or local anesthesia with mild sedation, compared with general anesthesia. However, there is evidence that preparation of the wound bed by surgical debridement is effective in assisting the wound-healing process.[13]

As further work is pursued in identifying the processes affecting healing in this group at the molecular level, so too must studies be pursued in the clinical context. Although wounds cannot be created, methods of treatment, including growth factors, human skin equivalents, and stem cells, can be studied in a prospective fashion.

DISCUSSION OF FINDINGS AND RELEVANT LITERATURE

Skin aging is a complex biological process that is a consequence of intrinsic or genetically programmed aging that occurs with time, and extrinsic aging caused by environmental factors. Collagen synthesis and deposition gradually decline with age and cellular dysfunction becomes increasingly pronounced. Fibroblasts isolated from chronic wounds have increased cell death and decreased proliferative capacity when compared with young adult cells.[14] This increase in cellular senescence has been attributed to several factors, such as telomerase erosion[15] and oxidative stress.[16] This dysfunction, and resultant decrease in collagen deposition, might partly explain the development of dermal atrophy and poor wound healing in the elderly.[17]

In addition to changes at the molecular level, the clinical appearance of medical comorbidities further delays the ability to heal. This is evident in mouse models, where aged diabetic mice displayed a 36% reduction in stiffness and a 42% reduction in breaking load postwounding when compared with age-matched controls. This finding is independent of hyperglycemic state or diabetic status in the young mouse.[18] This finding supports the idea of a synergistic effect between diabetes and aging.

Arterial insufficiency also poses a significant impediment to healing in the elderly. Physical examination or presence of Doppler signals does not ensure adequate blood supply, putting patients at increased risk of missed ischemia.[19] Although it may be possible to heal wounds arising from vascular insufficiency without correcting the underlying disorder, patients are prone to recurrence and placed at an increased risk for limb loss and chronic morbidity. Arterial insufficiency, especially in combination with infection, is a significant factor in nonhealing of wounds.[20] Surgical correction of this condition can promote healing and prevent limb loss.[21]

This risk also applies to venous ulcerations, as elderly patients have increased incidence of reflux, fibrosis, and clot formation. This condition has been shown to benefit from surgical correction as well, even in the presence of concomitant peripheral arterial disease.[22]

Mirroring clinical vascular dysfunction, impaired angiogenesis has been demonstrated experimentally in animal models[23] and the aged patient. Tissues from aged individuals display a substantially lower capillary density than do tissues from nonaged counterparts, and the neovascular response in aged tissues is delayed by ~40% when compared with the response of tissues from younger individuals. Diminished angiogenesis also impairs the migration and function of macrophages, which are essential to wound healing through their effects on the inflammatory response and secretion of essential growth factors.[24]

Several studies over the last decade have examined the role of supplementation of these growth factors either systemically or topically. Vascular endothelial growth factor (VEGF), transforming growth factor-1, basic fibroblast growth factor, platelet-derived growth factor, and others have been shown to be of benefit in various animal models.[25–28] When recombinant VEGF protein was administered to young and old rabbits, both groups exhibited a significant and similar increase in blood pressure ratio, angiographic score, and capillary density.[23] In human studies, recombinant human platelet-derived growth factor applied once daily to patients with diabetic foot ulcers resulted in a significant increase in complete healing. This finding was accompanied by a significant decrease in the time to complete healing by 30%.[29] This exemplifies that with the correct treatment, the aged patient has the potential to heal just as well as younger populations.

Delayed healing capacity makes the elderly much more susceptible to infection and the systemic complications that arise when it remains untreated. The vulnerability of these patients to infection is demonstrated by a recent study examining 984 intensive care patients. Results showed that although the incidence of nosocomial bloodstream infection is lower among very old (age >75) patients, the adverse impact of the infection is much higher.[30] All open wounds will become colonized, and impaired cellular function may allow this to become a nidus for an impending systemic infection. Additionally, the presence of infection may be a contributing factor in the delay in healing seen in this population by inhibiting already dysfunctional macrophages and prolonging the inflammatory phase.[31] Removal of this inhibitory factor, via sharp surgical debridement and antibiotic therapy, may prove to be invaluable to healing wounds in the elderly patient.

The use of human-derived bilayered skin substitutes provides cells and matrix on which healthy tissue can begin to develop after debridement and antibiotic therapy. These skin substitutes secrete increased levels of inflammatory and angiogenic mediators, which are often depressed in the elderly patient with a

TAKE-HOME MESSAGES

Basic science advances

- Delayed wound healing in the aged patient is related to multiple physiologic impairments.
- Fibroblast and endothelial cell proliferation are greatly reduced in elderly patients.
- Fibroblasts isolated from chronic wounds have increased cell death and decreased proliferative capacity when compared with young adult cells.
- Collagen and elastin syntheses, angiogenesis, growth factor synthesis, and macrophage function are greatly reduced in aged skin.
- Reduction in collagen and elastin levels may explain the dermal atrophy seen in the elderly.
- Decreased angiogenesis and subsequent delay of macrophage migration, in combination with medical comorbidities and/or infection, may explain the delayed healing response seen in the elderly.

Clinical science advances

- The elderly population is the most susceptible to the complications of chronic wounds, such as osteomyelitis, sepsis, and amputations.
- Underlying disorders, such as arterial or venous insufficiency, must be addressed and corrected to optimize the chances of healing the wound.
- Operative correction of venous insufficiency is safe even in the presence of concomitant peripheral arterial disease.
- Vascular insufficiency and infection have a synergistic effect in impeding wound healing.
- Optimal management of medical comorbidities, such as diabetes and cardiovascular disease, has been shown to positively affect the course of healing in chronic wounds.
- Early recognition and treatment of bacterial infection of a wound, especially in the elderly population, is essential for both healing and avoidance of systemic complications.
- Surgical debridement has proven to be safe and beneficial in the elderly, removing contaminated, deleterious tissue, while allowing healthy tissue to grow.
- In addition, surgical debridement allows for the clinician to obtain a deep tissue or bone culture, directing appropriate antibiotic therapy. This is limb and life saving, as infected wounds are much less likely to heal.
- Utilization of new molecular therapies, such as growth factors and human tissue substitutes, has provided exciting new avenues to accelerated healing.

chronic wound.[32] In small series, results have shown up to an 89% healing rate, including both surgical and nonsurgical wounds.[33] A separate study showed complete healing within 6 months in 72.5% (29/40) of patients after operative debridement.[34] However, such results, and the use of regenerative products, require careful patient selection for success.[35]

Future therapies, including stem cells and gene transfer, are currently being studied and hold great promise for the future.[36]

RELEVANCE TO CLINICAL CARE

The ultimate goal in treating an aged patient with wound is the same as in any patient—to promote healing and avoid amputations or related complications. However, it has been proven that the elderly patient needs to be treated with an increased level of intensity. This is achieved through the concerted efforts of both the clinician and surgeon providing a truly multidisciplinary approach to healing. Through the use of established protocols designed to address and decrease the impediments to healing, all providers can treat the patient with the highest level of care.[37] Working with constant communication, wounds in this population can be identified earlier, treated to eliminate correctable causes of impaired healing, and followed closely to ensure the best chance of healing. This coordination can also facilitate improved after care, prevention, and education of the patient. This care, combined with targeted therapies developed through our increasing understanding at the molecular level, will support the hypothesis that all wounds can heal in this population.

CAUTION, CRITICAL REMARKS, AND RECOMMENDATIONS

It is evident that there is no such thing as a simple wound in an elderly patient. The susceptibility of these patients to the complications related to wounds demands an increased level of care and extreme vigilance. Although much remains to be elucidated as to the exact mechanism of decreased healing potential in the elderly, and despite the fact that often lack of healing in this population is multifactorial, it should still be hypothesized that all wounds in the elderly will heal with intensive local care of the wound. Multiple forms of treatment, including topical therapies, growth factors, surgical debridement, and optimal management of medical comorbidities, must all be employed through a multidisciplinary approach. Additionally, care must extend beyond the inpatient or office setting, with careful evaluation of the patients' home situation and ability to care for the wound during the healing phase. Too often these patients present with an advanced wound, further decreasing their chance at healing. Visiting nurse services, frequent office visits, and home evaluations should all be employed in the care of the elderly, decreasing the chance of progression of an already extremely dangerous condition.

FUTURE DEVELOPMENT

As our understanding of the changes that occur in the human body with ageing grows and our realization that comorbid conditions greatly affect healing develops, future therapies targeting this population will continue to develop.

As previously mentioned, decreased angiogenesis in the elderly provides a target for treatment. Growth factors, such as VEGF in sustained release delivery, are actively being explored as potential therapies to promote healing in this population. Additionally, the advent of stem cell therapy has brought about a new, exciting potential therapy that could possibly change the entire field of wound care. Multiple current studies are ongoing in this area, with promising results in animal models.[38,39] Given the complex medical condition of the elderly population, further development of a focused electronic medical record of wounds may prove to be an essential informatics tool in managing these patients, providing a concise record of all essential medical data to multiple clinicians in real time.

AUTHOR DISCLOSURE STATEMENT

The authors have no commercial interests or competing financial interests to disclose.

REFERENCES

1. National intercensial estimates. Population Division, U.S. Census Bureau. www.census.gov. June 2009.

2. Centers for Disease Control: *The Burden of Chronic Disease and the Future of Public Health.* Atlanta, GA: U.S. Department of Health and Human Services, 2005.

3. Wicke C, Bachinger A, Coerper S, Beckert S, Witte MB, and Königsrainer A: Aging influences wound healing in patients with chronic lower extremity wounds treated in a specialized wound care center. Wound Repair Regen 2009; **17:** 25.

4. Beckrich K and Aronovitch SA: Hospital-acquired pressure ulcers: a comparison of costs in medical vs. surgical patients. Nurs Econ 1999; **17:** 263.

5. Stockl K, Vanderplas A, Tafesse E, and Chang E: Costs of lower-extremity ulcers among patients with diabetes. Diabetes Care 2004; **27:** 2129.

6. Vileikyte L: Diabetic foot ulcers: a quality of life issue. Diabetes Metab Res Rev 2001; **17:** 246.

7. Mouton CP, Bazaldua OV, Pierce B, and Espino DV: Common infections in older adults. Am Fam Physician 2001; **63:** 257.

8. Angus DC, Linde-Zwirble WT, Lidicker J, Clermont G, Carcillo J, and Pinsky MR: Epidemiology of severe sepsis in the United States: analysis of incidence, outcome, and associated costs of care. Crit Care Med 2001; **29:** 1303.

9. Suchyta MR, Clemmer TP, Elliott CG, Orme JF Jr., Morris AH, Jacobson J, and Menlove R: Increased mortality of older patients with acute respiratory distress syndrome. Chest 1997; **111:** 1334.

10. Thomas DR: Age-related changes in wound healing. Drugs Aging 2001; **18:** 607.

11. Swift ME, Kleinman HK, and DiPietro LA: Impaired wound repair and delayed angiogenesis in aged mice. Lab Invest 1999; **79:** 1479.

12. Plisko A and Gilchrest BA: Growth factor responsiveness of cultured human fibroblasts declines with age. J Gerontol 1983; **38:** 513.

13. Attinger C, Janis J, Steinberg J, Schwartz J, Al-Attar A, and Couch K. Clinical approach to wounds: debridement and wound bed preparation including the use of dressings and wound-healing adjuvants. Plast Reconstr Surg 2006; **117(suppl):** 72S.

14. Stanley AC, Park HY, Phillips TJ, Russakovsky V, and Menzoian JO: Reduced growth of dermal fibroblasts from chronic venous ulcers can be stimulated with growth factors. J Vasc Surg 1997; **26:** 994.

15. Kipling D and Faragher RG: Telomeres. Ageing hard or hardly ageing? Nature 1999; **398:** 191.

16. Walaschek M and Scharffetter-Kochanek K: Oxidative stress in chronic venous leg ulcers. Wound Repair Regen 2005; **13:** 452.

17. Uitto J and Bernstein EF: Molecular mechanisms of cutaneous aging: connective tissue alterations in the dermis. J Investig Dermatol Symp Proc 1998; **3:** 41.

18. Brem H, Tomic-Canic M, Entero H, Hanflik A, Wang V, Fallon J, and Ehrlich HP: The synergism of age and db/db genotype impairs wound healing. Exp Gerontol 2007; **42:** 523.

19. Teodorescu VJ, Chen C, Morrissey N, Faries PL, Marin ML, and Hollier LH: Detailed protocol of ischemia and the use of noninvasive vascular laboratory testing in diabetic foot ulcers. Am J Surg 2004; **187:** 75S.

20. Prompers L, Schaper N, Apelqvist J, Edmonds M, Jude E, Mauricio D, Uccioli L, Urbancic V, Bakker K, Holstein P, Jirkovska A, Piaggesi A, Ragnarson-Tennvall G, Reike H, Spraul M, Van Acker K, Van Baal J, Van Merode F, Ferreira I, and Huijberts M: Prediction of outcome in individuals with diabetic foot ulcers: focus on the differences between individuals with and without peripheral arterial disease. The Eurodiale Study. Diabetologia 2008; **51:** 747.

21. Hopf HW, Ueno C, Aslam R, Burnand K, Fife C, Grant L, Holloway A, Iafrati MD, Mani R, Misare B, Rosen N, Shapshak D, Benjamin Slade J Jr., West J, and Barbul A: Guidelines for the treatment of arterial insufficiency ulcers. Wound Repair Regen 2006; **14:** 693.

22. Obermayer A, Göstl K, Partsch H, and Benesch T: Venous reflux surgery promotes venous leg ulcer healing despite reduced ankle brachial pressure index. Int Angiol 2008; **27:** 239.

23. Rivard A, Fabre J, Silver M, Chen D, Murohara T, Kearney M, Magner M, Asahara T, and Isner J. Age-dependent impairment of angiogenesis. Circulation 1999; **99:** 111.

24. Cohen BJ, Danon D, and Roth GS: Wound repair in mice as influenced by age and antimacrophage serum. J Gerontol 1987; **42:** 295.

25. Broadley KN, Aquino AM, Woodward SC, Buckley-Sturrock A, Sato Y, Rifkin DB, and Davidson JM: Monospecific antibodies implicate basic fibroblast growth factor in normal wound repair. Lab Invest 1989; **61:** 571.

26. Mustoe TA, Pierce GF, Thomason A, Gramates P, Sporn MB, and Deuel TF: Accelerated healing of incisional wounds in rats induced by transforming growth factor-beta. Science 1987; **237:** 1333.

27. Mustoe TA, Pierce GF, and Deuel TF: Growth factor-induced acceleration of tissue repair through direct and inductive activities in a rabbit dermal ulcer model. J Clin Invest 1991; **87:** 694.

28. Fu X, Li X, Cheng B, Chen W, and Sheng Z: Engineered growth factors and cutaneous wound healing: success and possible questions in the past 10 years. Wound Repair Regen 2005; **13:** 122.

29. Steed DL: Clinical evaluation of recombinant human platelet derived growth factor for the treatment of lower extremity ulcers. Plas Reconstr Surg 2006; **117(suppl):** 143s.

30. Blot S, Cankurtaran M, Petrovic M, Vandijck D, Lizy C, Decruyenaere J, Danneels C, Vandewoude K, Piette A, Vershraegen G, Van Den Noortgate N, Peleman R, and Vogelaers D: Epidemiology and outcome of nosocomial bloodstream infection in elderly critically ill patients: a comparison between middle-aged, old, and very old patients. Crit Care Med 2009; **37:** 1634.

31. Schilling J: Wound healing. Surg Clin N Am 1976; **56:** 859.

32. Spiekstra S, Breetveld M, Rustemeyer T, Scheper R, and Gibbs S: Wound-healing factors secreted by epidermal keratinocytes and dermal fibroblasts in skin substitutes. Wound Repair Regen 2007; **15:** 708.

33. Shealy F and DeLoach E: Complicated surgical and nonsurgical wounds in a private practice setting. Adv Skin Wound Care 2006; **19:** 310.

34. Brem H, Tomic-Canic M, Tarnovskaya A, Ehrlich HP, Baskin-Bey E, Gill K, Carasa M, Weinberger S, Entero H, and Vladeck B. Healing of elderly patients with diabetic foot ulcers, venous stasis ulcers, and pressure ulcers. Surg Technol Int 2003; **11:** 161.

35. Zaulyanov L and Kirsner R: A review of a bilayered living cell treatment (Apligraf®) in the treatment of venous leg ulcers and diabetic foot ulcers. Clin Interv Aging 2007; **2:** 93.

36. Wu Y, Wang J, Scott PG, and Tredget EE: Bone marrow-derived stem cells in wound healing: a review. Wound Repair Regen 2007; **15(Suppl 1):** S18.

37. Robson MC and Barbul A: Guidelines for the best care of chronic wounds. Wound Repair Regen 2006; **14:** 647.

38. Altman AM, Yan Y, Matthias N, Bai X, Rios C, Mathur AB, Song YH, and Alt EU: IFATS collection: human adipose-derived stem cells seeded on a silk fibroin-chitosan scaffold enhance wound repair in a murine soft tissue injury model. Stem Cells 2009; **27:** 250.

39. Stappenbeck TS and Miyoshi H: The role of stromal stem cells in tissue regeneration and wound repair. Science 2009; **324:** 1666.

The Role of Stress in Wound Healing

Loretta Vileikyte[1,2,*] and Matthew Hardman[3]

[1]Cardiovascular Medicine Research Group, School of Clinical and Laboratory Sciences, University of Manchester, Manchester, United Kingdom.
[2]Division of Endocrinology, Diabetes and Metabolism, University of Miami, Miami, Florida.
[3]Faculty of Life Sciences, University of Manchester, Manchester, United Kingdom.

Background: Experimental studies in humans and rodents have demonstrated that stress-induced increases in cortisol levels result in the downregulation of the early inflammatory response leading to delayed acute wound healing.
The Problem: As chronic wounds are fundamentally different from acute wounds, available information on the effects of stress on acute wound healing may not be directly relevant to chronic ulcers and hence the need for studies that examine the ways by which stress affects chronic wound healing.
Basic/Clinical Science Advances: The hypothalamic–pituitary–adrenal and sympathetic–adrenal–medullary axes play the principal role in mediating the effects of stress on wound healing through hormones such as cortisol and epinephrine. A common theme in the effects of stress on delayed wound healing is immunomodulation. Several studies demonstrated that clinically significant depressive symptoms affect the healing of chronic wounds including diabetic and venous ulcers, though the potential endocrine immunologic mediators are yet to be explored.
Clinical Care Relevance: An increasing number of chronic nonhealing wounds in the elderly population represent a major drain on the global Health Services, associated with severe morbidity and high mortality rates. It is therefore possible that the alleviating patient stress may have a significant impact on this important area of unmet clinical need.
Conclusion: Although a variety of stress paradigms, wounding techniques, and methods of healing assessment make the interpretation of findings somewhat problematic, evidence suggests that stress impedes the healing of acute wounds. An understanding of the ways by which stress impacts chronic wound repair represents "area de rigueur" in wound research and care.

Abbreviations and Acronyms

HPA = hypothalamic–pituitary–adrenal

IL-1 = interleukin-1

*Correspondence: Manchester Diabetes Center, 193 Hathersage Road, Manchester M13 0JE, United Kingdom (e-mail: lvileikyte@med.miami.edu).

BACKGROUND

Folk wisdom has long suggested that stressful events take a toll on health, and numerous studies have now confirmed that the stress-induced disruption of the neuroendocrine immune equilibrium is detrimental to health.[1] Stress can provoke increases in proinflammatory cytokines that are associated with a variety of diseases, such as cardiovascular disease[2] and both type 1 and type 2 diabetes.[3,4] Moreover, several studies have provided convincing evidence linking stress-induced immune dysregulation with increased mortality.[5] Although the exact pathways linking stress to health outcomes have not yet been mapped, several plausible mechanisms have been identified. Stressors place demands on the body which are met by the activation of the hypothalamic–pituitary–adrenal (HPA) and the sympathetic–adrenal–medullary axes, leading to the upregulation of key stress hormones, cortisol, and

Printed in U.S.A.
DOI: 10.1089/awc.2009.0120

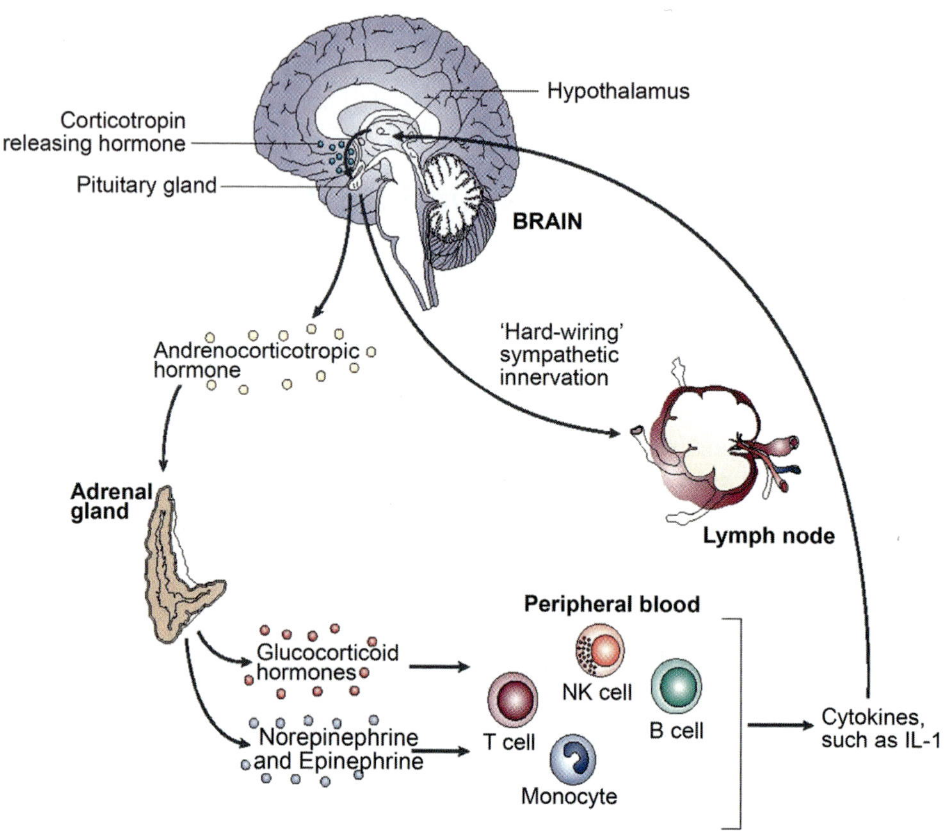

Fig. 1. Stress-induced neuroendocrine modulation of the immune system (adapted from Fig. 1 in Ref. 1). The two main components of the physiologic stress response are the hypothalamic–pituitary–adrenal (HPA) and the sympathetic–adrenal–medullary axes. The hypothalamus via hypophyseal portal system influences pituitary hormone release. The principal hypothalamic stimulus to HPA axis, corticotrophin-releasing hormone, stimulates release of adrenocorticotrophic hormone which then circulates in the bloodstream to the adrenal glands where it induces the production of glucocorticoids. The sympathetic–adrenal–medullary axis can be activated by stimulation of the adrenal medulla to produce the catecholamines, epinephrine and norepinephrine, as well as by hard-wiring, through sympathetic nervous system innervation of the organs of the immune system. Immune cells have receptors for stress hormones and immune modulation by these hormones might proceed either directly, through binding of the hormone to its receptor, or indirectly—by inducing dysregulation of cytokine production. The interactions between the central nervous and immune systems are bidirectional, in that cytokines can modulate the activity of the hypothalamus, influencing the production of corticotrophin-releasing hormone, which, in turn, can affect the HPA axis, resulting in dysregulation of the immune function.

epinephrine (physiologic stress response).[6] The skin itself has recently been shown to contain a stress response system analogous to the systemic HPA axis, centered around the hair follicle and able to synthesize cortisol.[7] In addition to their direct effects on endocrine and immune function, stressors can influence health indirectly, that is, by inducing negative emotional states (psychological stress response). Both anxiety and depression can substantially boost cortisol levels, and increases in the cortisol levels can provoke multiple immunologic changes.[8] Further, stress can impact health by triggering immunomodulatory behaviors, such as poorer sleep patterns, poorer nutrition, less exercising, and alcohol abuse.[9] Opposing the deleterious effects of stress are the beneficial effects of supportive social environment. Studies demonstrated that oxytocin, a neuropeptide known for promoting social behavior, is one of the links between positive social interactions and suppression of the HPA axis.[10] In view of the relative paucity of studies examining the effects of stress on chronic wounds, this chapter provides a critical overview of the experimental studies investigating the influence of stress on the acute wound healing and discusses how these findings could contribute to the development of a stress chronic wounds model (Fig. 1).

CLINICAL PROBLEM ADDRESSED

In a clinical setting, wounds to the skin or other external epithelia arise from a variety of causes, such as surgery, trauma, or burns. To repair this damage, an innate cutaneous wound healing response is invoked, a complex process defined by numerous overlapping stages: hemostasis (clotting), inflammation, proliferation and migration (including reepithelialization), and matrix remodeling. Under normal conditions these events lead to rapid and efficient restoration of tissue integrity and function (acute wound healing). However, a multitude of factors can detrimentally influence the efficiency with which a wound heals, such as older age or diabetes. If this delay is pronounced, the wound could transit into a chronic nonhealing state. In the case of diabetes, for example, evidence implicates that continued pressure on plantar neuropathic foot lesions is a major cause of ulcer chronicity.[11] Histologic examination of specimens from ulcers of patients receiving offloading before debridement indicated improved healing (angiogenesis and granulation tissue formation), as compared with a predominance of inflammatory elements in specimens from patients who did not receive offloading.[11] This suggests one possible path by which stress might contribute to the chronicity of such ulcers, that is, through nonadherence to prescribed offloading, as it is well established that distressed individuals are less likely to follow treatment recommendations.[12] The underlying molecular and cellular changes that result in the persistence of a chronic wound, and the role that stress plays in the pathology, are yet to be fully elucidated. Delayed acute wound healing and an increasing number of chronic nonhealing wounds in an ever expanding elderly population represent a major drain on the global Health Services, associated with severe morbidity and high mortality rates. It is therefore possible that the alleviating patient stress may have a significant impact on this important area of unmet clinical need.

RELEVANT BASIC SCIENCE CONTEXT

Emerging evidence highlights the importance of glucocorticoid upregulation in wound healing. It has been shown, for example, that increased levels of circulating glucocorticoids can downregulate local tissue levels of insulin-like growth factor-1 and lead to impaired fibroblast function.[13] Glucocorticoids may also influence the major leukocyte cell types involved in acute and chronic wound healing (macrophages and neutrophils), leading to alternatively activated macrophages and increased proinflammatory cytokine production.[14] In addition, glucocorticoids can impact angiogenesis by inhibiting vascular endothelial growth factor expression and can impair matrix deposition by downregulating transforming growth factor-β receptor levels.[15,16] Further, glucocorticoid responses are influenced by the local cytokine environment at sites of inflammation, such that changes in the glucocorticoid receptor expression and function may result in local cortisone resistance and susceptibility to tissue damage mediated by proinflammatory cytokines.[17] Bearing in mind the importance of glucocorticoids in wound healing and their pivotal role in the physiologic stress response, it was therefore expected that the upregulation of stress-induced glucocorticoid would modulate the healing of a variety of wounds. Indeed, both murine and human studies have demonstrated that stress-induced downregulation of the early inflammatory response by an increase in the cortisol levels results in delayed wound repair.[18] More recent studies have identified an additional wound healing modulator, the stress-induced hormone epinephrine. In mouse and human skin, high local epinephrine levels were demonstrated to inhibit keratinocyte migration.[19]

EXPERIMENTAL MODELS OR MATERIAL—ADVANTAGES AND LIMITATIONS

The impact of stress on wound healing has been studied almost exclusively in acute, experimentally induced wounds. The diversity of experimental models used, including among others punch biopsy wounds, mucosal wounds, suction blister wounds, and tape-stripping barrier disruption, severely complicates comparative analysis. Outcome measures also vary widely between studies, with wound healing quantified histologically, planimetrically, or even indirectly, by measuring the inflammatory biomarkers. Although histological analysis is the “gold standard,” the majority of studies have used planimetric measurements that are limited to assessing only a single aspect of the healing process (reepithelialization), often giving an inaccurate indication of acute wound healing. As a result, despite burgeoning research in stress and acute wound healing, existent methodological problems limit the potentially important role of these reports in guiding the design of studies in chronic wounds. Moreover, it is important to note that chronic wounds are fundamentally different entities from acute wounds. Specifically, chronic wounds are characterized by an unresolved inflammatory response, markedly delayed reepithelialization, and increased proteolysis.[20] An excessive inflammatory response contributes to increased levels of matrix metalloproteases, leading to a switch from tissue synthesis to matrix degradation with downstream impaired wound healing.[21] Matrix metalloprotease-9, for example, which is known to be upregulated in chronic wounds,[21] was found to be reduced in acute post-surgical wounds as a result of stress.[22] Therefore, the available information on the effects of stress on acute wound healing may not be directly relevant to chronic ulcers and hence the need for studies that examine the ways by which stress affects chronic wound healing. In contrast to the experimental research, conducted in a controlled laboratory setting, the design of studies in chronic wounds occurring in "real life" is fraught with difficulties. First, such studies have to be adequately powered to account for a myriad of potential confounders. In the case of diabetic foot ulcers, for example, in addition to well-established factors impeding wound healing, such as the presence of peripheral arterial disease and hyperglycemia, it is likely that this patient population would suffer from multiple comorbidities (*e.g.*, renal failure) and would be taking multiple medications (*e.g.*, steroids), known to affect wound healing. Second, adequate attention has to be given to the effects of adherence to treatment. The true impact of stress on chronic wound healing through physiologic mediators cannot be determined without accounting more adequately for the role of behavior. This is especially relevant to the study of diabetic foot ulcers, where continued pressure on plantar foot lesions as the result of nonadherence to offloading is a major cause of ulcer chronicity.

TAKE-HOME MESSAGE

Basic science advances

- The HPA and sympathetic–adrenal–medullary axes play the principal role in mediating the effects of stress on wound healing.
- The skin itself has recently been shown to contain a stress response system analogous to the systemic HPA axis.
- Stress-associated hormones, such as cortisol and epinephrine, delay wound healing.
- A common theme in the effects of stress on disease incidence and delayed wound healing is immunomodulation.
- Positive social interactions trigger the release of oxytocin, which alleviates the effects of stress on wound healing through suppression of the HPA axis.
- The wide range of experimental wound healing models used make it difficult to compare findings between studies.
- As chronic wounds are different entities from acute wounds, the mechanisms by which stress affects acute wound healing may not be directly applied to chronic wounds.

Clinical science advances

- The skin is particularly susceptible to the effects of acute and chronic stress.
- Although studies have shown that chronic stress is immunosuppressive, there is evidence to suggest that acute stress can enhance skin immunity.
- Stressors that are perceived as uncontrollable can lead to emotional distress, anxiety, and depression, which may in turn provoke multiple adverse immunologic changes.
- Stress can delay wound healing through nonadherence to prescribed treatment as well as by inducing maladaptive behaviors, such as poorer sleep, dietary habits, alcohol abuse, and smoking.
- Several studies demonstrated that clinically significant depression symptoms affect the healing of diabetic and venous ulcers, though the potential endocrine immunologic mediators have not been explored.

Relevance to clinical care

- The skin is the body's primary immune guard, preventing bacteria, viruses, and other exogenous antigens from entering. As such, the skin's ability to heal wounds effectively is essential to good health. Evidence from recently conducted studies, though somewhat limited by their methodology, indicates that stress negatively impacts acute wound healing. In agreement with laboratory findings, studies have also shown that greater psychological distress before surgery is associated with poorer outcomes, including longer hospitalization, more postoperative complications, and higher rates of rehospitalization. If confirmed by carefully designed studies in chronic wounds, this could potentially have significant implications in the context of such wounds, including diabetic foot ulceration and venous ulcers.

DISCUSSION OF FINDINGS AND RELEVANT LITERATURE

Evidence suggests that the stress-induced impairments in the early inflammatory response may be the origin of a dysregulated cascade of reparative processes that result in delayed wound healing.[1,18] In an early study, punch biopsy wound healing was shown to take 24% longer in women caring for a relative with Alzheimer's disease as compared with the age-matched controls,[23] correlating with a reduced response of peripheral monocytes to lipopolysaccharide stimulation. The same group assessed the effect of academic stress on oral mucosal wound healing.[24] Punch biopsy wounds to the hard palate healed on average 40% more slowly immediately before examinations as compared with summer vacation, correlating with a 70% reduction in wound interleukin (IL)-1β expression.[24] A number of studies have been carried out using a suction blister wound model. In this model, high perceived stress correlates with higher levels of salivary cortisol and lower levels of wound cytokines, such as IL-1α,[25] while subjects with lower anger control also display elevated cortisol and delayed healing.[26] Interestingly, microarray analysis suggests that skin blister-derived neutrophils from males subject to examination stress have a suppressed transcriptome compared with blister neutrophils from nonstressed individuals.[27] Following routine surgery, subjects with high perceived stress display an impaired wound inflammatory response, greater postsurgical pain, and delayed healing.[22,28]

Studies in rodents, using restraint as a reproducible stressor, have begun to reveal the mechanisms by which stress impacts wound healing, with defects noted in both inflammatory cell and fibroblast function. Delayed wound healing in mice exposed to restraint stress correlates with altered wound-specific expression of IL-1 and keratinocyte growth factor-1[29] and an increased incidence of opportunistic infection.[30] Overall healing is delayed in restrained mice correlating with a fourfold increase in serum corticosterone, which is functionally relevant, as blocking glucocorticoid receptor in restrained animals abolishes this delayed wound healing.[31] Further, latest studies indicate that stress also induces substantial hypoxia in the wound, thereby proposing an additional path by which stress may affect healing. In support of this hypothesis, restraint-stressed mice exposed to hyperbaric oxygen therapy twice daily healed at a rate nearly equal to unstressed mice.[32]

In contrast to the negative impact of stress on healing, social support plays a positive role on wound healing, and this effect was found to be in part mediated by oxytocin.[33,34] Detillion *et al.* demonstrated that treatment with oxytocin of Siberian hamsters, exposed to immobilization stress, blocked stress-induced increases in cortisol concentrations and facilitated wound healing.[33] In a rat burn injury model, exogenous oxytocin was also protective against tissue damage.[34] Personality traits can also buffer against the negative effects of stress on wound healing. In a study of healthy male adults, the "fast" wound healing group displayed higher dispositional optimism than the "slow" healing group.[35]

In contrast to acute wound studies, little is known about the effects of stress on healing of chronic wounds. To date, a single study has shown that clinically significant anxiety and depression adversely affect the healing of chronic venous ulcers.[36] A diabetic foot ulcer provides an excellent model for studying the effects of emotional distress on chronic wound healing, as increasing evidence suggests that neuropathy, a key risk factor for foot ulceration,[37] is also associated with an increased risk for depression.[38] A recent investigation of elderly diabetic patients showed that study participants with scores ≥ 10 on the geriatric depression scale had a significantly higher risk of not healing at 6 months as compared with those patients without clinically significant depressive symptoms, though the potential endocrine or immune modulators of the delayed healing were not explored.[39]

CAUTION, CRITICAL REMARKS, AND RECOMMENDATIONS

At present, the role of stress in modulating the chronic wound healing response is far from clear. Although numerous studies have been carried out to investigate the effects of stress on acute wound healing, the interpretation of findings has proved problematic. This is primarily due to poorly defined outcome measures, incomplete, or inaccurate measurement of wound healing. The few studies that have been carefully designed and analyzed do suggest that stress has a detrimental effect on the healing response. However, the molecular and cellular changes that are mediating these effects largely remain to be elucidated.

FUTURE DEVELOPMENTS

An understanding of the mechanisms by which stress affects chronic wound healing is in its infancy. Two published reports that examined the impact of depression on healing of venous and diabetic foot ulcers demonstrated that clinically significant depressive symptoms impede wound healing. However, the potential mechanisms by which depression and/or stress affects chronic ulcer healing were not explored. Our research group is conducting a National Institutes for Health–funded study that aims to examine two relatively independent pathways by which stress and associated negative affects are expected to delay the healing of diabetic foot ulcers. These include the physiologic path, through cortisol upregulation, and the behavioral path, through nonadherence to ulcer offloading. Foot ulcer healing rates are assessed using both planimetry and wound histology. Wound biopsies are being assayed histologically and immunocytochemically to determine precise markers of wound healing, such as deposition of extracellular matrix molecules, basement membrane formation, and the quantity and quality of the inflammatory response. The potential moderating role of social support and dispositional optimism is also being examined. The results from this study will allow the targeting of specific markers that may predict failure to heal diabetic foot ulcers and will therefore facilitate the tailoring of specific treatment and psychosocial behavioral interventions to the individual. Our data will provide an important insight into the cellular and molecular mechanisms underlying chronic impaired healing in patients with diabetes and why specific ulcers at the molecular level heal and others do not. Moreover, although not relevant to acute wounds, the results of our study may well be relevant to other chronic wounds such as venous ulcers.

ACKNOWLEDGMENT

Loretta Vileikyte is supported in part by an NIH/NIDDK grant 1R01 DK71066-01A2.

AUTHOR DISCLOSURE STATEMENT

No conflict of interest disclosed.

REFERENCES

1. Glaser R and Kiecolt-Glaser J: Stress-induced immune dysfunction: implications for health. Nat Rev Immunol 2005; **5:** 243.
2. Ridker PM, Rifai N, Stampfer MJ, and Hennekens CH: Plasma concentration of interleukin-6 and the risk of future myocardial infarction among apparently healthy men. Circulation 2000; **101:** 1767.
3. Falcone M and Sarvetnick N: The effect of local production of cytokines in the pathogenesis of insulin-dependent diabetes mellitus. Clin Immunol 1999; **90:** 2.
4. Pradhan AD, Manson JE, and Rifai N: C-reactive protein, interleukin 6, and risk of developing type 2 diabetes mellitus. JAMA 2001; **18:** 327.
5. Kiecolt-Glaser JK and Glaser R: Depression and immune function: central pathways to morbidity and mortality. J Psychosom Res 2002; **53:** 873.
6. Miller DB and O'Callaghan JP: Neuroendocrine aspects of the response to stress. Metabolism 2002; **51:** 5.
7. Ito N, Ito T, Kromminga A, Bettermann A, Takigawa M, Kees F, Straub RH, and Paus R: Human hair follicles display a functional equivalent of the hypothalamic-pituitary-adrenal axis and synthesize cortisol. FASEB J 2005; **19:** 1332.
8. Sherwood Brown E, Varghese FP, and McEwen BS: Association of depression with medical illness: does cortisol play a role? Biol Psychiatry 2004; **55:** 1.
9. Baum A and Posluszny DM: Health psychology: mapping biobehavioral contributions to health and illness. Annu Rev Psychol 1999; **50:** 137.
10. DeVries AC, Glasper ER, and Detillion CE: Social modulation of stress responses. Physiol Behav 2003; **79:** 399.
11. Piaggesi A, Viacava P, Rizzo L, Naccarato G, Baccetti F, Romanelli M, Zampa V, and Del Prato S: Semi-quantitative histological analysis of the histopathological features of the neuropathic foot ulcer-effects of pressure relief. Diabetes Care 2003; **26:** 3123.
12. DiMatteo MR, Lepper HS, and Croghan TW: Depression is a risk factor for non-compliance with medical treatment: meta-analysis of the effects of anxiety and depression on patient adherence. Arch Intern Med 2000; **160:** 2101.
13. Bitar MS: Insulin and glucocorticoid-dependent suppression of the IGF-I system in diabetic wounds. Surgery 2000; **127:** 687.
14. Song E, Ouyang N, Hörbelt M, Antus B, Wang M, and Exton MS: Influence of alternatively and classically activated macrophages on fibrogenic activities of human fibroblasts. Cell Immunol 2000; **204:** 19.
15. Roy SK: Regulation of transforming growth factor-beta-receptor type I and type II messenger ribonucleic acid expression in the hamster ovary by gonadotropins and steroid hormones. Biol Reprod 2000; **62:** 1858.
16. Nauck M, Karakiulakis G, Perruchoud AP, Papakonstantinou E, and Roth M: Corticosteroids inhibit the expression of the vascular endothelial growth factor gene in human vascular smooth muscle cells. Eur J Pharmacol 1998; **341:** 309.
17. Rook G, Baker R, Walker B, Honour J, Jessop D, Hernandez-Pando R, Arriaga K, Shaw R, Zumla A, and Lightman S: Local regulation of glucocorticoid activity in sites of inflammation. Insights from the study of tuberculosis. Ann NY Acad Sci 2000; **917:** 913.
18. Vileikyte L: Stress and wound healing. Clin Derm 2007; **25:** 49.
19. Sivamani RK, Pullar CE, Manabat-Hidalgo CG, Rocke DM, Carlsen RC, Greenhalgh DG, and Isseroff RR: Stress-mediated increases in systemic and local epinephrine impair skin wound healing: potential new indication for beta blockers. PLoS Med 2009; **6:** e12.
20. Falanga V: Wound healing and chronic wounds. J Cutan Med Surg 1998; **3:** 1.
21. Lobmann R, Ambrosch A, Schultz G, Waldmann K, Schiweck S, and Lehnert H: Expression of matrix metalloproteinses and their inhibitors in the wounds of diabetic and non-diabetic patients. Diabetologia 2002; **45:** 1011.
22. Broadbent E, Petrie KJ, Alley PG, and Booth RJ: Psychological stress impairs early wound repair following surgery. Psychosom Med 2003; **65:** 865.
23. Kiecolt-Glaser JK, Marucha PT, Malarkey WB, Mercado AM, and Glaser R: Slowing of wound healing by psychological stress. Lancet 1995; **346:** 1194.
24. Marucha PT, Kiecolt-Glaser JK, and Favagehi M: Mucosal wound healing is impaired by examination stress. Psychosom Med 1998; **60:** 362.
25. Glaser R, Kiecolt-Glaser JK, Marucha PT, MacCallum RC, Laskowski BF, and Malarkey WB: Stress-related changes in proinflammatory cytokine production in wounds. Arch Gen Psychiatry 1999; **56:** 450.
26. Gouin JP, Kiecolt-Glaser JK, Malarkey WB, and Glaser R: The influence of anger expression on wound healing. Brain Behav Immun 2008; **22:** 699.
27. Roy S, Khanna S, Yeh PE, Rink C, Malarkey WB, Kiecolt-Glaser J, Laskowski B, Glaser R, and Sen CK: Wound site neutrophil transcriptome in response to psychological stress in young men. Gene Expr 2005; **12:** 273.
28. McGuire L, Heffner K, Glaser R, Needleman B, Malarkey W, Dickinson S, Lemeshow S, Cook C, Muscarella P, Melvin WS, Ellison EC, and Kiecolt-Glaser JK: Pain and wound healing in surgical patients. Ann Behav Med 2006; **31:** 165.
29. Mercado AM, Quan N, Padgett DA, Sheridan JF, and Marucha PT: Restraint stress alters the expression of interleukin-1 and keratinocyte growth factor at the wound site: an *in situ* hybridization study. J Neuroimmunol 2002; **129:** 74.
30. Rojas I-G, Padgett DA, Sheridan JF, and Marucha PT: Stress-induced susceptibility to bacterial infection during cutaneous wound healing. Brain Behav Immunol 2002; **16:** 74.
31. Padgett DA, Marucha PT, and Sheridan JF: Restraint stress slows cutaneous wound healing in mice. Brain Behav Immunol 1998; **12:** 64.
32. Gajendrareddy PK, Sen CK, Horan MP, and Marucha PT: Hyperbaric oxygen therapy ameliorates stress-impaired dermal wound healing. Brain Behav Immunol 2005; **19:** 217.
33. Detillion CE, Craft TK, Glasper ER, Prendergast BJ, and DeVries AC: Social facilitation of wound healing. Psychoneuroendocrinology 2004; **29:** 1004.

34. Işeri SO, Gedik IE, Erzik C, Uslu B, Arbak S, Gedik N, and Yeğen BC: Oxytocin ameliorates skin damage and oxidant gastric injury in rats with thermal trauma. Burns 2008; **34:** 361.

35. Ebrecht M, Hextall J, Kirtley LG, Taylor A, Dyson M, and Weinman J: Perceived stress and cortisol levels predict speed of wound healing in healthy male adults. Psychoneuroendocrinology 2004; **29:** 798.

36. Cole-King A and Harding KG: Psychological factors and delayed healing in chronic wounds. Psychosom Med 2001; **63:** 216.

37. Boulton AJM, Kirsner RS, and Vileikyte L: Neuropathic diabetic foot ulcers. N Eng J Med 2004; **351:** 48.

38. Vileikyte L, Peyrot M, Gonzalez JS, Rubin RR, Garrow AB, Waterman C, Ulbrecht JS, Cavanagh PR, and Boulton JM: Predictors of depressive symptoms in persons with diabetic peripheral neuropathy: a longitudinal study. Diabetologia 2009; **52:** 1265.

39. Monami M, Longo R, Desideri CM, Masotti G, Marchionni N, and Mannucci E: The diabetic person without a foot ulcer: healing, recurrence and depressive symptoms. JAPMA 2008; **98:** 130.

Novel Mechanisms on the Pathophysiology of Venous Ulcers

Barbara Pieper,[1,*] Robert S. Kirsner,[2] and Thomas N. Templin[1]

[1]College of Nursing, Wayne State University, Detroit, Michigan.
[2]Department of Dermatology & Cutaneous Surgery, University of Miami Miller School of Medicine, Miami, Florida.

Abbreviations and Acronyms

CVD = chronic venous disorders

DVT = deep vein thrombosis

*Correspondence: College of Nursing, Wayne State University, 5557 Cass Ave., Detroit, Michigan 48202 (e-mail: bpieper@wayne.edu).

Background: Venous ulcers are a manifestation of chronic venous disorders (CVD). Superficial venous reflux and deep vein obstruction are the most common cause of CVD.

The Problem: Venous ulcers are associated with pain and decreased dorsiflexion. Walking intensity is lower, standing reduced, and sitting is often prolonged. Either initiating advanced venous disease or, as a result, gait abnormalities are present. Peripheral neuropathies may be a cofactor in the development of venous ulcers.

Basic/Clinical Science Advances: Recent advances include research on venous surgeries to decrease symptoms and aid ulcer healing; medications to decrease inflammation of venous disease; development of a symptoms diagnostic score; examination of CVD manifestations such as hemosiderin and telangiectasia; neuropathy with CVD; and renewed importance of arterial, nutrition, and psychological assessment. Persons who injected illicit drugs may serve as a model to study CVD/venous ulcers. Injection drug use intensifies typical CVD risk factors from vascular, nerve, and muscle damage from injecting and infections, unknown substances in the injected mixture, trauma, and deep vein thrombosis. Leg injecting has a direct effect on CVD and an indirect effect on ankle and walking mobility through CVD.

Clinical Care Relevance: Treatment is aimed at preventing venous hypertension and reflux, decreasing inflammation to alleviate symptoms, reducing risk of ulceration, reducing pain, and enhancing quality of life. This includes programs of activity/exercises, appropriate wound dressing, venous surgery, pain management, arterial flow assessment, and psychosocial assessment.

Conclusion: Venous disease is associated with many physical and psychosocial problems. Continued medical, surgical, and basic research holds promise for the best strategies for providing care.

BACKGROUND

Venous ulcers, active or healed, affect about 1% of the general population and are a manifestation of chronic venous disorders (CVD).[1] Ulcers typically occur in the medial malleolar region of the lower leg; they can be anywhere below the knee, but never on the plantar aspect of the foot. Risk factors for CVD include deep vein thrombosis (DVT), heredity, age, obesity, prolonged standing, pregnancy, lower extremity injection drug use, and greater height.[1–3] While not apparently causal, venous ulcers also occur with diabetes mellitus, lymphedema, and rheumatoid arthritis.

Superficial venous reflux and deep vein obstruction are the most common causes of CVD. Superficial venous reflux results from dysfunctional valves in the superficial or communicating veins that permit the high

ADVANCES IN WOUND CARE, VOLUME 1

Printed in U.S.A.
DOI: 10.1089/awc.2009.0001

pressure generated in the deep venous system during calf pump contraction to be transmitted to the superficial system (venous hypertension). Superficial venous reflux is present alone in 45% of venous leg ulcers.[2] Comparably, deep vein obstruction is primarily caused by DVT; valvular incompetence from trauma or DVT occurs in CVD about 18% to 20% of the time.[2] Venous hypertension causes distension of the capillary bed and leakage of fluid, red blood cells, and fibrinogen into the surrounding tissue and decreased oxygenation of the tissue. This fluid and cellular leakage leads to some of the manifestations of CVD, namely, edema, discoloration and hardening of the skin, and pain. Initial skin pigmentation changes appear to be melanin, but hemosiderin plays a role in the evolution of skin changes toward lipodermatosclerosis and ulceration.[4]

Apart from and in congruence with the venous system, the calf pump has a critical role in CVD. The calf pump from the contracting muscles of the leg leads to an increased deep vein pressure and emptying of the deep veins in a cephalic direction. There is a delicate interplay between the muscle-joint unit and intact veins and venous valves of the lower leg. Changes to the musculo-neuro-skeletal systems can adversely affect the dynamics of the calf pump.

While the exact pathophysiologic mechanisms that lead from venous disease to venous ulcers are not entirely known, proposed theories include pericapillary fibrin cuff formation leading to poor oxygen and nutrient exchange, trapping of growth factors within this cuff, and white blood cells plugging the capillaries.[1,2,5] Chronic leg inflammation is present in CVD and has been implicated as one of the causative factors leading to complications such as ulceration.[6] Matrix metalloproteinases in lipodermatosclerosis, venous ulcers, and venous ulcer drainage contributed to the breakdown of the extracellular matrix that promoted ulcer formation and impaired healing.[1] Ulcers tend to occur spontaneously (56%) or from trauma (44%); traumatic ulcers heal faster and recur less frequently than spontaneous ulcers.[7]

CLINICAL PROBLEM ADDRESSED

Normal ankle mobility and painless calf muscle movement are required for mobility. Decreased dorsiflexion is present in persons with venous ulceration. We reported dorsiflexion worsened with increasing CVD classes; mean values were about two-thirds of normal and less than that necessary for standing and stair ascent/descent.[8] Inversion values for ankle movement were slightly more than half normal.[8] Inversion during the toe-off phase of gait is necessary for speed needed in commu-

TAKE-HOME MESSAGE

Basic science advances

- Venous hypertension causes distension of the capillary bed and leakage of fluid, red blood cells, and fibrinogen into the surrounding tissue and decreased oxygenation of the tissue.
- Superficial venous reflux and deep vein obstruction can lead to CVD/venous ulcers.
- Inflammation of the leg may be measured with skin temperature. Inflammation is also noted at the cellular and histological level.
- Various antiinflammatory medications/substances have promise in the treatment of CVD inflammation.
- Unrestrained matrix metalloproteinase activity contributed to the breakdown of the extracellular matrix that promoted ulcer formation and impaired healing.
- The microcirculation of the skin of the legs with venous ulcers has anatomically altered capillaries that remain after ulcer closure.
- Tumor necrosis factor alpha was elevated in nonhealing venous ulcers.

Clinical science advances

- How the ulcer developed (spontaneous or trauma) may impact healing time and recurrence.
- An ulcerated leg severity assessment score is being developed for prediction of venous ulcer healing. Score components include patient age, ulcer chronicity, and venous refill time.[29]
- Venous surgery helps close venous ulcers and prevents recurrence. Various procedures are available, but need continued research.
- Decreased dorsiflexion is present in persons with venous ulcers.
- Walking intensity was lower in more severe CVD.
- Decreased heel rise test, decreased balance and gait testing, and slower walk speed were associated with worse CVD.
- Pain is present with venous ulcers and must be treated.
- Peripheral neuropathies occur and may be cofactors in venous ulcer development.
- A decrease in total nerve fibers of the epidermis is present in persons with venous ulcer; epidermal innervation may be important in healing.
- Illicit injection drug use in the groin, legs, and feet is the highest risk factor for venous ulcers as compared to injecting in the arms or noninjecting drug use and must not be ignored.

(continued)

Relevance to clinical care

- The damage from DVT must be prevented as early as possible.
- Leg injuries must be prevented or minimized as much as possible.
- Walking/activity must be encouraged.
- Compression bandages and stockings are cornerstones of venous ulcer care.
- Quality of life, pain, and mental health are critical concerns for persons/families with venous ulcers.
- Due to the chronicity and recurrence of venous ulcers, patient/family teaching is critical.
- Leg/ankle exercises may improve venous hemodynamics of the leg.
- Pentoxifylline was effective with compression bandages in venous ulcer care.
- Home-based exercise, such as with elastic bands, may help patients gain ankle range of motion and reduce pain.

nity mobility; thus, motion needed to generate force for subsequent steps is decreased.[8] Walking intensity was lower in the more severe clinical CVD, and prolonged sitting and reduced standing were associated with increased severity of CVD.[9,10] Older, overweight men with comorbid health conditions had the most restricted range of motion.[8] In contrast, others reported mobility patterns among patients with leg ulcers are not significantly different from age-matched controls.[11] Those with ulcers took fewer steps, but the groups were comparable in time spent standing, walking, and resting.[11] Movement dysfunction can lead to disability; thus, interventions to maintain ankle joint mobility for ambulation and stair use should be addressed.

Peripheral neuropathies may be a cofactor in the development of venous ulcers.[5] Neuropathic changes (*i.e.*, diabetes mellitus not present) include prolongation of distal motor latency, increased limits for warm and cold detection, and reduced vibration sense.[5] Light touch, vibratory sense, and deep tendon reflexes are significantly worse in persons with severe CVD.[5] Thus, sensory neuropathy is a feature of severe CVD and its distribution coincides with trophic changes. For persons with nonhealing ulcers, there may be decreased total nerve fibers of the epidermis and other abnormal fibers. Epidermal innervations may be important in healing. Neuropathic changes impact safety since impaired sensation, balance, and gait may increase the risk of falls and injury. In addition to having subjective and objective signs of neuropathy, patients with venous disease (*i.e.*, diabetes mellitus not present) also demonstrate gait abnormalities.[12] As a result of pain, muscle dysfunction, and changes in mobility and ankle range of motion, nerve involvement may affect calf muscle pump function.[5]

Venous leg ulcers are painful because of chemical, neuropathic, and fluid factors. Pain negatively impacts, mobility, sleep, mood, self-esteem, and quality of life.[3] Common pain descriptors were aching, stabbing, sharp, tender, and tiring. Pain was often stated as the worse symptom of a leg ulcer. Pain decreased and mobility improved when the leg ulcer healed.

RELEVANT BASIC SCIENCE CONTEXT

Venous ulceration begins by a spontaneous or traumatic stimulus that causes activation of the perivascular macrophages resulting in extensive tissue and blood vessel destruction. Leukocytes accumulate in the leg with leukocyte adhesion and migration through the endothelium of small vessels under conditions of high venous pressure.[1] The increased capillary pressure from venous hypertension results in loss of plasma proteins including fibrinogen. Fibrin deposits in venous ulcers are patchy and discontinuous around dermal vessels acting as a physiologic barrier under conditions of poor blood flow and impacting the exchange of oxygen and other nutrients.[13] Anatomically altered capillaries remain unchanged after re-epithelialization of the venous ulcer.

EXPERIMENTAL MODEL OR MATERIAL ADVANTAGES AND LIMITATIONS

Persons who inject illicit drugs may serve as a model to study CVD/venous ulcers; injected drugs intensifies typical CVD risk factors.[3] In methadone treatment, CVD point prevalence was 87%; 36% had healed or active ulcers.[3] They experience vascular, nerve, and muscle damage from injections and infections, substances mixed with the injected drug, trauma, and DVT. Injecting illicit drugs often begins in early adulthood; thus, venous ulcers occur in the person's 30s and 40s.[3]

We postulated that injection drug use, ankle mobility, general mobility, and pain impacted CVD. Years of injecting drugs were related to CVD when the injections were in the groin, legs, and feet.[3] In a study examining CVD in persons positive for human immunodeficiency virus, persons who injected illicit drugs had significantly more advanced CVD and worse ankle mobility than those who had not injected drugs.[14] In a study of venous disease in those in drug treatment, arm injectors were nine times more likely to have venous ulcers and leg and upper body injectors were 35 times more likely than persons who never injected drugs.[15] Ulcer size was related to greater current pain, worst pain in 24 h and higher pain intensity for injection users.[3]

For persons who injected illicit drugs, worsening CVD resulted in mobility restrictions.[8] The heel rise test as a measure of ankle mobility had the lowest performance in persons with venous ulcers.[16] Advanced CVD was associated with worse balance and gait, slower walk speed, and poorer composite score of walking, standing, stair ascent/descent, and working.[10] The calf muscles waste and weaken with disuse.

Persons who injected illicit drugs reported information accurately and were willing to participate in research.[17] Research challenges include developing a trusting relationship within the drug-use community, perceived bias in working with them, and under-recognized presence of CVD in this population.

DISCUSSION OF FINDINGS AND RELEVANT LITERATURE

The sequences of events that occur during the development and progression of venous disease have not been ascertained, but themes are disturbed venous flow and chronic inflammation (Fig. 1).[1,2] Triggers for ulceration include cellulitis, penetrating injury, contact dermatitis, rapidly aggravating leg edema, dry skin with scratching, insect

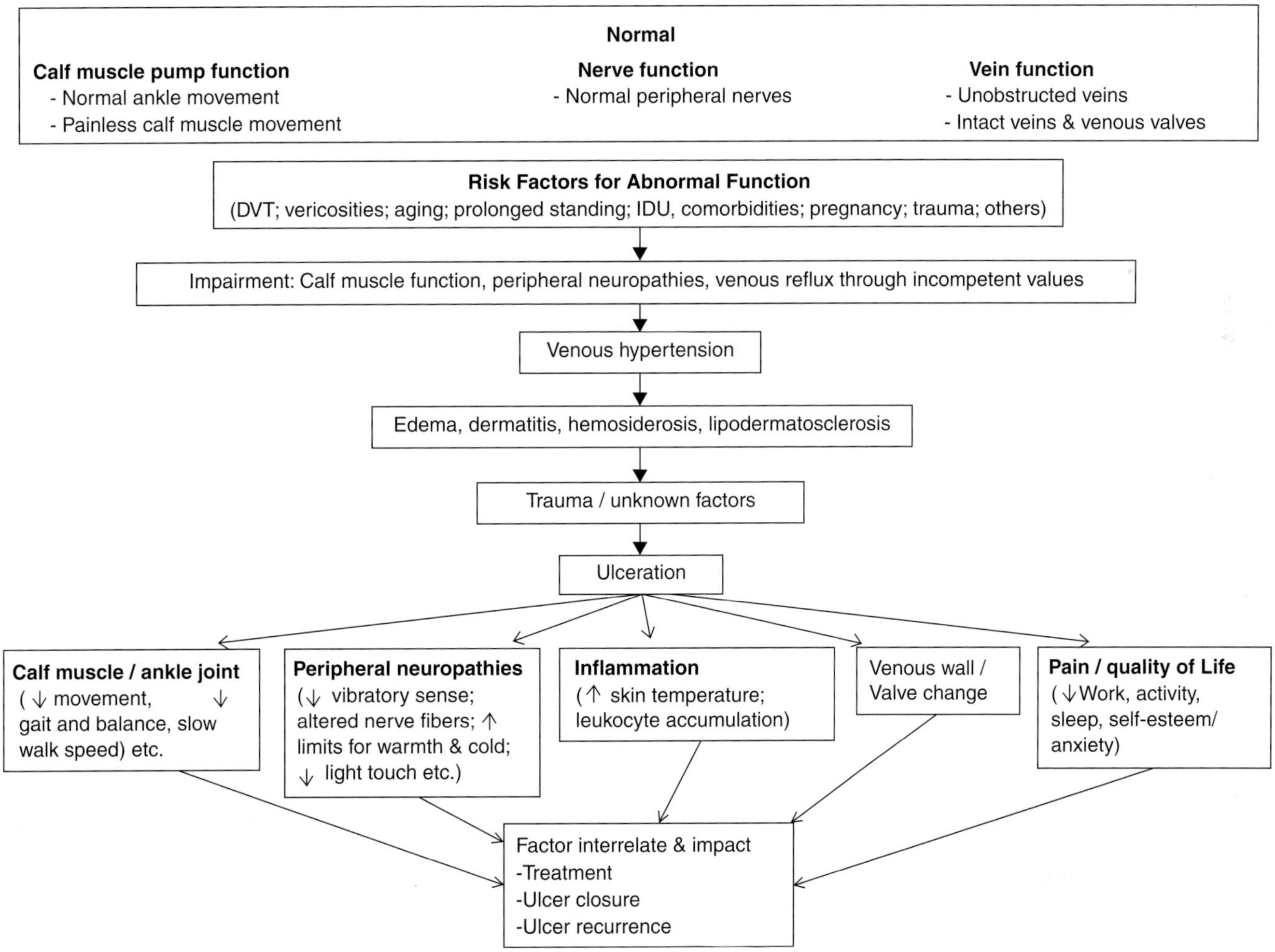

Figure 1. This diagram, modified from that proposed by Shiman and colleagues,[5] highlights normal, risk factors, abnormalities, and their effect on venous ulcers. Factors theorized as leading to venous ulcers also are impacted by the ulcer. Venous ulceration factors interrelate and impact care and wound closure.

bite, and bleeding from a superficial varicose vein. The cause–effect relationship between venous ulceration and physical activity remains unknown. The relationship may be reciprocal, with advancing disease reducing calf pump function and reduced calf pump function leading to increased venous hypertension.

Needless to say, physical activity research about CVD/venous ulcers is needed; patients should be encouraged to remain active. Although persons with advanced CVD have the lowest step continuous walking amplitude, they performed necessary activities at a slower pace.[9] Using elastic resistance bands, patients with venous ulcers achieved a gain in ankle range of motion and reduced pain.[18] The impact of neuropathies on activity and venous ulcer healing needs to be explored.

Treatment is aimed at preventing venous hypertension and reflux, decreasing inflammation to alleviate symptoms, and reducing risk of ulceration.[1] A high incidence and morbidity of postthrombotic syndrome occur after anticoagulation protocols. New strategies must focus on early and complete lysis of the thrombus load after DVT. Measurement and monitoring of skin temperature can augment clinical findings and guide treatment when localized inflammation is suspected.[6] Little is known about cooling the skin to decrease inflammation and prevent ulcers.[6] Medications to inhibit inflammation may be helpful.[1] Pentoxifylline, which helps blood flow and reduces inflammation, was found to be an effective adjunct to compression dressing for treating venous ulcers.[19] Although two substances with antiinflammatory properties (micronized purified flavonoid fraction and sulodexide) may have efficacy for CVD, they are not available in the United States and need further study.[20,21] The routine use of systemic antibiotics to promote healing of venous leg ulcers is not supported; antibiotics should be used for defined infection and not for bacterial colonization.[22] Adequate nutrition is critical since persons with venous ulcers were reported to have protein deficiency.[23] Arterial blood flow should be assessed in persons with venous ulcers. Increases in arterial inflow during a hyperemic limb challenge were less robust in patients with postthrombotic venous disease than normal volunteers and may be part of the pain experience present in venous disease.[24] Compression stockings improve venous hemodynamics and reduce edema and skin discoloration.[1,2] People wearing high rather than moderate compression stocking were less likely to develop a new venous ulcer, but moderate rather than high compression was more likely to be worn. Intermittent pneumatic compression helps ulcer healing when compared with no compression; it is unclear if it increases healing when added to compression bandages.

Venous surgery that prevents venous reflux is thought to aid venous ulcer healing and prevent recurrence.[1,2] Subfascial endoscopic perforator surgery combined with superficial venous surgery leads to a low recurrence rate of venous ulcers.[25] Endovascular laser ablation combined with high ligation was reported to be safe and effective with clinical-etiology-anatomic-pathophysiologic II–IV, but long-term results warrant further research.[26] Endovascular laser ablation was associated with faster ulcer healing and decreased ulcer recurrence.[27] Recent small trials suggest that vein ablation might be a preferred alternative, based on invasiveness and efficacy compared with subfascial endoscopic perforator surgery.[27] Bilayered living skin equivalent used with compression bandaging increased the chance of healing a venous ulcer compared with compression and a simple dressing.[2]

Venous ulcers impact quality of life in terms of body image, lifestyle, pain, itch, physical functioning and mobility, finding appropriate footwear, negative emotional reactions, and social isolation. Pain of venous leg ulcerations impacted sleep, movement, mood, and quality of life. Persons with venous leg ulcers tended to use analgesia for pain and reported it effective. Depression and anxiety, low self-esteem, and loss of self-control may occur; mental health counseling may be beneficial. A diagnostic score for CVD based on leg symptoms (*i.e.*, leg heaviness, itch, and phlebalgia; effect of environmental temperature and walking) is being developed.[28] The level of venous ulcer knowledge was related to coping; patients need to understand the chronicity of CVD/venous ulcers, interventions for care, dealing with the health care system, and handling personal self-care and emotional reactions.

In summary, venous ulcer research has included numerous designs and methods of data collection. Experimental studies have included control groups of persons without venous disease or comparisons of affected and unaffected legs. Tissue, cells, and wound fluid have been examined. Venous vascular studies, extremity temperature, effect of various venous surgeries, goniometry for ankle mobility, mobility tests such as the Tinetti gait and balance, walk speed, treadmill walking, and pedometer measurements have been explored. Research is needed to further understand the cause and treatment of venous ulcers.

CAUTION, CRITICAL REMARKS, AND RECOMMENDATIONS

Although occurring since ancient times, venous ulcers continue to negatively affect patients/families. Venous vascular studies and laboratory studies of venous ulcer tissue, cells, and fluid have aided in understanding the venous system, the ulcer, and the wound healing environment. Much remains to be learned. Ankle joint and physical activity are less in persons with venous ulcers, but how this lack of movement is related to venous ulcer occurrence is not known. Do more active people have fewer venous ulcers? Is wound healing enhanced with activity? Heinen and colleagues[30] found only 36% (9/25) of their subjects with CVD reported recommended levels of moderately strenuous physical activity defined as 30 min a day on at least 5 days per week. Although inflammation is part of the theory of CVD, the clinical impact of lowering this inflammation is not understood. Venous ulcers occur most commonly in the elderly, but researchers need to acknowledge and study other groups such as those who injected illicit drugs. Treatment of venous ulcers, surgical and medical, needs further study, especially long-term follow-up.

FUTURE DEVELOPMENT

Future research should continue to examine the cellular, microbiologic, and immunologic nature of venous ulcers as well as ankle joint movement and neuropathies for understanding venous ulcer development, treatment, and closure. Human models of venous disease exist, including persons who injected illicit drugs. As persons who injected drugs age, a greater understanding is needed of the effect of illicit drugs and cigarette use on the legs. Besides medications and surgery, physical activity protocols need to be developed.

AUTHOR DISCLOSURE STATEMENT

The authors have no disclosures to declare.

REFERENCES

1. Bergan JJ, Schmid-Schonbein GW, Coleridge Smith PD, Nicolaides AN, Boisseau MR, and Eklof B: Chronic venous disease. N Engl J Med 2006; **355:** 488.
2. de Araujo T, Valencia I, Federman DG, and Kirsner RS: Managing the patient with venous ulcers. Ann Intern Med 2003; **138:** 326.
3. Pieper B, Kirsner RS, Templin TN, and Birk TJ: Injection drug use—an understudied cause of venous disease. Arch Dermatol 2007; **143:** 1305.
4. Caggiati A, Rosi C, Franceschini M, and Innocenzi D: The nature of skin pigmentations in chronic venous insufficiency: a preliminary report. Eur J Endovasc Surg 2008; **35:** 111.
5. Shiman MI, Pieper B, Templin TN, Birk TJ, Patel AR, and Kirsner RS: Venous ulcers: a reappraisal. Analyzing the effects of neuropathy, muscle involvement, and range of motion upon gait and calf muscle function. Wound Repair Regen 2009; **17:** 149.
6. Kelechi TJ and Michel Y: A descriptive study of skin temperature, tissue perfusion, and tissue oxygen in patients with chronic venous disease. Biol Res Nurs 2007; **9:** 70.
7. Kullkarni SR, Gohel MS, Whyman MR, and Poskitt KR: Significance of limb trauma as an initiating factor in chronic leg ulceration. Phlebology 2008; **23:** 130.
8. Pieper B, Templin TN, Birk TJ, and Kirsner RS: Effects of injection-drug injury on ankle mobility and chronic venous disorders. J Nurs Sch 2007; **39:** 312.
9. Eifell RK, Ashour HY, Heslop PS, Walker DJ, and Lees TA: Association of 24-hour activity levels with the clinical severity of chronic venous disease. J Vasc Surg 2006; **44:** 580.
10. Pieper B, Templin TN, Birk TJ, and Kirsner RS: Chronic venous disorders and injection. Drug use: impact on balance, gait, and walk speed. J Wound Ostomy Continence Nurs 2008; **35:** 301.
11. Clarke-Moloney M, Godfrey A, O'Connor V, Meagher H, Burke PE, Kavanagh EG, Grace PA, and Lyons GM: Mobility in patients with venous leg ulceration. Eur J Vasc Endovasc Surg 2007; **33:** 488.
12. Newland MR, Patel AR, Prieto L, Boulton AJM, Pacheco M, and Kirsner RS: Neuropathy and gait disturbance in patients with venous disease: a pilot study. Arch Derm 2009; **145:** 467.
13. Kobrin KL, Thompson PJ, van de Scheur M, Kwak TH, Kim S, and Falanga V: Evaluation of dermal pericapillary fibrin cuffs in venous ulceration using confocal microscopy. Wound Repair Regen 2008; **16:** 503.
14. Pieper B, Templin T, and Ebright J: Ankle mobility in relation to chronic venous insufficiency in HIV-positive persons with and without a history of injection drug use. J Assoc Nurses AIDS Care 2006; **17:** 30.
15. Pieper B, Templin TN, Kirsner RS, and Birk TJ: Substance abuse and chronic venous disorders. 33rd Annual Midwest Nursing Research Conference, Minneapolis, MN, March 28, 2009.
16. Pieper B, Templin TN, Birk TJ, and Kirsner RS: The standing heel-rise test: relations to chronic venous disorders and balance, gait, and walk time in injection drug users. Ostomy Wound Manage 2008; **54:** 18.
17. Pieper B, Templin TN, Birk TJ, and Kirsner RS: Reliability and clinical validity of a technique to assess lifetime illicit drug use. Ostomy Wound Manage 2008; **54:** 16.
18. Davies JA, Bull RH, Farrelly IJ, and Wakelin MJ: A home-based exercise programme improves ankle range of motion in long term venous ulcer patients. Phlebology 2007; **22:** 86.
19. Jull A, Arroll B, Parag V, and Waters J: Pentoxifylline for treating venous leg ulcers. Cochrane Database Syst Rev 2007, Issue 3. Art. No.: CD001733. DOI: 10.1002/14651858.CD001733.pub2.
20. Katsenis K: Micronized purified flavonoid fraction (MPFF): a review of its pharmacological effects, therapeutic efficacy and benefits in management of chronic venous insufficiency. Curr Vasc Pharmacol 2005; **3:** 1.
21. Ciszewicz M, Polubinska A, Antoniewicz A, Suminska-Jasinska K, and Breborowicz A: Sulodexide suppresses inflammation in human endothelial cells and prevents glucose cytotoxicity. Transl Res 2009; **153:** 118.
22. O'Meara S, Al-Kurdi D, and Ovington LG: Antibiotics and antiseptics for venous leg ulcers. Cochrane Database Syst Rev 2008, Issue 1. Art. No.: CD003557. DOI: 10.1002/14651858.CD003557.pub2.
23. Legendre C, Debure C, Meaume S, Lok C, Golmard JL, and Senet P: Impact of protein deficiency on venous ulcer healing. J Vasc Surg 2008; **48:** 688.

24. Paolini DJ, Comerota AJ, and Jones LS: Lower extremity arterial inflow is adversely affected in patients with venous disease. J Vasc Surg 2008; **48:** 960.

25. Nelzen O and Fransson I: True long-term and recurrence of venous leg ulcers following SEPS combined with superficial venous surgery: a prospective study. Eur J Vasc Surg 2007; **34:** 605.

26. Kalteis M, Berger I, Messie-Werndl S, Pistrich R, Schimetta W, Polz W, and Hieller F: High ligation combined with stripping and endovenous laser ablation of the great saphenous vein: early results of a randomized controlled study. J Vasc Surg 2008; **47:** 822.

27. Viarengo LM, Poterio-Filho J, Poterio GM, Menezes FH, and Meirelles GV: Endovenous laser treatment for varicose veins in patients with active ulcers: measurement of intravenous and perivenous temperatures during the procedure. Dermatol Surg 2007; **33:** 1234.

28. Carpentier PH, Poulain C, Fabry R, Chleir F, Guias B, Bettarel-Binon C, and Venous Working Group of the Socíeté Française de Médccine Valsculaire: Ascribing leg symptoms to chronic venous disorders: the construction of a diagnostic score. J Vasc Surg 2007; **46:** 991.

29. Kulkarni SR, Gohel MS, Wakely C, Minor J, Poskitt KR, and Whyman MR: The ulcerated leg severity assessment score for prediction of venous leg ulcer healing. Br J Surg 2007; **94:** 189.

30. Neinen MM, Evers AW, Van Uden CJ, Van der Vleuten CJ, van de Kerkhof PC, and Van Achterberg T: Sedentary patients with venous or mixed leg ulcers: determinants of physical activity. J Adv Nurs 2007; **60:** 50.

Clinical Trials: The Use of Surrogate Endpoints

David J. Margolis*

Departments of Dermatology and Epidemiology, University of Pennsylvania, Philadelphia, Pennsylvania.

Background: Clinical trials are essential for the development of and ultimately the regulatory approval of a new therapy.
The Problem: Conducting clinical trials on patients with chronic wounds has always been very difficult. Difficulties are likely related to recruitment, time to reach a meaningful outcome, and costs of conducting these trials.
Basic/Clinical Science Advances: Surrogate endpoints occur sooner than the primary endpoint and help to diminish the cost of clinical trials. It is our contention that surrogate markers can be used in clinical trials such that shorter and smaller trials can be conducted with reasonable accuracy to determine which potentially new therapeutics should be studied in larger, longer trials. These markers have been validated in very large longitudinal cohort studies as well as cluster-randomized trials.
Clinical Care Relevance: As recommended in guidance documents, surrogate endpoints can be used to guide clinical care.
Conclusion: The use of surrogate endpoints has been validated in more than 20,000 subjects in both longitudinal cohort studies and randomized controlled trials as surrogate measures for chronic wound care studies. They will likely be most useful in early phase studies to help efficiently determine which therapeutics should be evaluated in later pivotal studies.

Abbreviations and Acronyms

aROC = area under the receiver operator characteristic curve

DNFU = diabetic neuropathic foot ulcer

FDA = Food and Drug Administration

VLU = venous leg ulcer

*Correspondence: Departments of Dermatology and Epidemiology, University of Pennsylvania, 815 Blockley Hall, 423 Guardian Drive, Philadelphia, Pennsylvania 19104 (e-mail: margo@mail.med.upenn.edu).

BACKGROUND

CLINICAL TRIALS ARE ESSENTIAL for the development of and ultimately the regulatory approval of a new therapy. In 2006 the Food and Drug Administration (FDA) finalized a guidance document on how to conduct a wound-healing study.[1,2] In this document they suggested that the only meaningful outcome was a healed wound. Conducting clinical trials on patients with chronic wounds has always been very difficult and this document did not suggest strategies to simplify these studies. Difficulties are likely related to recruitment, time to reach a meaningful outcome, and costs of conducting these trials. Most trials evaluating a healed wound require 12–24 weeks. However, it has never been apparent that all therapies that affect a wound and help it heal will necessarily be useful for an entire 16- to 20-week trial. For example, if the goal of using a new treatment is debridement, then one might only use it for a few weeks. While a new therapy may result in a wound being more likely to heal, ultimately getting that wound to heal may be dependent on many other factors. As of 2009, there were 110 wound-related clinical trials registered on clinical trials .gov, which is an international registry for clinical trials. Few were funded by major pharmaceutical companies and very few were truly innovative. By allowing only a healed wound as an acceptable outcome, the FDA may have hampered innovation. Trials evaluating this endpoint are limited by the prolonged time

Printed in U.S.A.
DOI: 10.1089/awc.2009.0076

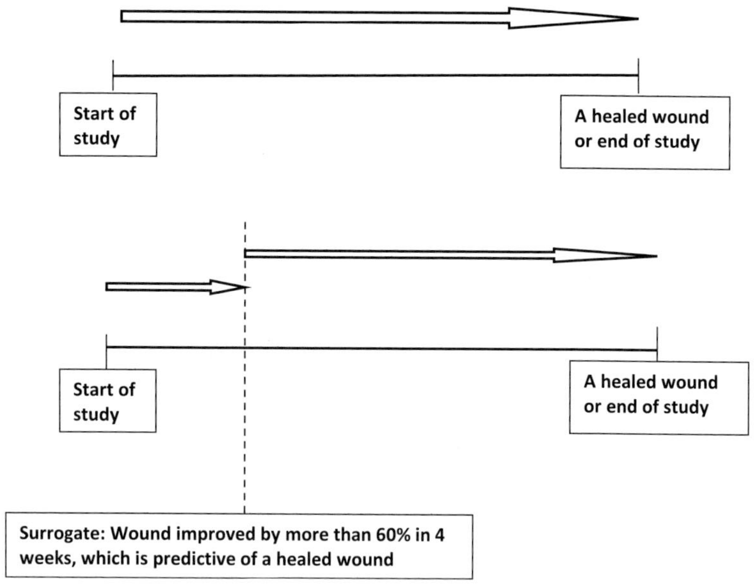

Figure 1. (**A**) In a conventional trial, a clinically meaningful endpoint is measured, and the trial length is sufficient so that the endpoint can occur. (**B**) When using a surrogate marker, the surrogate occurs before the clinically meaningful outcome but it must fully capture the net effect of the treatment on the clinical outcome. Therefore, a valid surrogate endpoint is related to the outcome of interest and is affected by the treatment of interest to the same degree and in a manner that accurately reflects the effect of the treatment on the true outcome.

period needed to allow for a wound to heal (*e.g.*, 12–24 weeks) and thereby the corresponding expense incurred to measure this outcome. A valid surrogate marker of complete wound healing would make early clinical trials (*i.e.*, trials designed to screen potentially therapeutic agents) more efficient in terms of cost, time, and number of subjects evaluated.

CLINICAL PROBLEM ADDRESSED

Surrogate endpoints occur sooner than the primary endpoint and help to diminish the cost of clinical trials (*e.g.*, less follow-up time, smaller sample size required for adequate power) (Fig. 1). Further, surrogate endpoints may allow a clinician to assess a patient's response to therapy during treatment. Several treatment guidelines have suggested reevaluating treatment goals every 4 weeks.

RELEVANT BASIC SCIENCE CONTEXT

Surrogate endpoints have been rigorously statistically defined by Prentice as "a response variable for which a test of the null hypothesis of no relationship to the treatment groups under comparison is also a valid test of the corresponding null hypothesis based on the true endpoint."[3] A surrogate endpoint has been defined in a clinical context by Temple as an "endpoint of a clinical trial that is a laboratory measurement or a physical sign used as a substitute for a clinically meaningful endpoint that measures directly how a patient feels, functions or survives."[4] Changes induced by a therapy on a surrogate endpoint are expected to reflect changes in a clinically meaningful endpoint. A surrogate endpoint must not be simply a correlate of the true clinical outcome, it must fully capture the net effect of the treatment on the clinical outcome. Therefore, a valid surrogate endpoint is related to the outcome of interest and is affected by the treatment of interest to the same degree and in a manner that accurately reflects the effect of the treatment on the true outcome. For example, agents used to treat diabetes use the surrogate of normoglycemia. While we often attribute medical importance to this clinical finding, we ultimately treat diabetes to prevent complications like cardiovascular disease, amputation, and renal disease. Controversy has recently surrounded this classic surrogate due to an unexpected increased risk of myocardial infarction believed to be associated with oral hypoglycemic agents, which received regulatory approval based on their ability to control hyperglycemia.[5,6] In any event, surrogate endpoints must be carefully evaluated before they are used in clinical trials.

EXPERIMENTAL MODEL

The validity of a surrogate endpoint is often supported by the biological plausibility of the relationship, the demonstration in epidemiological studies of the prognostic value of the surrogate endpoint for the clinical outcome, and evidence from clinical trials that the treatment effects on the surrogate endpoint correspond to effects on the outcome.[7,8] Study designs to estimate the validity of a surrogate endpoint are often longitudinal cohort studies, but surrogates have also been evaluated as part of randomized clinical trials.

Surrogate markers have been accepted by the FDA as proof of drug efficacy, provided that they were studied in large numbers of patients with appropriate follow-up periods.[4,9] However, a surrogate must always be carefully evaluated because the effect of a novel treatment on the surrogate does not always translate into a similar effect on the real outcome.

It is also important to put the context of their use in place. Surrogate endpoints may be helpful in early phase as well as late phase studies. Clinical trials are generally classified by the FDA in phases. The goal of this approach is to demonstrate that a new therapy is both safe and efficacious. First, each phase becomes progressively larger as the agent is demonstrated to be safe. Then, the goal of a phase 1 study is often human pharmacology. These studies often do not demonstrate that a new treatment is efficacious but in many ways prove concept in humans. Phase 2 studies are often conducted to help begin to demonstrate that a new compound may actually improve or cure a medical indication. Phase 3 studies are also called comparative efficacy studies. These are the studies that often show superiority of a new treatment as compared to another treatment. Although these studies are large enough to show efficacy, they are not large enough to ultimately prove that a treatment is safe. A final understanding of safety may not occur for several years until hundreds of thousands of individuals are exposed to a new treatment.

DISCUSSION OF FINDINGS AND RELEVANT LITERATURE

Several large studies have been conducted to evaluate potential surrogate markers based on wound improvement by the 4th week of care (Fig. 1). The goal of these studies was to determine if surrogate markers based primarily on changes in the size of a wound can be used to correctly predict who, with a diabetic neuropathic foot ulcer (DNFU) or venous leg ulcer (VLU), will heal.[10,11] Specifically in these retrospective cohort studies, the following surrogates were evaluated and shown to reasonably predict wound closure: log healing rate, log wound area ratio, and percentage change in wound area. Respectively, the formulas for these surrogates are $[\mathrm{Ln}(\mathrm{Area}_0)-\mathrm{Ln}(\mathrm{Area}_t)]/t$, $[\mathrm{Ln}(\mathrm{Area}_0)/\mathrm{Ln}(\mathrm{Area}_t)]$, and $[(\mathrm{Area}_0-\mathrm{Area}_t)/\mathrm{Area}_0]\times 100$, where Area_t is the wound area measured in mm^2 at week 4, Area_0 is the baseline wound area, and t is the time between the two measurements. A total of 56,488 wounds in 29,189 patients consistent with a standard definition of VLU were studied.[11] By the 4th week of standard care treatment, these markers could discriminate which patients will heal at 12 or 24 week of care (area under receiver operator characteristic curve [aROC]: 0.72–0.80).[11] An aROC estimate of 0.80 means that 80% of the time the surrogate will properly differentiate between a wound that will heal and one that will not. In a second study, using a standard definition of DNFU, 39,918 wounds on 20,213 individuals were evaluated using the same surrogates with respect to whether the wounds were healed by 12 or 20 weeks of care.[10] Again the surrogates could discriminate between those that healed and those that did not (aROC 0.76–0.80). Finally, we designed a cluster-randomized prospective clinical trial to begin to test the efficacy and feasibility of providing prognostic information on wound healing.[12] We did not provide healthcare providers with the 4-week surrogate information or with any guidance on wound care. The 4-week healing rates were evaluated for their ability to predict healing by the 24th week of care for VLU and 20th week of care for DNFU. With

TAKE-HOME MESSAGE

Basic science advances

- Surrogate markers are a valid endpoint for many clinical trials.
- A valid surrogate endpoint may allow for the identification of therapeutic agents for the treatment of chronic wounds expediting the discovery of new therapies.

Clinical science advances

- We have identified easy-to-measure surrogate endpoints for VLU and DNFU that occur by the 4th week of care.
- Clinical trials are generally classified by the FDA in phases. The goal of this approach is to demonstrate that a new therapy is both safe and efficacious. It is likely that using surrogate markers will expedite the early phase trial evaluation of new therapies. However, larger and longer studies will still be required to fully understand the safety profile of a new therapy.

Relevance to clinical care

- A valid surrogate endpoint may allow for the identification of patients who are not likely to heal by standard methods early in the patient's course of treatment, thereby allowing for expedited referral to specialty centers or the expedited initiation of more expensive, higher risk, or more novel therapies.
- It is also important to realize that recent guidance documents have suggested that 4-week response should be used to help with clinical decisions.[20–22]

respect to VLU, centers that had access to 4-week surrogate information were more likely to have healed patients, 1.43 (95% confidence interval: 1.05, 1.95) as compared those who did not.[12] With respect to DNFU, centers that had been randomized to receive only 4-week surrogate information were more likely to heal than individuals seen in centers that did not (odds ratio 1.50, 95% confidence interval: 1.05, 2.14).[12] Therefore, these surrogates were further validated by demonstrating that established risk factors for not healing, such as wound size, wound duration, and, for DNFU, anatomic grade, are also important risk factors for not achieving the surrogate endpoint, but these did not affect the ability of these surrogates to predict that a wound would heal.[12–15] To our knowledge this is the first and largest randomized evaluation of an administrative and educational intervention in wound care. It is our contention that these surrogate markers can be used in clinical trials such that shorter and smaller trials can be conducted with reasonable accuracy to determine which potentially new therapeutics should be studied in larger, longer trials.

Similarly in older and smaller studies, Margolis and colleagues found the initial rate of healing over 4 weeks to be predictive of complete healing in a study of 23 patients.[16] In a study of 14 patients, Tallman and colleagues found that the initial healing rate could predict complete healing as early as 3 weeks after starting therapy.[17] The percentage change in the VLU area over the initial 4 weeks of treatment has also been demonstrated to be a useful surrogate marker of complete healing in a dataset of 104 control subjects from a multi-centered, randomized clinical trial.[18] In this study, the percentage change in the ulcer area predicted complete healing independent of wound size. The percentage change in area from baseline to week 4 provided the best combination of positive and negative predictive values (68.2 and 74.7, respectively) and an aROC of 0.74. Others have also demonstrated that the rate of change or trajectory of change in wound size is an important predictor of healing.[19]

CAUTIONS AND CRITICAL REMARKS

The surrogates described above were developed in association with the use of standard therapy. As with all surrogates, it is possible that they may function differently in response to a new therapy. It is very important to realize that the surrogates may measure a different biological process than what occurs when a wound heals. However, because the surrogates described above are on the path toward a healed wound, it is unlikely that this will occur. As described in the cluster-randomized trial and recommended in several guidance documents, these surrogates can be used to guide patient care. However, no guidance was given to the healthcare providers in the randomized trial, so at this time while we know that receiving information about a surrogate correlated with a patient's wound healing, we ultimately do not know why. Finally, to the best of the author's knowledge, while early phase studies have begun to use the surrogates described in this report, we do not know how the FDA and other regulators will respond to this information. To date, no phase 3 studies have used a surrogate endpoint as the primary outcome with the approval of a regulatory body.

FUTURE DEVELOPMENTS

The FDA in their guidance to industry defines their efficacy endpoint as complete closure which ". . . is defined as skin re-epithelialization without drainage or dressing requirements confirmed at two consecutive study visits 2 weeks apart."[1,2] Further they note that, "Measurement of partial wound healing in early phase clinical trials, if prospectively defined, may indicate relevant biological activity and help guide subsequent trial design. Partial healing would not, however, suffice as a primary endpoint in phase 3 studies because the clinical benefit of incremental wound size changes has not been established."[1,2] It is important to note that while many of the surrogate measures described above are measures of partial healing, they are also associated with the efficacy endpoint described above. We are proposing the use of surrogate endpoints that have been validated in more than 20,000 subjects in both longitudinal cohort studies and randomized controlled trials as surrogate measures for chronic wound care studies. As noted by the FDA officials, they are certainly consistent with their current guidance for early phase studies.[23] Using them in these studies should help investigators to efficiently evaluate new therapeutics for phase 3 studies. However, they may also be adequate for phase 3 studies too.

AUTHOR DISCLOSURE STATEMENT

The author has no commercial associations that might create or seem to pose a conflict of interest in connection with this article.

REFERENCES

1. FDA Wound Healing Clinical Focus Group. Guidance for Industry: Chronic cutaneous ulcer and burn wounds—developing products for treatment (Draft—not for implementation). Wound Repair Regen 2001; **9:** 258.
2. Guidance for Industry: Chronic cutaneous ulcer and burn wounds—developing products for treatment. Food and Drug Administration. 2006 June. www.fda.gov/cber/gdlns/ulcburn.pdf.
3. Prentice RL: Surrogate endpoints in clinical trials: definitions and operational criteria. Stat Med 1989; **8:** 431.
4. Temple R: Are surrogate markers adequate to assess cardiovascular disease drugs? JAMA 1999; **282:** 790.
5. Nissen SE and Wolski K: Effect of rosiglitazone on the risk of myocardial infarction and death from cardiovascular causes [see comment]. New Engl J Med 2007; **356:** 2457.
6. Margolis DJ, Hoffstad O, and Strom BL: Association between serious ischemic cardiac outcomes and medications used to treat diabetes. Pharmacoepidemiol Drug Saf 2008; **17:** 753.
7. Fleming TR and DeMets DL: Surrogate end points in clinical trials: are we being misled? Ann Intern Med 1996; **125:** 605.
8. Pstay BM, Weiss NS, Furberg CD, *et al.*: Surrogate end points, health outcomes, and the drug-approval process for the treatment of risk factors for cardiovascular disease. JAMA 1999; **282:** 786.
9. FDA ICH E9: E9 Statistical Principles for Clinical Trials. www.fda.gov/downloads/Regulatory Information/Guidances/UCM129505.pdf. September 1998.
10. Margolis DJ, Gelfand JM, Hofstad O, and Berlin JA: Surrogate endpoints for the treatment of diabetic neuropathic foot ulcers. Diabetes Care 2003; **26:** 1696.
11. Gelfand JM, Hofstad O, and Margolis DJ: Surrogate endpoints for treatment of venous leg ulcers. J Invest Dermatol 2002; **119:** 1420.
12. Kurd SK, Hoffstad OJ, Bilker WB, and Margolis DJ: Evaluation of the use of prognostic information for the care of individuals with venous leg ulcers or diabetic neuropathic foot ulcers. Wound Repair Regen 2009; **17:** 318.
13. Margolis DJ, Berlin JA, and Strom BL: Risk factors associated with the failure of a venous leg ulcer to heal. Arch Dermatol 1999; **135:** 920.
14. Margolis DJ, Berlin JA, and Strom BL: Which venous leg ulcers will heal with a limb compression bandage? Am J Med 2000; **109:** 15.
15. Margolis DJ, Taylor LA, Hofstad O, and Berlin JA: Diabetic neuropathic foot ulcer: the association of wound size, wound duration, and wound grade. Diabetes Care 2002; **25:** 1835.
16. Margolis D, Gross E, Wood CR, and Lazarus GS: Planimetric rate of healing in venous ulcers of the leg treated with pressure bandage and hydrocolloid dressing. J Am Acad Dermatol 1993; **28:** 418.
17. Tallman P, Muscare E, Carson P, Eaglstein WH, and Falanga V: Initial rate of healing predicts complete healing of venous ulcers. Arch Dermatol 1997; **133:** 1231.
18. Kantor J and Margolis DJ: A multicentre study of percentage change in venous leg ulcer area as a prognostic index of healing at 24 weeks. Br J Dermatol 2000; **142:** 960.
19. Robson MC, Hill DP, Woodske ME, and Steed DL: Wound healing trajectories as predictors of effectiveness of therapeutic agents [see comments]. Arch Surg 2000; **135:** 773.
20. Robson MC, Cooper DM, Aslam R, *et al.*: Guidelines for the treatment of venous ulcers. Wound Repair Regen 2006; **14:** 649.
21. Steed DL, Attinger C, Colaizzi T, *et al.*: Guidelines for the treatment of diabetic ulcers. Wound Repair Regen 2006; **14:** 680.
22. Hinchliffe RJ, Apelqvist VJ, Armstrong DG, *et al.*: A systematic review of the effectiveness of interventions to enhance the healing of chronic ulcers in the foot in diabetes. Diabetes Metab Res Rev 2008; **24(Suppl):** S119.
23. Joint meeting of the skin diseases interagency coordinating committee and the diabetes mellitus interagency coordinating committee. National Institutes of Health. November 18;1–41. www.niddk.nih.gov/federal/dmicc/FINALNov-ICC-Summary.pdf.

Section 5

INFLAMMATION

Section Editors: Luisa Ann DiPietro and Sashwati Roy

WHS
Wound
Healing
Society

Neuroinflammatory Modulation of Cutaneous Responses to Injury

Anne N. Hocking, Lara A. Muffley, and Nicole S. Gibran*

Department of Surgery, University of Washington, Seattle, Washington.

Background: Neuroinflammation comprises a long-ignored humoral response to cutaneous injury. Both chronic nonhealing wounds due to diabetes mellitus and hypertrophic scars display abnormal nerve distribution and neuroinflammation. Patients with diabetes mellitus have diminished nerve numbers and nerve growth factor depletion in uninjured skin and cutaneous wounds.[1] Animal models suggest that restoration of substance P levels improves cellular inflammation and wound repair kinetics. In contrast, hypertrophic scars with excessive fibroproliferation have increased nerve numbers[2,3] with increased levels of substance P.

The Problem: How do neuropeptides regulate responses to cutaneous injury? Current evidence implicates neuropeptides in inflammation, angiogenesis, and fibroproliferation; however, the molecular mechanism needs to be elucidated.

Basic/Clinical Science Advances: A validated diabetic (db/db) mouse model of impaired wound healing suggests that exogenous modulation of substance P levels improves wound repair and that nerve growth factor restores sensory nerve numbers. Conversely, a promising model of fibroproliferative scar formation in the Duroc pig demonstrates statistically significant increased nerve numbers in the deep dermal scar.

Clinical Care Relevance: Understanding the contribution of neuropeptides to repair of cutaneous injury may provide novel therapeutic interventions for wounds that demonstrate excessive or inadequate healing.

Conclusion: Neuroinflammatory responses to cutaneous injury contribute to inflammation, angiogenesis, epithelialization, and fibroproliferation. Since nerve-derived mediators have both stimulatory and inhibitory effects on these processes, better understanding about the balance is necessary before therapeutic interventions are developed for clinical application.

Abbreviations and Acronyms

α-MSH = alpha melanocyte-stimulating hormone

MC1R = melanocortin 1 receptor

NEP = neutral endopeptidase

NF-κB = nuclear factor-kappa B

SNP = single-nucleotide polymorphism

*Correspondence: Department of Surgery, University of Washington, Harborview Medical Center, 325 Ninth Ave., P.O. Box 359796, Seattle, Washington 98104 (e-mail: nicoleg@u.washington.edu).

BACKGROUND

Normal wound repair involves an orderly cascade of events involving coagulation, inflammation, angiogenesis, epithelialization, and tissue remodeling. Whereas deficient early cellular responses and persistent inflammation lead to impaired wound healing such as chronic nonhealing wounds with diabetes mellitus, exuberant inflammation is associated with hypertrophic scar formation. Our long-term hypothesis has been that neuroinflammation comprises an essential role in the humoral response to injury.

Multiple resident cutaneous cell types contribute inflammatory mediators to the wound-healing milieu. One long-ignored source has been sensory neurons, which release both proinflammatory and antiinflammatory neuropeptides.[4–6] The skin is densely populated with sensory nerves, including C-fibers and δ-fibers, with axonal fibers extending

Printed in U.S.A.
DOI: 10.1089/awc.2009.0108

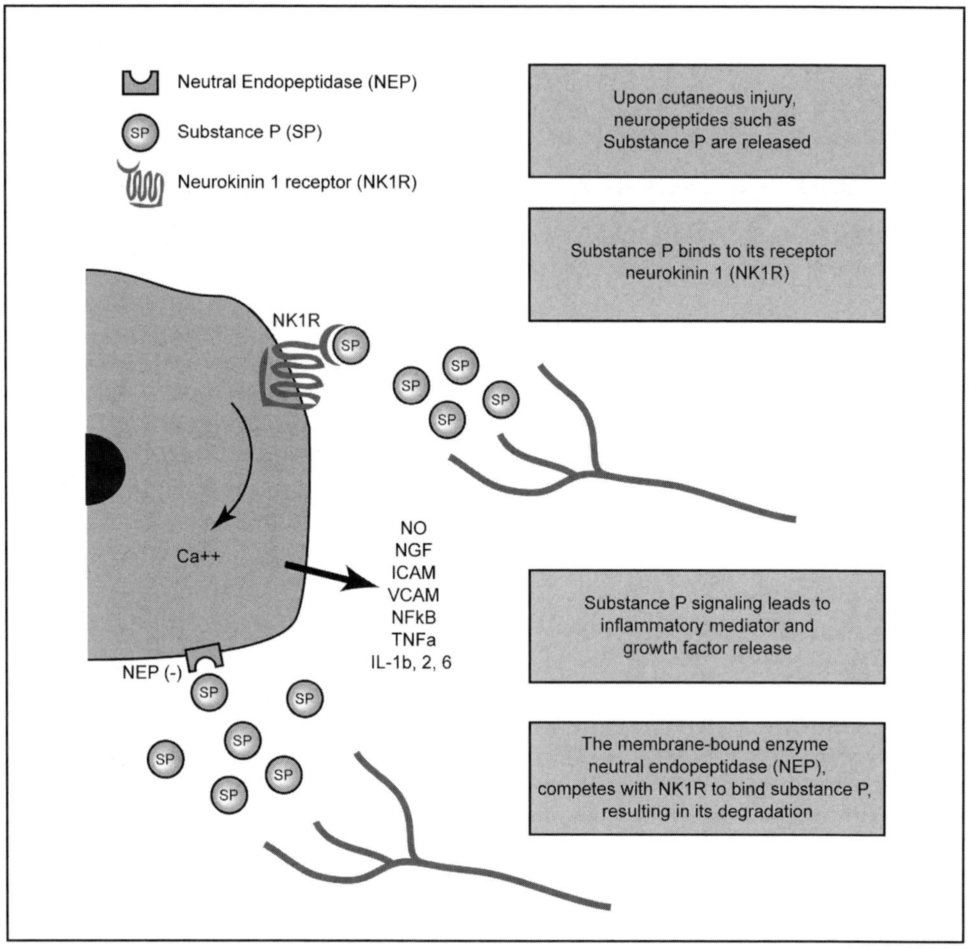

Figure 1. Neuropeptides contribute to all phases of cutaneous wound repair including inflammation, angiogenesis, and fibroproliferation. Substance P release from sensory nerves in skin is stimulated by cutaneous injury. This initiates a neuroinflammatory signaling cascade involving proinflammatory mediators and growth factors. Abnormal innervation and changes in substance P levels in diabetic wounds and hypertrophic scars may contribute to impaired responses to cutaneous injury.

to all layers of the skin including the epidermis.[7] Sensory nerves communicate tactile sensation (pain, temperature, itch, and proprioception) to the central nervous system and release neuropeptides into the local environment. The observation that nerve stimulation induces cutaneous vasodilatation and protein extravasation implicated nerves as important contributors to inflammation in the skin. Neuropeptides signal by binding to G protein–coupled receptors on target cells. Neuropeptide degradation by cell surface peptidases on target cells terminates signaling and regulates neuroinflammation[8] (Fig. 1).

There are numerous neuropeptides in the skin including substance P, calcitonin-gene-related peptide, neurokinin A, neurokinin Y, and alpha melanocyte-stimulating hormone (α-MSH).[6] Interestingly, nerves may not be the sole cellular source of neuropeptides in the skin because keratinocytes, microvascular endothelial cells, fibroblasts, and leukocytes also secrete neuropeptides.[9] The neuropeptide substance P has been shown to induce a classic wheal and flare response.[10] Other inflammatory responses regulated by substance P include degranulation of mast cells with histamine release, neutrophil chemotaxis, proliferation of macrophages, and production of growth factors and cytokines by keratinocytes and dermal microvascular endothelial cells.[11,12]

CLINICAL PROBLEM ADDRESSED

Both chronic nonhealing wounds due to diabetes mellitus and hypertrophic scar formation display abnormal nerve distribution and neuroinflammation. Patients with diabetes mellitus have diminished numbers of nerves and nerve growth factor depletion in both uninjured skin[13] and cutaneous wounds[1] with evidence of functional nerve die-back in patients with diabetes for 4 or more years, and in males more than females.[14] Also, in patients with diabetes, elevated neutral endopeptidase (NEP) activity leads to reduced neuropeptide levels that result in increased degradation.[15] Animal models suggest that restoration of substance P levels in healing wounds improves cellular inflammation and wound repair kinetics.[16–18]

In contrast, hypertrophic scars have increased nerve numbers with increased levels of substance P and significantly decreased NEP activity.[2,3] These results suggest that an imbalance in the neuroinflammatory response may impair cutaneous wound healing. From a clinical standpoint, itching is one of the most devastating complaints that patients with healing wounds and especially hypertrophic scars describe. Substance P is known to be associated directly and indirectly with itching. A common clinical remedy for patients with neuropathic pain is capsaicin, which depletes substance P from the terminal nerve endings. It has been used only sporadically in patients with hypertrophic scars due to the initial cutaneous burning sensation that patients experience for the first few applications.

Finally, increasing evidence that psychological states may be significant independent risk factors for postoperative outcomes suggests that we have underestimated how the central nervous system modulates physiologic responses to injury.[19]

BASIC SCIENCE CONTEXT

Neuropeptides are derived from the enzymatic cleavage of larger precursor proteins. Precursor proteins are packaged into secretory vesicles containing proteases specific for cleaving the precursor into mature neuropeptides. For example, the 11-amino acid proinflammatory peptide substance P is derived from preprotachykinin; likewise, the antiinflammatory peptide α-MSH derives from proopiomelanocortin after proteolytic cleavage catalyzed by the prohormone convertases 1 and 2. Secreted neuropeptides signal through G protein–coupled receptors on target cells; substance P binds neurokinin receptors and α-MSH binds the melanocortin-1 receptor. Downstream signaling by the neurokinin receptors leads to the activation of the proinflammatory mediators, phospholipase C and protein kinase C, which increase intracellular calcium and eventual nuclear factor-kappa B (NF-κB) activation.[20] Melanocortin receptors activate adenlylyl cyclase leading to cAMP accumulation and phosphorylation of cAMP-responsive element-binding protein with decreased NF-κB activation.[21] Signaling by both substance P and α-MSH is regulated by the metalloprotease, NEP, which degrades the neuropeptides at the cell membrane.

Substance P and α-MSH are both present in uninjured skin with precursor proteins expressed in resident skin cells; sensory nerves, keratinocytes, and endothelial cells secrete substance P, and keratinocytes, melanocytes, and dermal microvascular endothelial cells secrete α-MSH. The substance P receptor, neurokinin-1 receptor, is expressed in the skin by epidermal keratinocytes, dermal fibroblasts,[22] and dermal microvascular endothelial cells.[8] The α-MSH receptor, melanocortin 1 receptor (MC1R), localizes in skin to differentiating epidermal keratinocytes[23] and in murine excisional wounds to inflammatory cells, keratinocytes, and endothelial cells.

EXPERIMENTAL MODEL OR MATERIAL

Whereas *in vitro* observations about cellular responses to neuroinflammatory stimulation define mechanistic cellular events, they are irrelevant unless we can demonstrate differences in responses to cutaneous injury. Wound repair studies are often perceived as descriptive, but thorough characterization of healing is essential for establishing efficacy before expensive product development for clinical trial.

The db/db (BKS.Cg-m+/+*Lepr*^{db}/J) mouse represents one validated model of impaired wound healing due to diabetes mellitus. These mice have a spontaneous mutation in the leptin receptor and develop type 2 diabetes associated with hyperglycemia, hyperinsulinemia, hyperlipidemia, and obesity. Like patients with diabetes mellitus, the db/db mice develop peripheral neuropathy based on electrophysiology, morphometrics, and histology. The reduced number of sensory nerve fibers in db/db mice can be increased by topical administration of nerve growth factor suggesting that the nerves in the diabetic skin are responsive to neurotrophic factors if available.[16] Wounds in the db/db mice display delayed inflammation, granulation tissue formation, and wound closure compared with nondiabetic controls. After delayed infiltration of neutrophils and macrophages, the inflammatory response is sustained with prolonged expression of chemokines and persistence of inflammatory cells in the db/db wound.[24]

Absence of a well-validated animal model of fibroproliferative scarring has limited understanding of the pathophysiology of hypertrophic scarring. One promising model may be the thickened scars that form in deep partial-thickness wounds in the Duroc pig.[25,26] Unique to this pig breed is the formation of thick, hard, hyper/hypopigmented, hairless, contracted scars in deep dermal wounds. Unlike human hypertrophic scars, which may grow 1–2 cm above the surrounding skin, scar height in the Duroc wounds reaches 1–2 mm above the surface. Nevertheless, the Duroc deep dermal scars typically measure 11 mm from hypodermis to stratum corneum compared with normal porcine skin thickness of 3 mm. The deep dermal scars have a similar histology to human hypertrophic scars with large numbers of disorganized collagen fibers in some places forming whorls and nodules. The porcine scars demonstrate statistically significant increased nerve numbers.[27]

DISCUSSION OF FINDINGS AND RELEVANT LITERATURE

Current clinical and scientific evidence supports a role for neuropeptides in normal cutaneous wound repair and implicates them in the pathophysiology of chronic nonhealing wounds in diabetes mellitus and hypertrophic scar formation. Importantly, neuropeptides contribute to all phases of wound repair with effects on inflammation, angiogenesis, and fibroproliferation. Neuropeptides that have been implicated in wound repair include substance P, neuropeptide Y, calcitonin-gene-related peptide, and α-MSH. In this section, we focus on substance P, which elicits proinflammatory responses and α-MSH, which has antiinflammatory properties (Fig. 1).

Substance P

Substance P release from sensory nerves in skin is stimulated by cutaneous injury. In uninjured skin, substance P–positive nerves surround blood vessels, sweat glands, and extend into the epidermis.[28] Immediately after injury, substance P is detected in the epidermis and extracellular matrix of the acute burn wound. Four weeks after injury, substance P localizes to nerve fibers that have repopulated the healing dermis.

Abnormal innervation and changes in substance P levels in diabetic wounds and hypertrophic scars may contribute to impaired responses to cutaneous injury. Chronic nonhealing wounds have a reduced number of sensory nerves, diminished substance P levels,[13] and increased NEP activity.[15] The converse is observed in hypertrophic scars that have increased sensory nerve numbers,[2] increased substance P, and diminished NEP activity.[3] Importantly, restoration of substance P levels in murine diabetic wounds by application of either exogenous substance P[29] or thiorphan,[18] an inhibitor of NEP, improves wound-healing kinetics and the inflammatory responses.[17]

A number of *in vivo* and *in vitro* studies indicate that substance P induces inflammatory responses to cutaneous injury. Recently we have demonstrated that topical application of substance P increases the density of inflammatory cells such as leukocytes, macrophages, and endothelial cells in a diabetic murine wound model.[17] This observation that substance P is a chemoattractant for the inflammatory cells recruitment into the wound is supported by studies showing that substance P promotes migration of leukocytes and neutrophils.[30–32] Substance P also stimulates cytokine and growth factor production by cells that participate in wound repair. Macrophages and neutrophils increase production of tumor necrosis factor-α, interleukin-1b, interleukin-2, and interleukin-6 when exposed to substance P.[33,34] Substance P also upregulates nerve growth factor expression by both keratinocytes[35] and dermal microvascular endothelial cells,[12] suggesting that following injury, nerve-derived mediators trigger

TAKE-HOME MESSAGE

Basic science advances

- Neuropeptides contribute to all phases of wound repair with effects on inflammation, angiogenesis, and fibroproliferation.
- Sensory nerves are not the only source of neuropeptides in the cutaneous wound; almost all cell types resident in uninjured skin and cutaneous wounds produce neuropeptides.
- Neuropeptides implicated in wound repair include substance P, neuropeptide Y, calcitonin-gene-related peptide, and α-MSH.
- Substance P has been shown to induce inflammatory responses to cutaneous injury in both *in vitro* and *in vivo* studies. In contrast, αMSH decreases inflammatory signaling and fibroproliferative responses *in vitro*.

Clinical science advance

- Our evolving understanding of the contribution of nerve-derived mediators to proinflammatory and antiinflammatory signaling in cutaneous injury suggests that modulation of the local nervous system may provide novel therapeutic interventions for wounds that demonstrate excessive or inadequate healing.

Relevance to clinical care

- Modulating healing wounds with neurotrophins or neuropeptides should be based on scientific evidence that the mediators are safe and efficacious before being clinically adopted.
- Currently available topical agents such as capsaicin may alter neurogenic pain such as itching.

the humoral responses necessary for nerve regeneration. Endothelial inflammatory responses to substance P include nitric oxide–mediated vasodilatation and increased expression of the adhesion molecules, intercellular adhesion molecule-1, and vascular cell adhesion molecule required for leukocyte–endothelial cell interactions.[36]

Diabetes mellitus–related metabolic perturbations including hyperglycemia and hyperlipidemia reduce substance P–mediated migration and proliferation by *in vitro* endothelial cells.[37] Whether this is due to upregulation of NEP enzyme activity or glycation of substance P must be determined.

αMSH

The melanocortin system is comprised of melanocyte-stimulating hormones (αMSH, βMSH, γMSH), adrenocorticotrophic hormone, and β-endorphin, which derive from the common precursor hormone, proopiomelanocortin. The melanocortin peptides bind five homologous receptors, which are G protein–coupled receptors that activate adenylyl cyclase leading to phosphorylation of cAMP-responsive element-binding protein. MC1R and αMSH are best understood in relation to population genetics, pigmentation, and melanoma risk.[38]

Under normal circumstances, MSH binding to its receptor MC1R regulates human cutaneous pigmentation by increasing production of the photoprotective brown/black eumelanin at the expense of yellow/red pheomelanin. One-third of the general population has a single-nucleotide polymorphism (SNP) in the MC1R gene. Many of these mutations are associated with light skin and red hair due to increased production of pheomelanin. However, Asians, Hispanics, and Native Americans also have increased incidence of MC1R SNPs. Nonfunctional SNPs in MC1R have been determined to be independent risk factors for melanoma making the melanocortin system a widely studied, well-characterized signaling pathway.

A role for the melanocortin system in the other cutaneous morphogenetic responses has also begun to emerge. Just as substance P increases *in vitro* cellular inflammatory responses, αMSH decreases inflammatory signaling and fibroproliferative responses in several cell types. In immune cells including macrophages, T cells, and neutrophils, αMSH downregulates the endotoxin receptor CD14 and thereby reduces endotoxin-mediated NF-κB activation and tumor necrosis factor-α production.[39] Likewise, αMSH suppresses TGFβ1-mediated synthesis of collagen types I, III, and V *in vitro* and decreases the number of vimentin and α – smooth muscle alpha cells *in vivo*.[40]

CAUTION, CRITICAL REMARKS, AND RECOMMENDATIONS

In spite of encouraging *in vitro* and animal data regarding the role of neuropeptides in wound repair processes, the medical community is not ready for the development of therapeutic interventions. Too often in a rush to develop mechanistic explanations for cellular responses, we overlook the larger picture of how an intervention may influence responses. Early clinical studies with wound manipulation with growth factors may have been more successful if we had better characterized the wounds with regard to receptor or enzymatic status.

Given our observations that insufficient neuroinflammation contributes to impaired healing and excessive neuroinflammation is associated with fibroproliferative scarring, we need to carefully determine where the balance may be. Restoring depleted neuroinflammatory signaling may generate wound closure more efficiently, but may also lead to excessive scar formation, hardly an improved response. Only with careful documentation of long-term responses to interventional perturbations, will we be able to find the balance and avoid unexpected findings at clinical trial.

FUTURE DEVELOPMENTS

Modulating neuroinflammation in healing wounds has enormous potential for both chronic nonhealing wounds and fibroproliferative scars. Since substance P is directly associated with itching in patients with healing wounds, especially hypertrophic scars, modulating substance P cutaneous activity could contribute dramatically to improve patient satisfaction and comfort following injury or surgery.

Mutations in the αMSH and MC1R genes are common in the general population and represent independent risk factors for the development of melanoma and other cutaneous neoplasia. Therefore, considerable scientific work has already established a foundation for pharmacologic manipulation of the melanocortin system. As these advances in modulating responses to αMSH develop, they should be evaluated as means to manipulate abnormal responses to cutaneous injury.

ACKNOWLEDGMENTS

The authors have been funded by the NIGMS (GM56483) and the NIDDK (DK508007).

AUTHOR DISCLOSURE STATEMENT

No conflict of interest disclosed.

REFERENCES

1. Underwood RA, Gibran NS, Muffley LA, Usui ML, and Olerud JE: Color subtractive-computer-assisted image analysis for quantification of cutaneous nerves in a diabetic mouse model. J Histochem Cytochem 2001; **49:** 1285.
2. Crowe R, Parkhouse N, McGrouther D, and Burnstock G: Neuropeptide-containing nerves in painful hypertrophic human scar tissue. Br J Dermatol 1994; **130:** 444.
3. Scott JR, Muangman PR, Tamura RN, Zhu KQ, Liang Z, Anthony J, Engrav LH, and Gibran NS: Substance P levels and neutral endopeptidase activity in acute burn wounds and hypertrophic scar. Plast Reconstr Surg 2005; **115:** 1095.
4. McDonald DM, Bowden JJ, Baluk P, and Bunnett NW: Neurogenic inflammation. A model for studying efferent actions of sensory nerves. Adv Exp Med Biol 1996; **410:** 453.
5. Payan DG: Neuropeptides and inflammation: the role of substance P. Annu Rev Med 1989; **40:** 341.
6. Luger TA: Neuromediators—a crucial component of the skin immune system. J Dermatol Sci 2002; **30:** 87.
7. Dalsgaard CJ, Bjorklund H, Jonsson CE, Hermansson A, and Dahl D: Distribution of neurofilament-immunoreactive nerve fibers in human skin. Histochemistry 1984; **81:** 111.
8. Bowden JJ, Garland AM, Baluk P, Lefevre P, Grady EF, Vigna SR, Bunnett NW, and McDonald DM: Direct observation of substance P-induced internalization of neurokinin 1 (NK1) receptors at sites of inflammation. Proc Natl Acad Sci USA 1994; **91:** 8964.
9. Lotti T, Hautmann G, and Panconesi E: Neuropeptides in skin. J Am Acad Dermatol 1995; **33:** 482.
10. Foreman JC: The skin as an organ for the study of the pharmacology of neuropeptides. Skin Pharmacol 1988; **1:** 77.
11. Ansel JC, Armstrong CA, Song I, Quinlan KL, Olerud JE, Caughman SW, and Bunnett NW: Interactions of the skin and nervous system. J Investig Dermatol Symp Proc 1997; **2:** 23.
12. Gibran NS, Tamura R, Tsou R, and Isik FF: Human dermal microvascular endothelial cells produce nerve growth factor: implications for wound repair. Shock 2003; **19:** 127.
13. Anand P: Neurotrophins and peripheral neuropathy. Philos Trans R Soc Lond B Biol Sci 1996; **351:** 449.
14. Allen C, Shen G, Palta M, Lotz B, Jacobson R, and D'Alessio D: Long-term hyperglycemia is related to peripheral nerve changes at a diabetes duration of 4 years. The Wisconsin Diabetes Registry. Diabetes Care 1997; **20:** 1154.
15. Antezana M, Sullivan S, Usui M, Gibran N, Spenny M, Larsen J, Ansel J, Bunnett N, and Olerud J: Neutral endopeptidase activity is increased in the skin of subjects with diabetic ulcers. J Invest Dermatol 2002; **119:** 1400.
16. Muangman P, Muffley LA, Anthony JP, Spenny ML, Underwood RA, Olerud JE, and Gibran NS: Nerve growth factor accelerates wound healing in diabetic mice. Wound Repair Regen 2004; **12:** 44.
17. Scott JR, Tamura RN, Muangman P, Isik FF, Xie C, and Gibran NS: Topical substance P increases inflammatory cell density in genetically diabetic murine wounds. Wound Repair Regen 2008; **16:** 529.
18. Spenny ML, Muangman P, Sullivan SR, Bunnett NW, Ansel JC, Olerud JE, and Gibran NS: Neutral endopeptidase inhibition in diabetic wound repair. Wound Repair Regen 2002; **10:** 295.
19. Oxlad M, Stubberfield J, Stuklis R, Edwards J, and Wade TD: Psychological risk factors for increased post-operative length of hospital stay following coronary artery bypass graft surgery. J Behav Med 2006; **29:** 179.
20. Quinlan KL, Naik SM, Cannon G, Armstrong CA, Bunnett NW, Ansel JC, and Caughman SW: Substance P activates coincident NF-AT- and NF-kappa B-dependent adhesion molecule gene expression in microvascular endothelial cells through intracellular calcium mobilization. J Immunol 1999; **163:** 5656.
21. Haycock JW, Wagner M, Morandini R, Ghanem G, Rennie IG, and Mac Neil S: Alpha-melanocyte-stimulating hormone inhibits NF-kappaB activation in human melanocytes and melanoma cells. J Invest Dermatol 1999; **113:** 560.
22. Liu JY, Hu JH, Zhu QG, Li FQ, and Sun HJ: Substance P receptor expression in human skin keratinocytes and fibroblasts. Br J Dermatol 2006; **155:** 657.
23. Chakraborty AK, Funasaka Y, Pawelek JM, Nagahama M, Ito A, and Ichihashi M: Enhanced expression of melanocortin-1 receptor (MC1-R) in normal human keratinocytes during differentiation: evidence for increased expression of POMC peptides near suprabasal layer of epidermis. J Invest Dermatol 1999; **112:** 853.
24. Wetzler C, Kampfer H, Stallmeyer B, Pfeilschifter J, and Frank S: Large and sustained induction of chemokines during impaired wound healing in the genetically diabetic mouse: prolonged persistence of neutrophils and macrophages during the late phase of repair. J Invest Dermatol 2000; **115:** 245.
25. Gallant-Behm CL and Hart DA: Genetic analysis of skin wound healing and scarring in a porcine model. Wound Repair Regen 2006; **14:** 46.
26. Zhu KQ, Carrougher GJ, Gibran NS, Isik FF, and Engrav LH: Review of the female Duroc/Yorkshire pig model of human fibroproliferative scarring. Wound Repair Regen 2007; **15 Suppl 1:** S32.
27. Liang Z, Engrav LH, Muangman P, Muffley LA, Zhu KQ, Carrougher GJ, Underwood RA, and Gibran NS: Nerve quantification in female red Duroc pig (FRDP) scar compared to human hypertrophic scar. Burns 2004; **30:** 57.
28. Dunnick CA, Gibran NS, and Heimbach DM: Substance P has a role in neurogenic mediation of human burn wound healing. J Burn Care Rehabil 1996; **17:** 390.
29. Gibran NS, Jang YC, Isik FF, Greenhalgh DG, Muffley LA, Underwood RA, Usui ML, Larsen J, Smith DG, Bunnett N, Ansel JC, and Olerud JE: Diminished neuropeptide levels contribute to the impaired cutaneous healing response associated with diabetes mellitus. J Surg Res 2002; **108:** 122.
30. Helme RD, Eglezos A, and Hosking CS: Substance P induces chemotaxis of neutrophils in normal and capsaicin-treated rats. Immunol Cell Biol 1987; **65:** 267.
31. Roch-Arveiller M, Regoli D, Chanaud B, Lenoir M, Muntaner O, Stralzko S, and Giroud JP: Tachykinins: effects on motility and metabolism of rat polymorphonuclear leucocytes. Pharmacology 1986; **33:** 266.
32. Carolan EJ, and Casale TB: Effects of neuropeptides on neutrophil migration through noncellular and endothelial barriers. J Allergy Clin Immunol 1993; **92:** 589.
33. Ansel JC, Brown JR, Payan DG, and Brown MA: Substance P selectively activates TNF-alpha gene expression in murine mast cells. J Immunol 1993; **150:** 4478.
34. Delgado AV, McManus AT, and Chambers JP: Production of tumor necrosis factor-alpha, interleukin 1-beta, interleukin 2, and interleukin 6 by rat leukocyte subpopulations after exposure to substance P. Neuropeptides 2003; **37:** 355.
35. Burbach GJ, Kim KH, Zivony AS, Kim A, Aranda J, Wright S, Naik SM, Caughman SW, Ansel JC, and Armstrong CA: The neurosensory tachykinins substance P and neurokinin A directly induce keratinocyte nerve growth factor. J Invest Dermatol 2001; **117:** 1075.
36. Quinlan KL, Song IS, Bunnett NW, Letran E, Steinhoff M, Harten B, Olerud JE, Armstrong CA, Caughman SW, and Ansel JC: Neuropeptide regulation of human dermal microvascular endothelial cell ICAM-1 expression and function. Am J Physiol 1998; **275(6 Pt 1):** C1580.
37. Wang Q, Muffley LA, Hall K, Chase M, and Gibran NS: Elevated glucose and fatty acid levels impair substance P induced dermal microvascular endothelial cell migration and proliferation in an agarose gel model system. Shock 2009; **32:** 491.
38. Millington GW: Proopiomelanocortin (POMC): the cutaneous roles of its melanocortin products and receptors. Clin Exp Dermatol 2006; **31:** 407.
39. Luger TA, Brzoska T, Scholzen TE, Kalden DH, Sunderkotter C, Armstrong C, and Ansel J: The role of alpha-MSH as a modulator of cutaneous inflammation. Ann NY Acad Sci 2000; **917:** 232.
40. Bohm M, Raghunath M, Sunderkotter C, Schiller M, Stander S, Brzoska T, Cauvet T, Schioth HB, Schwarz T, and Luger TA: Collagen metabolism is a novel target of the neuropeptide alpha-melanocyte-stimulating hormone. J Biol Chem 2004; **279:** 6959.

Cytokines and Growth Factors in the Regulation of Wound Inflammation

Tim D. Eubank and Clay B. Marsh*

Division of Pulmonary, Allergy, Critical Care, and Sleep Medicine, Department of Internal Medicine, The Ohio State University, Columbus, Ohio.

Background: Cytokines and growth factors play regulatory roles in wound healing. As part of this process, inflammation initiates healing and its regulation is so important that homeostatic mechanisms evolved to control this activity. Normal wound inflammation involves platelet activation and recruitment of neutrophils, macrophages, and fibroblasts to the wound site in a regimented fashion. Correspondingly, cytokine release from these cells orchestrates successful wound closure.
The Problem: A dichotomy exists between physiological inflammation leading to wound healing and pathological inflammation obstructing it. Transitioning physiological inflammation to chronic inflammation is associated with poor wound healing. A basic understanding of pathological mechanisms blocking normal wound repair is essential in the clinical setting. This article reviews normal wound healing and physiological inflammation and how disruption of this orchestrated pathway interferes with wound healing.
Basic/Clinical Science Advances: Recent advances aimed at diminishing pathological inflammation focuses on regulating endogenous growth factors, cytokines, and chemokines via gene therapy, with delivery systems such as adenoviral vectors and gene-activated matrices.
Clinical Care Relevance: The production of gene delivery systems, enzymatic debriding products, and bioengineered materials shows promise in reversing pathological inflammation and is the focus of clinical therapeutic applications.
Conclusion: Pathological inflammation is the central miscreant in normal wound repair. Technological advances that optimize the orchestrated immunological events leading to normal wound healing are the next generation of wound healing therapies.

BACKGROUND

Inflammation is critical in effective wound repair. Upon injury, a cascade of events triggers platelet activation, resulting in effective hemostasis and the production of cytokines and growth factors important in normal wound healing. These mediators suppress infection and induce the recruitment of progenitor and mature cells to generate an effective environment to repair and remodel the wound. Evolutionarily defined, this inflammatory response may be somewhat antiquated today. In the absence of topical antibiotics and sterile surgical techniques, our primitive ancestors required a strong and sustained inflammatory response to alleviate infection in an open wound. Today, while we control infection with antibiotics, it may be this sustained inflammation that reduces effective wound healing. Many studies report that extended tissue inflammation leads to a nonhealing

Abbreviations and Acronyms

CXC = cysteine–any amino acid–cysteine binding chemokine
GM-CSF = granulocyte/macrophage colony-stimulating factor
IL-1β = interleukin-1 beta
IL-6 = interleukin-6
IL-10 = interleukin-10
IP-10 = interferon-inducible protein 10
JAK = janus kinase
KGF = keratinocyte growth factor
MCP-1 = monocyte chemotactic protein-1
MIP-2 = macrophage inflammatory protein-2
MMP = matrix metalloproteinase
PDGF = platelet-derived growth factor
SCID = severe combined immunodeficiency
SMAD = (*Caenorhabditis elegans* protein) "SMA" and (*Drosophila* protein) "mothers against decapentaplegic"
STAT = signal transducers and activators of transcription
TGF-α/β = transforming growth factor alpha/beta
TIMPs = tissue inhibitor of metalloproteinases

(continued)

Printed in U.S.A.
DOI: 10.1089/awc.2009.0122

Abbreviations and Acronyms *(continued)*

TNF-α = tumor necrosis factor-alpha

VEGF = vascular endothelial growth factor

*Correspondence: Division of Pulmonary, Allergy, Critical Care, and Sleep Medicine, Department of Internal Medicine, The Ohio State University, 473 W. 12th Ave., Columbus, Ohio 43210 (e-mail: clay.marsh@osumc.edu).

phenotype, while its absence supports conventional healing.

Cytokines, growth factors, and chemokines are small, soluble proteins that affect the behavior and recruitment of cells. These factors are released from platelets, infiltrating cells, or the local mesenchyme to instigate and sustain effective wound healing and then terminate the inflammatory response. Fortunately, these factors have short half-lives in the wound. This control mechanism reduces the tendency toward chronic inflammation. However, the abnormal presence or absence of any one of these factors during wound healing can lead to continuous inflammation. In the orchestration of normal inflammation, platelets and neutrophils are released passively from injured blood vessels to suppress initial infection. Cell recruitment to the wound is critical and must follow an explicit timetable for normal healing. Chemokines released by keratinocytes and macrophages not only orchestrate cellular traffic but also induce matrix metalloproteinases (MMPs) from various leukocyte subtypes and play a role in tissue remodeling. The profile of a successfully healed wound has low numbers of neutrophils and macrophages, a diminishing number of fibroblasts, and a balance between MMP collagenolysis and collagen synthesis (Fig. 1).

CLINIC PROBLEM ADDRESSED

There are no current gene therapy clinical trials reportedly underway targeting inflammatory cytokines, growth factors, or chemokines that directly influence inflammation or govern immune cell recruitment. However, there are trials underway to optimize recombinant cytokine delivery including adenovirus transfection that would be advantageous for instructing cells of the wound microenvironment to produce anti-inflammatory mediators. Also, genetic methods to manipulate bone marrow stem cells for implantation into wounds for similar cytokine expression are being evaluated.

BASIC SCIENCE CONTEXT

Reports illustrating the presence or absence of both pro- and anti-inflammatory mediators in the wounds of animal models have required the generation of an abundance of transgenic mice over the past decade. These mice have been used to knockout or overexpress cytokines or growth factors thought to be essential for normal wound healing. Further, these mice have facilitated the ability to predict the outcome of chronic wounds with attempts to emulate human pathologies. Porcine models are under development to emulate human wound treatment better than their murine counterparts as mice, unlike humans, have loose skin and heal using purse string contraction.

EXPERIMENTAL MODEL OR MATERIAL

Because wound inflammation results from both a delicate balance and timing of cytokine release, the type of treatment administered to these wounds is relevant to the regulation of these cytokines.

Debridement

Alternatives for surgical debridement are the papain-, urea-, and collagenase-based applications to reduce wound contact and limit damage to emerging granulation tissue. Also, biosurgery techniques such as maggot therapy have been shown to accelerate chronic wound healing by clearing the wound of inflammatory mediators.[1]

Topical treatments

Talactoferrin, an immunomodulatory protein and form of lactoferrin, activates dendritic cells. Topical

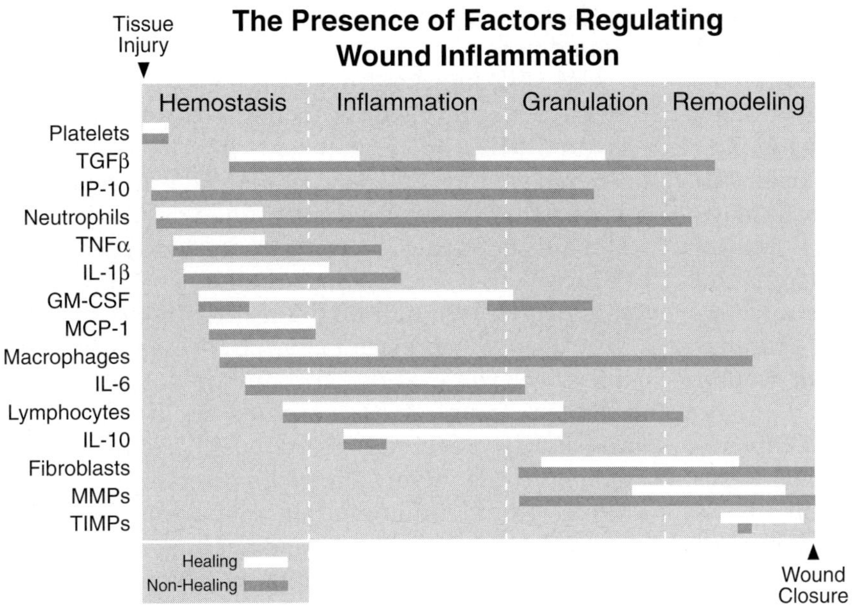

Figure 1. The presence of factors regulating wound inflammation. Chronic wounds persist due to dysregulation of a homeostasis between pro- and anti-inflammatory mediators. Overexpression of TGF-β, TNF-α, and MMPs prolongs the inflammatory phase of normal wound healing and delays granulation and vascularization, while aberrant expression of IL-10 and TIMPs further inhibits wound closure. Lastly, extended occupancy of immune cells like neutrophils and macrophages also contribute to a nonhealing phenotype. The duration of factors present during normal wound healing, white bars, or during the life of chronic wounds, dark bars. TGF-β = transforming growth factor beta; TNF-α = tumor necrosis factor-alpha; MMPs = matrix metalloproteinases; IL-10 = interleukin-10; TIMPs = tissue inhibitor of metalloproteinases.

treatment has significantly accelerated wound closure rates by enhancing the production of inflammatory mediators interleukin-8, interleukin-6 (IL-6), macrophage inflammatory protein-1α (MIP-1α), and tumor necrosis factor-alpha (TNF-α).[2] Propolis, a natural antibiotic produced by trees, improved healing in diabetic rats by controlling neutrophil infiltration into wounds by activation of antiinflammatory pathways.[3]

Nutrition

Polyunsaturated fats in fish oil, eicosapentaenoic acid, and docosahexaenoic acid affects the production of the proinflammatory cytokines associated with initiating and sustaining inflammation.[4]

DISCUSSION OF FINDINGS AND RELEVANT LITERATURE

Most nonhealing wounds fail to advance through the phases of normal tissue repair and remain in a state of inflammation. Over the years, leukocytes have been seen as essential in normal wound healing, but a recent consensus in the literature is to the contrary. Several mouse models illustrate the ability of cutaneous wounds to close without neutrophils and macrophages. Both of these cells are major sources of proinflammatory cytokines that regulate tissue inhibitor of metalloproteinases and MMPs that are elevated in chronic wounds. Consequently, mediators crucial for repair like α2-microgloblin and α1-antitrypsin as well as growth factors that stimulate angiogenesis such as vascular endothelial growth factor (VEGF) and platelet-derived growth factor (PDGF) are substrates for MMP activity. Further, neutrophils are a source of reactive oxygen species that regulate expression of proinflammatory cytokines like interleukin-1 beta (IL-1β), IL-6, and TNF-α. Spleen focus forming virus proviral integration oncogene spi1 (PU.1)–deficient mice, devoid of both neutrophils and macrophages, not only heal wounds effectively, but actually accelerate wound closure.[5] Dovi *et al*. also found accelerated wound closure in neutrophil-depleted mice and even diabetic neutropenic mice heal at a 50% faster rate than wild-type mice.[6]

TAKE-HOME MESSAGE

Basic science advances

- Many studies suggest that a chronic wound is the result of a sustained inflammatory response that prohibits subsequent re-epithelialization and granulation phases.
- A sustained presence of neutrophils and macrophages in wounds leads to a nonhealing phenotype.
- TGF-β is a multifunctional cytokine in wound healing and its expression both increases or reduces wound inflammation depending on the time and location of its expression.
- The process of physiological wound healing entails both the timely release and cessation of inflammatory modulators, namely, TNF-α, IL-1β, IL-6, and IL-10.

Depletion of circulating mononuclear cells in diabetic C57Bl/6J-ob/ob mice using antibodies against F4/80 also accelerates wound closure.[7] Interestingly, not all types of wounds fare better without macrophages. In other studies, macrophages play an important role in wound healing. For example, cryoinjury in mice inducing left ventricular damage in combination with clodronate impairs wound healing. This defect is thought to occur from the secretion of transforming growth factor beta (TGF-β) and VEGF-A, which lead to successful granulation.[8] This study highlights differences in wound types and need for further investigation.

Growth factors like TGF-β, granulocyte/macrophage colony-stimulating factor (GM-CSF), keratinocyte growth factor (KGF), VEGF, and PDGF play roles in both physiological and pathological healing. The number of reports of the pluripotent cytokine TGF-β in wound healing is immense and illustrates the schizophrenic nature of TGF-β. Produced in a latent form by platelets, TGF-β is activated upon proteolytic cleavage. Once activated, it binds receptors on fibroblasts and keratinocytes leading to extracellular matrix production in the wound. TGF-β's role in inflammation stems from its recruitment of inflammatory cells into the wound bed. Various animal studies indicate that active TGF-β in wounds is beneficial for wound closure. A hallmark study on TGF-β was performed by Brown *et al.*,[9] where full-thickness excisional wounds were created on TGF-β1 knockout mice 10 days postpartum. Early phases of wound repair were normal in these mice, demonstrating redundant roles of other TGF-β isoforms at this stage. Ultimately, the lack of TGF-β1 results in a severe inflammatory response accompanied by a marked inflammatory cell infiltrate into the wound, leading to severe late-stage wound-healing defects. Another study performed by Crowe *et al.*[10] removed the influence of the severe inflammatory response accompanying TGF-β knockout mice by crossing with scid$^{-/-}$ mice (where SCID is severe combined immunodeficiency). The absence of both TGF-β1 and T/B cells in these wounds impairs wound closure. The author suggests compensatory roles of TGF-β1 and lymphocytes in these wounds. On the contrary, Ashcroft *et al.*[11] used smad3-null mice (where [SMAD] is *Caenorhabditis elegans* protein] "SMA" and [*Drosophila* protein] "mothers against decapentaplegic") to study TGF-β effects on full-thickness incisional wounds interfering with downstream signaling after TGF-β receptor activation. These mice have reduced inflammation accompanied by accelerated wound closure due to lack of neutrophils and monocytes in the wound bed.

GM-CSF knockout mice were also used in a cutaneous wound-healing model. Fang *et al.*[12] discovered that mice deficient in GM-CSF have delayed wound closure accompanied by a reduction in neutrophils, macrophages, and vascularization. The author suggests that this effect may be due to reduced IL-6, monocyte chemotactic protein-1 (MCP-1/CCL2), and MIP-2 at the wound site and that GM-CSF induces factors that augment keratinocyte proliferation and inflammation. Other relevant growth factors studied are KGF, VEGF, and PDGF. Although essential in wound repair, none of these factors showed a direct role in regulating wound inflammation. For example, KGF-null mice show normal wound healing,[13] whereas a KGF dominant-negative mouse did not.[14] An explanation for this observation may lie in redundant ligand binding to the KGF family of receptors, namely, fibroblast growth factors in KGF-null mice. Although VEGF is observed in chronic wounds, its increase may be simply the result of tissue hypoxia and may not directly contribute to sustained inflammation. Lastly, PDGF-B chain does not show direct influence on wound inflammation, but recruits pericytes and smooth muscle cells to the wound for successful angiogenesis.[15]

To elucidate the specific mediators that orchestrate cell recruitment into wounds, various mouse models targeting specific chemokines have been investigated. IP-10/CXCL10 (where CXC is cysteine–any amino acid–cysteine binding chemokine) is detected at high levels in chronic wounds and recruits neutrophils and lymphocytes. IP-10–overexpressing mice exhibit more intense inflammation and have interrupted granulation and wound closure,[16] supporting the detrimental role of neutrophils. MCP-1/CCL2 is abundant in acute wounds and targets monocyte and fibrocyte recruitment to the wound. MCP-1/CCL2$^{-/-}$ mice exhibit delayed wound angiogenesis and collagen production, but surprisingly, there was no change in the wound macrophage population. These data indicate that other chemokines in the wound environment like MIP-1α/CCL3 and MIP-1β/CCL-4 can recruit macrophages to the wound site.[17]

Inflammation-regulating cytokines relevant in physiological wound healing include TNF-α, IL-1β, IL-6, and IL-10.[18] TNF-α is released by neutrophils upon tissue injury, initiating the early inflammation phase. Recently, Salanova *et al.*[19] reported that neutrophils acquire functional GPIIb/IIIa receptors from platelet-derived microparticles.

These receptors, not endogenously expressed on neutrophils, are incorporated into the cell membrane and lead to augmented TNF-α production when accompanied by the receptor complex for GM-CSF. Activation leads to nuclear factor kappa-light-chain-enhancer of activated B cells nuclear translocation and neutrophil-induced inflammation. Mori *et al.*[20] demonstrated that the absence of TNF-α signaling is beneficial to wound closure using TNF-Rp55 (receptor for TNF-α) knockout mice. Even though data showed a significant reduction of leukocyte migration into the wounds, increases in angiogenesis, collagen, re-epithelialization, and wound closure, most likely due to increases in growth factor production, are observed.

Hubner *et al.*[21] showed that the importance of IL-1 in wound healing as a strong and early induction of IL-1α and β was present after cutaneous injury to IL-1 receptor–deficient mice and wild-type littermates. The highest levels of these cytokines were seen around 12–24 h postwounding, and after completion of the proliferative phase of wound healing these cytokines returned to basal levels.

A role for IL-6, a mixed pro- and anti-inflammatory cytokine that signals through the janus kinase (Jak)/signal transducers and activators of transcription (Stat) pathway and is produced by keratinocytes, is suggested by Gallucci *et al.*[22] by wounding IL-6 knockout mice. The group reported a predictable inflammatory suppression but also a deceleration in wound closure. Recombinant IL-6 administered upon injury rescued wound healing by augmenting inflammation. This study supports the need for IL-6 and early phase inflammation to facilitate late-stage wound healing. This work was corroborated as stat3-deficient mice presented the same wound phenotype as the IL-6 knockout mice.

Finally, IL-10, an anti-inflammatory cytokine, was studied for its role in wound healing by Eming *et al.*[23] Wound closure was accentuated in IL-10–deficient mice as a result of increased myofibroblast differentiation. Interestingly, the number of macrophages in these wounds was significantly increased. This opposes other reports suggesting a suppressive role for macrophages in nonhealing wounds (see above). This study highlights that the mere presence of macrophages in wounds is not enough to predict outcome. The wound microenvironment is likely to play a role in macrophage phenotype and how these cells behave to support or suppress normal wound healing. Further illustrated in this study is the fact that IL-10, an anti-inflammatory cytokine, can impede wound healing.

CAUTION, CRITICAL REMARKS, AND RECOMMENDATIONS

Even though diagnosis and observation has exposed aberrant regulation of both pro- and anti-inflammatory mediators in patients with chronic wounds, the wound healing community, both basic and clinical scientists, must have the discipline and oversight to tread lightly when it comes to gene therapy. The mechanism of successful wound healing is far more complex than merely inducing the expression of an anti-inflammatory factor, or targeting cells for chemokine receptor deletion. Additionally, widening the scope of investigation into chronic wounds to understand the role of cell fragments or microvesicles in the wound bed may be beneficial. These particles are known to carry both proteins and nucleic acids to act on cell types in a paracrine fashion as well as deliver functional proteins to be used by cells in which they do not endogenously express.[19] These studies could lead to novel therapeutic targets.

FUTURE DEVELOPMENT

The elucidation of the regulatory mechanisms governing chronic inflammation in wounds seems to be on the horizon. Each day, reports are published optimizing novel methodologies focused on regulating the inflammatory process during tissue repair. Furthering advances in controlling inflammation at the cellular level, for example, improving the half-life of synthetic extracellular matrix as a new tissue scaffold, should be streamlined for practical application. Also, upgrading debridement reagents and investigating and improving topical treatments would be beneficial to wound clinics. However, probably the most important advances should be in methods of targeted gene expression of growth factors and cytokines that the literature has already established as essential in overcoming chronic wounds.

ACKNOWLEDGMENTS

Research in the author's laboratory is funded by internal support from both The Inflammation and Regenerative Medicine Thematic Groups in the Davis Heart & Lung Research Institute, as well as Battelle Industries and NIH/NHLBI award 2R01HL067176, and NIH/NCI 1 K99CA131552.

AUTHOR DISCLOSURE STATEMENT

No conflict of interests disclosed.

REFERENCES

1. Hunter S, Langemo D, Thompson P, Hanson D, and Anderson J: Maggot therapy for wound management. Adv Skin Wound Care 2009; **22:** 25.

2. Engelmayer J, Blezinger P, and Varadhachary A: Talactoferrin stimulates wound healing with modulation of inflammation. J Surg Res 2008; **149:** 278.

3. McLennan SV, Bonner J, Milne S, Lo L, Charlton A, Kurup S, *et al.*: The anti-inflammatory agent propolis improves wound healing in a rodent model of experimental diabetes. Wound Repair Regen 2008; **16:** 706.

4. McDaniel JC, Belury M, Ahijevych K, and Blakely W: Omega-3 fatty acids effect on wound healing. Wound Repair Regen 2008; **16:** 337.

5. Martin P, D'Souza D, Martin J, Grose R, Cooper L, Maki R, *et al.*: Wound healing in the PU.1 null mouse—tissue repair is not dependent on inflammatory cells. Curr Biol 2003; **13:** 1122.

6. Dovi JV, He LK, and DiPietro LA: Accelerated wound closure in neutrophil-depleted mice. J Leukoc Biol 2003; **73:** 448.

7. Goren I, Muller E, Schiefelbein D, Christen U, Pfeilschifter J, Muhl H, *et al.*: Systemic anti-TNFalpha treatment restores diabetes-impaired skin repair in ob/ob mice by inactivation of macrophages. J Invest Dermatol 2007; **127:** 2259.

8. van Amerongen MJ, Harmsen MC, van Rooijen N, Petersen AH, and van Luyn MJ: Macrophage depletion impairs wound healing and increases left ventricular remodeling after myocardial injury in mice. Am J Pathol 2007; **170:** 818.

9. Brown RL, Ormsby I, Doetschman TC, and Greenhalgh DG: Wound healing in the transforming growth factor-beta-deficient mouse. Wound Repair Regen 1995; **3:** 25.

10. Crowe MJ, Doetschman T, and Greenhalgh DG: Delayed wound healing in immunodeficient TGF-beta 1 knockout mice. J Invest Dermatol 2000; **115:** 3.

11. Ashcroft GS, Yang X, Glick AB, Weinstein M, Letterio JL, Mizel DE, *et al.*: Mice lacking Smad3 show accelerated wound healing and an impaired local inflammatory response. Nat Cell Biol 1999; **1:** 260.

12. Fang Y, Gong SJ, Xu YH, Hambly BD, and Bao S: Impaired cutaneous wound healing in granulocyte/macrophage colony-stimulating factor knockout mice. Br J Dermatol 2007; **157:** 458.

13. Werner S, Smola H, Liao X, Longaker MT, Krieg T, Hofschneider PH, *et al.*: The function of KGF in morphogenesis of epithelium and reepithelialization of wounds. Science 1994; **266:** 819.

14. Guo L, Degenstein L, and Fuchs E: Keratinocyte growth factor is required for hair development but not for wound healing. Genes Dev 1996; **10:** 165.

15. Buetow BS, Crosby JR, Kaminski WE, Ramachandran RK, Lindahl P, Martin P, *et al.*: Platelet-derived growth factor B-chain of hematopoietic origin is not necessary for granulation tissue formation and its absence enhances vascularization. Am J Pathol 2001; **159:** 1869.

16. Luster AD, Cardiff RD, MacLean JA, Crowe K, and Granstein RD: Delayed wound healing and disorganized neovascularization in transgenic mice expressing the IP-10 chemokine. Proc Assoc Am Phys 1998; **110:** 183.

17. Low QE, Drugea IA, Duffner LA, Quinn DG, Cook DN, Rollins BJ, *et al.*: Wound healing in MIP-1alpha(-/-) and MCP-1(-/-) mice. Am J Pathol 2001; **159:** 457.

18. Werner S, and Grose R: Regulation of wound healing by growth factors and cytokines. Physiol Rev 2003; **83:** 835.

19. Salanova B, Choi M, Rolle S, Wellner M, Luft FC, and Kettritz R: Beta2-integrins and acquired glycoprotein IIb/IIIa (GPIIb/IIIa) receptors cooperate in NF-kappaB activation of human neutrophils. J Biol Chem 2007; **282:** 27960.

20. Mori R, Kondo T, Ohshima T, Ishida Y, and Mukaida N: Accelerated wound healing in tumor necrosis factor receptor p55-deficient mice with reduced leukocyte infiltration. FASEB J 2002; **16:** 963.

21. Hubner G, Brauchle M, Smola H, Madlener M, Fassler R, and Werner S: Differential regulation of pro-inflammatory cytokines during wound healing in normal and glucocorticoid-treated mice. Cytokine 1996; **8:** 548.

22. Gallucci RM, Simeonova PP, Matheson JM, Kommineni C, Guriel JL, Sugawara T, *et al.*: Impaired cutaneous wound healing in interleukin-6-deficient and immunosuppressed mice. FASEB J 2000; **14:** 2525.

23. Eming SA, Werner S, Bugnon P, Wickenhauser C, Siewe L, Utermohlen O, *et al.* Accelerated wound closure in mice deficient for interleukin-10. Am J Pathol 2007; **170:** 188.

A Family of Small Cytokines Called Chemokines Is Important in Regulation of Wound Repair

Manuela Martins-Green* and Melissa Petreaca

Department of Cell Biology and Neuroscience, University of California, Riverside, California.

Background: Chemokines are small cytokines that chemoattract leukocytes and modulate angiogenesis and contribute to resolution of the granulation tissue. There are about 50 human chemokines that group into four families: CXC, CC, CX3C, and XC. These small cytokines activate G-protein–linked receptors that are expressed in a variety of cells in the wound tissue. Therefore, chemokine–chemokine receptor interactions are potentially very important in controlling repair.

The Problem: These small cytokines are promiscuous in their binding to receptors, and the receptors can bind to multiple chemokines. This complexity requires sophisticated approaches to understand how this network works in an integrated manner.

Basic/Clinical Science Advances: The major advance made in the field of chemokines and wound healing was the discovery that specific chemokines are expressed/produced in temporal and spatial patterns during wound healing. Clinically, the major contribution to date is the discovery that they bind to seven-transmembrane receptors amenable to small molecule therapy.

Clinical Care Relevance: Chemokines have potential as therapeutic agents in several ways. One can use modified antagonists of the proteins themselves or of their N-termini; use monoclonal antibodies directed either to a specific chemokine or to its receptor; and use small molecules that inhibit their receptors. Because the pertinent chemokines are produced in sequence during wound healing, it is possible to take advantage of this and apply treatments in a strategic manner.

Conclusion: Current knowledge of chemokine biology should propel the field toward a better understanding of the contribution that chemokine dysregulation makes to chronic inflammation, excess or impaired angiogenesis, and, equally important but more challenging, their role in pathological wound healing.

Abbreviations and Acronyms

AHA = American Heart Association

ECM = extracellular matrix

NIH = National Institute of Health

TRDRP = Tobacco-Related Disease Research Program

*Correspondence: Department of Cell Biology and Neuroscience, University of California, 900 University Ave., Riverside, California 92521 (e-mail: manuela.martins@ucr.edu).

BACKGROUND

Wound healing is a complex process in which proinflammatory cytokines recruit various types of leukocytes to the injured area, where they function as key players during the inflammatory phase of healing. These leukocytes arrive at the site of injury in a temporally defined manner and localize in spatially defined patterns in the repaired tissue. Neutrophils arrive first, then disappear when monocytes/macrophages arrive, and, finally, as the latter are disappearing, lymphocytes arrive. If the healing progresses normally, each of these cell types disappears in as orderly a fashion as they arrive. During their presence in the injured tissue, macrophages secrete a number of cytokines that set in motion the next phase of repair, which involves

Printed in U.S.A.
DOI: 10.1089/awc.2009.0123

cell proliferation, extracellular matrix (ECM) deposition, and development of blood vessels to knit the tissue together in a productive manner. Finally, during the remodeling phase, the lymphocytes disappear and much of the other cell types, ECM molecules, and blood vessels are eliminated.[1,2]

Chemokines are chemotactic cytokines that play critical functions not only in the regulation of immune cell networks, but also in inflammatory responses and in the development of new blood vessels from preexisting vessels, that is, angiogenesis. Therefore, these small cytokines are poised to act effectively in tissue repair.[3]

In humans, this family of cytokines is composed of about 50 different chemokines that bind to G-protein–linked seven-transmembrane receptors (Table 1). There are four subfamilies of chemokines, the CXC, the CC, the XC, and the CX3C, based on the number of amino acids present between the two first cysteines in the molecule.[4] Chemokines are small basic proteins (8–12 kDa) that in general act as monomers, but can also function as dimers or higher-order oligomers, and bind to their G-protein–linked receptors in regions of acidic amino acids. In addition, chemokines also bind to glycosaminoglycans that are present on the cell surface and in this manner can form haptotactic gradients that are essential for chemotaxis (directional movement) of the leukocytes to the site of injury.[5] CXC and CC chemokines make up the bulk of the chemokines. Although some are involved in the homeostatic traffic of leukocytes, most are primarily involved in inflammatory processes and in angiogenesis.[6] In this review, we will focus on the role of CXC and CC chemokines and their receptors in the various phases of wound healing.

Table 1. *Chemokine–chemokine receptor superfamily*

CXC Chemokines	CXC Receptors	CC Chemokines	CC Receptors
CXCL1	CXCR2	CCL1	CCR8
CXCL2	CXCR2	CCL2	CCR2
CXCL3	CXCR2	CCL3	CCR1, CCR5
CXCL4	N/A*	CCL4	CCR5
CXCL5	CXCR2	CCL5	CCR1, CCR3, CCR5
CXCL6	CXCR1, CXCR2	CCL6	N/A*
CXCL7	CXCR2	CCL7	CCR1, CCR2, CCR3
CXCL8	CXCR1, CXCR2	CCL8	CCR3, CCR5
CXCL9	CXCR3	CCL9/10	CCR1
CXCL10	CXCR3	CCL11	CCR3
CXCL11	CXCR3	CCL12	CCR2
CXCL12	CXCR4	CCL13	CCR2, CCR3
CXCL13	CXCR5	CCL14	CCR1, CCR5
CXCL14	N/A*	CCL15	CCR1, CCR3
CXCL15/16	CXCR6	CCL16	CCR1, CCR2
		CCL17	CCR4
XC Chemokines	**XC Receptors**	CCL18	N/A*
XCL1	XCR1	CCL19	CCR7
XCL2	XCR1	CCL20	CCR6
		CCL21	CCR7
CX3C Chemokines	**CX3 Receptors**	CCL22	CCR4
CX3CL1	CX3CR1	CCL23	CCR1
		CCL24	CCR3
		CCL25	CCR9
		CCL26	CCR3
		CCL27	CCR10
		CCL28	CCR3/CCR10

*N/A Non-Applicable

CLINICAL PROBLEM ADDRESSED

The clinical problem that needs to be addressed relates to situations in which inflammation becomes chronic and angiogenesis is either absent or excessive, leading to impaired healing and chronic wounds. Because chemokines are so closely involved in the regulation of both inflammation and angiogenesis, one could envision that manipulation of this network of cytokines could modulate either or both of these processes.[7] Further, because chemokines from the CXC and CC families are expressed throughout the wound-healing process in specific temporal and spatial patterns, this network of proteins lends itself to providing regulated control for proper healing.[3,8]

BASIC SCIENCE CONTEXT

Basic research performed to understand the role of chemokines in wound healing has revealed that the CXC are key players.[9,10] This subfamily can be further divided into those that contain the Glu-Leu-Arg (ELR) motif adjacent to the first two cysteines and those that do not contain this domain. The ELR+ chemokines are proinflammatory and play important roles in chemoattracting leukocytes. For example, CXCL8 and CXCL1 are produced within hours of injury and are strong chemoattractants of neutrophils, the first set of leukocytes arriving at the wound site.[3] In addition, CXCL8 stimulates endothelial cell permeability by co-opting the vascular endothelial growth factor receptor 2, thereby facilitating neutrophil extravasation through stimulation of endothelial permeability[11]; CXCL8 then binds to its receptors, CXCR1/CXCR2, on these leukocytes, promoting their chemoattraction to the site of injury, where they clear the wound of infection and cellular debris. These chemokines also function in angiogenesis early in granulation tissue formation,[12–14] and in the differentiation of fibroblasts to myofibroblasts that promote wound contraction.[15] Once at the site of injury, neutrophils produce CCL2, a monocyte chemoattractant protein, which in turn attracts monocytes that subsequently undergo differentiation into macrophages.[16] These leukocytes, along with the fibroblasts, are the workhorses of the healing process by playing major roles in development of the granulation tissue.

All chemokine receptors identified to date belong to the superfamily of G-protein–linked seven-transmembrane receptors, which are a type of receptors that are ideally suited for the development of small molecular inhibitors, making them highly amenable for drug therapy.[4] The fact that there are fewer receptors than there are chemokines indicates that at least some of the chemokine receptors have more than one ligand, leading to a complicated network of interactions, which must be taken into consideration when studying these molecules. These interactions depend not only on the presence of specific receptors on the cell surface, but also on the microenvironment that provides the context for presentation of the chemokines to their receptors.[5]

EXPERIMENTAL MODEL OR MATERIAL

The possibility of using models other than humans to study the function of chemokines in the processes involved in wound healing is problematic because the network of chemokines and receptors in humans differs from those in animal models, in particular, rodent models, which are the most commonly used model systems. Studies in normal healing in humans, using excision wounds, have provided insight into the temporal and spatial patterns of expression of chemokines during the healing process.[8,17] It was found that the recruitment of the various leukocyte types is regulated by chemokines and that chemokine receptors are expressed in cells resident in the wound and during wound healing. Unfortunately, mechanistic studies in humans are very difficult because of the inability to manipulate the system effectively. In general, healing in pigs and rabbits more closely resembles healing in humans. Not much is known about the chemokine network in pigs or in rabbits, but because the healing process is close to that of humans, inferences can be made from the human studies. The problem with these larger animal models is that, unlike mouse models, they do not lend themselves to genetic manipulation for functional studies. Mouse models, however, have the potential for inclusion or removal of chemokines and/or their receptors. Studies in mice defective in the CXCR2, a promiscuous receptor that binds many of the proinflammatory chemokines, have shown that healing is delayed.[9] The problem with these studies is that the mice are already immune-compromised before the wounds are generated; therefore, it is difficult to determine the contributions of this receptor and its ligands to healing.[9] Another mouse model that overexpresses CXCL10 shows delayed healing with defects in neovascularization,[18] whereas mice deficient in CXCL11 or CXCR3 exhibit abnormal re-epithelialization.[19,20] Despite these findings, we know that mice do not have the gene for a key proinflammatory chemokine in humans, CXCL8, and the functionality of the specific receptor for this chemokine, CXCR1, is controversial in mice.[21,22] The lack of this critical chemokine–receptor pair in mice may fundamentally change the chemokine–receptor network in these animals, limiting the applicability of data obtained from mouse models to our understanding of human chemokine–receptor networks in wound healing. We have recently developed a mouse line that is a conditional transgenic for the human CXCR1 receptor, which can be manipulated by crossing with specific Cre mice.[23,24] *In vivo*, when human CXCL8 is injected under the skin of a mouse that overexpresses CXCR1 only in lymphocytes, these cells are recruited to the site of injection, indicating that the receptor is functional and able to respond to its ligand.[24] These mice are otherwise normal in every way we have examined; thus, we expect to be able to address specific roles of human CXCL8 in healing by stimulating the expression of this receptor in specific cells by crossing with mice expressing Cre recombinase under the control of various tissue-specific promoters.

DISCUSSION OF FINDINGS AND RELEVANT LITERATURE

Chemokines have become an integral part of the network of cytokines operating during wound healing. The first evidence that chemokines are associated with healing was reported in 1990, when it was found that chicken CXCL8 (at that time named 9E3/cCAF [chicken chemotactic and angiogenic factor]) is overexpressed during wound healing. This chemokine is highly expressed in the first 4–48 hours after injury. It is primarily expressed by the fibroblasts of the tissue, especially where interstitial collagen is abundant, and by the endothelial cells of microvessels of the granulation tissue.[12,25,26]

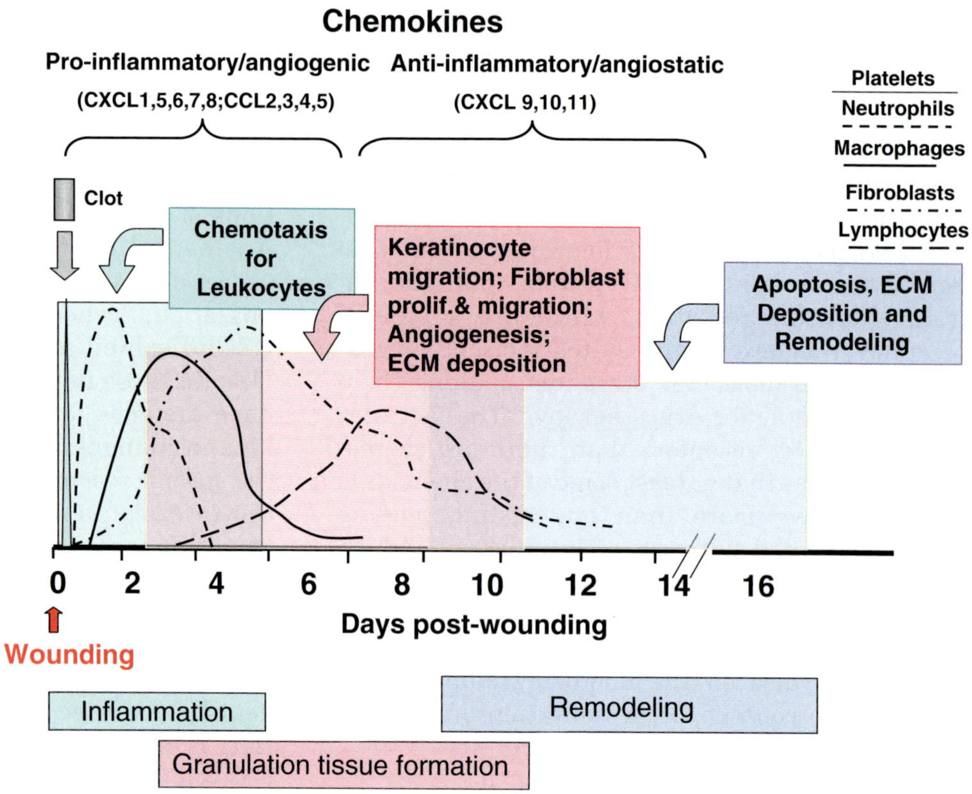

Figure 1. Chemokines and their roles in the various phases of wound healing. Immediately after wounding, formation of the clot initiates a series of events that lead to the inflammatory phase of wound healing. Platelet granules release a number of molecular mediators; among them is the chemokine CXCL4, which is antiangiogenic and ensures that blood vessels do not develop prematurely. CXCL1 and 8 are also produced shortly after wounding and chemoattract neutrophils, which rid the wound of bacteria and foreign materials.[31] Neutrophils, in turn, produce CCL2, a potent chemoattractant of monocyte/macrophages. These leukocytes clean up the debris and dead neutrophils, and, along with other cells in the wound (*e.g.*, fibroblasts), produce a plethora of growth factors and cytokines, among which are the chemokines CXCL8 and CCL2, 3, 4, and 5. CCL2 will continue to attract more macrophages until fibrinogen in the wound disappears, at which time macrophage arrival stops. At this time in the progression of the healing process, CXCL8, along with vascular endothelial growth factor, stimulates angiogenesis. CCL3, 4, and 5 are instrumental in bringing in lymphocytes that are the last major type of leukocytes present in the wound tissue. CXCL9, 10, and 11 are produced a bit later during healing and are known to be anti-inflammatory and anti-angiogenic or angiostatic. These chemokines are present in the right place at the right time to ensure that angiogenesis is terminated and inflammation is resolved.

Today we know that other chemokines are stimulated shortly after injury (Fig. 1) (*e.g.*, CXCL1, 4, 5, and 7; CCL2, 3, 4, and 5), and produced during the inflammatory phase (*e.g.*, CXCL1 and 8; CCL2) and in the granulation tissue (CCL3, 4, and 5; CXCL9, 10, and 11).[3,10] The injury response chemokines CXCL1, 5, 7, and 8 initiate neutrophil chemotaxis through the CXCR2 receptor, whereas CXCL4 participates in the coagulation process and prevents the premature development of blood vessels.[6] Of the inflammatory phase chemokines, CXCL8 is a key potent chemoattractant for neutrophils through both CXCR1 and CXCR2, and is a very effective activator of neutrophil activation through CXCR1.[27] CCL2, produced by neutrophils and fibroblasts, is the critical chemokine that chemoattracts the next wave of leukocytes coming to the wound site, the monocytes.[28] After arrival at the wound site, monocytes differentiate into macrophages, which then, along with fibroblasts, produce chemokines such as CXCL8, which with vascular endothelial growth factor and basic fibroblast growth factor stimulate angiogenesis.[1] During granulation tissue development, the CCL3, 4, and 5 chemokines attract lymphocytes, the next wave of leukocytes, which function in the final stages of development of this tissue. Finally, the angiostatic chemokines CXCL9, 10, and 11 are produced, in part stimulated by interferon γ and tumor necrosis factor α, and are instrumental in terminating angiogenesis. The effects of these three angiostatic chemokines are mediated by CXCR3, a receptor that is expressed in a cell cycle–dependent manner, leading to inhibition of endothelial cell proliferation when bound to its ligands. In addition to the receptor-mediated effects of chemokines, these proteins also affect the wound-healing process via receptor-independent events.[29]

Considerable knowledge has been obtained on the factors and mechanisms involved in the initiation of inflammation and angiogenesis, but little is known about the key players and the mechanisms involved in resolution of these processes. The chemokine network is a good candidate for controlling both the initiation of inflammation and for termination of angiogenesis. Lack of regulation of this complex network of cytokines can result in chronic inflammation, deregulation of blood vessel development, and establishment of a chronic wound environment. Because these chemokines are small proteins that do not have modifications other than the two disulfide bonds, are stable, and are amenable to large-scale production, it is possible to use these proteins or peptides corresponding to functional regions as adjuvants for wound therapy. Further, the fact that they bind G-protein–linked receptors increases the likelihood that their biological pathways can be controllable by small chemical molecules. Although chemokine-loaded dressings have not been used to deliver these proteins to wounds, the chemokine chicken CXCL8 has been delivered to excision wounds in chickens and found to accelerate wound healing,[15] stimulate fibroblasts to acquire a myofibroblastic phenotype,[15] and modulate ECM deposition.[30]

CAUTION, CRITICAL REMARKS, AND RECOMMENDATION

Although considerable knowledge has been acquired regarding expression and production of chemokines at the wound site, very little is known about their functions during healing, and much less is known about the integrated function of this network of small cytokines. In performing such studies, it is important to remember that many chemokines bind more than one receptor, and that the reverse is also true, making the elucidation of specific roles very complex. It is also critical that those performing studies on chemokines in wound healing carefully consider the model to be used, given that the most commonly used model system is the murine, which does not fully mimic human healing.[10] The best way to approach these problems is to use genetically modified models, and to verify these findings by using human organ cultures that mimic functional human tissues *in vivo*, and, when possible, confirming the results in humans.

FUTURE DEVELOPMENTS

Several studies have demonstrated the importance of chemokines in inflammation and in angiogenesis during normal wound healing. It is also important to note that the sequence of expression/production of chemokines during wound healing is known. This knowledge will facilitate modulation of the function of these small cytokines during healing and should propel the field toward a better understanding of the mechanisms whereby chemokine dysregulation may contribute to chronic inflammation and excessive or impaired angiogenesis. Equally important, but more challenging, the evidence presented above can contribute to the understanding of the role of chemokines in pathological wound healing. In addition, the development of models that mimic chronic wounds in humans is of para-

TAKE-HOME MESSAGE

Basic science advances

- Chemokines are small basic molecules (8–12 kDa) with a simple structure and two disulfide bonds (as their only modifications) that help fold the protein into its functional structure.
- They are highly conserved proteins.
- They bind to G-protein–linked receptors that cross the plasma membrane seven times (seven-transmembrane receptors).
- Chemokines bind to their receptor in acidic pockets, and many can bind different receptors, conferring redundancy and complexity to the system.
- Chemokine functions in wound healing are inducible.
- Chemokines are expressed in a temporal and spatial manner during wound healing.

Clinical science advances

- The activation of G-protein coupled receptors by chemokines is highly significant for the clinic because these receptors are very amenable to development of small molecules that control function.
- Chemokines are highly conserved in vertebrates.
- Because chemokines are small proteins without modifications, their agonist/antagonist peptides can be made by recombinant means and directed to fold properly.
- Chemokines are associated with impaired healing, with a variety of skin disorders, and with chronic inflammation.
- They are important in aspects of tumor development related to inflammation and angiogenesis.

Relevance to clinical care

- Although not much has been done in the clinic regarding the use of chemokines and/or their receptors as a basis for treatment, these molecules have a great deal of potential.
- Chronic inflammation can potentially be reduced or eliminated by interfering with proinflammatory chemokines and/or their receptors.
- A number of approaches can be used:
  - Small molecules that inhibit the receptors
  - Modified antagonists of chemokines or their N-termini
  - Neutralizing monoclonal antibodies directed to either the chemokine or its receptor
- More studies on the role of chemokines/receptors need to be performed to use them effectively in the clinic.

mount importance, and should be a focus of future studies.

ACKNOWLEDGMENTS

The research in wound healing and in chemokines has been funded by National Institutes of Health (NIH), American Heart Association (AHA), Tobacco-Related Disease Research Program (TRDRP), and Philip Morris to Manuela Martins-Green, and by numerous fellowships and awards.

AUTHOR DISCLOSURE STATEMENT

Author M.M.-G. holds a patent on the effects of the chicken CXCL8 in differentiation of fibroblasts into myofibroblasts (US Patent no. 09/811, 162).

REFERENCES

1. Singer AJ and Clark RA: Cutaneous wound healing. N Engl J Med 1999; **341:** 738.
2. Werner S and Grose R: Regulation of wound healing by growth factors and cytokines. Physiol Rev 2003; **83:** 835.
3. Gillitzer R and Goebeler M: Chemokines in cutaneous wound healing. J Leukoc Biol 2001; **69:** 513.
4. Rossi D and Zlotnik A: The biology of chemokines and their receptors. Annu Rev Immunol 2000; **18:** 217.
5. Proudfoot AE, Handel TM, Johnson Z, Lau EK, Li-Wang P, Clark-Lewis I, Borlat F, Wells TN, and Kosco-Vilbois MH: Glycosaminoglycan binding and oligomerization are essential for the *in vivo* activity of certain chemokines. Proc Natl Acad Sci USA 2003; **100:** 1885.
6. Zlotnik A, Yoshie O, and Nomiyama H: The chemokine and chemokine receptor superfamilies and their molecular evolution. Genome Biol 2006; **7:** 243.
7. Romagnani P, Lasagni L, Annunziato F, Serio M, and Romagnani S: CXC chemokines: the regulatory link between inflammation and angiogenesis. Trends Immunol 2004; **25:** 201.
8. Engelhardt E, Toksoy A, Goebeler M, Debus S, Brocker EB, and Gillitzer R: Chemokines IL-8, GROalpha, MCP-1, IP-10, and Mig are sequentially and differentially expressed during phase-specific infiltration of leukocyte subsets in human wound healing. Am J Pathol 1998; **153:** 1849.
9. Devalaraja RM, Nanney LB, Du J, Qian Q, Yu Y, Devalaraja MN, and Richmond A: Delayed wound healing in CXCR2 knockout mice. J Invest Dermatol 2000; **115:** 234.
10. Zaja-Milatovic S and Richmond A: CXC chemokines and their receptors: a case for a significant biological role in cutaneous wound healing. Histol Histop 2008; **23:** 1399.
11. Petreaca ML, Yao M, Liu Y, Defea K, and Martins-Green M: Transactivation of vascular endothelial growth factor receptor-2 (VEGFR2) by interleukin-8 (IL-8/CXCL8) is required for IL-8/CXCL8-induced endothelial permeability. Mol Biol Cell 2007; **18:** 5014.
12. Martins-Green M and Bissell MJ: Localization of 9E3/CEF-4 in avian tissues: expression is absent in Rous sarcoma virus-induced tumors but is stimulated by injury. J Cell Biol 1990; **110:** 581.
13. Koch AE, Polverini PJ, Kunkel SL, Harlow LA, DiPietro LA, Elner VM, Elner SG, and Strieter RM: Interleukin-8 as a macrophage-derived mediator of angiogenesis. Science 1992; **258:** 1798.
14. Strieter R, Polverini P, Kunkel SL, Arenberg DA, Burdick MD, Kasper J, Dzuiba J, Van Damme J, Walz A, Marriott D, Sham-Yen C, Roczniak S, and Shanafelt AB: The functional role of the ELR motif in CXC chemokine-mediated angiogenesis. J Biol Chem 1995; **270:** 27348.
15. Feugate JE, Li Q, Wong L, and Martins-Green M: The cxc chemokine cCAF stimulates differentiation of fibroblasts into myofibroblasts and accelerates wound closure. J Cell Biol 2002; **156:** 161.
16. DiPietro LA, Polverini PJ, Rahbe SM, and Kovacs EJ: Modulation of JE/MCP-1 expression in dermal wound repair. Am J Pathol 1995; **146:** 868.
17. Eming SA, Krieg T, and Davidson JM: Inflammation in wound repair: molecular and cellular mechanisms. J Invest Dermatol 2007; **127:** 514.
18. Luster AD, Cardiff RD, MacLean JA, Crowe K, and Granstein RD: Delayed wound healing and disorganized neovascularization in transgenic mice expressing the IP-10 chemokine. Proc Assoc Am Physicians 1998; **110:** 183.
19. Yates CC, Whaley, D, Y-Chen A, Kulesekaran P, Hebda PA, and Wells A: ELR-negative CXC chemokine CXCL11 (IP-9/I-TAC) facilitates dermal and epidermal maturation during wound repair. Am J Pathol 2008; **173:** 643.
20. Yates CC, Whaley D, Hooda S, Hebda PA, Bodnar RJ, and Wells A: Delayed reepithelialization and basement membrane regeneration after wounding in mice lacking CXCR3. Wound Repair Regen 2009; **17:** 34.
21. Moepps B, Nuesseler E, Braun M, and Gierschik P: A homolog of the human chemokine receptor CXCR1 is expressed in the mouse. Mol Immunol 2006; **43:** 897.
22. Fan X, Patera AC, Pong-Kennedy A, Deno G, Gonsiorek W, Manfra DJ, Vassileva G, Zeng M, Jackson C, Sullivan L, Sharif-Rodriguez W, Opdenakker G, Van Damme J, Hedrick JA, Lundell D, Lira SA, and Hipkin RW: Murine CXCR1 is a functional receptor for GCP-2/CXCL6 and interleukin-8/CXCL8. J Biol Chem 2007; **282:** 11658.
23. Zheng L, Njauw CN, and Martins-Green M: A hCXCR1 transgenic mouse model containing a conditional color-switching system for imaging of hCXCL8/IL-8 functions *in vivo*. J Leukoc Biol 2007; **82:** 1247.
24. Zheng L, Njauw CN, and Martins-Green M: A one-plasmid conditional color-switching transgenic system for multimodal bioimaging. Transgenic Res 2008; **17:** 741.
25. Martins-Green M, Aotaki-Keen A, Hjelmeland LM, and Bissell MJ: The 9E3 protein: immunolocalization *in vivo* and evidence for multiple forms in culture. J Cell Sci 1992; **101 (Pt 3):** 701.
26. Martins-Green M and Hanafusa H: The 9E3/CEF4 gene and its product the chicken chemotactic and angiogenic factor (cCAF): potential roles in wound healing and tumor development. Cytokine Growth Factor Rev 1997; **8:** 221.
27. Jones SA, Wolf M, Qin S, Mackay CR, and Baggiolini M: Different functions for the interleukin 8 receptors (IL-8R) of human neutrophil leukocytes: NADPH oxidase and phospholipase D are activated through IL-8R1 but not IL-8R2. Proc Natl Acad Sci USA 1996; **93:** 6682.
28. Yoshimura T, Yuhki N, Moore SK, Appella E, Lerman MI, and Leonard EJ: Human monocyte chemoattractant protein-1 (MCP-1). Full-length cDNA cloning, expression in mitogen-stimulated blood mononuclear leukocytes, and sequence similarity to mouse competence gene JE. FEBS Lett 1989; **244:** 487.
29. Rosenkilde MM and Schwartz TW: The chemokine system—a major regulator of angiogenesis in health and disease. APMIS 2004; **112:** 481.
30. Feugate JE, Wong L, Li QJ, and Martins-Green M: The CXC chemokine cCAF stimulates precocious deposition of ECM molecules by wound fibroblasts, accelerating development of granulation tissue. BMC Cell Biol 2002; **3:** 1.

Amplifying Healing: The Role of Antimicrobial Peptides in Wound Repair

Katherine A. Radek and Richard Louis Gallo*

Division of Dermatology, Department of Medicine, University of California, San Diego, California.

Background: Since discovering antimicrobial peptides (AMPs) in mammalian tissues during the 1990s, dramatic strides have been made toward elucidating their multifunctional roles during inflammatory processes, including tissue repair. With the emergence of antibiotic-resistant bacteria, these host defense peptides represent a promising alternative to minimize infection while stimulating cellular functions to maximize wound repair.
The Problem: A major obstacle hindering the development of AMP-based therapies for wound care is the limited number of effective animal model systems. Although many AMPs are active in *in vitro* systems, current *in vivo* models require supraphysiologic peptide concentrations that are often toxic to the host. The development of more effective topical therapies may help circumvent this clinical impediment. Further, many AMPs have been misclassified and studied as antimicrobials when their primary role is that of chemotactic, growth factor activation, or pro-angiogenic origin.
Basic/Clinical Science Advances: In 1994, initial evidence for mammalian AMPs was observed by identifying their role as inducers of proteoglycan expression during wound repair. Subsequent studies established that many AMPs exert their activity by modulating other aspects of wound healing, including keratinocyte migration, angiogenesis, and matrix synthesis.
Clinical Care Relevance: Therapeutic regimens consisting of multiple AMPs combined with conventional antibiotics, designed to reduce microbial colonization while concurrently stimulating host immunomodulatory functions, represent a promising approach to wound care.
Conclusion: As the spectrum of immunomodulatory functions of AMPs expands, we face the challenge of designing peptide treatment regimens that maintain their ability to stimulate wound repair processes, while minimizing host toxicity. Gaining further insight into mechanisms by which AMPs influence healing signifies the potential therapeutic strategies that can be applied to nonhealing wounds.

Abbreviations and Acronyms

AMPs = antimicrobial peptides

hBD = human beta defensins

HNP = human neutrophil peptides

VEGF = vascular endothelial growth factor

*Correspondence: Division of Dermatology, Department of Medicine, University of California, La Jolla, San Diego, California 92161 (e-mail: rgallo@vapop.ucsd.edu).

BACKGROUND

Our appreciation for the complexity of the innate immune system and its role in tissue defense and repair has expanded rapidly in the last decade. Although the acute inflammatory response was initially limited to growth factors and inflammatory cells, antimicrobial peptides (AMPs) are now deemed a fundamental component of the innate immune system. AMPs were initially identified during the 1980s in both insects and plants as small, gene-encoded peptides that contributed to their resistance to pathogens. Two major categories of AMPs, the defensins and the cathelicidins, were subsequently identified and

Printed in U.S.A.
DOI: 10.1089/awc.2009.0129

characterized across a multitude of species. Defensins were originally discovered as positively charged peptides in human and rabbit neutrophils that exerted antimicrobial activity against bacteria and viruses.[1] Cathelicidins were later identified in mammalian species, with the porcine cathelicidin PR-39 representing the first of many AMPs present in mammalian skin, specifically in porcine wound fluid.[2] The significance of AMPs to mammalian immunity was initially underestimated because of a popular bias toward study of adaptive cell-mediated immune defense systems. However, AMPs have since been found to be abundantly upregulated in a variety of epithelia under both physiologic and pathologic conditions, such as wound healing, and are now recognized as an essential component of the mammalian immune response. Further, recent studies have expanded the repertoire of functions for AMPs to include not only their capacity to function as peptide antibiotics, but also their ability to stimulate multiple elements of the wound healing response.

CLINICAL PROBLEM ADDRESSED

Infection and pathologic inflammation represent two daunting challenges associated with the treatment of acute and chronic wounds, contributing to substantial psychosocial and economic burdens. Pathogenic microbes have evolved sophisticated mechanisms to resist the actions of antibiotics through alterations in membrane protein composition, activation of energy-dependent transporters, or secretion of proteolytic enzymes.

Skin and soft tissue infections account for over 27% of hospital-acquired infections, many of which have methicillin-resistant *Staphylococcus aureus* as the etiologic agent.[3] Further, vancomycin-resistant *Enterococcus* and multidrug-resistant *Pseudomonas* are emerging pathogens frequently isolated from ducubiti and diabetic ulcers.[4,5] Chronic wounds are characterized by aberrant inflammatory responses and are highly prone to both functional restrictions and infection. Understanding the complex molecular mechanisms by which AMPs minimize invasive infections, while orchestrating normal progression of wound healing, is critical for developing therapeutic regimens that restore normal equilibrium in wounds.

BASIC SCIENCE CONTEXT

AMPs are short proteins (~10–50 amino acids) synthesized and stored in epithelial and immune tissues to serve as an immediate chemical impediment to invasive infection under normal homeostasis or after the physical barrier has been breached. Factors that impact the efficacy of AMPs include their size, charge, protein sequence, structural conformation, and degree of hydrophobicity. Cutaneous AMP expression is enhanced under physiologic or pathologic conditions after an increase in gene and protein expression in resident cells, as well as by deposition after degranulation of neutrophils.[6–8] Cathelicidins and defensins comprise the two main classifications of AMPs in humans, although a surplus of other AMPs also reside in a variety of tissues.

Humans possess a single cathelicidin gene that encodes for hCAP18/LL-37, a pro-protein with a highly conserved N-terminal cathelin domain and a variable antimicrobial C-terminal domain. Cathelicidin is constitutively expressed in some cell types, such as eccrine epithelia, while inducible in other types, such as keratinocytes, after infection and/or injury. The human cathelicidin peptide, LL-37, is comprised of 37 amino acids that conforms to a positively charged α-helical structure in physiologic solutions.[9] Processing of the LL-37 from the hCAP18 cathelin precursor domain is critical for maximal activation of both its antimicrobial activity and immunomodulatory functions.[10–12] Although LL-37 is often referred to as the sole human cathelicidin, in reality it represents only one of many potential peptides that can be proteolytically cleaved from the carboxy-terminus of the hCAP18 precursor protein.[12]

Defensins are also synthesized as pro-proteins that are proteolytically processed into small, cationic peptides. In humans they are classified into two major families, the α- and β-defensins, that contain individual characteristic disulfide bridges for the formation of a β-sheet structure, which facilitates their interactions with target microbial membranes. In humans, neutrophils express α-defensins 1–4 (human neutrophil peptides [HNP] 1–4), while intestinal Paneth cells express α-defensins 5 and 6 (human α-defensins 5 and 6). There are over 20 distinct mRNAs for the defensins dispersed throughout various tissues, with the β-defensins (human β-defensins [hBD] 1–4) being more extensively expressed in mucosal and cutaneous epithelia compared with α-defensins.[13] Similarly to cathelicidins, most α-defensins require proteolytic processing for their activation, with the exception of human α-defensins 5.[14] In contrast, most β-defensins exhibit short N-terminal sequences to maintain activity in their full-length forms.[15] Differential regulation and expression of defensins have been observed in wound-associated responses in various tissues, including skin, lung, and intestine.[15–17]

EXPERIMENTAL MODEL

To date, few AMP experimental model systems exist that are reminiscent of the human response to injury and infection. Cathelicidin was identified as an essential component of innate host defense in 2001. Mice encoding a disruption in the cathelicidin gene, *Camp*, were rendered highly susceptible to invasive Group A *Streptococcus* infection.[18] Although this mouse model allows for the study of both the antimicrobial and immunomodulatory role of cathelicidin, there are significant differences in cathelicidin regulation between human and mouse likely related to the evolutionary nocturnal adaptation of mice. In human keratinocytes, cathelicidin induced maximal upregulation (>100-fold) in the presence of $1,25(OH)_2$ vitamin D_3 compared with other hormones, cytokines, or microbial products.[19] Further, wounded human skin exhibited a significant increase in cathelicidin expression and 1,25 vitamin D_3 catabolic enzymes.[20] One major caveat with the cathelicidin mutant mouse model is that mice lack the vitamin D_3 responsive element within the *Camp* promoter, and thus their keratinocytes do not respond to $1,25(OH)_2$ vitamin D_3 normally obtained by exposure to sunlight and dietary nutrients. Mice deficient in β-defensin-1 also exhibited delayed lung clearance of *Haemophilus influenzae* and increased bladder colonization of *Staphylococcus* species.[21,22] Nonetheless, mice deficient in *Camp* and mouse β-defensin-1 have provided useful and significant information regarding the role of AMPs in innate immune defense and wound repair that has been extrapolated to human systems.

In vitro model systems have clearly demonstrated the killing capacity of AMPs against numerous microbes. However, many assays were not performed under physiologic conditions, which is critical for their optimal function. In 2006, a study found that carbonate that is present in most buffered aqueous solutions (such as blood and wound fluid) acts as a critical ionic factor that allows for cathelicidins and defensins to kill microbes at physiologic salt and serum concentrations.[9] Thus, the *in vivo* environment dictates how AMPs will impart their ability to function as antibiotics or cell signaling molecules.

DISCUSSION OF FINDINGS AND RELEVANT LITERATURE

The initial discovery of AMPs in mammalian skin was made when PR-39, a proline-rich porcine cathelicidin peptide, was identified in wound fluid.[2] PR-39 enhanced the expression of cell surface heparan sulfate proteoglycans syndecan-1 and -4 that enabled cells involved in wound repair to become more responsive to elements of the microenvironment and thus promote cell proliferation and migration. Further studies provided evidence for AMPs as direct cell signaling molecules during wound healing, irrespective of their antimicrobial and immunomodulatory functions (Fig. 1).

Two critical growth factors involved in wound healing, insulin-like growth factor-1 and transforming growth factor-α, induce distinct expression profiles of several keratinocyte AMPs that can then directly stimulate epithelial cells to both migrate and proliferate.[17] Treatment of organ-cultured human skin with antibodies against LL-37 exhibited a dose-dependent decrease in re-epithelialization and suppression of keratinocyte proliferation, suggesting that LL-37 may directly participate in keratinocyte proliferation and migration during normal wound repair.[23] Further studies confirmed that LL-37 promoted heparin-binding–mediated transactivation of epidermal

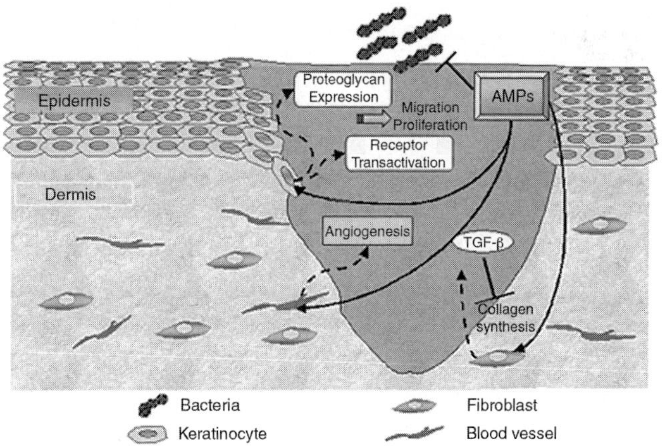

Figure 1. Major functions for antimicrobial peptides (AMPs) in wound healing. AMPs can impart microbicidal activity against invading microbes, while stimulating selective components of inflammation, re-epithelialization, angiogenesis, and matrix formation that are beneficial to the host. These peptides induce a multitude of responses in resident skin cells such as keratinocytes, fibroblasts, and endothelial cells. AMPs modify gene and protein expression of host proteins, increase production of chemokines and cytokines, induce receptor activation, influence matrix synthesis and degradation, and promote vascular proliferation. The consequence of this diverse cell signaling modulation is a well-orchestrated progression of tissue repair that restores normal functional capacity.

TAKE-HOME MESSAGE

Basic science advances

- In addition to their antibiotic activity, AMPs also enhance selective innate immune responses and manipulate precise immunomodulatory actions upon host signaling pathways.
- Reduced AMP expression is observed in multiple types of poorly healing wounds, including diabetic ulcers and burn wounds.
- Cathelicidins and defensins are dramatically upregulated at the wound edge after injury, and show a direct relationship between their expression and the rate of wound healing.
- AMPs enhance wound closure in skin and other tissues through specific cell signaling pathways in epithelial cells.
- AMPs are required for activating vessel regrowth during wound angiogenesis, which may implicate their role in chronic wounds resulting from poor vascularization.
- Cathelicidin-deficient mice exhibit defects in microbial host defense, but also show delayed wound closure and angiogenesis.
- AMPs contribute to the regulation of extracellular matrix proteins and enzymes to favor matrix deposition during the remodeling phase of tissue repair.
- AMPs are natural multifunctional peptides with the potential to manipulate several aspects of wound repair and represent an important component of innate immunity that warrants further investigation and characterization to yield promising treatments for wound care.

Clinical science advances

- AMPs embody an inspiring new approach to the treatment of infection and tissue repair, and may help surmount the emergent dilemma of antibiotic-resistant bacteria frequently observed in wound infections.
- Synthetically designed peptides have been recently engineered to enhance potency against a wide variety of pathogens and retain their immunomodulatory activity, with less cytotoxicity than those used in earlier trials.
- Manipulation of unique combinations of synthetic AMPs in conjunction with antibiotics may prove a successful treatment strategy to minimize bacterial antibiotic resistance while promoting immunomodulatory functions specific to each patient's distinct requirements to improve nonhealing wounds.

Relevance to clinical care

- During the last decade, numerous AMP regimens have been used in various clinical trials and have shown promise. Designer synthetic peptides such as proline-Novispirin G10™[35] (Novozymes, Denmark) and Demegel™[34] (Demegen, Pittsburgh, PA) were shown to exhibit minimal cytotoxicity while still providing sufficient microbicidal activity and chemotactic ability in burn injury models *in vivo.* Recently, the broad-spectrum magainin analog, Pexiganan™,[36] (Magainin Pharmaceuticals, Plymouth Meeting, PA [original] Now Manufactured by Macrochem) was used as a topical cream for the treatment of mild, superficially infected diabetic foot ulcers and shown to be comparable to treatment with oral antibiotics, and shown not to induce allergic sensitization as seen with other topical antibiotics. Future clinical trials using synthetic AMP regimens may yield promising results to not only reduce wound infection rates, but also improve the overall rate of healing to augment wound closure, reverse vascular insufficiency, and enhance matrix remodeling.

growth factor receptor via phosphorylation and subsequent activation of STAT proteins to enhance keratinocyte migration.[24,25] LL-37 was recently implicated in keratinocyte cytoskeletal rearrangement leading to enhanced wound closure *in vitro*.[26] Adenoviral transfer of LL-37 to excisional wounds significantly increased wound closure and granulation tissue formation in the healing-impaired diabetic ob/ob mouse, indicating the *in vivo* role for LL-37 in promoting wound closure.

The defensin family of AMPs was also shown to influence keratinocyte function and their response to injury. hBD 2–4 increased keratinocyte expression of multiple pro-inflammatory cytokines, while promoting intracellular mobilization of calcium that resulted in enhanced keratinocyte migration and proliferation.[24] Defensins NP-1 and NP-2 were also elevated in tear fluid after corneal epithelial abrasion, and appeared to directly correlate to wound closure.[27] Collectively, AMPs appear to be direct signaling molecules that enhance epithelial functions required for normal wound repair, particularly migration and proliferation of keratinocytes.

Angiogenesis is vital for wound revascularization and is both positively and negatively influenced by AMPs, linking inflammation and innate immune defense through angiogenesis. Administration of LL-37 induced neovascularization in both the chorioallantoic membrane assay and in a mouse model of hind-limb ischemia via the formyl peptide receptor-like 1 expressed on endothelial cells.[28] Further, cathelicidin-deficient mice exhibited a significant reduction in wound angiogenesis. PR-39 was later shown to act as an antiapoptotic factor in endothelial cells during hypoxia, which would be particularly critical during early tissue repair when wounds are considerably hypoxic.[29] hBD-2 was recently shown to stimulate chemotaxis and wound closure of human umbilical vein endothelial cells similarly to vascular endothelial growth factor (VEGF), while stimulating the formation of capillary networks on Matrigel even in the presence of a VEGF antibody, indicating a novel

VEGF-independent mechanism for vessel formation through hBD-2.[30] In contrast to cathelicidin and β-defensins, the α-defensins HNP-1–4 were determined to negatively regulate angiogenesis by diminishing the $\alpha5\beta1$-mediated endothelial cell adhesion and migration toward fibronectin, inhibited VEGF-induced proliferation, induced apoptosis, and blocked the formation of capillary tubes in three-dimensional fibrin matrices. Lactoferrin, a glycoprotein exhibiting antimicrobial properties, significantly increased VEGF-induced extracellular signal-related kinase mitogen–associated protein kinase phosphorylation in endothelial cells and correlated with an increase in cell proliferation and migration, suggesting a potential role for lactoferrin in angiogenesis.[31,32] Thus, AMPs may be of clinical value in promoting angiogenesis in wounds that exhibit vascular insufficiency, as frequently observed in diabetic patients with ischemic ulcers.

Synthesis of extracellular matrix molecules and proteolytic enzymes during wound repair is required for wound closure and restoration of wound strength and functional capacity. HNP-1, a member of the α-defensins, significantly increased the expression of neutrophil collagen type I mRNA and protein, while reducing the expression of the matrix degrading enzyme, matrix metalloproteinase-1.[33] Keratinocytes incubated with increasing concentrations of LL-37 exhibited an enhanced matrix metalloproteinase activation, and an increase in the urokinase-type plasminogen activator receptor that allows for cellular migration.[26] Further, LL-37 directly influenced dermal fibroblasts by inhibiting transforming growth factor-β–induced collagen expression through the activation of extracellular signal–related kinase, indicating an anti-fibrotic role for cathelicidin in wound healing.

Synthetically engineered AMPs have been designed to increase potency and activity against cutaneous pathogens associated with burn and chronic wounds, yet remain noncytotoxic. Such peptides include demegel, pexiganin, and proline novospirinG10 and have been efficient in reducing bacterial load in burns and diabetic wounds.[34–36] Potentially, these peptides may also be used to improve other aspects of wound repair to minimize the overall incidence of wound infection and dehiscence in nonhealing wounds.

CAUTION, CRITICAL REMARKS, AND RECOMMENDATIONS

The mounting obstacle of antibiotic-resistant bacteria and the requirement for alternative antimicrobial agents has rendered AMPs as potential candidates for the development of therapeutic molecules. AMPs can both inhibit microbial growth, while stimulating precise facets of inflammation, angiogenesis, and matrix formation that are beneficial to the host. One must also bear in mind that a particular function observed with one AMP might not necessarily be applied to other AMPs, even within the same family. The use of AMPs as therapeutics represents a double-edged sword when used as modulators of host cell signaling. Thus, a fine balance must be maintained to encourage host inflammatory signaling pathways without development of chronic inflammation, particularly relevant when dealing with systemic therapeutics. Topical therapy for treating sterile and infected chronic wounds appears to be a hopeful route for administration of AMPs, as it can circumvent potential undesirable systemic effects, has minimal risk for inducing antibiotic resistance, and encourages patients to assess their wound when applying daily topical treatment. However, some lingering obstacles exist for the treatment of infected and/or chronic skin wounds and include minimal tissue penetrability, unknown cytotoxicity, and high production costs, all of which may be surmounted in future clinical trials.

FUTURE DEVELOPMENTS

Further identification of ancillary mechanisms by which AMPs can exert selective modulatory effects on host tissue repair will yield additional treatment strategies for use with current AMP therapeutics. The use of AMPs to provide a prompt but provisional response in nonhealing wounds may promote tissue repair sufficient to prevent further colonization with invasive bacteria and restore barrier function to support cellular proliferation, while limiting the chronic inflammation. The expansion of safe, multifactorial treatments incorporating several AMPs designed to manipulate specific cellular processes that are defective in particular subsets of nonhealing wounds will vastly impact wound care management. Collectively, the conserved structural characteristics, in combination with the diverse array of tissue specificity and function, make AMPs exclusive candidates for the design of novel drug therapeutics that target nonhealing wounds.

ACKNOWLEDGMENTS

Wound healing research conducted in the author's laboratory is funded by a Veterans Affairs Merit Award and National Institutes of Health Grants: NIH/NIAID HHSN26620040029C, ADB contract nos. N01-AI-40029AI48176, AI052453, and AR45676 to Richard Louis Gallo; NIH/NIAMS F32AR054220 to Katherine A. Radek.

AUTHOR DISCLOSURE STATEMENT

No conflict of interest is disclosed.

REFERENCES

1. Ganz T, Selsted ME, Szklarek D, Harwig SS, Daher K, Bainton DF, and Lehrer RI: Defensins. Natural peptide antibiotics of human neutrophils. J Clin Invest 1985; **76:** 1427.
2. Gallo RL, Ono M, Povsic T, Page C, Eriksson E, Klagsbrun M, and Bernfield M: Syndecans, cell surface heparan sulfate proteoglycans, are induced by a proline-rich antimicrobial peptide from wounds. Proc Natl Acad Sci USA 1994; **91:** 11035.
3. Lipsky BA, Weigelt JA, Gupta V, Killian A, and Peng MM: Skin, soft tissue, bone, and joint infections in hospitalized patients: epidemiology and microbiological, clinical, and economic outcomes. Infect Control Hosp Epidemiol 2007; **28:** 1290.
4. Lee DC, Barlas D, Ryan JG, Ward MF, Sama AE, and Farber BF: Methicillin-resistant *Staphylococcus aureus* and vancomycin-resistant enterococci: prevalence and predictors of colonization in patients presenting to the emergency department from nursing homes. J Am Geriatr Soc 2002; **50:** 1463.
5. Tascini C, Gemignani G, Palumbo F, Leonildi A, Tedeschi A, Lambelet P, Lucarini A, Piaggesi A, and Menichetti F: Clinical and microbiological efficacy of colistin therapy alone or in combination as treatment for multidrug resistant *Pseudomonas aeruginosa* diabetic foot infections with or without osteomyelitis. J Chemother 2006; **18:** 648.
6. De Y, Chen Q, Schmidt AP, Anderson GM, Wang JM, Wooters J, Oppenheim JJ, and Chertov O: LL-37, the neutrophil granule- and epithelial cell-derived cathelicidin, utilizes formyl peptide receptor-like 1 (FPRL1) as a receptor to chemoattract human peripheral blood neutrophils, monocytes, and T cells. J Exp Med 2000; **192:** 1069.
7. Di Nardo A, Vitiello A, and Gallo RL: Cutting edge: mast cell antimicrobial activity is mediated by expression of cathelicidin antimicrobial peptide. J Immunol 2003; **170:** 2274.
8. Dorschner RA, Pestonjamasp VK, Tamakuwala S, Ohtake T, Rudisill J, Nizet V, Agerberth B, Gudmundsson GH, and Gallo RL: Cutaneous injury induces the release of cathelicidin anti-microbial peptides active against group A Streptococcus. J Invest Dermatol 2001; **117:** 91.
9. Dorschner RA, Lopez-Garcia B, Peschel A, Kraus D, Morikawa K, Nizet V, and Gallo RL: The mammalian ionic environment dictates microbial susceptibility to antimicrobial defense peptides. FASEB J 2006; **20:** 35.
10. Murakami M, Lopez-Garcia B, Braff M, Dorschner RA, and Gallo RL: Postsecretory processing generates multiple cathelicidins for enhanced topical antimicrobial defense. J Immunol 2004; **172:** 3070.
11. Sorensen OE, Follin P, Johnsen AH, Calafat J, Tjabringa GS, Hiemstra PS, and Borregaard N: Human cathelicidin, hCAP-18, is processed to the antimicrobial peptide LL-37 by extracellular cleavage with proteinase 3. Blood 2001; **97:** 3951.
12. Yamasaki K, Schauber J, Coda A, Lin H, Dorschner RA, Schechter NM, Bonnart C, Descargues P, Hovnanian A, and Gallo RL: Kallikrein-mediated proteolysis regulates the antimicrobial effects of cathelicidins in skin. FASEB J 2006; **20:** 2068.
13. Selsted ME and Ouellette AJ: Mammalian defensins in the antimicrobial immune response. Nat Immunol 2005; **6:** 551.
14. Ghosh D, Porter E, Shen B, Lee SK, Wilk D, Drazba J, Yadav SP, Crabb JW, Ganz T, and Bevins CL: Paneth cell trypsin is the processing enzyme for human defensin-5. Nat Immunol 2002; **3:** 583.
15. van Wetering S, Sterk PJ, Rabe KF, and Hiemstra PS: Defensins: key players or bystanders in infection, injury, and repair in the lung? J Allergy Clin Immunol 1999; **104:** 1131.
16. Otte JM, Werner I, Brand S, Chromik AM, Schmitz F, Kleine M, and Schmidt WE: Human beta defensin 2 promotes intestinal wound healing *in vitro*. J Cell Biochem 2008; **104:** 2286.
17. Sorensen OE, Cowland JB, Theilgaard-Monch K, Liu L, Ganz T, and Borregaard N: Wound healing and expression of antimicrobial peptides/polypeptides in human keratinocytes, a consequence of common growth factors. J Immunol 2003; **170:** 5583.
18. Nizet V, Ohtake T, Lauth X, Trowbridge J, Rudisill J, Dorschner RA, Pestonjamasp V, Piraino J, Huttner K, and Gallo RL: Innate antimicrobial peptide protects the skin from invasive bacterial infection. Nature 2001; **414:** 454.
19. Schauber J, Dorschner RA, Yamasaki K, Brouha B, and Gallo RL: Control of the innate epithelial antimicrobial response is cell-type specific and dependent on relevant microenvironmental stimuli. Immunology 2006; **118:** 509.
20. Schauber J, Dorschner RA, Coda AB, Buchau AS, Liu PT, Kiken D, Helfrich YR, Kang S, Elalieh HZ, Steinmeyer A, Zugel U, Bikle DD, Modlin RL, and Gallo RL: Injury enhances TLR2 function and antimicrobial peptide expression through a vitamin D-dependent mechanism. J Clin Invest 2007; **117:** 803.
21. Morrison G, Kilanowski F, Davidson D, and Dorin J: Characterization of the mouse beta defensin 1, Defb1, mutant mouse model. Infect Immun 2002; **70:** 3053.
22. Moser C, Weiner DJ, Lysenko E, Bals R, Weiser JN, and Wilson JM: beta-Defensin 1 contributes to pulmonary innate immunity in mice. Infect Immun 2002; **70:** 3068.
23. Heilborn JD, Nilsson MF, Kratz G, Weber G, Sorensen O, Borregaard N, and Stahle-Backdahl M: The cathelicidin anti-microbial peptide LL-37 is involved in re-epithelialization of human skin wounds and is lacking in chronic ulcer epithelium. J Invest Dermatol 2003; **120:** 379.
24. Niyonsaba F, Ushio H, Nakano N, Ng W, Sayama K, Hashimoto K, Nagaoka I, Okumura K, and Ogawa H: Antimicrobial peptides human beta-defensins stimulate epidermal keratinocyte migration, proliferation and production of proinflammatory cytokines and chemokines. J Invest Dermatol 2007; **127:** 594.
25. Tokumaru S, Sayama K, Shirakata Y, Komatsuzawa H, Ouhara K, Hanakawa Y, Yahata Y, Dai X, Tohyama M, Nagai H, Yang L, Higashiyama S, Yoshimura A, Sugai M, and Hashimoto K: Induction of keratinocyte migration via transactivation of the epidermal growth factor receptor by the antimicrobial peptide LL-37. J Immunol 2005; **175:** 4662.
26. Carretero M, Escamez MJ, Garcia M, Duarte B, Holguin A, Retamosa L, Jorcano JL, Rio MD, and Larcher F: *In vitro* and *in vivo* wound healing-promoting activities of human cathelicidin LL-37. J Invest Dermatol 2009; **128:** 223.
27. Zhou L, Beuerman RW, Huang L, Barathi A, Foo YH, Li SF, Chew FT, and Tan D: Proteomic analysis of rabbit tear fluid: defensin levels after an experimental corneal wound are correlated to wound closure. Proteomics 2007; **7:** 3194.
28. Koczulla R, von Degenfeld G, Kupatt C, Krotz F, Zahler S, Gloe T, Issbrucker K, Unterberger P, Zaiou M, Lebherz C, Karl A, Raake P, Pfosser A, Boekstegers P, Welsch U, Hiemstra PS, Vogelmeier C, Gallo RL, Clauss M, and Bals R: An angiogenic role for the human peptide antibiotic LL-37/hCAP-18. J Clin Invest 2003; **111:** 1665.
29. Wu J, Parungo C, Wu G, Kang PM, Laham RJ, Sellke FW, Simons M, and Li J: PR39 inhibits apoptosis in hypoxic endothelial cells: role of inhibitor apoptosis protein-2. Circulation 2004; **109:** 1660.
30. Baroni A, Donnarumma G, Paoletti I, Longanesi-Cattani I, Bifulco K, Tufano MA, and Carriero MV: Antimicrobial human beta-defensin-2 stimulates migration, proliferation and tube formation of human umbilical vein endothelial cells. Peptides 2009; **30:** 267.
31. Kim CW, Son KN, Choi SY, and Kim J: Human lactoferrin upregulates expression of KDR/Flk-1 and stimulates VEGF-A-mediated endothelial cell proliferation and migration. FEBS Lett 2006; **580:** 4332.
32. Weinberg ED: Antibiotic properties and applications of lactoferrin. Curr Pharm Des 2007; **13:** 801.

33. Oono T, Shirafuji Y, Huh WK, Akiyama H, and Iwatsuki K: Effects of human neutrophil peptide-1 on the expression of interstitial collagenase and type I collagen in human dermal fibroblasts. Arch Dermatol Res 2002; **294:** 185.

34. Chalekson CP, Neumeister MW, and Jaynes J: Improvement in burn wound infection and survival with antimicrobial peptide D2A21 (Demegel). Plast Reconstr Surg 2002; **109:** 1338.

35. Jacobsen F, Mohammadi-Tabrisi A, Hirsch T, Mittler D, Mygind PH, Sonksen CP, Raventos D, Kristensen HH, Gatermann S, Lehnhardt M, Daigeler A, Steinau HU, and Steinstraesser L: Antimicrobial activity of the recombinant designer host defence peptide P-novispirin G10 in infected full-thickness wounds of porcine skin. J Antimicrob Chemother 2007; **59:** 493.

36. Lipsky BA, Holroyd KJ, and Zasloff M: Topical versus systemic antimicrobial therapy for treating mildly infected diabetic foot ulcers: a randomized, controlled, double-blinded, multicenter trial of pexiganan cream. Clin Infect Dis 2008; **47:** 1537.

WHS
Wound
Healing
Society

Lipid Mediators: Important Regulators of Cutaneous Wound Inflammation

Traci A. Wilgus*

Department of Pathology, The Ohio State University, Columbus, Ohio.

Abbreviations and Acronyms

AA = arachidonic acid

AT = aspirin triggered

COX = cyclooxygenase

DHA = docosahexaenoic acid

EPA = eicosapentaenoic acid

LO = lipoxygenase

LT = leukotrienes

LX = lipoxins

NSAIDs = nonsteroidal anti-inflammatory drugs

PD = DHA-derived protectin

PG = prostaglandin

PUFAs = polyunsaturated fatty acids

RvD = DHA-derived resolvin

RvE = EPA-derived resolvin

TX = thromboxanes

*Correspondence: Department of Pathology, The Ohio State University, 129 Hamilton Hall, 1645 Neil Ave., Columbus, Ohio 43210 (e-mail: traci.wilgus@osumc.edu).

Background: Inflammation is an acute reaction to injury, but it has long-lasting effects on the repair process. Bioactive lipids, particularly those derived from polyunsaturated fatty acids, are important inflammatory mediators. Most lipid mediators are pro-inflammatory, but recent studies have identified a role for anti-inflammatory lipids during the resolution of inflammation. Both pro-inflammatory and anti-inflammatory lipids are likely involved in the regulation of wound inflammation.

The Problem: Inflammation is necessary for preventing wound infection, but persistent inflammation can delay healing and promote fibrosis. Lipid mediators are known to regulate inflammation, but their role in repair is not well studied and little is known about what controls the resolution of wound inflammation.

Basic/Clinical Science Advances: The recent identification of several anti-inflammatory and pro-resolving lipids suggests that the resolution of inflammation during wound healing is an active process. Determining how these pro-resolving lipids function during repair could be important for understanding the requirements for successful healing.

Clinical Care Relevance: Modulating the levels of bioactive lipids during the inflammatory phase of wound repair could be a promising approach for enhancing healing by optimizing bacterial killing, accelerating wound closure, or reducing scar formation.

Conclusion: While there is an established role for bioactive lipids in the control of inflammation, the function of these molecules in the context of wound healing must be clarified. New information could increase our understanding of what governs the induction and resolution of inflammation during repair, ultimately aiding in the development of new wound-healing therapies.

BACKGROUND

Inflammation is involved in many pathological processes, including carcinogenesis, atherosclerosis, and the response to injury. While a vigorous inflammatory response was once considered vital for the healing of cutaneous wounds, views on the relative importance of inflammation in wound healing have evolved. Recent studies have indicated that normal wounds may elicit a more robust inflammatory response than what is actually required for optimal healing. Experiments have shown that at early stages of development fetal skin can heal without a scar, but scarless healing can only occur in the absence of inflammation.[1–8] In adult wound-healing models, reducing inflammation can enhance repair by accelerating closure and reducing scar formation.[9–11] In addition, an overzealous inflammatory response can be detrimental, as improper or delayed resolution of inflammation is

ADVANCES IN WOUND CARE, VOLUME 1

Printed in U.S.A.
DOI: 10.1089/awc.2009.0040

often associated with chronic or poorly healing wounds.[12,13]

Bioactive lipids represent one of the many types of mediators that regulate inflammation. Classes of inflammatory lipid mediators include the endocannabinoids (anandamides, 2-arachidonoylglycerol, arachindonoyl ethanolamide), lysophospholipids (lysophosphatidic acid, sphingosine-1-phosphate), and polyunsaturated fatty acid (PUFA)-derived lipids (prostaglandins [PG], leukotrienes [LT], lipoxins [LX], resolvins, protectins). While some studies have suggested a role for endocannabinoids and lysophospholipids in response to injury,[14,15] the PUFA-derived lipids have been the focus of most wound-healing studies.

Various lipid mediators with diverse biological actions during inflammation are generated from PUFAs. They are derived largely from the omega-6 PUFA arachidonic acid (AA) and the omega-3 PUFAs docosahexaenoic acid (DHA) and eicosapentaenoic acid (EPA).[16] AA metabolites, collectively referred to as eicosanoids, are the most commonly studied. Due to the availability of the broad class of nonsteroidal anti-inflammatory drugs (NSAIDs), much is known about the role of PGs in inflammation. NSAIDs inhibit the conversion of AA to PGs by targeting cyclooxygenase (COX) enzymes and are effective in reducing PG-associated pain and inflammation.[17] While most lipid mediators are pro-inflammatory, anti-inflammatory lipid mediators also exist. The LXs, which are produced from AA by the lipoxygenase (LO) enzymes, are anti-inflammatory. Lipid mediators derived from DHA and EPA, including the resolvins and protectins, have anti-inflammatory functions and are thought to promote the resolution of inflammation.[16] In addition, novel pro-resolving lipids called maresins were recently identified in macrophages, suggesting that there is still much left to learn about the resolution of inflammation.[18]

CLINICAL PROBLEM ADDRESSED

Wound repair consists of a series of phases including periods of inflammation, proliferation, and scar formation/remodeling.[19,20] The inflammatory phase is induced rapidly upon injury and has long-lasting effects, influencing later wound-healing events such as reepithelialization, angiogenesis, and scar formation. Optimal healing relies on an effective inflammatory response that terminates in a timely manner. Ineffective inflammation or improper clearance of microbes can lead to infection, while an exaggerated inflammatory response can delay healing (as in the case of diabetic wounds) or lead to excessive scarring. PGs are one class of pro-inflammatory lipids that can influence healing, and their production is inhibited by NSAIDs. There is widespread use of NSAIDs in the general population, and they can be used to relieve pain postoperatively or during surgical wound debridement. NSAIDs have been shown to be effective for post-operative pain management when used alone and to have opioid-sparing effects when used as part of a combination therapy.[21] Despite the common use of NSAIDs, surprisingly little is known about how these drugs affect clinical healing outcomes.

BASIC SCIENCE CONTEXT

Bioactive lipids are critical mediators of inflammation and are involved in the induction, maintenance, and resolution of inflammation. PUFA-derived lipids are the most extensively studied class of lipids with respect to wound healing. Eicosanoids derived from AA make up the largest class of well-characterized inflammatory lipid mediators. Two distinct classes of enzymes are responsible for producing the majority of eicosanoids from AA during acute inflammation: the COX enzymes (COX-1; COX-2) and the LO enzymes (5-LO; 12-LO; 15-LO). PGs, thromboxanes (TXs), and prostacyclins are produced by the COX enzymes, whereas LTs and LXs are generated by the LO enzymes[22] (Fig. 1). With the exception of the LXs, eicosanoids are pro-inflammatory and help trigger classic acute inflammatory events, including vasoconstriction, vasodilation, vascular permeability, and innate immune cell recruitment.[23] Some eicosanoids, such as PGI_2 (prostacyclin) and PGE_2, have also been shown to regulate angiogenesis during wound healing.[24,25] While the majority of the lipid mediators are pro-inflammatory, anti-inflammatory lipids do exist and have been gaining attention recently. LXs were the first lipids recognized as having anti-inflammatory functions, and since then resolvins and protectins have also been identified. These anti-inflammatory lipids can block neutrophil transmigration and infiltration, increase phagocytosis of apoptotic neutrophils by macrophages, and stimulate the sequestration of chemokines by neutrophils.[16,26,27] The primary enzymes responsible for the synthesis of anti-inflammatory lipids are the LOs. LXs (LXA_4; LXB_4) are derived from AA, and anti-inflammatory lipids can also be generated from EPA (resolvin E1/RvE1; resolvin E2/RvE2) and DHA (resolvin D1/RvD1; protectin D1/PD1).[16] Recent studies suggest that resolvins undergo metabolic inactivation, which may facilitate the restoration of

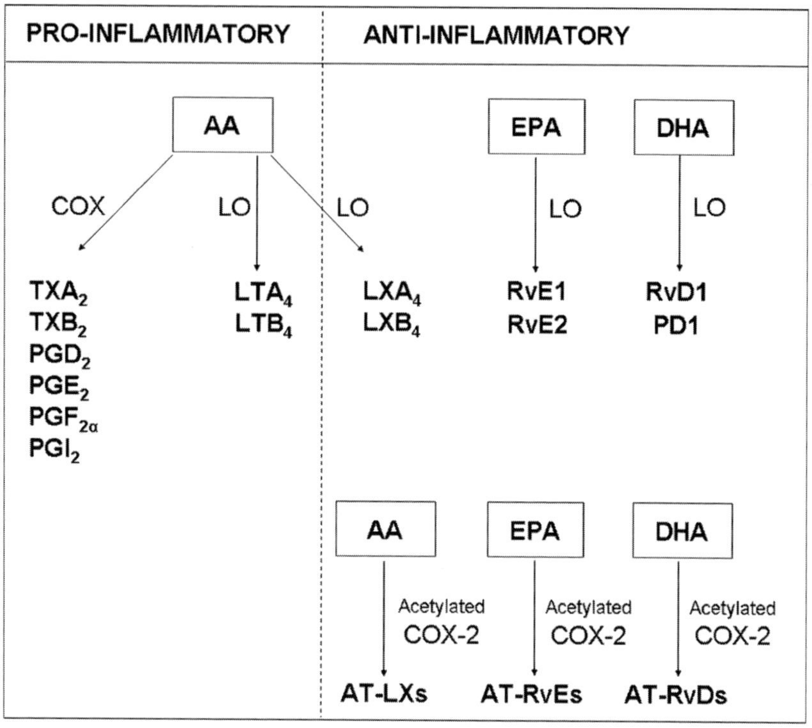

Figure 1. Schematic of inflammatory lipid synthetic pathways. Pro-inflammatory (left) and anti-inflammatory (right) lipid mediators regulate the induction and resolution of inflammation. These lipids are synthesized from polyunsaturated fatty acids, such as arachidonic acid (AA), eicosapentaenoic acid (EPA), and docosahexaenoic acid (DHA). The initial steps in a series of reactions converting precursor fatty acids to pathway end-products are catalyzed by the cyclooxygenase (COX) and lipoxygenase (LO) enzymes. AA is converted to pro-inflammatory thromboxanes and prostaglandins via the COX pathway. AA can also be converted to pro-inflammatory leukotrienes or anti-inflammatory lipoxins (LXs) via LO-mediated pathways. LO enzymes are also involved in the production of anti-inflammatory resolvins (RvEs and RvDs) and protectins from EPA and DHA. Anti-inflammatory lipids can also be generated via a different mechanism by COX-2 in the presence of aspirin. Aspirin-acetylated COX-2 can catalyze the formation of aspirin-triggered (AT) forms of the lipoxins (AT-LXs) and resolvins (AT-RvEs and AT-RvDs) from AA, EPA, or DHA. For more information about the structures of the bioactive lipids and their precursors, please see reviews by Serhan[22] and Gronert.[50]

homeostasis.[28] A new class of pro-resolving lipids derived from DHA via LO enzymes in macrophages termed maresins have also recently been identified.[18] In addition to LO-catalyzed reactions, anti-inflammatory lipids can also be produced through an alternate pathway by COX-2 in the presence of aspirin. Aspirin acetylates COX-2, allowing production of aspirin-triggered (AT) forms (epimers) of the LXs and resolvins.[23] Overall, the production of anti-inflammatory lipids suggests that the resolution of inflammation is an active process and not simply a passive process resulting from the gradual decline in the levels of pro-inflammatory lipids.[16] While there is some information about the importance of pro-inflammatory lipids in wound repair, the significance of the anti-inflammatory lipids is not known.

EXPERIMENTAL MODEL OR MATERIAL

The role of lipid mediators in inflammation has been shown in various models of acute and chronic inflammation. Although less is known about the role of lipid mediators in wound inflammation compared to other models of inflammation, there is evidence that they play a significant role in regulating the inflammatory phase of repair.[11,29,30] Much of the research to date has focused on the pro-inflammatory effects of the AA-derived eicosanoids, namely LTs and PGs. The eicosanoids have a wide range of effects during acute inflammation and are involved in the regulation of vasoconstriction (TXA_2, LTs), vasodilation (PGI_2, PGE_1, PGE_2, PGD_2), vascular permeability (LTs), and chemotaxis and adhesion of neutrophils (LTB_4).[23] The PGs have been studied extensively since the discovery that their production is reduced by NSAIDs. This class of pharmaceuticals, which includes the commonly used drugs ibuprofen, naproxen, and aspirin, block the conversion of AA to pro-inflammatory PGs by inhibiting the enzymatic activity of both cyclooxygenases (COX-1; COX-2). Based on the distinct biological roles of the COX enzymes, with COX-1 being involved in maintaining homeostasis and COX-2 contributing more significantly to inflammation, and the gastrointestinal toxicity associated with COX-1 inhibition, COX-2–selective NSAIDs were developed.[17] Systemic administration of selective COX-2 inhibitors, such as rofecoxib (Vioxx) and celecoxib (Celebrex), were effective in alleviating chronic pain and inflammation, but were found to have serious cardiovascular side effects.[17] Nevertheless, these drugs continue to be useful tools for studying the role of eicosanoids in inflammation and disease processes. The interest in the COX enzymes that grew after the development of COX-2 inhibitors also led to the generation of COX-1 and COX-2 knockout mice, which have been used to study the role of these enzymes and their PG products in wound repair.

DISCUSSION OF FINDINGS AND RELEVANT LITERATURE

The majority of published research investigating the role of lipid mediators in wound healing focuses on PGs. Several studies have shown that COX-1 expression remains relatively constant during healing in contrast to COX-2, which is present at low levels in uninjured skin but is highly expressed in wounded tissue.[31,32] COX-2 is produced in various cell types after injury, including keratinocytes, endothelial cells, fibroblasts, and macrophages,[31–33] and is thought to be the primary enzyme responsible for increased production of the pro-inflammatory mediator PGE_2 in wounded skin.[11,33] Studies have suggested that high COX-2 protein expression and PG production in chronic venous leg ulcers may contribute to the failure of these wounds to properly resolve inflammation and close efficiently.[33]

Both selective and nonselective NSAIDs as well as COX knockout mice have been used to study the role of the PGs in wound healing with varied results. One study showed that incisional wounds from COX-1 and COX-2 knockout mice display reduced tensile strength but no macroscopic healing abnormalities,[34] while another described alterations in wound architecture in COX-1 knockout mice.[35] Although COX knockout mice exhibit some alterations in healing, less severe healing differences have been described with COX inhibitors. Systemic treatment with diclofenac (nonselective NSAID) or SC-791 (COX-2 inhibitor) did not affect keratinocyte proliferation or differentiation, angiogenesis, or tensile strength in incisional mouse wounds.[32] Systemic administration of indomethacin (nonselective NSAID) or NS-398 (COX-2 inhibitor) in excisional rat wounds[31] and oral administration of valdecoxib (COX-2 inhibitor) or SC-560 (COX-1 inhibitor) in incisional mouse wounds[36] resulted in slight delays in early reepithelialization with no effect on tensile strength.

A role for COX-2 and PGE_2 in cutaneous scar formation has also been demonstrated. Topical treatment with the COX-2 inhibitor celecoxib significantly reduced neutrophil infiltration and scar formation in incisional mouse wounds without adversely affecting tensile strength.[11] PGE_2 has also been shown to promote fibrosis in several studies. One study used a mouse model of fetal wound healing in which E15 (embryonic day 15) skin wounds heal without a scar and E18 (embryonic day 18) wounds heal with a scar. In this system, COX-2 was expressed at higher levels and more PGE_2 was produced in scar-forming E18 wounds compared to scarless E15 wounds.[37] Further, injection of PGE_2 into E15 wounds, which normally heal without a scar, caused delayed healing and scar tissue production.[37] A pro-fibrotic role for PGE_2 has also been demonstrated in studies indicating that treatment with PGs increases collagen production and fibrosis.[38,39] Although PGE_2

TAKE-HOME MESSAGE

Basic science advances

- Inflammation can have beneficial or detrimental effects on wound healing; an effective inflammatory response can prevent infection, but persistent, nonresolving inflammation is associated with chronic wounds and excessive scar formation.
- Lipid mediators derived from the PUFAs (AA; DHA; EPA) are critical regulators of inflammation.
- Many bioactive lipids are pro-inflammatory (TXs; PGs; LTs), but anti-inflammatory lipids (LXs; resolvins; protectins) also exist, and are thought to limit inflammation and promote resolution.
- Both pro- and anti-inflammatory lipids likely regulate wound healing, but further studies are needed to fully characterize lipid profiles during wound healing and to determine how these molecules impact each phase of repair.

Clinical science advances

- Bioactive lipids play an important role in regulating the induction, maintenance, and resolution of inflammation.
- Modulating different classes of lipid mediators at specific times during healing could be used to stimulate effective removal of pathogens, accelerate resolution of the inflammatory phase, increase the rate of closure, or reduce fibrosis in healing wounds.
- Biosynthetic mimetics and agonists of the anti-inflammatory/pro-resolving lipids are being developed[22]; these compounds will be useful in determining the importance of these lipids during repair and could potentially be used therapeutically to enhance healing.

Relevance to clinical care

- Currently, little is known about the exact functions of bioactive lipids during cutaneous repair in a clinical setting, and the role of the recently identified anti-inflammatory lipids in wound healing has not yet been examined.
- Despite the widespread use of NSAIDs, the clinical effects of these drugs on wound healing have not been fully explored.
- Alterations in dietary PUFA intake can change the profile of bioactive lipids, but the clinical implications of these changes for wound healing are not known.

stimulates fibrosis in the skin, its effects appear to be organ specific.[40] This could be explained by the fact that fibroblast responses to PGE_2 are highly variable. Fibroblasts from different organs or even fibroblasts from the same organ at different ages respond differently to PGE_2.[37,41–44]

In normal wounds inflammation is self-resolving, but little is known about what controls the resolution of wound inflammation. Pro-resolving mediators could be particularly important in diabetic and other nonhealing wounds that exhibit prolonged, unresolved inflammation.[12,33] Future studies must fully characterize the lipids involved in the induction and resolution of inflammation during wound healing and identify factors that regulate the synthesis of these lipids. For example, in other systems the pro-inflammatory PGs PGE_2 and PGD_2 can induce a class switch by promoting the production of anti-inflammatory lipids,[45] suggesting that mechanisms are in place to limit and resolve the inflammatory response. It is not known whether this regulatory system is active during wound healing. If PGE_2 and PGD_2 can stimulate synthesis of the anti-inflammatory lipids during repair, this could add another layer of complexity with regard to NSAIDs. It has been suggested that by inhibiting PG production, NSAIDs may stifle the synthesis of anti-inflammatory/pro-resolving lipids, causing incomplete resolution of inflammation.[23] As research on anti-inflammatory lipids is in the initial stages, we do not know how altered levels of these mediators will affect wound inflammation or repair. Synthetic analogs and mimetics of the anti-inflammatory lipids are also being developed[22] and should help define the role of these lipids in the repair process. Another potential way to modulate levels of bioactive lipids is by altering dietary PUFA intake. Omega-3 PUFA intake has recently been shown to alter the profile of pro-resolving and pro-inflammatory lipid mediators.[46] However, reported effects of DHA and EPA on acute skin inflammation differ.[47,48] Wound-healing studies in animal models have shown that diets rich in omega-3 PUFAs may actually be harmful by reducing tensile strength.[49] While dietary PUFA supplementation may change circulating or tissue levels of bioactive lipids and alter inflammation or healing, information about the clinical effects on acute and chronic wound healing is lacking.

CAUTION, CRITICAL REMARKS, AND RECOMMENDATIONS

Despite the fact that bioactive lipids are likely involved to some degree in all phases of wound healing, very little is known about how they control repair in a clinical setting. NSAIDs are commonly used to treat PG-associated pain and inflammation. However, the ability of some pro-inflammatory PGs to trigger the production of anti-inflammatory/pro-resolving lipids suggests that by blocking the production of PGs, NSAIDs may inadvertently prohibit complete resolution of inflammation. Current strategies of using NSAIDs to inhibit inflammation may be enhanced or replaced in the future with therapies designed to promote resolution.

FUTURE DEVELOPMENTS

Given the importance of lipid mediators in inflammation, more work must be done to fully characterize lipid profiles during repair. A comprehensive analysis of the bioactive lipids could identify novel biomarkers used to recognize various stages of healing and to distinguish between healing and nonhealing wounds. The impact of NSAID use on repair in patients has not been fully explored, and their potential to adversely affect the resolution of inflammation has not been determined. The wide range of biological effects attributed to lipid mediators suggests that altering the levels of different lipids at precise times during repair may be a viable strategy to enhance healing.

AUTHOR DISCLOSURE STATEMENT

No conflict of interest disclosed.

REFERENCES

1. Armstrong JR and Ferguson MW: Ontogeny of the skin and the transition from scar-free to scarring phenotype during wound healing in the pouch young of a marsupial, Monodelphis domestica. Dev Biol 1995; **169:** 242.
2. Dixon JB: Inflammation in the foetal and neonatal rat: the local reactions to skin burns. J Pathol Bacteriol 1960; **80:** 73.
3. Frantz FW, Bettinger DA, Haynes JH, Johnson DE, Harvey KM, Dalton HP, Yager DR, Diegelmann RF, and Cohen IK: Biology of fetal repair: the presence of bacteria in fetal wounds induces an adult-like healing response. J Pediatr Surg 1993, **28:** 428; discussion 433–424.
4. Kumta S, Ritz M, Hurley JV, Crowe D, Romeo R, and O'Brien BM: Acute inflammation in foetal and adult sheep: the response to subcutaneous injection of turpentine and carrageenan. Br J Plast Surg 1994; **47:** 360.
5. Liechty KW, Adzick NS, and Crombleholme TM: Diminished interleukin 6 (IL-6) production during scarless human fetal wound repair. Cytokine 2000; **12:** 671.
6. Liechty KW, Crombleholme TM, Cass DL, Martin B, and Adzick NS: Diminished interleukin-8 (IL-8) production in the fetal wound healing response. J Surg Res 1998; **77:** 80.
7. Liechty KW, Kim HB, Adzick NS, and Crombleholme TM: Fetal wound repair results in scar formation in

interleukin-10-deficient mice in a syngeneic murine model of scarless fetal wound repair. J Pediatr Surg 2000; **35:** 866; discussion 872–863.

8. Somasundaram K and Prathap K: Intra-uterine healing of skin wounds in rabbit foetuses. J Pathol 1970; **100:** 81.
9. Dovi JV, He LK, and DiPietro LA: Accelerated wound closure in neutrophil-depleted mice. J Leukoc Biol 2003; **73:** 448.
10. Martin P, D'Souza D, Martin J, Grose R, Cooper L, Maki R, and McKercher SR: Wound healing in the PU.1 null mouse—tissue repair is not dependent on inflammatory cells. Curr Biol 2003; **13:** 1122.
11. Wilgus TA, Vodovotz Y, Vittadini E, Clubbs EA, and Oberyszyn TM: Reduction of scar formation in full-thickness wounds with topical celecoxib treatment. Wound Repair Regen 2003; **11:** 25.
12. Acosta JB, Del Barco DG, Vera DC, Savigne W, Lopez-Saura P, Guillen Nieto G, and Schultz GS: The pro-inflammatory environment in recalcitrant diabetic foot wounds. Int Wound J 2008; **5:** 530.
13. Goren I, Muller E, Schiefelbein D, Christen U, Pfeilschifter J, Muhl H, and Frank S: Systemic anti-TNFalpha treatment restores diabetes-impaired skin repair in ob/ob mice by inactivation of macrophages. J Invest Dermatol 2007; **127:** 2259.
14. Garcia-Ovejero D, Arevalo-Martin A, Petrosino S, Docagne F, Hagen C, Bisogno T, Watanabe M, Guaza C, Di Marzo V, and Molina-Holgado E: The endocannabinoid system is modulated in response to spinal cord injury in rats. Neurobiol Dis 2009; **33:** 57.
15. Kawanabe T, Kawakami T, Yatomi Y, Shimada S, and Soma Y: Sphingosine 1-phosphate accelerates wound healing in diabetic mice. J Dermatol Sci 2007; **48:** 53.
16. Ariel A and Serhan CN: Resolvins and protectins in the termination program of acute inflammation. Trends Immunol 2007; **28:** 176.
17. Khanapure SP, Garvey DS, Janero DR, and Letts LG: Eicosanoids in inflammation: biosynthesis, pharmacology, and therapeutic frontiers. Curr Top Med Chem 2007; **7:** 311.
18. Serhan CN, Yang R, Martinod K, Kasuga K, Pillai PS, Porter TF, Oh SF, and Spite M: Maresins: novel macrophage mediators with potent antiinflammatory and proresolving actions. J Exp Med 2009; **206:** 15.
19. Martin P: Wound healing—aiming for perfect skin regeneration. Science 1997; **276:** 75.
20. Singer AJ and Clark RA: Cutaneous wound healing. N Engl J Med 1999; **341:** 738.
21. Stephens JM, Pashos CL, Haider S, and Wong JM: Making progress in the management of postoperative pain: a review of the cyclooxygenase 2-specific inhibitors. Pharmacotherapy 2004; **24:** 1714.
22. Serhan CN: Systems approach with inflammatory exudates uncovers novel anti-inflammatory and pro-resolving mediators. Prostaglandins Leukot Essent Fatty Acids 2008; **79:** 157.
23. Serhan CN, Chiang N, and Van Dyke TE: Resolving inflammation: dual anti-inflammatory and pro-resolution lipid mediators. Nat Rev Immunol 2008; **8:** 349.
24. Kamoshita E, Ikeda Y, Fujita M, Amano H, Oikawa A, Suzuki T, Ogawa Y, Yamashina S, Azuma S, Narumiya S, Unno N, and Majima M: Recruitment of a prostaglandin E receptor subtype, EP3-expressing bone marrow cells is crucial in wound-induced angiogenesis. Am J Pathol 2006; **169:** 1458.
25. Yamamoto T, Horikawa N, Komuro Y, and Hara Y: Effect of topical application of a stable prostacyclin analogue, SM-10902 on wound healing in diabetic mice. Eur J Pharmacol 1996; **302:** 53.
26. Godson C, Mitchell S, Harvery K, Petasis NA, Hogg N, and Brady HR: Cutting edge: lipoxins rapidly stimulate nonphlogistic phagocytosis of apoptotic neutrophils by monocyte-derived macrophages. J Immunol 2000; **164:** 1663.
27. Ariel A, Fredman G, Sun YP, Kantarci A, Van Dyke TE, Luster AD, and Serhan CN: Apoptotic neutrophils and T cells sequester chemokines during immune response resolution through modulation of CCR5 expression. Nat Immunol 2006; **7:** 1209.
28. Hong S, Porter TF, Lu Y, Oh SF, Pillai PS, and Serhan CN: Resolvin E1 metabolome in local inactivation during inflammation-resolution. J Immunol 2008; **180:** 3512.
29. Lundberg C and Gerdin B: The inflammatory reaction in an experimental model of open wounds in the rat. The effect of arachidonic acid metabolites. Eur J Pharmacol 1984; **97:** 229.
30. Morykwas MJ, Perry SL, and Argenta LC: Effects of prostaglandins and indomethacin on the cellular inflammatory response following surgical trauma in fetal rabbits. Int J Tissue React 1993; **15:** 151.
31. Futagami A, Ishizaki M, Fukuda Y, Kawana S, and Yamanaka N: Wound healing involves induction of cyclooxygenase-2 expression in rat skin. Lab Invest 2002; **82:** 1503.
32. Blomme EA, Chinn KS, Hardy MM, Casler JJ, Kim SH, Opsahl AC, Hall WA, Trajkovic D, Khan KN, and Tripp CS: Selective cyclooxygenase-2 inhibition does not affect the healing of cutaneous full-thickness incisional wounds in SKH-1 mice. Br J Dermatol 2003; **148:** 211.
33. Abd-El-Aleem SA, Ferguson MW, Appleton I, Bhowmick A, McCollum CN, and Ireland GW: Expression of cyclooxygenase isoforms in normal human skin and chronic venous ulcers. J Pathol 2001; **195:** 616.
34. Laulederkind SJ, Thompson-Jaeger S, Goorha S, Chen Q, Fu A, Rho JY, Ballou LR, and Raghow R: Both constitutive and inducible prostaglandin H synthase affect dermal wound healing in mice. Lab Invest 2002; **82:** 919.
35. Kampfer H, Brautigam L, Geisslinger G, Pfeilschifter J, and Frank S: Cyclooxygenase-1-coupled prostaglandin biosynthesis constitutes an essential prerequisite for skin repair. J Invest Dermatol 2003; **120:** 880.
36. Muller-Decker K, Hirschner W, Marks F, and Furstenberger G: The effects of cyclooxygenase isozyme inhibition on incisional wound healing in mouse skin. J Invest Dermatol 2002; **119:** 1189.
37. Wilgus TA, Bergdall VK, Tober KL, Hill KJ, Mitra S, Flavahan NA, and Oberyszyn TM: The impact of cyclooxygenase-2 mediated inflammation on scarless fetal wound healing. Am J Pathol 2004; **165:** 753.
38. Talwar M, Moyana TN, Bharadwaj B, and Tan LK: The effect of a synthetic analogue of prostaglandin E2 on wound healing in rats. Ann Clin Lab Sci 1996; **26:** 451.
39. Lupulescu A: Effect of prostaglandins on protein, RNA, DNA and collagen synthesis in experimental wounds. Prostaglandins 1975; **10:** 573.
40. Charbeneau RP and Peters-Golden M: Eicosanoids: mediators and therapeutic targets in fibrotic lung disease. Clin Sci (Colch) 2005; **108:** 479.
41. Huang SK, Wettlaufer SH, Chung J, and Peters-Golden M: Prostaglandin E2 inhibits specific lung fibroblast functions via selective actions of PKA and Epac-1. Am J Respir Cell Mol Biol 2008; **39:** 482.
42. Parekh A, Sandulache VC, Lieb AS, Dohar JE, and Hebda PA: Differential regulation of free-floating collagen gel contraction by human fetal and adult dermal fibroblasts in response to prostaglandin E2 mediated by an EP2/cAMP-dependent mechanism. Wound Repair Regen 2007; **15:** 390.
43. Parekh A, Sandulache VC, Singh T, Cetin S, Sacks MS, Dohar JE, and Hebda PA: Prostaglandin E2 differentially regulates contraction and structural reorganization of anchored collagen gels by human adult and fetal dermal fibroblasts. Wound Repair Regen 2009; **17:** 88.
44. Sandulache VC, Parekh A, Li-Korotky HS, Dohar JE, and Hebda PA: Prostaglandin E2 differentially modulates human fetal and adult dermal fibroblast migration and contraction: implication for wound healing. Wound Repair Regen 2006; **14:** 633.
45. Levy BD, Clish CB, Schmidt B, Gronert K, and Serhan CN: Lipid mediator class switching during acute inflammation: signals in resolution. Nat Immunol 2001; **2:** 612.
46. Poulsen RC, Gotlinger KH, Serhan CN, and Kruger MC: Identification of inflammatory and proresolving lipid mediators in bone marrow and their lipidomic profiles with ovariectomy and omega-3 intake. Am J Hematol 2008; **83:** 437.
47. Danno K, Ikai K, and Imamura S: Anti-inflammatory effects of eicosapentaenoic acid on experimental skin inflammation models. Arch Dermatol Res 1993; **285:** 432.
48. McDaniel JC, Belury M, Ahijevych K, and Blakely W: Omega-3 fatty acids effect on wound healing. Wound Repair Regen 2008; **16:** 337.
49. Albina JE, Gladden P, and Walsh WR: Detrimental effects of an omega-3 fatty acid-enriched diet on wound healing. JPEN J Parenter Enteral Nutr 1993; **17:** 519.
50. Gronert K: Lipid autacoids in inflammation and injury responses: a matter of privilege. Mol Interv 2008; **8:** 28.

WHS
Wound
Healing
Society

Neutrophils and Mast Cells in Wound Healing

Luisa Ann DiPietro*

Center for Wound Healing and Tissue Regeneration, University of Illinois at Chicago, Chicago, Illinois.

*Correspondence: Center for Wound Healing and Tissue Regeneration, University of Illinois at Chicago, 801 S Paulina, Chicago, Illinois 60612 (e-mail: ldipiet@uic.edu).

Background: Neutrophils and mast cells have been assumed to be critically important for optimal wound healing. Neutrophils, one of the most abundant phagocytes of the immune system, decontaminate the wound. Neutrophils also produce toxic byproducts, such as free oxygen radicals, that may increase local damage. Mast cells, which reside in tissues in a resting state, can be activated by trauma or immune-mediated mechanisms. Activated mast cells promote inflammation by releasing granular contents that are vasoactive as well as other proinflammatory mediators. Mast cells have been associated with scar formation, leading to speculation about the role of these cells as promoters of tissue fibrosis.

The Problem: Both neutrophils and mast cells are prominent at sites of injury, and a functional significance has been ascribed to this observation. However, recent studies in specialized animal models demonstrated that healing proceeds very well in the absence of these cells. The major issue is the importance of these cells in wound decontamination versus a critical role in the repair process itself.

Basic/Clinical Science Advances: Wounds in mast cell-deficient mice have been shown to heal either normally or with a moderate delay in closure. Inhibition of mast cell function reduces scar formation in the Red Duroc pig, a well-described model of hypertrophic scarring. Neutrophil content differs in normal and poorly healing wounds. In the absence of infection, neutrophil depletion appears to improve healing outcomes.

Clinical Care Relevance: Modulation of inflammation is a potentially relevant clinical treatment paradigm. Modalities that specifically target neutrophils and/or mast cell function warrant more study as potential effective therapeutics.

Conclusion: As the roles of neutrophils and macrophages are clarified, targeted therapeutics to selectively modulate the function of these cells may be developed. The therapeutics could be personalized to the type of wound and likelihood of infective or fibrotic processes.

BACKGROUND

In 1922, Dr. Alexis Carrel demonstrated that leukocytes were capable of producing factors that stimulated cellular proliferation.[1] Dr. Carrel suggested that "The initiation of healing seems to depend on the coming of leucocytes to the wounded tissue.... Possibly the white cells bring substances which adult tissues require to cicatrize or regenerate." Since that time, the appropriate function of inflammatory cells has generally been considered indispensable for successful wound healing. The study of the role of inflammatory cells in wound-healing outcomes and tissue regeneration has received intense attention, with more than 1,000 articles on the topic published within the past 5 years. These studies demonstrate both negative and positive effects of inflammation on healing outcomes. Although the precise balance of inflammatory cells that might result in perfect healing are not yet known,

ADVANCES IN WOUND CARE, VOLUME 1

Printed in U.S.A.
DOI: 10.1089/awc.2009.0163

many studies point to specific key elements that either promote or discourage ideal tissue repair.

The pattern of leukocytic infiltration into wounds is similar in progression to other acute inflammatory conditions. Within seconds of injury, resident mast cells degranulate, releasing many proinflammatory mediators, including vasoactive amines. Some of the mast cell-derived mediators, such as histamine, activate the vascular endothelium, cause increased vascular permeability, and promote vasodilatation.[2] This activity of mast cells contributes to the generation of the four cardinal signs of inflammation: rubor (redness), dolor (pain), calor (heat), and tumor (swelling). Following mast cell degranulation, neutrophils are attracted to the wound sites by chemotactic mediators derived from platelets, mast cells, and resident innate immune cells, and perhaps by activation of complement.[3] If the wound is contaminated, microbial products may also serve as leukocyte chemoattractants. Within a day or two of injury, circulating monocytes enter the wound and differentiate into mature tissue macrophages.[4] During this time, the mast cell content increases in the wound bed, with most of the infiltrating mast cells originating in the adjacent tissue.[2] As the white cell density within the wound increases, the leukocytes that have been recruited into the wound produce large amounts of cytokines and chemoattractants, amplifying the inflammatory response. In the late inflammatory phase of wound repair, T lymphocytes appear in the wound bed and may support the resolution and remodeling of the wound.[5,6]

CLINICAL PROBLEM ADDRESSED

An appropriate inflammatory response is a critical element of successful wound healing. The importance of neutrophils in this response is highlighted by the well-accepted observation that neutropenic patients suffer from increased levels of wound infection. While the neutrophil may be important to wound decontamination, even a normal and limited neutrophilic infiltration seems capable of negatively influencing long-term outcomes, perhaps by creating bystander tissue damage. Moreover, an excessive and unrelenting neutrophilic presence is inhibitory to wound closure. Likewise, the mast cell plays an important role in modulating wound outcomes. An increased mast cell infiltration is associated with fibrosis and hypertrophic scar formation. Thus, an understanding of the role of neutrophils and mast cells at sites of injury has relevance to wound infection, wound closure, and scar formation.

BASIC SCIENCE CONTEXT

A large amount of evidence suggests that neutrophils might negatively influence repair, as this cell type is capable of destroying normal tissue. Neutrophils do produce a variety of growth factors that could promote revascularization and repair of injured tissue.[7] However, they also produce many enzymes that can induce substantial tissue damage (Fig. 1). Neutrophil proteases, such as elastase and cathepsin G, can degrade most components of the extracellular matrix as well as proteins as diverse as clotting factors, complement, immunoglobulins, and cytokines.[8–10] Importantly, the production of the collagenase matrix metalloproteinase-8 by neutrophils has been linked to the pathogenesis of nonhealing chronic ulcers.[11] Because the extracellular matrix serves as a supporting scaffold for infiltrating cells, modification of the extracellular matrix by neutrophils could have important consequences for repair. Neutrophils also produce a large number of free oxygen radicals, placing considerable oxidative stress on the wound. Mediators such as superoxide and hydrogen peroxide cause additional tissue damage, delaying the repair process and modifying healing outcomes.[12] Paradoxically, other studies demonstrated that neutrophils may release factors that support tissue growth, such as vascular

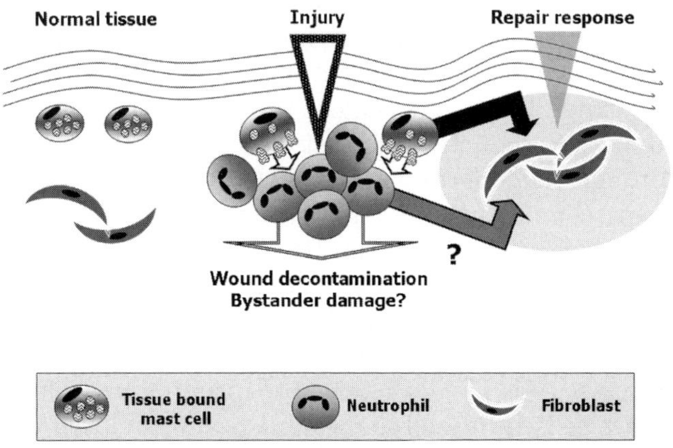

Figure 1. In normal tissue, quiescent mast cells reside passively. Following tissue injury, mast cell degranulation releases mediators that activate endothelium and enhance inflammation (small open arrows). Neutrophils are recruited to the wound site by both mediators from mast cells and other mediators; they quickly become the most abundant cell in the wound bed. Neutrophils are very effective at decontaminating the wound, but they may also cause bystander damage because of the release of bioactive mediators that can damage healthy cells and tissue (large open arrow). Both mast cells and neutrophils may also directly or indirectly influence the proliferative activity of fibroblasts within the wound (large solid arrows). In particular, mast cell activity is associated with greater scar formation in the wound.

endothelial growth factor, thus supporting tissue repair and revascularization.[13] This apparent dichotomy stresses the need for additional studies on neutrophil functionality at wound sites.

While neutrophils are often associated with delayed wound healing, an increased density of mast cells has been linked to excess fibrosis, or scar formation.[2,14,15] Mast cells have been shown to directly influence fibroblast function in several ways, including increased contraction *in vitro*, and are associated with altered collagen synthesis and wound remodeling *in vivo*[15–17] (Fig. 1). Mast cells contain several specific mediators that can modulate fibroblast activity. For example, both tryptase and chymase, which are found in mast cell granules, have been described to have many effects beyond their protease activity that could influence scar formation, including direct effects on fibroblast function and the proangiogenic activity of tryptase.[18,19] In addition to direct effects, resident mast cells are clearly involved in the initiation of inflammation that follows injury and are important to the recruitment of neutrophils.[20] Whether this modulation of inflammation is linked to the influence of mast cells on scar formation is not yet known.

EXPERIMENTAL MODEL OR MATERIAL

Several experimental models have been used to examine the role of neutrophils and mast cells in wound repair. Multiple studies have utilized antibody depletion strategies to reduce circulating neutrophils and subsequent wound neutrophil content. The reduction of mast cell activity in normal animals is generally accomplished with pharmacologic agents that prevent mast cell degranulation. Another strategy that has been employed is the use of either antibodies or neutralizing factors, to inhibit the function of inflammatory cytokines that recruit these cell types. Mice that are genetically deficient in mast cells have been used to examine the role of mast cells in numerous wound healing-related pathologies. More recently, mice with specific defects that more comprehensively reduce inflammatory responses (*e.g.*, transforming growth factor-beta–deficient mice and PU.1-deficient mice) have been developed and used to examine the overall role of inflammation in healing outcomes.

DISCUSSION OF FINDINGS AND RELEVANT LITERATURE

There is little argument that proper leukocyte activity assists in microbial decontamination of wounds. However, several recent studies support the concept that inflammation is dispensable for efficient tissue repair so long as microbial contamination is controlled. Studies on healing in the early to midgestation fetus showed that early fetal wounds exhibit very little, if any, inflammatory response while healing in a scarless fashion.[21,22] While intrinsic differences in growth factor production, levels of stem cells, and cellular proliferation capacity probably support the ideal response that occurs during fetal wound repair, the findings suggested that inflammation is not an essential feature of adequate repair. In support of this concept, scar formation appears to be accelerated when inflammation is provoked in fetal wounds.[23,24]

In adult mice, acute inflammation has also been described to be irrelevant or even detrimental to repair. In the PU.1 null mouse, which lacks both macrophages and functioning neutrophils, little inflammation occurs at the wound site and repair appears to be scar-free, similar to the fetus.[25] Mice with a deletion of the Smad3 gene, a molecule critical to the intracellular signaling of transforming growth factor-beta1, exhibited accelerated cutaneous wound healing and significantly reduced the influx of inflammatory cells.[26] Similarly, studies in a number of other systems have shown that soluble factors that reduce inflammation in wounds, such as the cytokine interferon-gamma-induced protein-10 and heparin-binding epidermal growth factor, are often beneficial to wound-healing outcomes in the adult organism.[27,28] These studies suggested that appropriate modulation of inflammation by therapeutics might facilitate regeneration rather than repair.

Neutrophils are thought to be dispensable to healing, and a single study, conducted by Simpson and Ross in 1972, was widely accepted to have shown that the loss of neutrophils had little effect on wound healing.[29] In their study, no discernable differences in fibrin content, connective tissue formation, macrophage content, or macrophage phagocytosis were seen between wounds of neutropenic and control guinea pigs. More recent studies[30] showed that dermal healing is not adversely affected by neutrophil depletion, as neither collagen deposition nor wound-breaking strength was significantly different between neutropenic and control mice. Remarkably, though, epidermal healing, measured by wound closure, proceeded significantly faster in neutropenic than control mice ($77.7 + 14.2\%$ vs. $41.2 + 0.9\%$, $p < 0.02$ at day 2). In a diabetic strain known to have delayed repair, neutropenic mice exhibited an astounding 50% acceleration of wound closure.

One important consideration is that the functional activity of the neutrophil may shift in response to systemic influences, such as stress.[31] This means that the simple number of neutrophils in the wound may be an insufficient indicator of their activity, and that functional shifts rather than quantity might dictate whether neutrophils play a beneficial or detrimental role. Recent studies suggested that certain therapeutic modalities may influence neutrophil accumulation and perhaps shift activity to phenotypes more supportive of repair. For example, the use of vacuum-assisted closure devices has been linked to increased neutrophil content and wound vascularity.[32] Another critical consideration is that neutrophils have also been shown to influence other immune cells in the wound. In particular, neutrophils appear to be capable of modulating macrophage phenotype. The capability of neutrophils to modulate cytokine production by macrophages has been documented in the context of wound healing.[33] Moreover, macrophages recognize and ingest senescent or apoptotic neutrophils; the phagocytosis of neutrophils has been suggested to modify the macrophage phenotype toward one that would favor repair.[34]

The degranulation of mast cells represents one of the earliest proinflammatory events after tissue damage. A commonly held assumption has been that the activity of these cells provides the initial stimulus for repair, jump-starting the healing process. This assumption was largely predicated upon the truth that mast cells contain proinflammatory mediators and growth factors. In several studies, wound-healing outcomes have been examined in mice that are genetically deficient for mast cells. In one study, the absence of mast cells had no effect on wound closure, collagen synthesis, or angiogenesis, with the only significant change being a decrease in neutrophil infiltration that occurred in the wounds of mast cell-deficient mice.[20] In a second study, larger wounds were shown to exhibit retarded closure in mast cell-deficient mice.[35] Thus, the influence and importance of mast cells may rely upon the size of the wound. More recently, the role of mast cells in wound healing and scar formation has been studied in pigs.[36] Red Duroc pigs are known to have shown significant wound contraction and scar formation. Treatment of these pigs with the mast cell stabilizer ketotifen resulted in reduced early but not late wound contraction and reduced the deposition of collagen. These results suggest that the inhibition of mast cell degranulation might favorably reduce contraction and scar formation without affecting the normal healing process in detrimental ways.

CAUTION, CRITICAL REMARKS, AND RECOMMENDATIONS

Our present understanding of the interplay of all of the molecules and cells that contribute to inflammation at sites of injury is wholly incomplete. This situation makes it quite difficult to predict what effect the perturbation of any specific aspect of the inflammatory response will have on wound-healing outcomes. Additional mechanistic information might allow mathematical modeling that could be predictive of outcomes following any proposed intervention. Such a model would accelerate progress by guiding therapeutic choices.

FUTURE DEVELOPMENTS

The inflammatory response is highly individualized, and ideal therapeutic approaches will ultimately need to be personalized. It will be important to learn more about types and variety of individual inflammatory responses at wound sites, as well as how systemic and local factors influence these responses, to customize treatments. The identification of reliable markers, whether genetic or systemic, will be needed to accomplish a personalized approach for manipulating inflammation. Such knowledge will

TAKE-HOME MESSAGE

Basic science advances

- Acute inflammatory cells such as mast cells and neutrophils are important to wound decontamination.
- Although important to the prevention of infection, neutrophil and mast cell activity in wounds negatively influences wound closure and promotes scar formation.

Clinical science advances

- Nonhealing wounds frequently exhibit excessive neutrophil content, whereas fibrosis and scar formation are associated with mast cell infiltration.
- A reduction in neutrophil activity in wounds could lead to improved and more regenerative repair. Such a reduction must be judicious, as neutrophils are important to the effective decontamination of wounds.
- The inhibition of mast cell degranulation could be a promising new therapeutic for the reduction of scar formation.

Relevance to clinical care

- At present, the utility of using inflammatory modulators to alter human wound-healing outcomes has not been tested.
- Several current therapies probably support optimal wound inflammation.

have applications both to wound care and in a substantial number of other disease states in which aberrant inflammation plays a role.

ACKNOWLEDGMENT

Wound-healing research in the author's laboratory was supported by grants RO1-GM50875 and P20-GM078426.

DISCLAIMER

The contents of this manuscript are solely the responsibility of the author and do not necessarily represent the official views of the NIGMS or NIH.

AUTHOR DISCLOSURE STATEMENT

No conflict of interest disclosed.

REFERENCES

1. Carrel A: Growth-promoting function of leucocytes. J Exp Med 1922; **36:** 385.
2. Artuc M, Hermes B, Steckelings UM, Grutzkau A, and Henz BM: Mast cells and their mediators in cutaneous wound healing—active participants or innocent bystanders? Exp Dermatol 1999; **8:** 1.
3. Park JE and Barbul A: Understanding the role of immune regulation in wound healing. Am J Surg 2004; **187:** 11S.
4. Ross R and Odland G: Human wound repair. II. Inflammatory cells, epithelial–mesenchymal interrelations, and fibrogenesis. J Cell Biol 1968; **39:** 152.
5. Barbul A, Shawe T, Rotter SM, Efron JE, Wasserkrug HL, and Badawy SB: Wound healing in nude mice: a study on the regulatory role of lymphocytes in fibroplasia. Surgery 1989; **105:** 764.
6. Barbul A, Breslin RJ, Woodyard JP, Wasserkrug HL, and Efron G: The effect of *in vivo* T helper and T suppressor lymphocyte depletion on wound healing. Ann Surg 1989; **209:** 479.
7. Taichman NS, Young S, Cruchley AT, Taylor P, and Paleolog E: Human neutrophils secrete vascular endothelial growth factor. J Leukoc Biol 1997; **62:** 397.
8. Briggaman RA, Schechter NM, Fraki J, and Lazarus GS: Degradation of the epidermal-dermal junction by proteolytic enzymes from human skin and human polymorphonuclear leukocytes. J Exp Med 1984; **160:** 1027.
9. Dovi JV, Szpaderska AM, and DiPietro LA: Neutrophil function in the healing wound: adding insult to injury? Thromb Haemost 2004; **92:** 275.
10. Li WY, Chong SS, Huang EY, and Tuan TL: Plasminogen activator/plasmin system: a major player in wound healing? Wound Repair Regen 2003; **11:** 239.
11. Nwomeh BC, Liang HX, Cohen IK, and Yager DR: MMP-8 is the predominant collagenase in healing wounds and nonhealing ulcers. J Surg Res 1999; **81:** 189.
12. Wilgus TA, Vodovotz Y, Vittadini E, Clubbs EA, and Oberyszyn TM: Reduction of scar formation in full-thickness wounds with topical celecoxib treatment. Wound Repair Regen 2003; **11:** 25.
13. Kasama T, Miwa Y, Isozaki T, Odai T, Adachi M, and Kunkel SL: Neutrophil-derived cytokines: potential therapeutic targets in inflammation. Curr Drug Targets Inflamm Allergy 2005; **4:** 273.
14. Hebda PA, Collins MA, and Tharp MD: Mast cell and myofibroblast in wound healing. Dermatol Clin 1993; **11:** 685.
15. Iba Y, Shibata A, Kato M, and Masukawa T: Possible involvement of mast cells in collagen remodeling in the late phase of cutaneous wound healing in mice. Int Immunopharmacol 2004; **4:** 1873.
16. Moyer KE, Saggers GC, and Ehrlich HP: Mast cells promote fibroblast populated collagen lattice contraction through gap junction intercellular communication. Wound Repair Regen 2004; **12:** 269.
17. Sasaki A, Mueller RV, Xi G, Sipe R, Buck D, and Hollinger J: Mast cells: an unexpected finding in the modulation of cutaneous wound repair by charged beads. Plast Reconstr Surg 2003; **111:** 1446.
18. Hiromatsu Y and Toda S: Mast cells and angiogenesis. Microsc Res Tech 2003; **60:** 64.
19. Garbuzenko E, Berkman N, Puxeddu I, Kramer M, Nagler A, and Levi-Schaffer F: Mast cells induce activation of human lung fibroblasts *in vitro*. Exp Lung Res 2004; **30:** 705.
20. Egozi EI, Ferreira AM, Burns AL, Gamelli RL, and Dipietro LA: Mast cells modulate the inflammatory but not the proliferative response in healing wounds. Wound Repair Regen 2003; **11:** 46.
21. Cowin AJ, Brosnan MP, Holmes TM, and Ferguson MW: Endogenous inflammatory response to dermal wound healing in the fetal and adult mouse. Dev Dyn 1998; **212:** 385.
22. Hopkinson-Woolley J, Hughes D, Gordon S, and Martin P: Macrophage recruitment during limb development and wound healing in the embryonic and foetal mouse. J Cell Sci 1994; **107(Pt 5):** 1159.
23. Wilgus TA, Bergdall VK, Tober KL, Hill KJ, Mitra S, Flavahan NA, and Oberyszyn TM: The impact of cyclooxygenase-2 mediated inflammation on scarless fetal wound healing. Am J Pathol 2004; **165:** 753.
24. Ozturk S, Deveci M, Sengezer M, and Gunhan O: Results of artificial inflammation in scarless foetal wound healing: an experimental study in foetal lambs. Br J Plast Surg 2001; **54:** 47.
25. Martin P, D'Souza D, Martin J, Grose R, Cooper L, Maki R, and McKercher SR: Wound healing in the PU.1 null mouse—tissue repair is not dependent on inflammatory cells. Curr Biol 2003; **13:** 1122.
26. Ashcroft GS, Yang X, Glick AB, Weinstein M, Letterio JL, Mizel DE, Anzano M, Greenwell-Wild T, Wahl SM, Deng C, and Roberts AB: Mice lacking Smad3 show accelerated wound healing and an impaired local inflammatory response [see comment]. Nat Cell Biol 1999; **1:** 260.
27. Luster AD, Cardiff RD, MacLean JA, Crowe K, and Granstein RD: Delayed wound healing and disorganized neovascularization in transgenic mice expressing the IP-10 chemokine. Proc Assoc Am Phys 1998; **110:** 183.
28. Xia G, Rachfal AW, Martin AE, and Besner GE: Upregulation of endogenous heparin-binding EGF-like growth factor (HB-EGF) expression after intestinal ischemia/reperfusion injury. J Invest Surg 2003; **16:** 57.
29. Simpson DM and Ross R: The neutrophilic leukocyte in wound repair: a study with antineutrophil serum. J Clin Invest 1972; **51:** 2009.
30. Dovi JV, He LK, and DiPietro LA: Accelerated wound closure in neutrophil-depleted mice. J Leukoc Biol 2003; **73:** 448.
31. Roy S, Khanna S, Yeh PE, Rink C, Malarkey WB, Kiecolt-Glaser J, Laskowski B, Glaser R, and Sen CK: Wound site neutrophil transcriptome in response to psychological stress in young men. Gene Expr 2005; **12:** 273.

32. Labler L, Rancan M, Mica L, Harter L, Mihic-Probst D, and Keel M: Vacuum-assisted closure therapy increases local interleukin-8 and vascular endothelial growth factor levels in traumatic wounds. J Trauma 2009; **66:** 749.

33. Daley JM, Reichner JS, Mahoney EJ, Manfield L, Henry WL Jr., Mastrofrancesco B, and Albina JE: Modulation of macrophage phenotype by soluble product(s) released from neutrophils. J Immunol 2005; **174:** 2265.

34. Meszaros AJ, Reichner JS, and Albina JE: Macrophage phagocytosis of wound neutrophils. J Leukoc Biol 1999; **65:** 35.

35. Weller K, Foitzik K, Paus R, Syska W, and Maurer M: Mast cells are required for normal healing of skin wounds in mice. FASEB J 2006; **20:** 2366.

36. Gallant-Behm CL, Hildebrand KA, and Hart DA: The mast cell stabilizer ketotifen prevents development of excessive skin wound contraction and fibrosis in red Duroc pigs. Wound Repair Regen 2008; **16:** 226.

WHS Wound Healing Society

The Role of Mesenchymal Stem Cells and Fibrocytes in Wound Healing and Hypertrophic Scar Formation: Recent Advances

Jie Ding[1] and Edward E Tredget[2,*]

[1]Plastic Surgery Laboratory, Department of Surgery, University of Alberta, Edmonton, Alberta, Canada.
[2]Firefighters' Burn Treatment Unit, Plastic Surgery Research Laboratory, Division of Plastic and Reconstructive Surgery, Division of Critical Care Medicine, Department of Surgery, University of Alberta, Edmonton, Alberta, Canada.

Abbreviations and Acronyms

Ang = angiopoietin

BM-MSCs = bone marrow–derived mesenchymal stem cells

CTGF = connective tissue growth factor

ECM = extracellular matrix

HTS = hypertrophic scar

IFN = interferon

IL = interleukin

LSP1 = leukocyte-specific protein 1

PBMC = peripheral blood mononuclear cells

αSMA = α smooth muscle actin

TGFβ = transforming growth factor β

Th = helper T cell

*Correspondence: Firefighters' Burn Treatment Unit, Plastic Surgery Research Laboratory, Division of Plastic and Reconstructive Surgery, Division of Critical Care Medicine, Department of Surgery, University of Alberta, 2D2.28 WMC, 8440-112 St., Edmonton, Alberta, Canada T6G 2B7 (e-mail: etredget@ualberta.ca).

Background: Hypertrophic scar (HTS) is a common and significant negative outcome of injury to the deep layers of the dermis where prolonged inflammation is common. It leads to increased health care costs but also causes significant psychological problems for burn survivors.

The Problem: Current forms of treatment for HTS include pressure garments, topically applied silicone and intralesional steroids; however, HTS responds to these current forms of therapy slowly over months or years, and often incompletely.

Basic/Clinical Science Advances: Basic studies of HTS have shown abnormalities in extracellular matrix composition, changes in cytokine and growth factor production, activation of a T lymphocyte-mediated immune response and delayed apoptosis. Recently, bone marrow-derived mesenchymal stem cells (BM-MSCs) were found to promote leukocyte and monocyte migration into wound sites where they are involved in re-epithelialization, granulation tissue formation and enhanced angiogenesis. One specific hematopoetic-derived circulating stem cell is the fibrocyte, which regulates fibroblast function and ultimately leads to the development of fibrotic conditions. Clinical improvement in scar quality in burn patients following interferon α2b treatment was associated with a decrease in the number and a down-regulation of the function of fibrocytes, as well as decreased angiogenesis mediated by vascular endothelium growth factor.

Clinical Care Relevance: The focus of wound care for burn patients includes not only the immediate treatment, but also prevention of sequelae including HTS. Effective care depends on an improved understanding of the mechanisms that cause HTS in patients with thermal injuries.

Conclusion: Investigating the role of bone marrow-derived stem cells may identify new HTS prevention and treatment methods.

BACKGROUND

The American Burn Association National Burn Repository 2007 Report reviewed a total of 181,836 records of acute burn admissions for the period 1998–2007. The mean age for all cases was 35 years, the mortality rate was 4.9%, and the average length of stay was 7 days.[1] Significant emotional and psychological difficulties often occur when patients survive large thermal injuries that result in inflammation, hypertrophic scarring, contractures, and pigmentation changes. Although wound healing research has made significant progress in recent years, further understanding of the mechanism of hypertrophic scar (HTS) formation, especially the contribution of stem cells and progenitors to wound healing, would enable us to find new therapies for the prevention

Printed in U.S.A.
DOI: 10.1089/awc.2009.0143

and treatment of HTS. The purpose of this review is to summarize the cellular and molecular advances with regard to the role of bone marrow–derived mesenchymal stem cells (BM-MSCs) and fibrocytes in fibrosis of the skin.

CLINICAL PROBLEM

HTS is a common and significant negative outcome of thermal injury to the deep dermal layers of the skin where prolonged inflammation is common. It not only leads to increased health-care costs but also causes significant psychological problems for burn survivors. Unfortunately, the current understanding of HTS pathogenesis is limited, and few effective therapies exist, as with other fibroproliferative disorders. Therefore, improving our understanding of the mechanisms that cause HTS would help us develop effective preventative and therapeutic therapies for patients with thermal injuries.

RELEVANT BASIC SCIENCE CONTEXT

Wound healing in mammals generally follows specific phases over time that include hemostasis, inflammation, proliferation, and maturation. To repair the injury, the body initially makes granulation tissue to revascularize the wound, before ultimately repairing the wound which involves extracellular matrix (ECM) synthesis that can lead to the development of scar tissue. Scarring is a natural part of the healing process. As one of the two types of abnormal scars, HTS is a red, raised mass of tissue in the skin which conventionally does not grow beyond the boundaries of the original wound.

HTS tissue has an altered ultrastructure, which is caused by changes in the ECM composition, including a high proportion of embryonic type III collagen,[2] a temporary absence of elastin,[3] increased water and high concentrations of the glycosaminoglycan components, uronic acid, hexosamine, and fibronection.[4] As well, there is an absence of glycosaminoglycan, decorin, and abnormally high levels of byglycan and versican.[5]

Longitudinal studies of the systemic and local immune responses in burn patients have suggested that HTS formation is associated with a polarized immune response including certain types of lymphocyte infiltration, related cytokine release, and specific antigen expression on lymphocytes. The presence of more immunocompetent CD3+ T cells was reported in active HTS compared with the normotrophic scar. There were increased numbers of macrophages and Langerhan's cells, but minimal numbers of B cells were seen in HTS tissue.[6] CD4+ T cells were more predominate in the dermis as well as in the epidermis in HTS, whereas CD8+ T cells were less represented.[7] In an animal model and in patients with burn injury, reduced type 1 T helper cell (Th1) cytokines, interleukin (IL) 12 and interferon (IFN)-γ, increased Th2 cytokines, IL-4, 5, 10, and 13, augmented Th3 cytokines, IL-2, 4, and 10, and overexpressed growth factors, platelet-derived growth factor, transforming growth factor β (TGF-β), and insulin-like growth factor (IGF) have been reported to possibly be involved in HTS formation.[8]

The hypercellularity of HTS, decreased gap junctional intercellular communication of HTS fibroblasts, and increased levels of the bcl-2 oncogene in the peripheral blood mononuclear cell (PBMC) fraction in burn patients suggests that decreased apoptosis of myofibroblasts leads to an imbalance between ECM deposition and degradation, which may be related to the high expression of p53 and caspase-3.[9]

EXPERIMENTAL MODEL OR MATERIAL ADVANTAGES AND LIMITATIONS

The development of useful experimental models is required to investigate the wound healing process, which will help us understand the mechanism of hypertrophic scarring and allow us to develop novel therapeutic methods. *In vitro* models including fibroblasts, keratinocytes, macrophages, and endothelial cells are often used for wound healing research. *In vivo* models include both animal and human models. Many different types of animal models have been used for wound healing research and include incisional, excisional, burn, and granulation tissue models. Animal models of hypertrophic scarring are heterologous hypertrophic scarring or keloid implants in immunodeficient animals including the athymic mice and rats, the immune privileged site of hamster cheek pouch, heterologous hypertrophic scarring, or keloid induction via chemically mediated injury in guinea pigs, anatomic specific sites in rabbit ears, and a porcine model.[10] The prominent advantage of *in vivo* models is that wounded tissue is similar to wounds found in clinical practice. The main disadvantage is the limited ability to examine a single-tissue component contribution in wound healing. Sullivan *et al.* reported the similarity between different models which were 78% between pig and human, 53% between human and small mammal, and 57% between human and *in vitro* studies.[11] There has been a trend to modify the commonly

TAKE-HOME MESSAGE

Basic science advances

- BM-MSCs enhance wound healing by regulating keratinocyte differentiation and paracrine-mediated angiogenesis.
- Fibrocytes contribute to wound healing by regulating fibroblasts which results in changes in collagen production, proliferation, migration, and differentiation of fibrocytes to functional myofibroblasts.
- Increased skin fibrosis of LSP1-deficient mice is associated with increased cytokine and chemokine secretion, leukocyte and fibrocyte recruitment, as well as granulation tissue formation.
- Fibrosis of the skin is associated with a polarized Th2 systemic response to injury that leads to increased T cells and their Th2 fibrogenic cytokines in tissue and the development of fibrosis and HTS.
- Deep dermal fibroblasts are critical to the formation of HTS.
- Experimental animal studies suggest that MSC-based therapeutics accelerate the wound healing process in part through the secretion of proangiogenic factors.

Clinical science advances

- The existing therapeutic approaches used to treat excessive dermal scarring include the application of antiinflammatory agents, antimetabolites, anti-TGFβ family protein reagents, and antifibrotic cytokines. Dressings effective in the reduction of HTS include hydrogel and silicone gel sheets. Induction of scar degradation by calcium antagonists and apoptosis inducers, and surgical interventions such as excision of scar tissue, autografts, laser therapy, radiation therapy, and cryosurgery are all used clinically.[28]
- Recently, more effective managements reported in the literature include the therapeutic effects of recombinant adenovirus vector-containing hepatocyte growth factor[29] and cyclin-dependent kinase inhibitor 1B (p27)[30] on scars that were investigated in a rabbit HTS model. The administration of avotermin (recombinant, active, human TGFβ3), a key protein involved in scar-free healing observed in embryos, improved scarring by intradermal injection in three double-blind, placebo-controlled phase I/II studies.[31]

Relevance to clinical care

- The primary role of wound care is to prevent infection, protect the wound, and prevent scar formation. One standard of care for the prevention of abnormal scarring after burn injury is pressure garment therapy. Anzarut *et al.*[32] reviewed six unique trials involving 316 patients with pressure garment therapy, and it appears to improve scar height, although this difference is small and of questionable clinical importance.
- Aside from standard wound care, biological dressings based on living cultured allofibroblasts and type I collagen with platelet-derived growth factor-BB stimulated epithelial regeneration of the third-degree burn wounds, and epithelialization was not associated with the formation of HTS.[33] A clinical study confirmed that chitin nanofibril-based gel with the main biochemical activities of polymorphonuclear cell activation, fibroblast activation, cytokine production, giant cell migration, and stimulation of type IV collagen synthesis promoted rapid and physiological healing of different types of wounds. Moreover, it seems to prevent hypertrophic scarring.[34]

used animal models or combine *in vivo* and *in vitro* models to examine a single system, cell type, or gene in an effort to determine which contribute to wound healing and the development of HTS. An example is the leukocyte-specific protein 1 (LSP1) null mouse excision model that is specific for determining the biological role of LSP1 in wound healing,[12] and a full-thickness human skin graft placed on a nude mouse represents an ideal hypertrophic scaring animal model.[13]

DISCUSSION OF FINDINGS AND RELEVANT LITERATURE

Using a splinted wound mouse model, the benefit of BM-MSCs in wound healing has been determined.[14] Compared with the dermal fibroblasts or vehicle medium-treated wounds, the application of green fluorescence protein–expressing allogenic BM-MSCs into excisional wounds significantly shortened the time to wound closure by enhancing reepithelialization, cellularity, and angiogenesis. An increase in the number of skin appendages was found in BM-MSC-treated wounds. Immunostaining for green fluorescence protein and epithelial cytokeratin provides evidence that BM-MSCs are involved in the cellular formation of keratinocytes. Some double-positive cells in the dermis formed structures that resembled developing sweat or sebaceous glands. All these suggest a direct contribution of BM-MSCs to cutaneous regeneration. Moreover, vessels and their fine branches were found extending into the BM-MSC-treated wounds. Immunohistological staining of tissue sections showed increased endothelial CD31 expression and capillary density. High levels of vascular endothelium growth factor and angiopoietin 1 (Ang1) were found in BM-MSC-treated wounds. *In vitro*, the BM-MSC-conditioned medium significantly enhanced tube formation of human umbilical vein endothelial cells, increased mRNA levels of Ang1 and 2, and augmented Ang1 protein expressions of human umbilical vein endothelial cells, suggesting that BM-MSCs promote wound healing through differentiation and release of proangiogenic factors.

As a newly identified leukocyte subpopulation originating from bone marrow, fibrocytes have been reported to contribute to tissue repair by several mechanisms such as recruitment into wound sites,[15] secretion of inflammatory cytokines,[16] antigen presentation,[17] angiogenesis,[18] differentiation into myofibroblast population,[19] and mediation of immune response by Th2 cells.[20]

Current studies showed that dermal fibroblasts treated *in vitro* with media conditioned by fibrocytes from burn patients significantly augmented hydroxyproline synthesis, cell proliferation, and migration compared with the dermal fibroblasts treated with media conditioned by fibrocytes from normal uninjured subjects. The increased cell proliferation and migration observed could be reversed by treatment with TGF-β antibody. These treated fibroblasts were larger with irregular projections and bundles of actin filaments and stress fibers, hallmark histological features of myofibroblasts. As well, they had increased α smooth muscle antigen (αSMA) staining, increased αSMA protein expression, and increased populations of αSMA-expressing cells. Additionally, they exhibited a significantly higher degree of contraction in collagen lattices that could be antagonized by adding TGF-β antibody. A significant increase in the amount of TGF-β1 was found in conditioned medium from burn patient fibrocytes as well as higher levels of mRNA and protein expression of connective tissue growth factor (CTGF) compared with medium from normal volunteers. Overall this indicates an indirect role for fibrocytes in hypertrophic scarring by regulating dermal fibroblasts.[21]

Persistent inflammation with infiltration of leukocytes and release of soluble mediators is a common problem in HTS formation. To investigate the role of T cells and their cytokines in the development of HTS, intracellular cytokine synthesis of circulating T cells was measured serially in burn patients who developed HTS. Low IFNγ-positive Th1 cells were found in association with low IL-12 and absent IFNγ cytokine levels in the serum; however, IL-4-positive Th2 cells were significantly increased compared with the normal controls. Serum IL-10 and TGFβ levels were significantly increased early after burn injury in patients who later developed HTS. Activated PBMCs demonstrated that IFNγ mRNA was present only in normal volunteers or patients without HTS. IL-4 mRNA levels were increased in the PBMCs of burn patients with HTS. In HTS tissues, IL-4 mRNA was increased, whereas, IFNγ mRNA was reduced. Increased CD3+ and CD4+ cells were present in HTS tissue and were coexpressed with TGFβ.[7] The incubation of PBMCs *in vitro* in serum-free medium containing IL-4 increased the number of fibrocytes, suggesting that the Th2 cytokine IL-4 is able to promote fibrocyte differentiation.[22] Further, a regulatory function of TGFβ-producing CD4+ T cells to fibroblasts was found by incubation of dermal fibroblasts *in vitro* with CD4+ T lymphocyte-conditioned media.[23] These studies suggest that fibrosis of the skin is associated with a polarized Th2 systemic response to injury that leads to increased T cells and their Th2 fibrogenic cytokines in tissue and the development of fibrosis and HTS. Figure 1 shows a hypothetical diagram of the role of Th1/Th2/Th3 fibrogenic growth factors in wound healing.

In our model of impaired wound healing using diabetic mice, the study results show that MSC-based therapeutics accelerated the wound healing process in part by secreting proangiogenic factors. However, in HTS where excessive ECM is associated with hypervascularity, improvement seen in scar quality following treatment with IFNα2b is associated with decreased angiogenesis, a reduction in bone marrow–derived fibrocytes. To date there is no evidence for a role of MSC-based therapeutics for the treatment of HTS.

The biological role of LSP1 as a new maker for fibrocytes was examined in the development of skin

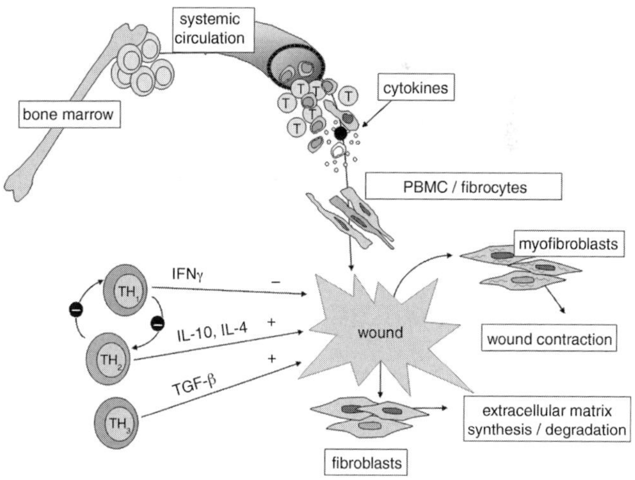

Figure 1. A hypothetical diagram of the role of helper T cell (Th)1/Th2/Th3 fibrogenic growth factors in wound healing. Fibrocytes are believed to be derived from the mesenchymal precursor cells of the bone marrow. Wound healing research suggests that fibrocytes have an important role during the inflammatory and proliferative phases of wound healing and are regulated by Th1/Th2/Th3 cytokines. Th1 cytokines, such as interferon (IFN)-γ inhibit, and Th2 cytokines, such as IL-10 and 14 as well as Th3 cytokines, such as transforming growth factor β (TGF-β), promote bone marrow–derived fibrocytes to differentiate into fibroblasts and myofibroblasts in the wounds, which stimulates extracellular matrix synthesis and wound contraction in hypertrophic scar.[8]

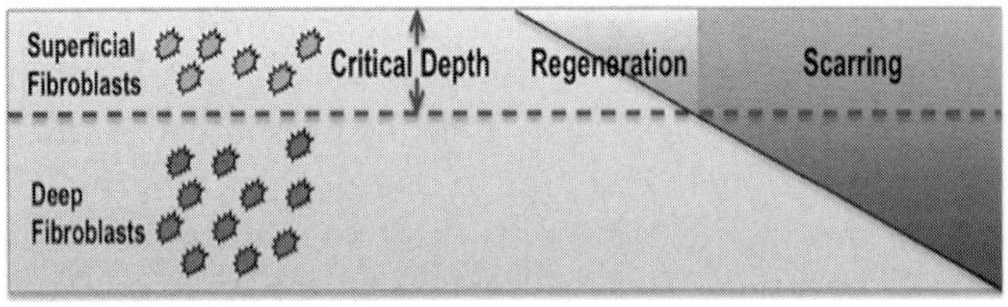

Figure 2. Regeneration occurs in superficial wounds, whereas scarring occurs in deeper wounds. From: Kwan P et al.: Scar and contraction: biological principles. Hand Burns 2009; **25:** 511.

fibrosis using bleomycin in LSP1 −/− mice. The absence of LSP1 promoted fibrosis with an increased thickness of skin and collagen content. The likely mechanism seems to be through an increased leukocyte infiltration through the endothelium into the wound, which led to locally elevated synthesis and release of chemokines and growth factors.[12]

Additionally, it has been recognized that regeneration occurs in superficial wounds, whereas scarring occurs in deeper wounds as shown in Fig. 2. Therefore, the importance of fibroblasts from the deeper layers of the skin in the formation of HTS has been identified. Fibroblasts from the deeper layer of skin incubated *in vitro* were larger in size, proliferated slowly, produced more collagen, versican, TGF-β, and less decorin, collagenase (matrix metalloproteinase 1), and upregulated the mRNA expression of heat-shock protein 47 and CTGF. CTGF mRNA levels were reversed by treating cells with TGF-β1-neutralizing antibodies. As well, fibroblasts from the deeper dermis expressed more αSMA and were associated with enhanced contraction of collagen lattices *in vitro*.[24]

Using current studies, the improvement of scar quality after treatment with IFNα2b is associated not only with an induction of myofibroblast apoptosis[25] but also with a decreased fibrocyte number and inhibition of fibrocyte function[26] as well as decreased angiogenesis mediated by vascular endothelium growth factor.[27]

CAUTION, CRITICAL REMARKS AND RECOMMENDATIONS

Effective prevention and treatment of HTS depends on a good understanding of the wound healing process and the mechanism of HTS formation. Therefore, establishing credible *in vivo* and *in vitro* models to investigate a single system, single type of cells, single fibrogenic growth factor, or single gene can be evaluated. Recent studies have shown that bone marrow–derived stem cells and progenitors seem to play a critical role in wound healing as well as HTS formation. Enhancement of research in this area, particularly to determine how the depth of injury and degree of inflammation relate to activation of bone marrow–derived cells, may be a breakthrough in understanding the mechanism of hypertrophic scarring. Moreover, activation of the immune system may also determine the outcome of wound healing since we know that prolonged inflammation and deep injury usually precede HTS.

FUTURE DEVELOPMENTS

The relative importance of bone marrow–derived cells such as fibrocytes and other hematopoetic cells as well as MSCs in wound healing and the development of fibrosis of the skin and other tissues is as yet unclear. Although it is clearly established that deep injuries to the skin predictably lead to the development of HTS, emerging evidence suggests that considerable heterogeneity of fibroblasts exists within the deeper layers of the dermis, and their features *in vitro* closely resemble HTS fibroblasts when compared with the site-matched normal controls. Increased awareness of both circulating stem cells as well as stem cell at rest in regions of the skin adds complexity to the understanding but offers exciting possibilities for the treatment of fibroproliferative disorders of the skin and other tissues in the future.

ACKNOWLEDGMENTS

The wound healing research in the author's laboratory is funded by the Canadian Institutes of Health Research, the Alberta Heritage Foundation for Medical Research, and Firefighters' Burn Trust Fund of the University of Alberta.

AUTHOR DISCLOSURE STATEMENT

The author has no conflict of interest.

REFERENCES

1. Miller SF, Bessey P, Lentz CW, Jeng JC, Schurr M, and Browning S: National Burn Repository 2007 Report: a synopsis of the 2007 call for data. J Burn Care Res 2007; **29:** 862.
2. Bailey AJ, Bazin S, Sims TJ, *et al.*: Characterization of the collagen of human hypertrophic and normal scars. Biochim Biophys Acta 1975; **405:** 412.
3. Linares HA, Kischer CW, Dobrkovsky M, and Larson DL: The histiotypic organization of the hypertrophic scar in humans. J Invest Dermatol 1972; **59:** 323.

4. Scott PG, Dodd CM, Tredget EE, Ghahary A, and Rahemtulla F: Chemical characterization and quantification of proteoglycans in human post-burn hypertrophic and mature scars. Clin Sci (Lond) 1996; **90:** 417.

5. Alexander SA and Donoff RB: The histochemistry of glycosaminoglycans within hypertrophic scars. J Surg Res 1980; **28:** 171.

6. Castagnoli C, Trombotto C, Ondei S, *et al.*: Characterization of T-cell subsets infiltrating post-burn hypertrophic scar tissues. Burns 1997; **23:** 565.

7. Tredget EE, Yang L, Delehanty M, Shankowsky H, and Scott PG: Polarized Th2 cytokine production in patients with hypertrophic scar following thermal injury. J Interferon Cytokine Res 2006; **26:** 179.

8. Armour A, Scott PG, and Tredget EE: Cellular and molecular pathology of HTS: basis for treatment. Wound Repair Regen 2007; **15:** 6.

9. van der Veer WM, Bloemen MC, and Ulrich MM, *et al.*: Potential cellular and molecular causes of hypertrophic scar formation. Burns 2009; **35:** 15.

10. Ramos MLC, Gragnani A, and Ferreira LM: Is there an ideal animal model to study hypertrophic scarring? J Burn Care Res 2008; **29:** 363.

11. Sullivan TP, Eaglstei WH, Davis SC, and Mertz P: The pig as a model for human wound healing. Wound Repair Regen 2001; **9:** 66.

12. Wang JF, Jiao HY, Stewart TL, *et al.*: Increased severity of bleomycin-induced skin fibrosis in mice with leukocyte-specific protein deficiency. J Invest Dermatol 2008; **128:** 2767.

13. Yang DY, Li SR, Wu JL, Chen YQ, *et al.*: Establishment of a hypertrophic scar model by transplanting full-thickness human skin grafts onto the backs of nude mice. Plast Reconstr Surg 2007; **119:** 104.

14. Wu Y, Chen L, Scott PG, and Tredget EE: Mesenchymal stem cells enhance wound healing through differentiation and angiogenesis. Stem Cells 2007; **25:** 2648.

15. Yang LJ, Scott PG, Dodd C, *et al.*: Identification of fibrocytes in postburn hypertrophic scar. Wound Repair Regen 2005; **13:** 398.

16. Chesney J, Metz C, Stavitsky AB, Bacher M, and Bucala R: Regulated production of type I collagen and inflammatory cytokines by peripheral blood fibrocytes. J Immunol 1998; **160:** 419.

17. Chesney J, Bacher M, Bender A, and Bucala R: The peripheral blood fibrocyte is a potent antigen-presenting cell capable of priming naive T cells *in situ.* Proc Natl Acad Sci USA 1997; **94:** 6307.

18. Hartlapp I, Abe R, and Saeed RW: Fibrocytes induce an angiogenic phenotype in cultured endothelial cells and promote angiogenesis *in vivo.* FASEB J 2001; **15:** 2215.

19. Mori L, Bellini A, Stacey MA, Schmidt M, and Mattoli S: Fibrocytes contribute to the myofibroblast population in wounded skin and originate from the bone marrow. Exp Cell Res 2005; **304:** 81.

20. Grab DJ, Salem ML, Dumler JS, and Bucala R: A role for the peripheral blood fibrocyte in leishmaniasis? Trends Parasitol 2004; **20:** 12.

21. Shao DD, Suresh R, Vakil V, Gomer RH, and Pilling D: Pivotal advance: Th-1 cytokines inhibit, and Th-2 cytokines promote fibrocyte differentiation. J Leukoc Biol 2008; **83:** 1323.

22. Wang JF, Jiao HY, Stewart TL, *et al.*: Fibrocytes from burn patients regulate the activities of fibroblasts. Wound Repair Regen 2007; **15:** 113.

23. Wang JF, Jiao HY, Stewart TL, *et al.*: Increased TGFβ-producing CD4+ T lymphocytes in postburn patients and their potential interaction with dermal fibroblasts in hypertrophic scarring. Wound Repair Regen 2007; **15:** 530.

24. Wang JF, Dodd C, Shankowsky HA, Scott PG, and Tredget EE: Deep dermal fibroblasts contribute to hypertrophic scarring. Lab Invest 2008; **88:** 1278.

25. Nedelec B, Shankowsky H, Scott PG, Ghahary A, and Tredget EE: Myofibroblasts and apoptosis in human hypertrophic scars: the effect of interferon-alpha 2b. Surgery 2001; **130:** 798.

26. Wang JF, Jiao H, Stewart TL, *et al.*: Improvement in postburn hypertrophic scar after treatment with IFN-alpha 2b is associated with decreased fibrocytes. J Interferon Cytokine Res 2007; **27:** 921.

27. Wang JF, Chen H, Shankowsky HA, Scott PG, and Tredget EE: Improved scar in postburn patients following interferon-α2b treatment is associated with decreased angiogenesis mediated by vascular endothelial cell growth factor. J Interferon Cytokine Res 2008; **28:** 423.

28. Roseborough IE, Grevious MA, and Lee RC: Prevention and treatment of excessive dermal scarring. J Natl Med Assoc 2004; **96:** 108.

29. Ha X, Yuan B, Li Y, Lao M, and Wu Z: Gene therapy for pathological scar with hepatocyte growth factor mediated by recombinant adenovirus vector. Sci China Ser C Life Sci 2003; **46:** 320.

30. Yang JG, Sun NX, Cui LJ, *et al.*: Adenovirus-mediated delivery of p27(KIP1) to prevent wound healing after experimental glaucoma filtration surgery. Acta Pharmacol Sin 2009; **30:** 413.

31. Ferguson MWJ, DuncanJ, Bond J, *et al.*: Prophylactic administration of avotermin for improvement of skin scarring: three double-blind, placebo-controlled, phase I/II studies. Lancet 2009; **373:** 1264.

32. Anzarut A, Olson J, Singh P, Rowe BH, and Tredget EE: The effectiveness of pressure garment therapy for the prevention of abnormal scarring after burn injury: a meta-analysis. J Plast Reconstr Aesthetic Surg 2009; **62:** 77.

33. Ermolov AS, Smirnov SV, Khvatov VB, *et al.*: The use of bioactive wound dressing, stimulating epithelial regeneration of IIIa-degree burn wounds. Bull Exp Biol Med 2008; **146:** 153.

34. Mezzana P: Clinical efficacy of a new chitin nanofibrils-based gel in wound healing. Acta Chir Plast 2008; **50:** 81.

Linking the Advanced Glycation Endproducts/ Receptor for Advanced Glycation Endproducts Pathway in Diabetics with Inflammation and Topical Antiinflammatory Treatments of Chronic Wounds

Gregory Schultz,[1,*] Jorge Berlanga Acosta,[2] Linda Cowan,[3] and Joyce Stechmiller[3]

[1]*Department of Obstetrics and Gynecology, Institute for Wound Research, University of Florida, Gainesville, Florida.*
[2]*Center for Genetic Engineering and Biotechnology, Havana City, Cuba.*
[3]*Department of Adult and Elderly Nursing, University of Florida, Gainesville, Florida.*

Abbreviations and Acronyms

AGE = advanced glycation endproducts
FDA = Food and Drug Administration
IgG1 = immunoglobulin
IL-1 = interleukin one
MMPs = matrix metalloproteinases
RAGE = receptor for advanced glycation endproducts
TACE = tumor necrosis factor alpha converting enzyme
TNF-α = tumor necrosis factor-alpha

*Correspondence: Department of Obstetrics and Gynecology, Institute for Wound Research, University of Florida, Gainesville, Florida 32610-0294 (e-mail: schultzg@ufl.edu).

Background: Chronic wounds are a major complication of diabetes, affecting approximately 15% of people with diabetes during their lifetime. If not properly treated, these ulcers can become infected, leading to amputation. The annual amputation rate among diabetic patients is approximately 50 per 10,000, and limb amputation is associated with higher risk of further amputation and a 5-year mortality rate approaching 50%.
The Problem: There is a need to better understand how alterations of cellular and extracellular molecules caused by diabetes contribute to the molecular pathologies identified in chronic wounds. Integration of this knowledge into a series of linked pathways that contribute to the failure of diabetic skin wounds to heal will indicate where new therapeutic strategies can be designed to correct biochemical imbalances in diabetic wound beds and promote healing.
Basic/Clinical Science Advances: Combining information on the roles of advanced glycation endproducts (AGE) and the receptor for AGE in multiple diseases like atherosclerosis, arthritis, and sepsis has provided insight into many of the molecular pathologies found in chronic diabetic wounds. The emerging hypothesis links chronic hyperglycemia associated with type 1 and 2 diabetes with elevated levels of AGE/receptor for AGE, which increases synthesis of proinflammatory cytokines that subsequently stimulate production of proteases in wounds, and ultimately impair healing by destroying proteins that are essential for healing.
Clinical Care Relevance: New topical therapies with inhibitors that block activation of protumor necrosis factor-alpha or inhibit matrix metalloproteinases or with antibodies that inhibit tumor necrosis factor-alpha are producing promising results in initial clinical studies.
Conclusion: Better understanding of the causes of molecular imbalances that prevent diabetic wounds from healing will lead to new therapeutic strategies.

BACKGROUND

Chronic hyperglycemia is a characteristic of both type 1 and type 2 diabetes, and it leads to large increases in the amounts of advanced glycation endproducts (AGE) that are produced by nonenzymatic glycation and oxidation of proteins and lipids in the extracellular matrix and cell membranes.[1,2] AGEs bind to the receptor for AGE (RAGE), which is a multiligand member of the immunoglobulin (IgG1) superfamily of cell surface molecules and is present on

ADVANCES IN WOUND CARE, VOLUME 1

Printed in U.S.A.
DOI: 10.1089/awc.2009.0096

numerous cell types, including endothelial cells, mononuclear phagocytes, smooth muscle cells, and fibroblasts. AGE binding to RAGE activates at least two major signal transduction pathways, one involving the small G-protein Ras, the protein kinase ERK-2, and ultimately leading to activation of the transcription factor AP-1.[1,2] The second signal transduction pathway activated by AGE/RAGE complex leads to activation of the transcription factor NF-κB. These two pathways converge at the transcriptional level to induce the expression of several proinflammatory cytokines, including tumor necrosis factor-alpha (TNF-α), interleukin one (IL-1), and interleukin six, which are potent chemotactic factors for neutrophils and macrophages.[3] TNF-α and IL-1 also directly down-regulate the synthesis of collagen by fibroblasts and up-regulate synthesis of matrix metalloproteinases (MMPs) by fibroblasts and inflammatory cells.[4,5] Chronic elevation of MMPs in wounds leads to degradation of proteins that are essential for wound healing, such as growth factors, receptors, and extracellular matrix.[6–8] Thus, as shown in Figure 1, in diabetics a molecular pathway links hyperglycemia with elevated levels of AGE/RAGE, which leads to increased synthesis of inflammatory cytokines like TNF-α and IL-1. These cytokines then directly stimulate production of proteases like MMPs and neutrophil elastase that eventually impair healing by degrading proteins that are essential for healing.

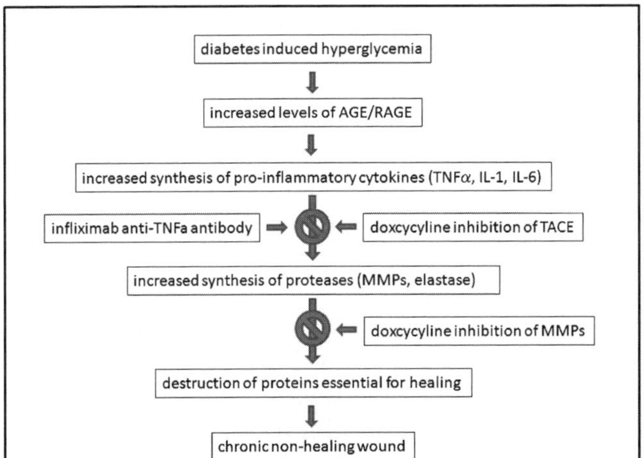

Figure 1. Linkage between diabetes-induced hyperglycemia, advanced glycation endproducts (AGE)/receptor for AGE (RAGE), inflammation, and proteases. Diabetes induces hyperglycemia, which increases the levels of AGE through nonenzymatic glycation reactions. AGE bind to the receptor (RAGE), which stimulates synthesis of proinflammatory cytokines that stimulate synthesis of proteases (matrix metalloproteinases [MMPs] and elastase). Chronic elevation of proteolytic activity in wounds leads to destruction of proteins that are essential for healing, which impairs healing and produces a chronic wound.

CLINICAL PROBLEM ADDRESSED

Chronic wounds are a major complication of diabetes, effecting approximately 15% of people with diabetes during their lifetime.[9] If not properly treated, these ulcers can become infected or gangrenous and can lead to amputation of the affected limb. The annual amputation rate among diabetic patients is approximately 50 per 10,000.[10] In addition to a significant economic burden, limb amputation is associated with higher morbidity, increased risk of further amputation, and a 5-year mortality rate of approximately 50%.[11] The principles of wound care that are outlined in the concept of "Wound Bed Preparation" integrate four important components that need to be optimized in the care of both acute and chronic wounds: appropriate tissue debridement, controlling infection and inflammation, establishing proper moisture balance, and enhancing epithelial cell migration.[12–14] Employing appropriate standard-of-care therapies will remove major barriers to healing in most chronic wounds and allow healing to proceed. However, adding advanced dressings or therapies to standard care may be necessary to stimulate healing of some chronic wounds. For example, dressings that reduce MMP activity in wound fluids by binding the proteases were reported to promote healing of long-term chronic venous ulcers.[15] Topical treatment with platelet-derived growth factor-BB was shown to significantly improve healing of chronic diabetic foot ulcers in four randomized clinical trials.[9] However, many patients do not have access to these therapies either because of cost or because their wound care provider is not skilled in debridement, which is essential to optimize the effects of platelet-derived growth factor treatment.[16] Thus, there is a need to develop new therapies that are less expensive and are able to be used broadly by wound care providers with minimal training. Ideally, these therapies would specifically target the molecular imbalances that prevent the wounds from healing. Simply stated, however, development of these new therapies requires sufficient knowledge about two key issues: (1) what molecules are either too high or too low to allow healing in the wound; (2) what causes the alterations and imbalances of these essential molecules. Armed with this knowledge, logical approaches can be developed to clinically correct these problems in wound beds.

RELEVANT BASIC SCIENCE CONTEXT

There is strong experimental and clinical evidence that elevated levels of AGE/RAGE promote inflammation and tissue damage in multiple diseases like atherosclerosis, arthritis, and sepsis by elevating inflammatory cytokines like TNF-α and IL-1 that increase synthesis of proteases, including MMPs and neutrophil elastase, that damage tissue and cause pathologies.[17–19] Establishing good glycemic control in diabetic patients is fundamentally important in resetting the AGE/RAGE system to more normal levels. However, once a chronic wound has developed in a diabetic patient, maintaining proper glycemic control is usually not sufficient to promote healing because the molecular environment in the wound is altered so extensively that spontaneous recovery is impaired. In most cases, therapeutic interventions in the wound bed are required to reestablish a molecular environment, that is adequate to support healing. Thus, new therapies that act downstream of the AGE/RAGE system are needed together with proper glycemic control to rapidly reestablish a molecular environment that promotes healing.

EXPERIMENTAL MODEL OR MATERIAL—ADVANTAGES AND LIMITATIONS

Two classes of drugs are being evaluated for topical treatment of chronic diabetic foot ulcers: (1) an inhibitor of metalloproteinases, doxycycline, which is also a synthetic antibiotic; (2) a TNF-α binding protein, infliximab, which is a chimeric IgG1 monoclonal antibody that binds and neutralizes soluble and membrane bound TNF-α with high affinity and specificity. Neither of these drugs directly target the AGE/RAGE system, but instead, they target the downstream inflammation and proteases that result in part from AGE/RAGE stimulation. All three of these drugs are well-known and are approved by Food and Drug Administration (FDA) for other indications.

Doxycycline is approved by the FDA and in Europe for use as an oral or intravenous antibiotic that has bacteriostatic activity against both Gram-positive and Gram-negative bacteria through blocking bacterial protein synthesis by binding to bacterial ribosome proteins. However, it is also a nonspecific, competitive inhibitor of metalloproteinases, and it is this property that enables doxycycline to inhibit two key subfamilies of proteases that are members of the metalloproteinase superfamily of enzymes, specifically the TNF-α converting enzyme (TACE) and the MMPs.[20–23] Thus, doxycycline has three actions that help to restore the proper molecular balance in wounds: (1) it inhibits TACE, which reduces the release of soluble, active TNF-α; (2) it inhibits MMPs that are up-regulated by TNF-α and IL-1; (3) its bacteriostatic action helps to reduce levels of planktonic bacteria in a wound bed.

The anti-TNF-α drug, infliximab, is approved by the FDA and in Europe for use in patients with rheumatoid arthritis. Infliximab is a monoclonal antibody that functions by binding soluble TNFa, thereby preventing it from binding to the TNF-α receptor in the plasmamembrane of target cells and activating intracellular signal transduction pathways that lead to multiple diverse effects of TNF-α in different cell types, including up-regulation of MMP synthesis, apoptosis of some cells, and proliferation of others.[24,25]

A major advantage for both of these drugs is that they are all approved by the FDA and in Europe. However, they are not approved for topical application to chronic diabetic ulcers. Thus, a disadvantage is that the FDA required an investigational new drug exemption for the topical use of doxycycline since both the formulation and route of administration are changed from the approved use. The anti-TNF-α drug is being used in Europe, which

TAKE-HOME MESSAGE

Basic science advances

- Hyperglycemia caused by diabetes increases the levels of AGE through nonenzymatic glycation reactions.
- AGE bind to the receptor (RAGE) stimulates synthesis of proinflammatory cytokines (TNF-α, IL-1, and interleukin six) that stimulate synthesis of proteases (MMPs and elastase).
- Chronic elevation of proteolytic activity in wounds leads to destruction of proteins that are essential for healing a chronic wound.

Clinical science advances

- Topical treatment of chronic diabetic foot ulcers with an inhibitor of TACE and MMPs (doxycycline) improved healing in a pilot, randomized, double-blinded, placebo-controlled clinical trial.
- Topical treatment of chronic wounds of various etiologies with an anti-TNF-α antibody improved healing in a case series of 8 patients with 12 chronic wounds.

Relevance to clinical care

- New therapies based on selectively inhibiting the downstream effects on inflammation and proteases of AGE/RAGE system may provide additional treatments that correct molecular imbalances in chronic wounds and improve healing.

requires different governmental clearance requirements than in the United States, but it is possible that an investigational new drug exemption would be required for topical use of infliximab in a clinical trial. An advantage for a topical doxycycline formulation is that it is a generic drug of relatively low cost. Although there is always a risk of bacteria developing resistance to an antibiotic, over 50 years of clinical use of doxycycline has not led to a serious loss of bacteriostatic efficacy against the major species of human pathogens. Further, 1% topical doxycycline gel (10 mg/g) probably provides a very high concentration of doxycycline in the wound bed, at levels that are approximately 300-times higher than the highest minimum inhibitory concentration of 32 μg/mL for representative bacteria listed in FDA-approved package inserts. The high concentration reduces the risk of selecting doxycycline-resistant bacteria in chronic wounds treated with topical 1% doxycycline.

DISCUSSION OF FINDINGS AND RELEVANT LITERATURE

TACE and MMP inhibition by topical doxycycline treatment

A pilot, randomized, double-blinded, placebo-controlled trial was performed using topical treatment with either 1% doxycycline gel or vehicle gel and standardized good wound care of chronic, full-thickness, lower extremity ulcers in diabetic patients.[26] After a thorough history and physical exam at the screening visit, patients who met the following criteria were enrolled: ulcer duration of 4 weeks to 2 years; ulcer dimensions between 1.7 and 12 cm^2; bacterial counts from punch biopsy of $\leq 1 \times 10^6$/g of tissue; transcutaneous oxygen saturation of $\geq$30 mm Hg; ankle brachial index $\geq$0.8; blood analyses within normal limits, including complete blood count, metabolic panel, and glycosylated hemoglobin A 1C of $\leq$ 6%. Patients were randomly assigned to one of the treatment arms by the pharmacy at the time the patient was enrolled. All four chronic ulcers of diabetic patients treated daily with topical 1% doxycycline healed in the 20-week treatment period, whereas only one of three patients treated with vehicle healed ($p = 0.05$ using χ^2-test). No adverse events were attributed to doxycycline treatment. Further, one of the two control patients who received standardized care elected at the end of the 20-week study to cross over and receive 1% doxycycline gel treatment. After 10 additional weeks of treatment, the wound area was reduced 80%. A larger randomized, double-blinded, placebo-controlled clinical trial is currently underway to determine the effect of topical treatment with doxycycline gel on healing of chronic diabetic foot ulcers.

TNF-α inhibition by topical infliximab treatment

In a case series, infliximab was applied topically to eight patients with chronic ulcers of more than a 4-month duration (range: 4 months to 30 years), and the wound size ranged from 1 to 300 cm.[2,27] The ulcers had multifactorial etiology, with chronic venous insufficiency in six cases being the most prominent factor. All the ulcers had failed to respond to any previous conventional treatment, including compression therapy. Infliximab was applied repeatedly to ulcers either as a 10 mg/mL solution after 3 to 4 weeks and covered with an adhesive sheet, or applied as a gel formulation (0.45, 1, or 4.5 mg/g) either once or twice a week under a hydrofiber dressing/adhesive sheet. Improvement was assessed by measuring the percentage of change in the ulcer surface area. Seven of the eight patients (12 of 14 ulcers) responded to treatment with infliximab. After 4 weeks of treatment, surface area was reduced by more than 50% in 6 of the 14 treated ulcers. Within 8 weeks, five ulcers completely healed, while another four were reduced by more than 75% in size. This case series suggested that chronic, therapy-resistant leg ulcers responded well to repeated topical administration of a solution or a gel containing the TNF-α antibody, infliximab. These results justify conducting randomized controlled studies to further evaluate the effect of topical infliximab on chronic wound healing. Further, laboratory data indicate that another anti-TNF-α drug, Etanercept, which is a recombinant fusion protein consisting of the soluble receptor TNF receptor (p75) and linked to the Fc portion of human IgG1, is able to inhibit TNF-α activity in chronic wound fluids.[28]

CAUTION, CRITICAL REMARKS, AND RECOMMENDATIONS

The linkage of a fundamental alteration of diabetes, hyperglycemia, with a cascading sequence of molecular alterations that ultimately results in a hostile molecular environment for healing provides an improved framework in which to develop new therapies. This has led recently to two different approaches using FDA-approved drugs that inhibit actions of two key components of the cascade, specifically TNF-α and MMPs. These two initial clinical studies present encouraging results, but they clearly do not prove the hypothesis, nor at this point, change the standard of care for chronic diabetic ulcers.

FUTURE DEVELOPMENT

The basic science experiments and the two initial clinical studies justify conducting additional, well-designed, clinical trials that will definitely determine if these new therapies promote healing of chronic diabetic ulcers.

AUTHOR DISCLOSURE STATEMENT

None of the authors have real or perceived conflicts of interest in connection with this chapter, and no competing financial interests exist.

REFERENCES

1. Yan SF, Ramasamy R, Naka Y, and Schmidt AM: Glycation, inflammation, and RAGE: a scaffold for the macrovascular complications of diabetes and beyond. Circ Res 2003; **93:** 1159.
2. Neumann A, Schinzel R, Palm D, Riederer P, and Munch G: High molecular weight hyaluronic acid inhibits advanced glycation endproduct-induced NF-kappaB activation and cytokine expression. FEBS Lett 1999; **453:** 283.
3. Meiners I, Hauschildt S, Nieber K, and Munch G: Pentoxyphylline and propentophylline are inhibitors of TNF-alpha release in monocytes activated by advanced glycation endproducts. J Neural Transm 2004; **111:** 441.
4. Solis-Herruzo JA, Brenners DA, and Chojkier M: Tumor necrosis factor alpha inhibits collagen gene transcription and collagen synthesis in cultured human fibroblasts. J Biol Chem 1988; **263:** 5841.
5. Unemori EN, Hibbs MS, and Amento EP: Constitutive expression of 92-kD gelatinse (type V collagenase) by rheumatoid synovial fibroblast and its induction in normal human fibroblasts by inflammatory cytokines. J Clin Investig 1991; **88:** 1656.
6. Tarnuzzer RW and Schultz GS: Biochemical analysis of acute and chronic wound environments. Wound Repair Regen 1996; **4:** 321.
7. Mast BA and Schultz GS: Interactions of cytokines, growth factors, and proteases in acute and chronic wounds. Wound Repair Regen 1996; **4:** 411.
8. Yager DR and Nwomeh BC: The proteolytic environment of chronic wounds. Wound Repair Regen 1999; **7:** 433.
9. Smiell JM, Wieman TJ, Steed DL, Perry BH, Sampson AR, and Schwab BH: Efficacy and safety of becaplermin (recombinant human platelet-derived growth factor-BB) in patients with nonhealing, lower extremity diabetic ulcers: a combined analysis of four randomized studies. Wound Repair Regen 1999; **7:** 335.
10. Larsson J, Apelqvist J, Agardh CD, and Stenstrom A: Decreasing incidence of major amputation in diabetic patients: a consequence of a multidisciplinary foot care team approach? Diabet Med 1995; **12:** 770.
11. Reiber GE, Boyko EJ, and Smith DG: Lower extremity foot ulcers and amputations in diabetes. In: *Diabetes in America*, edited by National Diabetes Data Group. Bethesda, MD: National Institutes of Health, 1995, pp. 409–427.
12. Schultz GS, Sibbald RG, Falanga V, Ayello EA, Dowsett C, Harding K, Romanelli M, Stacey MC, Teot L, and Vanscheidt W: Wound bed preparation: a systematic approach to wound management. Wound Repair Regen 2003; **11 Suppl 1:** S1.
13. Dowsett C and Ayello E: TIME principles of chronic wound bed preparation and treatment. Br J Nurs 2004; **13:** S16.
14. Schultz G, Mozingo D, Romanelli M, and Claxton K: Wound healing and TIME; new concepts and scientific applications. Wound Repair Regen 2005; **13:** S1.
15. Vin F, Teot L, and Meaume S: The healing properties of Promogran in venous leg ulcers. J Wound Care 2002; **11:** 335.
16. Steed DL, Donohoe D, Webster MW, and Lindsley L: Effect of extensive debridement and treatment on the healing of diabetic foot ulcers. Diabetic Ulcer Study Group. J Am Coll Surg 1996; **183:** 61.
17. Schmidt AM and Stern DM: RAGE: a new target for the prevention and treatment of the vascular and inflammatory complications of diabetes. Trends Endocrinol Metab 2000; **11:** 368.
18. Moser B, Hudson BI, and Schmidt AM: Soluble RAGE: a hot new biomarker for the hot joint? Arthritis Res Ther 2005; **7:** 142.
19. van Zoelen MA and van der PT: Targeting RAGE in sepsis. Crit Care 2008; **12:** 103.
20. Golub LM, Sorsa T, Lee HM, Ciancio S, Sorbi D, Ramamurthy NS, Gruber B, Salo T, and Konttinen YT: Doxycycline inhibits neutrophil (PMN)-type matrix metalloproteinases in human adult periodontitis gingiva. J Clin Periodontol 1995; **22:** 100.
21. Smith GN Jr., Mickler EA, Hasty KA, and Brandt KD: Specificity of inhibition of matrix metalloproteinase activity by doxycycline: relationship to structure of the enzyme. Arthritis Rheum 1999; **42:** 1140.
22. Bostanci N, Reddi D, Rangarajan M, Curtis MA, and Belibasakis GN: Porphyromonas gingivalis stimulates TACE production by T cells. Oral Microbiol Immunol 2009; **24:** 146.
23. Meli DN, Coimbra RS, Erhart DG, Loquet G, Bellac CL, Tauber MG, Neumann U, and Leib SL: Doxycycline reduces mortality and injury to the brain and cochlea in experimental pneumococcal meningitis. Infect Immun 2006; **74:** 3890.
24. Frater-Schroder M, Risau W, Hallmann R, Gautschi P, and Bohlen P: Tumor necrosis factor type alpha, a potent inhibitor of endothelial cell growth *in vitro*, is angiogenic *in vivo*. Proc Natl Acad Sci USA 1987; **84:** 5277.
25. Polunovsky VA, Wendt CH, Ingbar DH, Peterson MS, and Bitterman PB: Induction of endothelial cell apoptosis by TNF alpha: modulation by inhibitors of protein synthesis. Exp Cell Res 1994; **214:** 584.
26. Chin GA, Thigpin TG, Perrin KJ, Moldawer LL, and Schultz GS: Treatment of chronic ulcers in diabetic patients with a topical metalloproteinase inhibitor, doxycycline. Wounds 2003; **15:** 315.
27. Streit M, Beleznay Z, and Braathen LR: Topical application of the tumour necrosis factor-alpha antibody infliximab improves healing of chronic wounds. Int Wound J 2006; **3:** 171.
28. Cowin AJ, Hatzirodos N, Rigden J, Fitridge R, and Belford DA: Etanercept decreases tumor necrosis factor-alpha activity in chronic wound fluid. Wound Repair Regen 2006; **14:** 421.

Resolution of Inflammation in Wound Healing: Significance of Dead Cell Clearance

Sashwati Roy*

Department of Surgery, Comprehensive Wound Center, The Ohio State University Medical Center, Columbus, Ohio.

Background: Wound inflammation is driven by several mediators that are tightly controlled in space–time. Successful repair after tissue injury requires timely resolution of the inflammatory response. This response is self-limiting and resolves through the release of endogenous antiinflammatory mediators and the clearance of inflammatory cells.

The Problem: Whereas the knowledge about mechanisms and molecules inducing and perpetuating the inflammatory response is constantly increasing, mechanisms that resolve inflammation remain poorly understood, especially in the context of wound healing. Most chronic wounds have dysregulated inflammatory response. This chapter describes some of the latest key concepts in resolution of inflammation that are relevant for the etiology of inflamed nonhealing wounds.

Basic/Clinical Science Advances: Recent data indicate that the resolution of inflammation is an active process controlled by endogenous mediators that suppress proinflammatory gene expression and cell trafficking, as well as induce inflammatory-cell apoptosis and subsequent clearance of these apoptotic cells.

Clinical Care Relevance: The goal in the treatment of chronic inflamed wounds must be to inhibit persistent inflammation and restore tissue function. To achieve this goal, an understanding of the mechanisms that regulate resolution of inflammation is critical.

Conclusions: Apoptosis of inflammatory cells followed by successful clearance of the cell corpse, or cellular debridement, is essential for resolution of inflammation. Development of therapeutics directed to promote cellular debridement may switch the ongoing inflammation into resolution.

Abbreviations and Acronyms

ELMO = engulfment and motility protein

Gas6 = growth arrest–specific gene

LPC = lysophosphatidylcholine

MFG-E8 = milk-fat-globule-epidermal growth factor 8

PMN = polymorphonuclear neutrophil

PS = phosphatidylserine

PVA = polyvinyl alcohol

TGF-β1 = transforming growth factor-β1

*Correspondence: Department of Surgery, Comprehensive Wound Center, The Ohio State University Medical Center, Columbus, Ohio 43210 (e-mail: sashwati.roy@osumc.edu).

BACKGROUND

INFLAMMATION (LATIN, *INFLAMATIO*, to set on fire) was first coined by a Roman scientist, Celsus, more than 2000 years ago. The defining clinical cardinal signs of inflammation are rubor (redness), calor (warmth), tumor (swelling), dolor (pain), and *functio laesa* (loss of function). Acute inflammation is the initial response of the body to a harmful stimulus such as irritation, foreign material infection, or other injury. The overall function of inflammation is to neutralize and destroy any toxic agents at the site of injury and to restore tissue homeostasis.

The inflammatory response involves the sequential release of mediators and the recruitment of circulating leukocytes, which become activated at the inflammatory site and release further mediators. It is generally believed that once the inflammatory response has neutralized an injurious stimulus, inflammation somehow fades out, possibly from proinflammatory mediator catabolism. On the contrary, the inflammatory response resolves through the release

Printed in U.S.A.
DOI: 10.1089/awc.2009.0158

of endogenous antiinflammatory mediators and the clearance of inflammatory cells.[1] There are a number of routes available for the efficient clearance of inflammatory cells; the most desirable for successful resolution is death by apoptosis followed by phagocytosis.[2] Apoptosis, or programmed cell death, is a constitutive suicide program expressed in most, if not all, cells and can be triggered by a variety of extrinsic and intrinsic signals.[3] Apoptosis allows for the elimination of inflammatory cells that are no longer required at the injury site or cells that are too damaged to contribute to the healing process.[4] Subsequent to apoptosis, successful clearance of the inflammatory cell corpse, or cellular debridement, is essential for resolution of inflammation. In addition to performing a purely garbage disposal function, recognition of the apoptotic cell results in enhanced production of antiinflammatory mediators by the phagocytes.[5–7] Failed or delayed clearance of apoptotic cells may result in chronic inflammation. In the clinical treatment of wound healing, debridement is commonly practiced and mostly refers to the surgical removal of dead, damaged, or infected tissue to improve the healing potential of the remaining healthy tissue. Successful healing depends on the efficient removal of dead or dying cells that are either no longer required at the injury site or too damaged to contribute to the healing process. Diabetic human wounds are stalled at the inflammatory phase because of insufficiencies in the inflammation and debridement processes.[8] Current developments posit that at the wound site successful debridement at the cellular level is a prerequisite to the resolution of inflammation and successful healing. This review will primarily focus on the mechanisms and significance of apoptotic cell clearance in the resolution of wound inflammation.

CLINICAL PROBLEM ADDRESSED

Dysregulated inflammatory phase or impairment in the resolution of inflammation is one of the major factors that underlie most chronic wounds such as diabetic ulcers.[9] In the clinical treatment of chronic wounds, debridement is commonly practiced and refers to the removal of dead, damaged, or infected tissue to improve the healing potential of the remaining healthy tissue. Often, this removal is surgical, but other methods exist such as mechanical, chemical, autolytic (self-digestion), and even maggot therapy. Current developments indicate that at the wound site successful debridement at the cellular level, or cellular debridement, is a prerequisite to the resolution of inflammation and successful healing.

RELEVANT BASIC SCIENCE CONTEXT

During the early inflammatory phase of wound healing, a large number of polymorphonuclear neutrophils (PMN) (nearly 50% of all cells at the wound site) are recruited to the injury site.[10] After completion of their tasks, PMN must be eliminated to begin the next stage of wound healing. Persistent presence of inflammatory cells will result in nonhealing wounds. Accumulation of mononuclear phagocytes invariably occurs at sites where a large number of apoptotic cells are generated in tissues after injury and/or inflammation. The timely removal of the apoptotic cells before they undergo secondary necrosis necessitates macrophage migration.[11] Apoptosis of inflammatory cells followed by engulfment of such cells by macrophages results in potent antiinflammatory and immunosuppressive effects by production of antiinflammatory cytokines such as transforming growth factor-β1 (TGF-β1), interleukin-10, and interleukin-4.[5–7] These cytokines, on the other hand, suppress production of proinflammatory cytokines, suggesting a potential role of apoptotic cell clearance in resolution of wound inflammation.

Because of the high efficiency and rapidity of apoptotic cell removal and digestion, visual evidence of dead cell clearance histologically represents only a tiny snapshot of what may be a large and often under-appreciated ongoing process.[12] Only when such clearance is defective, the extent of these processes becomes apparent.[12] Inappropriate clearance of cell corpses may lead to autoimmune diseases and chronic inflammation. A number of studies have produced compelling evidence to support that binding or uptake of apoptotic cells by macrophages stimulate these cells to release mediators that suppress the inflammatory response.[13,14] In particular, strong *in vitro* and *in vivo* evidence points to the secretion of the antiinflammatory cytokine TGF-β1 from macrophages, which can suppress proinflammatory signals from toll-like receptors.[15,16] After apoptotic cell engulfment a requirement for TGF-β1 was also shown in the inhibition of thromboxane synthase and thromboxanes, of 5-lipoxygenase and sulfidopeptide leukotrienes, as well as of inducible nitric-oxide synthase and nitric oxide.[17]

EXPERIMENTAL MODELS OR MATERIALS—ADVANTAGES AND LIMITATIONS

Inflammatory cells and fluids harvested from wounds are relevant experimental materials/models to study the inflammatory response in acute or chronic wounds. Polyvinyl alcohol (PVA) sponge–derived macrophages and PMN from rodents have been used in the past to study mechanisms of wound inflammatory cell clearance by macrophages.[4] Harvesting fluids and cells from human wounds is more challenging than collecting these samples from experimental animal wounds. The use of negative-pressure wound therapy, also known as V.A.C.® (KCI, Inc.), has been shown to be an effective way to accelerate healing of various wounds.[18] Our laboratory and others routinely use the fluids from the V.A.C. canisters for assessment of wound inflammatory or antiinflammatory environments.[19] Other models to collect fluid and cells from human wounds are the use of blister chambers, implanted Silastic catheter, and tube drains. These samples can then be used to study proteolytic activity and cytokine and growth factor balance, as well as wound cell genome and macrophage phagocytosis activity.[20,21]

DISCUSSION OF FINDINGS AND RELEVANT LITERATURE

Because the phagocytosis of apoptotic cells has distinctive morphologic features and unique downstream consequences, deCathelineau and Henson[22] coined the term *efferocytosis* (taken from the Latin *effero* meaning to take to the grave or to bury). Phagocytic clearance of apoptotic cells, or efferocytosis, consists of at least four distinct steps: (i) secreted ("find-me") signals causing accumulation of phagocytes at the site where apoptotic cells are located; (ii) recognition ("eat-me") of dying cells through a number of bridge molecules and receptors; (iii) engulfment by a unique uptake process; and (iv) processing of engulfed cells within phagocytes[11] (Fig. 1).

Find-me

Apoptotic cells release attraction signals that direct phagocytes to their location.[23] The supernatant of several types of apoptotic cells contains chemoattractant activity for monocytes and primary human macrophages.[23] Caspase-3–mediated activation of Ca^{2+}-independent phospholipase A2 in apoptotic cells is linked to the release of chemoattractant signals, which, using several approaches (including mass spectrometry), was shown to be lysophosphatidylcholine.[23]

Recognition ("eat-me")

Cells undergoing apoptosis flag themselves for removal by presenting "eat-me" signals at the cell surface.[23] These flags on the corpse differentiate them from viable cells for recognition by macrophages. Phosphatidylserine (PS) externalization is a general feature and hallmark of apoptosis.[24,25] Selective NADPH oxidase–dependent oxidation of PS and subsequent externalization has been demonstrated in a wide range of apoptotic models.[26] Externalization of oxidized PS, in conjunction with its nonoxidized counterpart, serves as an "eat-me" signal.[23] The significance of PS oxidation and

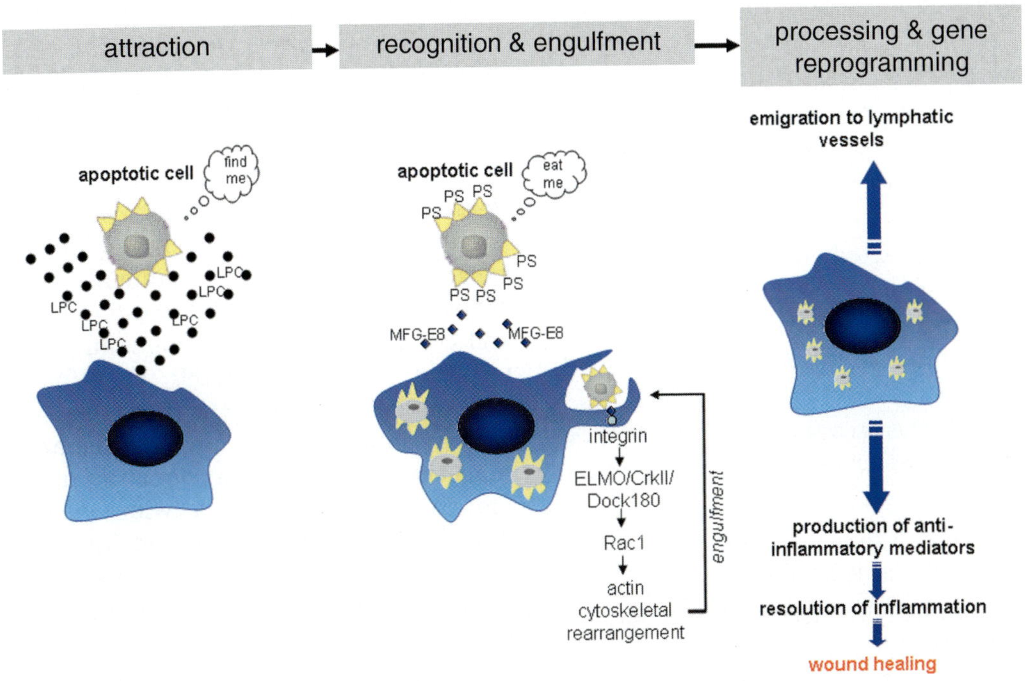

Figure 1. Mechanisms of efferocytosis and significance in resolution of wound inflammation. Distinct steps of efferocytosis are shown: (i) attraction of phagocytes at the site where apoptotic cells are located because of "find-me" signals (*e.g.*, LPC) produced by the apoptotic cells; (ii) recognition ("eat-me" signals; *e.g.*, PS externalization) of dying cells through a number of bridge molecules (*e.g.*, MFG-E8) and receptors (*e.g.*, integrins) (see text for details of these and other such molecules), and engulfment of apoptotic cells by a unique uptake process involving binding of MGF-E8 with integrins, activating ELMO/CrkII/Dock 180, and Rac1 proteins that are known to regulate rearrangements of the actin cytoskeleton and phagocytosis/engulfment; and (iii) processing of apoptotic cells by macrophages results in macrophages to either emigrate to lymphatic vessels or reprogram their gene expression to start production of antiinflammatory cytokines. These cytokines will help resolve inflammation. Resolution of inflammation is essential for successful healing of a wound. LPC = lysophosphatidylcholine; PS = phosphatidylserine; MFG-E8 = milk fat globulin E8; ELMO = engulfment and motility protein.

externalization in apoptotic cell clearance during wound healing remains to be examined. NADPH oxidase plays a critical and specific role in PS oxidation and externalization.[26] Patients with chronic granulomatous disease, an inherited condition in humans characterized by impairment of NADPH oxidase activity,[27] frequently develop disorders of autoimmunity against inadequately cleared dead tissue.[28]

Bridging molecules and phagocyte receptors

Most receptors on phagocytes do not bind to phospholipids directly, but rather via soluble bridging proteins.[29] An increasing number of these soluble factors are emerging whose role is to opsonize apoptotic cells and create molecular bridges between components of the apoptotic cells and phagocyte surfaces. This family of specialized proteins includes annexin I (Anx I or lipocortin), thrombospondin, milk-fat-globule-epidermal growth factor 8 (MFG-E8), Del-1, β2-glycoprotein I, protein S, and growth arrest–specific gene 6 (Gas6).[29,30] MFG-E8 (also known as lactadehrin), one of the key bridging molecule proteins, was identified as a protein secreted by activated macrophages.[31] *In vivo* studies have recognized the significance of MFG-E8 in apoptotic cell clearance.[31] MFG-E8 is capable of binding to PS on apoptotic cells as well as integrins on macrophages.[31] Mice lacking MFG-E8 suffer late-onset autoimmune disorder, a disease often associated with impaired clearance of apoptotic cells.[28] MFG-E8 binds to either $\alpha v\beta 3$ or $\alpha v\beta 5$ integrin receptor on the macrophage surface via a typical tripeptide Arg-Gly-Asp motif located within its two EGF repeats.[31]

TAKE-HOME MESSAGE

Basic science advances

- The inflammatory response is self-limiting and resolves through the release of endogenous antiinflammatory mediators and the clearance of inflammatory cells.
- Apoptosis of inflammatory cells followed by phagocytic removal of these cells is a prerequisite for the restoration of normal tissue function and resolution of inflammation. Failed or delayed clearance of apoptotic cells may result in chronic inflammation.
- Clearance of apoptotic cells by macrophages results in potent antiinflammatory and immunosuppressive effects by production of antiinflammatory mediators, which in turn switch off the inflammatory signals resulting in resolution of inflammation.
- Specific mechanisms of efferocytosis include (i) accumulation of phagocytes at the site where apoptotic cells are located; (ii) recognition ("eat-me") of dying cells through a number of bridge molecules and receptors; (iii) engulfment by a unique uptake process; and (iv) processing of engulfed cells within phagocytes.

Clinical science advance

- Dysregulated inflammatory phase or impairment in the resolution of inflammation is one of the major factors that underlies most chronic wounds, such as diabetic ulcers.
- In the clinical treatment of chronic wounds, debridement is commonly practiced and refers to the removal of dead, damaged, or infected tissue to improve the healing potential of the remaining healthy tissue.
- Removal of apoptotic cells can be accomplished by debridement at cellular levels.
- Recent studies indicate that cellular debridement is a prerequisite to the resolution of inflammation and successful healing.

Relevance to clinical care

- The goal in the treatment of chronic inflamed wounds must be to inhibit persistent inflammation and restore tissue function.
- To achieve this goal, understanding of the mechanisms that regulate resolution of inflammation is critical.
- Modulation of wound inflammation and healing outcomes by regulating specific aspects of the physiological cellular debridement process represent potentially important therapeutic opportunities that remain untapped at present.

Engulfment and processing of engulfed cells

Not much is known about how the final step of apoptotic cell clearance, that is, processing of apoptotic bodies, is regulated and how it differs from the processing of classically opsonized or microbial cells that employ a route of degradation from phagosomes to lysosomes. The genes identified in genetic screens of *Caenorhabditi elegans* that is defective in apoptotic cell clearance are also associated with cell adhesion and migration events in species ranging from worms to mammals. The genes in *C. elegans* (*ced-2*, *ced-5*, *ced-10*, and *ced-12*) and their mammalian counterparts (CrkII, DOCK180, engulfment and motility protein, and Rac1) encode proteins that comprise an evolutionarily conserved Rho–GTPase signaling module that functions in a wide variety of cells.[30] Crk, DOCK180, and Rac1 are downstream of adhesion receptors (*i.e.*, integrin) and receptor tyrosine kinases.[30] In a general model of MFG-E8–mediated binding and internalization of apoptotic cell by phagocytes, a central role of $\alpha v\beta 5$ integrin was noted. $\beta 5$ Cytoplasmic tail and engagement of the $\alpha v\beta 5$ heterodimer result in recruitment of the p130cas–

CrkII–Dock180 molecular complex, which in turn triggers Rac1 activation and phagosome formation.[32]

Interactions with apoptotic cells: functional consequences for immunity

Phagocytosis of apoptotic cells is actively antiinflammatory and antiimmunogenic with generation of antiinflammatory mediators such as TGF-β and antiinflammatory eicosanoids.[17] Evidence from mouse studies demonstrates a central role of Mer receptor tyrosine kinase in suppressing proinflammation signals from toll-like receptors.[30]

CAUTION, CRITICAL REMARKS, AND RECOMMENDATIONS

A range of therapies exist for the treatment of inflammation-driven diseases such as asthma, rheumatoid arthritis, psoriatic arthritis, systemic lupus erythematosus, Crohn's disease, multiple sclerosis, and systemic vasculitis. However, these therapeutics have undesirable side effects. For instance, steroids can cause osteoporosis and impair wound healing. Novel compounds based on the mechanism of action of a given proresolving mediator will be specific in their activity and likely to produce a lower burden of side effects.[2]

FUTURE DEVELOPMENT

At present, the treatment of inflammatory diseases is primarily based on interrupting the synthesis or action of mediators that drive the host's response to injury. Developing drugs that drive resolution will be critical to treating diseases with chronic inflammation. Such therapeutics might be based on factors that promote macrophage phagocytosis of apoptotic cells. In doing so, it might be possible to switch the ongoing inflammation into resolution. Unfortunately, due to relative immaturity of this area of research, the therapeutics that can promote resolution are far from the clinic. Understanding the mediators and mechanisms that are central to resolution will bring us into a new age of inflammation research, which, if approached with vision and perseverance, might provide benefit to healing of chronic wounds.

ACKNOWLEDGMENTS

Wound-healing research in the author's laboratory is funded by NIDDK R01 DK076566.

AUTHOR DISCLOSURE STATEMENT

No conflict of interest disclosed.

REFERENCES

1. Lawrence T, Gilroy DW, Colville-Nash PR, and Willoughby DA: Possible new role for NF-kappaB in the resolution of inflammation. Nat Med 2001; **7:** 1291.
2. Gilroy DW, Lawrence T, Perretti M, and Rossi AG: Inflammatory resolution: new opportunities for drug discovery. Nat Rev Drug Discov 2004; **3:** 401.
3. Hetts SW: To die or not to die: an overview of apoptosis and its role in disease [see comment]. JAMA 1998; **279:** 300.
4. Meszaros AJ, Reichner JS, and Albina JE: Macrophage phagocytosis of wound neutrophils. J Leukoc Biol 1999; **65:** 35.
5. Savill J: Apoptosis in resolution of inflammation. Kidney Blood Press Res 2000; **23:** 173.
6. Savill J, Dransfield I, Gregory C, and Haslett C: A blast from the past: clearance of apoptotic cells regulates immune responses. Nat Rev Immunol 2002; **2:** 965.
7. Savill J and Fadok V: Corpse clearance defines the meaning of cell death. Nature 2000; **407:** 784.
8. Loots MA, Lamme EN, Zeegelaar J, Mekkes JR, Bos JD, and Middelkoop E: Differences in cellular infiltrate and extracellular matrix of chronic diabetic and venous ulcers versus acute wounds. J Invest Dermatol 1998; **111:** 850.
9. Falanga V: Wound healing and its impairment in the diabetic foot. Lancet 2005; **366:** 1736.
10. Singer AJ and Clark RA: Cutaneous wound healing. N Engl J Med 1999; **341:** 738.
11. Erwig LP and Henson PM: Clearance of apoptotic cells by phagocytes. Cell Death Differ 2007. [Epub ahead of print.]
12. Erwig LP and Henson PM: Immunological consequences of apoptotic cell phagocytosis. Am J Pathol 2007; **1:** 2.
13. Fadok VA, Bratton DL, Konowal A, Freed PW, Westcott JY, and Henson PM: Macrophages that have ingested apoptotic cells *in vitro* inhibit proinflammatory cytokine production through autocrine/paracrine mechanisms involving TGF-beta, PGE2, and PAF. J Clin Invest 1998; **101:** 890.
14. Savill J, Gregory C, and Haslett C: Cell biology. Eat me or die. Science 2003; **302:** 1516.
15. Huynh ML, Fadok VA, and Henson PM: Phosphatidylserine-dependent ingestion of apoptotic cells promotes TGF-beta1 secretion and the resolution of inflammation. J Clin Invest 2002; **109:** 41.
16. Lucas M, Stuart LM, Savill J, and Lacy-Hulbert A: Apoptotic cells and innate immune stimuli combine to regulate macrophage cytokine secretion. J Immunol 2003; **171:** 2610.
17. Freire-de-Lima CG, Xiao YQ, Gardai SJ, Bratton DL, Schiemann WP, and Henson PM: Apoptotic cells, through transforming growth factor-beta, coordinately induce anti-inflammatory and suppress pro-inflammatory eicosanoid and NO synthesis in murine macrophages. J Biol Chem 2006; **281:** 38376.
18. Venturi ML, Attinger CE, Mesbahi AN, Hess CL, and Graw KS: Mechanisms and clinical applications of the vacuum-assisted closure (VAC) device: a review. Am J Clin Dermatol 2005; **6:** 185.
19. Hopf HW, Humphrey LM, Puzziferri N, West JM, Attinger CE, and Hunt TK: Adjuncts to preparing wounds for closure: hyperbaric oxygen, growth factors, skin substitutes, negative pressure wound therapy (vacuum-assisted closure). Foot Ankle Clin 2001; **6:** 661.
20. Trengove NJ, Stacey MC, MacAuley S, Bennett N, Gibson J, Burslem F, Murphy G, and Schultz G: Analysis of the acute and chronic wound environments: the role of proteases and their inhibitors. Wound Repair Regen 1999; **7:** 442.
21. Roy S, Khanna S, Yeh PE, Rink C, Malarkey WB, Kiecolt-Glaser J, Laskowski B, Glaser R, and Sen CK: Wound site neutrophil transcriptome in response to psychological stress in young men. Gene Expression **12:** 273.

22. deCathelineau AM and Henson PM: The final step in programmed cell death: phagocytes carry apoptotic cells to the grave. Essays Biochem 2003; **39:** 105.

23. Grimsley C and Ravichandran KS: Cues for apoptotic cell engulfment: eat-me, don't eat-me and come-get-me signals. Trends Cell Biol 2003; **13:** 648.

24. Bratton DL, Fadok VA, Richter DA, Kailey JM, Guthrie LA, and Henson PM: Appearance of phosphatidylserine on apoptotic cells requires calcium-mediated nonspecific flip-flop and is enhanced by loss of the aminophospholipid translocase. J Biol Chem 1997; **272:** 26159.

25. Fadok VA, de Cathelineau A, Daleke DL, Henson PM, and Bratton DL: Loss of phospholipid asymmetry and surface exposure of phosphatidylserine is required for phagocytosis of apoptotic cells by macrophages and fibroblasts. J Biol Chem 2001; **276:** 1071.

26. Kagan VE, Borisenko GG, Serinkan BF, Tyurina YY, Tyurin VA, Jiang J, Liu SX, Shvedova AA, Fabisiak JP, Uthaisang W, and Fadeel B: Appetizing rancidity of apoptotic cells for macrophages: oxidation, externalization, and recognition of phosphatidylserine. Am J Physiol Lung Cell Mol Physiol 2003; **285(1):** L1–L7.

27. Roos D and Curnutte JT: Chronic granulomatous disease. In: *Primary Immunodeficiency Diseases a Molecular and Genetic Approach*, edited by Ochs H, Smith CI, and Puck JM. New York: Oxford University Press, 1999, pp. 353–374.

28. Gaipl US, Franz S, Voll RE, Sheriff A, Kalden JR, and Herrmann M: Defects in the disposal of dying cells lead to autoimmunity. Curr Rheumatol Rep 2004; **6:** 401.

29. Zullig S and Hengartner MO: Cell biology. Tickling macrophages, a serious business. Science 2004; **304:** 1123.

30. Wu Y, Tibrewal N, and Birge RB: Phosphatidylserine recognition by phagocytes: a view to a kill. Trends Cell Biol 2006; **16:** 189.

31. Hanayama R, Tanaka M, Miyasaka K, Aozasa K, Koike M, Uchiyama Y, and Nagata S: Autoimmune disease and impaired uptake of apoptotic cells in MFG-E8-deficient mice [see comment]. Science 2004; **304:** 1147.

32. Albert ML, Kim JI, and Birge RB: Alphavbeta5 integrin recruits the CrkII-Dock180-rac1 complex for phagocytosis of apoptotic cells. Nat Cell Biol 2000; **2:** 899.

WHS Wound Healing Society

Chronic Wounds and Inflammation

Sebastian Willenborg,[1] Johanna Knipper,[1] Rajeev Ranjan,[1] Thomas Krieg,[1,2] and Sabine A. Eming[1,*]

[1]Department of Dermatology, University of Cologne, Cologne, Germany.
[2]Cologne Excellence Cluster on Cellular Stress Responses in Aging-Associated Diseases (CECAD), University of Cologne, Cologne, Germany.

Background: Restoration of tissue integrity and homeostasis after injury requires a complex and dynamic interplay of numerous cell types, including tissue-resident cells and hematopoietic cells recruited to the site of tissue damage, to accomplish the sequential stages of repair: inflammation, tissue formation, and tissue maturation.
The Problem: Experimental studies established the dogma that inflammation is essential to the establishment of cutaneous homeostasis after injury, and in recent years information about specific subsets of inflammatory cell lineages and the cytokine network orchestrating inflammation associated with tissue repair has increased. Recently, this dogma has been challenged, and reports have raised questions on the validity of the essential prerequisite of inflammation for efficient tissue repair.
Basic/Clinical Science Advances: Indeed, in experimental models of repair, inflammation has been shown to delay healing and to result in increased scarring. Further, chronic inflammation, a cardinal feature of the nonhealing wound, predisposes tissue to cancer development. The role that different subsets of the inflammatory cells play in wound repair and tissue growth has, until today, not been clearly defined.
Clinical Care Relevance: Modulation of the local immune response may prove an effective therapeutic strategy in situations of impaired healing.
Conclusion: A more detailed understanding in mechanisms controlling the inflammatory response during repair and how inflammation directs the outcome of the healing process will serve as a significant milestone in the therapy of pathological tissue repair.

Abbreviations and Acronyms

ER-b = estrogen receptor-beta
FGF = fibroblast growth factor
HGF = hepatocyte growth factor
IL-1 = interleukin-1
IL-6 = interleukin-6
IL-8 = interleukin-8
INF-γ = interferon-γ
MMPs = matrix metalloproteinases
PDGF = platelet-derived growth factor
PIGF = placental growth factor
ROS = reactive oxygen species
TGF-β = transforming-growth factor-β
TNF-α = tumor necrosis factor-α
VEGF = vascular endothelial growth factor

*Correspondence: Department of Dermatology, University of Cologne, Joseph-Stelzmann Str. 9, Cologne 50931, Germany (e-mail: sabine.eming@uni-koeln.de).

BACKGROUND

Tissue injury causes leakage of blood constituents into the wound site as well as release of vasoactive factors resulting in the activation of the clotting cascade. Clotted blood provides a matrix that determines cell adhesion and migration.[1] Platelets trapped in the clot are not only important for homeostasis but also provide a source of growth factors and proinflammatory cytokines that mediate the recruitment of inflammatory cells and fibroblasts into the wound site (Fig. 1). The early inflammatory phase of repair is characterized by local activation of the innate immune system, resulting in an early influx of polymorphonuclear leukocytes (neutrophils), followed by invasion of blood monocytes, which differentiate into tissue macrophages. Functional consequences of the innate immune response of the resident cells as well as the recruited inflammatory cells are not completely understood.[2,3] They combat invading microbes but may also critically support the repair

Printed in U.S.A.
DOI: 10.1089/awc.2009.0063

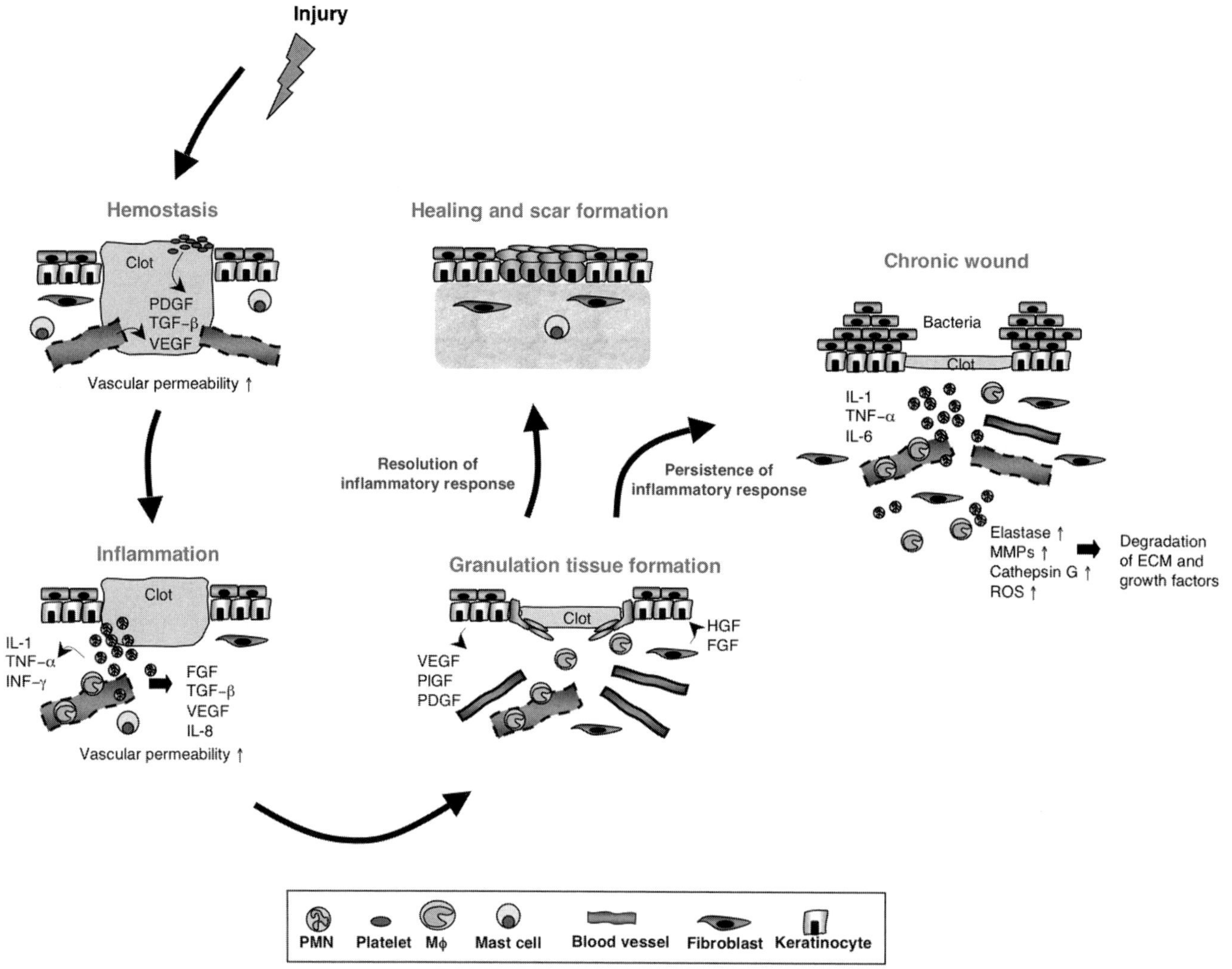

Figure 1. Model depicting outcomes of the repair response. Hemostasis is caused by leak of blood constituents and vasoactive factors into the wound site. Increased vascular permeability contributes to leak of blood constituents into the wound environment. The hemostatic plug consists of platelets and extracellular matrix molecules that facilitate invasion and migration of endothelial cells. Influx of polymorphonuclear leukocytes and macrophages (MΦ) characterizes the inflammatory phase of repair; different subsets of leukocytes release angiogenic growth factors and proinflammatory cytokines, which control the recruitment of inflammatory and endothelial cells into the wound site. During granulation tissue formation–activated MΦ, endothelial cells and fibroblasts form a functional unit essential for efficient blood vessel growth. Fibroblasts deposit a complex provisional wound matrix consisting of glycosaminoglycans, proteoglycans, collagen III, thrombospondin, fibronectin, and vitronectin, which promote endothelial tube formation and vessel growth. Transformation of granulation tissue into scar tissue is characterized by regression of capillaries and differentiation of newly formed blood vessels into mature vascular structures. This process is associated with a decrease in inflammation, presence of myofibroblasts, and substitution of the provisional wound matrix into a collagenous matrix. Chronic wounds fail to progress through the normal pattern of wound repair, but instead remain in a state of chronic inflammation predominantly characterized by abundant polymorphonuclear leukocyte and MΦ infiltration. Persisting inflammatory cells play a major role in the generation of proinflammatory cytokines, a protease-rich and prooxidant hostile microenvironment. Increased proteolytic activity (MMPs; elastase and cathepsin G) leads to degradation of growth factors and structural proteins of the extracellular matrix crucial for repair. Increased ROS can lead to direct damage of cells or extracellular matrix molecules, or contribute to increased expression of MMPs. Bacterial components may contribute to impaired repair mechanisms of the host by interference with cell–matrix interactions or stimulating the inflammatory response. MMPs = matrix metalloproteinases; ROS = reactive oxygen species; PDGF = platelet-derived growth factor; TGF-β = transforming-growth factor-β; VEGF = vascular endothelial growth factor; IL-1 = interleukin-1; IL-8 = interleukin-8; TNF-α = tumor necrosis factor-α; FGF = fibroblast growth factor; INF-γ = interferon-γ; PIGF = placental growth factor; HGF = hepatocyte growth factor; IL-6 = interleukin-6.

process by releasing a spectrum of cytokines and growth factors, which initiate the phase of tissue formation. In particular, invading macrophages are considered a rich source of growth-promoting mediators. In diverse model systems distinct macrophage activation states have been described (paradigm of M1/M2 polarization),[4] and future studies will have to clarify whether a specific macrophage activation state might be favorable in promoting the healing response and which of the microenvironmental cues direct macrophage activation.

An imbalanced and prolonged inflammatory response, on the other hand, may be detrimental to repair. During the phase of tissue formation, newly formed granulation tissue, consisting of invading endothelial cells, macrophages, and fibroblasts, covers and fills the wound area, followed by epithelialization to restore tissue integrity. Fibrin, fibronectin, vitronectin, and tenascin are components of the provisional extracellular wound matrix that facilitate cell adhesion, migration, and proliferation. At the wound edge, complex epidermal–mesenchymal interactions stimulate keratinocyte proliferation and migration.[5] Upon completion of epithelialization, cell proliferation and neovascularization cease, scar tissue forms, and the wound enters the maturation phase, which lasts several months. During this last phase, a balance is reached between synthesis of new components of scar matrix and their degradation by proteases. The mechanisms determining granulation tissue regression and its transformation into scar tissue at the stage of tissue maturation are largely unknown. Typical features of these events include regression of vascular structures, transformation of fibroblasts into myofibroblasts, substitution of provisional extracellular matrix by a permanent collagenous matrix, and, importantly, resolution of the inflammatory response. Mechanisms that terminate the inflammatory response at the wound site are not well understood and may involve increased production of antiinflammatory mediators, downregulation of proinflammatory factors, the normalization of microvascular permeability, and induction of apoptosis of inflammatory cells and their efflux from the tissue.

CLINICAL PROBLEM ADDRESSED

Impaired wound-healing conditions (*e.g.*, associated with diabetes mellitus, venous or arterial insufficiency, vasculitis, or hypertrophic scarring) are leading causes of morbidity and mortality. In Western countries, the incidence of nonhealing wounds is estimated 1%, with a prevalence of 3–5% in the population over 65 years of age.[6] It has been estimated that the economic burden of the European Community for treatment of wounds accounts for about 2% of the total health care costs. The incidence and prevalence of chronic wounds is increasing as a result of the ageing population and increased risk factors such as atherosclerosis, obesity, and diabetes. The advanced understanding of the molecular link between inflammation and repair will hopefully lead to the development of efficient therapeutic approaches to improve the quality of repair.

A cardinal feature of chronic skin ulcers is an exaggerated and prolonged inflammatory response at the wound site.[3,7] The mechanisms leading to the persistent inflammatory response in nonhealing wounds and the role that the inflammatory cells play in the pathology of chronic wounds have not been clearly defined. Therefore, a more thorough understanding of the underlying molecular and cellular mechanisms is an important task and will lead to the development of innovative strategies to improve tissue repair and regeneration.

BASIC SCIENCE CONTEXT

Restoration of tissue integrity and homeostasis after injury requires a complex and dynamic interplay of numerous cell types, extracellular matrix molecules, and soluble cytokines. Over the past decades basic science has made a tremendous contribution to a better understanding of the molecular basis of the events involved. Genetically modified mouse models have proven to be of immense help to dissect the contribution of specific immune modulators in tissue repair.[3] For example, a critical role of proinflammatory mediators in leukocyte function is evident in skin wounds of mice deficient for the tumor necrosis factor-α (TNF-α) receptor TNF-α-Rp55. Despite a significant reduction in leukocyte infiltration at the wound site, wounds showed an increase in angiogenesis, collagen content, reepithelialization, and expression of various growth factors and their receptors.[8] Ultimately, TNF-α-Rp55 deficiency and, presumably, lack of TNF-α signaling resulted in accelerated wound closure. In contrast to the generation of mouse models to identify the role of a single mediator coordinating inflammation during repair, Martin and Leibovich posed the more complex question whether the influx of neutrophils and macrophages is essential for cutaneous healing. These studies investigated perinatal repair in the PU.1 null mouse, which lacks cells of the myeloid lineage (macrophages, neutrophils, mast cells, and eosinophils) and B cells.[2] In newborn mutants, little inflammation occurred at the wound site. In contrast to the prevailing dogma, the healing occurred with a similar time course to wild-type siblings, and repair appeared scar-free, resembling fetal wound repair.

EXPERIMENTAL MODEL AND LIMITATIONS

There is substantial evidence of different model organisms that the immune system is of primary importance in determining the quality of the repair response, including the extent of scarring, and the restoration of organ structure and function. Findings in diverse species (amphibian, fish, xenopus, and mouse) support a correlation between the loss of regeneration capacity and maturation of immune competence.[9] However, in recent years, there is increasing evidence on conditions where the immune response promotes repair and ensures local tissue protection. Hence, the relationship between repair and the immune response is complex and there is evidence for both negative and positive roles. Complementary molecular analysis of the functional impact of the immune response on repair in diverse model systems will unravel complex interrelations among these events and in long term, advancing the development of therapies aiming to improve the quality of repair.

DISCUSSION OF FINDINGS AND RELEVANT LITERATURE

Diabetes-impaired healing

Diabetes mellitus is the most prevalent metabolic disease associated with an impaired capacity of tissue repair. The most common clinical picture of impaired wound healing associated with diabetes is the diabetic foot ulcer. Among diabetic patients, 2–3% will develop a foot ulcer each year and 15% will develop a foot ulcer during their lifetime.[10] Despite standard therapies, a significant percentage of diabetic foot ulcers follow a progressive course, are complicated by infection, and ultimately require amputation. The molecular mechanisms that lead to a reduced healing capacity in diabetes mellitus are not completely understood. It is generally accepted that skin ulceration and healing impairment is caused by a combination of directly diabetes-related factors (neuropathy and vascular disease) and external factors (excessive mechanical load, callus formation, and wound infection). Abnormal functions and gene expression patterns of wound-resident and nonresident hematopoietic cells have been described in diverse diabetes disease models and might contribute to the impairment of wound healing.[11] In this regard, it will be important to understand to which extent impaired reparative cell functions are due to direct effects of insulin resistance or its metabolic sequelae, including hyperglycemia, hyperlipidemia, or obesity.

During the past decade, several rodent models of diabetes and obesity have been extensively studied to unravel the functional link between the diabetes phenotype and impaired healing capacity. These studies highlight increased inflammation, altered angiogenesis, unbalanced protease activities, and advanced-glycation-end products as major pathomechanisms leading to an impaired healing phenotype.[12–14] More recently, the interrelation between proinflammatory pathways, obesity, and insulin resistance have been identified, and future studies will have to clarify whether these mechanisms are also functionally connected to diabetes-impaired healing. In these studies, the adipose tissue has been identified as an important initiator of the chronic inflammatory response in diabetes.[15] As the adipose tissue expands during the progression to obesity, the enlarging adipocytes become relatively hypoperfused, which creates regional areas of microhypoxia with increased expression of hypoxia-inducible-factor-1. Hypoxic adipose tissue displays enhanced activation of the JNK1 and IKK/NF-kB pathways as well as increased expression of genes involved in inflammation and endoplasmatic reticulum stress.[16] Activation of these pathways leads to chemokine release and subsequent recruitment of macrophages into the adipose tissue. Beside phagocytosis and tissue remodeling, these macrophages release proinflammatory cytokines, such as TNF-α, interleukin-6, and C-reactive protein, which can induce insulin resistance in neighboring adipocytes via paracrine effects. Indeed, TNF-α neutralization improves insulin sensitivity.[17] Recent studies provided a deeper mechanistic insight into the understanding of how macrophages link inflammation to insulin resistance. These studies showed that myeloid cell–specific knockouts of IKKb or JNK1 protected mice from high-fat-diet–induced glucose intolerance, hyperinsulinemia, and insulin resistance.[18] In the future, it would be important to find out whether the proinflammatory phenotype of macrophages contributes to the impairment of healing in diabetes and to clarify the efficacy of antiinflammatory therapy for diabetic-impaired wounds.

Molecular link between venous ulcers and inflammation

Venous leg ulcers represent the final outcome of lower extremity chronic venous hypertension. These ulcers can be defined as deep skin wounds, which sometimes even involve the subdermal tissues and are characterized by poor healing. Venous leg ulcers are common, with a prevalence of 3–5% in the population over 65 years of age, they cause considerable morbidity, and create persistent and substantial demands on health care resources.[6] During the past decades, major efforts to accelerate tissue repair in chronic venous leg ulcers have been only of limited success. This may at least be partly due to the lack of knowledge of the pathophysiology of chronic wounds and the role of their microenvironment. It is well accepted that due to the venous insufficiency, blood cells are trapped in the venous microcirculation secondary to venous hypertension and release toxic metabolites that lead to tissue damage. Further, increased hydrostatic pressure was shown to upregulate and activate a variety of cellular adhesion molecules and their counter receptors, thus enhancing the continuous extravasation of activated leukocytes, specifically neutrophils and macrophages. The persistence of these inflammatory cells at the wound site leads to an unrestricted proteolytic activity, which is commonly considered the final executor of a pathogenetic chain leading to matrix disruption, proteolysis of growth factors, and their receptors, which are essential for healing.[3,19–21] Many current therapeutic strategies aim at counteracting high-protease levels in the chronic wound environment. However, with increasing knowledge on the inflammatory pathways involved in the physiology and pathology of repair, potentially also anti-inflammatory strategies might be promising therapies to disrupt tissue damage–causing pathways in venous leg ulcers.

It is striking that although the prevalence of venous insufficiency is 20–50%, the incidence of disease progression in skin ulceration is relatively low (3–5%).[22] These data lead to the assumption that an impairment of venous hemodynamics is necessary but not sufficient for ulcer development. Indeed, recent studies indicated that a genetic component is relevant in disease progression to a recalcitrant venous ulcer. Along these lines, Zamboni *et al.* reported that in patients with primary venous disease the presence of a hemochromatosis gene mutation (C282Y) increases the risk of developing a skin ulcer.[22] Venous hypertension results in increased erythrocyte diapedesis, which causes local iron overload of skin tissue. Several authors have hypothesized that this iron could be released to generate free radicals because of excessive oxidative stress, thereby perpetuating the proinflammatory and highly proteolytic microenvironment. In patients affected by the C282Y mutation, mechanisms controlling the iron overload are disturbed, which leads to an increased risk of free iron and free radicals, which ultimately cause persistent inflammation, matrix breakdown, and skin lesions.

Recently, another study was published that provides an indirect genetic link between impaired healing and enhanced inflammation. The group of Ashcroft and colleagues reported that polymorphisms of upstream parts of the estrogen receptor-beta (ER-b) gene *ESR2*, are associated with ulceration in venous insufficiency.[23] The ER proteins, ER-a and ER-b, mediate the actions of estrogens important for wound repair through the activation or repression of genes associated with matrix production, protease inhibition, and inflammation. Estrogens have been shown to promote repair by the downregulation of the proinflammatory cytokine macrophage migration inhibitory factor.[24] It is intriguing to speculate that defective ER activation may result in proinflammatory conditions, promoting the development of venous ulcers. Increasing knowledge on inflammation might enable future research on the existence of additional indirect and/or direct genetic links between an altered immune responsiveness and venous leg ulcers. The identification of risk factors for the development of difficult-to-heal skin ulcers would be a milestone in tissue repair research and would open new prospects for the treatment and, even more important, also for prevention of chronic wounds.

TAKE-HOME MESSAGE

Basic science advance

- Complementary molecular analysis of the functional impact of the immune response on repair in diverse model systems will unravel complex interrelations among these events and, in long term, advance the development of therapies aiming to improve the quality of repair.

Clinical science advance

- Wound-healing disorders in the clinic present as hypertrophic scars or as nonhealing chronic wounds (ulcers), the latter presenting the most prevalent wound-healing problems in humans. Most chronic wounds are associated with well-defined clinical entities—in particular, venous insufficiency, diabetes mellitus, pressure necrosis, and vasculitis. Most nonhealing wounds fail to progress through the normal phases of wound repair, but instead remain in a chronic inflammatory state. Both underlying systemic defects and local stimuli might contribute to prolong the inflammatory phase of the local healing response, thereby generating a cascade of tissue responses that generate and amplify the hostile microenvironment.

Relevance to clinical care

- The advanced understanding of the molecular link between inflammation and repair will hopefully provide a rationale for targeting the inflammatory phase to modulate the outcome of the healing response.

SUMMARY ILLUSTRATION

Substantial evidence in different model organisms indicates that the immune system is of primary importance in determining the quality of the repair response, including the extent of scarring, and the restoration of organ structure and function. Findings in experimental models and disease conditions support a correlation between the loss of regeneration capacity and maturation of immune competence.

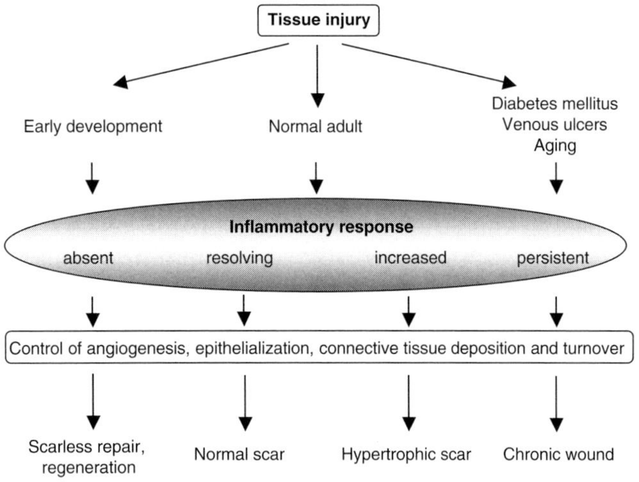

Functional impact of the inflammatory response on the quality of repair.

CAUTION, CRITICAL REMARKS, AND RECOMMENDATIONS

There is strong evidence that the immune response has fundamental impact on the quality of the tissue response to injury. Evidence for negative but also positive roles of the immune response in restoration of tissue homeostasis and organ function after injury was found in many species. An important challenge will be to dissect cell type–specific functions and pathways of the inflammatory response that are beneficial and/or harmful for repair. This knowledge will yield, hopefully, novel pharmacological targets to provide protection against inflammatory tissue damage and to promote tissue recovery.

FUTURE DEVELOPMENT

Certain types of chronic wounds, in particular, those with underlying vasculitis, respond to the classical antiinflammatory compounds, including glucocorticoids, azathioprin, and nonsteroidal antiinflammatory drugs. Recent reports indicate that chronic wounds also benefit from some of the new immune-modifying drugs, which are currently successfully used for other immune-mediated diseases. These include anti-TNF strategies, which have been proven to be most efficient in chronic inflammatory diseases, such as psoriasis, arthritis, and inflammatory bowel disease.[25] So far, there are few case reports highlighting its effectiveness in inflammatory ulcerative skin lesions such as in pyoderma gangrenosum or vasculitis,[25] and further studies are needed to verify these observations. Further, microvascular endothelial cells at the site of inflammation are both active participants and regulators of inflammatory processes.[26] Consequently, the endothelium has become an important target for the development of novel antiinflammatory therapies, including selectin blocking strategies.[27] Clinical studies will have to assess their potential therapeutic benefit in inflammation-mediated tissue injury that results in chronic wounds.

ACKNOWLEDGMENTS

Wound-healing research in the authors' laboratory is funded by DFG (SFB829), EU (Angioscaff), and CECAD.

AUTHOR DISCLOSURE STATEMENT

The authors (S.W., J.K., R.R., T.K., and S.A.E.) have no commercial associations that might create or seem to pose a conflict of interest in connection with this article.

REFERENCES

1. Gurtner GC, Werner S, Barrandon Y, and Longaker MT: Wound repair and regeneration. Nature 2008; **453:** 314.
2. Martin P and Leibovich SJ: Inflammatory cells during wound repair: the good, the bad and the ugly. Trends Cell Biol 2005; **15:** 599.
3. Eming SA, Krieg T, and Davidson D: Inflammation on wound repair: molecular and cellular mechanisms. J Invest Dermatol 2007; **127:** 514.
4. Gordon S: Alternative activation of macrophages. Nature 2003; **3:** 23.
5. Werner S, Krieg T, and Smola H: Keratinocyte-fibroblast interactions in wound healing. J Invest Dermatol 2007; **127:** 998.
6. Etufugh CN and Phillips TJ: Venous ulcers. Clin Dermatol 2007; **25:** 121.
7. Chen WY and Rogers AA: Recent insights into the causes of chronic leg ulceration in venous diseases and implications on other types of chronic wounds. Wound Repair Regen 2007; **15:** 434.
8. Mori R, Kondo T, Ohshima T, Ishida Y, and Mukaida N: Accelerated wound healing in TNF receptor p55-deficient mice with reduced leukocyte infiltration. FASEB J 2002; **16:** 963.
9. Brockes JP and Kumar A: Comparative aspects of animal regeneration. Annu Rev Cell Dev Biol 2008; **24:** 525.

10. Boulton AJ: The diabetic foot—an update. Foot Ankle Surg 2008; **14:** 120.

11. Brem H and Tomic-Canic MT: Cellular and molecular basis of wound healing in diabetes. J Clin Invest 2007; **117:** 1219.

12. Falanga V: Wound healing and its impairment in the diabetic foot. Lancet 2005; **366:** 1736.

13. Dovi JV, He LK, and DiPietro LA: Accelerated wound closure in neutrophil-depleted mice. J Leukoc Biol 2003; **73:** 448.

14. Goren I, Müller E, Pfeilschifter J, and Frank S: Severely impaired insulin signaling in chronic wounds of diabetic ob/ob mice: a potential role of tumor necrosis factor-alpha. Am J Pathol 2006; **168:** 765.

15. Schenk S, Saberi M, and Olefsky JM: Insulin sensitivity: modulation by nutrients and inflammation. J Clin Invest 2008; **118:** 2992.

16. Hosogai N, Fukuhara A, Oshima K, Miyata Y, Tanaka S, Segawa K, Furukawa S, Tochino Y, Komuro R, Matsuda M, and Shimomura I: Adipose tissue hypoxia in obesity and its impact on adipocytokine dysregulation. Diabetes 2007; **56:** 901.

17. Hotamisligil GS, Shargill NS, and Spiegelman BM: Adipose expression of tumor necrosis factor-alpha: direct role in obesity-linked insulin resistance. Science 1993; **259:** 87.

18. Solinas G, Vilcu C, Neels JG, Bandyopadhyay GK, Luo JL, Naugler W, Grivennikov S, Wynshaw-Boris A, Scadeng M, Olefsky JM, and Karin M: JNK1 in hematopoietically derived cells contributes to diet-induced inflammation and insulin resistance without affecting obesity. Cell Metab 2007; **6:** 386.

19. Lauer G, Sollberg S, Cole M, Flamme I, Stürzebecher J, Mann K, Krieg T, and Eming SA: Expression and proteolysis of vascular endothelial growth factor is increased in chronic wounds. J Invest Dermatol 2000; **115:** 12.

20. Eming SA, Smola-Hess S, Kurschat P, Hirche D, Krieg T, and Smola H: A novel property of povidon-iodine: inhibition of excessive protease levels in chronic non-healing wounds. J Invest Dermatol 2006; **126:** 2731.

21. Eming S, Smola H, Hartmann B, Malchau G, Wegner R, Krieg T, and Smola-Hess S: The inhibition of matrix metalloproteinase activity in chronic wounds by a polyacrylate superabsorber. Biomaterials 2008; **29:** 2932.

22. Zamboni P, Tognazzo S, Izzo M, Pancaldi F, Scapoli GL, Liboni A, and Gemmati D: Hemochromatosis C282Y gene mutation increases the risk of venous leg ulceration. J Vasc Surg 2005; **42:** 309.

23. Ashworth JJ, Smyth JV, Pendleton N, Horan M, Payton A, Worthington J, Ollier WE, and Ashcroft GS: Polymorphisms spanning the 0N exon and promoter of the estrogen receptor-beta (ERbeta) gene ESR2 are associated with venous ulceration. Clin Genet 2008; **73:** 55.

24. Feldmann M: Translating molecular insights in autoimmunity into effective therapy. Annu Rev Immunol 2009; **27:** 1.

25. Alexis AF and Strober BE: Off-label dermatologic uses of anti-TNF-a therapies. J Cutan Med Surg 2005; **9:** 296.

26. Pober JS and Sessa WC: Evolving functions of endothelial cells in inflammation. Nat Rev Immunol 2007; **7:** 803.

27. Ley K: The role of selectins in inflammation and disease. Trends Mol Med 2003; **9:** 263.

WHS
Wound
Healing
Society

The Role of Fibrocytes in Wound Healing

Adriana Blakaj and Richard Bucala*

Department of Medicine, Pathology, Epidemiology and Public Health, Yale University School of Medicine, New Haven, Connecticut.
Department of Cell Biology, Yale University School of Medicine, New Haven, Connecticut.

Abbreviations and Acronyms

α-SMA = alpha smooth muscle actin

CCR = chemokine receptor

EGFP = enhanced green fluorescent protein

IL = interleukin

LSP1 = leukocyte-specific protein 1

PDGF = platelet-derived growth factor

SAP = serum amyloid P

TGF-β1 = transforming growth factor β1

*Correspondence: Department of Medicine, Pathology, Epidemiology and Public Health, Yale University School of Medicine, The Anlyan Center, S525, P.O. Box 208031, 300 Cedar St., New Haven, Connecticut 06520-8031 (e-mail: richard.bucala@yale.edu).

Background: Fibrocytes, which are a group of bone marrow–derived mesenchymal progenitor cells, were first described in 1994 as fibroblast-like, peripheral blood cells that migrated to the regions of tissue injury. These cells are unique in their expression of extracellular matrix proteins concomitantly with markers of hematopoietic and monocyte lineage.
The Problem: The involvement of fibrocytes and the specific role they play in the process of wound repair has been a focus of study since their initial description. This article is a compilation of selected current reports that have elucidated the pivotal role of fibrocytes in wound healing, remodeling, and maintenance of tissue integrity.
Basic/Clinical Science Advances: Fibrocytes contribute to the healing repertoire via several mechanisms; they produce a combination of cytokines, chemokines, and growth factors to create a milieu favorable for repair to occur; they serve as antigen-presenting cells; they contribute to wound closure; and they promote angiogenesis. Further, regulatory pathways involving serum amyloid P, leukocyte-specific protein 1, and adenosine A_{2A} receptors have emphasized the significant role that fibrocytes have in wound healing.
Clinical Care Relevance: The clinical relevance of fibrocytes has focused on wound repair and inflammatory fibrosis. The relevance of fibrocytes to wound repair also can be applied to aberrant wound repair in disease processes that include systemic fibroses, interstitial pulmonary fibroses, airway remodeling in asthma, atherosclerosis, the stromal response to tumor invasion, and hypertrophic scarring.
Conclusion: It is evident from recent literature that fibrocytes likely play an important role in wound healing and fibrosis. The precise mechanisms by which they mediate pathologic processes await future examination. The therapeutic targeting of fibrocytes holds promise for the augmentation of wound repair and the treatment of different fibrosing disorders.

BACKGROUND

Fibrocytes were first described in 1994 as fibroblast-like, peripheral blood cells that migrated to the regions of tissue injury.[1] Since their original description, the wealth of information regarding fibrocyte biology has grown steadily and implicated this cell in wound healing and in many disease states that can be regarded as aberrant wound healing, including hypertrophic scars and keloids, airway remodeling in asthma, interstitial pulmonary fibroses, systemic fibroses, atherosclerosis, and the stromal response to tumor invasion.[2,3]

Phenotypic examination of these cells revealed a unique cytokine and chemokine profile distinct from monocytes, dendritic cells, Langerhans cells, T lymphocytes, fibroblasts, endothelial cells, and epithelial cells. Fibrocytes express fibroblast compo-

ADVANCES IN WOUND CARE, VOLUME 1

Printed in U.S.A.
DOI: 10.1089/awc.2009.0029

nents such as vimentin, collagen I, collagen III, and fibronectin, and they express the hematopoietic stem cell marker (CD34) and the leukocyte common antigen (CD45).[1] Moreover, fibrocytes exhibit unique cytoplasmic extensions that are intermediate in size between microvilli and pseudopodia.[1] Fibrocytes comprise approximately 0.5% of nonerythrocytic cells in the peripheral blood, and they differentiate from CD14+ cells in culture into a phenotype with wound-healing potential.

Initial observations of their recruitment to wound sites were found to be due to specific chemokine–chemokine receptor interactions. Namely, it was shown that fibrocytes migrate to wounds in response to secondary lymphoid chemokine, which is the ligand for chemokine receptor (CCR)7.[4] The fibrocyte chemokine expression profile also revealed other chemokine receptors on the surface of fibrocytes, such as CCR3, CCR5, CCR7, and CXC chemokine receptor 4,[4] which also likely function in fibrocyte signaling and trafficking pathways.

CINICAL PROBLEM ADDRESSED

A wound is caused by the physical disruption of normal tissue architecture. Wound healing necessitates a full ensemble of mediators and connective tissue components to provide a synchronized biological response that is requisite for optimal repair. A disruption in normal cellular architecture initiates a dynamic sequence of events that occur in three temporally overlapping phases: inflammation, tissue repair, and tissue remodeling.[5]

We review current literature that has emphasized the role of fibrocytes in wound healing. In addition, their clinical role in fibrosing diseases as well as in impaired wound healing is important.

RELEVANT BASIC SCIENCE CONTEXT

Fibrocytes produce a combination of cytokines, chemokines, and growth factors that create a milieu favorable for repair (Fig. 1). In cutaneous wounds, the CD34 hematopoietic marker initially expressed by fibrocytes decreases over time. This decrease in CD34 occurs in concert with the increased expression of prolyl-4-hyrdoxylase, an enzyme that is necessary for the stabilization of the collagen triple helix.[6] Aiba *et al.* hypothesize that CD34 expression reflects the inflammatory state of the wound, which is downregulated as fibrocytes differentiate into a more mature connective tissue cell. The leukocyte common antigen (CD45) displays a similar decrease in expression as fibrocytes differentiate.[7] This phenotypic transition of fibrocytes is also evident in the context of an increase in expression of transforming growth factor $\beta 1$ (TGF-$\beta 1$) in the wound.[6] TGF-$\beta 1$, a cytokine that plays an important role in tissue repair and fibrosis, was found to accelerate fibrocyte differentiation to cells that are phenotypically similar to mature fibroblasts and myofibroblasts, *in vitro*.[4] Further, fibrocytes were found to be an important source of cytokines and type I collagen during the inflammatory and repair phase of wound healing. High levels of interleukin (IL)-1 were observed to induce the fibrocyte secretion of chemokines (macrophage inflammatory protein-1α and 1β), fibrogenic cytokines including tumor necrosis factor-α, and hematopoietic growth factors (macrophage colony-stimulating factor, IL-6, IL-10).[8]

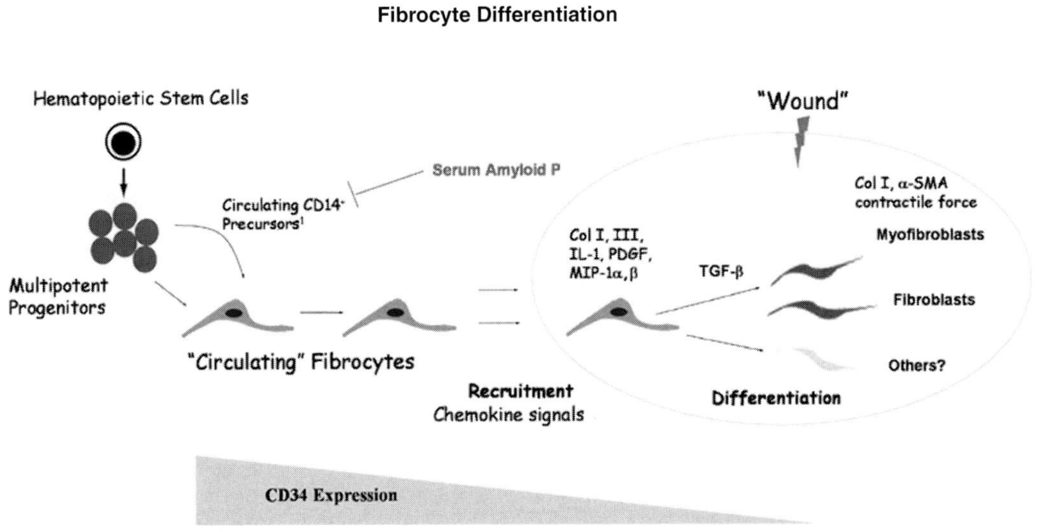

Figure 1. Known features of the differentiation pathway for fibrocytes. Fibrocytes are bone marrow-derived cells. Once fibrocytes differentiate from their CD14+ precursors, they are recruited to areas of wound repair, where they can further differentiate into more mature mesenchymal cells. The differentiation of fibrocytes into mature fibroblasts or myofibroblasts is stimulated by a number of factors and is also associated with a loss of the surface marker, CD34.

Fibrocytes are potent antigen-presenting cells that are capable of initiating and promoting T-cell immunity. They constitutively express surface proteins required for antigen presentation including class II major histocompatability complex molecules (HLA-DP, HLA-DQ, and HLA-DR) and the costimulatory molecules CD80 and CD86.[9] In addition, fibrocytes express the adhesion molecules CD11a, CD54, and CD58.[9] Further, human fibrocytes were found to induce a tetanus-toxoid-specific T-cell response that was greater than that induced by peripheral blood monocytes and nearly equivalent to that produced by dendritic cells.[9] In confirmation of the *in vitro* studies, *in vivo* studies showed that mouse fibrocytes pulsed with foreign antigen and injected in skin migrate to regional lymph nodes and prime naive T cells.[9] Fibrocytes, therefore, exhibit a potent antigen-presenting capability, indicating their likely role in the initiation of immunity during injury, wound repair, and in fibrotic responses associated with inflammation, such as granulomas and scleroderma.

Wound closure is an essential part of wound healing, in which myofibroblasts play an active role. Fibrocytes have been shown to express alpha smooth muscle actin (α-SMA) and contract collagen gels *in vitro*, revealing their potential to differentiate into myofibroblasts and contribute to wound contraction.[4] Indeed, fibrocytes also were found to differentiate to a myofibroblast phenotype *in vivo* and express α-SMA, thereby confirming that these circulating cells contribute to a subset of myofibroblasts in wounds and are integral mediators of wound healing.[7]

Fibrocytes have been shown to promote angiogenesis, which is a requisite for the development and maintenance of new granulation tissue, allowing wound closure and restoration of tissue integrity. Cultured fibrocytes participate in all aspects of neovascularization. They are involved in the proteolysis of the basement membrane by constitutively secreting extracellular matrix-degrading enzymes, namely matrix metalloproteinase 9, thus allowing for endothelial cell invasion. Fibrocytes are involved in the proliferation, migration, and tube formation of endothelial cells *in vitro* by their secretion of vascular endothelial growth factor, basic fibroblast growth factor (bFGF), IL-8, platelet-derived growth factor (PDGF), and hematopoietic growth factors. Moreover, these results were supported by *in vivo* studies using the Matrigel implant model, where the introduction of fibrocytes promoted the formation of new blood vessels.[10] The proangiogenic properties of fibrocytes are clearly vital for wound repair, and these findings may provide therapeutic opportunities in the promotion of wound repair.

EXPERIMENTAL MODEL OR MATERIAL

Several *in vitro* and many *in vivo* experimental models are currently being used in the study of fibrocytes.

The first study of fibrocytes was performed in a murine model of wound repair, which relied on surgical implantation of wound chambers in subcutaneous tissues. Subsequent examination of peripheral blood cells within 2 days of wound chamber implantation revealed a fibroblast-like circulating $CD34^+$/collagen type I^+ cell that was in the exudate fluid—adherent and spindle shaped—and thus termed a fibrocyte.[1]

Isolation of fibrocytes for further growth and characterization also can be achieved from $CD14^+$-enriched mononuclear cell population isolated from the buffy coat of peripheral blood.[4] *Ex vivo*–cultured fibrocytes from the mononuclear cells of peripheral blood can then be harvested for further analysis via methods such as flow cytometry.[11]

One of the first studies of fibrocyte chemotaxis in a *de novo* wound was accomplished by labeling fibrocytes *ex vivo* with a membrane-inserting dye, PKH-26, and administering these labeled cells in mice to observe the homing of fibrocytes to wounded regions, and thus physically linking fibrocytes to the process of wound repair.[4]

To determine whether these unique cells, indeed, had their origins in the bone marrow, experimental murine models of sex-mismatched bone marrow chimera mice were used. In this model, female mice, after total body irradiation, received a male whole bone marrow transplant. Further analysis by *in situ* hybridization of the wounded tissue in these mice revealed that circulating fibrocytes and fibrocytes isolated from the wounded tissue were male cells from the transplanted donor bone marrow, thus solidifying their hematopoietic origin.[7] In another model, bone marrow from enhanced green fluorescent protein (EGFP) transgenic mice was transplanted into the normal mice. The injured skin of this murine model was found to contain numerous EGFP+, bone marrow–derived cells. Most of these EGFP+ cells expressed CD45 and were phenotypically similar to fibrocytes, further creating a case for the hematopoietic, stem-cell origin of fibrocytes.[12]

In addition to the already mentioned experimental models, the advent of knock-out murine models along with various animal models of renal, pulmonary, and vascular diseases has further facilitated fibrocyte study in terms of the mediators and signaling pathways necessary for their regulation and trafficking.[13–17]

DISCUSSION OF FINDINGS AND RELEVANT LITERATURE

The regulation of fibrocytes is a dynamic process governed by many factors, each harboring its own therapeutic potential. The profibrotic cytokines, IL-4 and IL-13, along with PDGF promote the differentiation of CD14+ precursors to fibrocytes.[18] Further, the proinflammatory cytokines, IL-12 and IFN-γ, along with serum amyloid P (SAP) and aggregated immunoglobulin G inhibit the maturation of CD14+ precursors into fibrocytes.[18–20] The subsequent differentiation of fibrocytes into mature mesenchymal cells is stimulated with TGF-β1, as stated previously, as well as with endothelin-1, a peptide that plays an important role in vascular homeostatis.[21] Moreover, fibrocytes can also transform into adipocytes when cultured in adipogenic conditions,[22] indicating the potential of this cell to differentiate into more than one mesenchymal cell type.

Recent studies implicating leukocyte-specific protein 1 (LSP1), adenosine A_{2A} receptors, and SAP in fibrocyte regulation have further elucidated the role that fibrocytes play, specifically, in the process of wound repair, and they also provide promising therapeutic potential.

LSP1, a cytoskeletal protein reported to be important for leukocyte chemotaxis, may also play a regulatory role in wound healing and fibrocyte biology. Both leukocytes and fibrocytes express LSP1; however, fibroblasts do not. Moreover, LSP1 expression persists in fibrocytes and is more upregulated in fibrocytes than it is in leukocytes.[23] Interestingly, $LSP1^{-/-}$ null mice show accelerated healing of skin wounds, along with enhanced collagen synthesis, reepithelialization, and angiogenesis. Further, the number of fibrocytes in these mice is substantially higher than in the wild-type mice; thus, the accelerated wound healing observed in $LSP1^{-/-}$ mice could, partly, be associated with elevated fibrocyte levels.[24] In using this same mouse model and injecting bleomcyin to induce a fibrotic response, the numbers of fibrocytes in LSP1-deficient mice were increased in comparison to WT. Fibrocytes, therefore, are not only implicated in the increased fibrosis that is noticed with these mice but also they are likely a result of an increased mononuclear infiltrate.[25] Thus, elevated fibrocyte levels may accelerate wound healing as well as contribute to pathologic fibrosis.

Adenosine has long been associated with a role in the inflammatory response, which is important for wound healing. It has been shown that adenosine A2 receptor agonists play a beneficial role in wound healing in normal and diabetic animals.[26] Recently, it has become evident that adenosine A_{2A} receptors may function in the proliferation and differentiation of mouse bone marrow–derived mesenchymal stem cells.[27] Consistent with these results, the deletion or the blockade of adenosine

TAKE-HOME MESSAGE

Basic science advances

- Fibrocytes secrete various chemokines, cytokines, and growth factors that provide a suitable environment for their wound-healing capabilities.
- Fibrocytes are potent antigen-presenting cells, capable of initiating and promoting T-cell immunity.
- Fibrocytes are capable of differentiating to a phenotype that expresses α-SMA that promotes wound closure and contraction. Also, a subpopulation of myofibroblast has their origin in fibrocytes.
- Fibrocytes possess the ability to initiate angiogenesis in facilitating wound repair both *in vitro* and *in vivo* in a Matrigel angiogenesis murine model. They secrete matrix metalloproteinase 9, vascular endothelial growth factor, basic fibroblast growth factor, IL-8, and PDGF to promote angiogenesis.

Clinical science advances

- LSP1 is a cytoskeletal protein that has been reported to be important for leukocyte chemotaxis and may be important in fibrocyte biology. LSP1-deficient mice show accelerated wound healing as well as increased fibrocytes.
- LSP1-deficient mice subjected to bleomycin, an experimental model of scleroderma, showed increased number of fibrocytes in comparison to the wild-type mice.
- Adenosine A_{2A} receptor agonists are important in wound healing.
- Adenosine A_{2A} receptor may play a role in the differentiation and proliferation of mouse bone marrow–derived mesenchymal stem cells.
- Both local and systemic administration of SAP, an inhibitor of fibrocytes, compromises dermal wound healing in mice.

Clinical care advances

- Enhanced understanding of fibrocytes may help develop novel therapies for wound healing as well as disease states that can be regarded as aberrant wound healing, including hypertrophic scars and keloids, airway remodeling in asthma, interstitial pulmonary fibroses, systemic fibroses, atherosclerosis, and the stromal response to tumor invasion.

A_{2A} receptors results in less fibrocyte accumulation in the dermis of a bleomycin-treated murine model of scleroderma. Fibrocyte accumulation, therefore, is somehow regulated by adenosine A_{2A} receptors.[28] Whether fibrocytes are directly recruited by adenosine A_{2A} receptors to tissue, or whether the adenosine A_{2A} receptors stimulate the differentiation of precursors to fibrocytes, remains to be further studied. However, the implication that adenosine A_{2A} receptors may represent a therapeutic target for treating fibrosing diseases is an exciting one.

SAP, which is a member of the pentraxin family of proteins, is a critical factor in plasma that inhibits fibrocyte differentiation from monocytes *ex vivo*.[19] In a recent study, it has been shown that the administration of exogenous SAP, either locally or systemically, compromises dermal wound healing.[29] SAP-treated wounds showed a decreased rate of wound closure and a decreased number of myofibroblasts at 7 days postwounding.[29] These results are most likely a consequence of an inhibition of fibrocyte differentiation into myofibroblasts. SAP, therefore, represents a potential tool to either ameliorate the efficiency of normal wound healing or prevent aberrant wound-healing processes through their regulation of fibrocytes.

In general, adult wound healing results in scar formation, typified by a dysregulated reconstitution of the collagen matrix. Hypertrophic scars represent one form of an aberrant and exuberant wound-healing process. Fibrocytes were detected in greater numbers in postburn hypertrophic scar tissue as compared with mature scar tissue and normal dermis, therefore fortifying the hypothesis that they are involved in the development and perpetuation of aberrant wound healing.[23] It has been shown that fibrocytes from either burn patients or normal patients have a much lower ability to synthesize collagen *in vitro* than do dermal fibroblasts. This finding raises the possibility that the primary role of fibrocytes in the healing of burn wounds may not be in deposition of ECM and may instead be by the regulation of dermal fibroblasts.[30] Dermal fibroblasts, when conditioned with medium from burn patient fibrocytes, possess a heightened ability to proliferate and migrate, to express α-SMA, and to contract collagen lattices *in vitro*.[30] Further, the profibrotic factors, TGF-β1 and connective tissue growth factor, are produced in greater quantities by the fibrocytes of burn patients, and these cytokines may be integral regulators of fibroblast activity in response to thermal injury.[30] Thus, as indicated by this example, the regulation of fibrocytes in pathologic contexts also awaits further refinement.

CAUTION, CRITICAL REMARKS, AND RECOMMENDATIONS

Since their first description in 1994, the biology of fibrocytes has been expanded considerably. In wound repair, they have been shown to produce a combination of cytokines, chemokines, and growth factors necessary for the healing process. In addition, their role in antigen presentation, wound closure, and angiogenesis has been demarcated. Fibrocyte regulation via LSP1, adenosine A_{2A} receptors, and SAP has also been shown and awaits further characterization. In general, a more detailed view of how fibrocytes mobilize and the trafficking signals they require, as well as how they differentiate, must be further elucidated. It is imperative to create an even more refined picture of fibrocyte biology so as to best understand the role of fibrocytes in wound healing and pathologic conditions.

FUTURE DEVELOPMENT

As indicated in the aforementioned text, the role of fibrocytes in accelerating wound healing is being intricately defined, as is their role in fibrosing diseases. There is currently no Food and Drug Administration–approved therapy for fibrosing diseases, and so a better understanding of fibrocytes and their regulation marks these bone marrow–derived progenitors as potential therapeutic modalities to not only augment normal wound healing but also potentially reverse fibrosis in many disease states. The promise that fibrocytes could be expanded *ex vivo* and readministered to patients to treat disease, or that they may be used to construct therapeutic targets, is unmistakable and exciting. The careful balance of wound healing versus pathologic properties of fibrocytes must be further studied to manipulate these cells for therapeutic benefit.

AUTHOR DISCLOSURE STATEMENT

Adriana Blakaj: No competing financial interests exist. Richard Bucala: Dr. Bucala serves on the Scientific Advisory Board of Promedior, which is developing therapies to combat fibrosis. Dr. Bucala also is a coinventor on a patent describing the therapeutic use of fibrocytes.

REFERENCES

1. Bucala R, Spiegel LA, Chesney J, Hogan M, and Cerami A: Circulating fibrocytes define a new leukocyte subpopulation that mediates tissue repair. Mol Med 1994; **1:** 71.
2. Bucala R: *Fibrocytes: New Insights into Tissue Repair and Systemic Fibrosis.* Vol. xviii. Hackensack, NJ: World Scientific, 2007, p. 249.
3. Bellini A and Mattoli S: The role of the fibrocyte, a bone marrow-derived mesenchymal progenitor, in reactive and reparative fibroses. Lab Invest 2007; **87:** 858.
4. Abe R, Donnelly SC, Peng T, Bucala R, and Metz CN: Peripheral blood fibrocytes: differentiation pathway and migration to wound sites. J Immunol 2001; **166:** 7556.
5. Singer AJ and Clark RA: Cutaneous wound healing. N Engl J Med 1999; **341:** 738.
6. Aiba S and Tagami H: Inverse correlation between CD34 expression and proline-4-hydroxylase immunoreactivity on spindle cells noted in hypertrophic scars and keloids. J Cutan Pathol 1997; **24:** 65.
7. Mori L, Bellini A, Stacey MA, Schmidt M, and Mattoli S: Fibrocytes contribute to the myofibroblast population in wounded skin and originate from the bone marrow. Exp Cell Res 2005; **304:** 81.
8. Chesney J, Metz C, Stavitsky AB, Bacher M, and Bucala R: Regulated production of type I collagen and inflammatory cytokines by peripheral blood fibrocytes. J Immunol 1998; **160:** 419.
9. Chesney J, Bacher M, Bender A, and Bucala R: The peripheral blood fibrocyte is a potent antigen-presenting cell capable of priming naive T cells *in situ.* Proc Natl Acad Sci USA 1997; **94:** 6307.
10. Hartlapp I, *et al.*: Fibrocytes induce an angiogenic phenotype in cultured endothelial cells and promote angiogenesis *in vivo.* Faseb J 2001; **15:** 2215.
11. Quan TE and Bucala R: Culture and analysis of circulating fibrocytes. Methods Mol Med 2007; **135:** 423.
12. Fathke C, *et al.*: Contribution of bone marrow-derived cells to skin: collagen deposition and wound repair. Stem Cells 2004; **22:** 812.
13. Haudek SB, *et al.*: Bone marrow-derived fibroblast precursors mediate ischemic cardiomyopathy in mice. Proc Natl Acad Sci USA 2006; **103:** 18284.
14. Phillips RJ, *et al.*: Circulating fibrocytes traffic to the lungs in response to CXCL12 and mediate fibrosis. J Clin Invest 2004; **114:** 438.
15. Sakai N, *et al.*: Secondary lymphoid tissue chemokine (SLC/CCL21)/CCR7 signaling regulates fibrocytes in renal fibrosis. Proc Natl Acad Sci USA 2006; **103:** 14098.
16. Moore BB, *et al.*: CCR2-mediated recruitment of fibrocytes to the alveolar space after fibrotic injury. Am J Pathol 2005; **166:** 675.
17. Ishida Y, *et al.*: Essential roles of the CC chemokine ligand 3-CC chemokine receptor 5 axis in bleomycin-induced pulmonary fibrosis through regulation of macrophage and fibrocyte infiltration. Am J Pathol 2007; **170:** 843.
18. Shao DD, Suresh R, Vakil V, Gomer RH, and Pilling D: Pivotal advance: Th-1 cytokines inhibit, and Th-2 cytokines promote fibrocyte differentiation. J Leukoc Biol 2008; **83:** 1323.
19. Pilling D, Buckley CD, Salmon M, and Gomer RH: Inhibition of fibrocyte differentiation by serum amyloid P. J Immunol 2003; **171:** 5537.
20. Pilling D, Tucker NM, and Gomer RH: Aggregated IgG inhibits the differentiation of human fibrocytes. J Leukoc Biol 2006; **79:** 1242.
21. Schmidt M, Sun G, Stacey MA, Mori L, and Mattoli S: Identification of circulating fibrocytes as precursors of bronchial myofibroblasts in asthma. J Immunol 2003; **171:** 380.
22. Hong KM, Burdick MD, Phillips RJ, Heber D, and Strieter RM: Characterization of human fibrocytes as circulating adipocyte progenitors and the formation of human adipose tissue in SCID mice. Faseb J 2005; **19:** 2029.
23. Yang L, *et al.*: Identification of fibrocytes in postburn hypertrophic scar. Wound Repair Regen 2005; **13:** 398.
24. Wang J, *et al.*: Accelerated wound healing in leukocyte-specific, protein 1-deficient mouse is associated with increased infiltration of leukocytes and fibrocytes. J Leukoc Biol 2007; **82:** 1554.
25. Wang J, *et al.*: Increased severity of bleomycin-induced skin fibrosis in mice with leukocyte-specific protein 1 deficiency. J Invest Dermatol 2008; **128:** 2767.
26. Montesinos MC, *et al.*: Wound healing is accelerated by agonists of adenosine A2 (G alpha s-linked) receptors. J Exp Med 1997; **186:** 1615.
27. Katebi M, Soleimani M, and Cronstein BN: Adenosine A2A receptors play an active role in mouse bone marrow-derived mesenchymal stem cell development. J Leukoc Biol 2008; **85:** 438.
28. Katebi M, Fernandez P, Chan ES, and Cronstein BN: Adenosine A2A receptor blockade or deletion diminishes fibrocyte accumulation in the skin in a murine model of scleroderma, bleomycin-induced fibrosis. Inflammation 2008; **31:** 299.
29. Naik-Mathuria B, *et al.*: Serum amyloid P inhibits dermal wound healing. Wound Repair Regen 2008; **16:** 266.
30. Wang JF, *et al.*: Fibrocytes from burn patients regulate the activities of fibroblasts. Wound Repair Regen 2007; **15:** 113.

Postoperative Peritoneal Adhesion Formation: An Update

Richard Peter ten Broek and Harry van Goor*

Department of Surgery, Radboud University Nijmegen Medical Centre, Nijmegen, The Netherlands.

Abbreviations and Acronyms

ASBO = adhesive small bowel obstruction

FH = ferric hyaluronate

HA/CMC = hyaluronic acid/carboxymethyl cellulose

HBO = hyperbaric oxygen

INF-γ = interferon-γ

MMP = matrix metalloproteinase

NK-1R = neurokinin-1 receptor

ORC = oxidized-regenerating cellulose

PAI = plasminogen activator inhibitor

RCT = randomized controlled trial

SBO = small bowel obstruction

tPA = tissue plasminogen activator

*Correspondence: Department of Surgery, Radboud University Nijmegen Medical Centre, P.O. Box 9101, 6500 HB Nijmegen, The Netherlands (e-mail: h.vangoor@chir.umcn.nl).

Background: The abdominal cavity is covered by a thin serous membrane called the peritoneum. The healing of peritoneum after surgical trauma often leads to the formation of permanent adhesions. In the past decade the understanding of the pathogenesis of adhesion formation has grown rapidly.
The Problem: Adhesions are the most common cause of late postoperative complications such as inadvertent enterotomy at reentry, small bowel obstruction (SBO), chronic pain, and secondary female infertility. SBO often requires emergency reoperation, with high operative risks and a high risk for recurrence of adhesions. In this article we discuss selected recent studies on advances in the prevention of adhesion formation and treatment of adhesive SBO (ASBO).
Basic/Clinical Science Advances: Recent meta-analysis of registered adhesion prevention products showed that a hyaluronic acid/carboxymethyl cellulose barrier effectively reduces adhesion formation. A significant reduction in the incidence of ASBO requiring reoperation was demonstrated. A new target for pharmacologic adhesion prevention, the neurokinin-1 receptor, was studied, and results on prevention of *de novo* adhesion formation and adhesion reformation are promising. Hyperbaric oxygen therapy seems to be a useful adjunct to the conservative management of ASBO.
Clinical Care Relevance: ASBO is a serious condition with high morbidity and mortality. Prevention of adhesions and advances in conservative treatment will lower morbidity and mortality and improve quality of life for large numbers of patients.
Conclusion: Barrier agents can effectively reduce adhesion formation in gastrointestinal surgery. The growing understanding of the mechanisms of adhesion formation reveals promising targets for both adhesion prevention and the treatment of mature adhesions.

BACKGROUND

Each time the abdomen is opened during surgery a wound is created in a thin serous membrane called peritoneum. The peritoneum covers both the entire abdominal wall (parietal peritoneum) and all the organs and structures (visceral peritoneum) inside the abdominal cavity. The peritoneum consists of a thin monocellular layer of mesothelial cells resting upon a loose network of connective tissue composed of glycoproteins, glycosaminoglycans, proteoglycans, several types of collagen, and a variety of cells (fibroblasts, macrophages, mast cells, and fat). Each manipulation in the abdominal cavity potentially injures the peritoneum, leading to inflammation and mesothelial cell loss. Peritoneal healing consists of a complex cascade of events with the intention of rapid remesothelialization. Unlike the healing of the skin, which becomes gradually epithelialized

Printed in U.S.A.
DOI: 10.1089/awc.2009.0164

from the borders, peritoneal healing occurs by mesothelialization of the entire surface of the defect. There are four hypotheses on the origin of these cells colonizing the defect[1]: (1) growth from peripheral cells, (2) transformation of underlying mesenchymal (stem) cells, (3) transplantation of mesothelial cells from adjacent structures or free-floating mesenchymal cells, and (4) transformation of cells from the peritoneal fluid.

Recently Gómez-Gil *et al.* demonstrated the existence of a pluripotent mesenchymal cell population in the omentum.[2] Further, they demonstrated that these mesenchymal cells undergo a phenotypical transition into fibroblasts, the major cell type in the production of extracellular matrix.

This extracellular matrix forms fibrous bands connecting opposing areas of damaged peritoneum. Such bands can be resolved by the fibrinolytic system only in their early fibrinous phase. The fibrinolytic system is activated by peritoneal tissue plasminogen activator (tPA) (Fig. 1). tPA turns plasminogen into the active plasmin that splits fibrin into fibrin degradation products, resulting in adhesion-free peritoneal healing.[3] However, when fibrinolysis is insufficient, the fibrin is gradually replaced by more permanent components of extracellular matrix, such as collagen, and adhesions are formed. Fibrinolysis is inhibited by plasminogen activator inhibitor (PAI) that is released during and after injury, and the amount of PAI correlates with the degree of inflammation[4] (Fig. 1). The net plasminogen activating activity determines adhesion-free peritoneal healing. Many factors in the peritoneal fluid and tissue influence fibrinolysis and the development of fibrinous networks and fibrous bands; inflammatory cytokines, growth factors, and enzymes like matrix metalloproteinase contribute to the formation of adhesions (Fig. 1). Precise mechanisms and the relative contribution of these factors and enzymes need to be further unraveled.

Postoperative peritoneal adhesions develop in as many as 95% of the patients undergoing a laparotomy.[5] Laparoscopy seems to be associated with less adhesions; however, convincing evidence still lacks.[6–8] Given the almost 100% incidence, adhesions might be considered as part of normal peritoneal healing. Others call adhesions the most frequent complication of intraperitoneal surgery.

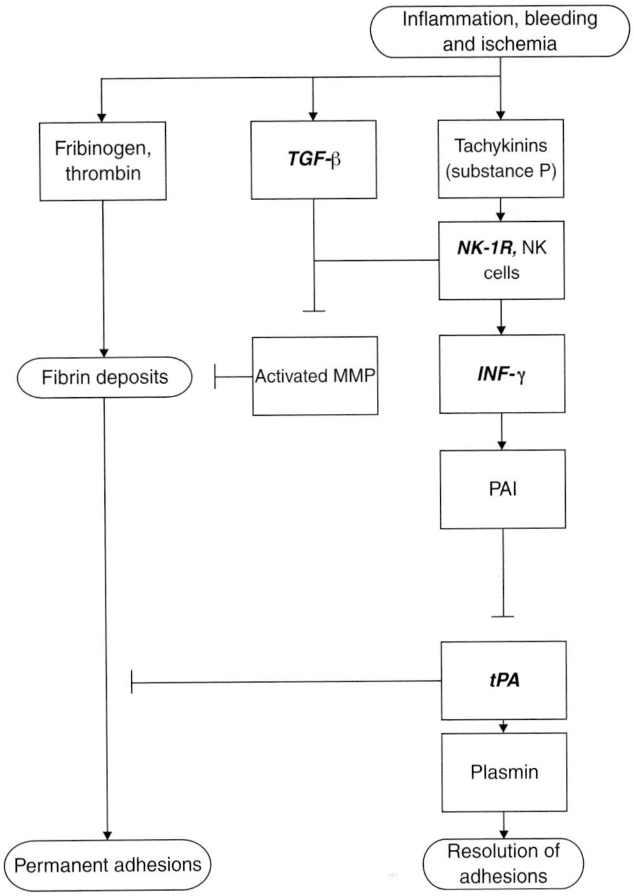

Figure 1. Scheme of important steps in adhesion formation. In the first 3 postoperative days fibrin deposits accumulate. In normal peritoneal healing plasminogen is converted by tPA into active plasmin resulting in fibrin resolution. PAI inhibits tPA. MMPs remodel extracellular matrix. Inflammation, bleeding, and ischemia induced by surgical trauma stimulate the release of numerous adhesion molecules, chemotactic cytokins, tachykinins, interleukins, and growth factors that regulate the modeling of the extracellular matrix and the net fibrinolytic activity. Substance P and TGF-*β* have recently been identified as two important factors in the formation of adhesions. TGF-*β* inhibits MMP leading to an altered remodeling of extracellular fibrin deposits that favor adhesion formation. Substance P favors adhesion formation by both inhibition of MMPs as well as stimulating the release of PAI by binding to the NK-1R. Antagonizing NK-1R, TGF-*β*, and INF-*γ*, and administration of recombinant tPA prevent adhesion formation and may be a novel targeted systemic therapy for adhesions. INF-*γ* = interferon-*γ*; MMP = matrix metalloproteinase; NK-1R = neurokinin-1 receptor; PAI = plasminogen activator inhibitor; TGF-*β* = transforming growth factor-beta; tPA = tissue plasminogen activator.

CLINICAL PROBLEM

Postsurgical adhesions prolong operation time at abdominal reentry and cause inadvertent enterotomy during adhesiolysis, secondary female infertility, and chronic pain, impacting the lives of millions of patients worldwide.[9] The most frequently addressed complication in general surgery is adhesive small bowel obstruction (ASBO). ASBO causes significant morbidity and mortality and has large socioeconomic impact. In a population-based study, Kössi *et al.* estimated that each year 3.0 patients per 10,000 inhabitants are admitted to hospital for ASBO and that, on average, the treatment for each ASBO patient costs 8.3 hospital-days and 0.3 operations.[10] Based on these estimates, total annual cost of ASBO approximated $85,000 per 10,000 inhabitants. In-hospital mortality from ASBO ranged between 5.2 and 7.0 in two large studies.[11,12]

To reduce the burden of ASBO, the clinician faces at least two major challenges. The first challenge is to prevent the formation of postoperative adhesions. In addition to a reduction of ASBO this might also benefit safe access to the peritoneal cavity in case of reentry. The second challenge is improving the therapeutic management of ASBO.

The initial management of ASBO is conservative, namely intravenous fluid administration and nasogastric decompression. However, ASBO requires surgery when conservative treatment fails to rapidly improve signs of bowel obstruction. Indication and timing of surgery is difficult even for the experienced clinician; studies on the management of ASBO clearly demonstrate a higher mortality in patients who had prolonged conservative treatment before the decision was made to reoperate.[11,12] The reoperation itself can cause inadvertent enterotomies and initiate new adhesions.[13–15] Thus, more successful conservative management and better tools to decide to operate in an earlier phase of SBO would be advantageous.

SCIENTIFIC CONTEXT

Since 1980 many agents have been developed to reduce adhesions. These agents can grossly be divided into three groups: (1) systemic agents, (2) local (intraperitoneal) barrier agents, and (3) intraperitoneal broad coverage liquid barriers.

The use of systemic agents to reduce adhesions has quickly been abandoned because these had limited antiadhesive capacity, were nonsite specific, and had serious adverse effects. For example, corticosteroids compromised wound healing while having only little effect on adhesion formation.[16] For a number of local barrier agents, a significant reduction in adhesions has been demonstrated in randomized controlled trials (RCTs).[16,17] However, there is little evidence of reduction of clinically relevant endpoints such as SBO and pregnancies, and most RCTs have been performed in clean, relatively bloodless gynecologic surgery. It is questionable if barriers are also effective in contaminated major gastrointestinal surgery.[18,19]

With regard to the improvement of conservative management of ASBO, the use of an radioopaque oral water-soluble contrast, named gastrografin, has become of interest because of its diagnostic and therapeutic potency. A recent meta-analysis of clinical trials on the use of gastrogafin demonstrated that gastrografin accurately predicts the need for surgery and reduces hospital stay without an operation. However, gastrografin did not reduce the need for surgery.[20] More recently hyperbaric oxygen (HBO) therapy has been proposed as a treatment for ASBO in patients who fail responding to standard conservative treatment.[21]

ENDPOINTS IN CLINICAL RESEARCH

Scoring the incidence of adhesions at a reoperation or "second-look surgery" is the gold standard in adhesion prevention research. This has great impact for the recruitment of patients for such studies, as it is not ethical to do an invasive procedure only for scientific purpose. Thus, testing of adhesion preventive agents can only be done in patients undergoing a planned second-stage surgery such as ileoanalpouch procedure with temporary loop ileostomy or fertility surgery. These are relatively small groups of patients worldwide.

Taking ASBO as a primary endpoint, however, means large numbers of patients who have to be included with a long follow-up. Most researchers do not have the resources to conduct these types of large complicated studies. Another methodological difficulty lies in the evaluation of ASBO. Adhesions as cause of SBO is only certain when diagnosed during operation or autopsy. So diagnosis of ASBO cannot be 100% accurate in patients who are successfully managed by conservative means. This might not be relevant for clinical practice, but is important when evaluating the efficacy of anti-adhesion agents.

DISCUSSION OF RELEVANT RECENT LITERATURE

The most extensively researched adhesion barrier is oxidized-regenerating cellulose (ORC, Interceed®; Ethicon, Sommerville, NJ).[17] There is strong evidence for its efficacy in reducing adhesions from multiple RCTs. Sawada *et al.* also demonstrated a significantly higher pregnancy rate following fertility surgery using an ORC adhesion barrier.[17,22] The use of ORC is limited to clean gynecologic surgery because it evokes an adverse, adhesiogenic, response in the presence of blood.[23]

Only few RCTs have been conducted evaluating the efficacy of adhesion barriers in gastrointestinal surgery. A recent systematic review by the Cochrane collaboration included seven RCTs evaluating the efficacy and adverse events of adhesion prevention in intestinal surgery.[24] The RCTs addressed two types of agents: hyaluronic acid/carboxymethyl cellulose (HA/CMC; Seprafilm® Adhesion Barrier, Genzyme Corporation, Cambridge, MA; six RCTs) and ferric hyaluronate (FH) gel (Intergel®, Lifecore Biomedial Inc, Chaska, MN; one RCT). In one RCT, a modified type of HA/CMC was used; glycerol was added to the HA/CMC to improve handling properties.[25] This modified type of HA/CMC film showed a trend toward more infectious complications that were not known from large RCTs with unmodified HA/CMC. Recalculating the data, this RCT did not have a significant effect on the final outcome of the analysis.

The RCT on FH gel did not report on the incidence of adhesions.[26] This study was prematurely stopped because of a significantly higher number of complications in the FH gel group, especially prolonged postoperative ileus.

Most studies on HA/CMC described the incidence and extent of adhesions at second look in patients having a planned stoma closure. Only one large RCT of 1,701 patients was designed to evaluate ASBO and one RCT reported on ASBO.[18,27] HA/CMC effectively reduced both the incidence and extent of adhesions, and there was a small but significant reduction in patients who had to undergo surgery for ASBO.

In the study of Fazio *et al.*, patients with a wide variety of operations were included.[18] In a recent RCT, not included in the Cochrane review, only gastric cancer patients were randomized to have HA/CMC or nothing. This RCT showed a small, nonsignificant reduction in SBO of all causes with the use of HA/CMC.[28]

The convincing evidence of HA/CMC barrier effectively reducing adhesions is in contrast with the little evidence reducing the incidence of ASBO. Part of this is explained by the local application of this barrier. Adhesion barriers are placed at peritoneal sites that are visibly injured, while a single adhesive band may have developed from an unrecognized injury. It is technically impossible, time consuming, and costly to cover the entire peritoneal cavity with a local adhesion barrier. Adding a broad coverage barrier as an adjunct to a local barrier might overcome the possibility of leaving difficult to reach damaged areas uncovered. There is, however, no evidence for the efficacy of broad coverage liquids and gels in intestinal surgery. As an alternative to broad coverage barriers, recombinant tPA could be administered in the peritoneal cavity. Thus far there has been reluctance using fibrinolytics because of fear for bleeding complications and impaired wound healing, despite numerous experimental data showing that tPA is safe and effective.[29,30] In a recent pilot RCT in humans it was demonstrated that low doses of recombinant TPA can safely be administered.[31]

It is striking to notice that many agents were very promising in experimental studies but did not enter the clinical arena, and from the agents that were tested in humans, only few successfully demonstrated a significant reduction in the incidence of adhesion in RCTs. One explanation is the type of animal models used by most investigators. Only mild damage to the serosal layer and parietal peritoneum is made in animals without previous oper-

TAKE-HOME MESSAGE

Basic science advances

- Animal models that better mimic clinical situations should be used to test antiadhesion agents.
- To prevent time-consuming, expensive, and complicated clinical trials with low efficacy agents, antiadhesives should be tested in animal models of *de novo* adhesion formation and adhesion reformation, and safety should be evaluated under contaminated conditions and in a bowel anastomosis model.
- NK-1R antagonists show promising results on preventing both adhesion formation and adhesion reformation.
- Further understanding of the continuous remodeling of adhesions and the regulation of peritoneal fibroblasts might help to find therapies against mature adhesions and lysed adhesions.

Clinical science advances

- Adhesion barrier agents effectively reduce adhesion formation.
- Adhesion barriers are effective in fertility surgery.
- Effects on ASBO reduction still are limited.
- Better clinical results might be achieved by combined use of a local barrier and a broad coverage barrier.
- More research is needed to study the effects of antiadhesion agents in patients undergoing reoperation.
- HBO therapy seems a promising addition to the present noninvasive therapy for ASBO.

Relevance to clinical care

- Adhesion barriers reduce adhesion formation and should be considered in fertility surgery and in case of a planned second-stage surgery, a high probability of reoperation, and a high risk of ASBO.
- HBO therapy for ASBO should be considered in patients at high predicted risk of perioperative morbidity and mortality.
- Imaging is helpful in predicting the need for reoperation.

ation. This leads to relatively mild *de novo* adhesion formation that are easy to prevent. Many patients already have adhesions from prior surgery, infection, or tumors and these adhesions have great propensity to reform after lysis, and in patients dissection is more extensive with bowel resection, damage to mesenterial vascularization, blood loss, and risk of fecal spill.[32] To increase the translational value of animal studies, adhesion models should better mimic the clinical situation and comprise both *de novo* and reforming adhesions.

Continuing research slowly unravels the pathogenesis of adhesions and provides new formulas of antiadhesive agents. Recently the role of the neurokinin-1 receptor (NK-1R) in adhesion formation has been delineated.[33] This receptor promotes adhesion formation by modulating tPA, PAI, matrix metalloproteinase, and reactive oxygen species. Tachykinins, primarily substance P, are ligands to this receptor.[33] A highly specific antagonist has been synthesized preventing stimulation of the NK-1R by tachykinins. This NK-1R antagonist, called CJ-12,255, demonstrated a reduction of both *de novo* adhesion formation and adhesion reformation after lysis in a second operation. The antagonist did not compromise anastomotic bursting pressure, an important finding for intended use in gastrointestinal surgery. Kosaka *et al.* found that tachykinins also stimulate the release of interferon-γ from natural killer cells. Interferon-γ independently promotes PAI release, a known strong inhibitor of fibrinolysis.[34]

Wilkosz *et al.* gave new insights into the role of fibroblasts in human adhesion formation and adhesion remodeling. They demonstrated that fibroblasts undergo differentiation to myofibroblasts and even to a smooth muscle–like phenotype. Most interesting was the finding of proliferating and collagen-producing fibroblasts present in mature adhesions, indicating that adhesions are a continuously regenerating tissue and not a static scar. While most antiadhesion agents have their window of opportunity in the first phase of adhesion formation, agents antagonizing this dynamic phase might provide a novel approach for mature adhesions and adhesion reformation.[35]

In spite of all efforts to reduce adhesion formation, surgeons will be confronted with ASBO patients for whom reoperation is not an attractive option. Especially in patients with multiple previous episodes of ASBO or severe comorbidity, it would be helpful if the risk of a next, adhesiogenic laparotomy could be avoided. Ambiru *et al.* demonstrated that addition of HBO therapy to standard conservative treatment with nasogastric decompression significantly increased the success rate of conservative treatment (85.9% *vs.* 79.8%; $p = 0.011$) in patients with clinical and radiological confirmation of ASBO.[21] HBO therapy started after more than 7 days of failed conservative treatment resulted in a resolution of ASBO in 81.7% of the patients.

CRITICAL REMARKS

NK-1R antagonist demonstrated promising and specific effects on adhesion formation in animal models. No safety profile for use in humans is yet available.

FUTURE DEVELOPMENTS

Adhesions are the most common complication of peritoneal surgery. More awareness is needed among surgeons, urologists, and gynecologists on the long-term negative effects of adhesions on patient well-being and the available means to reduce adhesions. The growing insight into the pathogenesis of adhesions reveals promising mechanisms for novel therapies. For a safe and effective introduction of novel therapies, a battery of animal models should be applied mimicking clinical scenarios.

AUTHOR DISCLOSURE STATEMENT

No competing financial interests exist.

REFERENCES

1. Duron JJ: Postoperative intraperitoneal adhesion pathophysiology. Colorectal Dis 2007; **9 (Suppl 2):** 14.

2. Gómez-Gil V, Pascual G, Garcia-Honduvilla N, Rodriguez M, Bujan J, and Bellon JM: Characterizing omental adhesions by culturing cells isolated from a novel *in vivo* adhesion model. Wound Repair Regen 2009; **17:** 51.

3. Hellebrekers BW, Emeis JJ, Kooistra T, Trimbos JB, Moore NR, Zwinderman KH, *et al.*: A role for the fibrinolytic system in postsurgical adhesion formation. Fertil Steril 2005; **83:** 122.

4. Vipond MN, Whawell SA, Thompson JN, and Dudley HA: Peritoneal fibrinolytic activity and intra-abdominal adhesions. Lancet 1990; **335:** 1120.

5. Menzies D and Ellis H: Intestinal obstruction from adhesions—how big is the problem? Ann R Coll Surg Engl 1990; **72:** 60.

6. Gutt CN, Oniu T, Schemmer P, Mehrabi A, and Buchler MW: Fewer adhesions induced by laparoscopic surgery? Surg Endosc 2004; **18:** 898.

7. Levrant SG, Bieber EJ, and Barnes RB: Anterior abdominal wall adhesions after laparotomy or laparoscopy. J Am Assoc Gynecol Laparosc 1997; **4:** 353.

8. Wiseman DM, Trout JR, and Diamond MP: The rates of adhesion development and the effects of crystalloid solutions on adhesion development in pelvic surgery. Fertil Steril 1998; **70:** 702.

9. van Goor H: Consequences and complications of peritoneal adhesions. Colorectal Dis 2007; 9 Suppl **2:** 25.

10. Kössi J, Salminen P, Rantala A, and Laato M: Population-based study of the surgical workload and economic impact of bowel obstruction caused by postoperative adhesions. Br J Surg 2003; **90:** 1441.

11. Fevang BT, Fevang J, Stangeland L, Soreide O, Svanes K, and Viste A: Complications and death after surgical treatment of small bowel obstruction: a 35-year institutional experience. Ann Surg 2000; **231:** 529.

12. Foster NM, McGory ML, Zingmond DS, and Ko CY: Small bowel obstruction: a population-based appraisal. J Am Coll Surg 2006; **203:** 170.

13. Fevang BT, Fevang J, Lie SA, Soreide O, Svanes K, and Viste A: Long-term prognosis after operation for adhesive small bowel obstruction. Ann Surg 2004; **240:** 193.

14. Van Der Krabben AA, Dijkstra FR, Nieuwenhuijzen M, Reijnen MM, Schaapveld M, and van Goor H: Morbidity and mortality of inadvertent enterotomy during adhesiotomy. Br J Surg 2000; **87:** 467.

15. Moran BJ: Adhesion-related small bowel obstruction. Colorectal Dis 2007; 9 Suppl **2:** 39.

16. Metwally M, Watson A, Lilford R, and Vandekerckhove P: Fluid and pharmacological agents for adhesion prevention after gynaecological surgery. Cochrane Database Syst Rev 2006; **2:** CD001298.

17. Farquhar C, Vandekerckhove P, Watson A, Vail A, and Wiseman D: Barrier agents for preventing adhesions after surgery for subfertility. Cochrane Database Syst Rev 2000; **2:** CD000475.

18. Fazio VW, Cohen Z, Fleshman JW, van Goor H, Bauer JJ, Wolff BG, *et al.*: Reduction in adhesive small-bowel obstruction by Seprafilm adhesion barrier after intestinal resection. Dis Colon Rectum 2006; **49:** 1.

19. Vrijland WW, Tseng LN, Eijkman HJ, Hop WC, Jakimowicz JJ, Leguit P, *et al.*: Fewer intraperitoneal adhesions with use of hyaluronic acid-carboxymethylcellulose membrane: a randomized clinical trial. Ann Surg 2002; **235:** 193.

20. Abbas SM, Bissett IP, and Parry BR: Meta-analysis of oral water-soluble contrast agent in the management of adhesive small bowel obstruction. Br J Surg 2007; **94:** 404.

21. Ambiru S, Furuyama N, Kimura F, Shimizu H, Yoshidome H, Miyazaki M, *et al.*: Effect of hyperbaric oxygen therapy on patients with adhesive intestinal obstruction associated with abdominal surgery who have failed to respond to more than 7 days of conservative treatment. Hepatogastroenterology 2008; **55:** 491.

22. Sawada T, Nishizawa H, Nishio E, and Kadowaki M: Postoperative adhesion prevention with an oxidized regenerated cellulose adhesion barrier in infertile women. J Reprod Med 2000; **45:** 387.

23. Wiseman DM, Gottlick-Iarkowski L, and Kamp L: Effect of different barriers of oxidized regenerated cellulose (ORC) on cecal and sidewall adhesions in the presence and absence of bleeding. J Invest Surg 1999; **12:** 141.

24. Kumar S, Wong PF, and Leaper DJ: Intra-peritoneal prophylactic agents for preventing adhesions and adhesive intestinal obstruction after non-gynaecological abdominal surgery. Cochrane Database Syst Rev 2009; **1:** CD005080.

25. Cohen Z, Senagore AJ, Dayton MT, Koruda MJ, Beck DE, Wolff BG, *et al.*: Prevention of postoperative abdominal adhesions by a novel, glycerol/sodium hyaluronate/carboxymethylcellulose-based bioresorbable membrane: a prospective, randomized, evaluator-blinded multicenter study. Dis Colon Rectum 2005; **48:** 1130.

26. Tang CL, Jayne DG, Seow-Choen F, Ng YY, Eu KW, and Mustapha N: A randomized controlled trial of 0.5% ferric hyaluronate gel (Intergel) in the prevention of adhesions following abdominal surgery. Ann Surg 2006; **243:** 449.

27. Kusunoki M, Ikeuchi H, Yanagi H, Noda M, Tonouchi H, Mohri Y, *et al.*: Bioresorbable hyaluronate-carboxymethylcellulose membrane (Seprafilm) in surgery for rectal carcinoma: a prospective randomized clinical trial. Surg Today 2005; **35:** 940.

28. Hayashi S, Takayama T, Masuda H, Kochi M, Ishii Y, Matsuda M, *et al.*: Bioresorbable membrane to reduce postoperative small bowel obstruction in patients with gastric cancer: a randomized clinical trial. Ann Surg 2008; **247:** 766.

29. Van Goor H., Bom VJ, van der Meer J., Sluiter WJ, Geerards S, and van der Schaaf W. *et al.*: Pharmacokinetics of human recombinant tissue-type plasminogen activator, administered intra-abdominally, in a rat peritonitis model. Eur Surg Res 1996; **28:** 287.

30. Buyne OR, Van GH, Bleichrodt RP, Verweij PE, and Hendriks T: Both tissue-type plasminogen activator and urokinase prevent intraabdominal abscess formation after surgical treatment of peritonitis in the rat. Surgery 2008; **144:** 66.

31. Hellebrekers BW, Trimbos-Kemper TC, Boesten L, Jansen FW, Kolkman W, Trimbos JB, *et al.*: Preoperative predictors of postsurgical adhesion formation and the Prevention of Adhesions with Plasminogen Activator (PAPA-study): results of a clinical pilot study. Fertil Steril 2009; **4:** 1204.

32. Beck DE, Cohen Z, Fleshman JW, Kaufman HS, van Goor H, and Wolff BG: A prospective, randomized, multicenter, controlled study of the safety of Seprafilm adhesion barrier in abdominopelvic surgery of the intestine. Dis Colon Rectum 2003; **46:** 1310.

33. Reed KL, Stucchi AF, Leeman SE, and Becker JM: Inhibitory effects of a neurokinin-1 receptor antagonist on postoperative peritoneal adhesion formation. Ann NY Acad Sci 2008; **1144:** 116.

34. Kosaka H, Yoshimoto T, Yoshimoto T, Fujimoto J, and Nakanishi K: Interferon-gamma is a therapeutic target molecule for prevention of postoperative adhesion formation. Nat Med 2008; **14:** 437.

35. Wilkosz S, Epstein J, de Giorgio-Miller A, McLean W, Ireland G, and Herrick S: Remodelling of adipose tissue during experimental omental adhesion formation. Br J Surg 2008; **95:** 387.

Section 6

BIOFILM

Section Editors: Philip S. Stewart and Gregory Schultz

New Frontiers of Molecular Microbiology in Wound Healing

Swetha Kandula,[1] Jonathan Mark Zenilman,[2] Johan Humberto Melendez,[2] and Gerald Sylvan Lazarus[1,*]

[1]Dermatology and Johns Hopkins Wound Center at Bayview, Johns Hopkins Medical Institutions, Baltimore, Maryland.
[2]Division of Infectious Diseases, Department of Medicine, Johns Hopkins Bayview Medical Center, Johns Hopkins Medical Institutions, Baltimore, Maryland.

Background: Chronic lower extremity wounds are a major health problem, especially in older patients with chronic illnesses.
The Problem: Nonhealing of wounds is often attributed to infection, but the relationships between commensalism, surface bacteria, delayed wound healing, and invasive infection are not well defined. It is critical to define the full inventory of the organisms, characterize their location within the wound, determine whether the organisms are in the planktonic form or in biofilms, and correlate these with clinical parameters.
Basic/Clinical Science Advances: Studies have shown that only a minority of bacteria can be grown in culture.[1] Genomic tools such as polymerase chain reaction, fluorescent *in situ* hybridization, and metagenomic analysis using rapid DNA sequencing by pyrosequencing have improved our ability to define the microbiology of chronic wounds, and to census fastidious organisms within these wounds. Confocal and scanning electron microscopy permits the localization of bacteria within wounds and biofilms.
Clinical Care Relevance: Noncultivable and fastidious organisms are increasingly appreciated as pathogens and/or cofactors in chronic inflammatory conditions such as wounds. In chronic wounds classic bacterial pathogens, such as *Staphylococcus aureus* and Gram-negative bacilli, may grow in biofilms, which alters their growth characteristics, pathogenicity, and response to therapy. We are entering a new era of wound microbiology that could profoundly influence our use of antimicrobial therapy in delayed or nonhealing wounds.
Conclusion: Robust new analytic and morphological methods can establish the spectrum, density, three-dimensional location, and status of organisms as either planktonic or within a biofilm. Correlating these microbiological data with comprehensive clinical parameters can formulate testable hypothesis on the role of bacteria in healing of chronic wounds and revolutionize our approach to the use of antimicrobial agents in wound care.

Abbreviations and Acronyms

CFU = colony-forming unit

EPS = extracellular polymeric substance

FISH = fluorescent *in situ* hybridization

MRSA = methicillin-resistant *Staphylococcus aureus*

PCR = polymerase chain reaction

RT-PCR = real-time polymerase chain reaction

*Correspondence: Dermatology and Johns Hopkins Wound Center at Bayview, Johns Hopkins Medical Institutions, MFL Center Tower, Suite 2500, 5200 Eastern Ave., Baltimore, Maryland 21224-2780 (e-mail: glazaru1@jhmi.edu).

BACKGROUND

Chronic wounds cause substantial morbidity and have estimated direct medical costs in 2004 of $10 billion.[2] The etiology of chronic wounds is multifactorial. Presence of bacteria is postulated to inhibit wound healing.[3] Differentiating surface commensal colonization, which would not require therapy, from invasive infection is empiric, and not based on scientifically supported concepts. Consequently, topical and systemic antimicrobials are widely used, despite minimal evidence basis for these therapies; they also cause untoward reactions in patients, are costly, and promote growth of antibiotic-resistant

Printed in U.S.A.
DOI: 10.1089/awc.2009.0106

organisms such as methicillin-resistant *Staphylococcus aureus* (MRSA) and *Pseudomonas*.[4]

One of the leading hypotheses that explain the limited effectiveness of antimicrobials in wounds is that bacteria are in biofilm that leads to persistent infection and inflammation.[5,6] Biofilms are complex multicellular bacterial communities that arise on mucosal or other exposed surfaces. These bacterial communities are embedded in a matrix of extracellular polymeric substance (EPS). The chronic wound, which is a nutrient-rich environment for bacteria, contains a mixture of proteins, glycolipids, polysaccharides, and extracellular DNA that furnishes a nearly perfect milieu for biofilm development. The EPS contains polysaccharides and glycoproteins secreted by bacteria in response to environmental cues.[7] Biofilms are complex structures that are dynamic, change in response to the environment, and possess specific channels to facilitate cell–cell communication, including pili-facilitated conjugation and gene exchange. They have chemical mediators such as quorum-sensing compounds, and even nanowires, which are small protein wire-like structures that can directly connect different bacterial cells.[8,9]

Compared to the planktonic bacteria typically found in culture systems, biofilm-associated bacteria have different phenotypic characteristics and genetic expression profiles. Biofilm-associated bacteria have longer doubling times,[10,11] dramatically reduced antimicrobial susceptibility, altered host immunological responses,[12] and slow mobility of invading host inflammatory cells.[13] For example, *Pseudomonas* mucosal infection is typically associated with presence of a visible biofilm and the production of virulence factors, such as rhamnolipids that induce host leukocyte necrosis that further amplifies inflammation.[14] By contrast, other bacterial species and/or combinations may in fact potentially facilitate wound healing by inhibiting colonization and invasion by competing pathogenic organisms (probiotic effect).[15]

Antimicrobial resistance in biofilm bacteria occurs because of decreased penetration of antibiotics through the biofilm, altered microbial metabolism, and increased doubling time. Doubling (generation) time is especially important since the effect of all B-lactam antibiotics, and many other antimicrobials are dependent on bacterial replication to maximize bactericidal effect. Biofilm-associated bacteria are thought to play a major role in the chronicity of chronic wounds, implanted prosthetic devices, endocarditis, and osteomyelitis.

CLINICAL PROBLEM ADDRESSED

We define wound infection clinically as a constellation of clinical signs and symptoms such as fever, redness, heat, pain, and leukocytosis, which imply that bacteria are overcoming host defenses and spreading beyond the wound border.[16,17] By contrast, slowed or nonhealing is defined by persistence of the clinical lesion and has multiple causes including poor vascular supply, aging, cachexia, and toxic drugs.

The role of bacteria in retarded healing is difficult to define; ascertainment of the bacterial population in wounds is challenging since only a minority of bacteria can be cultured.[18] Bacterial cultures, even when carefully performed, have a number of practical problems. These include the difficulty of identifying multiple organisms in a single specimen, and the challenge in culturing obligate anaerobes. Wound swabs, the most widely used culture material, are plagued by poor reproducibility and sampling bias issues. For example, we found, in a prospective series of patients that data from qualitative wound swabs were highly discordant with results obtained from quantitative cultures.[19–21] Nevertheless, clinical practice in most wound care settings bases treatment decisions on identification of cultivable organisms from wound swabs.

Deep tissue biopsy has been the gold standard because superficial swabs do not provide information on the bacteria invading deep tissues.[22,23] However, tissue biopsies are invasive, and technically demanding. In response to this need, we explored a variety of tissue sampling techniques. We demonstrated using a single brisk harvest with a 3 mm curette from the undermining advancing border of the wound that one can reliably and reproducibly harvest 20 mg of tissue, an amount sufficient to perform multiple analyses. Further, we found that the ecology of large wounds was similar in different intrawound sampling sites. We found that 100% (25/25) of the time, the same organisms were cultured from the contralateral positions (180°) across the rim of the wound and the center,[19,20] and these findings were confirmed by real-time polymerase chain reaction (RT-PCR).[24] Curettage correlates better with deep tissue biopsy than swab or aspirate, is relatively noninvasive, and is more sensitive and specific than swab culture, and the technique can be used to reliably isolate anaerobic bacteria. In addition, the procedure probably disrupts the biofilm in the area where it is performed and might accelerate wound healing.

RELEVANT BASIC SCIENCE CONTEXT

Most approaches to identify bacterial DNA use identification and isolation of 16s ribosomal DNA, which is unique to bacterial species and is a universal bacterial primer. The 16s sequences are then used as the initiator to amplify the species-specific DNA that flanks the 16s site. The flanking areas are then sequenced and the products are called clones. These sequences are compared to large libraries and databases that can match the experimental result with the species-specific sequence. In a mixed environment such as a wound, separating the various clones, sequencing, and identifying them are highly labor intensive and time consuming. More recent automated sequencing technologies, such as pyrosequencing, rapidly analyze the samples directly and perform rapid sequencing. These methods, which are fully computerized and automated, offer the benefit of high-throughput and rapid turnaround, but are costly and require highly sophisticated genetic and informatics resources. Such technology is presently restricted to research settings, but rapid advances may allow it to become clinically useful in the next 5 years.

EXPERIMENTAL MATERIAL—ADVANTAGES AND LIMITATIONS

Even when reference quality samples are utilized, current culture technology is limited. Specimen transport issues can reduce sensitivity. Many hospitals and clinics require microbiology be performed by outside labs, often in distant cities. The turnaround time for bacterial cultures is often >2 days, especially when multiple organisms are found. Identification of some organisms, such as *Acinetobacter*, may take up to 4 days.

Molecular microbiological diagnostics offer substantial promise in addressing these problems, and can revolutionize approaches. These methods offer increased sensitivity, rapid turnaround, ability to identify fastidious organisms, and there is minimal impact of transport since we are analyzing for DNA. As these methods are developed, there are important challenges, including defining sensitivity and specificity, and translating these techniques from the research to clinical and applied settings.

An initial approach is nucleic acid amplification by PCR. PCR methods are highly sensitive and can detect as few as 10 copies of DNA per sample. PCR

Table 1. *The various methodologies utilized to detect the bacteria in wounds are outlined below in tabular format*

Method	Technique—Description	Processing Time and Costs	Advantages	Disadvantages	Practice Implications
Qualitative cultures	Swab culture of wound taken from debrided surface; standard bacteriology culture	1 h for Gram stain; 1–3 days for culture results	Inexpensive, widely available	Low sensitivity, especially for fastidious organisms; not quantitative	Useful to identify presence of specific organisms, such as MRSA or *Pseudomonas*
Quantitative culture	Tissue specimen homogenized; organisms identified and quantitated. About 10^5 CFU/g is empiric threshold for invasive infection.	3–4 days for speciation and quantitation; requires rapid processing expensive	Provides accurate and reproducible measure of organism burden within wound	Labor intensive, requires specialized facilities, long lag time until results are available, which impacts clinical utility; unknown if infection threshold varies by organism	Widely used in Burn units, but clinical correlation not well-defined
Nucleic acid amplification-PCR	DNA is extracted from specimens and amplified, using organism-specific primers.	Processing time can be 4–6 h; moderate cost	Rapid turnaround; assays can be highly sensitive	Requires testing against probes for known organisms; not useful for identifying unknowns; not clinically standardized; will also identify DNA from nonviable organisms	Research settings largely; increasing use to quantify organisms load and to identify MRSA in surveillance settings
Metagenomic methods	DNA is extracted from wound specimens, amplified, and sequenced. Different sequencing approaches include clone libraries and pyrosequencing.	Multiple steps involved; processing takes several days; requires extensive lab and informatics support; expensive	Method can identify all of the bacterial sequences within a specimen, including fastidious organisms, organisms in low numbers; can identify unknown organisms	Expensive, long turnaround time, not standardized; sequences identified may include surface contaminants, and nonviable organisms.	Research settings, to particularly identify nonviable organisms

MRSA = methicillin-resistant *Staphylococcus aureus*; CFU = colony-forming unit; PCR = polymerase chain reaction.

methods target identification of specific organisms. In clinical settings where PCR is widely used, such as assessment of sexually transmitted mucosal infection or rapid diagnosis of meningitis, specific limited organism panels are used, precluding detection of unsuspected bacteria. RT-PCR has turnaround times of <4 h, and can be multiplexed so that multiple assays can be run simultaneously. Therefore, this technique can rapidly identify the presence or absence of specific organisms, which can be particularly valuable in settings where treatment decisions for bacteria such as MRSA and *Pseudomonas* are required. In our clinic, we have been able to successfully use PCR with high sensitivity to identify the 12 most commonly found organisms, including *S. aureus*, MRSA, Group B streptococci, *Pseudomonas*, and a variety of enteric species.[24]

Metagenomic approaches[18,25] identify all bacterial sequences within a sample and speciate through correlation with known large sequence databases. This approach is highly complex and technically demanding, but can be used to identify previously unknown or unidentified species within a wound (Table 1). Preliminary data from a series of over 20 patients from our center revealed an average of 10 different bacterial families in the wounds four times more than culture-based analyses.[4] Fastidious anaerobic pathogens such as *Mobiluncus*, *Gardnerella*, and *Atobopium* species, which are also associated with bacterial vaginosis, were often isolated. This suggests that combinations of previously underidentified organisms may cause inflammatory states seen in chronic wounds as they do in bacterial vaginosis.

Dowd studied diabetic foot ulcers with bacterial tag–encoded FLX amplicon pyrosequencing and proposed that aerobes and anaerobes coexist producing profound biological effects that cannot be caused by individual species alone.[26] This highlights the importance of studying the ecobiology of wounds to determine the difference between healing wounds versus nonhealing wounds.

TAKE-HOME MESSAGE

Basic science advances

- Qualitative cultures are useful to detect planktonic bacteria that overcome the host (infection) but not in establishing the census of all organisms within the wound.
- Quantitative culture although considered the gold standard for studying wound microbiology is incomplete in assessing the full spectrum of microbial agents.
- RT-PCR analysis for specified organisms is more sensitive than standard culture but still does not identify the full spectrum of bacteria within the wound.
- Metagenomic analysis with pyrosequencing demonstrates a high diversity of previously undetected microorganisms present within the wound.
- Our data suggest that we can morphologically detect the organisms at the rim of the wound by FISH technology, and density is similar to results obtained using quantitative microbiology.[29]

Clinical science advances

- Chronic wounds are colonized by a much wider diversity of organisms than previously suspected.
- Biofilms are multicellular communities that are embedded in a matrix of EPS partly derived from the sessile cells in the community and may play a major role in the persistence of infection in chronic wounds.

Relevance to clinical care

- Curettage for collection of tissue is relatively noninvasive and can be used to reliably isolate bacterial population.
- Previously unidentified organisms detected by metagenomic analysis may play a major pathophysiological role in wound healing either as a pathogen or filling an ecological niche to promote healing.

DISCUSSION

Current DNA-based identification technologies cannot differentiate between live and nonviable organisms, which can be confusing especially if assessment is being done to monitor treatment efficacy. Newer approaches probably will approach wounds from the standpoint of identifying the transcriptome, which identifies active RNA transcription and therefore by definition, viable organisms. These methods have the potential to provide critical information on the role of specific microorganisms and bacterial communities on chronic wound pathogenesis.

Fluorescent *in situ* hybridization (FISH) is a morphological technique using bacterial-specific fluorescent-labeled genome probes. Tissue biopsies are carefully taken and the organisms are pinpointed within the macroorganization of the wound or biofilm. FISH is especially useful in associating specific organisms and organism types within biofilm, since biofilm-associated organisms have characteristic aggregation patterns, and can be identified within the EPS matrix. Lawrence *et al.* demonstrated that aggregation of bacteria within a biofilm differs based on their species. For example, *Pseudomonas aeruginosa* biofilms were characterized by a dense cell mass located near the biofilm base, whereas *Vibrio parahaemolyticus* biofilms exhibited an inverted pyramid structure, with the most biofilm biomass located near the biofilm–liquid interface.[27]

Confocal microscopy is a method where fluorescent-tagged organisms can be identified within three-dimensions within a wound. By serially focusing up and down a specimen in increments as small as 5 μm, these images can be integrated and reconstructed to provide a three-dimensional picture. Confocal microscopy can also be performed on live tissue and, with serial observations, can track bacteria within a wound. Additional fluorescent stains can be used to assess viability and for specific structural components.

These methods have been used by James *et al.*, who found that 60% of chronic wounds contained biofilm on light and scanning electron microscopy compared to only 6% of acute wounds.[28]

CAUTION, CRITICAL REMARKS, AND RECOMMENDATIONS

New molecular analytic methods can establish the spectrum and density of organisms within a wound.

These robust analytic and morphological methods can establish the spectrum, density, three-dimensional location, and status of organisms as either planktonic or within a biofilm. Correlating these microbiological data with comprehensive clinical parameters can permit formulation of testable hypothesis on the role of bacteria in healing of chronic wounds and revolutionize our approach to the use of antimicrobial agents in wound care.

FUTURE DEVELOPMENT: NEW MOLECULAR TECHNIQUES

The microflora of chronic wounds is far more complicated than previously suspected. Not only do a large number of species inhabit the wounds, but also organisms live in complex structures within biofilms.

The development of molecular diagnostics and their application to clinical medicine may revolutionize the approach to assessing the role of bacteria in chronic wounds. Although these have not yet been widely used in practice, as testing techniques become validated, they may have enormous utility to the clinicians.

There are a number of important challenges, including developing techniques to identify multiple organisms, and determining the sensitivity and specificity of these techniques. Nevertheless, the past several years have seen the development of incredibly powerful new methods that may better define the role of bacteria in delayed wound healing.

ACKNOWLEDGMENTS

We would like to thank Dr. Mark Shirtliff, University of Maryland Schools of Dentistry and Medicine, Baltimore, MD, for the peptide nucleic acid–FISH photomicrographs; Dr. Lance Price, Translational Genomics Research Institute & Northern Arizona University, Flagstaff, AZ, for the metagenomic data; Yelena Frankel M.D., M.P.H., Department of Dermatology, Johns Hopkins University School of Medicine, Baltimore, MD, for wound sampling and studying the clinical correlations; and Jo Martin, Johns Hopkins University School of Medicine, Baltimore, MD, for the comprehensive review of the literature.

AUTHOR DISCLOSURE STATEMENT

There are no conflicts of interest for Mr. Johan Melendez and Drs. Kandula, Zenilman, and Lazarus.

REFERENCES

1. Kaeberlein F, Lewis K, and Epstein SS: Isolating "uncultivable" microorganisms in pure culture in a simulated natural environment. Science 2002; **296:** 1127.
2. Bickers DR, Lim HW, Margolis D, Weinstock MA, Goodman C, and Faulkner E: The burden of skin diseases: 2004 a joint project of the American Academy of Dermatology Association and the Society for Investigative Dermatology. J Am Acad Dermatol 2006; **55:** 490.
3. Madsen SM, Westh H, Danielsen L, and Rosdahl VT: Bacterial colonization and healing of venous leg ulcers. APMIS 1996; **104:** 895.
4. Price LB, Liu CM, Melendez JH, Frankel YM, Engelthaler D, Aziz M, Bowers J, Rattray R, Ravel J, Kingsley C, Keim PS, Lazarus GS, and Zenilman JM: Community analysis of chronic wound bacteria using 16S rRNA gene-based pyrosequencing: impact of diabetes and antibiotics on chronic wound microbiota. PLoS One 2009; **4:** e6462.
5. Bjarnsholt T, Kirketerp-Moller K, Jensen PO, *et al.*: Why chronic wounds will not heal: a novel hypothesis. Wound Repair Regen 2008; **16:** 2.
6. Kirketerp-Møller K, Jensen PØ, Fazli M, Madsen KG, Pedersen J, Moser C, Tolker-Nielsen T, Høiby N, Givskov M, and Bjarnsholt T: Distribution, organization, and ecology of bacteria in chronic wounds. J Clin Microbiol 2008; **46:** 2717.
7. Whitchurch CB, Tolker-Nielsen T, Ragas PC, and Mattick JS: Extracellular DNA required for bacterial biofilm formation. Science 2002; **295:** 1487.
8. Gorby YA, Yanina S, McLean JS, Rosso KM, Moyles D, Dohnalkova A, Beveridge TJ, Chang IS, Kim BH, Kim KS, Culley DE, Reed SB, Romine MF, Saffarini DA, Hill EA, Shi L, Elias DA, Kennedy DW, Pinchuk G, Watanabe K, Ishii S, Logan B, Nealson KH, and Fredrickson JK: Electrically conductive bacterial nanowires produced by *Shewanella one-*

idensis strain MR-1 and other microorganisms. Proc Natl Acad Sci USA 2006; **103:** 11358.

9. Moller S, Korber DR, Wolfaardt GM, Molin S, and Caldwell FR: Impact of nutrient composition on a degradative biofilms community. Appl Environ Microbiol 1997; **63:** 2432.

10. Tam K, Kinsinger N, Ayala P, Qi F, Shi W, and Myung NV: Real-time monitoring of *Streptococcus mutans* biofilm formation using a quartz crystal microbalance. Caries Res 2007; **41:** 474.

11. Yang L, Haagensen JA, Jelsbak L, Johansen HK, Sternberg C, Høiby N, and Molin S: *In situ* growth rates and biofilm development of *Pseudomonas aeruginosa* populations in chronic lung infections. J Bacteriol 2008; **190:** 2767.

12. Ramsey MM and Whiteley M: Polymicrobial interactions stimulate resistance to host innate immunity through metabolite perception. Proc Natl Acad Sci USA 2009; **106:** 1578.

13. Bjarnsholt T, Jensen PØ, Burmølle M, Hentzer M, Haagensen JA, Hougen HP, Calum H, Madsen KG, Moser C, Molin S, Høiby N, and Givskov M: *Pseudomonas aeruginosa* tolerance to tobramycin, hydrogen peroxide and polymorphonuclear leukocytes is quorum-sensing dependent. Microbiology 2005; **151(Pt 2):** 373.

14. Jensen PØ, Bjarnsholt T, Phipps R, Rasmussen TB, Calum H, Christoffersen L, Moser C, Williams P, Pressler T, Givskov M, and Høiby N: Rapid necrotic killing of polymorphonuclear leukocytes is caused by quorum-sensing controlled production of rhamnolipid by *Pseudomonas aeruginosa*. Microbiology 2007; **153(Pt 5):** 1329.

15. Costerton JW: *The Biofilm Primer*. New York: Springer Science and Business Media, 2007.

16. Lazarus GS and Zenilman J: Microbial bioburden and chronic wounds: role of new molecular methodologies in assessing and treating wounds. Technical Advisory Conference and Wound Biofilm Retreat, Montana State University, Bozeman, MO. February 3–4, 2009.

17. Martin JM, Zenilman JM, and Lazarus GS: Molecular microbiology: new dimensions for cutaneous biology and wound healing. J Invest Dermatol 2009 [Epub ahead of print].

18. Davies CE, Hill KE, Wilson MJ, Stephens P, Hill CM, Harding KG, *et al.*: Use of 16S ribosomal DNA PCR and denaturing gradient gel electrophoresis for analysis of the microfloras of healing and nonhealing chronic venous leg ulcers. J Clin Microbiol 2004; **42:** 3549.

19. Frankel YM, Melendez JH, Price LB, Wang NY, Zenilman JM, and Lazarus GS: Diagnosing chronic wound infection: comparison of routine cultures, quantitative microbiology and molecular techniques. J Am Acad Dermatol 2008; **58 Suppl 2:** AB142.

20. Frankel YM, Melendez JH, Wang NY, Price LB, Zenilman JM, and Lazarus GS: Defining wound microbial flora: molecular microbiology opening new horizons. Arch Dermatol 2009; **10:** 1193.

21. Price LB, Melendez JH, Frankel YM, Wang NY, Bowers J, Ravel J, Keim P, Lazarus GS, and Zenilman JM: 16S-based molecular characterization of chronic wound microflora to improve future therapies. Presented at 48th Annual ICAAC/IDSA 46th Annual Meeting scheduled on October 25–28, 2008, Washington, DC.

22. Davies CE, Hill KE, Newcombe RG, Stephens P, Wilson MJ, Harding KG, *et al.*: A prospective study of the microbiology of chronic venous leg ulcers to reevaluate the clinical predictive value of tissue biopsies and swabs. Wound Repair Regen 2007; **15:** 17.

23. Robson MC and Heggers JP: Bacterial quantification of open wounds. Mil Med 1969; **134:** 19.

24. Melendez JH, Frankel YM, Price LB, Wang NY, Lazarus GS, and Zenilman JM: Microbial analysis of chronic wounds by qualitative culture, quantitative microbiology and molecular methods. Presented at the 108th General Meeting of the American Society for Microbiology, June 1–5, 2008. Boston, MA.

25. Dowd SE, Sun Y, Secor PR, Rhoads DD, Wolcott BM, James GA, *et al.*: Survey of bacterial diversity in chronic wounds using pyrosequencing, DGGE, and full ribosome shotgun sequencing. BMC Microbiol 2008; **8:** 43.

26. Dowd SE, Wolcott RD, Sun Y, McKeehan T, Smith E, and Rhoads D: Polymicrobial nature of chronic diabetic foot ulcer biofilm infections determined using bacterial tag encoded FLX amplicon pyrosequencing (bTEFAP). PLoS ONE 2008; **8:** e3326.

27. Lawrence JR, Korber DR, Hoyle BD, Costerton JW, and Caldwell DE: Optical sectioning of microbial biofilms. J Bacteriol 1991; **173:** 6558.

28. James GA, Swogger E, Wolcott R, *et al.*: Biofilms in chronic wounds. Wound Repair Regen 2008; **16:** 37.

29. Kandula S, Melendez JH, Shirtliff ME, Zenilman JM, and Lazarus GS: Molecular techniques: role in diagnosing microbial bioburden within a wound. Presented at the 69th SID Annual Meeting held at the Palais de congrès Convention Center, May 6–9, 2009, Montreal, Canada.

Ecology of Biofilms in Chronic Wounds

Thomas Bjarnsholt[1,2,*] and Michael Givskov[1]

[1]Department of International Health, Immunology, and Microbiology, Faculty of Health Sciences, University of Copenhagen, Copenhagen, Denmark.
[2]Department of Clinical Microbiology, Rigshospitalet, Copenhagen, Denmark.

Background: Between 1% and 2% of the population in the developed world experiences a nonhealing or chronic wound, characterized by an apparent arrest in a stage dominated by inflammatory processes.

The Problem: Bacteria are present in these wounds. Does this interfere with the wound healing and does the bacterial mode of growth play a role?

Basic/Clinical Science Advances: Research groups have proposed that bacteria might be involved in and contribute to the lack of healing of these wounds. Wound samples have been investigated by standard culturing methods, molecular methods, and peptide nucleic acid–based fluorescence *in situ* hybridization (PNA FISH) for direct identification of bacteria. By means of the classic culturing methods, *Staphylococcus aureus* has been detected in the majority of the wounds, whereas *Pseudomonas aeruginosa* has been observed less frequently. In contrast, using PNA FISH, a large fraction of wounds have been observed to contain *P. aeruginosa*. Further, PNA FISH has revealed the structural organization of bacteria in the samples. It appeared that *P. aeruginosa* aggregated as microcolonies imbedded in the matrix component alginate, which is a characteristic hallmark of the biofilm mode of growth. These microcolonies were detected inside the wound bed, whereas *S. aureus*, when present, are detected on the surface of the wound.

Clinical Care Relevance: Biofilms are extremely tolerant to antimicrobials and components of the host defense. This tolerance becomes particularly evident for the clinician. To achieve a beneficial effect, treatments require high concentrations of antimicrobial compounds, for a prolonged time. Especially *P. aeruginosa* biofilm eliminate neutrophiles by excreted rhamnolipids.

Conclusion: We hypothesize that the presence of *P. aeruginosa* in the biofilm mode of growth and its concomitant elimination of neutrophiles is the main cause of inefficient eradication by antibiotic treatment and activity of the innate immune system, respectively.

Abbreviations and Acronyms

CF = cystic fibrosis

FISH = fluorescence *in situ* hybridization

MMP = matrix metalloproteinase

PMN = polymorphonuclear leucocyte

PNA = peptide nucleic acid

QS = quorum sensing

*Correspondence: Department for Clinical Microbiology, H:S Rigshospitalet, afsnit 9301, Juliane Maries Vej 22, Copenhagen Ø DK-2100, Denmark (e-mail: tbjarnsholt@sund.ku.dk).

BACKGROUND

After the advent of antibiotics, the spectrum of infectious diseases has changed dramatically, particularly in the developed world. The majority of infections are still acute and generally treatable with antibiotics; however, patients suffering from a disease causing deficiencies in the primary defense barriers (the innate immunity) are often at risk of developing a chronic infection. This includes disruption of the anatomic (skin, mucous membranes, cilia), physiologic (temperature, low pH), inflammatory barriers (lactoferrin etc.), and the phagocytic barriers (neutrophiles polymorphonuclear leucocytes [PMNs], macrophages, etc.). These deficiencies can be divided into genetic abnomalities, presence of foreign bodies, and acquired chronic diseases. The classic example of a genetic disorder is cystic fibrosis (CF).

Printed in U.S.A.
DOI: 10.1089/awc.2009.0091

These patients have thickened mucus that impairs the normal mucociliary clearing of the lungs, enabling persistent bacterial infections in the lungs. The presence of foreign bodies includes artificial limbs or body parts and catheters, but also injection of tissue fillers are now being reported as a cause for chronic infections.[1] The acquired chronic diseases include patients suffering from diabetes, immunological malfunctions due to inborn defects or cancer, malnutrition, obesity, drug abuse, alcoholism, and smoking. These patients may be prone to the development of a nonhealing wound chronically infected with bacteria.

A common denominator in the above problems is believed to be a lifestyle bacteria adapt to, referred to as the biofilm mode of growth. In this state the bacteria aggregate in clumps and numerous studies of *in vitro* and *in vivo* biofilms have demonstrated an extreme tolerance to the bulk of antimicrobial agents and components of the human defense including the inflammatory processes. Biofilm antibiotic tolerance is not to be mistaken with antibiotic resistance, since the bacteria when being in biofilm survive antibiotic treatment, but if the biofilm is disrupted the bacteria become susceptible to the treatment.[2] This tolerance becomes particularly evident for the clinician because to achieve a beneficial effect, treatments require high concentrations of antimicrobial compounds, such as antibiotics, silver, and detergents, for a prolonged time. The failure to successfully treat such infections often results in surgical removal, like debridement of the dead tissue of wounds. In extreme cases, the entire infected area has to be removed, such as amputation of limbs, removal of the inserted foreign body, or transplantation of the lungs of CF patients. Another important characteristic of chronic infections (in addition to the presence of bacterial biofilms) is that the inflammatory response seems to be arrested in a semi-acute process, with a continued influx of PMNs.

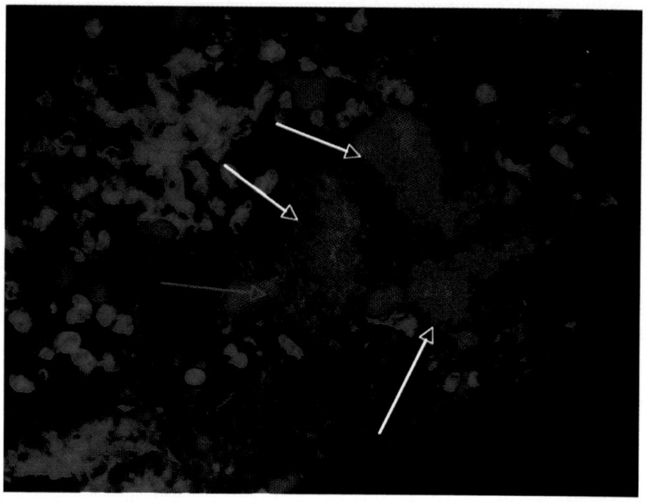

Figure 1. Bacterial biofilms in a chronic, infected wound, collected with the permission of the patient and in accordance with the biomedical project protocol (KA-20051011) approved by the Danish scientific ethical board. Bacteria were examined by PNA fluorescence *in situ* hybridization (AdvanDx, Woburn, MA), using a mixture of Texas Red-labeled, Pseudomonas aeruginosa–specific PNA probe and fluorescein-labeled universal bacterium PNA probe. The tissue section was counterstained with 4′,6-diamidino-2-phenylindole for viewing of host cells (blue). White arrows point at P. aeruginosa biofilm and red arrow points at a biofilm of an unidentified bacterium. The two bacterial species do not form mixed biofilms, and the host cells (white blood cells) are unable to penetrate the large P. aeruginosa biofilms, supporting our shield model. PNA = peptide nucleic acid–based.

CLINICAL PROBLEM: BIOFILMS IN CHRONIC WOUNDS

The newest considered patient group linked to bacterial biofilms is the nonhealing wounds including venous leg, pressure, and diabetic ulcers (Fig. 1). The first direct evidence of biofilm involvement in chronic wounds was based on microscopic identification of bacterial aggregates (Fig. 1) by Bjarnsholt *et al.*,[3] Davis *et al.*,[4] and James *et al.*,[5] accepted for publication in the order shown, though published in the same issue of Wound Repair and Regeneration 2008. These three publications were preceded by a number of reports suggesting the presence of biofilms in wounds and have been preceded by articles elaborating on and expanding the observations of biofilms in chronic wounds.[6,7]

In a study by Kirketerp-Møller *et al.*,[8] the authors collected and examined chronic wound samples obtained from 22 different patients, all allegedly infected by *Pseudomonas aeruginosa*. The focus on *P. aeruginosa* was derived from the hypothesis that *P. aeruginosa* play a major role in chronic wounds. These wound samples were investigated by both standard culturing methods and peptide nucleic acid–based fluorescence *in situ* hybridization (PNA FISH) for direct identification of bacteria. PNA FISH allows illuminating of specific target cells directly inside a sample. By means of the classic culturing methods, *Staphylococcus aureus* was detected in the majority of the wounds, whereas *P. aeruginosa* was observed less frequently. In contrast, using PNA FISH, the authors found that a large fraction of the wounds in fact harbored *P. aeruginosa*. Further, PNA FISH revealed the structural organization of bacteria in the samples (Fig. 1). It appeared that *P. aeruginosa* aggregated as microcolonies imbedded in the matrix component alginate. Presence of the matrix is one of the hallmarks of the biofilm mode of growth. These microcolonies were detected inside the wound bed, whereas *S. aureus*, when present, was detected on the surface of the wounds. This is supported by the observations by Davis *et al.*,[4] who demonstrated that *S. aureus* form microcolonies encased in an extracellular matrix on the surface of the wound bed. In the study by James *et al.*,[5] the authors established an elevated presence of microbial aggregates in chronic wounds compared to acute wounds by usage of scanning electron microscopy. Additionally it has been reported that *P. aeruginosa*–infected wounds appear significantly larger in terms of area than wounds that did not contain *P. aeruginosa*.[9–11]

BASIC SCIENCE: THE INFLAMMATORY CELLS AND THEIR CONTRIBUTION

Both cellular and humoral responses take part in the inflammatory process of chronic wounds. Similar to any other infection, PMNs (the majority of white blood cells) are detected in high amounts in chronic wounds as described by Lobmann *et al.*[12] The humoral response involves release of matrix metalloproteinases (MMPs), growth factors, and cytokines. In the present context, excess amounts of MMPs are of special interest. MMPs belong to a family of zinc-dependent endoproteinases that are involved in the degradation of extracellular matrix components. They are produced by several different cells, including fibroblasts, macrophages, eosinophils, but in particular the PMNs. The MMPs participate in the first phase of the wound-healing process, by removing devitalized tissue, and are therefore believed to play an important role in normal wound healing and remodeling. As for the repair phase, MMPs are necessary for angiogenesis, wound matrix contraction, migration of fibroblasts and keratinocytes, and reepithelialization. However, several papers suggest that elevated levels of active MMPs impair wound healing.[12–14] In particular, infections with *P. aeruginosa* show altered levels of MMPs and MMP-regulating cytokines.[13,15]

The lack of efficient eradication of *P. aeruginosa* resembles the chronic bacterial infection found in the lungs of patients suffering from CF.[16] The inflammatory response in chronic *P. aeruginosa* infection of the CF lung is dominated by PMNs; chronic *P. aeruginosa* infection follows infections with other bacteria, for example, *S. aureus*; there are elevated MMP levels, and antimicrobial therapy has little or no effect.[17–19]

EXPERIMENTAL MATERIAL—ADVANTAGES AND LIMITATIONS: WHICH BACTERIA ARE PRESENT AND WHAT IS THEIR ROLE?

The presence of a bacterial diversity in chronic wounds was established several years ago. In one such study, Gjødsbol *et al.*[9] investigated the bacterial flora by standard culturing. They found chronic venous leg ulcers to harbor *S. aureus* (in 93.5% of the investigated ulcers), *Enterococcus faecalis* (71.7%), *P. aeruginosa* (52.2%), coagulase-negative staphylococci (45.7%), *Proteus* species (41.3%), and anaerobic bacteria (39.1%). James *et al.*[5] also investigated the flora in chronic wounds by culturing and found the most common bacteria to be *Staphylococcus* (65%), *Enterococcus* (62%), and *Pseudomonas* (35%) (for complete list see James *et al.*[5]). Other groups have used molecular techniques to establish the bacterial flora (16s sequencing and denaturing gradient gel electrophoresis). In one such approach, Dowd *et al.*,[20] similar to Kirketerp-Møller *et al.*,[8] established that standard culturing of bacteria from wound samples does not reveal the true bacterial diversity in the wounds. Dowd *et al.* concluded as many others that *S. aureus* and *P. aeruginosa* were among the major bacterial species present in the wounds. Additionally Dowd identified a large population of anaerobic bacteria in the wounds. Using these fairly new molecular techniques, even small populations of a specific bacterium can be detected. This has resulted in a large number of microbes having been identified in wounds. These techniques are qualitative, which means that they do

TAKE-HOME MESSAGE

Basic science advance

- Evidence is accumulating that bacteria are present as biofilms in chronic wounds.

Clinical science advances

- The mere observation of biofilms in wounds alone does not illuminate the role biofilms play in the complicated process of wound healing.
- A bacterial diversity exists in chronic wounds.
- The authors of this chapter describe the important role of *P. aeruginosa* biofilms in persistence, chronic inflammation, and collateral tissue damage.

Relevance to clinical care

- The presence of biofilms in chronic wounds demands a search for novel diagnostic tools and treatment strategies.

not reveal the proportions of different bacteria or how they are organized and distributed in the wounds. Another key concern is that these techniques cannot be used to identify which bacteria play a key role in the impairment of the wound-healing process.

A common denominator of previous studies describing the bacteriology of chronic wounds is that they agree on the almost universal presence of *S. aureus*.[9,21,22] Also most studies agree on the *P. aeruginosa* being present in around half of the investigated wounds and that the deep dermal tissues of all chronic wounds harbor multiple bacterial species.[5,9] The organization and distribution of these two bacteria was proposed by Kirketerp-Møller *et al.*,[8] who employed two specific PNA probes for FISH analysis, one for *S. aureus* and one for *P. aeruginosa* in combination with a universal bacterial probe. Their observations revealed that the different bacterial species might be present in the same wound but they do not amalgamate. They observed very few aggregates of different bacteria in close proximity of each other and never as part of a truly mixed population. One example of aggregates of mixed species was observed by James *et al.*,[5] they detected rod- and cocci-shaped bacteria within close proximity in one wound. Based on the available evidence in the literature it seems that bacteria in chronic infections aggregate mostly as single species,[3,4,8] Bjarnsholt *et al.*, in press. This is in contrast to bacterial aggregation in other natural environments such as the flocks in waste water treatment plants and the soil where several species coaggregate. This coaggregation is explained by the beneficial catabolism and anabolism of compounds among the different bacteria. The plausible reason why multispecies biofilms are not common in chronic infections is that the nutrient availability is high, that is, symbiosis is not a crucial requisite for growth. The key challenge for colonizing bacteria is rather if they can they survive the encounter with the defense system.

DISCUSSION: THE SHIELD HYPOTHESIS

Our latest investigations suggest that *P. aeruginosa* produce a shield of excreted rhamnolipids, a detergent, against incoming inflammatory cells. It was demonstrated by Jensen *et al.* that *P. aeruginosa* biofilms are capable of eliminating human neutrophiles by excreted rhamnolipids.[23] Bjarnsholt *et al.* proposed[3] that this elimination also occurs in infected wounds. The consequences are a chronic inflammatory condition, a continuous influx of neutrophiles, and an efflux of intracellular degradation enzymes from the dead neutrophils such as reactive oxygen species and MMPs. This could explain the imbalance of MMPs seen in the chronic wound fluid. In the study by Kirketerp-Møller *et al.*,[8] the authors showed that the presence of microcolonies was connected to a massive gathering of leukocytes; however, when the microcolonies consisted of *P. aeruginosa*, no penetration of leukocytes into the microcolonies could be detected (Fig. 1). The rhamnolipid production is regulated by a cell-to-cell bacterial signaling system in a process denoted quorum sensing (QS).[24] For *P. aeruginosa* the QS regulatory system is the major regulator of virulence, and most of the regulated genes encode gene products that play a role in the infection process.[25] QS regulation depends on the buildup of the signal molecules produced by each individual cell, and the regulatory cascade is initiated when a certain threshold of the signal molecules has been reached. Biofilms are the perfect place for QS regulation to be initiated since many bacteria are together in close proximity. Interestingly, QS regulation is also involved in the increased tolerance to a variety of antibiotics.[26,27]

CAUTION, CRITICAL REMARKS, AND RECOMMENDATIONS

The question is to the importance of the bacterial flora whether this also contributes to the delayed healing of the wounds. Observations from wounds indicate that the presence of *P. aeruginosa* is preceded by the presence of *S. aureus*. It is likely that the eradication regime for common pathogens such as *S. aureus* opens the door for infecting opportunistic pathogens such as *P. aeruginosa*. This phenomenon is observed in the progress of different infections of the CF lung. Here the patients become infected with *Haemophilus influenzae*, *Streptococcus pneumonia*, and especially with *S. aureus*; they are treatable, but eventually the CF lung "succumbs" to a chronic *P. aeruginosa* infection. We do not suggest that *S. aureus* or any other bacteria should not be treated, but care should be taken to keep *P. aeruginosa* off the wound. Due to this we stress that hygiene has top priority at wound ward as well as everywhere in hospital and healthcare systems to avoid cross infections between patients.

Additionally we recommend that the clinicians sample from within the wound bed and not only superficial, and the clinical microbiologists initiate identification of anaerobic bacteria and not only the most common aerobic human pathogens.

FUTURE DEVELOPMENT: NEW TREATMENT STRATEGIES

Successful treatment of a nonhealing wound depends on identifying and treating the factors that cause the arrest of the healing process. Until recently, it has not been fully explained why chronic wounds have elevated MMPs or why PMNs exist in vast numbers in the chronic wound. Our hypothesis could explain this and we put forward several possibilities that might help tip the balance in favor of healing. Adaptations from the CF clinic might prove to be resourceful. For many years, it has been known that an early, aggressive eradication therapy against *P. aeruginosa* and other bacteria prevents the onset of chronic infection.[28] This could be achieved by developing ways to increase antibiotic levels within the local wound bed and/or to disrupt the biofilms within the local wound bed. Boosting of the cellular immune system, for example, using growth factors and MMP inhibitors as well as local modulation of the invading bacteria by the topical application of silver ions, might also promote healing. However, if our hypothesis is correct, new treatment scenarios are within reach. Lately, a number of studies have proven the concept of QS inhibitors as a relevant antimicrobial treatment.[29–32] Since the production of rhamnolipids is regulated by QS, the application of QS inhibitor compounds will prevent the buildup of the PMN shield and consequently enable proper antimicrobial activities of the PMNs. Because PMN lysis is likely to be restored to a more moderate level, local tissue destruction is kept at a minimum and the MMP levels will be lowered as well. These effects will be expected to tip the balance in favor of bacterial clearance and subsequent healing. Effective QS blockers have been designed,[25,30,33,34] but further clinical tests including their relevance in wound-healing therapy are required.

ACKNOWLEDGMENTS

M.G. has received financial support from the Det Frie Forskningsråd/Teknologi og Produktion supported "A new approach to the control of microbial activity," the Biomedical Consortium "Biomed," and Mölnlycke Health Care. T.B. has received financial support from The Carlsberg Foundation and Lundbeck Foundation "The implication of bacterial biofilms in chronic infections."

AUTHOR DISCLOSURE STATEMENT

No conflict of interest disclosed.

REFERENCES

1. Bjarnsholt T, Tolker-Nielsen T, Givskov M, Janssen M, and Chrsitensen LH: Detection of bacteria by FISH in culture-negative soft tissue filler lesions. Dermatol Surg 2009; **Suppl 2 35:** 1620.
2. Bayles KW: The biological role of death and lysis in biofilm development. Nat Rev Microbiol 2007; **5:** 721.
3. Bjarnsholt T, Kirketerp-Moller K, Jensen PO, Madsen KG, Phipps R, Krogfelt K, Høiby N, and Givskov M: Why chronic wounds will not heal: a novel hypothesis. Wound Repair Regen 2008; **16:** 2.
4. Davis SC, Ricotti C, Cazzaniga A, Welsh E, Eaglstein WH, and Mertz PM: Microscopic and physiologic evidence for biofilm-associated wound colonization *in vivo*. Wound Repair Regen 2008; **16:** 23.
5. James GA, Swogger E, Wolcott R, Pulcini ED, Secor P, Sestrich J, Costerton JW, and Stewart PS: Biofilms in chronic wounds. Wound Repair Regen 2008; **16:** 37.
6. Percival SL and Bowler PG: Biofilms and their potential role in wound healing. Wounds 2004; **16:** (7).
7. Mertz PM: Cutaneous biofilms: friend or foe? Wounds 2003; **15:** 129.
8. Kirketerp-Møller K, Jensen PO, Fazli M, Madsen KG, Pedersen J, Moser C, Tolker-Nielsen T, Høiby N, Givskov M, and Bjarnsholt T: Distribution, organization, and ecology of bacteria in chronic wounds. J Clin Microbiol 2008; **46:** 2717.
9. Gjødsbol K, Christensen JJ, Karlsmark T, Jorgensen B, Klein BM, and Krogfelt KA: Multiple bacterial species reside in chronic wounds: a longitudinal study. Int Wound J 2006; **3:** 225.
10. Madsen SM, Westh H, Danielsen L, and Rosdahl VT: Bacterial colonization and healing of venous leg ulcers. APMIS 1996; **104:** 895.
11. Halbert AR, Stacey MC, Rohr JB, and Jopp-McKay A: The effect of bacterial colonization on venous ulcer healing. Australas J Dermatol 1992; **33:** 75.
12. Lobmann R, Schultz G, and Lehnert H: Proteases and the diabetic foot syndrome: mechanisms and therapeutic implications. Diabetes Care 2005; **28:** 461.
13. de BS, Polette M, Zahm JM, Hinnrasky J, Kileztky C, Bajolet O, Klossek JM, Filloux A, Lazdunski A, and Puchelle E: *Pseudomonas aeruginosa* virulence factors delay airway epithelial wound repair by altering the actin cytoskeleton and inducing overactivation of epithelial matrix metalloproteinase-2. Lab Investig 2000; **80:** 209.
14. Ikema K, Matsumoto K, Inomata Y, Komohara Y, Miyajima S, Takeya M, and Tanihara H: Induction of matrix metalloproteinases (MMPs) and tissue inhibitors of MMPs correlates with outcome of acute experimental pseudomonal keratitis. Exp Eye Res 2006; **83:** 1396.
15. Dong Z, Ghabrial M, Katar M, Fridman R, and Berk RS: Membrane-type matrix metalloproteinases in mice intracorneally infected with *Pseudomonas aeruginosa*. Invest Ophthalmol Vis Sci 2000; **41:** 4189.
16. Koch C and Høiby N: Diagnosis and treatment of cystic fibrosis. Respiration 2000; **67:** 239.
17. Gaggar A, Li Y, Weathington N, Winkler M, Kong M, Jackson P, Blalock JE, and Clancy JP: Matrix metalloprotease-9 dysregulation in lower airway secretions of cystic fibrosis patients. Am J Physiol Lung Cell Mol Physiol 2007; **293:** L96.
18. Høiby N, Frederiksen B, and Pressler T: Eradication of early *Pseudomonas aeruginosa* infection. J Cyst Fibros 2005; **4 Suppl 2:** 49.
19. Hansen CR, Pressler T, and Hoiby N: Early aggressive eradication therapy for intermittent *Pseudomonas aeruginosa* airway colonization in cystic fibrosis patients: 15 years experience. J Cyst Fibros 2008; **7:** 523.
20. Dowd SE, Sun Y, Secor PR, Rhoads DD, Wolcott BM, James GA, and Wolcott RD: Survey of

bacterial diversity in chronic wounds using pyrosequencing, DGGE, and full ribosome shotgun sequencing. BMC Microbiol 2008; **8:** 43.

21. Colsky AS, Kirsner RS, and Kerdel FA: Microbiologic evaluation of cutaneous wounds in hospitalized dermatology patients. Ostomy Wound Manag 1998; **44:** 40–42, 44, 46.

22. Valencia IC, Kirsner RS, and Kerdel FA: Microbiologic evaluation of skin wounds: alarming trend toward antibiotic resistance in an inpatient dermatology service during a 10-year period. J Am Acad Dermatol 2004; **50:** 845.

23. Jensen PO, Bjarnsholt T, Phipps R, Rasmussen TB, Calum H, Christoffersen L, Moser C, Williams P, Pressler T, Givskov M, and Høiby N: Rapid necrotic killing of polymorphonuclear leukocytes is caused by quorum-sensing-controlled production of rhamnolipid by *Pseudomonas aeruginosa.* Microbiology 2007; **153(Pt 5):** 1329.

24. Fuqua C, Parsek MR, and Greenberg EP: Regulation of gene expression by cell-to-cell communication: acyl-homoserine lactone quorum sensing. Annu Rev Genet 2001; **35:** 439.

25. Hentzer M, Wu H, Andersen JB, Riedel K, Rasmussen TB, Bagge N, Kumar N, Schembri MA, Song Z, Kristoffersen P, Manefield M, Costerton JW, Molin S, Eberl L, Steinberg P, Kjelleberg S, Høiby N, and Givskov M: Attenuation of *Pseudomonas aeruginosa* virulence by quorum sensing inhibitors. EMBO J 2003; **22:** 3803.

26. Bjarnsholt T, Jensen PO, Burmolle M, Hentzer M, Haagensen JA, Hougen HP, Calum H, Madsen KG, Moser C, Molin S, Høiby N, and Givskov M: *Pseudomonas aeruginosa* tolerance to tobramycin, hydrogen peroxide and polymorphonuclear leukocytes is quorum-sensing dependent. Microbiology 2005; **151(Pt 2):** 373.

27. Bjarnsholt T and Givskov M: The role of quorum sensing in the pathogenicity of the cunning aggressor *Pseudomonas aeruginosa.* Anal Bioanal Chem 2007; **387:** 409.

28. Valerius NH, Koch C, and Høiby N: Prevention of chronic *Pseudomonas aeruginosa* colonisation in cystic fibrosis by early treatment. Lancet 1991; **338:** 725.

29. Bjarnsholt T and Givskov M: Quorum sensing inhibitory drugs as next generation antimicrobials: worth the effort? Curr Infect Dis Rep 2008; **10:** 22.

30. Bjarnsholt T, Jensen PO, Rasmussen TB, Christophersen L, Calum H, Hentzer M, Hougen HP, Rygaard J, Moser C, Eberl L, Høiby N, and Givskov M: Garlic blocks quorum sensing and promotes rapid clearing of pulmonary *Pseudomonas aeruginosa* infections. Microbiology 2005; **151(Pt 12):** 3873.

31. Rasmussen TB, Skindersoe ME, Bjarnsholt T, Phipps RK, Christensen KB, Jensen PO, Andersen JB, Koch B, Larsen TO, Hentzer M, Eberl L, Hoiby N, and Givskov M: Identity and effects of quorum-sensing inhibitors produced by *Penicillium* species. Microbiology 2005; **151(Pt 5):** 1325.

32. Rasmussen TB, Bjarnsholt T, Skindersoe ME, Hentzer M, Kristoffersen P, Kote M, Nielsen J, Eberl L, and Givskov M: Screening for quorum-sensing inhibitors (QSI) by use of a novel genetic system, the QSI selector. J Bacteriol 2005; **187:** 1799.

33. Givskov M, de Nys R, Manefield M, Gram L, Maximilien R, Eberl L, Molin S, Steinberg PD, and Kjelleberg S: Eukaryotic interference with homoserine lactone-mediated prokaryotic signalling. J Bacteriol 1996; **178:** 6618.

34. Rasmussen TB, Skindersoe ME, Bjarnsholt T, Christensen KB, Andersen JB, Ostenfeld-Larsen T, Hentzer M, and Givskov M: Idendity and effects of quorum sensing inhibitors produced by *Penicillum* species. Microbiology 2005; **151:** 1325.

In Vitro Models for the Growth and Analysis of Chronic Wound Biofilms

Garth A. James,* Alessandra Marçal Agostinho, and Elinor de Lancey Pulcini

Center for Biofilm Engineering, Montana State University, Bozeman, Montana.

Background: Chronic wounds are a major health problem in the United States and throughout the world. Increasing evidence suggests that bacteria inhabiting these wounds exist as biofilms. A biofilm consists of aggregated populations of microorganisms enmeshed in an extracellular matrix and attached to a surface. Biofilm communities show tolerance to antimicrobial agents as well as host immune defenses. Exacerbating this situation is the emergence of drug-resistant bacteria.
The problem: Traditional development and testing of antibacterial agents over the past century has focused on free-floating (planktonic) bacteria in culture. In addition to the emergence of drug-resistant strains, research over the past 20 years has clearly demonstrated that bacteria growing in biofilms differ considerably, particularly with respect to increased antimicrobial tolerance, from their planktonic counterparts. A number of *in vitro* biofilm models have been developed, but only few are relevant to biofilms growing on the surface of the wounds.
Basic/Clinical Science Advances: The development of models for the *in vitro* study of chronic wound biofilms is a key step for targeting antimicrobial treatment against these microbial communities. These models promise to provide a useful tool for chronic wound research and for developing novel therapies.
Clinical Care Relevance: Improved techniques for evaluating biofilm response to antimicrobial treatment will help the development of new therapies.
Conclusion: Although all *in vitro* biofilm models provide valuable data, an *in vitro* biofilm model of a chronic wound should have an air–liquid–solid interface and be suitable for robust treatment regimes. Both the colony model and the drip flow reactor model fit these criteria.

Abbreviations and Acronyms

ASTM = American Society for Testing and Materials
CBD = Calgary biofilm device
CBM = colony biofilm model
CDC-BR = Centers for Disease Control-biofilm reactor
DFR = drip flow reactor
FC = flow cell
LCW = Lubbock chronic wound biofilm model
MTP = 96-well microtiter plate

*Correspondence: Center for Biofilm Engineering, Montana State University, 366 EPS Building, Bozeman, Montana 59717 (e-mail: gjames@erc.montana.edu).

BACKGROUND

CHRONIC WOUNDS, which include venous, pressure, and diabetic ulcers, are a major health problem in the United States and throughout the world. Approximately 67% of all the lower extremity amputations (75,000 in 2003) are performed in diabetic patients who have a chronic diabetic ulcer.[1] In 2006, in the United States, 503,300 patients had a hospital stay that resulted in a pressure ulcer, an 80% increase since 1993. Between $9 and $11.6 million are spent on pressure ulcer care each year and over 60,000 patients die each year as a direct or indirect result of their pressure ulcer.[2] Wounds are susceptible to microbial contamination from both exogenous and endogenous sources, including nose, skin, mouth, and gut, and it is likely that these microorganisms are involved in the development of biofilms.[3] It has been suggested that infections can interrupt the normal

Printed in U.S.A.
DOI: 10.1089/awc.2009.0105

sequence of wound healing. The presence of biofilms in the wound bed may cause an increased inflammatory response.[4] Of further concern is the enhanced tolerance of biofilms to antibiotics and other antimicrobial agents. Bacteria in biofilms are a hundred to thousand times more tolerant than free-floating (planktonic) bacteria to a variety of agents.[5] Traditionally, research, development, and testing of antimicrobial agents have focused on the more susceptible free-floating bacteria, although over the past 20 years of biofilm research a number of *in vitro* biofilm models have been developed.

CLINICAL PROBLEM ADDRESSED

In addition to the emergence of multidrug-resistant bacterial strains such as methicillin-resistant *Staphylococcus aureus*, vancomycin-intermediate *S. aureus*, and vancomycin-resistant *Enterococcus*, increasing evidence suggests that microorganisms inhabiting wounds exist as biofilm communities.[4,6,7] Microorganisms growing as biofilms are much more tolerant to antimicrobial agents than free-floating bacteria. However, antimicrobial treatments have traditionally been developed and tested using free-floating bacteria. New methods are needed to evaluate the effectiveness of treatments against biofilms and to develop new therapies. Chronic wounds support a diverse microflora that is protected from host immune responses and antibiotic treatments through multiple mechanisms.[4,8] Trengove *et al.* demonstrated that wounds with four or more bacterial species had a significantly lower rate of healing, indicating that the various bacteria have a synergistic effect, increasing their pathogenicity in chronic wounds.[9]

As stressed by Percival *et al.*, "every effort must be taken to ensure that *in vitro* models are both as stringent and realistic as possible."[10] Although it is recognized that *in vitro* data cannot be directly extrapolated to clinical outcomes, *in vitro* models can be valuable for testing of antimicrobial agents. Specific characteristics of a biofilm develop in response to growth conditions and environmental stresses. A good *in vitro* model must produce repeatable and reproducible biofilms. Development of relevant models of chronic biofilm wound infection will ultimately lead to the understanding of specific mechanisms by which biofilms impair healing and the development of new therapies.

RELEVANT BASIC SCIENCE CONTEXT

The development of model systems necessary to investigate the role of biofilms in delayed wound healing and to develop strategies for combating these microbial communities will likely require relevant animal models, tissue and cell culture models, as well as biofilm growth models. *In vitro* biofilm models allow for the study of complex phenomena that are not observed using traditional culture methods and that may be difficult to evaluate *in vivo*. The impaired susceptibility to antibiotics, reduced microbial growth rates, altered microenvironments, gene expression, interspecies microbial interactions, and cell-to-cell communication (quorum sensing) are some of the biofilm characteristics that need to be analyzed in chronic wound models.

EXPERIMENTAL MODELS OR MATERIALS NOTE

Several biofilm models, some of which have used clinically relevant microbial communities for various applications, include static reactors,[11] chemostats,[12] capillary flow cells (FCs),[13] perfused biofilm fermenters,[14] rotating disk reactors,[15] the colony biofilm model (CBM),[16] the modified Robbin's device,[17] the Calgary biofilm device (CBD),[18] the annular reactor,[19] the Centers for Disease Control-biofilm reactor (CDC-BR),[20] the drip flow reactor (DFR),[21] the Lubbock chronic wound biofilm model (LCW),[22] and the 96-well microtiter plate (MTP).[23] Some of these models are described in more detail in "Discussion of Findings and Relevant Literature" and brief descriptions are given below. Diagrams of each model discussed are shown in Figure 1.

- MTP: A high-throughput system that has been used for screening purposes. Biofilms are grown within the wells of the plate.
- CBD/minimum biofilm eradication concentration: This device consists of lid with 96 pegs that fit into the wells of a standard MTP. Biofilms are grown on the pegs.
- DFR: Biofilms are grown on a microscope slide placed in an inclined chamber; a continuously supplied nutrient medium drips onto the slide and runs down the surface. An American Society for Testing and Materials (ASTM)-approved standard method (E 2647-08) for growing *Pseudomonas aeruginosa* biofilms under low shear conditions was developed using this model.
- CDC-BR: Biofilms are grown on 24 coupons held in eight separate holders that are submerged in a vessel with mixing and continuous nutrient flow. This model forms the

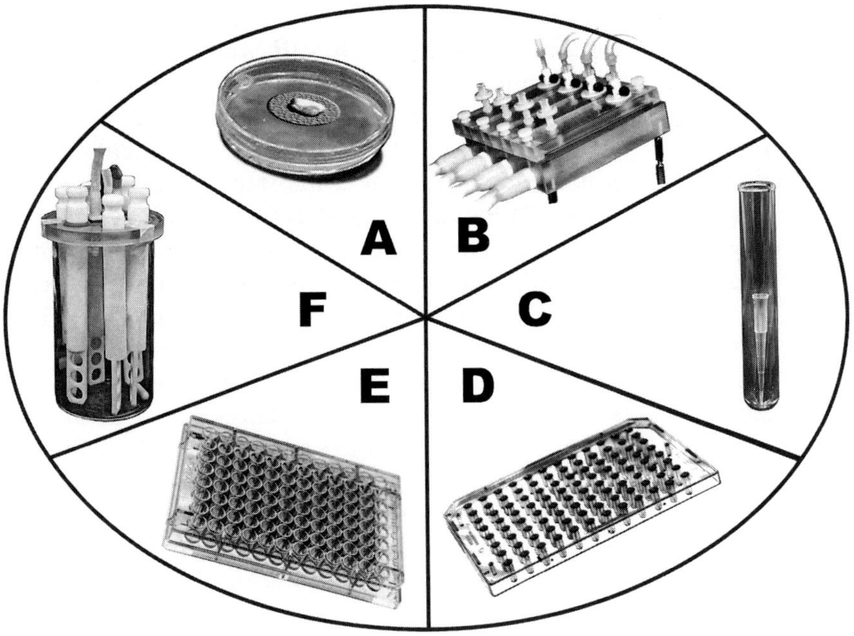

Figure 1. Biofilm reactors/models. A = colony biofilm model; B = drip flow reactor; C = Lubbock chronic wound biofilm model; D = Calgary biofilm device; E = 96-well microtiter plate; F = CDC reactor.

basis of ASTM-approved standard method (#E 2562-07) for the growth of *P. aeruginosa* biofilms.

- CBM: Biofilm is grown on a polycarbonate membrane placed on an agar plate.
- LCW: Biofilm is grown on a pipette tip within a test tube containing growth medium.
- FC: Biofilm is grown within a glass capillary or chamber with continuous flow of nutrient medium.

DISCUSSION OF FINDINGS AND RELEVANT LITERATURE

The growth of biofilms using an MTP was first described by Christensen *et al.* for evaluating the adherence of staphylococci.[23] Biofilm and planktonic cells are grown within the wells of the plate, and the planktonic cells are then rinsed away. Biofilm is quantified by staining with a reagent, such as crystal violet, and then the bound stain is extracted and measured spectrophotometrically. This model is a relatively simple high-throughput system that uses common laboratory equipment.

CBD (www.innovotech.ca) also uses the 96-well plate format in which biofilm is grown on a custom lid with 96 pegs that fit into the plate wells. This model was developed in 1999 for the determination of antibiotic susceptibilities of bacterial biofilms, the minimum biofilm eradication concentration.[18] Similar to a traditional minimum bactericidal concentration assay, based on turbidity due to regrowth following antibiotic treatment, this assay may have clinical applications.

The DFR (www.biofilms.biz) was first described by Xu *et al.* for the evaluation of oxygen distribution on *P.aeruginosa* biofilms.[21] The DFR is unique in that biofilms are grown over a gas (air)–liquid–solid interface by a constant flow of fluid across a surface. This model has been used to evaluate chemical and hydrodynamic treatments for removal of biofilms formed by chronic rhinosinusitis isolates of *P. aeruginosa* and *S. aureus* on hydroxyapatite surfaces.[24] This model provides a large sample area (c.a.18.75 cm^2) allowing an adequate sample for a variety of analyses.

The CDC-BR (www.biofilms.biz) is a rugged and repeatable method for growing biofilms.[25] We have used this model to evaluate the use of asiatic acid and corosolic acid to enhance the susceptibility of *P. aeruginosa* biofilms to tobramycin[26] and to evaluate the susceptibility of a *P. aeruginosa* chronic wound isolate to treatment with lactoferrin and xylitol.[27] Biofilm is grown on 24.5-inch diameter removable coupons immersed in a continuous-flow stirred tank reactor.

The CBM was first described by Anderl *et al.* (2000) to evaluate the penetration of antibiotics into *Klebsiella pneumoniae* biofilms.[16] Biofilm is grown on a polycarbonate membrane placed on a nutrient agar plate. The membrane is periodically transferred to fresh plates. Unlike a bacterial colony growing on a traditional agar plate, the colonies produced show the enhanced antimicrobial tolerance associated with biofilms. This technically simple model has produced valuable insight into biofilm physiology and response to antimicrobial agents.[28,29]

The LCW is a relatively new model specifically developed to grow a multispecies biofilm consisting of the three species of bacteria most commonly isolated from chronic wounds, *P. aeruginosa*, *Enterococcus faecalis*, and *S. aureus*.[22] Biofilms grown in this model have been shown by polymerase chain reaction to contain all three species and exhibit antimicrobial tolerance.

FC enables real-time microscopic analyses of bacteria growing under continuous-flow conditions. FCs have been used to study bacterial attachment, surface colonization,[30] and antibiotic penetration.[31] We have recently used FC to evaluate the susceptibility of a *P. aeruginosa* chronic wound isolate to treatment with the potential antibiofilm agents, lactoferrin and xylitol.[27] Observation of FC biofilms using a variety of fluorescent probes and comparison of mutant to wild-type bacteria have provided insight into the function and complexity of these communities.

Each of the biofilm models described above has specific benefits and shortfalls for the study of biofilms. The MTP and CBD both use 96-well formats that enable high-throughput screening, although conclusions regarding biofilm growth and physiology should be confirmed in more dynamic systems. The DFR, CDC-BR, and FC all grow biofilms under dynamic continuous-flow conditions, and the former two models form the basis of ASTM-approved standard methods. FC is the only model that enables real-time microscopic analysis of biofilms, but collection of samples for other analyses is limited. The CBM is a simple model but mimics a wound environment where bacteria are growing at an air interface with nutrients supplied from below. The CBM is particularly amenable to microscopic analysis after cryosectioning, and the membrane biofilms can be transferred to *in vivo* models. The LCW is the only model described to date that was specifically developed for the analysis of wound biofilms. With the exception of the LCW, the models described above have been used to study single-species biofilms. Due to the polymicrobial nature of wound biofilms, the further development of multispecies models is important to further our understanding of these complex communities.

CAUTION, CRITICAL REMARKS, AND RECOMMENDATIONS

The models presented herein are relatively simple *in vitro* systems for growing biofilms. A chronic wound is a complex environment involving a variety of host, microbial, and environmental factors. Nonetheless, *in vitro* models enable relatively rapid and inexpensive screening of potential antibiofilm agents. Some of these models with modifications, which better reproduce the conditions present in chronic wounds, could be used as important tools for the study of the impact of these microbial community biofilms in the normal process of healing. Promising treatment strategies identified using biofilm models should be further evaluated in more sophisticated systems that incorporate host factors. Models are currently being developed to investigate biofilm–host interactions in wounds using biofilm/cell culture, biofilm/tissue culture, and a variety of animal models.

TAKE-HOME MESSAGE

Basic science advances

- *In vitro* models can help the understanding of how biofilms affect wound healing.
- *In vitro* models allow the rapid and inexpensive screening of antimicrobial compounds before further testing in more complex systems.
- *In vitro* biofilm models lack the host factors involved in wound colonization and infection, but may provide a better screening method for treatments that can be subsequently evaluated in cell and tissue culture as well as animal models, and ultimately human trials.
- Both the DFR and the CDC-BR models have been approved by ASTM as standard methods for the growth of biofilms.

Clinical science advances

- Existing models allow the selection of promising treatments for further evaluation.
- New, improved models will help identify biofilm-targeted agents for wound treatment.
- Specific characteristics of a biofilm develop in response to growth conditions and environmental stresses.

Relevance to clinical care

- Improved efficacy testing of traditional wound care products and novel treatments will aid in selection of appropriate therapies.
- Evaluation of biofilm-targeted agents may lead to the discovery of novel wound care approaches.

FUTURE DEVELOPMENT

There is a need for future research with focus on the development of an *in vitro* model that better mimics the wound environment. A suitable model will allow the evaluation of commercial wound care products as well as experimental antimicrobial compounds. Some characteristics of a promising *in vitro* model are as follows:

- growth of biofilms in an air–solid–liquid interface
- ability to transfer the biofilms from the reactor without disturbance for analysis such as microscopy
- ability to grow multispecies biofilms as well as complex anaerobic biofilms
- use of liquid growth medium that more closely resembles wound exudates
- suitable for robust treatment regimes.

ACKNOWLEDGMENTS

Wound healing research in the authors' laboratory is funded by an Exploratory Research Center Grant (#5P20GM078445-02) from the National Institute of General Medical Science.

AUTHOR DISCLOSURE STATEMENT

No conflict of interest disclosed.

REFERENCES

1. Amputee Coalition of America Fact Sheet. 2008. Diabetes and Lower Extremity Amputations. http://www.amputee-coalition.org/fact_sheets/diabetes_leamp.html#ref4
2. Russo CA, Steiner C, and Spector W: Hospitalizations related to pressure ulcers among adults 18 years and older, 2006. HCUP Healthcare cost and utilization project of the Agency for Healthcare Research and Quality, 2006.
3. Davies CE, Wilson MJ, Hill KE, Stephens P, Hill MC, Harding KG, and Thomas DW: Use of molecular techniques to study microbial diversity in the skin: chronic wounds reevaluated. Wound Rep Reg 2001; **9:** 332.
4. Bjarnsholt T, Kirketerp-Møller K, Jensen PØ, Madsen KG, Phipps R, Krogfelt K, Høiby N, and Givskov M: Why chronic wounds will not heal: a novel hypothesis. Wound Repair Regen 2008; **16:** 2.
5. Costerton JW, Cheng KJ, Geesey GG, Ladd TI, Nickel JC, Dasgupta M, and Marrie TJ: Bacterial biofilms in nature and disease. Annu Rev Microbiol 1987; **41:** 435.
6. Davis SC, Ricotti C, Cazzaniga A, Welsh E, Eaglstein WH, and Mertz PM: Microscopic and physiologic evidence for biofilm-associated wound colonization *in vivo*. Wound Repair Regen 2008; **16:** 23.
7. James GA, Korber DR, Caldwell DE, and Costerton JW: Digital image analysis of the growth and starvation responses of a surface colonizing *Acinetobacter* spp. J Bacteriol 1995; **177:** 907.
8. Edwards R and Harding KG: Bacteria and wound healing. Curr Opin Infect Dis 2004; **7:** 91.
9. Trengove NJ, Stacey MC, McGechie DF, and Mata S: Qualitative bacteriology and leg ulcer healing. J Wound Care 1996; **5:** 277.
10. Percival SL, Bowler PG, and Dolman J: Antimicrobial activity of silver-containing dressings on wound microorganisms using an *in vitro* dental model. Int Wound J 2007; **4:** 186.
11. O'Toole GA and Kolter R: Initiation of biofilm formation in *Pseudomonas fluorescens* WCS365 proceeds via multiple, convergent signaling pathways: a genetic analysis. Mol Microbiol 1998; **28:** 449.
12. Anwar H, Van Biesen T, Dasgupta M, Lam K, and Consterton W: Interaction of biofilm bacteria with antibiotics in a novel *in vitro* chemostat system. Antimicrobiol Agents Chemother 1989; **33:** 1824.
13. Mittelman MW, Kohring LL, and White DC: Multipurpose laminar-flow adhesion cells for the study of bacterial colonization and biofilm formation. Biofouling 1992; **6:** 39.
14. Allison D, Maira-Litran T, and Gilbert P: Perfused biofilm fermenters. Methods Enzymol 1999; **310:** 232.
15. Zelver N, Hamilton M, Pitts B, Goeres D, Walker D, Sturman P, and Heersink J: Measuring antimicrobial effects on biofilm bacteria: from laboratory to field. Methods Enzymol 1999; **310:** 608.
16. Anderl JN, Franklin MJ, and Stewart PS: Role of antibiotic penetration limitation in *Klebsiella pneumoniae* biofilm resistance to ampicillin and ciprofloxacin. Antimicrobiol Agents Chemother 2000; **44:** 1818.
17. Nickel JC, Wright JB, Ruseska I, Marrie TJ, Whitfield C, and Costerton JW: Antibiotic resistance of *Pseudomonas aeruginosa* colonizing a urinary catheter *in vitro*. Eur J Clin Microbiol 1985; **4:** 213.
18. Ceri H, Olson ME, Stremick C, Read RR, Morck D, and Buret A: The Calgary biofilm device: a new technology for rapid determination of antibiotic susceptibilities of bacterial biofilms. J Clin Microbiol 1999; **37:** 1771.
19. Camper A, Jones WL, and Hayes JT: Effect of growth conditions and substratum composition on the persistence of coliforms in mixed-population biofilms. Appl Environ Microbiol 1996; **62:** 4014.
20. Donlan RM, Murga R, Carpenter J, Brown E, Besser R, and Fields B: Monochloramine disinfection of biofilm associated *Legionella pneumophila* in a potable water model system. In: *Legionella*, Marre, R. ed. Washington, DC: American Society for Microbiology, 2001; pp. 406–410.
21. Xu KD, Stewart PS, Xia F, Huang CT, and McFeters GA: Spatial physiological heterogeneity in *Pseudomonas aeruginosa* biofilm is determined by oxygen availability. Appl Environ Microbiol 1998; **64:** 4035.
22. Sun Y, Dowd SE, Smith E, Rhoads DD, and Wolcott RD: *In vitro* multispecies Lubbock chronic wound biofilm model. Wound Repair Regen 2008; **16:** 805.
23. Christensen GD, Simpson WA, Younger JJ, Baddour LM, Barret FF, Melton DM, and Beachey EH: Adherence of coagulase-negative *Staphylococci* to plastic tissue culture plates: a quantitative model for the adherence of *Staphylococci* to medical devices. J Clin Microbiol 1985; **22:** 996.
24. Desrosiers M, Myntti M, and James G: Methods for removing bacterial biofilms: *in vitro* study using clinical chronic rhinosinusitis specimens. Am J Rhinol 2007; **21:** 527.
25. Goeres DM, Loetterle LR, Hamilton MA, Murga R, Kirby DW, and Donlan RM: Statistical assessment of a laboratory method for growing biofilms. Microbiology 2005; **151(Pt 3):** 757.
26. Garo E, Eldridge GR, Goering MG, Delancey-Pulcini E, Hamilton M, Costerton JW, and James GA: Asiatic acid and corosolic acid enhance the susceptibility of *P. aeruginosa* biofilm to tobramycin. Antimicrob Agents Chemother 2007; **51:** 1813.
27. Ammons MCB, Ward LS, Fisher ST, Wolcott RD, and James GA: *In vitro* susceptibility of established biofilms composed of a clinical wound isolate of *Pseudomonas aeruginosa* treated with lactoferrin and xylitol. Int J Antimicrob Agents 2009; **33:** 230.

28. Rani SA, Pitts B, Beynal H, Veluchamy RA, Lewandowski Z, Davison WM, Buckingham-Meyer K, and Stewart P: Spatial patterns of DNA replication, protein synthesis, and oxygen concentration within bacterial biofilms reveal diverse physiological states. J Bacteriol 2007; **189:** 4223.

29. Zheng Z and Stewart PS: Penetration of rifampin through *Staphylococcus epidermidis* biofilms. Antimicrob Agents Chemother 2002; **46:** 900.

30. Lawrence JR, Delaquis PJ, Korber DR, and Caldwell DE: Behavior of *Pseudomonas fluorescences* within the hydrodynamic boundary layer of solid-liquid interfaces. Microb Ecol; **14:** 1987.

31. Korber DR, James GA, and Costerton JW: Evaluation of fleroxacin activity against established *Pseudomonas fluorescens* biofilms. Appl Environ Microbiol 1994; **60:** 1663.

Effects of Antimicrobial Agents on an *In Vitro* Biofilm Model of Skin Wounds

Priscilla L. Phillips,[1,*] Qingping Yang,[1] Edith Sampson,[2] and Gregory Schultz[1]

[1]Institute of Wound Research, Department of Obstetrics and Gynecology and [2]Department of Otolaryngology, College of Medicine, University of Florida, Gainesville, Florida.

Background: The presence of persistent bacterial biofilms contributes to the molecular pathologies of many diseases, causes pathological inflammation, and is proposed to contribute to development of chronic wounds.
The Problem: Biofilm development is a complex process, and its composition is greatly influenced by the microflora involved, the environment, and especially its maturity and the substrate to which it attaches. The assessment of the efficacy of antimicrobial treatments on immature biofilm or biofilm established on inert nonbiological surfaces may not accurately reflect the susceptibility of bacterial biofilm found in chronic wounds. The study of biofilms in chronic wound healing would benefit from models that more closely mimic the physiology of human wounds.
Basic/Clinical Science Advances: Regardless of their location or diversity, all microbial biofilms have a typical common pattern of developmental process including attachment, microcolony formation, maturation, and dispersion. Recent studies have shown that there are significant differences in gene expression between biofilm cultured on nonbiological surfaces compared to biological surfaces (i.e., tissue).
Clinical Care Relevance: The exopolymeric substance structure and metabolic status of bacteria in mature biofilms provides substantial protection for bacteria to environmental stresses and produces extreme resistance to antibiotics, antimicrobials, antibodies, and phagocytic cells.
Conclusion: An *in vitro* porcine skin explant biofilm model was developed and used to assess efficacy of antimicrobial dressings on mature biofilm. This model suggests that cadexomer iodine, but not antibiotics, silver, povidone iodine, and polyhexamethylene biguanide, is an effective antimicrobial agent in killing/reducing existing mature *Pseudomonas aeruginosa* PAO1 biofilm.

Abbreviations and Acronyms

ddH_2O = double-distilled water

PHMB = polyhexamethylene biguanide

PPM = parts per million

Tween 80 = Polysorbate 80, a nonionic surfactant and emulsifier

*Correspondence: Institute for Wound Research, Department of Obstetrics and Gynecology, University of Florida, Gainesville, Florida 32610 (e-mail: prislp@ufl.edu).

BACKGROUND

Many species of bacteria are important pathogens causing human diseases. Even benign bacterial species (commensal or derived from the environment), when found on intact skin, often become opportunistic pathogens when they are found on skin compromised by trauma (*e.g.*, surgical, burn, and laceration) or disease (*e.g.*, diabetes, dermatitis, and ischemia). Persistent bacterial biofilm is known to contribute to molecular pathologies of many diseases (*e.g.*, cystic fibrosis, periodontitis, and chronic otitis media) and is believed to be the source of chronic infections associated with medical devices.[1] It is believed that the increased production and release of pro-inflammatory molecules and enzymes into the tissues around the biofilms, along with the release of bacterial toxins, lead to the collateral tissue damage (*e.g.*, necrosis) that promotes biofilms to enlarge into adjacent tissues.[2] Treatment and

Printed in U.S.A.
DOI: 10.1089/awc.2009.0059

prevention of infection caused by the presence of biofilm on medical devices have been based on *in vitro* or *in vivo* studies of biofilm formation and the response of biofilm to various antimicrobial agents. The more recently established link of bacterial biofilm to the development of chronic wounds[1–3] has lead to the desire to assess the efficacy of antimicrobial treatments (*e.g.*, topical agents and dressings) to eradicate bacterial biofilm and/or prevent the establishment of bacterial biofilm in wounds.

CLINICAL PROBLEM ADDRESSED

Chronic wounds recalcitrant to healing are an increasingly severe worldwide problem to both human health and healthcare costs. They include predominantly diabetic foot ulcers, pressure ulcers, and venous leg ulcers, which lead to pain, impaired mobility, reduced quality of life, frequent amputations, and morbidity. More than 1% of people in developed countries have been estimated to experience a chronic wound during their lifetime, which increases as the prevalence of lifestyle diseases such as obesity, diabetes, and cardiovascular diseases increases.[4] Chronic wound healing is a complex biochemical and cellular process related to the general phenomenon of growth and tissue regeneration. A number of causative factors, including poor perfusion, white cell dysfunction, age-impaired stress response, poor nutrition, and repetitive pressure, among others, contribute to the delay in healing of chronic wounds.[5–7] These factors have been extensively investigated through various established wound healing models. Biofilms in chronic wounds are proposed to also be a major contributor interrupting the normal process of healing.[3,8] James *et al.*[3] showed that 60% of chronic wounds and 6% of acute wounds contained biofilm structures. However, many basic questions concerning this barrier to healing remain unaddressed. For example, what is the precise role of biofilms in delaying wound healing? If the presence of bacterial biofilm is one of the major contributors to nonhealing of wounds, how can biofilm-infected wounds be effectively treated considering the inherent tolerance of bacterial biofilm to many commonly used antimicrobial agents? Ethical and/or experimental restrictions often lead to the unacceptability of investigating new substances or wound dressings in humans. Thus, applicable wound models outside of humans are required.

BASIC SCIENCE CONTEXT

Although bacterial biofilms can be formed on a variety of surface interfaces, they develop preferentially on inert surfaces and dead tissues.[9] Bacteria embedded in biofilms are physiologically different from planktonic (free floating) ones. Planktonic bacteria reversibly adhere to surfaces, such as open wounds or medical devices. In response to environmental signals, they become sessile (irreversibly attached) and secrete a protective matrix consisting of self-synthesized extracellular polymeric substance, differentiate and form microcolonies, and finally build up to form complex biofilms.[1,10] Mature biofilms are dynamic microbial populations that respond to various environmental signals through various molecular mechanisms, including quorum sensing molecules, that result in changes in gene expression patterns.[11,12] These changes in mature biofilm may result in induction of highly regulated bacterial cell death,[13] or dispersion where single motile cells are produced or biofilm fragments break off and are dispersed into the surrounding environment.[1,10] These dispersed cells seed other surfaces, re-initiating the process. The highly dense cell populations of biofilms are able to overcome the potential limitation of nutrients and oxygen as well as toxicity of metabolic products[14,15] due to the biofilm's complex three-dimensional structure[16,17] thought to be analogous to tissues of higher organisms. The bacteria within biofilms are notoriously resistant to host defenses, antibiotics, disinfectants, and biocides, which leads to difficulty in eradication of the biofilm by conventional antimicrobial treatments.[2,10]

EXPERIMENTAL MODEL OR MATERIAL

In vitro model systems are generally more rapid and simple with less expense and minimal ethical considerations, compared to *in vivo* wound models.[18] The effects of different agents or factors at various concentrations can be studied simultaneously without the added complication of the broad heterogenicity found using *in vivo* models.[18] Finally, the study of the mechanisms of action of chemical agents is complicated under *in vivo* compared to *in vitro* conditions. The established *in vitro* biofilm models used to evaluate various antimicrobial agents are based on culturing biofilm on various inert nonbiological materials (e.g., plastics and metals): examples include the modified Robbins device, Calgary biofilm device, disk reactor, CDC biofilm reactor, perfuse biofilm fermentor, and model bladder.[1] These models are typically used to culture 24–48 h immature biofilm. While exceptions such as the continuous culture chemostat model[19] have been designed to grow mature old biofilm (up to 7 days), it uses inert nonbiological substrata for biofilm attachment. Considering that biofilm development has clearly been shown to be regulated by environmental signals, including the type of substrata to which it attaches,[20–22] the data resulting from *in vitro* assessments using these models and other commonly used biofilm culturing methods (*e.g.*, agar or poloxamer solid media) can only be translated as the effects these test agents may have on immature biofilm and/or biofilm found on such nonbiological material.

Alternatively, an *ex vivo* wound healing model has one of the advantages of an *in vivo* wound healing model in that the tissue explants are viable and can be used to evaluate growth and healing to some extent. Porcine skin has been used as a model system for human wound healing and has shown the greatest similarity to human skin.[23,24] A porcine *ex vivo* tissue model for wound healing has been used for investigation of growth effects (wound closure) to evaluate different types of dressings, dermal substitutes, cell and tissue transplantation, and pharmacological agents.[18] A porcine *ex vivo* model has also been used as a bacterial infection wound healing model, but it has not been tested as a model suitable for biofilm growth and assessment. Whether or not tissue viability can be maintained remains unknown while establishing a mature bacterial biofilm. Regardless, if the specific aim of the study is to determine the effect of antimicrobial treatments on mature bacterial biofilm rather than the effect of antimicrobial treatments on tissue growth and healing, such an *ex vivo* wound healing model is not necessary. When considering that the substrate to which biofilm attaches has significant effect on biofilm growth and development and with a desire for a cost-effective, relatively rapid, and reproducible model, an *in vitro* (nonviable) porcine explant biofilm model was determined to be a suitable model system for development and was used in this study.

An *in vitro* porcine explant biofilm model was used to assess the efficacy of commercially available antimicrobial and moisture wound dressings (premoistened with sterile double-distilled water [ddH_2O]) on mature 3-day *Pseudomonas aeruginosa* PAO1 biofilm. *P. aeruginosa* is a major clinically relevant Gram-negative bacterium that forms biofilm commonly associated with the pathologies of several diseases (*i.e.*, otitis media, cystic fibrosis, chronic bacterial prostatitis, chronic wounds, etc.) as well as device-related chronic infections.[1,25] Before dressing exposure, the mature biofilm on the explants was treated for 24 h with 200 μg/mL gentamicin in tryptic soy broth to kill all planktonic bacteria (Fig. 1). This pretreatment exposure to antibiotic is essential to produce functionally defined biofilm for the assessment of test antimicrobial

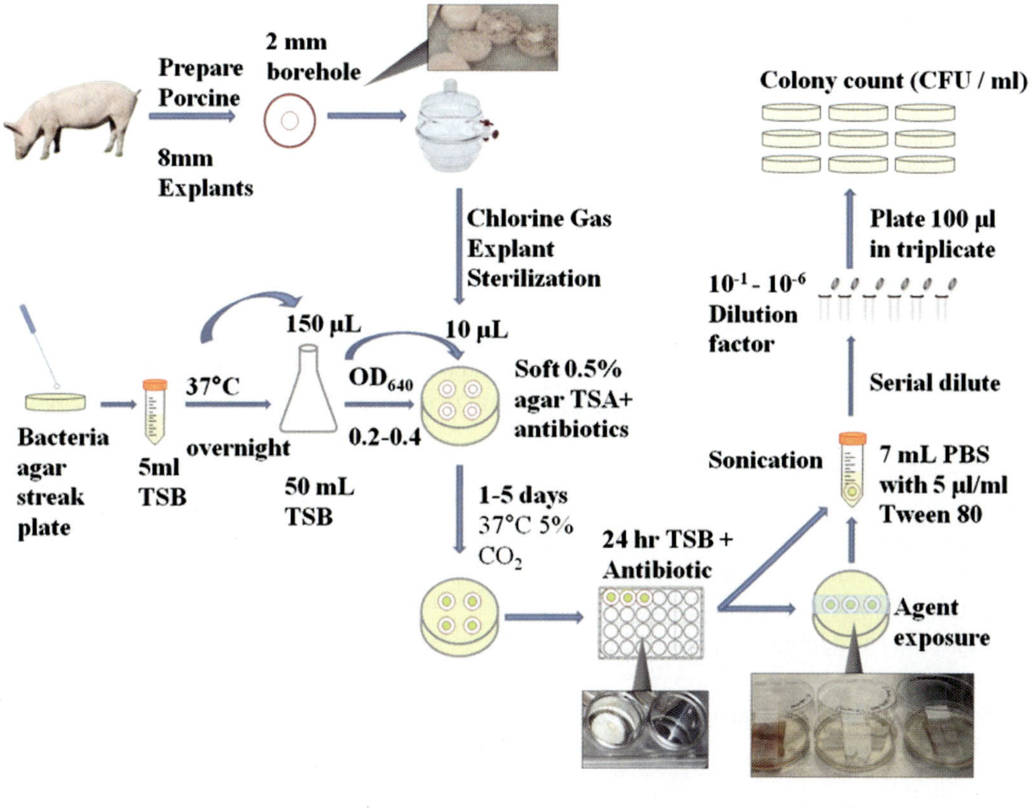

Figure 1. The overview of the key parameters of the in vitro porcine explant biofilm model. Chlorine gas–sterilized fresh 8 mm porcine skin explants with mechanically created 2 mm partial-thickness wound beds were prepared and inoculated with early logarithmic-phase bacterial culture. The explants with 1 to 5 day cultured biofilm to be used in mature biofilm studies are treated overnight in liquid media containing ≥100 minimal inhibitory concentration of appropriate antibiotic to kill remaining planktonic bacteria. Colony-forming units per mL was determined from serial dilutions and spread plating onto tryptic soy agar of sonicated explant bacterial suspension in sterile 7 mL phosphate-buffered saline with 5 μg/mL Tween-80.

agents against mature biofilm in this model. Biofilm growth curves showed that gentamicin-sensitive PAO1 formed mature biofilm with maximal antimicrobial tolerance in 3 days in this model system.

MATERIALS LIST

- Acticoat™ absorbent (Smith&Nephew, Hull, UK)—calcium alginate coated with Silcryst Nanocrystals™ antimicrobial moisture dressing designed to absorb wound exudates (of full- and partial-thickness wounds) and steadily release silver ions (70–100 parts per million [ppm] continuously available) for up to 7 days (with an antimicrobial effect minimum of 3 days)
- Acticoat™-7 (Smith&Nephew)—two layers of an absorbent inner core sandwiched between three layers of Silcryst Nanocrystals™ silver–coated polyethylene net is an antimicrobial, low adherent, moisture dressing designed for use on full- and partial-thickness wounds with steady release of silver ions (70–100 ppm continuously available) for up to 7 days
- Algisite™ M (Smith&Nephew)—calcium alginate moisture dressing designed to absorb wound exudates (of full- and partial-thickness wounds) for up to 3 days (or changed daily for heavily exuding or infected wound)
- Aquacel® Ag (ConvaTec®, Skillman, NJ)—antimicrobial hydrofiber® sodium carboxymethylcellulose moisture dressing designed to absorb wound exudates and steadily release silver ions (1 ppm continuously available) for up to 7 days
- Aquacel® hydrofiber® 177902 (ConvaTec®)—sodium carboxymethlcellulose moisture dressing design to absorb wound exudates for up to 7 days
- Curity™ AMD™—0.2% polyhexamethylene biguanide (PHMB) (Covidien, Mansfield, MA) gauze wound packing strip designed to resist bacterial colonization within the dressing and act as a prophylactic barrier to prevent penetration of external invading/contaminating bacteria
- Gauze sponge (16 ply USP Type VII) wetted with 3 mL sterile ddH_2O
- Iodoflex™—cadexomer iodine (Smith&Nephew) is an antimicrobial moisture dressing designed to absorb wound exudate, lower wound pH, and time-release iodine from cadexomer beads
- NanoDox™ hydrogel—3% doxycycline monohydrate (Nanotherapeutics, Alachua, FL) is designed to provide a moist wound environment and deliver the broad spectrum antibiotic doxycycline, which also inhibits matrix metalloproteinases
- 10% (w/v) povidone iodine (3 mL, filtered)–soaked gauze sponge (16 ply USP Type VII) slowly releases polyvinyl-pyrrolidone iodophore
- Tegaderm™ AgMesh (3M Health Care, St. Paul, MN)—antimicrobial nonwoven cotton dressing that contains silver sulfate and is designed to release ionic silver on moist or moistened wounds for up to 7 days

TAKE-HOME MESSAGE

- Biofilm development is a complex process and its composition is greatly influenced by the microflora involved, the environment, and especially its maturity and the substrate to which it attaches.
- An *in vitro* porcine skin explant biofilm model was developed and used to assess efficacy of antimicrobial dressings to more accurately reflect the susceptibility of mature bacterial biofilm found in chronic wounds.
- This model suggests that antibiotics, silver, povidone iodine, and PHMB are ineffective antimicrobial agents in killing/eliminating existing mature *P. aeruginosa* PAO1 biofilm.
- Cadexomer iodine appears to be an effective antimicrobial wound dressing against mature *P. aeruginosa* PAO1 biofilm.

DISCUSSION OF FINDINGS AND RELEVANT LITERATURE

Iodine is an essential trace element and a broad-spectrum antimicrobial agent. At physiological pH at low concentrations, the only important species are I^-, I_2, and I_3^-, where hydrated molecular iodine (I_2) has the highest antimicrobial potential.[26] Iodine is the most effective antimicrobial agent tested against mature 3-day *P. aeruginosa* PAO1 biofilm in this *in vitro* porcine explant biofilm model system, and cadexomer iodine is the most effective form. Cadexomer iodine reduces mature PAO1 biofilm ~8 logs (from ~10^8 to <100 colony-forming units/mL, the detection limit of the spread plate quantification method used) after 1 and 3 days exposure to dressing completely hydrated with sterile ddH_2O. Povidone iodine–saturated gauze only reduced mature PAO1 biofilm ~1.5–2 logs after 1-day exposure compared to no dressing or wet gauze sponge. Cadexomer iodine has been shown to accelerate wound healing, particularly chronic venous leg ulcers.[26]

Silver is a broad-spectrum antimicrobial agent and is generally recognized as safe with minimal side effects.[27] Silver-resistant bacteria have been reported since the 1950s, but are currently relatively rare.[26,27] This model showed that silver is not an effective antimicrobial agent against mature PAO1 biofilms. The results show that Acticoat™–Absorbant significantly reduces biofilm compared to its direct counterpart dressing Algisite™-M by ~3 logs (but <1 log reduction compared to wet gauze), suggesting that nanocrystalline silver is the most effective form of antimicrobial silver tested. This antimicrobial effect was not observed when comparing Aquacel-Ag/Aquacel, Acticoat™-7/Gauze, or Tegaderm-Ag/Gauze dressing pairs (where each showed no significant biofilm reduction).

Doxycycline is a broad-spectrum semisynthetic tetracycline antibiotic developed in the 1960s and has been shown to have low toxicity.[6] It is commonly used in the treatment of many bacterial infections such as Lyme disease, *Yersinia pestis* (bubonic plague), syphilis, chlamydia, rosacea, anthrax, and the like, by inhibiting bacterial protein synthesis and has been used as a prophylaxis against malaria by inhibiting development of the protozoan parasite.[6] *P. aeruginosa* is less sensitive but generally susceptible to tetracyclines such as doxycycline.[28] Doxycycline also inhibits matrix metalloproteinases that have been found to be elevated in chronic wounds, contributing to the delay in wound healing.[29] In this model, 3% doxycycline showed a ~1 log reduction of mature PAO1 biofilm compared to moisture dressings (similar to Acticoat™–Absorbant silver dressing).

PHMB is not considered cytotoxic and acts by associating with the acidic lipid components of microbial membranes to cause phase separation, disrupting microbial membranes at high concentrations.[30] This model showed that 0.2% PHMB does not significantly reduce mature PAO1 biofilm compared to moisture dressings.

Advanced moisture dressings designed to absorb wound exudates and/or maintain a moist wound environment may be changed daily, most commonly three times a week, up to the length of time prescribed by the manufacturer, depending on the level of wound drainage. Moisture dressings, particularly calcium alginate, appears to promote biofilm growth to some extent in this model compared to no dressing, suggesting that dressing changes should be performed daily rather than maintained for extended periods of time. Due to less available moisture and nutrients (the dressing absorbed nutrients and antibiotic from the media), the antimicrobial dressings used are most appropriately compared to their corresponding dressing lacking the antimicrobial rather than no dressing.

CAUTION, CRITICAL REMARKS, AND RECOMMENDATIONS

While this model suggests that cadexomer iodine is an effective antimicrobial wound dressing, the efficacy of this dressing has yet to be assessed against clinically relevant microbial species other than *P. aeruginosa* PAO1 biofilm. This model was specifically established to more closely mimic wound attachment/substrata factors that influence biofilm development. Chronic wound bed biofilms also face both cellular and humoral immune defenses. How bacterial biofilms specifically interact with these and other host-related processes or factors involved in wound healing, which may or may not influence (help or hinder) the efficacy of specific antimicrobial treatments, cannot be determined with this model system.

FUTURE DEVELOPMENTS

Further developments of this model will include improved growth conditions to more closely mimic the nutritional conditions found in wounds (*e.g.*, blood and serum), and assessment of single species and polymicrobial biofilm with additional clinically relevant bacterial species. Other topical antimicrobial treatments, like medical honey and nitrous oxide gas exposure, need to be evaluated. The effect of cadexomer bead vehicle on bacterial biofilm should also be assessed.

AUTHOR DISCLOSURE STATEMENT

No conflict of interest to disclose.

REFERENCES

1. Donlan RM and Costerton JW: Biofilms: survival mechanisms of clinically relevant microorganisms. Clin Microbiol Rev 2002; **15:** 167.
2. Edwards R and Harding KG: Bacteria and wound healing. Curr Opin Infect Dis 2004; **17:** 91.
3. James GA, Swogger E, Wolcott R, Pulcini E, Secor P, Sestrich J, Costerton JW, and Stewart PS: Biofilms in chronic wounds. Wound Repair Regen 2008; **16:** 37.
4. Kirketerp-Moller K, Jensen PO, Fazli M, Madsen KG, Pedersen J, Moser C, Tolker-Nielsen T, Hoiby N, Givskov M, and Bjarnsholt T: Distribution, organization, and ecology of bacteria in chronic wounds. J Clin Microbiol 2008; **46:** 2717.
5. Blakytny R and Jude E: The molecular biology of chronic wounds and delayed healing in diabetes. Diabet Med 2006; **23:** 594.

6. Falanga V, Brem H, Ennis WJ, Wolcott R, Gould LJ, and Ayello EA: Maintenance debridement in the treatment of difficult-to-heal chronic wounds—a compendium of clinical research and practice recommendations of an expert panel. Wounds 2008; **(20 Suppl):** 2.

7. Schultz GS, Sibbald RG, Falanga V, Ayello EA, Dowsett C, Harding K, Romanelli M, Stacey MC, Teot L, and Vanscheidt W: Wound bed preparation: a systematic approach to wound management. Wound Repair Regen 2003; **11 (Suppl 1):** S1–S28.

8. Percival SL and Bowler PG: Biofilms and their potential role in wound healing. Wounds A Compend Clin Res Pract 2004; **16:** 234.

9. Hall-Stoodley L, Costerton JW, and Stoodley P: Bacterial biofilms: from the natural environment to infectious diseases. Nat Rev Microbiol 2004; **2:** 95.

10. Costerton JW, Stewart PS, and Greenberg EP: Bacterial biofilms: a common cause of persistent infections. Science 1999; **284:** 1318.

11. Tolker-Nielsen T and Molin S: Spatial organization of microbial biofilm communities. Microb Ecol 2000; **40:** 75.

12. Reading NC and Sperandio V: Quorum sensing: the many languages of bacteria. FEMS Microbiol Lett 2006; **254:** 1.

13. Rice KC and Bayles KW: Molecular control of bacterial death and lysis. Microbiol Mol Biol Rev 2008; **72:** 85.

14. Parsek MR and Greenberg EP: Sociomicrobiology: the connections between quorum sensing and biofilms. Trends Microbiol 2005; **13:** 27.

15. Xu KD, Stewart PS, Xia F, Huang CT, and McFeters GA: Spatial physiological heterogeneity in *Pseudomonas aeruginosa* biofilm is determined by oxygen availability. Appl Environ Microbiol 1998; **64:** 4035.

16. de Beer D, Stoodley P, Roe F, and Lewandowski Z: Effects of biofilm structures on oxygen distribution and mass transport. Biotechnol Bioeng 2004; **43:** 1131.

17. Stoodley P, Debeer D, and Lewandowski Z: Liquid flow in biofilm systems. Appl Environ Microbiol 1994; **60:** 2711.

18. Gottrup F, Agren MS, and Karlsmark T: Models for use in wound healing research: a survey focusing on *in vitro* and *in vivo* adult soft tissue. Wound Repair Regen 2000; **8:** 83.

19. Keevil CW: Continuous culture models to study pathogens in biofilms. Microb Growth Biofilms B 2001; **337:** 104.

20. Ren D, Bedzyk LA, Thomas SM, Ye RW, and Wood TK: Gene expression in *Escherichia coli* biofilms. Appl Microbiol Biotechnol 2004; **64:** 515.

21. Cho KH and Caparon MG: Patterns of virulence gene expression differ between biofilm and tissue communities of *Streptococcus pyogenes*. Mol Microbiol 2005; **57:** 1545.

22. Luppens SB and ten Cate JM: Effect of biofilm model, mode of growth, and strain on *Streptococcus mutans* protein expression as determined by two-dimensional difference gel electrophoresis. J Proteome Res 2005; **4:** 232.

23. Schmook FP, Meingassner JG, and Billich A: Comparison of human skin or epidermis models with human and animal skin in *in-vitro* percutaneous absorption. Int J Pharm 2001; **215:** 51.

24. Sullivan TP, Eaglstein WH, Davis SC, and Mertz P: The pig as a model for human wound healing. Wound Repair Regen 2001; **9:** 66.

25. Bjarnsholt T, Kirketerp-Moller K, Jensen PO, Madsen KG, Phipps R, Krogfelt K, Hoiby N, and Givskov M: Why chronic wounds will not heal: a novel hypothesis. Wound Repair Regen 2008; **16:** 2.

26. Cooper RA: Iodine revisited. Int Wound J 2007; **4:** 124.

27. Brett DW: A review of moisture-control dressings in wound care. J Wound Ostomy Continence Nurs 2006; **33 (6 Suppl):** S3.

28. Shanmuganathan S, Shanumugasundaram N, Adhirajan N, Lakshmi TSR, and Babu M: Preparation and characterization of chitosan microspheres for doxycycline delivery. Carbohydr Polym 2008; **73:** 201.

29. Sapadin AN and Fleischmajer R: Tetracyclines: nonantibiotic properties and their clinical implications. J Am Acad Dermatol 2006; **54:** 258.

30. Cazzaniga A, Serralta V, Davis S, Orr R, Eaglstein W, and Mertz PM: The effect of an antimicrobial gauze dressing impregnated with 0.2-percent polyhexamethylene biguanide as a barrier to prevent *Pseudomonas aeruginosa* wound invasion. Wounds A Compend Clin Res Pract 2002; **14:** 169.

Animal Models of Biofilm-Infected Wound Healing

Anandev N. Gurjala,[1] Clark F. Schierle,[1] Robert D. Galiano,[1] Kai P. Leung,[2] and Thomas A. Mustoe[1,*]

[1]Laboratory for Wound Repair and Regenerative Medicine, Division of Plastic Surgery, Department of Surgery, Northwestern Feinberg School of Medicine, Chicago, Illinois.
[2]Microbiology Branch, Walter Reed Army Research Institute, Great Lakes, Illinois.

*Correspondence: 675 North St. Clair, Suite 19-250, Chicago, Illinois 60611 (e-mail: tmustoe@nmh.org).

Background: The presence of bacterial biofilms in chronic wounds has emerged as a major potential etiology in their pathogenesis. The ability of bacterial biofilms to induce localized inflammatory states with clinically significant effects has been confirmed in other disease states and is an attractive hypothesis for the inflammatory arrest observed in diabetic foot ulcers, pressure ulcers, and venous stasis ulcers.
The Problem: *In vitro* biofilm models will continue to provide valuable information especially in the areas of bacterial genetics and mechanisms of resistance and treatment. Due to the complex interaction between bacterial biofilms and host factors such as the local wound environment and the immune response, *in vivo* biofilm wound models will also be necessary for conducting clinically relevant studies.
Basic/Clinical Science Advances: Biofilms have been positively identified in human chronic wounds, and similar techniques have now been used to identify experimentally induced biofilm in the wounds of murine, rat, and porcine animal models. Assessment of wound-healing kinetics in the presence of biofilm has confirmed causality between biofilm and impaired wound healing using animal models.
Clinical Care Relevance: The possibility that bacterial biofilms are a common etiology in the impaired healing of all types of chronic wounds makes them an obvious therapeutic target with the potential for large clinical impact.
Conclusion: Although still in their early stages, recently developed animal models will be essential in answering fundamental questions about biofilm behavior *in vivo*, the host response to biofilm, and the effectiveness of antibiofilm treatment strategies.

BACKGROUND

Bacterial biofilms have emerged as likely playing a major causal role in the pathogenesis of chronic wounds, including pressure ulcers, diabetic foot ulcers, and venous stasis ulcers. A significant body of literature describing the pathology of bacterial biofilms in other disease systems, including endocarditis, cystic fibrosis, periodontitis, osteomyelitis, and foreign body infections, demonstrates that bacteria in biofilm phase can find harbor in many parts of the body, rendering significant and destructive effects due to the resistance of biofilm to host defenses and conventional antibiotics.[1,2] In fact the success of the pharmaceutical bias toward treating planktonic-phase bacterial infections has uncovered a new class of insidious, difficult-to-treat disease states that find their basis in biofilm biology. With the ability of planktonic bacteria to adhere to, thrive as a biofilm community on, and mediate local

Printed in U.S.A.
DOI: 10.1089/awc.2009.0094

destruction to various surfaces on the body such as damaged heart valves and poorly functioning respiratory tract, the potential role of biofilm infection on compromised skin offers an enticing parallel to such pathology.

Indeed, persistent low-grade inflammation—characteristic of biofilm–host pathophysiology as a result of an endless cycle in which host defenses are rendered unable to fully clear the biofilm infection, but are constantly stimulated by its release of virulence factors and shedding of planktonic bacteria—has been a hallmark of chronic wounds, observed long before biofilm theory had gained traction. Many studies have shown that chronic wounds characteristically have a persistent inflammatory profile, seen both clinically by excessive granulation tissue and at the molecular level by high levels of inflammatory cytokines. Suppression of growth factors, oxidative damage from the neutrophil respiratory burst, and degradative metalloproteinases effect a wound-healing milieu that is not conducive to healing, resulting in arrest of the wound in the inflammatory phase of healing.[3] Biofilm theory offers a simple and powerful explanation for both the cause and persistence of the low-grade inflammation thought to be critical to the nonprogression of chronic wounds.[4]

CLINICAL PROBLEM ADDRESSED

The possibility that biofilm plays a significant role in all types of chronic wounds makes it an obvious therapeutic target with potential for tremendous clinical impact. Due to the limited ability to study biofilm in human subjects imposed by ethical and logistic factors, development of experimental biofilm wound models is requisite. Recent *in vitro* models have yielded essential information, especially in the areas of bacterial quorum sensing,[5] mechanisms of bacterial resistance,[6] and effectiveness of microbicidal dressings.[7] The extremely large number of variables at play, including bacterial genetics and host factors—especially the effects of the immune response and wound bed components—however, makes extrapolation of these results to the clinical setting extremely difficult, and necessitates that they be verified *in vivo*. Although in their infancy, *in vivo* biofilm wound models will be essential in the study of biofilm-infected wound healing.

RELEVANT BASIC SCIENCE CONTEXT

Bill Costerton has defined biofilm as a sessile community of bacteria that are irreversibly attached to a surface or to each other, live in clusters embedded within a matrix of extracellular polymeric substance that they have produced, and exhibit an altered phenotype with respect to gene transcription. Bacterial biofilms are extremely complex in morphology and functionally heterogeneic, conferring unique properties distinct from their planktonic counterparts.[8] The biofilm phenotype has been shown to not only protect bacteria mechanically by extracellular polymeric substance but also to aid in the transfer of resistance plasmids and production of leukocyte-inactivating substances.[9] It is believed that biofilms may exhibit commensal relationships with their hosts, as in the intestinal gut, but when present in unfamiliar tissues become pathologic once a certain level of "biofilm burden" is reached.

Emergence of the biofilm hypothesis for chronic wounds as propagated by Stewart, Bjarnsholt, and others has led to a flurry of activity in trying to verify the presence or absence of biofilm in chronic wounds.[10] Using conventional planktonic culture techniques, Gjodsbol *et al.* demonstrated that chronic wounds are colonized by multiple bacterial species (including *Staphylococcus aureus*, *Pseudomonas aeruginosa*, *Proteus* species, and anaerobes) and that these bacteria persist over time within the wound.[11] More recently, James *et al.* convincingly demonstrated using light and scanning electron microscopy that bacteria in chronic wounds of all types (diabetic foot ulcers, pressure ulcers, and venous stasis ulcers) are actually present in biofilm phase and confirmed that chronic wounds are host to polybacterial biofilms using DNA sequencing and gel electrophoresis techniques.[12] Work by Frankel *et al.* expands on the polybacterial nature of chronic wounds, showing an even richer variety of as many as 20 or more commonly found flora.[17] These studies have been instrumental in establishing the correlation between nonhealing chronic wounds and the presence of bacterial biofilm.

EXPERIMENTAL MODEL—ADVANTAGES AND LIMITATIONS

Development of an *in vivo* biofilm wound-healing model is essentially a superimposition of bacterial microbiologic techniques onto existing, well-established animal models that have been used throughout the study of cutaneous wound healing, primarily in mouse, rat, rabbit, and pig. While interspecies differences between these animal models and human are of obvious concern, wound-healing mechanisms on a molecular level have proven largely conserved, with many examples of successful translation from animal model to the clinic. Each species enjoys its own advantages: mouse offering a full complement of genetic and molecular tools and rat nearly as much, along with low cost, and quick turnaround times; the rabbit ear offering robust wound-healing metrics; and pig offering the most human-like skin. Mouse and rat models, however, must contend with unhuman-like wound contraction due to a subcutaneous muscle layer, rabbit with a dearth of genetic and molecular resources, and porcine with extremely high cost, increased turnover times, and an almost complete absence of genetic and molecular tools.

Establishing clinically relevant bacterial biofilm infections in these animal models presents myriad challenges, foremost of which is distinguishing between active, acute, planktonic-phase bacterial infection and chronic biofilm-phase infection within the artificially created wound. Creating a predominantly biofilm-phase animal wound is essential to isolating the effects of biofilm on wound healing, as opposed to acute infection.[13] Moreover, diversity of bacteria and their biofilms mean that there is no one biofilm marker, making it difficult to specifically label and visualize biofilm in wounds; current methods are limited to establishing presence of biofilm on the basis of morphology and nonspecific labels that cross-react with host components.

DISCUSSION OF FINDINGS AND RELEVANT LITERATURE

Although a multitude of infected animal models exist, especially in the implant and orthopedic literature, efforts to develop models for biofilm in partial- or full-thickness open wounds have been more nascent. A review of the literature yields contributions from three principal groups to date, including the present authors.

Schaber *et al.* first demonstrated in 2007 by confocal and scanning electron microscopy that *P. aeruginosa* could form biofilm in thermally injured mice.[18] Mertz *et al.* went on to systematically establish biofilm in wounds with the goal of fulfilling the aforementioned criteria for a biofilm-phase infection.[14] Employing their previously established porcine model, partial-thickness wounds were created on the backs of pigs, inoculated with a clinical isolate of *S. aureus*, and covered with a polyurethane dressing for 48 h. Wounds were then assessed for presence of biofilm using light, scanning electron, and epifluorescence microscopy. Using this multimodal imaging, the authors were able to clearly exhibit laboratory-induced biofilm living on the surface of the partial-thickness open wounds.

To more fully distinguish between planktonic- and biofilm-phase bacteria, Mertz *et al.* also studied the effect of topical antibiotics on inoculated wounds, hypothesizing that biofilm-phase bacteria would demonstrate increased resistance. *S. aureus*–inoculated wounds were divided into a group treated with antibiotics within 15 min of inoculation (to assess microbicidal activity against planktonic bacteria) and a second group treated with antibiotics following 48 h of incubation (to assess microbicidal activity against biofilm-phase bacteria). Indeed, bacterial colony counts from the planktonic group demonstrated significant bacterial kill within 24–48 h after antibiotic treatment, while bacterial counts from the biofilm group persisted for as many as 120 h after antibiotic treatment. Using antibiotic resistance as another criterion, then, the Mertz group took an important first step in demonstrating conclusively that biofilm can be generated in an open-wound animal model.

The present authors undertook to adapt biofilm to two of our laboratory's established wound-healing models, the splinted mouse model (originally developed by Galiano in 2004) and the rabbit dermal ulcer model (developed by Mustoe in 1990). Full-thickness cutaneous punch wounds on the dorsal aspect of mice were stabilized with an adhesive silicone ring to eliminate the contribution of contraction to wound closure and then inoculated with *Staphylococcus* species. Light microscopy confirmed the presence of biofilm on the surface of the wound beds. Seven days following wound creation, healing of control wounds versus biofilm wounds was compared by analysis of epithelialization rates, whereas control wounds demonstrated near complete reepithelialization across the wound bed, biofilm-infected wounds demonstrated severely impaired re-epithelialization, with epithelial gaps over four times greater than controls.

Next we examined the impact on wound healing of our *Staphylococcus* strains' capacity to form biofilm or not. Mouse wounds were either inoculated with a nonbiofilm-forming *Staphylococcus* mutant ($TRAP^-$) or treated with RNAIII-inhibiting peptide, an antimicrobial capable of disrupting *Staphylococcal* quorum sensing and thus the ability to form biofilm. $TRAP^-$ wounds demonstrated epithelialization kinetics much closer to those of controls, and treating with RNAIII-inhibiting peptide was able to successfully restore essentially uninfected wound-healing kinetics. Infection with a TRAP$^+$ knock-in mutant once more led to *in vivo* biofilm formation and severely impaired reepithelialization. In further support of the biofilm hypothesis, using our mouse model we were therefore able to present the first direct evidence for a causal relationship between bacterial biofilms and impairment of wound healing.[15]

We have also been able to take advantage of our rabbit dermal ulcer model's robust ability to distinguish fine differences in wound healing using a variety of wound-healing parameters (unpublished results). Employing light, scanning electron, and epifluorescence microscopy, we have been able to establish our ability to reliably create bacterial biofilm in full-thickness rabbit dermal punch wounds. Histological analysis of *S. aureus*–infected biofilm wounds has not only confirmed a near total abrogation of epithelialization but also interestingly an increase in overall granulation tissue area and volume, but without any meaningful wound closure (Fig. 1). These characteristics model very closely the impaired epithelialization and overabundant granulation tissue well known to human chronic wounds. Gene expression analysis of tissue from our rabbit model shows a marked inflammatory profile, also highly consistent with human chronic wounds. We believe the biofilm rabbit dermal ulcer model to be comprehensive in its ability to capture multiple aspects of human chronic wounds, and that combined with its precise wound-healing metrics will serve as a useful tool in the study of biofilm-infected wound healing.

TAKE-HOME MESSAGE

Basic science advances

- Biofilm theory in wounds offers a powerful and parsimonious explanation for the inflammatory arrest of human chronic wounds.
- Study of biofilms in wound healing will require a dual approach involving both *in vitro* and *in vivo* experiments. Due to the large number of both bacterial and host variables at play, development of *in vivo* models will be essential for acquisition of clinically relevant results.
- Although currently few in number, animal models of biofilm-infected wound healing have been developed.
- Biofilm has been shown causally to impair wound healing in mouse and rabbit, as evidenced by delayed epithelialization and exuberant granulation tissue.

Clinical science advances

- Biofilm pathophysiology has been shown to be of significance in many other disease states, cutaneous wounds offering another setting for biofilm–host interaction.
- Studies of human wounds have established that in a majority of chronic wounds biofilm can be visualized, with molecular analyses revealing diverse polymicrobial communities.
- Debridement as a mainstay of wound therapy, having been proven as one of the few reliable methods to spur chronic wounds toward healing, makes sense in the context of biofilm theory and supports the notion of biofilm clearance as a viable strategy for restoring the wound-healing phenotype.

Relevance to clinical care

- Bacterial biofilms represent a promising new target with significant potential for addressing all types of chronic wounds, regardless of underlying etiology (venous hydrostatic pressure, ischemia-reperfusion injury, and diabetes). The ability to address a common factor contributing to the nonhealing of all chronic wounds would allow for considerable clinical impact.
- Development of animal models offers a platform for high-throughput testing of anti-biofilm therapies, speeding implementation of novel treatments to human trials.

CAUTION, CRITICAL REMARKS, AND RECOMMENDATIONS

Having biopsied biofilm from chronic wounds and demonstrated causality between biofilm and impaired healing in animal models, evidence for biofilm theory in chronic wounds is much less circumstantial than even one year ago. Despite this significant progress, we are still at the precipice of our undertaking, and many fundamental questions remain before a bedside treatment eradicating biofilm can become a reality. Regarding bacterial biofilm behavior in wounds, it is still unknown how bacteria become established in chronic wounds. What is their source? What determines the polybacterial makeup of the biofilm, and how do polyspecies interact with one another in the same wound? How does bacterial makeup of a wound change over time? Which species are the most detrimental to wound healing? And what is the mechanism of their wound-healing impairment? Moreover, much is unknown about the host response to biofilm: as all wounds are known to become colonized by bacteria, why do some wounds heal normally while others progress to become chronic? Are some hosts intrinsically compromised? What level of biofilm burden overwhelms host defenses and pushes the wound into a chronic inflammatory state? Last, what is the best strategy for clearing biofilm

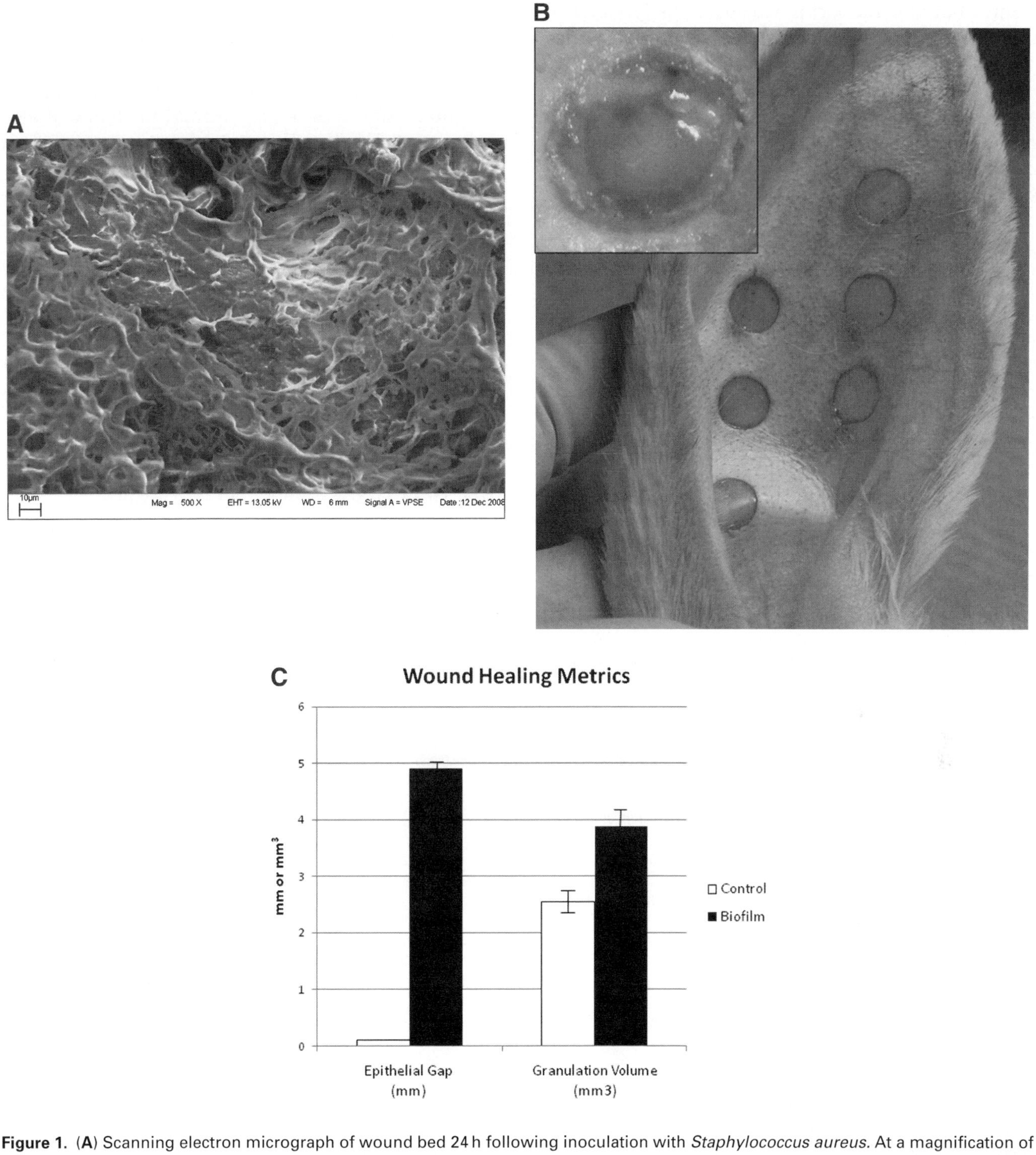

Figure 1. (**A**) Scanning electron micrograph of wound bed 24 h following inoculation with *Staphylococcus aureus.* At a magnification of 500×, a mature biofilm can be seen with its characteristic complex architecture (individual bacteria cannot be seen at this magnification). (**B**) Rabbit ear with freshly created full-thickness dermal punch wounds. Inset shows view of a single wound following a 7-day healing period with biofilm present. A filmy layer can be seen over the wound bed, which has completely failed to epithelialize. There is abundant granulation tissue heaped up at the wound perimeter, but without any ingrowth or progression toward a healed wound; (**C**) measures of wound-healing reflect a significant impairment in biofilm wounds. Whereas control wounds have fully reepithelialized resulting in a 0-mm epithelial gap, biofilm wounds have maintained a 4.9-mm epithelial gap. Granulation tissue volume also reflects the exuberant granulation tissue growth in biofilm versus control wounds.

from wounds? Bacterial variation, polybacterial biofilms, and intrinsic differences in host response present significant therapeutic challenges and make an anti-biofilm monotherapy less likely. In each of these three areas—biofilm behavior, host response, and treatment—animal models will aid us in answering many of these questions, and a systematic approach will be necessary.

FUTURE DEVELOPMENT

As stated, key experiments in the future will entail determining which bacterial species are the most potent inhibitors of wound healing along with their mechanisms of impairment, and developing polybacterial biofilm models, especially including anaerobic species. Moreover, in our effort to create increasingly relevant models, it will be essential to combine biofilm with the other pillars of chronic wound pathogenesis—ischemia, ischemia-reperfusion injury, venous stasis, diabetes, age, and other host factors.[16] The influence of biofilm-infected foreign bodies on wound healing will be another important and clinically relevant aspect to consider. Biofilm in combination with these factors may be the key to generating a true chronic wound model in animals. Animal models will also prove useful on the diagnostic front, as a variety of methods are developed to detect the presence or absence of biofilm in wounds to direct appropriate therapies.

ACKNOWLEDGMENTS

Wound-healing research in the author's laboratory was supported by internal funding. We would like to thank Kai P. Leung from the Walter Reed Army Institute of Research, Great Lakes, IL, for supplying us with bacterial strains and assistance with scanning electron microscopy.

AUTHOR DISCLOSURE STATEMENT

No competing financial interests exist for any authors of this paper.

REFERENCES

1. Hall-Stoodley L, Costerton JW, and Stoodley P: Bacterial biofilms: from the natural environment to infectious diseases. Nat Rev Microbiol 2004; **2:** 95.

2. Parsek MR and Singh PK: Bacterial biofilms: an emerging link to disease pathogenesis. Annu Rev Microbiol 2003; **57:** 677.

3. Menke NB, Ward KR, Witten TM, Bonchev DG, and Diegelmann RF: Impaired wound healing. Clin Dermatol 2007; **25:** 19.

4. Wolcott RD, Rhoads DD, and Dowd SE: Biofilms and chronic wound inflammation. J Wound Care 2008; **17:** 333.

5. Kong KF, Vuong C, and Otto M: *Staphylococcus quorum* sensing in biofilm formation and infection. Int J Med Microbiol 2006; **296:** 133.

6. Anderson GG and O'Toole GA: Innate and induced resistance mechanisms of bacterial biofilms. Curr Top Microbiol Immunol 2008; **322:** 85.

7. Sun Y, Dowd SE, Smith E, Rhoads DD, and Wolcott RD: *In vitro* multispecies Lubbock chronic wound biofilm model. Wound Repair Regen 2008; **16:** 805.

8. Stoodley P, Sauer K, Davies DG, and Costerton JW: Biofilms as complex differentiated communities. Annu Rev Microbiol 2002; **56:** 187.

9. Fux CA, Costerton JW, Stewart PS, and Stoodley P: Survival strategies of infectious biofilms. Trends Microbiol 2005; **13:** 34.

10. Bjarnsholt T, Kirketerp-Moller K, Jensen PO, Madsen KG, Phipps R, Krogfelt K, Hoiby N, and Givskov M: Why chronic wounds will not heal: a novel hypothesis. Wound Repair Regen 2008; **16:** 2.

11. Gjodsbol K, Christensen JJ, Karlsmark T, Jorgensen B, Klein BM, and Krogfelt KA: Multiple bacterial species reside in chronic wounds: a longitudinal study. Int Wound J 2006; **3:** 225.

12. James GA, Swogger E, Wolcott R, Pulcini E, Secor P, Sestrich J, Costerton JW, and Stewart PS: Biofilms in chronic wounds. Wound Repair Regen 2008; **16:** 37.

13. Edwards R and Harding KG: Bacteria and wound healing. Curr Opin Infect Dis 2004; **17:** 91.

14. Davis SC, Ricotti C, Cazzaniga A, Welsh E, Eaglstein WH, and Mertz PM: Microscopic and physiologic evidence for biofilm-associated wound colonization *in vivo*. Wound Repair Regen 2008; **16:** 23.

15. Schierle CF, De la Garza M, Mustoe TA, and Galiano RD: Staphylococcal biofilms impair wound healing by delaying reepithelialization in a murine cutaneous wound model. Wound Repair Regen; 2009: 354.

16. Mustoe TA, O'Shaughnessy K, and Kloeters O: Chronic wound pathogenesis and current treatment strategies: a unifying hypothesis. Plast Reconstr Surg 2006; **117(7 Suppl):** 35S.

17. Frankel YM, Melendez JH, Wang NY, Price LB, Zenilman JM, and Lazarus GS: Defining wound microbial flora: microbiology opening new horizons. Arch Dermatol 2009; **145:** 1193.

18. Schaber JA, Triffo WJ, Sang SJ, Oliver JW, Hastert MC, Griswold JA, Auer M, Hamood AN, Rumbaugh KP: Pseudomonas aeruginosa forms biofilms in acute infection independent of cell-to-cell signaling. Infect Immun 2007; **75:** 3715.

WHS Wound Healing Society

Biofilm-Based Wound Care

Randall D. Wolcott,[1,*] Scot Dowd,[2] John Kennedy,[3] and Curtis E. Jones[3]

[1]Southwest Regional Wound Care Center, Lubbock, Texas.
[2]Research and Testing Laboratories of the Southwest, Lubbock, Texas.
[3]Department of Pharmaceutical Sciences, South University School of Pharmacy, Savannah, Georgia.

Background: Chronic infections produced by polymicrobial biofilms are responsible for the majority of human infections. Biofilm has been demonstrated to infect most of the different tissues of the body, and the chronic infection of skin may be chronic nonhealing wounds. Robert Koch developed our current clinical culturing techniques 150 years ago to avoid dealing with polymicrobial infections.
The Problem: If all biofilm infections were considered a single disease, much like cancer encompassing all malignancies, we would find up to 16 million new biofilm infections in the United States each year. More importantly many people die from their biofilm infections such as chronic pulmonary obstructive disease (COPD), ventilator-acquired pneumonia and wounds. The problem is an outdated view of bacterial infections, their diagnosis, and treatment.
Basic/Clinical Science Advances: New diagnostic tools, such as quantitative polymerase chain reaction, along with other molecular methods, and a new treatment paradigm, biofilm-based wound care, have been demonstrated to improve clinical outcomes for the management of chronic wounds.
Clinical Care Relevance: The use of molecular methods for diagnosis and changing treatments to specifically target biofilm have made a significant impact on how wound care practitioners treat patients. More accurate diagnoses along with more effective treatment options offer better patient outcomes.
Conclusion: When multiple strategies are used simultaneously to suppress biofilm below a level that causes disease, the host is able to clear the chronic infection and heal the chronic wound.

Abbreviations and Acronyms

COPD = chronic pulmonary obstructive disease

EPS = extracellular polymeric substance

*Correspondence: Southwest Regional Wound Care Center, 2002 Oxford Ave., Lubbock, Texas 79413 (e-mail: randy@randallwolcott.com).

BACKGROUND

One hundred and fifty years ago Robert Koch developed pure cultures. From this he devised his famous postulates that associated one germ with one disease. However, other scientists of his day found it very difficult to duplicate his pure culture experiments. "No matter how ingenious their machinery, how careful the researchers, they kept ending up with beakers of mixed bacteria. The inability to get anything but mixed cultures lead many scientist to believe that bacteria had to be in mix groups to thrive."[1] However, Koch's one-germ-equals-one-disease precept won out. His method is still extremely important when managing single-species acute (planktonic) infections and remains a foundational principle in infectious disease.

With the new millennium came the realization that 65–80% of human infectious disease is caused by biofilm phenotype bacteria.[2] Multiple studies in cystic fibrosis,[3] chronic rhinosinusitis, and in wounds[4,5] have demonstrated that these biofilm infections have amazing microbial

Printed in U.S.A.
DOI: 10.1089/awc.2009.0104

diversity. It has become clear that the genetic diversity as well as the phenotypic diversity within biofilms are very potent survival strategies and reasons for the persistence of chronic infections.

If all biofilm infections were considered a single disease, much like cancer encompassing all malignancies, we would find up to 16 million new biofilm infections in the United States each year. More importantly, up to 500,000 people die from their biofilm infections such as COPD (50,000), ventilator-acquired pneumonia (67,000), and wounds (100,000). The patients who die from biofilm disease suffer just as much as those who die from cancer. Biofilm infections are extremely important to the medical community.

CLINICAL PROBLEM ADDRESSED

Biofilm infections are manifested clinically as chronic infections.[2] Chronic infections wax and wane, respond incompletely to antibiotics only to reemerge when the antibiotics are withdrawn. Counter intuitively, corticosteroids demonstrate a clinical benefit to treating chronic infections produced by biofilm possibly by reducing inflammation and inhibiting nutrition to the biofilm by decreasing exudate. Many chronic infections are never eradicated because of these treatment limitations, and the infection is "managed" until there is such degradation of the tissue that the body part has to be removed. Treating chronic infections produced by biofilm, by removal of body parts (tonsillectomy, sinus surgery, and heart valve replacement), must be replaced by an *in situ* solution.

Chronic wounds have the same clinical pattern as chronic infections. Chronic wounds respond to antimicrobial agents such as antibiotics, selective topical biocides, and heavy metals such as silver and gallium. These treatments will suppress the biofilm for a short duration, and then the biofilm reemerges. This trial-and-error method is pursued through several iterations until there is enough tissue loss that the leg is amputated. This follows the clinical pattern seen in many other chronic infections.

Because of the clinical evidence to suggest that biofilm could explain many of the wound phenomena witnessed by wound care clinicians, James *et al.* set out to determine the presence of biofilm in chronic wounds. Using tissue gram stains, denaturing gradient gel electrophoresis, and electron microscopy, it was clear that a majority of chronic wounds possess identifiable biofilm on their surface,[6] whereas the 16 acute wounds that were simultaneously studied showed little evidence of biofilm. However, it was still unclear whether biofilm was interfering with healing or was just filling a nutrient niche opened by an impaired host process maintaining the chronic wound. In an effort to understand biofilm's role in the nonhealing of chronic wounds, but more importantly to offer hope to the individual patient who suffers from a chronic wound, our group began to pursue biofilm-based wound care. To develop a treatment regimen that specifically targets wound biofilm, we had to seek answers from the experts in the field.

BASIC SCIENCE CONTEXT

Diagnosing the bacteria on a wound is incredibly important in figuring out what treatment should be used. The Koch model for years seemed like an effective way of diagnosing the right bacteria, but developments in the last couple decades have found that wound bacteria may not be planktonic. That is to say, a single-cell bacteria might not be causing the problems. Survival of the fittest tells us that if multiple bacteria start out on in the same place (a wound for example) that one bacteria species should emerge dominant and manipulate all the resources for itself to the detriment of any other bacteria. The new discovery of biofilm throws that notion on its side. Several bacteria may work together synergistically in a community, sharing resources. The result is a more advanced, more difficult to eradicate type of healing barrier to wounds. Like plaque, this biofilm comes back almost every 24 h and needs constant care. Our current techniques are not a strong-enough opponent to biofilm. New diagnostic tools, such as quantitative polymerase chain reaction, and other molecular methods are helping improve clinical outcomes for the management of chronic wounds. Proper treatment starts with the proper diagnosis of the complicated bacterial properties of the wound—specifically, a biofilm-based approach.

EXPERIMENTAL MODEL OR MATERIAL

Biofilm-based wound care was evaluated at the Southwest Regional Wound Care Center by examining 190 patients with a full-thickness wound on an extremity with critical ischemia (TCpO2 less than 20).[7] These wounds were evaluated over a 2-year period using retrospective analysis. All wounds were subjected to frequent debridement, high-dose and long-duration antibiotics, selective biocides, and multiple antibiofilm agents. The best outcomes reported in the literature for full-thickness wounds in limbs with critical limb ischemia was 65% of patients getting better during the study.[8] Our study demonstrated that 76% of these wounds in patients with critical limb ischemia healed completely, which was statistically significant difference.[7] This demonstrates that not only is biofilm present in a majority of chronic wounds, but also by specifically targeting wound biofilm, wound healing outcomes are improved. This suggests that wound biofilm is indeed an important barrier to the nonhealing of wounds.

DISCUSSION OF FINDINGS AND RELEVANT LITERATURE

Bill Costerton, possibly because of his extended experience with dental disease, was very instrumental in helping us develop the framework for biofilm-based wound care. In dentistry, when plaque causes disease such as cavities or periodontal disease, it becomes important to increase the aggressiveness of removal. Therefore, twice a day brushing is augmented with flossing, professional cleaning, ultrasonics, or other plaque removal methods. It cannot be overstated that physical removal or debridement of wound biofilm therefore becomes the most important element to biofilm-based wound care.

One of the most advanced treating agents known to dentistry, that is, toothpaste, brings up another important management strategy. Once the biofilm is debrided it must become metabolically active to reconstitute itself, and it is during this phase in its growth cycle that it becomes much more susceptible to treating agents. By targeting multiple biofilm vulnerabilities during reconstitution, biofilm can be further suppressed. It became important then to identify clinically relevant actives that could target wound biofilm postdebridement.

Phil Stewart has documented that early, young biofilm is relatively susceptible to antibiotics and biocides and that this susceptibility significantly declines as the biofilm matures.[9,10] Once mature biofilm is established there are very few strategies that can be successful in diminishing it. Also, biofilm is known for its ability to make rapid phenotypic changes, pursue horizontal gene transfer, and alter quorum-sensing mechanisms and many of its colony defenses to adapt to any single stress. Therefore, multiple concurrent strategies, which change frequently, seem to be the best approach to such a determined foe.

This has led to us developing the following principles for biofilm-based wound management. First, biofilm-based wound care must be composed of multiple concurrent dynamic strategies that are targeted at the specific wound biofilm. To accomplish this, diagnostics had to first be developed. Pure cultures were developed by Robert Koch over 150 years ago as a workaround for polymicrobial infections. It was only by growing the bacteria on the thick liquid agar that the planktonic phenotype could be selected that was more amenable to being cultivated into a pure culture. Agar cultures select against 99% of known bacteria, are incapable of quantifying the bacteria that do grow, and only yield planktonic sensitivities to antibiotics. Agar cultures often yield misleading information and the information is not produced in real-time.

Molecular cultures have many advantages. Quantitative polymerase chain reaction is able to, through utilization of bacterial-specific primers, and comparison to universal standards, rapidly identify the relative amount of the targeted bacteria in the wound. By using specific primers and probes, major pathogens can rapidly be identified within 2 h. This gives the ability to understand the bacterial bioburden and the contribution of common pathogens to the wound biofilm.[11] For many wounds this is the only test necessary to institute specific targeted therapy.

In some wounds, however, other pathogens constitute the majority of bacteria composing the wound biofilm. By adapting pyrosequencing technology,[4] a universal diagnostic tool has been developed that can identify the vast majority of microorganisms, including fungi and bacteria. Within 2 days a wound sample can be prepared, the DNA extracted, and bacterial genetic information sequenced, allowing a relatively quantitative assessment of each microbial species present in the wound biofilm with DNA certainty. This sets a new gold standard for pathogen diagnostics. Again, this type of diagnostic allows for targeted therapy of the specific wound biofilm. The problem then becomes resolving how to treat some of these bacteria that may never have been isolated in pure form according to Koch's postulates. It opens up the door for polymicrobial infections and bacterial synergistic infections.

Molecular methods have ushered in a new treatment paradigm for chronic wounds, which should extrapolate to all chronic infections. Maybe the most important benefit to wound care is that using these molecular diagnostic methods, we can understand the genetic makeup of the biofilm, and specific treatments can be instituted and then reevaluated for efficacy again by molecular methods. This is a huge step away from the blind trial-and-error management of chronic wounds toward a more scientifically based treatment regimen.

With the ability to diagnose, biofilm-based wound care has become more effective. The major strategies of biofilm-based wound care include frequent aggressive debridement, use of systemic antibiotics in high doses for long duration, use of selective biocides, and the use of combinations of antibacterial biofilm agents.

Debridement is the most important aspect of biofilm-based wound care. Aggressive, frequent debridement, removing all adherent slough can be accomplished by mechanical, biologic, enzymatic, or sharp debridement. Sharp debridement offers the advantage of being able to remove the interface of the biofilm and the host by removing 1–2 mm into viable tissue. Also, any anatomy that favors biofilm development such as surfaces that touch, tunneling, and undermining must be removed. The purpose is to produce a wound bed that is open with no overlapping surfaces or irregularities so that the wound environment favors the host and not the biofilm.[12]

By utilizing the information from molecular diagnostics, systemic antibiotics can be chosen that target the predominant bacterial species constituting the wound biofilm. Instituting antibiotics postdebridement while the wound biofilm is reconstituting itself, biofilm becomes more vulnerable to antibiotic therapy. By utilizing antibiotics in high doses for long durations, as is done in other biofilm-based diseases (endocarditis, osteomyelitis, etc.), the biofilm can be more completely suppressed. Antibiotics rarely eradicate wound biofilm and the goal is to utilize antibiotics as an adjunct to suppress wound biofilm below a level that prevents healing.

Over 25 years ago now, nonselective biocides such as Dakin's solution, acetic acid, and peroxide were studied relative to wet-to-dry dressings. Although clinicians strongly suspected bacteria's role in the nonhealing of wounds, these nonselective biocides actually decreased healing outcomes. Most wound care societies recommend against the use of harsh agents that cause damage to host proteins and cells.

Selective biocides such as ionic silver, cadexomer iodine, and low-dose methylene blue have been demonstrated to improve healing outcomes. These selective biocides have a broad antimicrobial spectrum and yet have very little host toxicity. Wound biofilm is the best explanation why harsh nonselective biocides impair healing, while selective biocides improve healing. Nonselective biocides do very little damage to the wound biofilm, which quickly reconstitutes itself, yet host cells and proteins are damaged and not so easily replaced. In the impaired host, such as the older diabetic, this tips the balance in favor of the biofilm, whereas selective biocides do not produce host damage and the damage that they do to the biofilm adds to the collective suppression of the multiple concurrent strategy approach to wound care.

The final category includes agents that can be used individually or in combination to suppress different aspects of wound biofilm. Naomi Balaban has reported that naturally occurring hamamelitannin may act as a quorum-sensing inhibitor at the same site as RNA III inhibitory peptide, which appears to directly inhibit biofilm activity in *Staphylococcus* spp.[13] Dispersin B, mutanase, and dextranase have the ability to degrade the extracellular polymeric substances composed of sugar subunits, whereas xylitol, a five-carbon alcohol sugar, may act as a false metabolite producing degraded extracellular polymeric substance.[14] Lactoferrin may block attachment of biofilm back on the surface of a freshly debrided wound.[15] Citric

TAKE-HOME MESSAGE

Basic science advances

- Biofilm phenotype bacteria have been demonstrated to have great genotypic and phenotypic diversity.
- Pure cultures, the technology used for clinical cultures, is not adequate to evaluate polymicrobial biofilm infections. Molecular methods have been developed and validated.

Clinical science advances

- Chronic wounds are now considered to be chronic infections.
- Molecular methods can aid in the proper diagnosis and treatment of wound biofilm.
- Multiple concurrent strategies, including sharp/surgical debridement, high-dose and long-duration antibiotics, selective biocides, and multiple antibiofilm agents, improve wound healing outcomes.

Relevance to clinical care

- By diagnosing the correct bacterial diversity of a wound, the more targeted treatments can be implemented.
- Using multiple concurrent strategies is the best approach to treating wound biofilm.
- Frequent, aggressive debridements disrupt the biofilm, making it more vulnerable to treatments while it is reconstituting itself.

Table 1. *Topical antibiofilm agents*

Antibiotics		Quorum-Sensing Inhibitors		Enzymes		False Metabolites		Surfactants	
Agent	Proposed Mode of Action	Agent	Proposed Mode of Action	Agent	Proposed Mode of Action	Agent	Proposed Mode of Action	Agent	Proposed Mode of Action
Doxycycline	(1) Inhibition of protein synthesis via binding to 30s ribosomal subunit; (2) Inhibition of MMPs	Furanones	Interference of Lux system due to structural similarity to AHLs	Dextranase	Inhibition of bacterial adhesion[17]	Xylitol	Impaired metabolic function and EPS production[18]	Nonionic Surfactants (Polysorbates)	Inhibition of bacterial adhesion[19]
Tetracycline	Inhibition of protein synthesis via binding to 30s ribosomal subunit	Hamamelitannin	Inhibition of RNA III synthesis and inhibition of bacterial adhesion[20]	DNAase	Cleavage of extracellular DNA in biofilm EPS. Reduction in total mass of EPS;[21] Inhibition of bacterial adhesion[22]	Gallium (III) nitrate	Interference of iron metabolism Increased keratinocyte motility[23]; Decreased MMP activity[23]	Quaternary Ammonium Compounds	Alterations of cell wall permeability, metabolism and adhesion[24]
Amionglycosides Streptomycin Kanamycin Gentamycin	Inhibition of protein synthesis via binding to 30s ribosomal subunit	RNA III inhibiting peptide	Competitive inhibitor of RAP;[25] decreases epithelial adhesion and biofilm mass[26]	Proteinase K	Inhibition of bacterial adhesion[22,27]	Erythritol Maltitol	False metabolic substrate	Farnesol	Inhibition of filamentation of candida albicans;[28] direct antimicrobial effects; synergy with other antimicrobials[29]
Triclosan	Inhibition of fatty acid synthesis and FAB pathway producing AHLs (Quorum sensing)[30]	Salicylic acid	Alterations in AHL production;[31] Alteration in bacterial adhesion;[32] Possible iron chelation	Dispersin B	Degradation of NAG in EPS mediating cellular adhesion[33]	Innate immunityLactoferrin	Iron chelator and inhibition of bacterial attachment[34–37]	Bacteriophage Therapy	Viral infection of bacterial host resulting in cell wall lysis

This table includes just a few examples of categories (groups) and agents mentioned in the literature to control biofilm. Antibiotics although 2–3 orders of magnitude less potent against biofilm phenotype remains a valuable adjunct in biofilm suppression. Quorum-sensing inhibitors promise to give us the ability to disrupt the command language of the biofilm community. Enzymes that attack the different EPS components (polysaccharides, DNA, and proteins) have the ability to degrade the protective matrix. False metabolites can attack individual bacteria by disrupting metabolic pathways or produce defective secreted products. Surfactants are a combination of surface acting agent. These agents have the ability to emulsify biofilm products and lift them from the wound. Innate immunity factors may augment host immunity for the suppression of biofilm. Bacteriophage therapy has several advantages, including the ability to adapt to the bacteria as it changes, strategies to degrade the EPS, and the ability to amplify itself in the biofilm infection.

EPS, extracellular polymeric substance.

acid zwitterion has been demonstrated to chemically degrade the polysaccharide bonds, which deteriorates the extracellular polymeric substance and impairs biofilm defenses.[16] Table 1 is a list of antibacterial biofilm agents and their proposed mechanisms of action.

CAUTION, CRITICAL REMARKS, AND RECOMMENDATIONS

This information and clinical recommendations are based on limited clinical data and no randomized control trials.

FUTURE DEVELOPMENTS

Molecular methods that have been optimized and validated for the diagnosis of clinical wound samples need to be expanded to all clinical infections. Now that molecular methods have identified new organisms, new diversity, new synergies, and other previously unknown bacterial barriers, novel treatment options for chronic infections must be developed.

ACKNOWLEDGMENT

The authors thank Lorna Wolcott Cooper, MA, for her help in the editing of this article.

AUTHOR DISCLOSURE STATEMENT

Dr. Randall Wolcott is a codeveloper and coowner of PathoGenius, which is a for-profit molecular laboratory.

Dr. Scot Dowd is a codeveloper and coowner of PathoGenius, which is a for-profit molecular laboratory.

Dr. John Kennedy is a faculty member of South University School of Pharmacy and a founder/principal of Southeastern Medical Technologies, LLC, which is an unaffiliated, for-profit development laboratory with primary focus in oncology, wound care, and surgical applications.

Dr. Curtis Jones is a faculty member of South University School of Pharmacy and a founder/principal of Southeastern Medical Technologies, LLC, which is an unaffiliated, for-profit development laboratory with primary focus in oncology, wound care, and surgical applications.

REFERENCES

1. Hager T: *The Demon Under the Microscope*. New York: Harmony Books, 2006.
2. Costerton W, Veeh R, Shirtliff M, Pasmore M, Post C, and Ehrlich G: The application of biofilm science to the study and control of chronic bacterial infections. J Clin Invest 2003; **112:** 1466.
3. Harris JK, De Groote MA, Sagel SD, Zemanick ET, Kapsner R, Penvari C, Kaess H, Deterding RR, Accurso FJ, and Pace NR: Molecular identification of bacteria in bronchoalveolar lavage fluid from children with cystic fibrosis. Proc Natl Acad Sci USA 2007; **104:** 20529.
4. Dowd SE, Sun Y, Secor PR, Rhoads DD, Wolcott BM, James GA, and Wolcott RD: Survey of bacterial diversity in chronic wounds using Pyrosequencing, DGGE, and full ribosome shotgun sequencing. BMC Microbiol 2008; **8:** 43.
5. Dowd SE, Wolcott RD, Sun Y, McKeehan T, Smith E, and Rhoads D: Polymicrobial nature of chronic diabetic foot ulcer biofilm infections determined using bacterial tag encoded FLX amplicon pyrosequencing (bTEFAP). PLoS ONE 2008; **3:** e3326.
6. James GA, Swogger E, Wolcott R, Pulcini ED, Secor P, Sestrich J, Costerton JW, and Stewart PS: Biofilms in chronic wounds. Wound Repair Regen 2008; Jan–Feb; **16:** 37.
7. Wolcott RD and Rhoads DD: A study of biofilm-based wound management in subjects with critical limb ischemia. J Wound Care 2008; **17:** 145, 154.
8. Fife CE, Buyukcakir C, Otto GH, Sheffield PJ, Warriner RA, Love TL, and Mader J: The predictive value of transcutaneous oxygen tension measurement in diabetic lower extremity ulcers treated with hyperbaric oxygen therapy: a retrospective analysis of 1,144 patients. Wound Repair Regen 2002; **10:** 198.
9. Stewart PS and Costerton JW: Antibiotic resistance of bacteria in biofilms. Lancet 2001; **358:** 135.
10. Stewart PS, Rayner J, Roe F, and Rees WM: Biofilm penetration and disinfection efficacy of alkaline hypochlorite and chlorosulfamates. J Appl Microbiol 2001; **91:** 525.
11. Wolcott RD and Dowd SE: A rapid molecular method for characterising bacterial bioburden in chronic wounds. J Wound Care 2008; **17:** 513.
12. Wolcott R and Dowd SE: Wound debridement. J Wound Care 2009.
13. Balaban N, Cirioni O, Giacometti A, Ghiselli R, Braunstein JB, Silvestri C, Mocchegiani F, Saba V, and Scalise G: Treatment of *Staphylococcus aureus* biofilm infection by the quorum-sensing inhibitor RIP. Antimicrob Agents Chemother 2007; **51:** 2226.
14. Tapiainen T, Sormunen R, Kaijalainen T, Kontiokari T, Ikaheimo I, and Uhari M: Ultrastructure of *Streptococcus pneumoniae* after exposure to xylitol. J Antimicrob Chemother 2004; **54:** 225.
15. Singh PK, Parsek MR, Greenberg EP, and Welsh MJ: A component of innate immunity prevents bacterial biofilm development. Nature 2002; **417:** 552.
16. Desrosiers M, Myntti M, and James G: Methods for removing bacterial biofilms: *in vitro* study using clinical chronic rhinosinusitis specimens. Am J Rhinol 2007; **21:** 527.
17. Dall L, Barnes WG, and Lane JW: Enzymatic modification of glycocalyx in the treatment of experimental endocarditis due to viridins streptococci. J Infect Dis 1987; **156:** 736.
18. Tapiainen T, Sormunen R, Kaijalainen T, *et al.*: Ultrastructure of *Streptococcus pneumoniae* after exposure to xylitol. J Antimicrob Chemother 2004; **54:** 225.
19. Toutain-Kidd CT, Kadivar SC, and Bramante CT: Polysorbate 80 inhibition of *Pseudomonas aeruginosa* biofilm formation and its cleavage by the secreted lipase LipA. Antimicrob Agents Chemother 2009; **53:** 136.
20. Kiran MD, Adikesavan NV, and Cirioni O: Discovery of a quorum-sensing inhibitor of drug-resistant staphylococcal infections by structure-based virtual screening. Mol Pharmacol 2008; **73:** 1578.
21. Hall-Stoodley L, Nistico L, and Sambanthamoorthy K: Characterization of biofilm matrix, degradation by DNase treatment and evidence of capsule downregulation in Streptococcus pneumoniae clinical isolates. BMC Microbiol 2008; **8:** 173.
22. Fredheim EG, Klingenberg C, and Rohde H: Biofilm formation by *Staphylococcus haemolyticus*. J Clin Microbiol 2009; **47:** 1172.

23. Goncalves J, Wasif N, and Esposito D: Gallium nitrate accelerates partial thickness wound repair and alters keratinocyte integrin expression to favor a motile phenotype. J Surg Res 2002; **103:** 134.

24. Ciancio SG: Dental products. In: *Encyclopedia of Pharmaceutical Technology*. Vol. 2, edited by Swarbrick J and Boylan JC. New York: Marcel Dekker, 2002.

25. Fux C, Stoodley P, and Hall-Stoodley L: Bacterial biofilms: a diagnostic and therapeutic challenge. Expert Rev Anti-Infect Ther 2003; **1:** 667.

26. Balaban N, Cirioni O, and Giacometti A: Treatment of *Staphylococcus aureus* biofilm infection by the quorum-sensing inhibitor RIP. Antimicrob Agents Chemother 2007; **51:** 2226.

27. Patterson JL, Girerd PH, Karjane NW, and Jefferson KK: Effect of biofilm phenotype on resistance of Gardnerella vaginalis to hydrogen peroxide and lactic acid. Am J Obstet Gynecol 2007; **197:** 170.

28. Ramage G, Saville SP, and Wickes BL: Inhibition of *Candida albicans* biofilm formation by farnesol, a quorum-sensing molecule. Appl Environ Microbiol 2002; **68:** 5459.

29. Jabra-Rizk MA, Meiller T F, and James CE: Effect of farnesol on *Staphylococcus aureus* biofilm formation and antimicrobial susceptibility. Antimicrob Agents Chemother 2006; **50:** 1463.

30. Hoang TT and Schweizer HP: Characterization of *Pseudomonas aeruginosa* Enoyl-Acyl carrier protein reductase (FabI): a target for the antimicrobial triclosan and its role in acylated homoserine lactone synthesis. J Bacteriol 1999; **181:** 5489.

31. Bandara MB, Zhu H, and Sankaridurg PR: Salicylic acid reduces the production of several potential virulence factors of *Pseudomoas aeruginosa* associated with microbial keratitis. Invest Ophthalmol Vis Sci 2006; **47:** 4453.

32. Bandara BM, Sankaridurg PR, and Willcox MDP: Non-steroidal anti inflammatory agents decrease bacterial colonisation of contact lenses and prevent adhesion to human corneal epithelial cells. Curr Eye Res 2004; **29:** 245.

33. Ramasubbu N, Thomas LM, and Ragunath C: Structural analysis of dispersin B, a biofilm-releasing glycoside hydrolase from the periodontopathogen actinobacillus actinomycetemcomitans. J Mol Biol 2005; **349:** 475.

34. Psaltis AJ, Ha KR, Beule AG, *et al.*: Confocal scanning laser microscopy evidence of biofilms in patients with chronic rhinosinusitis. Laryngoscope 2007; **117:** 1302–6.

35. Singh PK, Parsek MR, Greenberg EP, and Welsh MJ: A component of innate immunity prevents bacterial biofilm development. Nature 2002; **417:** 552.

36. Ward PP, Uribe-Luna S, and Conneely OM: Lactoferrin and host defense. Biochem Cell Biol 2002; **80:** 95.

37. Weinberg ED: Antibiotic properties and applications of lactoferrin. Curr Pharm Des 2007; **13:** 801.

Section 7

Oxygen and Angiogenesis

Section Editors: Omaida C. Velazquez and Gayle M. Gordillo

The Impact of Hyperbaric Oxygen on Cutaneous Wound Repair

Stephen R. Thom*

Department of Emergency Medicine, Institute for Environmental Medicine, University of Pennsylvania Medical Center, Philadelphia, Pennsylvania.

Background: The goal of this chapter is to outline recent advances addressing the role that hyperbaric oxygen (HBO_2) therapy plays in refractory wound healing.
The Problem: Basic science has lagged behind clinical trials and improved understanding of HBO_2 mechanisms should assist clinical decisions on its utilization.
Basic/Clinical Science Advances: The discussion will focus on how elevated production of reactive chemical species appears to be the basis for therapeutic mechanisms of HBO_2. Reactive species of oxygen and nitrogen are recognized to play major roles in cell signal transduction cascades that are a part of normal wound healing. Neovascularization is enhanced by HBO_2 because it increases production of oxidizing species. HBO_2 enhances local growth factor production to improve angiogenesis and it activates a physiological redox-active autocrine loop in circulating vasculogenic stem/progenitor cells that stimulate vasculogenesis.
Conclusion: HBO_2 causes a therapeutic oxidative stress and careful attention to its dosing limits development of adverse effects.

Abbreviations and Acronyms

DFU = diabetic foot wound
EPC = endothelial progenitor cells
HBO_2 = hyperbaric oxygen
HIF = hypoxia-inducible factor
MMP-9 = matrix metallo-proteinase-9
NADPH = nicotine adenine dinucleotide phosphate
•NO = nitric oxide
NOS = nitric oxide synthase
RNS = reactive nitrogen species
ROS = reactive oxygen species
SDF-1 = stromal cell–derived factor-1
SPCs = stem/progenitor cells
Trx-1 = thioredoxin-1
TrxR = thioredoxin reductase
Trx-S_2 = oxidized thioredoxin
Trx-SH_2 = reduced thioredoxin
VEGF = vascular endothelial growth factor

*Correspondence: Department of Emergency Medicine, Institute for Environmental Medicine, University of Pennsylvania Medical Center, 1 John Morgan Building, 3620 Hamilton Walk, Philadelphia, Pennsylvania 19104 (e-mail: sthom@mail.med.upenn.edu).

BACKGROUND

POSTNATAL NEOVASCULARIZATION occurs by two processes, angiogenesis and vasculogenesis. Angiogenesis is the well-recognized formation of vascular channels mediated by local endothelial cells and the alternative is vasculogenesis, which involves recruitment and differentiation of circulating stem/progenitor cells (SPCs) to form vessels *de novo*. The bone marrow is the major reservoir of SPCs—including vasculogenic SPCs, some of them termed as endothelial progenitor cells (EPC). Over the past several years our laboratory has been engaged in an investigation of vasculogenic SPCs. Our findings indicate that a general moniker, SPC, is more accurate than EPC because these cells will differentiate into more than just the endothelium when recruited to target sites.[1–3]

Therapeutic mechanisms of action for hyperbaric oxygen (HBO_2) are based on elevation of both the partial pressure of O_2 and hydrostatic pressure. Events relevant to cutaneous wound healing occur because tissue O_2 tension is elevated and values of approximately 220 mmHg can be expected in humans exposed to typical treatment protocols.[4] Attenuated blood flow to tissues diminishes oxygenation, of course, and whether this can be corrected is always an element of clinical management.

The traditional rationale for HBO_2 has been that it may improve the physiological state of hypoperfused, hypoxic tissues by providing metabolic substrate and possibly by limiting edema formation due to hyperoxic vasoconstriction. While provision of O_2 may offer some transient improvements, recent findings

Printed in U.S.A.
DOI: 10.1089/awc.2009.0093

demonstrate a more sophisticated basis that is focused on oxidative stress. The toxicity of O_2 is based on free radical formation, which is typically viewed as posing an adverse environmental influence. It is quite clear, however, that appropriate intracellular levels of reactive oxygen species (ROS) and reactive nitrogen species (RNS) play a vital role in regulating many biological processes.[5–8]

ROS are generated as natural by-products of metabolism and it is well accepted that agents such as superoxide, hydrogen peroxide, and hydroxyl are elevated in tissues as a consequence of exposure to HBO_2. RNS such as nitric oxide (·NO) and products generated by reactions between ROS and ·NO, or its oxidation products such as nitrite, are also elevated by HBO_2. HBO_2 can activate nitric oxide synthase enzymes and it can also increase production of RNS capable of nitrosylation reactions through involvement of enzymes such as myeloperoxidase.[3,9–13]

ROS and RNS serve as signaling molecules in transduction cascades, or pathways, for a variety of growth factors, cytokines, and hormones.[14,15] As such, reactive species can generate either "positive" or "negative" effects depending on their concentration and intracellular localization. Clearly, production of reactive species by HBO_2 mediates O_2 toxicity, which encompasses pulmonary injuries, central nervous system effects manifested by grand mal seizures, and ocular effects such as reversible myopia. Because exposure to hyperoxia in clinical HBO_2 protocols is rather brief (typically $\sim 2\,h/day$), studies show that antioxidant defenses are adequate so that biochemical stresses are reversible.[16–18]

CLINICAL PROBLEM ADDRESSED

HBO_2 is used in current practice to treat refractory diabetic wounds and delayed radiation injuries. A typical treatment protocol is daily exposures to 2.0 to 2.4 atmospheres absolute for 90 to 120 min for 20 or more days. Treatments often include the so-called air breaks, where a patient breathes just air for 5 min once or twice through the course of a treatment. This intervention has been demonstrated to enhance pulmonary O_2 tolerance.

HBO_2 is considered when standard clinical management fails to resolve wound problems. In the context of diabetic wounds, this poses a daunting potential for HBO_2 utilization once selection criteria are established. About 20% of the diabetic lower extremity ulcers have arterial flow insufficiency as their primary etiology, approximately 50% will have primary diabetic neuropathy, and about 30% will have both conditions.[19] Even after correction of large blood vessel dysfunction, only about 47% of the patients will heal promptly with standardized treatment including glycemic control, debridement of necrotic tissue, control of infection, use of moist dressings, and protection from pressure or trauma related to ambulation.[20] These are the individuals for whom HBO_2 may be considered. The effectiveness of HBO_2 as an adjuvant therapy for the treatment of diabetic lower extremity ulcerations is supported by six randomized trials and evaluations from a number of independent evidence-based reviews.[21–25] These are briefly outlined in Table 1 and further discussion of citations can be found in Kranke *et al.*[22]

The benefit of HBO_2 for radiation injuries also has been shown in randomized trials and its utilization supported by independent evidence-based reviews.[26–28] In the context of this chapter it is important to point out that the citations listed include several conditions that do not involve cutaneous wounds. These clinical findings have relevance in this chapter because mechanisms of action for HBO_2 are pertinent to many forms of radiation injury (to be discussed below). We think that it is also imperative to state that for both diabetic wounds and radiation injuries, HBO_2 is used in conjunction with standard surgical management techniques. If used only in a postoperative period, or if no surgical intervention is undertaken, HBO_2 is frequently inadequate treatment.[29,30]

RELEVANT BASIC SCIENCE

A detailed discussion on the pathophysiology of diabetic wounds and delayed radiation injuries is beyond the scope of this review, and the reader is referred to several recent publications.[31,32] Common elements shared by both disorders include depletion of epithelial and stromal cells, chronic inflammation, fibrosis, an imbalance or abnormalities in extracellular matrix components and remodeling processes, and impaired keratinocyte function. Diabetic wound healing is also impaired by deceased growth factor production, while in postradiation tissues there appears to be an imbalance between factors mediating fibrosis versus normal tissue healing.

HBO_2 reduces circulating levels of proinflammatory cytokines under stress conditions (*e.g.*, endotoxin challenge), but HBO_2 does not alter circulating levels of insulin, insulin-like growth factors, or proinflammatory cytokines in normal healthy humans.[33,34] In wounded tissues or isolated cells, HBO_2 increases synthesis of many growth

Table 1. *Summary of six randomized trials involving hyperbaric oxygen and diabetic lower extremity wounds*

Author citation	Study design	Patient number	Condition	Results	Benefit (HBO_2 vs. Std Care)
Doctor, *et al.*[44]	RCT	30 (15 HBO_2, 15 control)	Hospitalized DFU	Above ankle amputations—HBO_2: 2/15; control: 7/15, $p < 0.05$; minor amputations: NS; number + cultures decreased in HBO_2 group, $p < 0.05$	86% versus 27%
Faglia, *et al.*[45]	RCT	70 (35 HBO_2, 33 control); 2 lost to follow-up	Severe, infected, ischemic DFU	Major amputations: HBO_2: 3/35 (8.6%); control: 11/33 (33.3%), $p = 0.016$	91% versus 66%
Abidia, *et al.*[46]	RCT, double-blind, sham	18 (8 HBO_2, 8 control); 2 lost to follow-up	Ischemic DFU, 1–10 mm diameter	Healing at 12 week follow-up point: HBO_2: 5/8; control: 1/8	63% versus 13%
Kalani, *et al.*[47]	RCT	38 (17 HBO_2, 21 control)	DFU	Healing at 3 year follow-up point: HBO_2: 13/17 (76%); control: 10/21 (48%); amputations—HBO_2: 2/17 (12%); control: 7/21 (33%)	76% versus 48%
Kessler, *et al.*[48]	RCT	28 (15 HBO_2, 13 control)	Wagner 1–3 DFU	Wound size at 2 weeks—HBO_2 group 42% reduction; control 22% reduction; At 4 weeks complete healing—HBO_2: Control: 0	Wound size reduction hastened
Lin, *et al.*[49]	RCT	29 (17 HBO_2, 12 control)	Ischemic diabetic feet	With 30 HBO_2 treatments improved $TcPO_2$ (57.7 vs. 35.8 mmHg in control) and laser Doppler flow (35.6 vs. 25.8 in control)	~30% improvement in wound characteristics

HBO_2 = hyperbaric oxygen; DFU = diabetic foot wound; RCT = randomized controlled clinical trial; NS = nonsignificant; $TcPO_2$ = transcutaneous oxygen tension.

factors.[35–38] HBO_2 improves clonal cell growth of SPCs from humans and animals.[3] Functional enhancements of SPCs by HBO_2, including increased synthesis of growth factors, are related to augmentation of hypoxia-inducible factor 1 (HIF-1) and HIF-2 levels.[2] This clearly sounds paradoxical because expression and activation of HIF-α subunits are tightly regulated, and their degradation by the ubiquitin-proteasome pathway typically occurs when cells are replete with O_2. Whether hypoxic or normoxic conditions prevail, however, free radicals are required for HIF expression and there are many normoxic pathways for augmenting HIF-α expression and activity.[5]

The influence HBO_2 has on HIF isoforms may differ between SPCs and other cells, and further work is required to elucidate what are likely to be the variations based on tissue-specific responses. Higher or lower concentrations of HIF isoforms at a site also may vary based on chronology (*e.g.*, looking early or late after wounding or an ischemic insult). One recent model showing accelerated wound healing by HBO_2 reported lower HIF-1 levels at wound margins, along with reduced inflammation and fewer apoptotic cells.[35] This contrasts with higher levels of HIF-1 in response to hyperoxia that have been linked to elevated vascular endothelial growth factor (VEGF) in wounds.[38]

Bone marrow nitric oxide synthase activity is required to move SPCs out of the bone marrow.[39] SPC mobilization is compromised by diabetes, radiation, and chemotherapy, as well as other factors such as advanced age, female gender, and coronary artery disease.[40,41] By stimulating ·NO synthesis in bone marrow, HBO_2 mobilizes SPCs in normal humans and patients previously exposed to radiation,[3] and preliminary observations suggest the same is true for diabetic patients. In animal models SPCs mobilized by HBO_2 migrate to wounds and accelerate healing.[12,13]

EXPERIMENTAL APPROACHES

Work on human SPCs and HBO_2 has enumerated and characterized circulating cells using flow cytometry techniques and *ex vivo* culturing.[3] Improvements of SPC vasculogenesis by HBO_2 were shown using subcutaneous Matrigel as an avascular SPC "target" in a mouse model. These trials have shown that SPCs influence their own fate and promote vasculogenesis rather than merely responding to chemical gradients established by other cells.[2] Chimeric animals with ischemic wounds were exposed to HBO_2 where it was shown that the mobilized SPCs are recruited to peripheral sites and accelerated wound healing.[12,13] Fluid from experimental wounds was analyzed to document VEGF elevations in response to hyperoxia. Ischemic flaps in rats and *ex vivo* cell culture were used to evaluate effects of hyperoxia on wound margin HIF-1 and growth factor synthesis by specific human and animal cell types.[35–37]

DISCUSSION OF FINDINGS

Growth factors coordinate local angiogenesis and they stimulate the recruitment and differentiation of circulating SPCs to form vessels by *de novo* vasculogenesis.[1–3,12,13] VEGF and angiopoietin, as well as stromal cell–derived factor-1 (SDF-1), influence SPCs homing to wounds and SPC's differentiation to endothelial cells. Hence, there is a clear overlap between the two neovascularization processes. Growth factors are synthesized by local endothelial cells, perivascular myofibroblasts, keratinocytes, macrophages, bone marrow–derived hemangiocytes, and EPC. Moreover, by stimulating protein kinases, growth factors influence synthesis of HIFs.[1,2]

HBO_2 increases the number of circulating SPCs and improves SPC clonal cell growth in humans and animals.[2,3] At least one aspect of the mechanism for these effects is an oxidative stress response. By enhancing production of ROS in SPCs, HBO_2 accelerates vascular channel development, cell differentiation based on cell surface marker expression and cell cycle entry, and effects of HBO_2 are additive with those of lactate. SPCs exhibit augmented production of the antioxidant thioredoxin-1 (Trx1) and one of its regulatory enzymes, thioredoxin reductase.[2] Among other actions, Trx1 has been shown to promote the expression and activity of HIFs. HIF-1 and −2 can then secondarily stimulate transcription of many genes involved in neovascularization including SDF-1 and its counterpart ligand, CXCR4, as well as VEGF. Therefore, $CD34^+$ SPCs exhibit an oxidative stress response to HBO_2 that involves increases in Trx1, thioredoxin reductase, all three HIFs, phosphorylated mitogen-activated protein kinases, VEGF, and SDF-1.[1,2]

TAKE-HOME MESSAGE

Molecular mechanisms of neovascularization involve production of reactive species and HBO_2 functions through the same pathways. By limiting duration and number of HBO_2 exposures, beneficial actions of "oxidative stress" emerge without high risk of adverse effects. HBO_2 has been shown in randomized trials to improve healing of refractory wounds related to diabetes and radiation injury. This chapter has focused on wound-healing aspects of HBO_2 but augmentation of neovascularization is not the sole mechanism of HBO_2 action. For example, some antiinflammatory effects of HBO_2 were mentioned above.[33,34] Production of reactive species will also temporarily impede activated neutrophil adherence that can ameliorate some injuries.[10]

Basic science advances

- HBO_2 increases local growth factor production—this may involve •NO production in endothelium, and for SPCs, it involves oxidants such as hydrogen peroxide.
- HBO_2 activates SPC mobilization from marrow, cell cycle entry, growth factor production, and formation of vascular channels.

Clinical science advance

- Randomized trials support efficacy of HBO_2—the most obvious limitation is that trial sizes have been small.

Relevance to clinical care

- HBO_2 works and it is cost effective based on assessments from independent reviews.[23–25] Improvements in patient selection criteria should be sought to assist decisions on when/where its utilization is most effective.

SUMMARY ILLUSTRATION

Figure 1 outlines sites of action and the events associated with HBO_2 enhancement of neovascularization. Reactive species are required for normal cell transduction cascades and normal mobilization of SPCs from the bone marrow.[14,15] Reactive species are also required for maintaining bone marrow SPC's ability for self-renewal, but excessive production can cause bone marrow failure. Our findings indicate that the term "excessive" requires better definition. Oxidative stress from very different stimuli (lactate and HBO_2) exerts a trophic effect on SPCs.[1,2] HBO_2-mediated oxidative stress will also augment SPC's mobilization from the bone marrow.[3,12,13] By enhancing growth factor synthesis, HBO_2 can have complex effects on angiogenesis as well as vasculogenesis. Recent studies indicate that a redox-activated autocrine loop provides a feedback process that augments neovascularization.

CRITICAL REMARKS

With better definition of basic mechanisms, it is becoming clearer that HBO_2 can stimulate healing in refractory wounds and irradiated tissues. The biochemical lesions present due to diabetes

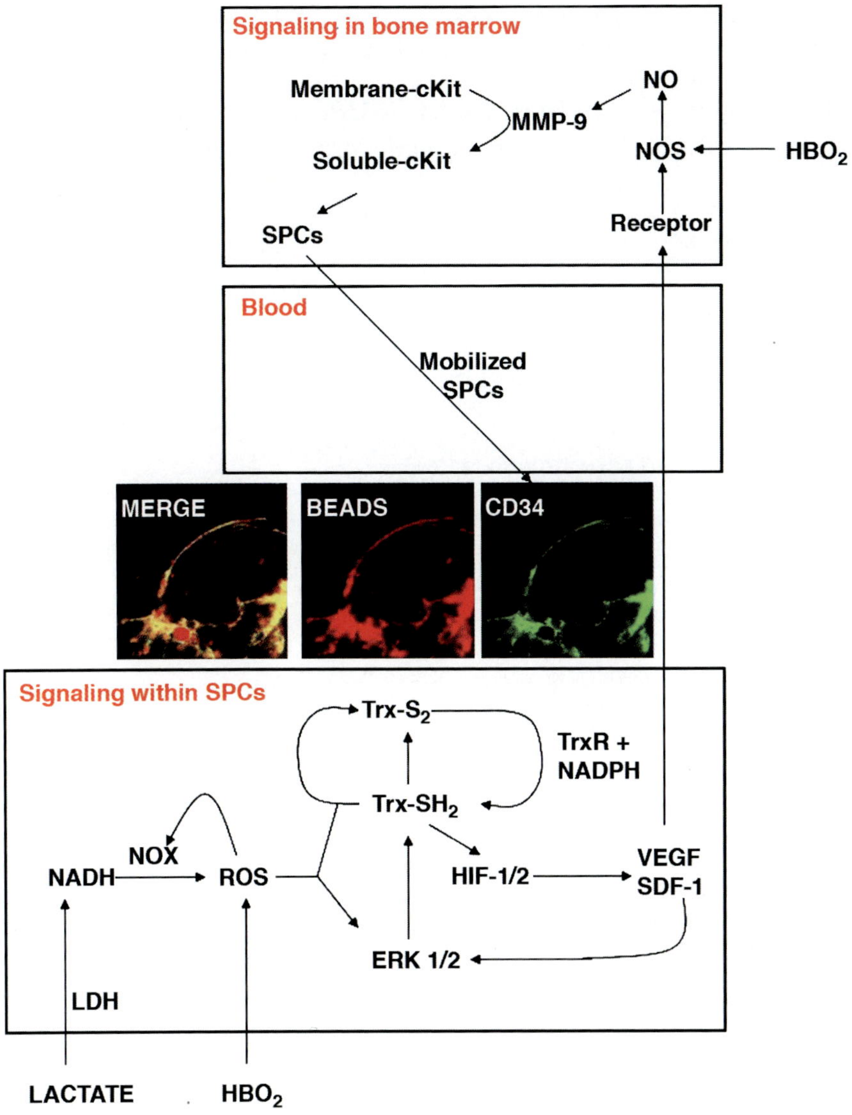

Figure 1. Schematic showing various sites where hyperbaric oxygen (HBO_2) can augment neovascularization. HBO_2 activates bone marrow endothelial nitric oxide synthase and nitric oxide (•NO) then will nitrosylate and thus activate matrix metalloproteinase-9(MMP-9). MMP-9 cleaves inactive, membrane-bound cKit ligand (*aka*—stem cell factor) and once unbound this factor will stimulate stem/progenitor cell's (SPCs) cell cycle progression and liberation into the blood stream. SPCs will home to peripheral sites and this process is enhanced by local synthesis of agents such as stromal cell–derived factor-1 (SDF-1) and vascular endothelial growth factor (VEGF). SPCs can be stimulated by lactate and also HBO_2 via synthesis of reactive oxygen species (ROS). ROS pose an oxidative stress that is in part countered by the thioredoxin (Trx) system. The Trx system includes reduced thioredoxin ($Trx-SH_2$), oxidized thioredoxin ($Trx-S_2$), thioredoxin reductase (TrxR), and reducing power for the system is supplied by nicotine adenine dinucleotide phosphate (NADPH). Trx-1 will stimulate synthesis of hypoxia-inducible factors 1 and 2 (HIF-1/2), that in turn stimulate production of SDF-1 and VEGF. A feedback process comes into play due to activation of the extracellular-regulated protein kinases 1 and 2 (Erk 1/2) that, among other things, can augment Trx synthesis. Growth factors liberated from peripheral sites appear to diffuse back to bone marrow where, with time, elevations of marrow SPCs number can be demonstrated. The color insert demonstrates findings when Matrigel is injected to provide an avascular SPC "target." Peripherally recruited SPCs (shown by staining for $CD34^+$ cells) can form vascular channels (demonstrated by intracardiac infusion of Nile red beads). *Bona fide* vasculogenesis—the formation of vascular channels by SPCs—is demonstrated by the merged confocal microscope image.

no doubt impede some therapeutic responses, and better definition of these variables should improve selection of patients who will benefit from HBO_2. Standard use of HBO_2 encompasses prophylactic administration when surgery is considered in an irradiated field and use as an adjunctive intervention combined with surgical reconstruction to resolve cutaneous and underlying tissue radiation necrosis. The incidence of clinical problems without use of HBO_2 is hotly debated, which rightly raises questions pertaining to relative value of HBO_2.[42] Reasons for the variable estimations of risk may relate to how one defines successful recovery/rehabilitation, differences in radiation dose and fractionation patterns, inconsistent definitions of the primary problem, and myriad host factors including comorbidities and nutritional status. In the two oral extraction prophylaxis trials that included a control group, the incidence of osteoradionecrosis when HBO_2 was included was 5% (2 of 37; all patients had received >6000 cGy)[26] and 3% (1 of 29; patients received 5000 to 6600 cGy)[43]; versus an incidence in the control group of 29.9% (11 of 37)[26] and 15% (1 of 7).[43] These analyses provide insight because the same selection criteria were used for both treatment groups. Without question, however, better clarification of risks and benefits to interventions without—and with—HBO_2 are needed.

FUTURE DEVELOPMENT

While there have been substantial advancements in the field of Undersea and Hyperbaric

Medicine in recent years, more work is required to establish the breadth of HBO_2 utilization in 21st century medicine. Investigations of fundamental mechanisms are still needed and on the clinical front, patient selection criteria must be clarified to truly make HBO_2 a cost-effective treatment modality.

ACKNOWLEDGMENT

This work was supported by funds provided by the Office of Naval Research and the NIH (DK080376).

AUTHOR DISCLOSURE STATEMENT

There was no nonfederal sponsorship provided to the author.

REFERENCES

1. Milovanova T, Bhopale VM, Sorokina EM, Moore JS, Hunt TK, Velazquez OC, *et al.*: Lactate stimulates vasculogenic stem cells via the thioredoxin system and engages an autocrine activation loop involving hypoxia inducible factor-1. Mol Biol Cell 2008; **28:** 6248.
2. Milovanova T, Bhopale VM, Sorokina EM, Moore JS, Hunt TK, Velazquez OC, *et al.*: Hyperbaric oxygen stimulates vasculogenic stem cell growth and differentiation *in vivo*. J Appl Physiol 2008; **106:** 711.
3. Thom S, Bhopale V, Velazquez O, Goldstein L, Thom L, and Buerk D: Stem cell mobilization by hyperbaric oxygen. Am J Physiol Heart Circ Physiol 2006; **290:** H1378.
4. Wells CH, Goodpasture JE, Harrigan DJ, and Hart GB: Tissue gas measurements during hyperbaric oxygen exposure. In: *Proceedings of the 6th International Conference on Hyperbaric Medicine*, edited by Smith, G. Aberdeen: University Press, 1977, pp. 118–124.
5. Chandel N, McClintock D, Feliciano C, Wood T, Melendez J, Rodriguez A, *et al.*: Reactive oxygen species generated at mitochondrial complex III stabilizes hypoxia-inducible factor-1 alpha during hypoxia. J Biol Chem 2000; **275:** 25130.
6. Kunsch C and Medford RM: Oxidative stress as a regulator of gene expression in the vasculature. Circ Res 1999; **85:** 753.
7. Xia C, Meng Q, Liu LZ, Rojanasakul Y, Wang XR, and Jiang BH: Reactive oxygen species regulate angiogenesis and tumor growth through vascular endothelial growth factor. Cancer Res 2007; **67:** 10823.
8. Piao YJ, Seo YH, Hong F, Kim JH, Kim YJ, Kang MH, *et al.*: Nox 2 stimulates muscle differentiation via NF-kappaB/iNOS pathway. Free Radic Biol Med 2005; **38:** 6653.
9. Thom SR, Fisher D, Zhang J, Bhopale VM, Ohnishi ST, Kotake Y, *et al.*: Stimulation of perivascular nitric oxide synthesis by oxygen. Am J Physiol Heart Circ Physiol 2003; **284:** H1230.
10. Thom S, Bhopale V, Mancini J, and Milovanova T: Actin S-nitrosylation inhibits neutrophil beta-2 integrin function. J Biol Chem 2008; **283:** 10822.
11. Thom SR, Bhopale V, Fisher D, Manevich Y, Huang PL, and Buerk DG: Stimulation of nitric oxide synthase in cerebral cortex due to elevated partial pressures of oxygen: an oxidative stress response. J Neurobiol 2002; **51:** 85.
12. Goldstein LJ, Gallagher KA, Bauer SM, Bauer RJ, Baireddy V, Liu ZJ, *et al.*: Endothelial progenitor cell release into circulation is triggered by hyperoxia-induced increases in bone marrow nitric oxide. Stem Cells 2006; **24:** 2309.
13. Gallagher KA, Goldstein LJ, Buerk DG, Nedeau A, Xaio M, Chen H, *et al.*: Diabetic impairments in NO-mediated endothelial progenitor-cell mobilization and homing are reversed by hyperoxia and SDF-1a. J Clin Investig 2007; **117:** 1249.
14. Maulik N: Redox signaling and angiogenesis. Antioxid Redox Signal 2002; **4:** 805.
15. Ushio-Fukai M and Alexander R: Reactive oxygen species as mediators of angiogenesis signaling. Mol Cell Biochem 2004; **264:** 85.
16. Narkowicz CK, Vial JH, and McCartney PW: Hyperbaric oxygen therapy increases free radical levels in the blood of humans. Free Radic Res Commun 1993; **19:** 71.
17. Dennog C, Gedik C, Wood S, and Speit G: Analysis of oxidative DNA damage and HPRT mutations in humans after hyperbaric oxygen treatment. Mutation Res 1999; **431:** 351.
18. Rothfuss A, Radermacher P, and Speit G: Involvement of heme oxygenase-1 (HO-1) in the adaptive protection of human lymphocytes after hyperbaric oxygen (HBO) treatment. Carcinogenesis 2001; **22:** 1979.
19. Reiber GE, Vileikyte L, and Boyko EJ: Causal pathways for incident lower-extremity ulcers in patients with diabetes from two settings. Diabetes Care 1999; **22:** 157.
20. Kantor J and Margolis DJ: Expected healing rates for chronic wounds. Wounds 2000; **12:** 155.
21. Hess CL, Howard MA, and Attinger CE: A review of mechanical adjuncts in wound healing: hydrotherapy, ultrasound, negative pressure therapy, hyperbaric oxygen, and electrostimulation. Ann Plast Surg 2003; **51:** 210.
22. Kranke P, Bennett M, Roeckl-Wiedmann I, and Debus S: Hyperbaric oxygen therapy for chronic wounds. Cochrane Database Syst Rev 2004: CD004123.
23. Consensus Development Conference on Diabetic Foot Wound Care. 7–8 April 1999, Boston, Massachusetts. American Diabetes Association. J Am Podiatr Med Assoc 1999; **89:** 475.
24. Hyperbaric oxygen therapy for wound healing. Tecnologica MAP Suppl 1999; 7.
25. Hailey D, Jacobs P, Perry D, Chuck A, Morrison A, and Bondreau R: *Technology Report: Adjunctive Hyperbaric Oxygen Therapy for Diabetic Foot Ulcer: An Economic Analysis.* Ottawa: Canadian Agency for Drugs and Technologies in Health, 2007, Report No. 75:1–32.
26. Marx RE, Johnson RP, and Kline SN: Prevention of osteoradionecrosis: a randomized prospective clinical trial of hyperbaric oxygen versus penicillin. JADA 1985; **111:** 49.
27. Clarke R, Tenorio C, Hussey J, Toklu A, Cone D, Hinojosa J, *et al.*: Hyperbaric oxygen treatment of chronic radiation proctitis: a randomized and controlled double blind crossover trial with long-term follow-up. Int J Radiat Oncol Biol Phys 2008; **72:** 134.
28. Bennett M, Feldmeier J, Hampson N, Smee R, and Milross C: Hyperbaric oxygen therapy for late radiation tisue injury (Cochrane review). Cochrane Libr 2005; Issue 3 CD005005.
29. Annane D, Depondt J, Aubert P, Villart M, Gehanno P, Gajdos P, *et al.*: Hyperbaric oxygen therapy for radionecrosis of the jaw: a randomized, placebo-controlled, double-blind trial from the ORN96 study group. J Clin Oncol 2004; **22:** 4893.
30. Maier A, Gaggl A, Klemen H, Santler G, Anegg U, Fell B, *et al.*: Review of severe osteoradionecrosis treated by surgery alone or surgery with postoperative hyperbaric oxygenation. Br J Oral Maxillofac Surg 2000; **38:** 173.
31. Denham J and Hauer-Jensen M: The radiotherapeutic injury—a complex "wound". Radiother Oncol 2002; **63:** 129.
32. Falanga V: Wound healing and its impairment in the diabetic foot. Lancet 2005; **366:** 1736.
33. Chen S-J, Yu C-T, Cheng Y-L, Yu S-Y, and Lo H-C: Effect of hyperbaric oxygen therapy on circulating interleukin-8, nitric oxide, and insulin-like growth factors in patients with type 2 diabetes mellitus. Clin Biochem 2006; **40:** 30.
34. Fildissis G, Venetsanou K, Myrianthefs P, Karatzas S, Zidianakis V, and Baltopoulos G: Whole blood pro-inflammatory cytokines and adhesion molecules post-lipopolysaccharides exposure in hyperbaric conditions. Eur Cytokine Netw 2004; **15:** 217.
35. Zhang Q, Chang Q, Cox R, Gong X, and Gould L: Hyperbaric oxygen attenuates apoptosis and decreases inflammation in an ischemic wound model. J Invest Dermatol 2008; **128:** 2102.

36. Kang TS, Gorti GK, Quan SY, Ho M, and Koch RJ: Effect of hyperbaric oxygen on the growth factor profile of fibroblasts. Arch Fac Plast Surg 2004; **6:** 31.

37. Lin S, Shyu KG, Lee CC, Wang BW, Chang CC, Liu YC, *et al.*: Hyperbaric oxygen selectively induces angiopoietin-2 in human umbilical vein endothelial cells. Biochem Biophys Res Commun 2002; **296:** 710.

38. Hunt T, Aslam R, Beckert S, Wagner S, Ghani Q, Hussain M, *et al.*: Aerobically derived lactate stimulates revascularization and tissue repair via redox mechanisms. Antioxid Redox Signal 2007; **9:** 1115.

39. Aicher A, Heeschen C, Mildner-Rihm C, Urbich C, Ihling C, Technau-Ihling K, *et al.*: Essential role of endothelial nitric oxide synthase for mobilization of stem and progenitor cells. Nat Med 2003; **9:** 1370.

40. Du XL, Edelstein D, Obici S, Higham N, Zou MH, and Brownlee M: Insulin resistance reduces arterial prostacyclin synthase and eNOS activities by increasing endothelial fatty acid oxidation. J Clin Investig 2006; **116:** 1071.

41. Platzbecker U, Bornhauser M, Zimmer K, Lerche L, Rutt C, Ehninger G, *et al.*: Second donation of granulocyte-colony-stimulating factor-mobilized peripheral blood progenitor cells: risk factors associated with a low yield of CD34 + cells. Transfusion 2005; **45:** 11.

42. Clayman L: Management of dental extractions in irradiated jaws: a protocol without hyperbaric oxygen therapy. J Oral Maxillofac Surg 1997; **55:** 275.

43. Vudiniabola S, Pirone C, Willaimson J, and Goss AN: Hyperbaric oxygen in the prevention of osteoradionecrosis of the jaws. Aust Dent J 1999; **44:** 243.

44. Doctor N, Pandya S, and Supe A: Hyperbaric oxygen therapy in diabetic foot. J Postgrad Med 1992; **38:** 112.

45. Faglia E, Favales F, Aldeghi A, Calia P, Quarantiello A, Oriani G, Michael M, Campagnoli P, and Morabito A: Adjunctive systemic hyperbaric oxygen therapy in treatment of severe prevalently ischemic diabetic foot ulcer. A randomized study. Diabetes Care 1996; **19:** 1338.

46. Abidia, A, Laden G, Kuhan G, Johnson BF, Wilkinson AR, Renwick PM, Masson EA, and McCollum PT: The role of hyperbaric oxygen therapy in ischemic diabetic lower extremity ulcers: a double-blind randomized-controlled trial. Eur J Vasc Endovas Surg 2003; **25:** 513.

47. Kalani M, Jörneskog G, Naderi N, Lind F, and Brismar K: Hyperbaric oxygen (HBO) therapy in treatment of diabetic foot ulcers. Long-term follow-up. J Diab Comp 2002; **16:** 153.

48. Kessler L, Bilbault P, Ortéga F, Grasso C, Passemard R, Stephan D, Pinget M, and Schneider F: Hyperbaric oxygenation accelerates the healing rate of non-ischemic chronic diabetic foot ulcers: a prospective randomized study. Diab Care 2003; **26:** 2378.

49. Lin TF, Chen SB, and Niu KC: The vascular effects of hyperbaric oxygen therapy in treatment of early diabetic foot. Undersea Hyperbaric Med 2001; **28** (Suppl) 67.

Angiogenesis in Wound Healing: The Role of Oxygen

Zhao-Jun Liu[1,2] and Omaida C. Velazquez[1,2,*]

[1]The DeWitt Daughtry Family Department of Surgery, Leonard M. Miller School of Medicine, University of Miami, Miami, Florida.
[2]Sylvester Comprehensive Cancer Center, University of Miami, Miami, Florida.

Background: Diabetic foot disease is a major health problem. Diminished peripheral blood flow and decreased local neovascularization are critical factors in these patients. The correction of impaired local angiogenesis may be a key component in developing therapeutic protocols for treating chronic wounds of the lower extremity and diabetic foot ulcers.
The Problem: Endothelial progenitor cells (EPCs) are the key cellular effectors of postnatal neovascularization and play a central role in wound healing, but their circulating and wound level numbers are decreased in diabetes, implicating an abnormality in EPC mobilization and homing mechanisms.
Basic/Clinical Science Advances: Hyperoxia, induced by hyperbaric oxygen therapy protocol, can significantly enhance the mobilization of EPC from the bone marrow into peripheral blood. However, increased circulating EPCs failed to reach to wound tissues. This is partly as a result of down-regulated stromal cell–derived factor-1α in local wound lesions with diabetes. Administration of exogenous stromal cell–derived factor-1α into wounds reversed the EPC homing impairment and, with hyperoxia, synergistically enhanced EPC mobilization, homing, neovascularization, and wound healing.
Clinical Care Relevance: Our novel approach serves a potential solution to correct the impairment and to increase homing of EPC to wound tissues. It provides a scientific basis for the establishment of combination treatment protocols that include systemic hyperoxia and wound chemokine replacement.
Conclusion: Angiogenesis plays a critical role in wound repair. Our findings bring new insights into the problem of delayed wound healing and offer novel therapeutic options in the treatment of wounds, in particular, chronic and nonhealing wounds, and would thus have tremendous benefit to both individual patients and society.

Abbreviations and Acronyms

BM = bone marrow

CXCR4 = chemokine receptor 4

ECs = endothelial cells

eNOS = endothelial nitric oxide synthase

EPC = endothelial progenitor cell

HBO = hyperbaric oxygen

PDGF = platelet-derived growth factor-BB

SDF = stromal cell–derived factor

*Correspondence: The DeWitt Daughtry Family Department of Surgery, Leonard M. Miller School of Medicine, University of Miami, 1611 NW 12th Ave., East Tower 3016, Miami, Florida 33136 (e-mail: ovelazquez@med.miami.edu).

BACKGROUND

A CHRONIC WOUND IS any interruption in the continuity of the skin and integrity of the tissue that requires a prolonged time (>8 weeks) to heal, does not heal, or recurs. The most prevalent forms of chronic wounds are leg ulcers caused by vascular insufficiency, and foot ulcerations associated with diabetic complications.[1] In diabetes, a myriad of factors, including intrinsic factors (neuropathy, vascular problems, and other complicating systemic effects due to diabetes) and extrinsic factors (wound infection, callus formation, and excessive pressure to the site), can impair wound healing. It is well known that peripheral vascular disease (macroangiopathy), along with diabetic neuropathy, plays a major role in diabetic foot ulceration. Recently, microangiopathy has also been implicated in the pathogenesis of diabetic foot ulcers.[2] Some of these vascular complications in diabetes, as well as the healing defects, have been associated with a decrease in number

ADVANCES IN WOUND CARE, VOLUME 1

Printed in U.S.A.
DOI: 10.1089/awc.2009.0092

and function of circulating endothelial progenitor cell (EPC).[3,4]

EPCs are embedded in a microenvironment (niche) of bone marrow (BM) and can be mobilized to the circulation.[5] The contribution of BM EPC to neovascularization in wounds results from a multistep process, involving sensing the ischemia signal from the remote tissue, releasing EPCs from BM niche into circulation, homing of circulating EPCs to the target tissues, the integration of the EPCs into blood vessels, and the *in situ* differentiation/maturation of EPCs into matured, functional endothelial cells (ECs). Therefore, novel methods to enhance mobilization of EPC from BM to increase amount of circulating EPCs, and to facilitate efficient recruitment of these cells to the target tissue can potentially be developed into therapeutic options to promote neovascularization and improve chronic wound healing.

CLINICAL PROBLEM ADDRESSED

Impaired wound healing is a major clinical problem in diabetic patients. Poor healing of diabetic wounds is characterized by impaired angiogenesis, yet current therapies have a limited success rate and fall short in addressing the microvascular pathology present in diabetics.[6] In diabetics, circulating and wound level numbers of EPCs are decreased, implicating an abnormality in EPC mobilization and/or homing mechanisms. We hypothesized that diabetes results in reduced mobilization of EPCs from BM into circulation, and down-regulates tissue levels of EPC-homing chemokines at wound lesions. We tested the potential synergistic effects of increasing EPC mobilization and facilitating EPC homing on promoting angiogenesis and reversing impaired wound healing.

RELEVANT BASIC SCIENCE CONTEXT

Restoring blood flow to the site of injured tissue is a prerequisite for mounting a successful repair response. Until recently, neovascularization was thought to arise solely from preexisting vessels. However, recent studies have proven that EPC can contribute to neovascularization as well.[7] Under normal conditions, the number of circulating EPCs is relatively small but is increased in response to trauma or ischemia, which mobilizes these cells from the BM (EPC mobilization). The recruitment of circulating EPCs to the sites of neovascularization (EPC homing) is subject to regulation by many factors, including chemokines and growth factors. The precise mechanisms of EPC mobilization and homing are not entirely elucidated. Many chemokines and cytokines trigger stem/progenitor cell release by endothelial nitric oxide synthase (eNOS)–dependent and NO-mediated paracrine signaling pathways to induce activation of matrix metallopeptidase-9, which releases the stem cell active cytokine, soluble Kit ligand in BM (Fig. 1). This cascade has been previously proposed to be essential for EPC mobilization.[8,9] Chemokines also play critical roles in regulating the trafficking of circulating EPCs from the bloodstream to ischemic tissues. Stromal cell–derived factor (SDF)-1α is the predominant chemokine that is upregulated in ischemic tissue and acts as a homing signal for EPCs.[10] SDF-1α mediates BM-derived EPC homing through its receptor chemokine receptor 4 (CXCR4). Inhibition of the SDF-1α-CXCR4 axis partially blocks the homing of progenitor/stem cells to the ischemic myocardium.[11] Likewise, suppression of CXCR4 by anti-CXCR4 neutralizing antibodies significantly reduced SDF-1α-induced adhesion of EPC to EC monolayers, the migration of EPC *in vitro*,[12] and the *in vivo* homing of myeloid EPC to the ischemic limb in a model of hind limb ischemia.[13]

In diabetics, however, there is functional impairment of this dynamic cascade, and the main physiologic stimulus for EPC mobilization and recruitment (*i.e.*, ischemia) fails to induce therapeutic EPC-mediated neovascularization and healing in wounds. We have recently demonstrated that both the eNOS pathway in the BM and the local concentration of SDF-1α in the cutaneous wound are impaired and significantly decreased in diabetic mice[14] (Fig. 2).

EXPERIMENTAL MODEL OR MATERIAL—ADVANTAGES AND LIMITATIONS

Recent investigations from our laboratory and collaborators have demonstrated that EPC mobilization into circulation is triggered by hyperbaric oxygen (HBO) through increasing BM NO levels with resulting enhancement in ischemic limb perfusion and wound healing.[15–17] Using ischemic and diabetic murine models, we have determined that hyperoxia, induced by a clinically relevant HBO protocol, increases NO levels within the hindlimb femur BM, accelerates the spontaneous revascularization of surgically induced hind limb ischemia, and increases the number of BM-derived EPCs in circulation and within cutaneous hind limb ischemic incisional wounds and diabetic excisional wounds.[14] These effects appear to be specific to the release of BM-derived EPC, but not lymphocytes, and responsive to the cytokine milieu of the wound.

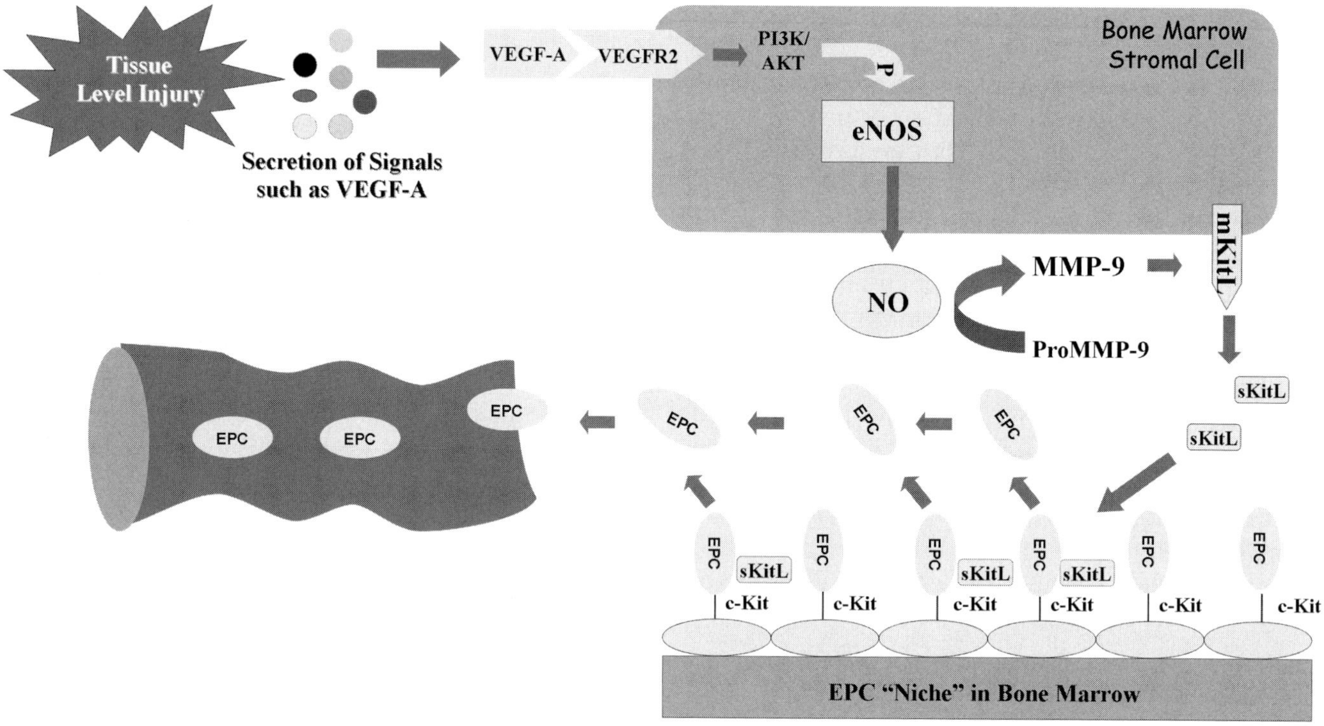

Figure 1. Endothelial nitric oxide synthase (eNOS)-NO-matrix metallopeptidase (MMP)-9-KitL cascade–mediated mobilization of bone marrow (BM) endothelial progenitor cell (EPC). Injured tissue releases signal molecules, such as vascular endothelial growth factor (VEGF)-A, that can be sensed by BM stromal cells. VEGF-A and other mobilizing stimuli might signal through their cognate receptors to activate the eNOS within the BM stromal cells. eNOS induces production of NO that stimulates and/or maintains MMP-9 activity resulting in cleavage of soluble kit ligand (sKitL) from membrane-bound kit ligand (mKitL) to mobilize c-Kit^{+} EPCs from BM niche into the circulation.

In the ischemic and diabetic murine models that were used, therapeutic wound-healing effects of increased BM-derived EPC mobilization into circulation and recruitment into wounds were observed in association with enhancement of neovascularization of the wounds and improved spontaneous recovery of hind limb perfusion. HBO is noninvasive and appears to be a potent and safe clinically applicable therapeutic choice. Systemic hyperoxia induced by HBO is a treatment approved by the United States Food and Drug Administration as a safe, adjunctive therapy to stimulate wound healing in diabetic patients.

However, the observed clinical effects of HBO treatment on wound healing are variable. We have found that mobilized EPCs fail to reach the injured tissue, implicating the EPC homing mechanism is impaired in the diabetic wound. Further study demonstrated that the local concentration of SDF-1α in diabetic wound is significantly decreased and that epithelial cells and myofibroblasts appeared to be responsible for the down-regulation of SDF-1α in diabetic wounds[14] We have observed that the exogenous administration of SDF-1α to diabetic wounds increases the wound-level EPC recruitment (homing). Since SDF-1α is a well-studied chemokine and local application of an optimal amount and form of this soluble factor is technically easy and carries a theoretical low-risk, its advantage can be obviously appreciated. However, the potential clinical efficacy and/or side effects of local application of SDF-1α remains unknown and need to be investigated by formal clinical trials.

DISCUSSION OF FINDINGS AND RELEVANT LITERATURE

It is increasingly evident that wound healing occurs because of events in two compartments. Within the BM, various signaling pathways lead to mobilization of BM-derived EPCs and other progenitor/stem cells involved in the healing cascade. Within the wound, neovascularization occurs because of local factors that stimulate adjacent cells (angiogenesis) and because of recruited circulating EPCs that contribute to existing and new vascular channels (vasculogenesis). Vascular maintenance, repair, and wound-healing cellular

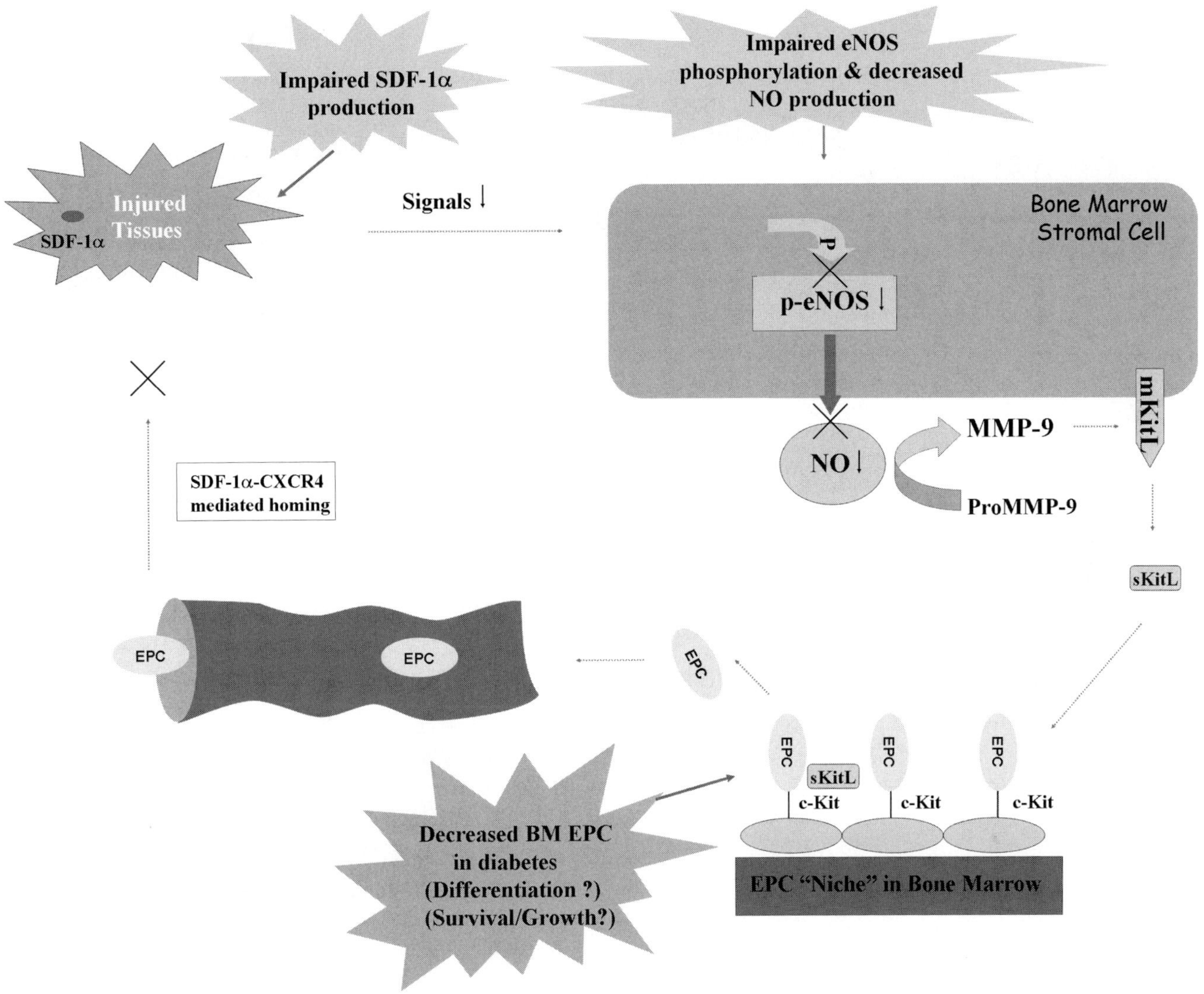

Figure 2. Impaired eNOS-NO cascade in the BM and down-regulated stromal cell–derived factor (SDF)-1α production at the injured tissues in diabetic mouse. Impaired eNOS phosphorylation results in decreased production of NO in BM, which affects downstream pathway leading to EPC mobilization. In the injured tissues, production of SDF-1α is down-regulated, resulting in decreased recruitment/homing of circulating EPCs. EPC number in diabetic BM is diminished due to unknown mechanisms. These factors contribute to the impaired neovascularization and delayed or nonhealing of wounds in diabetes.

and molecular cascades at the level of both the BM and within the peripheral wound are compromised by diabetes as a result of BM-derived EPC impairments.[3,4]

The number and function of EPCs is down-regulated in diabetes mellitus. Reduced levels and impaired function of EPCs have been described in both type 1 and type 2 diabetic patients.[18,19] EPC recruitment for reendothelialization after vascular injury is also impaired in diabetes.[20] These alterations are likely to be involved in the pathogenesis of vascular disease in diabetes. The mechanisms responsible for decreased circulating and wound level EPCs in diabetes have not been previously determined. We have demonstrated that phosphorylation of eNOS in BM is impaired and that SDF-1α expression by epithelial cells and myofibroblasts in the granulation tissue of cutaneous wounds is decreased in our diabetic murine model. Impaired phosphorylation of eNOS in the BM and decreased wound expression of SDF-1α have a direct impact on EPC mobilization from BM into circulation and EPC homing to wounds, respectively, and can be therapeutically reversed to enhance EPCs available in peripheral wound tissue and improve wound healing. By utilizing HBO to induce tissue-level hyperoxia, we have shown that multiple BM NOS isoforms may be activated,

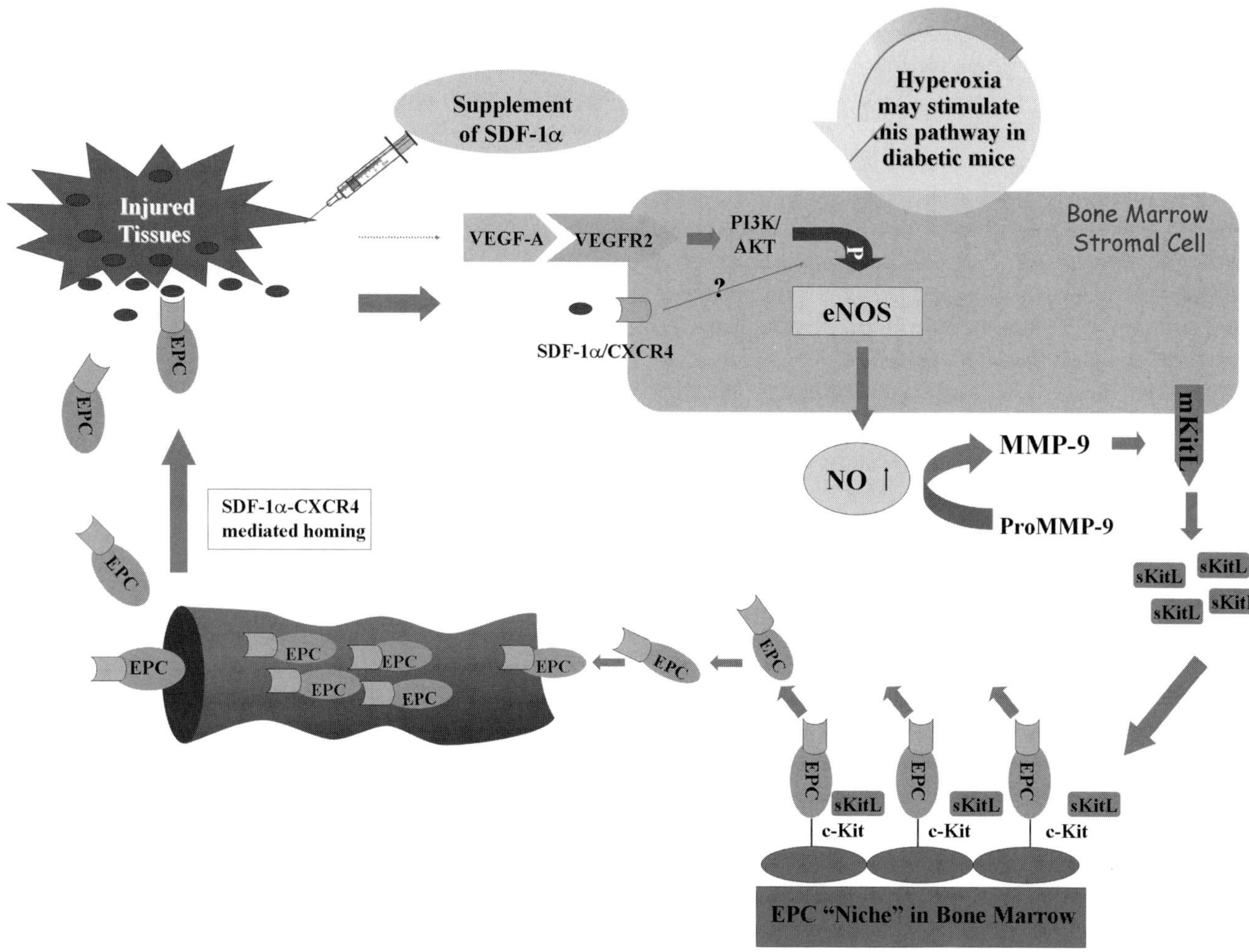

Figure 3. Synergistic effects of hyperoxia and exogenous SDF-1α on regulating EPC mobilization and homing. Hyperoxia increases NO levels, likely through stimulating NOS/NO pathway, in BM to promote EPC mobilization. EPC expresses chemokine receptor 4 (CXCR4) on the cell surface. Local supplement of SDF-1α enhances EPC homing to the wound tissues via the interaction mediated by SDF-1α–CXCR4. SDF-1α might also function as a signal to stimulate BM EPC mobilization.

leading to increased NO levels in the BM and hence enhanced mobilization of EPCs into the circulation, thus partially reversing the defect in eNOS activation and EPC release caused by diabetes. In addition, by increasing wound levels of SDF-1α, we have shown that not only is the diabetic EPC homing impairment reversed, but also a synergistic increase in EPC mobilization, homing, and wound healing may be achieved when used in conjunction with HBO (Fig. 3). The novel targets identified by our study (HBO-mediated EPC release by NOS activation and SDF-1α–mediated EPC homing), along with knowledge about the timing for the initiation of these therapies and the effect of lactate in recruitment of EPCs,[21] carry important clinical relevance for advancement in the field of diabetic wound healing. These data provide the foundation for significant improvements on existing clinical protocols for this significant unsolved medical problem.

The process of EPC homing to sites of ischemia includes detachment from the BM niche, rolling into blood vessels and traveling within the circulation, adhesion to the EC monolayers, and incorporation into neovessels. Recent studies support the idea that EPC and progenitor cells utilize adhesion molecules for homing to sites of neovascularization similar to the adhesion molecules engaged by leukocytes for recruitment to sites of inflammation.[22] Chemokines play critical roles in the regulation of this trafficking of circulating EPCs from the bloodstream to ischemic tissues. SDF-1α is the predominant chemokine that is upregulated in ischemic tissue and acts as a homing signal for EPCs. While the role of SDF-1α in EPC homing to ischemic tissue is known, the effect of SDF-1α expression at the tissue level in diabetic wounds had not been previously studied. We have demonstrated that the local concentration of SDF-1α in diabetic wound is significantly decreased. The exogenous administration of SDF-1α to wounds of diabetic mice increases the wound-level EPC recruitment and healing when given within first 48 h after wounding, suggesting that in a clinical setting the chronic would require debridement first and then chemokine application. Since debridement is already part of standard clinical practices, applicability of this new concept would seem highly feasible. More importantly, in combination with HBO therapy that brings increased amount of circulating EPCs, raising SDF-1α levels by local injection of recombinant SDF-1α protein significantly enhances EPC recruitment to wound tissues and improves wound healing in a diabetic animal model.

CAUTION, CRITICAL REMARKS, AND RECOMMENDATIONS

Oxygen plays a key role in wound healing. Low oxygen tension (hypoxia) around the wound is one of several critical factors that mutually enhance the progression of a chronic ulcer, while a plentiful supply of oxygen is essential for a variety of the healing processes. Oxygen tension is positively correlated with collagen production,[23] bacterial killing,[24] epithelialization,[25] and angiogenesis.[26]

Hyperoxia appears to involve a signal cascade similar to the sequence of events detailing hypoxia-induced EPC release. The reasons for this seemingly paradoxical response to hyperoxia are unclear, but based on our findings and the reported effects of hypoxia, both hypoxia and hyperoxia result in NOS activation and a subsequent increase in BM NO level. One possible explanation for this response involves the possibility that an oxygen tension sensor, triggered by any perturbation in the oxygen levels, results in NO production and EPC release. Another potential explanation is that both high and low local oxygen concentrations act via distinct mechanisms that ultimately converge on NOS activation. Whatever the reason, it is clear that with hypoxia, systemic effects of vascular endothelial growth factor A via vascular endothelial growth factor R2 mediate NOS activation, whereas with hyperoxia, NO levels rise within minutes and the effects are quickly reversible upon withdrawal of the stimulus, suggesting a direct activation of NOS by a change in oxygen tension. Further studies are needed to more specifically examine this question.

FUTURE DEVELOPMENT

The identification of hyperoxia as an efficient tool in the mobilization of BM-derived EPC is of great significance. Understanding the limitations of HBO in modulating only the EPC mobilization step but not the homing of the increased circulating EPC to the target tissue provides useful guidance for the development of new clinical protocols to treat diabetic wounds. In addition to SDF-1α, other strategies for modifying the wound environment, such as platelet-derived growth factor-BB (PDGF-BB),[27] fibroblasts delivered in an absorbable mesh,[28] or in type 1 collagen,[29] which, at least partially, function directly or indirectly through accelerating recruitment of EPC, are under investigation. A better understanding of the molecular and cellular etiologies of nonhealing, diabetic wounds in combination with development of efficient approaches for correcting EPC deficits and functional impairments will eventually result in the development of clinically efficient and feasible therapies that prevent wound progression, eliminate amputations, and promote rapid healing in patients with diabetes.

ACKNOWLEDGMENT

This study is funded by NIH award GM081570-01A1.

TAKE-HOME MESSAGE

- EPCs are the newest cellular target to influence postnatal angiogenesis.
- The number of circulating EPCs in diabetic mice is decreased, presumably due to the impairment of eNOS/NO pathway in the BM.
- Systemic hyperoxia induced by HBO protocols is able to enhance BM EPC mobilization into circulation with minimal if any side effects.
- Effect of HBO on EPC mobilization is likely mediated by up-regulating eNOS/NO pathway.
- However, increased circulating EPC induced by HBO treatment fail to be recruited to wound lesion. An additional homing signal(s) is required.
- SDF-1α is a potent cell homing factor. However, tissue levels of SDF-1α are down-regulated in diabetic wounds.
- Local supplement of SDF-1α enhances mobilized EPCs homing to the diabetic wound tissue and promotes neovascularization.
- A combination of systemic HBO treatment and local supplement of SDF-1α synergistically promotes EPC mobilization and homing.
- Therefore, combined therapeutic approaches to target individual impairments and to correct diabetes-related EPC deficits will likely synergize and lead to a more successful treatment outcome for diabetic wounds.

AUTHOR DISCLOSURE STATEMENT

The authors disclose that there are no commercial associations related with this work and no commercial conflict of interest in connection with this manuscript. No competing financial interests exist. A provisionary patent on HBO and SDF-1α treatments for wound healing has been filed.

REFERENCES

1. Wu SC, Driver VR, Wrobel JS, and Armstrong DG: Foot ulcers in the diabetic patient, prevention and treatment. Vasc Health Risk Manag 2007; **3:** 65.
2. La Fontaine J, Harkless LB, Davis CE, Allen MA, and Shireman PK: Current concepts in diabetic microvascular dysfunction. J Am Podiatr Med Assoc 2006; **96:** 245.
3. Fadini GP, Miorin M, Facco M, *et al.*: Circulating endothelial progenitor cells are reduced in peripheral vascular complications of type 2 diabetes mellitus. J Am Coll Cardiol 2005; **45:** 1449.
4. Loomans CJ, De Koning EJ, Staal FJ, Rabelink TJ, and Zonneveld AJ: Endothelial progenitor cell dysfunction in type 1 diabetes: another consequence of oxidative stress? Antioxid Redox Signal 2005; **7:** 1468.
5. Kaplan RN, Psaila B, and Lyden D: Niche-to-niche migration of bone-marrow-derived cells. Trends Mol Med 2007; **13:** 72.
6. Ngo BT, Hayes KD, DiMiao DJ, Srinivasan SK, Huerter CJ, and Rendell MS: Manifestations of cutaneous diabetic microangiopathy. Am J Clin Dermatol 2005; **6:** 225.
7. Rafii S, Meeus S, Dias S, *et al.*: Contribution of marrow-derived progenitors to vascular and cardiac regeneration. Semin Cell Dev Biol 2002; **13:** 61.
8. Heissig B, Hattori K, Dias S, *et al.*: Recruitment of stem and progenitor cells from the bone marrow niche requires MMP-9 mediated release of kit-ligand. Cell 2002; **109:** 625.
9. Aicher A, Heeschen C, Mildner-Rihm C, *et al.*: Essential role of endothelial nitric oxide synthase for mobilization of stem and progenitor cells. Nat Med 2003; **9:** 1370.
10. Lapidot T: Mechanism of human stem cell migration and repopulation of NOD/SCID and B2mnull NOD/SCID mice. The role of SDF-1/CXCR4 interactions. Ann NY Acad Sci 2001; **938:** 83.
11. Abbott JD, Huang Y, Liu D, Hickey R, Krause DS, and Giordano FJ: Stromal cell-derived factor-1alpha plays a critical role in stem cell recruitment to the heart after myocardial infarction but is not sufficient to induce homing in the absence of injury. Circulation 2004; **110:** 3300.
12. Ceradini DJ, Kulkarni AR, Callaghan MJ, *et al.*: Progenitor cell trafficking is regulated by hypoxic gradients through HIF-1 induction of SDF-1. Nat Med 2004; **10:** 858.
13. Walter DH, Haendeler J, Reinhold J, *et al.*: Impaired CXCR4 signaling contributes to the reduced neovascularization capacity of endothelial progenitor cells from patients with coronary artery disease. Circ Res 2005; **97:** 1142.
14. Gallagher KA, Liu ZJ, Xiao M, *et al.*: Diabetic impairments in NO-mediated endothelial progenitor cell mobilization and homing are reversed by hyperoxia and SDF-1 alpha. J Clin Invest 2007; **117:** 1249.
15. Goldstein LJ, Gallagher KA, Bauer SM, *et al.*: Endothelial progenitor cell release into circulation is triggered by hyperoxia-induced increases in bone marrow nitric oxide. Stem Cells 2006; **24:** 2309.
16. Thom SR, Bhopale VM, Velazquez OC, Goldstein LJ, Thom LH, and Buerk DG: Stem cell mobilization by hyperbaric oxygen. Am J Physiol Heart Circ Physiol 2006; **290:** H1378.
17. Milovanova TN, Bhopale VM, Sorokina EM, *et al.*: Hyperbaric oxygen stimulates vasculogenic stem cell growth and differentiation *in vivo.* J Appl Physiol 2009; **106:** 711.
18. Loomans CJ, de Koning EJ, Staal FJ, *et al.*: Endothelial progenitor cell dysfunction: a novel concept in the pathogenesis of vascular complications of type 1 diabetes. Diabetes 2004; **53:** 195.
19. Tepper OM, Galiano RD, Capla JM, *et al.*: Human endothelial progenitor cells from type II diabetics exhibit impaired proliferation, adhesion, and incorporation into vascular structures. Circulation 2002; **106:** 2781.
20. Ii M, Takenaka H, Asai J, *et al.*: Endothelial progenitor thrombospondin-1 mediates diabetes-induced delay in reendothelialization following arterial injury. Circ Res 2006; **98:** 697.
21. Milovanova TN, Bhopale VM, Sorokina EM, *et al.*: Lactate stimulates vasculogenic stem cells via the thioredoxin system and engages an autocrine activation loop involving hypoxia-inducible factor 1. Mol Cell Biol 2008; **28:** 6248.
22. Ley K, Laudanna C, Cybulsky MI, and Nourshargh S: Getting to the site of inflammation: the leukocyte adhesion cascade updated. Nat Rev Immunol 2007; **7:** 678.
23. Hunt TK and Pai MP: The effect of varying ambient oxygen tensions on wound metabolism and collagen synthesis. Surg Gynecol Obstet 1972; **135:** 561.
24. Hohn DC, MacKay RD, Halliday B, and Hunt TK: Effect of O2 tension on microbicidal function of leukocytes in wounds and *in vitro.* Surg Forum 1976; **27:** 18.
25. Uhl E, Sirsjo A, Haapaniemi T, Nilsson G, and Nylander G: Hyperbaric oxygen improves wound healing in normal and ischemic skin tissue. Plast Reconstr Surg 1994; **93:** 835.
26. Knighton DR, Silver IA, and Hunt TK: Regulation of wound-healing angiogenesis-effect of oxygen gradients and inspired oxygen concentration. Surgery 1981; **90:** 262.
27. Smiell JM: Clinical safety of becaplermin (rhPDGF-BB) gel. Becaplermin Studies Group. Am J Surg 1998; **176:** 68S.
28. Marston WA, Hanft J, Norwood P, and Pollak R: The efficacy and safety of dermagraft in improving the healing of chronic diabetic foot ulcers: results of a prospective randomized trial. Diabetes Care 2003; **26:** 1701.
29. Brem H, Balledux J, Bloom T, Kerstein MD, and Hollier L: Healing of diabetic foot ulcers and pressure ulcers with human skin equivalent: a new paradigm in wound healing. Arch Surg 2000; **135:** 627.

Spinal Cord Injury and Repair: Role of Blood Vessel Loss and Endogenous Angiogenesis

Martin Oudega*

Departments of Physical Medicine & Rehabilitation and Neurobiology, University of Pittsburgh School of Medicine, Pittsburgh, Pennsylvania.

Background: After spinal cord injury (SCI), endogenous degenerative events cause ongoing loss of nervous tissue. There is no clinical therapy available resulting in significant, biologically meaningful recovery of function; thus, the prognosis is poor and SCI results in permanent functional impairments.

The Problem: The involvement of blood vessel loss in tissue destruction after SCI is often underappreciated. The role of the endogenous angiogenic response in spinal cord repair is poorly understood.

Basic/Clinical Science Advances: In animal models of SCI, some recent therapies that make use of angiogenesis for spinal cord repair approaches have emerged. These new approaches are reviewed here to increase our overall understanding of their role in the degenerative and regenerative events after injury.

Clinical Care Relevance: In the United States, approximately 12,000 people suffer an injury to their spinal cord each year. There is no treatment on hand that reverses the neurological impairments, resulting in a steadily growing group of chronically spinal cord–injured patients. At present there may be over 500,000 spinal cord–injured people who need full-time care. The personal and societal costs are high.

Conclusion: The loss of blood vessels after SCI contributes significantly to the final (functional) outcome. Animal models of SCI and repair have revealed that restoration of blood vessels within damaged tissue needs to be well-timed and include mechanisms to promote vessel maturity.

Abbreviations and Acronyms

MMP = matrix metalloproteinase

PARP-1 = poly(adenosine 5′-diphosphate-ribose) polymerase-1

SCI = spinal cord injury

VEGF = vascular endothelial growth factor

*Correspondence: Departments of Physical Medicine & Rehabilitation and Neurobiology, University of Pittsburgh School of Medicine, W1452 Biomedical Science Tower, 200 Lothrop St., Pittsburgh, Pennsylvania 15213-2536 (e-mail: moudega@pitt.edu).

BACKGROUND

Spinal cord injury (SCI) has a devastating impact on the life of the patient. The most obvious consequence of SCI is the immediate loss of motor and sensory function.[1] Additional impairments such as bladder, bowel, and sexual dysfunction, and chronic pain syndrome are less apparent but have an enormous impact on daily life. In the acute phase of SCI, neurons, astrocytes, and oligodendrocytes at and near the lesion die because of the impact forces.[1] Passing axons are severed resulting in an interruption of the flow of information between brain and periphery (Fig. 1A). Other (spared) axons may have their insulating myelin sheaths damaged, leaving them dysfunctional. These instant effects are substantiated by the loss of motor and sensory function.[1] Damage to blood vessels at the injury site results in hemorrhages in the central gray matter. Death cells, blood, and invading immune and inflammatory cells create together a toxic milieu causing additional cell death and axon damage and demyelination (secondary damage; Fig. 1A). Soon after injury (minutes–hours), T-lymphocytes

Printed in U.S.A.
DOI: 10.1089/awc.2009.0078

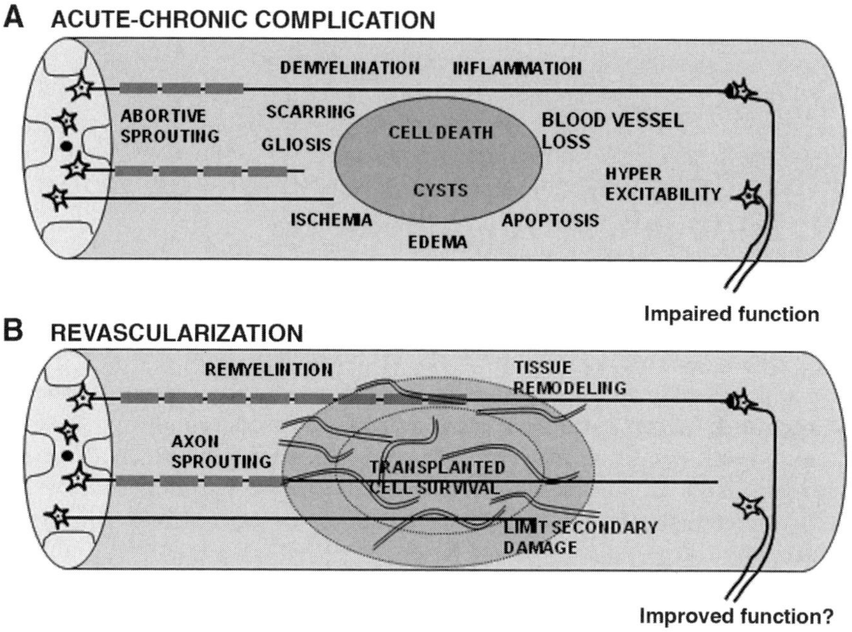

Figure 1. Schematic representation of (**A**) the acute and chronic events in the injured spinal cord that contribute to the overall tissue destruction and (**B**) the possible events that could be initiated after endogenous and therapy-induced revascularization and could contribute to overall repair.

invade the damaged tissue. Within hours–days they are followed by monocytes and macrophages, which often remain in the damaged area for years, and contribute significantly to secondary damage.[2] A glial scar forms around the impact epicenter consisting mainly of invading meningeal fibroblasts and surviving reactive astrocytes (Fig. 1A). A protective role has been ascribed to the scar, but its ability to obstruct endogenous or therapy-induced axon growth is most imperious.

In the chronic phase of SCI, the acute and subacute events continue ultimately resulting in atrophy of the spinal cord. Clearance of dead tissue leads to the formation of one or several fluid-filled cysts at the site of injury, which can expand into the rostral and caudal direction of the spinal cord (Fig. 1A). Some cells and molecules present at the injury site contribute to some degree to protection and repair, but the ultimate outcome of SCI is loss of tissue and function.

CLINICAL PROBLEM ADDRESSED

Endogenously there are several attempts within the damaged spinal cord to repair itself, but they do not result in significant improvements in function. Many severed axons form sprouts (*i.e.*, abortive sprouting) that grow over only a short distance before being retracted. Neurons from which the axon has been damaged express transiently[3] regeneration-associated genes and proteins that are involved in axonal extension. A number of molecules are present that could support axon regeneration such as fibroblast growth factor-2, glial cell–derived neurotrophic factor, ciliary neurotrophic factor, nerve growth factor, and brain-derived neurotrophic factor. Invading inflammatory cells may also contribute to regenerative sprouting.[4] Intact axons can grow (collateral) sprouts that contribute to the spontaneous functional recovery that is sometimes observed after SCI.[5,6] Remyelination of intact but demyelinated axons occurs by Schwann cells that migrate from adjacent dorsal roots or by newly generated oligodendrocytes.

However, these repair efforts do not result in life-changing functional improvements. Moreover, clinically there are no treatments available that would lead to such functional changes. Thus, SCI patients are in need of life-long and often around-the-clock care. In the United States about 40 people per million suffer from SCI per year; about 95% survive the initial hospitalization. Clinical care during the acute phase includes stabilization of the patient, possibly treatment with anti-inflammatory drugs to support tissue sparing, and on a case-by-case basis decompression surgery. Complications that may occur during the acute phase of SCI are listed in Table 1. During the chronic phase, complications such as pain, autonomic dysreflexia, septicemia, respiratory insufficiency, and pneumonia may occur (Table 1). Because these may lead to clinical deterioration, it is recommended that SCI patients receive annual screenings and long-term follow-ups. SCI patients should be given regular pneumococcal and influenza vaccines to prevent opportunistic infections. The onset of pressure ulcers and urinary tract

Table 1. *Possible acute and chronic complications associated with spinal cord injury in humans*

Acute (First Year)	Chronic
Urinary tract infection	Infertility
Autonomic dysreflexia	Infectious disease
Pain	Pressure sores
Wound infections	Eye/ear disorders
Chills/fever	Heart/circulatory problems
Pneumonia	Chronic pain syndrome
Renal malfunction	Muscle/joint pain
Heterotopic ossification	Muscle atrophy
Spasticity	Renal failure
Pressure sores	Bone fractures
	Spasticity

infections should be monitored and immediately treated.

BASIC SCIENCE CONTEXT

A less emphasized degenerative event that occurs in the injured spinal cord is the loss of blood vessels or devascularization at the impact epicenter and the accompanying hemorrhages, edema (swelling), and systemic consequences (Fig. 1A). The effects of blood vessel loss on the continuation of tissue destruction were shown clearly in animal models of SCI.[7]

Devascularization

Forces generated during an insult result in immediate death of endothelial cells of blood vessels. This results in vessel damage and consequently a sharp decrease or total lack of oxygen and nutrients. This ischemic period results in the accumulation of cytotoxic proteolytic enzymes and reactive oxygen species that contribute to the loss of nervous tissue. Reactive oxygen species, and other free radicals, lead to the formation of peroxides through lipid peroxidation that causes cell membrane damage and ultimately death.[8]

Hemorrhage

Hemorrhages (bleedings) are located first within the central gray matter, but soon expand into the white matter at the periphery and into the rostral and caudal spinal cord. Areas of hemorrhage can often be found away from the actual impact site. Bleedings contain many monocytes and macrophages that are known contributors to the destruction of spinal cord nervous tissue.[1,2]

Edema

Edema (swelling) of the injured spinal cord segment occurs, as drainage of extracellular fluid does not take place. The swollen tissue may become compressed against fractured vertebra, resulting in additional damage.

Systemic consequences

SCI affects the autoregulation, resulting in a decrease in blood flow, and thus ischemia, which results in loss of initially spared nervous tissue.[9] Nitric oxide may play an important role in the maintenance of arteriolar tone in the injured spinal cord.[10] An injury to the spinal cord can also cause neurogenic shock,[11] bradycardia, and hypotension. All these have negative effects on blood supply to the spinal cord and thus contribute to the overall damage. Importantly, their effects can also affect organs[12] as they decrease the mean arterial blood pressure, which may result in decreased microvascular blood flow and, as a consequence, organ dysfunction.

EXPERIMENTAL MODEL OR MATERIAL

About 75% of all human SCIs are contusive injuries caused by blunt objects that typically leave the surrounding dura intact. In about 25% of all cases, the spinal cord and dura are lacerated by penetrating sharp objects. There are three types of contusive injuries: massive compression (44% of all cases), contusion (31%), and solid cord injury (25%). The amount of tissue loss is most with a massive contusion and least with solid cord injury. Anatomically, contusive injuries are typically incomplete and present clinically as central cord syndrome with variable, but often complete, motor and sensory loss. In the laboratory, a complete or partial laceration of the spinal cord can be modeled using a surgical microknife or microscissors. A complete transection injury model allows for unambiguous reading of axonal regeneration responses, but it is also surgically the most challenging model. A contusion injury can be modeled by temporarily compressing the spinal cord using devices known as impactors. With a contusion injury, the analysis of axonal regeneration is complex due to spared axons and their collateral sprouts. Animal models that mimic SCI in humans have contributed to our understanding of mechanisms underlying endogenous degenerative and regenerative processes after SCI. The use of these models eventually may lead to the identification of target molecules and the development of repair approaches.

DISCUSSION OF FINDINGS AND RELEVANT LITERATURE

After SCI, many growth factors are expressed within the damaged and still intact nearby nervous tissue. Among these is vascular endothelial growth factor (VEGF),[13] which has immediate consequences for the vascularization in the injury site and its surroundings. Normally, after SCI, an angiogenic response is initiated resulting in the formation of new blood vessels in the injury site during the first week (Fig. 1B).[14,15] However, this response is transient; the new blood vessels retract from the damaged tissue. In a rat model of contusive SCI, it was demonstrated that new blood vessels are formed in a biphasic response[15] in which the first phase was accompanied by changes in locomotor function. Whether and how the new blood vessels are involved in the improvements in motor function is poorly understood. The initial but ultimately failed attempt to revascularize damaged cord tissue contributes to secondary degeneration after SCI.[11,16]

The endogenous angiogenic response is an indication of an attempt of self-repair by the damaged spinal cord. However, this response does not have a significant effect on the final outcome of SCI. Possible reasons, other than its transient character, that need to be kept in mind are that newly formed immature blood vessels are permeable for some time and therefore leaking molecules and cells into the revascularized region, which could contribute to further tissue destruction.

When newly formed blood vessels mature and adequately function, it is possible, although somewhat counterintuitive, that the reintroduction of oxygen (reperfusion) leads to apoptotic cell death (reperfusion injury) of neurons that survived the initial injury.[17] At the basis of this type of apoptotic neuronal death is poly(adenosine 5′-diphosphate-ribose) polymerase-1 (PARP-1), a nuclear enzyme that catalyzes the formation of (adenosine 5′-diphosphate-ribose)$_n$ chains from oxidized nicotinamide-adenine dinucleotide on acceptor proteins. Re-oxygenation after a period of oxygen and glucose deprivation, as could occur after maturing of newly formed blood vessels, may result in high activation of PARP-1 and therefore rapid consummation of oxidized nicotinamide-adenine dinucleotide, which may induce apoptotic neuronal death. This can be suppressed with B-cell lymphoma-2, indicating PARP-1–induced mitochondrial impairment as a critical step in the neuronal apoptosis after re-oxygenation.[17]

The formation of new mature blood vessels after SCI would allow re-establishing blood supply, and thus oxygen and nutrients delivery to the damaged area and its surroundings, and this could support tissue remodeling (Fig. 1B). There are risks involved that could result in additional damage (see above). Nevertheless, as evidenced in several studies using different injury and repair models, angiogenesis remains a potential therapeutic for repair of the injured spinal cord.[18]

It is likely that VEGF will play an important role in promoting revascularization and consequently in restoring vascular perfusion of damaged tissue.[16,19] After injury, VEGF and its receptors, fms-related tyrosine kinase-1 and flk-1 (a kinase insert domain receptor [also known as KDR or CD309]) (tyrosine kinase) receptors are rapidly upregulated on neurons and astrocytes near the impact site,[20] possibly induced by hypoxia, which could result in binding of the hypoxia-inducible factor to the hypoxia-response element of VEGF.[21] As described above, the presence of high levels

TAKE-HOME MESSAGE

Basic science advances

- SCI results in immediate loss of tissue and sensory and motor function.
- SCI initiates a series of pathophysiological events that contribute to secondary tissue loss resulting in cyst formation.
- Blood vessel loss results in ischemia, that is, lack of oxygen and nutrients, and consequently additional neural cell death.
- Blood vessel loss contributes significantly to the damage after SCI.
- Endogenous angiogenesis results in transient presence of blood vessels.
- Newly formed blood vessels are immature and contribute to tissue loss.

Clinical science advances

- SCI patients have permanent functional impairments and are in need of full-time care. The social and economic costs are large.
- There are no therapies that restore function with life-changing consequences.
- Promoting the formation of new blood vessels after SCI may support reparative events. Therapies aimed at promoting angiogenesis must include approaches to support blood vessel maturation. Therapies need to be well timed.
- VEGF is likely to play an important role in therapies focused on promoting angiogenesis.

Relevance to clinical care

- SCI patients have permanent functional impairments and are in need of full-time care. The social and economic costs are large.
- There are no therapies that restore function with life-changing consequences.
- SCI patients need annual screenings and long-term follow-ups as their overall health may deteriorate due to acute and chronic complications.

of VEGF may result in an adverse effect through promoting blood vessel permeability. In a rat model of SCI, the administration of VEGF significantly increased the blood vessel permeability in the spinal cord and caused tissue damage.[22]

Besides VEGF-based treatments, other approaches to increase revascularization have also shown to be effective. Administration of the chemoattractant chemokine (C-X-C motif) ligand 10[23] or matrix metalloproteinase inhibition[24] results in improved angiogenesis at an injury site and this was also shown to improve functional outcome.

It has to be kept in mind that the impact of blood vessel loss is larger than its contribution to tissue destruction; it also drastically limits the efficacy of repair-promoting treatments based on cell transplantation, as survival of grafted cells is seriously compromised due to lack of oxygen and nutrients. Thus, an alternative way to profit from promoting the formation of new blood vessels in and nearby the injury site is that it may increase the survival and thus the efficacy of cell transplants to support overall repair (Fig. 1B). In general, the survival of cells grafted into the injured spinal cord is low. Hill and colleagues[25] demonstrated that over 80% of Schwann cells transplanted into the contused adult rat spinal cord died within 7 days postinjection. This cell loss was independent of the density of cells injected.[25] Improving the vascularization of the damaged area before cell transplantation may improve their survival and thus their reparative effects.[26]

CAUTION, CRITICAL REMARKS, AND RECOMMENDATIONS

It is thought that the development of treatments that increase angiogenesis and restore normal blood flow would be supportive directly or indirectly for repair of the spinal cord.[15] It is clear, however, from our experiences in animal models of SCI that any therapy that focuses on restoring blood vessel presence in a damaged spinal cord should be well-timed and include approaches to promote the maturation of the new vessels.

FUTURE DEVELOPMENTS

Continuation of developing and employing models of human SCI focused on the role of blood vessel loss and formation is absolutely critical to increase our understanding of the role of blood vessel loss and formation to the overall damage after SCI. With that additional knowledge, it may be possible to develop strategies that include promoting angiogenesis that would result in biologically significant functional improvements after SCI.

ACKNOWLEDGMENTS

The author is indebted to laboratory members who diligently contributed to some of the work reviewed here.

AUTHOR DISCLOSURE STATEMENT

No conflict of interest disclosed.

REFERENCES

1. Hagg T and Oudega M: Degenerative and spontaneous regenerative processes after spinal cord injury. J Neurotrauma 2006; **23:** 264.

2. Popovich PG: Immunological regulation of neuronal degeneration and regeneration in the injured spinal cord. Prog Brain Res 2000; **128:** 43.

3. Tetzlaff W, Alexander SW, Miller FD, and Bisby MA: Response of facial and rubrospinal neurons to axotomy: changes in mRNA expression for cytoskeletal proteins and GAP-43. J Neurosci 1991; **11:** 2528.

4. Batchelor PE, Porritt MJ, Nilsson SK, Bertoncello I, Donnan GA, and Howells DW: Periwound dopaminergic sprouting is dependent on numbers of wound macrophages. Eur J Neurosci 2002; **15:** 826.

5. Hagg T: Collateral sprouting as a target for improved function after spinal cord injury. J Neurotrauma 2006; **23:** 281.

6. Raineteau O and Schwab ME: Plasticity of motor systems after incomplete spinal cord injury. Nat Rev Neurosci 2001; **2:** 263.

7. Mautes AE, Weinzierl MR, Donovan F, and Noble LJ: Vascular events after spinal cord injury: contribution to secondary pathogenesis. Phys Ther 2000; **80:** 673.

8. Carmeliet P: Angiogenesis in life, disease and medicine. Nature 2005; **438:** 932.

9. Krassioukov AV, Furlan JC, and Fehlings MG: Autonomic dysreflexia in acute spinal cord injury: an under-recognized clinical entity. J Neurotrauma 2003; **20:** 707.

10. Matsumoto M, Iida Y, Wakamatsu H, Ohtake K, Nakakimura K, Xiong L, and Sakabe T: The effects of N(G)-nitro-L-arginine-methyl ester on neurologic and histopathologic outcome after transient spinal cord ischemia in rabbits. Anesth Analg 1999; **89:** 696.

11. Tator CH and Fehlings MG: Review of the secondary injury theory of acute spinal cord trauma with emphasis on vascular mechanisms. J Neurosurg 1991; **75:** 15.

12. Guízar-Sahagún G, Velasco-Hernández L, Martínez-Cruz A, Castañeda-Hernández G, Bravo G, Rojas G, and Hong E: Systemic microcirculation after complete high and low thoracic spinal cord section in rats. J Neurotrauma 2004; **21:** 1614.

13. Leung DW, Cachianes G, Kuang WJ, Goeddel DV, and Ferrara N: Vascular endothelial growth factor is a secreted angiogenic mitogen. Science 1989; **246:** 1306.

14. Casella GT, Marcillo A, Bunge MB, and Wood PM: New vascular tissue rapidly replaces neural parenchyma and vessels destroyed by a contusion injury to the rat spinal cord. Exp Neurol 2002; **173:** 63.

15. Loy DN, Crawford CH, Darnall JB, Burke DA., Onifer SM, and Whittemore SR: Temporal progression of angiogenesis and basal lamina deposition after contusive spinal cord injury in the adult rat. J Comp Neurol 2002; **445:** 308.

16. Widenfalk J, Lipson A, Jubran M, Hofstetter C, Ebendal T, Cao Y, and Olson I: Vascular endothelial growth factor improves functional outcome and decreases secondary degeneration in

experimental spinal cord contusion injury. Neurosci 2003; **120:** 951.

17. Tanaka S, Takehashi M, Iida S, Kitajima T, Kamanaka Y, Stedeford T, Banasik M, and Ueda K: Mitochondrial impairment induced by poly(ADP-ribose) polymerase-1 activation in cortical neurons after oxygen and glucose deprivation. J Neurochem 2005; **95:** 179.

18. Zachary I: Neuroprotective role of vascular endothelial growth factor: signalling mechanisms, biological function, and therapeutic potential. Neurosignals 2005; **14:** 207.

19. Choi UH, Ha Y, Huang X, Park SR, Chung J, Hyun DK, Park H, Park HC, Kim SW, and Lee M: Hypoxia-inducible expression of vascular endothelial growth factor for the treatment of spinal cord injury in a rat model. J Neurosurg Spine 2007; **7:** 54.

20. Marti HH and Risau W: Systemic hypoxia changes the organ-specific distribution of vascular endothelial growth factor and its receptors. Proc Natl Acad Sci USA 1998; **95:** 15809.

21. Shweiki D, Itin A, Soffer D, and Keshet E: Vascular endothelial growth factor induced by hypoxia may mediate hypoxia-initiated angiogenesis. Nature 1992; **359:** 843.

22. Benton RL and Whittemore SR: VEGF165 therapy exacerbates secondary damage following spinal cord injury. Neurochem Res 2003; **28:** 1693.

23. Glaser J, Gonzalez R, Perreau VM, Cotman CW, and Keirstead HS: Neutralization of the chemokine CXCL10 enhances tissue sparing and angiogenesis following spinal cord injury. J Neurosci Res 2004; **77:** 701.

24. Noble LJ, Donovan F, Igarashi T, Goussev S, and Werb Z: Matrix metalloproteinases limit functional recovery after spinal cord injury by modulation of early vascular events. J Neurosci 2002; **22:** 7526.

25. Hill CE, Hurtado A, Blits B, Bahr BA, Wood PM, Bartlett Bunge M, and Oudega M: Early necrosis and apoptosis of Schwann cells transplanted into the injured rat spinal cord. Eur J Neurosci 2007; **26:** 1433.

26. Hurtado A, Moon LD, Maquet V, Blits B, Jérôme R, and Oudega M: Poly (D,L-lactic acid) macroporous guidance scaffolds seeded with Schwann cells genetically modified to secrete a bi-functional neurotrophin implanted in the completely transected adult rat thoracic spinal cord. Biomaterials 2006; **27:** 430.

Design of a Novel Protease-Resistant Vascular Endothelial Growth Factor-A Protein for Angiogenic Therapy

Stephanie Traub,[1] Tina Lucas,[1] Daniel Hoffmann,[1] Thomas Krieg,[1,2] and Sabine A. Eming[1,*]

[1]Department of Dermatology, University of Cologne, Cologne, Germany.
[2]Cologne Excellence Cluster on Cellular Stress Responses in Aging-Associated Diseases (CECAD), University of Cologne, Cologne, Germany.

Background: Normal tissue function requires adequate supply of oxygen through blood vessels. Understanding how blood vessels form is a challenging objective because angiogenesis is vital to many physiological and pathological processes. Unraveling mechanisms of angiogenesis would offer therapeutic options to ameliorate disorders that are currently leading causes of mortality and morbidity, including cardiovascular diseases, cancer, diabetic retinopathy, excessive tissue defects, and chronic nonhealing wounds.
The Problem: Restoring blood flow to the site of injured tissue is a prerequisite for mounting a successful repair response. Regardless of the underlying pathology, a typical feature of chronic nonhealing wounds is the reduced granulation tissue formation, hence the growth of vascular structures. Therefore, treatment modalities that normalize endothelial cell function and promote tissue vascularization provide a central strategy to normalize and accelerate the healing response and tissue regeneration.
Basic/Clinical Science Advances: In recent studies, we and others provided evidence that proteolytic processing of vascular endothelial growth factor-A (VEGF-A), a key mediator of angiogenesis, might be an important event controlling its activity in tissue repair and inflammatory conditions. Indeed, our data indicate that increased proteolysis of VEGF-A in the highly proteolytic microenvironment of the chronic wound leads to VEGF-A inactivation and reduced VEGF165 availability at the wound site, which might contribute to chronic wound pathology and impaired healing.
Clinical Care Relevance: These observations might have clinical impact. In the highly proteolytic environment of the nonhealing human wound, a protease-resistant VEGF165 mutant might be more effective in stimulating wound angiogenesis and in improving wound closure.
Conclusion: Protecting VEGF-A protein proteolysis and rescuing loss of VEGF-A activity in chronic wounds might provide a treatment modality that normalizes endothelial cell function and promotes tissue vascularization ultimately ameliorating tissue repair.

Abbreviations and Acronyms

ECM = extracellular matrix
MMP = matrix metalloproteinase
SDS-PAGE = sodium dodecyl sulfate polyacrylamide gel electrophoresis
VEGF = vascular endothelial growth factor

*Correspondence: Department of Dermatology, University of Cologne, Joseph-Stelzmann St. 9, Cologne, Germany 50931 (e-mail: sabine.eming@uni-koeln.de).

BACKGROUND

Angiogenesis is a vital component of normal wound healing. The precise control of blood vessel regeneration during repair is still not clearly understood. Several features characterize wound angiogenesis in skin: first, there is increasing evidence that this process occurs through both angiogenesis (sprouting of capillaries from existing blood vessels) and vasculogenesis (mobilization of bone marrow–derived endothelial stem cells). Second, the event is highly complex and requires a dynamic, temporally and spatially regulated

Printed in U.S.A.
DOI: 10.1089/awc.2009.0074

interaction between endothelial cells, soluble angiogenic growth factors, and extracellular matrix (ECM) molecules.

In recent years several mediators have been identified that are crucial for vessel formation, and new insight has been gained into their specific functions in controlling vascular remodeling and angiogenesis. In particular, genetically engineered mouse models provided substantial evidence that wound angiogenesis requires a dynamic interaction among endothelial cells, pro- and anti-angiogenic growth factors, and the ECM environment. Because of a complex network of numerous mediators controlling angiogenesis, a high functional redundancy in this process is assumed. Nevertheless, in the past 15 years, the family of vascular endothelial growth factor (VEGF) proteins and their receptors has emerged as key mediators in embryonic vascular development, physiological and pathological angiogenesis in the adult.[1] Although the general role of VEGF ligands and their receptors during angiogenesis has been intensively studied, their specific function in wound angiogenesis is not yet completely understood.

VEGF-A levels are regulated through transcriptional control and mRNA stability. Moreover, by differential mRNA splicing, the single human VEGF-A gene gives rise to at least eight isoforms ($VEGF_{121,\ 145,\ 148,\ 162,\ 165,\ 183,\ 189,\ \text{and}\ 206}$) whose relative abundance varies among different tissues[2]; the 165-amino acid isoform is the major gene product found in human tissues. The domains encoded by exons 1–5 of the VEGF-A gene are present in all VEGF splice variants and contain information required for the recognition of the tyrosine kinase VEGF receptors 1 (VEGFR-1/Flt-1) and 2 (VEGFR-2/KDR/Flk-1).[3] The isoforms are distinguished by the presence or absence of the domains encoded by exons 6 and 7 of the VEGF-A gene that code for two independent heparin-binding domains. Substantial evidence indicates that differences in the expression of the heparin-binding domains are crucially involved in the diverse biochemical and functional properties of the VEGF-A splice forms, including binding to cell surfaces and ECM,[4] receptor binding characteristics,[5] endothelial cell adhesion and survival,[4] and vascular branch formation.[6]

CLINICAL PROBLEM ADDRESSED

A typical feature of chronic nonhealing wounds is the reduced granulation tissue formation, hence the growth of vascular structures. In specific entities of impaired healing conditions, functional and organic changes involving the macrocirculatory and microcirculatory system have been defined, which ultimately might lead to tissue ischemia and tissue damage.[7] Functional and ultrastructural analysis of the microcirculation on the wound edge of patients with wound healing defects caused by venous insufficiency documents endothelial alterations that might lead to slow and insufficient capillary growth.[8] Therefore, treatment modalities that normalize endothelial cell function and promote tissue vascularization provide a central strategy to normalize and accelerate the healing response and tissue regeneration.

RELEVANT BASIC SCIENCE CONTEXT

In addition to mRNA-splicing, proteolytic mechanisms also generate VEGF-A variants with different biological activities.[9] This observation suggests that the proteolytic microenvironment should be considered as a critical determinant controlling VEGF-A–mediated activities. Initial evidence supporting the hypothesis that VEGF-A proteolytic processing regulates its activity was derived from studies analyzing the activity of the VEGF189 isoform.[10] Whereas native VEGF189 binds to VEGFR-1 but not VEGFR-2, maturation of native VEGF189 by urokinase plasminogen activator within the exon 6 encoded sequence resulted in its VEGFR-2 binding and exerted a mitogenic effect on endothelial cells. Whether VEGF189, in particular its urokinase plasminogen activator–mediated activation, plays a role *in vivo* has not been analyzed so far.

Recently, Lee and colleagues described additional matrix metalloproteinase (MMP) cleavage sites in the VEGF-A protein.[11] This group identified MMP-3, −7, −9, and −19, which efficiently cleaved the murine VEGF164 isoform; MMP-1 and −16 were less effective. MMP cleavage appeared to occur in sequential steps at residues 135, 120, and finally at residue 113. MMP cleavage resulted in dissociation of the VEGF165/164 heparin-binding motif. The biological impact of MMP processing of VEGF-A was assessed in an *in vivo* tumor model. Carcinoma cells were transfected with different VEGF-A variants and injected subcutaneously into a mouse model. Tumors that expressed the MMP-cleaved VEGF fragment VEGF1–113 grew poorly and showed capillary dilation of existing vessels. In contrast, tumors expressing the MMP-resistant VEGF-A variant displayed faster growth kinetics and the vasculature was characterized by increased capillary density with multiple and frequent branch points. Altered structural–functional properties of MMP-resistant VEGF164 might account for the accelerated tumor angiogenesis observed.

A cardinal feature of chronic nonhealing wounds is an unbalanced proteolytic microenvironment where disintegrating inflammatory cell subsets release active peptidases and overwhelm local antipeptidase tissue protective mechanisms. Substantial experimental evidence indicates that this process leads to uncontrolled destruction of factors promoting wound healing. Further, uncontrolled protease activity might counteract growth factor–based therapies due to digestion and inactivation of the therapeutic protein.

EXPERIMENTAL MODEL OR MATERIAL—ADVANTAGES AND LIMITATIONS

We investigated the hypothesis whether there exists a causative link between impaired angiogenesis and decreased VEGF-A activity in chronic nonhealing wounds. To test this hypothesis we analyzed VEGF-A expression and protein integrity in chronic nonhealing wounds (Fig. 1). VEGF-A mRNA and protein expression was highly upregulated in nonhealing wounds, and levels were comparable to normal-healing wounds.[12] Thus, these data prompted us to focus on the degradation pathway of VEGF165 protein. Our data demonstrated that in contrast to healing wounds, VEGF165 protein is a target of proteolytic processing in chronic nonhealing wounds. Sodium dodecyl sulfate polyacrylamide gel electrophoresis (SDS-PAGE) analysis and protease inhibitor studies strongly indicated that serine proteases—in particular, plasmin—are involved in VEGF165 processing in the context of the chronic wound environment. In contrast, inhibitors of MMPs, of cysteine proteinases, and of acidic proteases had no effect on VEGF165 degradation in wound fluid collected from nonhealing wounds. This observation is different from proteolytic cleavage of VEGF165 in tumors by MMPs[11] and indicates that in the hostile microenvironment of chronic wounds MMP-mediated cleavage of VEGF165 is not the primarily proteolytic pathway.

To further investigate the biological consequence of plasmin-mediated VEGF165 cleavage, we identified the plasmin cleavage site in the VEGF165 molecule. Plasmin digestion of VEGF165 yielded two fragments: an amino-terminal homodimer (VEGF1–110) that was resistant to further cleavage and a carboxyl-terminal polypeptide (VEGF111–165).[9,12,13] Plasmin digestion reduced significantly the mitogenic activity on endothelial cells.[9,13] By the introduction of amino acid alterations at the plasmin-sensitive cleavage site Arg110/Ala111, we generated plasmin-resistant VEGF165 mutants (Fig. 1). Substitutions at either site resulted in VEGF165 products that, while maintaining growth

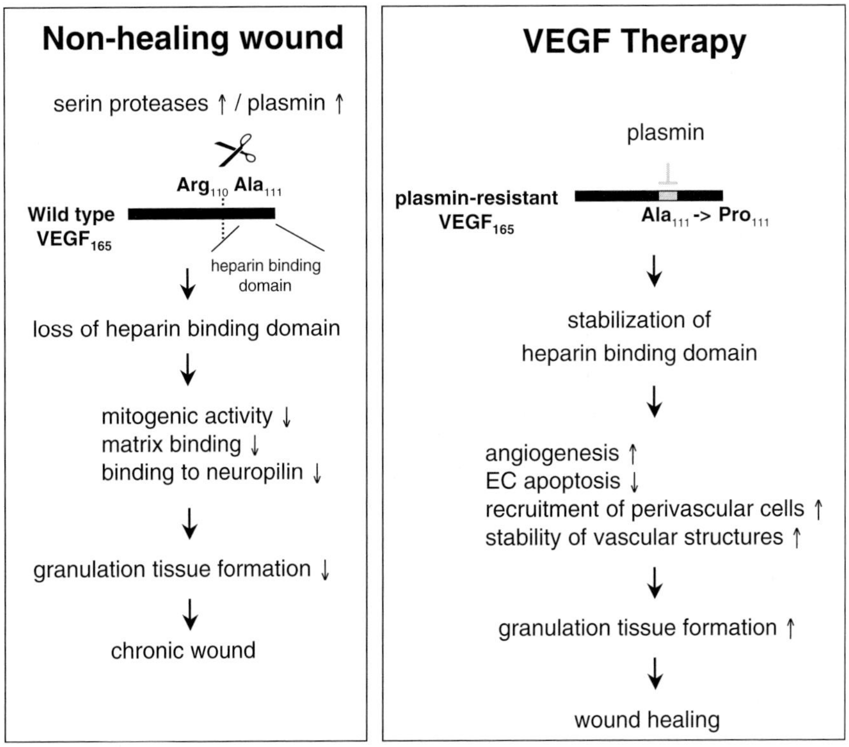

Figure 1. Schematic representation of functional consequences of proteolytic processing of vascular endothelial growth factor-A165 (VEGF-A165) in the hostile microenvironment of nonhealing wounds. VEGF-A165 protein is a target of serine proteases, in particular plasmin. Proteolytic cleavage of VEGF-A165 in wound fluid obtained from chronic venous stasis ulcers results in the degradation of the VEGF-A165 protein with loss of the heparin-binding domain and attenuated activity. Substitution of Ala111 with Pro111 yielded a plasmin-resistant VEGF-A165 mutant with substantial stabilization in wound fluid of chronic wounds. The plasmin-resistant VEGF-A165 mutant is biological active and increases the angiogenic response and the stability of vascular structures in a diabetic mouse model of impaired healing.

promoting properties, were fully plasmin resistant. A plasmin-resistant VEGF165 mutant (Ala111 → Pro111) (VEGF165^{A111P}) showed significantly increased stability when incubated in wound fluid derived from nonhealing wounds.[13] Taken together, our data demonstrated that in the highly proteolytic environment of human nonhealing skin ulcers, VEGF165 degradation is increased as compared to normal-healing wounds and VEGF-A processing can be partially rescued by inactivation of the plasmin-sensitive cleavage site Arg110/Ala111. Further, our data propose that reduced VEGF165 availability at the wound site may contribute to impaired healing.

DISCUSSION OF FINDINGS AND RELEVANT LITERATURE

To characterize the biological relevance of the protease sensitivity of VEGF165 *in vivo*, in particular during cutaneous repair, we investigated the stability and activity of locally applied VEGF165 wild-type (VEGF165-Wt) or a VEGF165 mutant resistant to plasmin proteolysis (VEGF165^{A111P}) in a genetic mouse model of impaired healing (*db/db* mouse)[14] (Fig. 1). Diabetic wounds have been shown to lack VEGF protein activity, not necessarily caused by increased proteolytic degradation, but most likely caused by decreased VEGF gene expression. Therefore, the diabetic-impaired wound healing model provided an ideal model system to test the functional impact of locally applied VEGF protein to normalize pathological repair. Our experiments provided the first *in vivo* data indicating that plasmin-catalyzed cleavage is critical to regulate VEGF165-mediated angiogenesis. We chose the particle-mediated gene transfer technology, a physical means of gene delivery, to overexpress VEGF165 variants at the wound site. Histological and functional data indicated that the improved healing response after VEGF165-Wt application was based on the induction of a highly vascularized granulation tissue as well as an accelerated reepithelialization process. Wounds transfected with the cDNA coding for VEGF165^{A111P} provoked an early granulation tissue formation, which in regard to the vessel density and cellular composition was similar to that induced by the wild-type molecule. However, vessel size was significantly increased in mutant versus wild-type-treated wounds 8 and 12 days after wounding. Nevertheless, differences in vessel size did not affect wound closure rate, which was similar in VEGF165-Wt- and VEGF165^{A111P}-transfected wounds. However, we found significant differences regarding vessel regression in VEGF165-Wt- and mutant-transfected wounds during later stages in the repair process. Whereas in wild-type-transfected wounds capillary density resolved rapidly upon completion of wound reepithelialization, VEGF165^{A111P}-transfected wounds were characterized by a significant delayed involution of capillary density after wound closure. This finding was consistent with a delayed and decreased number of apoptotic endothelial cells in VEGF165^{A111P}-transfected wounds when compared to VEGF165-Wt-transfected wounds, and it suggested an increased stability of vascular structures in VEGF165-mutant- versus VEGF165-Wt-treated wounds.

VEGF-A is a critical survival factor for vascular endothelium, in particular for immature vessels.[15] The decreased endothelial cell apoptosis observed in mutant-treated wounds may therefore have resulted from an increased stability and prolonged local activity of the VEGF165 mutant. This assumption was supported by Western blot analysis and CD31/TUNEL analysis, which demonstrated increased stability and activity of the VEGF165 mutant within a highly proteolytic wound environment. In addition, our data indicated that capillaries induced by the VEGF mutant were characterized by an increased coating of perivascular cells. VEGF165 is chemotactic for pericytes, and in various models of angiogenic remodeling ectopic application of VEGF-A has been shown to accelerate pericyte coverage of newly formed blood vessels, which ultimately increased vessel maturation.[16] Therefore, the prolonged vessel persistence in VEGF165^{A111P}-transfected wounds might result from a combination of prolonged local VEGF165 mutant activity and increased pericyte coating.

Different structural–functional properties of the VEGF165 mutant and the wild-type protein could account for the prolonged and enhanced activity of the mutant. We and others have demonstrated that plasmin-catalyzed cleavage of VEGF165 results in loss of its heparin-binding domain,[9,12,13] which is crucially involved in diverse biochemical and functional properties. Inactivation of the plasmin cleavage site leads to the preservation/integrity of the heparin-binding domain in the VEGF165 molecule, which enhances VEGF receptor affinity and/or ECM interactions. The VEGF-A heparin-binding domain has been identified as the epitope for Nrp-1 binding.[5] Although, endothelial VEGF-A signaling described to date is largely mediated via VEGFR-1 and/or −2, its mitogenic, migratory, and survival signaling can be significantly facilitated by signaling through the membrane-bound coreceptor Nrp-1.[17] In addition, the heparin-binding domain of VEGF-A isoforms is crucial for determining its binding to ECM molecules. Recent data have demonstrated that the angiogenic potential of matrix-associated isoforms is superior to soluble isoforms.[18] Overall, effects mediated by the heparin-binding domain may act separately and/or in concert to enhance and prolong the activity of the plasmin-resistant VEGF165 molecule in the *db/db* wound environment. Our present data provided experimental evidence that a plasmin-resistant VEGF165 variant exerts increased stability in the highly proteolytic environment of an impaired healing wound with significant consequences to blood vessel persistence.

CAUTION, CRITICAL REMARKS, AND RECOMMENDATIONS

It is a well-accepted concept that common cellular and molecular mechanisms are active during tissue repair and malignant tumor growth.[19] Indeed, cancer often develops at the site of chronic injury, and tissue injury has an important role in the pathogenesis of malignant disease. Therefore, the treatment of chronic wounds with growth factors is inevitably linked to the risk of malignant tumor development. Patients undergoing growth factor therapy should therefore be closely controlled for local and/or systemic malignant tumor development. Further, protein delivery systems that maximize the local effects of growth factors at the wound site and minimize systemic release or distribution of the topical applied molecules might contribute to eliminate deleterious systemic side effects. Finally, beside stimulating vascular growth, VEGF has been identified as one of the most potent mediators of vascular permeability.[1] In fact, clinical trials using systemic VEGF therapies to improve blood perfusion in vascular disease were limited to significant tissue edema.[2] Therefore, additional research is required to understand how this "local side effect" in VEGF therapy can be controlled.

FUTURE DEVELOPMENT

As for growth factors, regulation through proteolytic cleavage can also be observed for ECM proteins. Several matrix protein fragments exhibit an anti-angiogenic response in tumors. It will be interesting to see which fragments are involved not only in tumor angiogenesis but potentially also in anti-angiogenesis during wound healing. Recent studies have demonstrated that a set of axonal guidance molecules also plays an important role for the development of the vasculature as well as in angiogenesis. These molecules participate in the directional outgrowth of axons and are essential to attain the functional anatomy of the nervous system. Analyses of mutant mice deficient for these molecules, such as semaphorin III, neuropilins, ephrins, and netrin-1, revealed such multifunctionality. Comparing angiogenesis with axonal guidance, several similarities are obvious. Both processes rely upon directional outgrowth, induced either by growth factors or by other soluble proteins. Netrin-1, a protein identified for the guidance of commissural axons, plays a similar role in angiogenesis. In addition, it was shown that one of the netrin-1 receptors is expressed at the tip cells of growing small capillaries. It will be interesting to study this new group of molecules, for example, netrins, slits, and

TAKE-HOME MESSAGE

Basic science advance

- VEGF-A165 is a target of plasmin, and plasmin-mediated VEGF-A165 cleavage adds an additional control for VEGF-A–mediated processes. Different structural–functional properties might account for the altered VEGF activities of plasmin-processed VEGF-A165. Presented studies suggest that, in particular, loss of the heparin-binding domain results in a protease-resistant VEGF-A1–110 core fragment with attenuated angiogenic properties.

Clinical science advance

- Our data demonstrated that in the highly proteolytic environment of human nonhealing skin ulcers, VEGF-A165 degradation is increased as compared to normal-healing wounds and VEGF-A processing can be partially rescued by inactivation of the plasmin-sensitive cleavage site Arg110/Ala111. Further, our data propose that reduced VEGF165 availability at the wound site may contribute to impaired healing. Local therapy of chronic wounds lacking an angiogenic response with a protease-resistant VEGF165 molecule might be considered as a therapeutic option to stimulate vascularization and ultimately tissue growth. Diverse modalities of VEGF delivery into the wound might be discussed including direct protein application and cell- or gene-based delivery systems.

Relevance to clinical care

- Rendering the VEGF-A165 molecule resistant to proteolytic cleavage might increase the portion of matrix-bound VEGF-A165 molecules that are more efficient in supporting a more functional angiogenic response than soluble VEGF-A.

neuropilin, in the future with respect to angiogenesis in wound healing.

ACKNOWLEDGMENTS

Vascular research in the authors' laboratory is funded by DFG (SFB829), EU (Angioscaff), and CECAD.

AUTHOR DISCLOSURE STATEMENT

S.T., T.L., and D.H. disclose commercial associations that might create or seem to pose a conflict of interest in connection with the submitted manuscript. S.A.E. and T.K. hold a patent on the plasmin-resistant VEGF-A165 mutant (US 7,491,696 B2; EP 1 485 483 B1).

REFERENCES

1. Olsson AK, Dimberg A, Kreuger J, and Claesson-Welsh L: Nat Rev 2006; **7:** 359.
2. Ferrara N: VEGF: basic science and clinical progress. Endocr Rev 2004; **25:** 581.
3. Keyt BA, Nguyen HV, Berleau LT, Duarte CM, Park J, Chen H, and Ferrara N: Identification of vascular endothelial growth factor determinants for binding KDR and FLT-1 receptors. J Biol Chem 1996; **271:** 5638.
4. Hutchings H, Ortega N, and Plouet J: Extracellular matrix-bound VEGF promotes endothelial cell adhesion, migration, and survival through integrin ligation. FASEB J 2003; **17:** 1520.
5. Soker S, Takashima S, Miao HQ, Neufeld G, and Klagsbrun M: Neuropilin-1 is expressed by endothelial and tumor cells as isoform-specific receptor for VEGF. Cell 1998; **92:** 735.
6. Ruhrberg C, Gerhardt H, Golding M, Watson R, Ioannidou S, Fujisawa H, Betsholtz C, and Shima DT: Spatially restricted patterning cues provided by heparin-binding VEGF-A morphogenesis. Gene Dev 2002; **16:** 2684.
7. Luetolf O, Bull RH, Bates DO, and Mortimer PS: Capillary underperfusion in chronic venous insufficiency: a cause for leg ulceration? Br J Dermatol 1993; **128:** 249.
8. Leu AJ, Leu HL, Franzeck UK, and Bollinger A: Microvascular changes in chronic venous insufficiency—a review. Cardiovasc Surg 1995; **3:** 237.
9. Keyt BA, Berleau LT, Nguyen HV, Chen H, Heinsoh H, Vandlen R, and Ferrara N: The carboxyl-terminal domain (111–165) of VEGF is critical for its mitogenic potency. J Biol Chem 1996; **271:** 7788.
10. Plouet J, Moro F, Bertagnolli S, Coldeboeuf N, Mazarguil H, Clamens S, and Bayard F: Extracellular cleavage of the VEGF189-amino acid form by urokinase is required for its mitogenic effect. J Biol Chem 1997; **272:** 13390.
11. Lee S, Jilani SM, Nikolova GV, Carpizo D, and Iruela-Arispe ML: Processing of VEGF-A by MMPs regulates bioavailability and vascular patterning in tumors. J Cell Biol 2005; **169:** 681.
12. Lauer G, Sollberg S, Cole M, Flamme I, Stürzebecher J, Mann K, Krieg T, and Eming SA: Expression and proteolysis of VEGF is increased in chronic wounds. J Invest Dermatol 2000; **15:** 12.
13. Lauer G, Sollberg S, Cole M, Krieg T, and Eming SA: Generation of a novel proteolysis resistant VEGF 165 variant by a site-directed mutation at the plasmin sensitive cleavage site. FEBS Lett 2002; **531:** 309.
14. Roth D, Piekarek M, Christ H, Bloch W, Paulsson M, Krieg T, Davidson J, and Eming SA: Plasmin modulates VEGF-A mediated angiogenesis during wound repair. Am J Pathol 2006; **168:** 670.
15. Dor Y, Djonov V, Abramovitch R, Itin A, Fishman GI, Carmeliet P, Goelman G, and Keshet E: Conditional switching of VEGF provides new insights into adult neovascularization and pro-angiogenic therapy. EMBO J 2002; **21:** 1939.
16. Alon T, Hemo I, Itin A, Peer J, Stone J, and Keshet E: VEGF acts as a survival factor for newly formed retinal vessels and has implications for retinopathy of prematurity. Nat Med 1995; **10:** 1024.
17. Whitaker GB, Limberg BJ, and Rosenbaum JS: VEGF receptor-2 and neuropilin-1 form a receptor complex that is responsible for the differential signaling potency of VEGF165 and VEGF121. J Biol Chem 2001; **276:** 25520.
18. Zisch AH, Lutolf MP, Ehrbar M, Raeber GP, Rizzi SC, Davies N, Schmokel H, Bezuidenhout D, Djonov V, Zilla P, and Hubbell JA: Cell-demanded release of VEGF from synthetic, biointeractive cell ingrowth matrices for vascularized tissue growth. FASEB J 2003; **17:** 2260.
19. Schäfer M and Werner S: Cancer as an overhealing wound: an old hypothesis revisited. Nat Rev Mol Cell Biol 2008; **9:** 628.

WHS Wound Healing Society

Angiogenesis in Chronic Wounds

Tengjiao Cui, Robert S. Kirsner, and Jie Li*

Department of Dermatology and Cutaneous Surgery, University of Miami Miller School of Medicine, Miami, Florida.

Background: New blood vessel formation, or angiogenesis, is a critical event in wound healing process. This process involves not only cells but also a variety of growth factors and cytokines, which regulate the activities of their target cells. Normal angiogenesis is characterized by highly orchestrated cell–cell and cell–extracellular matrix interactions, leading to the formation of new vascular structures from their nearby intact blood vessels.

The Problem: In chronic wounds, the process of angiogenesis is impaired, resulting in defective granulation tissue formation, which eventually causes failure of the wound healing to progress through the proliferation phase.

Basic/Clinical Science Advances: Despite significant advance in knowledge regarding normal angiogenesis and wound healing, our understanding of angiogenesis in chronic wounds is still limited. Although some factors, including abnormal growth factor activities, excessive extracellular matrix degradation, and sustained hypoxia, are proposed to be related to impaired angiogenesis in chronic wounds, the details on how these factors affect angiogenesis remain unclear.

Clinical Care Relevance: Growth factor–derived products have been recently applied in treatment of neovascular deficiency in chronic wounds. Research efforts in this field will no doubt benefit our treatment of chronic wounds in the future.

Conclusion: Angiogenesis in chronic wounds is complicated and impaired. Using growth factor–derived substances in treatment of chronic wounds has shown positive, if not overwhelming, results. However, advance in treatment and clinic care of chronic wounds will significantly depend on our knowledge about the biological mechanisms, including angiogenic mechanisms, involved in chronic wound healing.

Abbreviations and Acronyms

ALK = activin receptor–like kinase

BM = basement membrane

ECM = extracellular matrix

EPC = endothelial progenitor cell

FGF = fibroblast growth factor

HBO = hyperbaric oxygen therapy

MMPs = matrix metalloproteinases

rhPDGF-BB = recombinant human platelet–derived growth factor-B homodimer

TGF-β = transforming growth factor-β

VEGF = vascular endothelial growth factor

*Correspondence: Department of Dermatology and Cutaneous Surgery, University of Miami Miller School of Medicine, 1600 NW 10th Ave., RMSB 2049 Miami, Florida 33136 (e-mail: jli@med.miami.edu).

BACKGROUND

Wound angiogenesis refers to the formation of new microvascular blood vessels from adjacent preexisting vessels during wound healing. It is a complicated and highly organized biological process that features growth of new blood vessels from established vessels into wound areas. In adults, endothelial cells of blood vessels are usually quiescent. Immediately after early inflammatory responses, the microvascular endothelial cells are activated by pro-angiogenic factors such as vascular endothelial growth factor (VEGF),[1] fibroblast growth factor (FGF),[2] transforming growth factor-β (TGF-β),[3] and platelet-derived growth factor (PDGF),[4] leading to expression of their target genes, which are critical for endothelial cell migration and proliferation.[5] The migrating endothelial cells follow chemotactic attractions, forming a capillary sprout.[6] Subsequently, endothelial cells align and rearrange along the re-established basement membrane (BM); pericytes

Printed in U.S.A.
DOI: 10.1089/awc.2009.0037

are recruited to stabilize newly formed tubes, resulting in mature and functional capillaries. In normal angiogenesis, interactions between cell–cell, cell–extracellular matrix (ECM), and cell–growth factors are well orchestrated. Disruption of any of these interactions usually results in a nonhealing or chronic wound. Besides, a balance between pro- and anti-angiogenic factors is also important for normal angiogenesis. Soluble VEGF receptor-1, endostatin fragment from type XVIII collagen, angiostatin fragment from plasminogen, and thrombospondin-1 and −2 are well-known endogenous angiogenic inhibitors.[7] Inflammatory cells such as macrophages are involved in angiogenic process by secreting mediators, including pro- and anti-angiogenic factors. Imbalance of pro- and anti-angiogenic factors contributes to healing problems in chronic wounds. In clinic, major chronic wounds include leg ulcers caused by vascular insufficiency and diabetic foot ulcers.[8] It has been estimated that up to 2 million Americans have nonhealing lower extremity wounds. Today, pharmaceutical products and clinic protocols for treatment of angiogenic deficiency–induced chronic wounds are still limited. Advances in this field significantly depend on our understanding about the mechanisms by which a normal angiogenic process is inhibited. Answers to this will provide us future directions for a better prevention and treatment of chronic wounds.

CLINICAL PROBLEM ADDRESSED

Chronic wounds are usually the results of impeded neovascularization. They occur frequently in patients with diabetes, venous, and arterial diseases. Diabetic foot ulcers, for example, heal slowly because of neuropathy, repeated trauma, and, in many cases, insufficient blood supply and dysfunction of blood vessels.[8] Normal angiogenesis depends mainly on endothelial cell migration and proliferation, and appropriate matrix deposition by fibroblasts. In chronic wounds, however, the cell functions are altered by harmful microenvironment at the wounds.[9] It has been reported that wound fluid from chronic ulcers failed to stimulate cell proliferation.[10] Specific mechanisms that are possibly involved in the causal relationship between aberrant angiogenesis and chronic wounds include inadequate ECM/BM degradation, imbalanced growth factor and cytokine activities, and signal transduction problems. For instance, matrix metalloproteinase (MMP) activities were found significantly increased in chronic wounds, which are believed to be correlated with an abnormal ECM/BM degradation in angiogenesis.[11] Further, decreased levels of pro-angiogenic factors, such as VEGF, and increased expression of anti-angiogenic factors, such as soluble VEGF receptor-1, were found associated with human chronic wounds.[7] It should be, however, noted that the pathways that lead to impaired angiogenesis in chronic wounds are not truly known. It is not clear how much of a wound's chronicity is caused by a primary impairment in angiogenesis. Because of the complexity resulted from multiple causal factors in the microenvironment, including infection, hypoxia, and abnormal activities of proteinases, and various comorbidities, such as diabetes and venous stasis, understanding healing process in chronic wounds is therefore challenging. Available treatments of chronic wounds include both standard wound cares, such as debridement, infection control, and endovascular revascularization, as well as adjunctive treatments by hyperbaric oxygen therapy (HBO), electrical stimulation, and recombinant human PDGF-BB (rhPDGF-BB).[12] However, responsiveness and effectiveness are often not satisfactory. Future developments in treatment will mainly depend on our knowledge about healing on the cellular and molecular level, as well as certain pathological conditions associated with chronic wounds.

BASIC SCIENCE CONTEXT

Angiogenesis happens in the proliferation phase of wound healing, in which vascular network extended on collagenous scaffold, leading to the formation of granulation tissue. In this process, growth factors stimulate the release of proteinases, such as MMPs, from endothelial cells, as well as keratinocytes, fibroblasts, and macrophages (Fig. 1). MMPs digest the BM, allowing endothelial cells to sprout from their parent vessels.[6] Subsequently, endothelial cells elongate and align along newly formed BM to form capillary, extending into wound bed. Meanwhile, pericytes are recruited to stabilize the new vessels. This process is highly regulated by growth factors and is disrupted in chronic wounds.

EXPERIMENTAL MODEL

Computational mathematical modeling provides us independent insights into a biological process, which otherwise need time-consuming, technically difficult, often costly experiments to elucidate. The mathematical models that describe the numerous components of the wound healing process, together with their synergistic or antagonistic interactions, give researchers an insight into the mechanisms

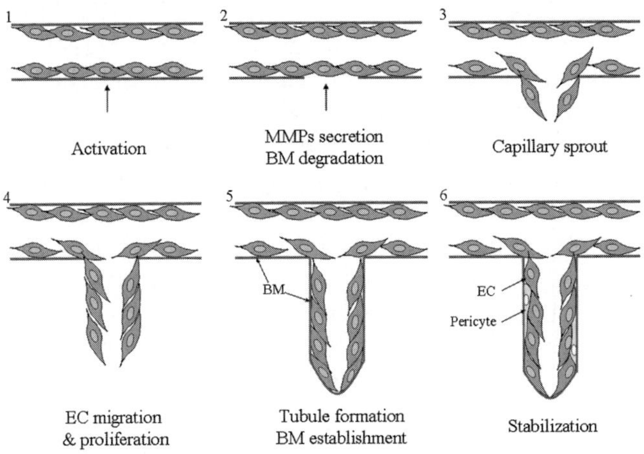

Figure 1. Schematic diagram of angiogenesis and potential points for therapeutic intervention. In an early stage of angiogenesis, quiescent endothelial cells (EC) are stimulated by pro-angiogenic factors, such as vascular endothelial growth factor (VEGF), transforming growth factor-β, fibroblast growth factor (FGF), and platelet-derived growth factor (PDGF). Endothelial cells, fibroblasts, and macrophages produce proteases, such as MMPs, which digest the BM, allowing endothelial cells escape from blood vessels (sprout). Endothelial cells then migrate and proliferate toward chemotactic attractions. Later on, endothelial cells elongate and align with each other along newly formed BM to form new blood vessels. Pericytes and smooth muscle cells (in arteries and veins) are recruited, which help to stabilize newly formed vascular structure and initiate the maturation of the vessels. The whole process of angiogenesis is strictly regulated. Any interruption within the angiogenic process may cause chronic wounds, so that each step of angiogenesis may be a potential point for therapeutic intervention: (i) decreased expression of pro-angiogenic factors, such as VEGF and PDGF, or increased expression of anti-angiogenic factors such as soluble VEGF, inhibits the activation in step 1; (ii) insufficient or excessive proteolytic activities may lead to inadequate extracellular matrix (ECM)/BM degradation in step 2, and prevent EC sprout and migration in steps 3–5; (iii) deficiency of PDGF or FGF may prevent pericyte recruitment in step 6, resulting in impairment of blood vessel stabilization and maturation; (iv) insufficiency of growth factors, such as VEGF, FGF, and transforming growth factor-β, may cause angiogenic inhibition in any step of angiogenesis.

involved. This information is also useful to medical staff for development of treatment methodologies. Today, a few mathematical models of chronic wounds have been developed. For example, Pettet *et al.* were able to simulate wound chronicity by assuming that capillary budding is downregulated.[13] Schugart *et al.* developed a model to address tissue oxygen tension in angiogenesis and wound healing.[14]

Compared to mathematical models, animal models are more widely accepted. Chick chorioallantoic membrane and rabbit corneal have been two common *in vivo* models for angiogenesis. Recently, a number of animal models for chronic wounds have been described. For instance, to study growth factor effects on chronic wounds, growth factor–derived materials are externally applied to animal wounds; in other cases, a transgene encoding a specific growth factor was injected into the wounds.[15] Animal models that mimic human comorbidities, including ischemia, aging, neuropathy, and diabetes, have been created. In another aspect, genetically engineered mice that have either missing genes (knockout) or overexpressing genes for specific factors in wound healing furthered our understanding of the mechanisms, by which these factors regulate the healing process.[16,17]

Last but not least, *in vitro* models, which are relatively easy, rapid, and cost effective, have been widely used to study the cell–cell and cell–matrix interactions, and effects of pro- and anti-angiogenic factors on wound angiogenesis. In addition to commonly used cell proliferation and migration assays, new assays were developed based on the ability of endothelial cells to form tubes in three-dimensional matrices.[18,19]

DISCUSSION OF FINDINGS AND RELEVANT LITERATURE

Usually, the treatment of chronic wounds starts with a sharp debridement to remove dead tissue debris, foci of infection, and senescent cells. The tissue removed may also contain harmful proteinases and growth factor–trapping factors. The purpose of the surgery, in fact, is to reestablish the dynamic process of normal wound healing. However, complete healing of chronic wounds cannot be realized by surgery itself. The associated comorbidities frequently cause healing impairment. Angiogenesis is the central step for wound healing, and has been demonstrated to be associated with almost all chronic wounds. Therefore, it is necessary to understand the mechanisms by which major biological events during angiogenesis are regulated.

Angiogenesis is a complicated and highly regulated process in which many different cells, growth factors, cytokines, and small molecules interact. The commonly recognized growth factors important in angiogenesis include VEGF,[1] FGF,[2] TGF-β,[3] angiopoietins, and PDGF.[4] Among them, angiopoietins are endothelial cell specific, whereas others have a broad range of target cells, such as fibroblasts, keratinocytes, and macrophages in addition to endothelial cells. VEGF is expressed at low levels in normal quiescent endothelium and keratinocytes; its expression can be significantly upregulated in response to the hypoxia after injury. However, the expression of VEGF was found decreased in diabetic wounds, and topical application of VEGF accelerates angiogenesis and wound healing, suggesting that a defect in VEGF regulation might be associated with the impaired angiogenesis.[20] VEGF is a potent mitogen to endothelial cells and stimulates cell proliferation,[21] and has been shown to induce cell migration.[22] VEGF also induces hyperpermeability of blood vessels,[23] which may facilitate endothelial cell migration at the initiation of angiogenesis.

TAKE-HOME MESSAGE

Basic science advances

- Angiogenesis refers to the growth of new blood vessels from preexisting parental vessels during wound healing.
- Angiogenesis is a highly regulated dynamic process, which is characterized by interactions between a variety of cells, growth factors and cytokines, enzymes, and ECM.
- Major cells involved in angiogenesis are endothelial cells, fibroblasts, and inflammatory cells. Stimulated by inflammatory responses, endothelial cells migrate and proliferate from preexisting blood vessels to form new vascular structures. Pericytes are later recruited to help stabilize the newly formed microvessels.
- Dysregulation of growth factors and excess activities of proteinases may contribute to the impairment of angiogenesis in chronic wounds.

Clinical science advances

- Chronic wounds are significantly delayed or sometimes nonhealing wounds. It can happen in any stage during wound healing process. In most cases, chronic wounds are found associated with impaired angiogenesis.
- Factors that cause chronic wounds are still unclear. Several commonly recognized factors include prolonged infections, abnormal activities of growth factors and proteinases, persistent hypoxia, and the like. The complexity of angiogenic problems in chronic wounds is furthered by a variety of comorbidities, such as diabetes mellitus, venous stasis, and arterial diseases that are frequently coexisted.
- Current treatments are mainly developed from our knowledge on normal angiogenesis. To elucidate the fact that specifically control the angiogenic process in chronic wounds will, therefore, provide us more specific and effective solution to solve particular angiogenic problems in chronic wounds.

Relevance to clinical care

- To date, a few growth factor–derived substances have been tested for the treatment of chronic wounds. However, the only Food and Drug Administration–approved product is rhPDGF-BB, or becaplermin. Becaplermin gel has been shown to significantly increase the angiogenesis and healing rate in diabetic foot ulcers.
- Gene therapies, in which a vector carrying specific genes is introduced into wound areas, are undergoing early clinic trials at this moment. These pioneering works show some promising results. For example, the effect of a transgene for human PDGF-B was tested in rabbit ischemic model, and researchers found that PDGF-B application resulted in better granulation tissue formation and wound closure rate.
- Wound hypoxia stimulates angiogenesis. However, sustained high level of hypoxia, as commonly noted in chronic wounds, may block wound angiogenesis. It has been shown that hypoxia inhibits collagen deposition, and oxygen is required for normal activities of fibroblasts, bacteria killing, and angiogenesis. HBO has been used in clinic to systemically increase oxygen level in chronic wounds.[29]

FGF2 has been shown to induce an angiogenic phenotype consisting of increased endothelial cell proliferation and migration, proteinase production, and expression of specific integrins.[24] *Fgf2* knockout mice demonstrated delayed wound repair.[16] FGF2 may also indirectly control angiogenesis in association with other growth factors, such as VEGF and PDGF. FGF2-induced angiogenesis can be inhibited by a neutralizing antibody against VEGF.[25] Besides, FGF2 has been implied to function in vessel maturation via its interaction with PDGF,[26] which displays potent biological activities on mural cells, including pericytes and vascular smooth muscle cells (in arteries and veins). Association of mural cells with newly formed blood vessels contributes to vessel stabilization and maturation. Different from VEGF and FGF, TGF-β was found to stimulate endothelial cell migration while inhibiting proliferation. Studies revealed that endothelial cells express two major TGF-β type I receptors: activin receptor–like kinase 1 (ALK1), involved in pro-angiogenic pathway, and ALK5, associated with anti-angiogenic pathway. TGF-β regulates endothelial cell migration and proliferation via a fine balance between ALK1 and ALK5 signaling.[27]

With regard to the important role of growth factors in angiogenesis, extensive efforts have been executed on developing growth factor therapies for chronic wound-associated angiogenic problems. While a few growth factors have been used in animal or preclinic trials, PDGF-derived rhPDGF-BB, or becaplermin gel, is so far, the only growth factor approved by the Food and Drug Administration for the treatment of diabetic neuropathic foot ulcers. Becaplermin is a homodimeric protein produced by DNA recombination technique. Its biological activity, similar to that of endogenous PDGF, specifically stimulates chemotatic migration and proliferation of endothelial cells, as well as recruits mural cells.[4] In diabetic ulcers, becaplermin was reported to significantly increase the complete healing rate and decrease the healing time.[12] However, the cost of becaplermin ($600/tube) and requirement for twice-a-day dressing changes raise questions about its practical value. Recently, Liechty *et al.* introduced a weakened adenoviral vector carrying human PDGF-B transgene into the wound of a rabbit ischemic model.[15] They found that the wound healing effect was long lasting and dramatic. The granulation tissue and wound closure rate of the treated group significantly exceeded those of the controls. Encouraged by this success, Margolis *et al.* initiated a phase 1 study of rhPDGF-BB injection as an adenoviral transgene into chronic ulcers,[28] and Tissue Repair Company has an ongoing phase 2 trial of PDGF expressed from an adenoviral vector. These pioneer works represent a future direction in treatment of chronic wounds using growth factor–derived protocols.

CAUTION, CRITICAL REMARKS, AND RECOMMENDATIONS

In most cases, a disrupted angiogenesis leads to an impaired wound repair. Therefore, advancement in treatment of chronic wounds will greatly depend on our understanding of the mechanisms that regulate wound angiogenesis at cellular and molecular levels. The more we understand the biological details involved in this process, the more possible that a novel therapeutic product can be developed. Further, it is already known that multiple harming factors, such as a prolonged hypoxia, overproduction of proteinases, inhibited cell proliferation and migration, and persistent infection, are major causes of angiogenic deficiency in chronic wounds. To know how these factors change a normal angiogenic process to an abnormal one will also provide us clues on blocking biological pathways induced by these harmful factors. In consideration of the complexity of angiogenesis in chronic wound, it is therefore not surprising that a combination of different treatments may be applied to achieve a complete healing. At this time, our choices for treatment of angiogenic deficiency in chronic wound are still limited. However, new pharmaceutical products and wound care protocols are expected in the future as our knowledge grows.

FUTURE DEVELOPMENT

In addition to growth factor–derived treatment, other researches in treatment of chronic wounds include gene and stem cell therapies. With gene therapy, plasmid DNA carrying a gene that encodes desired pro-angiogenic growth factors or cytokines is introduced into the wound bed. The rationale of stem cell therapy is based on the finding that bone marrow–derived endothelial progenitor cells (EPCs) also contribute to wound neovascularization. EPCs in bone marrow can be mobilized to the circulation and to the wound upon injury stimulation. In fact, a systematic hyperoxia induced by HBO enhanced the mobilization of EPCs and the neovascularization.[30] In addition, biomaterials, such as hydrogel matrices, have been shown promising for wound treatment. These materials may provide an extracellular scaffold for cells, and function in storing and releasing angiogenic factors. Finally, excessive activities of proteinases are found to be associated with angiogenic defects, which may result in abnormal digestion of growth factors and ECM components. Therefore, controlling the activities of proteinases will be a key factor in managing chronic wounds.

ACKNOWLEDGMENTS

This work was supported in part by grants from the NIH (AR048648 and GM079025) and the Dermatology Foundation of South Florida.

AUTHOR DISCLOSURE STATEMENT

No conflict of interest disclosed.

REFERENCES

1. Roya H, Bhardwaja S, and Yla-Herttuala S: Biology of vascular endothelial growth factors. FEBS Lett 2006; **580:** 2879.

2. Presta M, Dell'Era P, Mitola S, Moroni E, Ronca R, and Rusnati M: Fibroblast growth factor/fibroblast growth factor receptor system in angiogenesis. Cytokine Growth Factor Rev 2005; **16:** 159.

3. Goumans MJ, Liu Z, and Dijke P: TGF-β signaling in vascular biology and dysfunction. Cell Res 2009; **19:** 116.

4. Andrae J, Gallini R, and Betsholtz C: Role of platelet-derived growth factors in physiology and medicine. Genes Dev 2008; **22:** 1276.

5. Gerritsen ME and Bloor CM: Endothelial cell gene expression in response to injury. FASEB J 1993; **7:** 523.

6. van Hinsbergh VW and Koolwijk P: Endothelial sprouting and angiogenesis: matrix metalloproteinases in the lead. Cardiovasc Res 2008; **78:** 203.

7. Eming SA, Lauer G, Cole M, Jurk S, Christ H, Hornig C, Krieg T, and Weich HA: Increased levels of the soluble variant of the vascular endothelial growth factor receptor VEGFR-1 are associated with a poor prognosis in wound healing. J Invest Dermatol 2004; **123:** 799.

8. Dinh T and Veves A: Microcirculation of the diabetic foot. Curr Pharm Des 2005; **11:** 301.

9. Falanga V: Chronic wounds: pathophysiologic and experimental considerations. J Invest Dermatol 1993; **100:** 721.

10. Bucalo B, Eaglstein WH, and Falanga V: Inhibition of cell proliferation by chronic wound fluid. Wound Repair Regen 1993; **1:** 181.

11. Trengove NJ, Stacey MC, Macauley S, Bennett N, Gibson J, Burslem F, Murphy G, and Schultz G: Analysis of the acute and chronic wound environments: the role of proteases and their inhibitors. Wound Repair Regen 1999; **7:** 442.

12. Steed DL: Clinical evaluation of recombinant human platelet-derived growth factor for the treatment of lower extremity ulcers. Plast Resconstr Surg 2006; **117 (Suppl):** 143.

13. Pettet GJ, Byrne HM, Mcelwain DLS, and Norbury J: A model of wound-healing angiogenesis in soft tissue. Math Biosci 1996; **136:** 35.

14. Schugart RC, Friedman A, Zhao R, and Sen CK: Wound angiogenesis as a function of tissue oxygen tension: a mathematical model. PNAS 2008; **105:** 2628.

15. Liechty KW, Nesbit M, Herlyn M, Radu A, Adzick NS, and Crombleholme TM: Adenoviral-mediated overexpression of platelet-derived growth factor-B corrects ischemic impaired wound healing. J Invest Dermatol 1999; **113:** 375.

16. Ortega S, Ittmann M, Tsang SH, Ehrlich M, and Basilico C: Neuronal defects and delayed wound healing in mice lacking fibroblast growth factor 2. PNAS 1998; **95:** 5672.

17. Magnusson P, Rolny C, Jakobsson L, Wikner C, Wu Y, Hicklin DJ, and Welsh LC: Deregulation of Flk-1/vascular endothelial growth factor receptor-2 in fibroblast growth factor receptor-1-deficient vascular stem cell development. J Cell Sci 2004; **117:** 1513.

18. Crabtree B and Subramanian V: Behavior of endothelial cells on Matrigel and development of a method for a rapid and reproducible *in vitro* angiogenesis assay. In Vitro Cell Dev Biol Anim 2007; **43:** 87.

19. Li J, Zhou L, Tran HT, Chen Y, Nguyen N, Karasek MA, and Marinkovich MP: Overexpression of laminin-8 in human dermal microvascular endothelial cells promotes angiogenesis-related functions. J Invest Dermatol 2006; **126:** 432.

20. Galiano RD, Tepper OM, Pelo CR, Bhatt KA, Callaghan M, Bastidas N, Bunting S, Steinmetz HG, and Gurtner GC: Topical vascular endothelial growth factor accelerates diabetic wound healing through increased angiogenesis and by mobilizing and recruiting bone marrow-derived cells. Am J Pathol 2004; **164:** 1935.

21. Wu LW, Mayo LD, Dunbar JD, Kessler KM, Baerwald MR, Jaffe EA, Wang DF, Warren RS, and Donner DB: Utilization of distinct signaling pathways by receptors for vascular endothelial cell growth factor and other mitogens in the induction of endothelial cell proliferation. J Biol Chem 2000; **275:** 5096.

22. Senger DR, Claffey KP, Benes JE, Perruzzi CA, Sergiou AP, and Detmar M: Angiogenesis promoted by vascular endothelial growth factor: regulation through $\alpha1\beta1$ and $\alpha2\beta1$ integrins. PNAS 1997; **94:** 13612.

23. Nagy JA, Benjamin L, Zeng HY, Dvorak AM, and Dvorak HF: Vascular permeability, vascular hyperpermeability and angiogenesis. Angiogenesis 2008; **11:** 109.

24. Klein S, Giancotti FG, Presta M, Albelda SM, Buck CA, and Rifkin DB: Basic fibroblast growth factor modulates integrin expression in microvascular endothelial cells. Mol Biol Cell 1993; **4:** 973.

25. Seghezzi G, Patel S, Ren CJ, Gualandris A, Pintucci G, Robbins ES, Shapiro RL, Galloway AC, Rifkin DB, and Mignatti P: Fibroblast growth factor-2 (FGF-2) induces vascular endothelial growth factor (VEGF) expression in the endothelial cells of forming capillaries: an autocrine mechanism contributing to angiogenesis. J Cell Biol 1998; **141:** 1659.

26. Cao R, Brakenhielm E, Pawliuk R, Wariaro D, Post MJ, Wahlberg E, Leboulch P, and Cao Y: Angiogenic synergism, vascular stability and improvement of hind-limb ischemia by a combination of PDGF-BB and FGF-2. Nat Med 2003; **9:** 604.

27. Goumans MJ, Valdimarsdottir G, Itoh S, Rosendahl A, Sideras P, and Dijke P: Balancing the activation state of the endothelium via two distinct TGF-beta type I receptors. EMBO J 2002; **21:** 1743.

28. Margolis DJ, Crombleholme T, and Herlyn M: Clinical protocol: phase I trial to evaluate the safety of H5.020CMV.PDGF-B for the treatment of a diabetic insensate foot ulcer. Wound Repair Regen 2000; **8:** 480.

29. Thackham JA, McElwain DLS, and Long RJ: The use of hyperbaric oxygen therapy to treat chronic wounds: a review. Wound Repair Regen 2008; **16:** 321.

30. Liu ZJ and Velazquez OC: Hyperoxia, endothelial progenitor cell mobilization, and diabetic wound healing. Antioxid Redox Signal 2008; **10:** 1869.

WHS
Wound
Healing
Society

Tiny New Genes Called MicroRNAs Regulate Blood Vessel Formation

Chandan K. Sen*

Comprehensive Wound Center, The Ohio State University Medical Center, Columbus, Ohio.

Background: The recent discovery of microRNAs (miRs), recognized by Nobel Prize in 2006 and Lasker Award in 2008, caused a major shift in our understanding of the central dogma in molecular biology. Previously, genes that did not code proteins were summarily discarded as junk genes. Now, a small fraction of these junk genes—known as miRs—have emerged as key regulators of numerous aspects of tissue biology and function.
The Problem: Encoding genes make proteins. How is this process regulated? This is a major issue because such fundamental information is likely to be implicated in all aspects of human health and disease. Specifically, this article is a digest of select current reports describing how miRs regulate new blood vessel formation or angiogenesis. Impaired angiogenesis is recognized as a key limitation in several types of problem wounds.
Basic/Clinical Science Advances: In 2005–2008, the first series of observations establishing key significance of miRs in the regulation of vascular biology came from experimental studies involved in arresting miRNA biogenesis to deplete the miR pools of vascular tissues and cells. Dicer-dependent biogenesis of miRNA is required for blood vessel development during embryogenesis and wound healing.
Clinical Care Relevance: miR-based therapeutics represents one of the major commercial hotspots in today's biotechnology and clinical therapeutics market space.
Conclusion: As specific miRs are recognized for their ability to regulate specific biological functions, miR delivery and silencing technologies will emerge as a major therapeutic tool in the clinic. Understanding of the mechanism involved in the regulation of wound healing and angiogenesis by miRs therefore represents one of the most promising emergent areas in wound research and care.

Abbreviations and Acronyms

EGFR = epidermal growth factor receptor
HMECs = human microvascular endothelial cells
miR = microRNA
miRNA = microRNA
NADPH = nicotinamide adenine dinucleotide phosphate
ncRNA = noncoding RNA
nt = nucleotide
ROS = reactive oxygen species
siRNA = short interfering RNA
UTR = untranslated region
VEGF = vascular endothelial growth factor

*Correspondence: Comprehensive Wound Center, The Ohio State University Medical Center, 473W 12 Ave., Columbus, Ohio 43210 (e-mail: chandan.sen@osumc.edu.).

BACKGROUND

GENES MAKE PROTEINS, and proteins have a function that in turn makes life possible—this central dogma of biology had to be revisited in light of the discovery of microRNAs (miRs). We have known that DNA replicates its genetic information contained within nucleotide (nt) sequences and transcribes it to RNA, where it codes for the production of mRNA. Do the vast majority of nts in RNA carry the code to synthesize protein? No. However, almost all means of gene identification assume that genes encode proteins. The central dogma ignored a significant part of the genetic code, which remained under veils for decades. Noncoding RNA (ncRNA) genes produce functional RNA molecules rather than encoding proteins. Several different systematic screens have identified a surprisingly large number of ncRNA genes.[1] These RNAs (including those derived from introns) appear to comprise a

Printed in U.S.A.
DOI: 10.1089/awc.2009.0165

heretofore hidden layer of internal signals that control various levels of gene expression in physiology and development. This hidden layer of internal signals is now emerging to be of such critical significance that lack of consideration of that layer poses the serious risk of clouding our ability to understand the molecular basis of health and disease.[1–4] In all forms of life, ncRNA includes ribosomal RNA, transfer RNA, small nuclear RNA, small nucleolar RNA, interference RNA, short interfering RNA (siRNA), and micro RNA (miRNA). miRNAs are powerful regulators of gene expression. It is estimated that about 3% of human genes encode for miRNAs.[5] An miRNA is approximately 22 ribonucleotides-long non-coding RNA, with a potential to recognize multiple mRNA targets guided by sequence complementarity and RNA-binding proteins (Fig. 1). Recent evidence suggests that the number of unique miRNA genes in humans exceeds 1000.[6] The numbers of miRNAs and their targets turn out to be much greater than what we previously thought.[7] miRNAs are functionally versatile, with the capacity to specifically inhibit translation initiation or elongation, and induce mRNA destabilization, through predominantly targeting the 3′-untranslated regions (UTR) of mRNA.[8]

CLINICAL PROBLEM ADDRESSED

Wound vascularization represents a critical component of the successful wound healing process.[9] It is marked by endothelial cell migration and capillary formation where the migration of capillaries into the wound bed is critical for proper wound healing. The granulation phase and tissue deposition require nutrients supplied by the capillaries, and failure of this to occur will result in a chronically unhealed wound. The significant role of angiogenesis can be demonstrated in diseases like diabetes, or experimental models where this healing mechanism is impaired.[10–13]

BASIC SCIENCE CONTEXT

How do miRs function? miRNAs are functionally versatile, with the capacity to specifically inhibit translation initiation or elongation, and induce mRNA destabilization, through predominantly targeting the 3′-UTRs of mRNA. Briefly, miRNAs

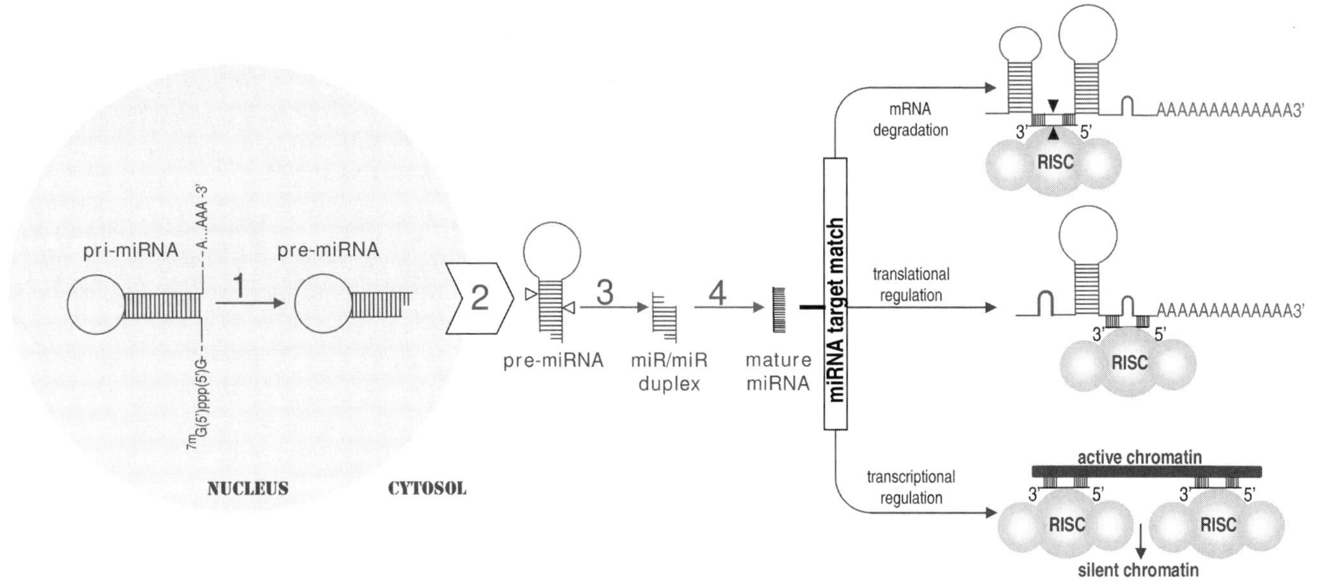

Figure 1. Overview of the major mechanisms involved in the generation and function of miRNAs. Primary transcripts of miRNAs (pri-miRNAs) are generated by polymerase II and possess a 5′ 7-methyl guanosine cap and are polyadenylated. Processing of pri-miRNAs in the nucleus is mediated by a microprocessor complex (1) including Pasha and Drosha. Drosha is an RNase III endonuclease that asymmetrically cleaves both strands of the hairpin stem at sites near the base of the primary stem loop, thus releasing a 60- to 70-nucleotide pre-miRNA that has a 5′ phosphate and a 2-nucleotide 3′ overhang. Specific RNA cleavage by Drosha predetermines the mature miRNA sequence and provides the substrate for subsequent processing events. The pre-miRNAs are transported to the cytoplasm by Exportin-5 (2). Once in the cytosol, a second RNase III endonuclease, Dicer (3), cleaves the pre-miRNA. Dicer releases a 22-nucleotide mature double-stranded miRNA with 5′ phosphates and 2-nucleotide 3′ overhangs. One strand of the miRNA duplex is subsequently incorporated into an effector complex termed RNA-induced silencing complex (4) or RNA-induced silencing complex (RISC) that mediates target gene expression. miRNA-induced mRNA degradation is commonly seen in plants. Translational regulation by miRNA is common in animals. Regulation of transcription by miRNA is common in yeast and plants. This mechanism is possibly functional in animals as well.

are transcribed in the nucleus by conventional mechanisms and are exported to the cytoplasm,[8] where after biological processing they form mature miRNAs that can interact with matching mRNAs by RNA–RNA binding. This binding, with the assistance of the RNA-induced silencing complex, leads to modes of action resulting in mRNA degradation or translational inhibition.[14] This mechanism of action is termed as posttranscriptional gene regulation. In animals, in contrast to plants, there is not 100% nt match between miRNA and its target mRNA, leading to a mode of action causing mRNA translational inhibition and not mRNA degradation.[15] The interaction between the miRNA and its matching mRNA occurs between the 5′ UTR of the miRNA to the 3′ UTR region of the mRNA by a matching seed element in the miRNA. Utilizing these data, computational prediction approaches estimate that miRNAs can target 30% of the human genome.[5,16–18] Other estimates claim that over 50% of human protein-coding genes might be regulated by miRNAs.[19] Further, one miRNA can regulate hundreds of genes,[19] and that one gene can be regulated by a number of miRNAs.

EXPERIMENTAL MODEL OR MATERIAL

In 2005–2008, the first series of observations establishing key significance of miRNAs in the regulation of mammalian vascular biology came from experimental studies involved in arresting miRNA biogenesis to deplete the miRNA pools of vascular tissues and cells.[20–23] Dicer, a member of the ribonuclease III family of enzymes, processes double-stranded RNA substrates into approximately 21- to 27-nt products that trigger sequence-directed gene silencing by RNA interference. The mechanism of RNA recognition and length-specific cleavage by Dicer has been established. Dicer represents a key enzyme involved in miRNA biogenesis.[24] In the study of embryonic angiogenesis it has been reported that the Dicer gene is significantly expressed in 11-day embryos and remains constant through day 17, evenly expressed throughout the embryonic tissues.[20] The *dicer*$^{ex1/2}$ mutant mouse model has been investigated.[20] Support for the involvement of miRNAs in angiogenesis also comes from *in vitro* studies investigating human umbilical vein endothelial cells or human microvascular endothelial cells (HMECs).[23,25]

DISCUSSION OF FINDINGS AND RELEVANT LITERATURE

The *dicer*$^{ex1/2}$ mutant mouse lacking the first two exons of *dicer* that are essential for the function of the protein represents a tool that has shed light on embryonic angiogenesis. Homozygous mutant mice were not viable; therefore, the embryos were examined. Starting from embryonic day 11.5, virtually all *dicer*$^{ex1/2}$ embryos were growth and developmentally retarded compared with their wild-type or heterozygous litter mates. The embryos that were still viable at this stage had thin and suboptimally developed blood vessels, providing first evidence for the involvement of miRNAs in angiogenesis.[20] Microscopic examination of the yolk sacs from the mutant embryos revealed that there were fewer blood vessels in the *dicer*$^{ex1/2}$ yolk sacs and that these vessels were thin, small, and less organized than those of control yolk sacs. These observations indicate that Dicer-dependent biogenesis of miRNA is required for blood vessel development during embryogenesis.

Support for the involvement of miRNAs in angiogenesis also comes from *in vitro* studies.[25] Large-scale analysis of miRNA expression in human umbilical vein endothelial cells led to the observation that among those miRNAs that are highly expressed, there are 15 that may target the receptors of angiogenic factors. In particular, miR-221 and miR-222 were identified as regulating c-Kit expression as well as the angiogenic properties of the c-kit ligand Stem Cell Factor. The miR-221/2 and c-Kit interaction represents an integral component of a complex circuit that controls the ability of endothelial cells to form new capillaries.[25] Inhibition of c-kit results in reduced vascular endothelial growth factor (VEGF) expression.[26] Further, we know that c-kit is involved in neovascularization.[27,28] In addition to Dicer, Drosha is an miRNA-processing enzyme that is required for the maturation of miRNAs. The maintenance and regulation of endogenous miRNA levels via Dicer-mediated processing is critical for endothelial cell gene expression and functions *in vitro*.[22] The significance of both Dicer and Drosha in driving angiogenesis *in vitro* has been reported.[21,22] Silencing of Dicer and Drosha significantly attenuated capillary sprouting of endothelial cells and tube-forming activity. Migration of endothelial cells was significantly decreased in Dicer siRNA–transfected cells, whereas Drosha siRNA had no effect. Silencing of Dicer, but not of Drosha, reduces angiogenesis *in vivo*. The let-7 family and mir-27b are recognized as key regulators of the angiogenic responses of endothelial cells.

Several studies have demonstrated a central role of nicotinamide adenine dinucleotide phosphate (NADPH) oxidase–derived reactive oxygen species (ROS) as signaling messengers in driving angiogenesis.[29–32] Whether such redox control of angiogenesis is subject to regulation by miRNA remains unknown. A recent study in our laboratory presents first evidence that cellular redox state, a key driver of cell signaling, is regulated by miRNAs. In this work, a Dicer knockdown approach was used to test the significance of miRNAs in regulating the redox state and angiogenic response of HMECs. Lowering of miRNA content by Dicer knockdown induced VEGF expression but diminished the angiogenic response of HMECs as determined by cell migration and Matrigel tube formation. Such impairment of angiogenic response in the Matrigel was rescued by exogenous low micromolar H_2O_2. Dicer knockdown HMECs demonstrated lower inducible production of ROS when activated with phorbol ester, tumor necrosis factor-α, or VEGF. Limiting the production of ROS by antioxidant treatment or NADPH oxidase knockdown approaches impaired angiogenic responses. Experiments to identify how ROS production is limited by Dicer knockdown identified lower expression of p47phox protein in these cells. This lowering of cellular miRNA content induced expression of the transcription factor HBP1, a suppressor transcription factor that negatively regulates p47phox expression. Knockdown of HBP1 restored the angiogenic response of miRNA-deficient HMECs.[23,33] Results of this study lead to the hypothesis that miRNAs regulate wound angiogenesis and may therefore influence wound healing outcomes. That miRNA may be implicated in wound healing is observed from another independent line of investigation examining the function of argonaute proteins. The argonautes represent a cadre of evolutionarily conserved proteins that directly associate with and are required for miRNA function. The core miRNA–ribonucleic–protein complex, composed of the miRNA and an Ago protein, functions as a highly modifiable scaffold that associates with specific mRNAs via the bound miRNA and facilitates the localized activity of a variety of accessory proteins.[34] The expression of Ago-2, critically important in mammalian RNAi, is regulated by the epidermal growth factor receptor (EGFR)/mitogen-activated protein kinase signaling pathway. The pharmacological inhibitor of mitogen-activated protein kinase kinase, U0126, or a siRNA directed against EGFR limits Ago-2

TAKE-HOME MESSAGE

Basic science advances

- miRs comprise a class of small endogenous ncRNAs that posttranscriptionally repress gene expression by base-pairing with their target mRNAs.
- Coding genes may or may not express proteins depending on miR regulation.
- Dicer-dependent miR biogenesis is required to enable angiogenesis.
- Understanding the molecular pathways leading to angiogenesis is incomplete without consideration of the role of miR.
- miR regulates cellular redox signaling and may therefore regulate numerous aspects of cell biology and function relevant to wound healing.
- National Institutes of Health (NIH) has earmarked grants to support small businesses developing technologies that can detect, isolate, and characterize disease-relevant miR.

Clinical science advances

- miR-based therapeutics now represents one of the major commercial hotspots. For example, in 2008 GlaxoSmithKline and Regulus Therapeutics formed strategic alliance to develop microRNA-targeted therapeutics to treat inflammatory diseases.
- The discovery of miRs as regulators of gene expression has created new options for the design of therapeutic agents that could modify gene expression in disease.
- Functional outcomes *in vivo* are often regulated by a large number of gene products that act in concert. Modulating one miR is likely to regulate the expression of a variety of functionally related genes.
- The ability to modulate miRNA activity *in vivo* is promising to induce wound angiogenesis.

Relevance to clinical care

- At present, miR therapy has not been tested for effects on wound healing. Trials addressing several other disorders are in progress, however. For example, the feasibility of miR delivery agents and inhibitors is supported by preclinical models and ongoing clinical trials with oligo-based therapeutics. Macugen (Pegaptinib) developed by Eyetech (now OSI Pharmaceuticals, Melville, NY) is an FDA-approved RNA-based drug that treats patients with age-related macular degeneration by binding to VEGF. Sirna (now Merck, Whitehouse Station, NJ) developed siRNA-027, an siRNA targeting VEGFR-1, which has entered a phase II clinical trial for the treatment of age-related macular degeneration. Alnylam has initiated a phase I human clinical trial of an inhaled formulation of ALN-RSV01, an siRNA-based drug for the treatment of respiratory syncytial virus (RSV) infections. The inhaled formulation of ALN-RSV01 used in this phase I study is delivered via a nebulizer and advances previous clinical work for ALN-RSV01 administered as an intranasal spray. The company previously completed two phase I human clinical trials of ALN-RSV01 using an intranasal formulation and demonstrated that ALN-RSV01 was safe and well tolerated in healthy volunteers.

expression.[35] Ago-2 overexpression enhances cell proliferation, attenuates cell–cell adhesion, and increases cell migration in an *in vitro* wound healing setting.[35]

CAUTION, CRITICAL REMARKS, AND RECOMMENDATIONS

At this time, the miR field is in its infancy, requiring thorough understanding of the underlying mechanisms before therapeutic applications may be concerned. Because each miR may have numerous gene targets, appropriate safety tests are needed to ensure that any beneficial outcome of miR-directed therapies is not dwarfed by risks that may present on a long-term basis. Understanding how each miR may influence the gene network in any given tissue and its functional consequences should provide lucrative returns.

FUTURE DEVELOPMENTS

First and foremost, it is critically important that studies to uncover miR-dependent biological mechanisms are undertaken in the field of wound healing. It would be important to delineate the significance of miR in different aspects of the biology of wound healing. From a therapeutic standpoint, the development of safe molecular tools to specifically manipulate miR expression *in vitro* as well as *in vivo* should have tremendous impact.

ACKNOWLEDGMENTS

Wound healing research in the author's laboratory is funded by National Institutes of Health awards GM 077185 and GM 069589.

AUTHOR DISCLOSURE STATEMENT

No conflict of interest disclosed.

REFERENCES

1. Mattick JS and Makunin IV: Non-coding RNA. Hum Mol Genet 2006; **15 Spec No 1:** R17.

2. Goodrich JA and Kugel JF: Non-coding-RNA regulators of RNA polymerase II transcription. Nat Rev Mol Cell Biol 2006; **7:** 612.

3. Tomaru Y and Hayashizaki Y: Cancer research with non-coding RNA. Cancer Sci 2006; **97:** 1285.

4. Racz Z and Hamar P: Can siRNA technology provide the tools for gene therapy of the future? Curr Med Chem 2006; **13:** 2299.

5. Sassen S, Miska EA, and Caldas C: MicroRNA: implications for cancer. Virchows Arch 2008; **452:** 1.

6. Perera RJ and Ray A: MicroRNAs in the search for understanding human diseases. BioDrugs 2007; **21:** 97.

7. Ro S, Park C, Young D, Sanders KM, and Yan W: Tissue-dependent paired expression of miRNAs. Nucleic Acids Res 2007; **35:** 5944.

8. Yi R, Qin Y, Macara IG, and Cullen BR: Exportin-5 mediates the nuclear export of pre-microRNAs and short hairpin RNAs. Genes Dev 2003; **17:** 3011.

9. Roy S, Khanna S, and Sen CK: Redox regulation of the VEGF signaling path and tissue vascularization: hydrogen peroxide, the common link between physical exercise and cutaneous wound healing. Free Radic Biol Med 2008; **44:** 180.

10. Cox L: Present angiogenesis research and its possible future implementation in wound care. J Wound Care 2003; **12:** 225.

11. Eming SA, Brachvogel B, Odorisio T, and Koch M: Regulation of angiogenesis: wound healing as a model. Prog Histochem Cytochem 2007; **42:** 115.

12. Rattan SI, Sejersen H, Fernandes RA, and Luo W: Stress-mediated hormetic modulation of aging, wound healing, and angiogenesis in human cells. Ann NY Acad Sci 2007; **1119:** 112.

13. Tonnesen MG, Feng X, and Clark RA: Angiogenesis in wound healing. J Investig Dermatol Symp Proc 2000; **5:** 40.

14. Tang G: siRNA and miRNA: an insight into RISCs. Trends Biochem Sci 2005; **30:** 106.

15. Carrington JC and Ambros V: Role of microRNAs in plant and animal development. Science 2003; **301:** 336.

16. Lewis BP, Burge CB, and Bartel DP: Conserved seed pairing, often flanked by adenosines, indicates that thousands of human genes are microRNA targets. Cell 2005; **120:** 15.

17. Kruger J and Rehmsmeier M: RNAhybrid: microRNA target prediction easy, fast and flexible. Nucleic Acids Res 2006; **34:** W451.

18. Smalheiser NR and Torvik VI: Complications in mammalian microRNA target prediction. Methods Mol Biol 2006; **342:** 115.

19. Wu W, Sun M, Zou GM, and Chen J: MicroRNA and cancer: current status and prospective. Int J Cancer 2007; **120:** 953.

20. Yang WJ, Yang DD, Na S, Sandusky GE, Zhang Q, and Zhao G: Dicer is required for embryonic angiogenesis during mouse development. J Biol Chem 2005; **280:** 9330.

21. Kuehbacher A, Urbich C, Zeiher AM, and Dimmeler S: Role of Dicer and Drosha for endothelial microRNA expression and angiogenesis. Circ Res 2007; **101:** 59.

22. Suarez Y, Fernandez-Hernando C, Pober JS, and Sessa WC: Dicer dependent microRNAs regulate gene expression and functions in human endothelial cells. Circ Res 2007; **100:** 1164.

23. Shilo S, Roy S, Khanna S, and Sen CK: Evidence for the involvement of miRNA in redox regulated angiogenic response of human microvascular endothelial cells. Arterioscler Thromb Vasc Biol 2008; **28:** 471.

24. Jaskiewicz L and Filipowicz W: Role of Dicer in posttranscriptional RNA silencing. Curr Top Microbiol Immunol 2008; **320:** 77.

25. Poliseno L, Tuccoli A, Mariani L, Evangelista M, Citti L, Woods K, Mercatanti A, Hammond S, and Rainaldi G: MicroRNAs modulate the angiogenic properties of HUVEC. Blood 2006; **108:** 3068.

26. Litz J and Krystal GW: Imatinib inhibits c-Kit-induced hypoxia-inducible factor-1alpha activity and vascular endothelial growth factor expression in small cell lung cancer cells. Mol Cancer Ther 2006; **5:** 1415.

27. Strumberg D: Preclinical and clinical development of the oral multikinase inhibitor sorafenib in cancer treatment. Drugs Today (Barc) 2005; **41:** 773.

28. Roboz GJ, Giles FJ, List AF, Cortes JE, Carlin R, Kowalski M, Bilic S, Masson E, Rosamilia M, Schuster MW, Laurent D, and Feldman EJ: Phase 1 study of PTK787/ZK 222584, a small molecule tyrosine kinase receptor inhibitor, for the treatment of acute myeloid leukemia and myelodysplastic syndrome. Leukemia 2006; **20:** 952.

29. Cave AC, Brewer AC, Narayanapanicker A, Ray R, Grieve DJ, Walker S, and Shah AM: NADPH

oxidases in cardiovascular health and disease. Antioxid Redox Signal 2006; **8:** 691.

30. Roy S, Khanna S, Nallu K, Hunt TK, and Sen CK: Dermal wound healing is subject to redox control. Mol Ther 2006; **13:** 211.

31. Sen CK, Khanna S, Babior BM, Hunt TK, Ellison EC, and Roy S: Oxidant-induced vascular endothelial growth factor expression in human keratinocytes and cutaneous wound healing. J Biol Chem 2002; **277:** 33284.

32. Ushio-Fukai M: VEGF signaling through NADPH oxidase-derived ROS. Antioxid Redox Signal 2007; **9:** 731.

33. Shilo S, Roy S, Khanna S, and Sen CK: MicroRNA in cutaneous wound healing: a new paradigm. DNA Cell Biol 2007; **26:** 227.

34. Hammell CM: The microRNA-argonaute complex: a platform for mRNA modulation. RNA Biol 2008; **5:** 123.

35. Adams BD, Claffey KP, and White BA: Argonaute-2 expression is regulated by EGFR/MAPK signaling and correlates with a transformed phenotype in breast cancer cells. Endocrinology 2009; **150:** 14.

Section 8

Gene- and Protein-Based Therapies

Section Editors: Jeffrey M. Davidson and Sabine A. Eming

Gene Transfer Techniques for Therapeutic Angiogenesis

Sundeep G. Keswani and Timothy M. Crombleholme*

Division of General, Thoracic, and Fetal Surgery, Center for Molecular Fetal Therapy, Cincinnati Children's Hospital Medical Center and the University of Cincinnati College of Medicine, Cincinnati, Ohio.

Background: The goal of therapeutic angiogenesis is to improve neovascularization in impaired tissue with the expectation that it will produce improved cellular, nutrient, and oxygen delivery resulting in enhanced wound healing. Gene transfer of proangiogenic growth factors to the wound has been demonstrated to achieve this goal.

The Problem: There are numerous candidate transgenes and several gene delivery systems that have been examined. In this article, we review the most significant candidate transgenes, and the advantages and disadvantages of the currently available gene transfer techniques.

Basic/Clinical Science Advances: Neovascularization is a complex process that is regulated by families of angiogenic growth factors, the most potent one being vascular endothelial growth factor. Vascular endothelial growth factor is primarily responsible for new vessel formation. Recently, new targets of angiogenesis have been elucidated. Stromal cell–derived factor-1, endothelial nitric oxide synthase, and the upstream transcription factor, hypoxia inducible factor-1 alpha, form a complex system that controls the wound's response to injury and represent new candidate vulnerary transgenes for therapeutic angiogenesis. To deliver these transgenes, there are both viral and nonviral gene transfer systems that can be used for *in vivo* or *ex vivo* gene transfer.

Clinical Care Relevance: Effective and efficient growth factor–induced neovascularization delivered by gene transfer techniques would represent a significant advance in the care of patients with chronic nonhealing wounds.

Conclusion: Gene transfer techniques of proangiogenic growth factors can positively influence the wound's neovascularization and wound repair response to tissue injury. The ideal candidate vulnerary transgene and gene delivery techniques are in the process of being determined.

Abbreviations and Acronyms

AAV = adeno-associated virus

Ad = adenovirus

EPC = endothelial progenitor cell

HIF-1α = hypoxia inducible factor-1 alpha

NOS = nitric oxide synthase

PDGF = platelet-derived growth factor

SDF-1 = stromal cell–derived factor-1

VEGF = vascular endothelial growth factor

*Correspondence: Division of General, Thoracic, and Fetal Surgery, The Center for Molecular Fetal Therapy, Cincinnati Children's Hospital Medical Center and the University of Cincinnati College of Medicine, 3333 Burnet Ave., Cincinnati, Ohio 45229-3039 (e-mail: timothy.crombleholme@cchmc.org).

BACKGROUND

CHRONIC NONHEALING WOUNDS represent a significant healthcare issue. Many of these wounds are found in patients with comorbidities such as diabetes, peripheral vascular disease, and chronic venous stasis and pressure ulcers. It has been demonstrated that these wounds are characterized by decreased growth factor and cytokine levels that result in an altered neovascularization and wound repair response to tissue injury. An initial strategy to correct this deficit was the topical supplementation of soluble growth factors to the wound that results in enhanced wound healing and neovascularization and provides proof of concept that therapeutic administration of select growth factors can favorably influence the wound milieu.[1] However, *in vivo* results with exogenous growth factor administration have been less than optimal.[2] For effective therapy, the delivery of growth factors to the wound would have to be more efficient and have

Printed in U.S.A.
DOI: 10.1089/awc.2009.0111

more sustained action to overcome natural barriers presented by the chronic wound. Given the limitations of topically applied growth factors, the concept of using viral and nonviral vector–mediated induction of transgene expression of essential growth factors by cells contributing to the wound healing response is particularly attractive.

Over the last several years, the model of therapeutic angiogenesis has evolved.[3] This model includes therapies that aim to restore blood vessels to ischemic tissue to increase cellular, nutrient, and oxygen delivery to the affected tissue. Gene transfer of proangiogenic growth factors to the wound can result in therapeutic angiogenesis.[4–15] However, because the wound healing and neovascularization response is mediated by numerous growth factors and cytokines that orchestrate diverse cellular functions, which vulnerary transgene would potentially be the most effective? This has been an active area of research in selecting the most efficient growth factor to employ. The development of transgenic mice, gene silencing, and overexpression technology have identified several candidates and coupled with their gene transfer techniques will be the focus of this chapter (Fig. 1).

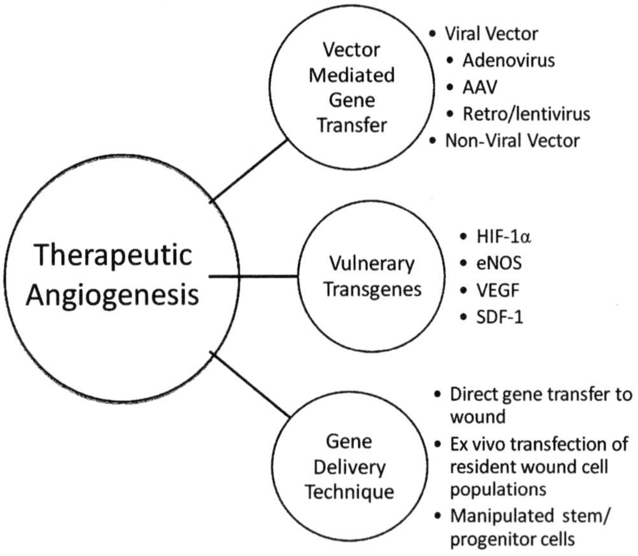

Figure 1. Gene transfer techniques for therapeutic angiogenesis. The goals of therapeutic angiogenesis are to improve neovascularization in impaired tissue with the expectation that it will produce improved cellular, nutrient, and oxygen delivery resulting in enhanced wound healing. There are three basic components needed to achieve this goal using gene transfer techniques. First, the ideal vector for gene transfer must be determined; currently, there are viral and nonviral vectors. Second, active investigations have demonstrated several new promising candidate vulnerary transgenes, but the ideal transgene or combination has yet to be determined. Last, gene transfer can be achieved by direct application to the wound, ex vivo transfection of resident wound cell populations such as fibroblast or keratinocytes and then administered to the wound, and finally stem and progenitor cells can be genetically manipulated and then administered to the wound to either differentiate into specific cell types or act as growth factor production units.

CLINICAL PROBLEM ADDRESSED

Tissue repair represents a dynamic, complex interactive sequence of events. Wound neovascularization is a critical component of this process. This has been shown to be deficient in several chronic disease states such as diabetes, peripheral vascular disease, and venous stasis ulcers, for which the subsequent clinical treatment accounts for billions in healthcare spending. Effective and efficient growth factor–induced neovascularization delivered by gene transfer techniques would represent a significant advance in the care of these patients.

RELEVANT BASIC SCIENCE CONTEXT

Neovascularization is the growth of newly formed blood vessels that is required for the delivery of oxygen and nutrients to regenerating tissue. Multiple growth factors released locally in the wound have direct or indirect angiogenic effects and include transforming growth factor-beta 1 (TGF-β1), platelet-derived growth factor (PDGF-B), basic fibroblast growth factor, and particularly vascular endothelial growth factor (VEGF).[14] The principal cell type traditionally thought to be involved in the process of angiogenesis is the microvascular endothelial cell. Intense investigation into new vessel formation has led to a model of understanding of angiogenesis controlled by families of angiogenic growth factors (including VEGF, TGF-β1, and PDGF-B), which are responsible for the formation of new vessels. Cutaneous injury results in the upregulation of VEGF, with keratinocytes and macrophages accounting for the majority of VEGF production.[15,16] This has been supported by studies where reduced expression of VEGF, or its accelerated degradation, has been found to be associated with impaired wound healing.[17,18] Ischemic and chronic nonhealing wounds that are treated with VEGF have improved wound healing and enhanced neovascularization.[4–7] The important role of VEGF in wound healing is further demonstrated by application of VEGF antibodies that results in a reduction in wound angiogenesis and granulation tissue in a porcine wound model.[19]

Recent investigation has focused on the role of hypoxia inducible factor-1 alpha (HIF-1α) in the role of wound repair and neovascularization. Hypoxia is a critical stimulus for normal tissue repair. This cellular response to hypoxia is mediated by HIF-1α. Hypoxic wound conditions result in the stabilization of HIF-1α and protection against degradation, which results in the induction of a variety of proangiogenic growth factors. This transcription factor is pivotal in wound healing, neovascularization, and progenitor cell recruitment. Further, HIF-1α has been shown to be deficient in the diabetic state, and restoration of HIF-1α function can result in enhanced neovascularization and wound healing.[8–10] HIF-1α or any of these proangiogenic compounds are candidate vulnerary transgenes for gene therapy applications for enhanced neovascularization and tissue repair.

EXPERIMENTAL MODEL OR MATERIAL

Gene transfer techniques can be separated into viral- and nonviral-mediated gene transfer. Viral-mediated gene transfer has been accomplished using adenovirus (Ad), adeno-associated virus (AAV), and retro-lentiviral vectors. Adenoviral constructs are commonly utilized because of their ease of construction with the capability of producing high titers and have the highest transduction efficiency to both dividing and nondividing cells. Second-generation Ad vectors can yield a suitable transgene capacity for wound healing applications. After administration, transgene expression can be seen maximally at 2–3 days and can be sustained for 2–3 weeks. While this may seem a limitation, for application in wound healing, a transient effect may be all that is desired and reports of insertional mutagenesis have been rare. The major disadvantage is the intense inflammatory response induced by the Ad vector that actually impedes wound healing in the absence of a vulnerary transgene.[20]

AAV is a nonpathogenic, nonenveloped virus. The wild-type virus specifically integrates into chromosome 19. However, when the virus has the recombination function deleted, it randomly integrates at a very low frequency, if it does so at all. A main advantage of the AAV vector is low immunogenicity with a greatly reduced inflammatory effect when administered to the wound and its ability to produce sustained transgene expression for several months. The disadvantages of AAV are the small transgene capacity, the slight potential for insertional mutagenesis, and the possibility that prolonged transgene expression might result in untoward effects in the wound bed.[21]

Viral vectors based on the retrovirus were the first class of vectors to be developed. The molecular biology of these vectors is well studied and results in dependable and controllable manipulation of the vector. The advantages are its ability to produce stable expression *ex vivo* in a wide variety of cells. However, there are some disadvantages for wound healing applications, including a limited transgene capacity, a finite risk of insertional mutagenesis, the inability to produce high titers, and a short half-life *in vivo*.[22] Retroviral vectors based on lentivirus have a 10 times greater transduction efficiency than retroviruses.[23] Additionally, they can transduce cells within the wound bed similar to adenoviral constructs but without the intense inflammatory response.[12,13]

Nonviral methods of gene transfer have made improvements in both delivery and efficacy. Cationic liposomes are positively charged lipids that form complexes with DNA, which then undergo endocytosis. They have variable transgene transfer efficiency rates. There are a variety of other methods, including the gene gun, microseeding, electroporation, and nanoparticle technology. Nanoparticle gene transfer, direct plasmid application, lipofection, and receptor-mediated delivery vectors demonstrate the most potential among the nonviral systems.[21,22]

DISCUSSION OF FINDINGS AND RELEVANT LITERATURE

The goals of therapeutic angiogenesis are to improve neovascularization in impaired tissue with the expectation that it will produce improved cellular, nutrient, and oxygen delivery resulting in enhanced wound healing. Gene transfer techniques to accomplish this goal can be implemented in three different ways: (1) direct delivery of vulnerary transgenes to the wound bed via injection, an aqueous solution or suspended in a matrix,[22] (2) *ex vivo* transfection of a resident wound population of cells or cell matrices that are then administered to the wound, and (3) the genetic manipulation of stem/progenitor cells that are then administered to the wound.

In initial studies, direct delivery of PDGF-B using an adenoviral construct in an ischemic rabbit ear model demonstrated improved wound healing and neovascularization.[24] This was also demonstrated in multiple mouse models of diabetes.[11] Interestingly, in the absence of the vulnerary transgene, the Ad vector actually impeded wound healing and neovascularization, making the positive effect of the Ad-*PDGF* all the more impressive. PDGF-B has also been overexpressed using a lenitviral construct with similarly enhanced neovascularization but with longer transgene expression and less inflammation.[12]

TAKE-HOME MESSAGE

Basic science advances

Advantages and disadvantages of individual vectors

- Adenoviral vectors
  - Advantages: excellent transduction efficiency, transduce nondividing cells, relative ease of production, and limited duration of transgene expression
  - Disadvantages: incites marked inflammatory response and limited duration of transgene expression
- Adeno-associated viral vectors
  - Advantages: durable transgene expression and low immunogenicity
  - Disadvantages: small transgene capacity and slight potential for insertional mutagenesis
- Retro/lenitviral vectors
  - Advantages: easily manipulated, stable expression in a variety of cells transduce nonreplicating cells, and minimal inflammatory response
  - Disadvantages: limited transgene capacity, short half-life *in vivo* (retrovirus), and slight potential for insertional mutagenesis
- Nonviral vectors
  - Advantages: improved safety profile
  - Disadvantages: variable transgene transfer efficiency

Hypoxia-induced neovascularization

- Hypoxia is critical stimulus for normal tissue repair
- The cellular response to hypoxia is mediated by HIF-1α.
- HIF-1α is upstream to SDF-1, NOS, and VEGF.
- HIF-1α is pivotal in wound healing, neovascularization, and progenitor cell recruitment.
- HIF-1α is deficient in the diabetic state, and restoration of HIF-1α function can result in enhanced neovascularization and wound healing.

Clinical science advances

- Goals of therapeutic angiogenesis are to improve neovascularization in tissue to produce improved blood, nutrient, and oxygen delivery resulting in enhanced wound healing.
- Gene transfer techniques to enhance neovascularization can be accomplished via three methods.
  - Direct delivery of vulnerary transgenes to the wound bed resulting in neovascularization
  - *Ex vivo* transfection of resident wound population of cells or cell matrices that are then administered to the wound
  - The genetic manipulation of stem/progenitor cells that are then administered to the wound

Relevance to clinical care

- Currently, of all the gene therapy trials that are registered, 63.2% are conducted in the United States, 9.3% of those are for cardiovascular indications, and nearly half of all studies are utilizing either an adenoviral (24.9%) or retroviral construct (21.7%).[32]

Similarly, VEGF has been overexpressed using both Ad- and AAV-based vectors in several chronic wound models.[4–7] Insight into the overexpression of VEGF can come from the transgenic mouse model that constitutively overexpresses VEGF. These mice are hypervascular but have leaky microvasculature.[25] Both Ad and AAV *VEGF* gene transfer in diabetic mice improved wound healing through the stimulation of angiogenesis, re-epithelization, synthesis, and maturation of extracellular matrix.[4–7] The delivery of angiopoietin-1 along with VEGF appears to stabilize the neovascularization and improves the leaky capillaries that results in improved tissue repair.[26]

Studies using overexpression of angiogenic growth factors have also resulted in increased endothelial progenitor cell (EPC) recruitment to the wound.[9–11] These cells may contribute to bone marrow–derived neovascularization or vasculogenesis, although the significance of these cells is not clearly understood. However, diminished numbers of EPCs have been associated with chronic disease states. Stromal cell–derived factor-1 (SDF-1) is a chemokine that plays a central role in the mobilization and recruitment of progenitor cells to injured and hypoxic tissues. Hiasa *et al.* used a plasmid DNA encoding *SDF-1* in ischemic mouse hind limbs that resulted in enhanced neovascularization and EPC recruitment. This effect was abrogated with the blockade of either VEGF or endothelial nitric oxide synthase (NOS), suggesting that SDF-1 worked through a VEGF/endothelial NOS pathway.[27] Upstream from SDF-1 activation is the transcription factor HIF-1α. HIF-1α is the key modulator of the wounds' response to hypoxia and has been shown to be deficient in diabetes as well as aged models.[8–10] Adenoviral overexpression of *HIF-1α* in the diabetic mouse model results in thick granulation tissue, enhanced neovascularization, and an increase in EPCs that corrects the diabetic wound and neovascularization impairment.[10]

An alternative to direct gene transfer is isolation of resident cell populations of wounds, such as fibroblasts or keratino-

- Several small clinical trials have been completed using gene transfer techniques to enhance neovascularization in limb ischemia with positive results.
- Plasmid gene transfer of fibroblast growth factor-1 to patients with critical limb ischemia in a multinational study was well tolerated. However, there was no improvement in chronic ulcer healing rates, but there was a significant reduction in amputation rates and a trend toward improved survival.[33]
- Two phase I clinical trials of adenoviral-mediated gene transfer of *PDGF-B* gene in chronic venous stasis ulcers and in diabetic ulcers show the adenoviral gene transfer to be safe and the effect on wound healing appears to be significant. Currently, a phase 2b trial is in progress evaluating transfer of the *PDGF-B* gene in diabetic ulcers.[32].

cytes, that can then be genetically manipulated *ex vivo* and then be returned to the wound to facilitate wound repair likely through a mechanism that involves functioning as a growth factor production platform. Dickens *et al.* expanded cultured keratinocytes and transfected them with a plasmid encoding for *VEGF* under the control of a tetracycline regulator. In porcine excisional wounds treated with these keratinocytes there was significantly enhanced neovascularization, matrix formation, and wound repair.[28] Additionally, the *VEGF* production could be controlled with the tetracycline regulator. Eming *et al.* used a retrovirus base vector to modify keratinocytes to express PDGF-A and subsequently cultured them onto a cellular dermis that was then transplanted into immunocompromised mice. The treated grafts demonstrated significantly more fibrovascular in growth compared to controls.[29] Fibroblasts have also been cultured and genetically modified to enhance wound repair and neovascularization.[30]

The third method of gene transfer to the wound is the least studied, that is, gene transfer to stem and progenitor cells to either use them as a growth factor production platform or to influence the differentiation pathway of pluripotent cells. Bone marrow–derived stromal cells have been shown to enhance neovascularization in a diabetic murine animal model.[31] The mechanism of the neovascularization is believed to be a paracrine effect of angiogenic growth factor production.

CAUTION, CRITICAL REMARKS, AND RECOMMENDATIONS

The rationale for and goals of therapeutic angiogenesis are clearly worth pursuing. These small clinical trials have yielded some encouraging data. However, safety in gene therapy must be paramount. Likely, the vectors that we have at our disposal today will not be the ones we use in the future. The ideal vector is the one that is minimally immunogenic, has high transduction efficiency, and is the one that has no risk of insertional mutagenesis.

FUTURE DEVELOPMENTS

Continued investigations will need to be carried out to not only develop the ideal gene transfer technique, but also elucidate the pathogenic mechanisms of these chronic disease states to continue to identify model candidate transgenes. It may be that a mixture of transgenes will be required to fully restore the wound healing impairment in many of these diseases. As these pathways and vulnerary transgenes are revealed, larger multicenter trials will be required to determine the true efficacy of this therapy.

ACKNOWLEDGMENTS

Wound healing research in the author's laboratory (T.M.C.) is supported by NIH awards DK072446 and DK074055.

AUTHOR DISCLOSURE STATEMENT

No conflict of interest disclosed for S.G.K. and T.M.C.

REFERENCES

1. Robson MC, Phillips LG, Thomason A, Robson LE, and Pierce GF: Platelet-derived growth factor BB for the treatment of chronic pressure ulcers. Lancet 1992; **339:** 23.
2. Steed DL: Clinical evaluation of recombinant human platelet-derived growth factor for the treatment of lower extremity ulcers. Plast Reconstr Surg 2006; **117:** 143S.
3. Madeddu P: Therapeutic angiogenesis and vasculogenesis for tissue regeneration. Exp Physiol 2005; **90:** 315.
4. Romano Di Peppe S, Mangoni A, Zambruno G, Spinetti G, Melillo G, Napolitano M, and Capogrossi MC: Adenovirus-mediated VEGF (165) gene transfer enhances wound healing by promoting angiogenesis in CD1 diabetic mice. Gene Ther 2002; **9:** 1271.
5. Vranckx JJ, Yao F, Petrie N, Augustinova H, Hoeller D, Visovatti S, Slama J, and Eriksson E: *In vivo* gene delivery of Ad-VEGF121 to full-thickness wounds in aged pigs results in high levels of VEGF expression but not in accelerated healing. Wound Repair Regen 2005; **13:** 51.
6. Deodato B, Arsic N, Zentilin L, Galeano M, Santoro D, Torre V, Altavilla D, Valdembri D, Bussolino F, Squadrito F, and Giacca M: Recombinant

AAV vector encoding human VEGF165 enhances wound healing. Gene Ther 2002; **12:** 777.

7. Brem H, Kodra A, Golinko MS, Entero H, Stojadinovic O, Wang VM, Sheahan CM, Weinberg AD, Woo SL, Ehrlich HP, and Tomic-Canic M: Mechanism of sustained release of vascular endothelial growth factor in accelerating experimental diabetic healing. J Invest Dermatol 2009; **129:** 2275.

8. Mace KA, Yu DH, Paydar KZ, Boudreau N, and Young DM: Sustained expression of Hif-1alpha in the diabetic environment promotes angiogenesis and cutaneous wound repair.Wound Repair Regen 2007; **15:** 636.

9. Liu L, Marti GP, Wei X, Zhang X, Zhang H, Liu YV, Nastai M, Semenza GL, and Harmon JW: Age-dependent impairment of HIF-1alpha expression in diabetic mice: correction with electroporation-facilitated gene therapy increases wound healing, angiogenesis, and circulating angiogenic cells. J Cell Physiol 2008; **217:** 319.

10. Botusan IR, Sunkari VG, Savu O, Catrina AI, Grünler J, Lindberg S, Pereira T, Ylä-Herttuala S, Poellinger L, Brismar K, and Catrina SB: Stabilization of HIF-1alpha is critical to improve wound healing in diabetic mice. Proc Natl Acad Sci 2008; **105:** 19426.

11. Keswani SG, Katz AB, Lim FY, Zoltick P, Radu A, Alaee D, Herlyn M, and Crombleholme TM: Adenoviral mediated gene transfer of PDGF-B enhances wound healing in type I and type II diabetic wounds. Wound Repair Regen 2004; **12:** 497.

12. Lee JA, Conejero JA, Mason JM, Parrett BM, Wear-Maggitti KD, Grant RT, and Breitbart AS: Lentiviral transfection with the PDGF-B gene improves diabetic wound healing. Plast Reconstr Surg 2005; **116:** 532.

13. Badillo AT, Chung S, Zhang L, Zoltick P, and Liechty KW: Lentiviral gene transfer of SDF-1alpha to wounds improves diabetic wound healing. J Surg Res 2007; **143:** 35.

14. Doukas J, Blease K, Craig D, Ma C, Chandler LA, Sosnowski BA, and Pierce F: Delivery of FGF genes to wound repair cells enhances arteriogenesis and myogenesis in skeletal muscle. Mol Ther 2002; **5:** 517.

15. Bao P, Kodra A, Tomic-Canic M, Golinko MS, Ehrlich HP, and Brem H: The role of vascular endothelial growth factor in wound healing. J Surg Res 2009; **153:** 347.

16. Werner S and Grose R: Regulation of wound healing by growth factors and cytokines. Physiol Rev 2003; **83:** 835.

17. Frank S, Hübner G, Breier G, Longaker MT, Greenhalgh DG, and Werner S: Regulation of vascular endothelial growth factor expression in cultured keratinocytes. Implications for normal and impaired wound healing. J Biol Chem 1995; **270:** 12607.

18. Swift ME, Kleinman HK, and DiPietro LA: Impaired wound repair and delayed angiogenesis in aged mice. Lab Investig 1999; **79:** 1479.

19. Howdieshell TR, Callaway D, Webb WL, Gaines MD, Procter CD Jr., Sathyanarayana, Pollock JS, Brock TL, and McNeil PL: Antibody neutralization of vascular endothelial growth factor inhibits wound granulation tissue formation. J Surg Res 2001; **96:** 173.

20. Crombleholme TM: Adenoviral-mediated gene transfer in wound healing. Wound Repair Regen 2000; **8:** 460.

21. Hirsch T, Spielmann M, Yao F, and Eriksson E: Gene therapy in cutaneous wound healing. Front Biosci 2007; **12:** 2507.

22. Eming SA, Krieg T, and Davidson JM: Gene therapy and wound healing. Clin Dermatol 2007; **25:** 79.

23. Indraccolo S, Habeler W, Tisato V, Stievano L, Piovan E, Tosello V, Esposito G, Wagner R, Uberla K, Chieco-Bianchi L, and Amadori A: Gene transfer in ovarian cancer cells: a comparison between retroviral and lentiviral vectors. Cancer Res 2002; **62:** 6099.

24. Liechty KW, Nesbit M, Herlyn M, Radu A, Adzick NS, and Crombleholme TM: Adenoviral-mediated overexpression of platelet-derived growth factor-B corrects ischemic impaired wound healing. J Invest Dermatol 1999; **113:** 375.

25. Thurston G, Suri C, Smith K, McClain J, Sato TN, Yancopoulos GD, and McDonald DM: Leakage-resistant blood vessels in mice transgenically overexpressing angiopoietin-1. Science 1999; **286:** 2511.

26. Yamauchi A, Ito Y, Morikawa M, Kobune M, Huang J, Sasaki K, Takahashi K, Nakamura K, Dehari H, Niitsu Y, Abe T, and Hamada H: Pre-administration of angiopoietin-1 followed by VEGF induces functional and mature vascular formation in a rabbit ischemic model. J Gene Med 2003; **5:** 994.

27. Hiasa K, Ishibashi M, Ohtani K, Inoue S, Zhao Q, Kitamoto S, Sata M, Ichiki T, Takeshita A, and Egashira K: Gene transfer of stromal cell-derived factor-1alpha enhances ischemic vasculogenesis and angiogenesis via vascular endothelial growth factor/endothelial nitric oxide synthase-related pathway: next-generation chemokine therapy for therapeutic neovascularization. Circulation 2004; **109:** 2454.

28. Dickens S, Vermeulen P, Hendrickx B, Van den Berge S, and Vranckx JJ: Regulable vascular endothelial growth factor165 overexpression by *ex vivo* expanded keratinocyte cultures promotes matrix formation, angiogenesis, and healing in porcine full-thickness wounds. Tissue Eng Part A 2008; **14:** 19.

29. Eming SA, Medalie DA, Tompkins RG, Yarmush ML, and Morgan JR: Genetically modified human keratinocytes overexpressing PDGF-A enhance the performance of a composite skin graft. Hum Gene Ther 1998; **9:** 529.

30. Mueller CK, Thorwarth MW, and Schultze-Mosgau S: Angiogenic gene-modified fibroblasts for induction of localized angiogenesis. J Surg Res 2009 [Epub ahead of print PMID:19394654].

31. Javazon EH, Keswani SG, Badillo AT, Crombleholme TM, Zoltick PW, Radu AP, Kozin ED, Beggs K, Malik AA, and Flake AW: Enhanced epithelial gap closure and increased angiogenesis in wounds of diabetic mice treated with adult murine bone marrow stromal progenitor cells. Wound Repair Regen 2007; **15:** 350.

32. Gene Therapy Clinical Trials: The Journal of Gene Medicine. Available at www.wiley.co.uk/genetherapy/clinical/, accessed 2009 March 1.

33. Nikol S, Baumgartner I, Van Belle E, Diehm C, Visoná A, Capogrossi MC, Ferreira-Maldent N, Gallino A, Wyatt MG, Wijesinghe LD, Fusari M, Stephan D, Emmerich J, Pompilio G, Vermassen F, Pham E, Grek V, Coleman M, and Meyer F; TALISMAN 201 investigators: Therapeutic angiogenesis with intramuscular NV1FGF improves amputation-free survival in patients with critical limb ischemia. Mol Ther 2008; **16:** 972.

Smart Growth Factor Gene Delivery for Impaired Wound Healing

María José Escámez,[1] Marta Carretero,[2] Marta García,[1] Lucía Martínez-Santamaría,[1] Alvaro Meana,[1,2] Fernando Larcher,[2] and Marcela Del Río[1,*]

[1]Regenerative Medicine Unit and [2]Cutaneous Diseases Modeling Unit, Epithelial Biomedicine Division, Basic Research Department, CIEMAT-CIBERER U714, Madrid, Spain.

Background: Acute and chronic wounds of diverse origins remain a chief clinical problem. Tissue engineering and gene therapy come into sight as novel therapeutic tools.
The Problem: Testing novel therapeutic strategies requires reliable wound-healing models and gene delivery systems.
Basic/Clinical Science Advances: Our recent studies address such troublesome matters. Our contribution comprises the development of a bioengineered human skin substitute suitable for clinical applications including acute and chronic wound management, a preclinical skin-humanized mouse model based on permanent human skin regeneration on immunodeficient animals upon grafting of the bioengineered skin equivalent. The humanized model appears to be a useful tool to perform acute healing studies and to design novel gene and protein delivery methods and the characterization of healing-promoting activities of some antimicrobial peptides.
Clinical Care Relevance: Benefits of clinical relevance could be achieved using smart bioengineered products combining cell and gene therapy aiming to enhance tissue repair and control infection concomitantly.
Conclusion: These avenues merge into the development of effective wound-healing management approaches.

Abbreviations and Acronyms

AMP = antimicrobial peptide
EMEA = European Medicine Agency
HBD = human beta defensins
hKGF = human keratinocyte growth factor
KGF = keratinocyte growth factor
VEGF = Vascular endothelial growth factor

*Correspondence: Regenerative Medicine Unit, Epithelial Biomedicine Division, Basic Research Department, CIEMAT-CIBERER U714, Avda. Complutense, 22, 28040 Madrid, Spain (e-mail: marcela.delrio@ciemat.es).

BACKGROUND

Nonhealing acute and chronic skin wounds are a diverse group of lesions of different etiology and manifestation. The most common cause of acute wounds is thermal injury. Chronic wounds include arterial, diabetic, pressure, and venous ulcers. Within this category, we may also include persistent wounds associated to inherited mechano-bullous skin disorders such as Epidermolysis Bullosa. Management of these wounds remains a major clinical challenge involving novel therapeutic strategies such as cell and gene therapy.[1,2] Several more or less complex tissue-engineered skin products aimed at wound-healing enhancement[2] are currently on the market. However, most of these products have limited applications. Our group has developed a tissue-engineered human skin equivalent[3] suitable for a broad spectrum of clinical applications, including permanent skin engraftment and regeneration and chronic wound-healing aid.[4–7] The development of smart bioengineered products acting concomitantly as tissue substitute and a source of soluble factors to improve the healing of wounds and prevent infection has been put forward by various laboratories, including ours.[8–11] Testing these therapeutic strategies requires reliable wound-healing models. Recently, our group has devoted a major effort to

Printed in U.S.A.
DOI: 10.1089/awc.2009.0044

establishing both a preclinical humanized wound-healing system and optimized methods for transient delivery of genes encoding wound healing–promoting factors.[12,13] Robust validation of these approaches has been achieved with keratinocyte growth factor (KGF) and the cathelicidin antimicrobial peptide (AMP) LL-37.

CLINICAL PROBLEM ADDRESSED

Burn injuries and chronic wounds are associated with diminished quality of life, frequent hospitalizations, and increased morbidity and mortality and still represent a major public health problem. The appropriate management of wounds is a standing clinical challenge.[2,14] Although significant progress has been made with state-of-the-art treatments, additional improvements could prove relevant in terms of efficacy. The lack of an appropriately vascularized wound bed and infection are clearly detrimental to the tissue repair process. Several strategies have been proposed by different groups, including ours, to solve these problems.[15–17] A comprehensive understanding of the mechanisms involved in normal and impaired wound healing could lead to smart combinations of tissue engineering with genetic modification of the cells to overproduce key therapeutic factors for satisfactory wound handling and care. Thus, novel approaches combining cell and gene therapy, coupled to the availability of clinically reliable wound-healing models, could be pivotal to the advancement of this field.[2,14,15,17,18]

RELEVANT BASIC SCIENCE CONTEXT

In vivo wound-healing studies in human skin are limited by ethical and practical issues. Current knowledge mainly stems from the use of murine models, including knockout and transgenic strategies. These studies have provided evidence of the relevance of targeted genes and the modulatory effects of many growth factors *in vivo*.[16,19,20] However, based on the significant differences existing between human and murine skin architecture, the question remains as to how far the results can be extrapolated to the human scenario. Studies in large animals such as pigs, whose skin architecture and dynamics resemble that of humans, are an alternative, but troublesome and expensive.[21] Human skin organotypic cultures represent a valid alternative to native skin *in vivo* studies, particularly those endowed with long-term culture life span.[22,23] However, they are restricted, among other constraints, by faulty pivotal mesenchymal responses such as angiogenesis. To circumvent these problems, researchers have often used xenogenic transplantation of donor skin biopsies to immunodeficient mice to perform relevant *in vivo* experimentation in a human context.[23–25] However, in addition to difficulties in sourcing, a major concern for this type of experiments is the big heterogeneity of the grafting material. As a result, regenerating human skin on immunodeficient mice by grafting a bioengineered skin substitute appears to be a balanced compromise between practicality and model fidelity. This methodology enables the generation of numerous mice engrafted with a significant area of single donor–derived human skin, known as skin-humanized mouse model.[7,12,25] This model is suitable as a platform to perform wound-healing studies and to test gene therapy approaches in a humanized context.

EXPERIMENTAL MODEL OR MATERIAL

The contribution of our group to the tissue regeneration field focused on three pivotal points.

Development of a skin equivalent for clinical purposes

The skin equivalent (Fig. 1) is based on a tridimensional fibrin-rich dermal scaffold containing live fibroblasts that supports, mechanically and metabolically, the establishment and maintenance of the epidermal component.[3] The dermal composition of this skin equivalent presents unique characteristics compared to other dermal equivalents, allowing for high proliferation rates of keratinocytes. This skin equivalent (World Patent WO/2002/072800) is being successfully used in clinics in its autologous version for permanent skin regeneration[3,5,6] and, lately, in its allogenic version for treating chronic wounds.[4] In addition, a new chimerical version of this substitute (a skin equivalent composed of autologous patient-derived keratinocytes and allogenic healthy donor–derived fibroblasts) has been awarded the Orphan Drug designation by the European Medicines Agency (EMEA) for the treatment of chronic wounds in patients affected with the rare inherited skin disorder Epidermolysis Bullosa (orphan designation number EU/306/369), and it is currently being tested in a phase I–II clinical trial in Spain (http://es.cellerix.com/index.php/Productos/Cx501).

Improvement of graft performance by promoting vascularization and fighting infections

We have proposed a combination of tissue engineering and gene therapy approaches for the treatment of chronic and acute wounds. Vascular endothelial growth factor (VEGF) promotes

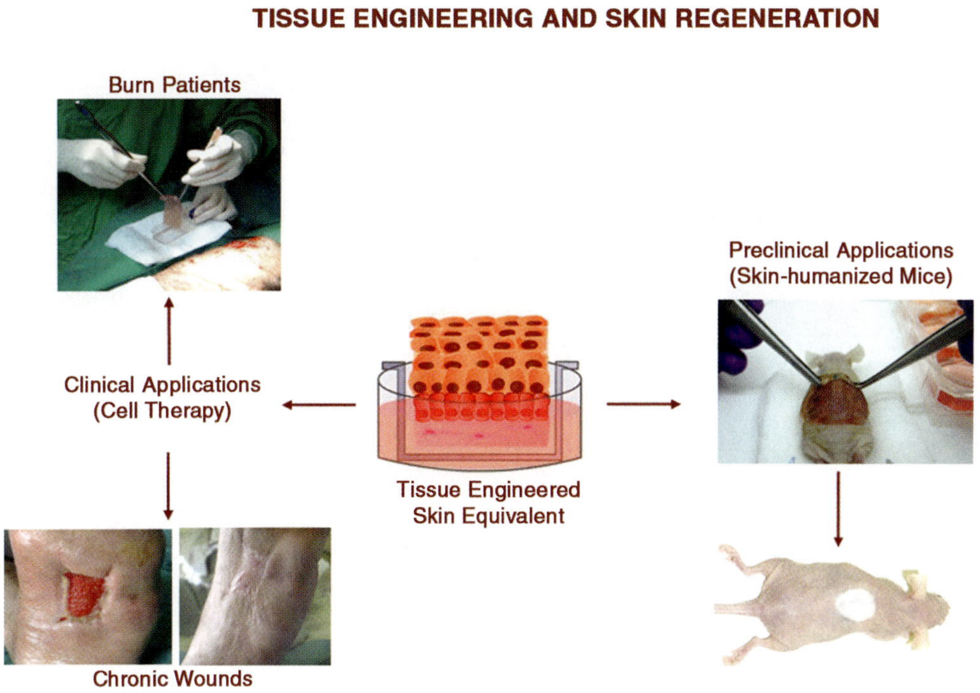

Figure 1. The tissue bioengineered skin equivalent is based on a fibrin matrix containing live fibroblasts as a dermal component and keratinocytes as the epidermal component. This bioengineered human skin has been successfully applied as a cell therapy approach aiming either permanent or temporary cover to treat burn patients and chronic nonhealing wounds, respectively. A skin-humanized mouse model based on the stable engraftment of this setting has been used as a platform for evaluating pharmacological, cell, and gene therapy strategies for wound healing.

cutaneous angiogenesis by inducing potent proliferation and migration of endothelial cells.[16,26] Using *in vivo* models, different laboratories have explored the effect of VEGF as a part of an angiogenic bioengineered material that might improve wound bed conditioning and engraftment.[8,11,27]

Infection is the other major setback for regeneration after skin grafting (either split-thickness or tissue-engineered autografts). The increasing appearance of multidrug-resistant microbes points to the need of using alternative therapies to conventional antibiotics. AMPs appear as good candidates as they present a broad spectrum of activity against microorganisms and, usually, a low induced-resistance due to their mechanism of action.[28] In addition, some AMPs have been suggested to elicit not only bacteria-killing activity but also healing-promoting effects.[29,30]

We have demonstrated the efficacy of adenoviral-mediated gene transfer by overexpressing human beta defensins (HBD)-2 and -3 and cathelicidin LL-37 in a skin equivalent setting.[9] Moreover, using an *in vivo* approach based on LL-37 adenoviral-mediated delivery to diabetic wounds in ob/ob mice, we have provided early evidence for the potential benefits of using AMP gene therapy in a healing impaired situation.[10] In this model, *in vivo LL-37* gene transfer increased the re-epithelialization rate and granulation tissue formation. These results evidence a realistic therapeutic option that might contribute to an efficient tissue repair as well as infection control at the wound site[10,31] (Fig. 2).

Development of a skin-humanized model to test gene-mediated factor delivery approaches

A reliable preclinical model to validate the efficacy of these and other factors for the treatment of wounds is mandatory. We have generated a skin-humanized mouse model based on the straightforward grafting of a bioengineered human skin equivalent onto the back of immunodeficient mice.[6,25] Once permanent human skin regeneration has been achieved (epidermal maturation and dermal matrix remodeling is accomplished within 9–10 weeks after grafting), the humanized mice are ready to be used in healing experiments. This model also offers the possibility of using genetically modified human keratinocytes and/or fibroblasts. After transplantation, a hybrid system is generated with a skin of human origin that is vascularized and innervated by mouse vessels and nerves. Probably, the main advantage of our system is that full-thickness wounds are performed in a context of a mature, quiescent, homogeneous human skin avoiding the need for volunteers and major differences in tissue architecture and kinetics found in mouse skin. Under these experimental conditions, we have provided *in vivo* evidence that either the native or a green fluorescent protein

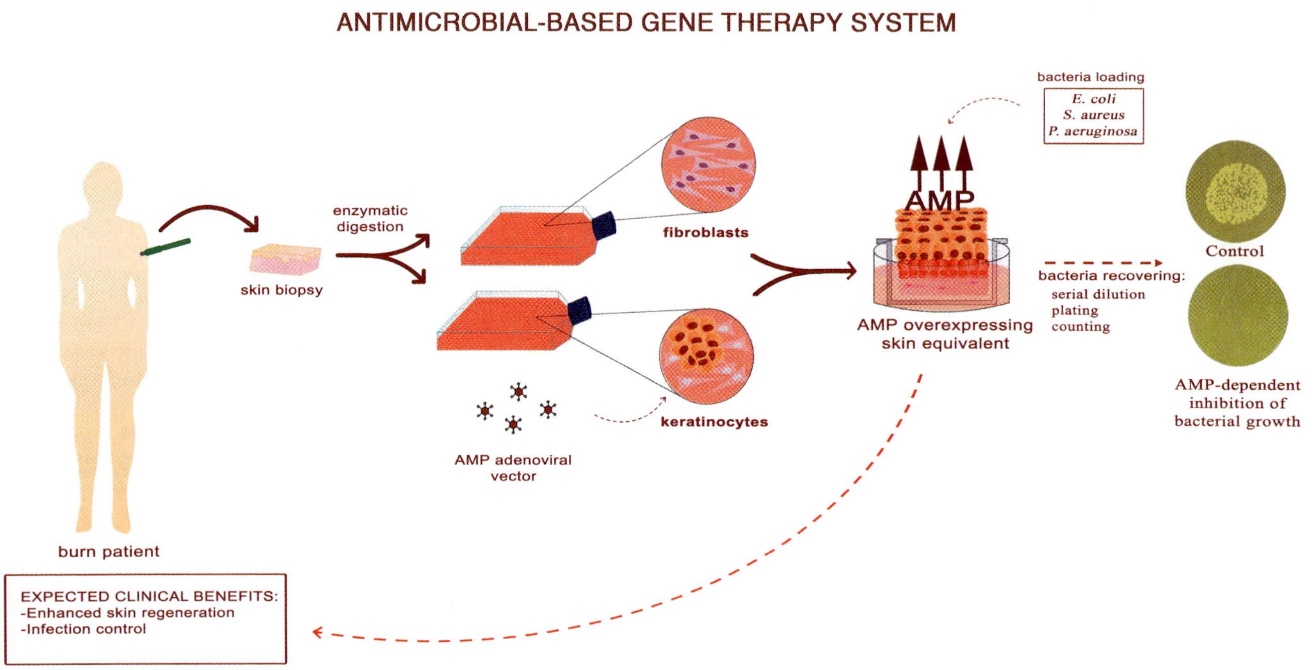

Figure 2. *In vitro* studies demonstrated efficient antimicrobial activity of adenoviral antimicrobial peptide (AMP) gene-transduced keratinocytes as a part of a skin equivalent by inhibiting the growth of different bacterial strains, usually associated to burn wounds. Combined cutaneous tissue engineering in conjunction with antimicrobial gene therapy emerges as a potential therapeutic approach for wound coverage and concomitantly combating infection in burn patients.

genetically modified skin-humanized mouse model recapitulates the main features of human wound healing.[12] Further, our wound-healing model allowed us to compare the efficacy of different transient gene transfer strategies aimed at delivering growth factors such as KGF to promote skin repair[13,32] (Fig. 3).

DISCUSSION OF FINDINGS AND RELEVANT LITERATURE

The skin equivalent developed by our team allows for generation of large bioengineered skin surfaces, restoration of both the epidermal and dermal skin compartments, and functional epidermal stem-cell preservation. Further, it has been successfully used, in its autologous version, for permanent skin regeneration in different situations: extensive burns, necrotizing fascitis, removal of giant nevi, and graft-versus-host disease.[3,5,6] In its allogenic version it has also been used as a healing aid to treat chronic wounds.[4]

Growth factors that play a critical role in normal wound healing and in addition are often deficient or inactive in chronic wounds have been highlighted as attractive therapeutic agents.[16–18] Among these, factors with a well-known angiogenic potential are main candidates to improve wound bed preparation.[2,14,33] We and others have thus explored the effect of VEGF overexpression by *ex vivo* gene transfer to keratinocytes.[8,27] *VEGF* delivered by gene-targeted endothelial cells embedded in a fibrin matrix was also successfully used in the ischemic distal pedicle flap rabbit model.[11]

A critical condition for an efficient engraftment is also the preservation of a sterile wound bed environment. To avoid infection, AMPs have been suggested as an alternative to the use of conventional antibiotics. Besides their role in innate host defense, other activities have been described for some of these AMPs that might positively influence the wound-healing response. In fact, the human cathelicidin LL-37 has been shown to induce an angiogenic response, to enhance adaptive immune responses by recruiting different immune cells, to induce the expression of syndecan in fibroblasts, to induce the production of cytokines and chemokines by keratinocytes, and to enhance the re-epithelialization process.[28] We have provided further evidence for the LL-37–mediated signaling pathways in keratinocytes that are involved in the migratory activity of these cells.[10] We demonstrated that overexpression of this peptide induced

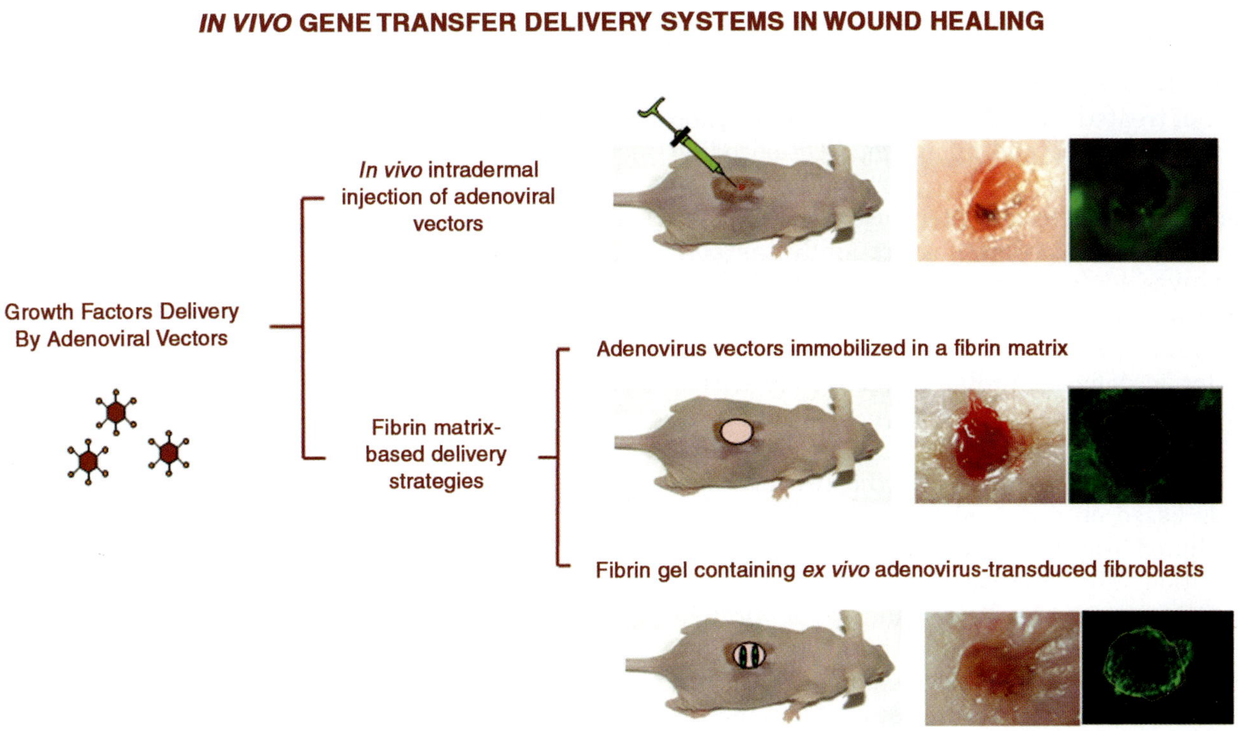

Figure 3. Different *in vivo* growth factor delivery approaches mediated by adenoviral vectors aiming to improve wound healing have been explored using the skin-humanized mouse model. Transient delivery of keratinocyte growth factor to wounds was achieved through direct intradermal adenoviral injection or through fibrin matrix strategies, containing either immobilized adenoviral vector or embedded adenoviral gene-transferred human fibroblasts.

phenotypic changes related to actin dynamics and was associated to augmented tyrosine phosphorylation of proteins involved in focal adhesion complexes. We have also demonstrated that events involved in the epithelial–mesenchymal transition are observed in the presence of the LL-37, such as induction of the Snail transcription factor, presence of discontinuous cell–cell contacts (adherens junctions and desmosomes), activation of matrix metalloproteinases, and activation of the mitogen-activated protein kinase and phosphoinositide 3-kinase/Akt signaling pathways. These signaling events could be mediated not only through the transactivation of epidermal growth factor receptor but also through the induction of G-protein-coupled receptor formyl peptide receptor like-1 expression in these cells. Using an *in vivo* approach based on LL-37 adenoviral-mediated delivery to diabetic wounds in ob/ob mice, we have provided evidence for the potential benefits of using AMP gene delivery for a healing-impaired situation. LL-37 increased the re-epithelialization rate and granulation tissue formation when administered around wound margins. In summary, we showed that gene delivery of factors such as VEGF and AMPs may have a positive impact on wound repair by promoting vascularization and/or controlling infection.

Another important contribution of our group is the development of a reliable *in vivo* tool that allows for preclinical studies to evaluate the benefits of delivering potential therapeutic factors to the wound site.[12,13] The validation of this wound-healing skin-humanized model has been performed by careful examination of a wide spectrum of parameters at different times post-wounding, including migration, proliferation, stratification, and differentiation, dermal remodeling, and dermo–epidermal junction reconstitution. In conclusion, the model mimics the different phases of the human wound-healing process. The biological validity of the model was further confirmed by probing its ability to respond to a known wound healing–promoting factor, such as KGF added exogenously as a recombinant protein.

Using the skin-humanized mouse system, we have compared the efficacy of different *in vivo* approaches involving transient delivery of *KGF* to wounds by using adenoviral vectors. In the first approach, human keratinocyte growth factor (*hKGF*) was delivered to wounds by intradermal injection of an adenoviral suspension. Although wound acceleration was achieved, the effect of hKGF was unreliable both in terms of the number of successfully targeted animals (versus the total number of treated animals) and re-epithelialization efficiency. In the second approach, *KGF*-encoding adenoviral vectors were immobilized in a fibrin gel carrier and applied immediately after wounding. In this case, the proportion of successfully targeted animals was higher than that achieved with the adenoviral injection method, and wound closure rose significantly. A third strategy was explored consisting in delivering hKGF protein from *ex vivo* adenoviral-transduced fibroblasts that were, in turn, embedded in a fibrin matrix and used to treat the wound. In contrast to the two previous methods based on direct adenovirus delivery, this cell-mediated system did not depend on *in vivo* cell transduction. This method depends on the direct transfer of exogenous KGF therapeutic protein from gene-targeted fibroblasts that was, in fact, achieved in all treated wounds, leading to a significant improvement in wound closure. Although all delivery systems achieved KGF protein overproduction at the wound site, with a concomitant re-epithelialization enhancement, only the use of genetically modified fibroblast-containing matrix as an *in situ* protein bioreactor was highly reproducible. This method appears the most reliable means to deliver growth factors to wounds avoiding the potential danger of scoring cases of faulty administration as therapeutic failures and direct exposure to viral vectors. The tissue engineering–based skin-humanized mouse model system emerges as a unique platform for evaluating pharmacological, cell, and gene therapy strategies for wound healing.

CAUTION, CRITICAL REMARKS, AND RECOMMENDATIONS

While cell-based therapy approaches have been successfully used for skin repair, particularly in severe skin losses and most recently for chronic wounds, the combination with genetic modification of cellular components needs to be carefully addressed in appropriate models. In spite of its complexity, normal skin wound healing is an efficient process that is difficult to accelerate or enhance through the activity of exogenous growth factors. Thus, healing-impaired models may better reveal the actual repair-promoting activities of healing-acting molecules. To better mimic a chronic skin repair–deficient condition, it seems worthy to develop new *in vivo* models of impaired wound healing. In fact, we are currently conducting experiments to establish models of impaired wound healing such as diabetic pigs and skin-humanized mice.[34]

TAKE-HOME MESSAGE

Basic science advances

- Testing cell–gene therapy approaches require valid surrogate markers in the context of appropriate wound-healing preclinical models. The skin-humanized mouse model represents one of such experimental platforms, and its ability to recapitulate physiologic acute human excisional wounds has been extremely useful to design new growth factor delivery strategies.

Clinical science advances

- With relatively few variations, our bioengineered skin equivalent has been shown to be capable of engraftment in cases of large skin acute losses (using autologous epidermal stem cells) or greatly enhancing the patient's own healing in chronic wounds. However, some defiant features such as infection or impaired vascularization compromise the therapeutic efficacy of skin substitutes. A further turn into the enhanced performance of skin substitutes may be the use of genetically modified keratinocytes and/or fibroblasts to provide a favorable niche for regeneration. Pleiotropic factors such as cathelicidin LL-37 appear in sight as potential candidates to perform such a role.

Relevance to clinical care

- Clinical management of skin wounds, from life-threatening acute (*e.g.*, severe burns) to highly prevalent ones such as chronic ulcers, represents a major challenge. Smart bioengineered products should provide both the cellular and soluble factors enabling wound closure for each situation.

FUTURE DEVELOPMENT

A large body of evidence now demonstrates that many currently available cell-based wound therapies are effective in achieving or accelerating cutaneous wound repair and/or regeneration. However, potential technologic improvements may further enhance the applications of this approach. For example, more effective cell preservation techniques could enhance shelf life and minimize problems related to storage and shipping. Issues related to the dermal matrix, important in providing a scaffold for mesenchymal cell homing and allowing better tissue regeneration, have not been properly addressed. Thus, poor durability due to degradation or, conversely, difficulties in matrix remodeling may limit effectiveness of certain cell-based wound therapies and cellular skin substitutes. As mentioned, fibroblast-populated fibrin matrices support keratinocyte growth and are easily remodeled into collagenous (human) dermal tissue *in vivo*, allowing their use for both allogenic and autologous grafting purposes. Due to costs, commercially available live allogenic bilayered products that are a few square centimeters in area are only suitable for treating small wound areas.

Among those working in the field of skin replacement there is a feeling that current use of bioengineered skin products is underdeveloped. Challenges remain regarding the abilities of skin bioengineering to improve cosmetic/esthetic situations such as burn sequels.

A comprehensive understanding of the mechanisms involved in normal and impaired healing could lead to smart combinations with genetic modification of the cells to overproduce various growth factors and cytokines. As many other young therapeutic modalities, skin bioengineering and cutaneous gene therapy will certainly meet further improvements as basic and applied science continue to nourish the field.

ACKNOWLEDGMENTS

This work was supported by Grants SAF2007-61019 from Ministerio de Ciencia e Innovación (Spain), PSE-090100-2006-3 from Ministerio de Educación y Ciencia (Spain), and LSHB-CT-512102 from European Framework Program (UE).

AUTHOR DISCLOSURE STATEMENT

No competing financial interests exist.

REFERENCES

1. Eming SA, Smola H, and Krieg T: Treatment of chronic wounds: state of the art and future concepts. Cells Tissues Organs 2002; **172:** 105.
2. Auger FA, Lacroix D, and Germain L: Skin substitutes and wound healing. Skin Pharmacol Physiol 2009; **22:** 94.
3. Meana A, Iglesias J, Del Rio M, *et al.*: Large surface of cultured human epithelium obtained on a dermal matrix based on live fibroblast-containing fibrin gels. Burns 1998; **24:** 621.
4. Camblor-Santervás L, Meana-Infiesta A, Llaneza-Coto JM, *et al.*: Treatment of chronic vascular ulcers with skin equivalent obtained by tissue engineering. Angiologia 2003; **55:** 21.
5. Llames S, Garcia E, Garcia V, *et al.*: Clinical results of an autologous engineered skin. Cell Tissue Bank 2006; **7:** 47.
6. Llames SG, Del Rio M, Larcher F, *et al.*: Human plasma as a dermal scaffold for the generation of a completely autologous bioengineered skin. Transplantation 2004; **77:** 350.
7. Garcia M, Escamez MJ, Carretero M, *et al.*: Modeling normal and pathological processes through skin tissue engineering. Mol Carcinog 2007; **46:** 741.
8. DelRio MD, Larcher F, Meana A, Segovia J, Alvarez A, and Jorcano J: Nonviral transfer of genes to pig primary keratinocytes. Induction of angiogenesis by composite grafts of modified keratinocytes overexpressing VEGF driven by a keratin promoter. Gene Ther 1999; **6:** 1734.
9. Carretero M, Del Rio M, Garcia M, *et al.*: A cutaneous gene therapy approach to treat infection through keratinocyte-targeted overexpression of antimicrobial peptides. FASEB J 2004; **18:** 1931.
10. Carretero M, Escamez MJ, Garcia M, *et al.*: *In vitro* and *in vivo* wound healing-promoting activities of human cathelicidin LL-37. J Invest Dermatol 2008; **128:** 223.
11. Lasso JM, Del Rio M, Garcia M, *et al.*: Improving flap survival by transplantation of a VEGF-secreting endothelised scaffold during distal pedicle flap creation. J Plast Reconstr Aesthet Surg 2007; **60:** 279.
12. Escamez MJ, Garcia M, Larcher F, *et al.*: An *in vivo* model of wound healing in genetically modified skin-humanized mice. J Invest Dermatol 2004; **123:** 1182.
13. Escamez MJ, Carretero M, Garcia M, *et al.*: Assessment of optimal virus-mediated growth factor gene delivery for human cutaneous wound healing enhancement. J Invest Dermatol 2008; **128:** 1565.
14. Macri L and Clark RA: Tissue engineering for cutaneous wounds: selecting the proper time and space for growth factors, cells and the extracellular matrix. Skin Pharmacol Physiol 2009; **22:** 83.
15. Carretero M, Escamez MJ, Prada F, *et al.*: Skin gene therapy for acquired and inherited disorders. Histol Histopathol 2006; **21:** 1233.
16. Werner S and Grose R: Regulation of wound healing by growth factors and cytokines. Physiol Rev 2003; **83:** 835.
17. Davidson JM, Whitsitt JS, Pennington B, Ballas CB, Eming S, and Benn SI: Gene therapy of wounds with growth factors. Curr Top Pathol 1999; **93:** 111.
18. Eming SA, Krieg T, and Davidson JM: Gene therapy and wound healing. Clin Dermatol 2007; **25:** 79.
19. Scheid A, Meuli M, Gassmann M, and Wenger RH: Genetically modified mouse models in studies on cutaneous wound healing. Exp Physiol 2000; **85:** 687.
20. Davidson J: Experimental Animal Wounds Models. Wounds 2001; **13:** 9.
21. Sullivan TP, Eaglstein WH, Davis SC, and Mertz P: The pig as a model for human wound healing. Wound Repair Regen 2001; **9:** 66.
22. Garlick JA and Taichman LB: Fate of human keratinocytes during reepithelialization in an organotypic culture model. Lab Invest 1994; **70:** 916.
23. Demarchez M, Sengel P, and Prunieras M: Wound healing of human skin transplanted onto the nude mouse. I. An immunohistological study of the reepithelialization process. Dev Biol 1986; **113:** 90.
24. Demarchez M, Hartmann DJ, Herbage D, Ville G, and Prunieras M: Wound healing of human skin transplanted onto the nude mouse. II. An immunohistological and ultrastructural study of the epidermal basement membrane zone reconstruction and connective tissue reorganization. Dev Biol 1987; **121:** 119.
25. Del Rio M, Larcher F, Serrano F, *et al.*: A preclinical model for the analysis of genetically modified human skin *in vivo*. Hum Gene Ther 2002; **13:** 959.
26. Larcher F, Murillas R, Bolontrade M, Conti CJ, and Jorcano JL: VEGF/VPF overexpression in skin of transgenic mice induces angiogenesis, vascular hyperpermeability and accelerated tumor development. Oncogene 1998; **17:** 303.
27. Supp DM, Supp AP, Bell SM, and Boyce ST: Enhanced vascularization of cultured skin substitutes genetically modified to overexpress vascular endothelial growth factor. J Invest Dermatol 2000; **114:** 5.
28. Braff MH and Gallo RL: Antimicrobial peptides: an essential component of the skin defensive barrier. Curr Top Microbiol Immunol 2006; **306:** 91.

29. Niyonsaba F, Ushio H, Nakano N, *et al.*: Antimicrobial peptides human beta-defensins stimulate epidermal keratinocyte migration, proliferation and production of proinflammatory cytokines and chemokines. J Invest Dermatol 2007; **127:** 594.

30. Otte JM, Werner I, Brand S, *et al.*: Human beta defensin 2 promotes intestinal wound healing *in vitro*. J Cell Biochem 2008; **104:** 2286.

31. Thomas-Virnig CL, Centanni JM, Johnston CE, *et al.*: Inhibition of multidrug-resistant *Acinetobacter baumannii* by nonviral expression of hCAP-18 in a bioengineered human skin tissue. Mol Ther 2009; **17:** 562.

32. Davidson JM: First-class delivery: getting growth factors to their destination. J Invest Dermatol 2008; **128:** 1360.

33. Eming SA, Brachvogel B, Odorisio T, and Koch M: Regulation of angiogenesis: wound healing as a model. Prog Histochem Cytochem 2007; **42:** 115.

34. Martinez-Santamaria L, Escamez MJ, Carretero M, *et al.*: Analysis of NGF effects in a humanized model of impaired wound healing. 21st World Congress of Dermatology, Buenos Aires, 2007.

WHS Wound Healing Society

Platelet-Derived Growth Factor Delivery via Nanofibrous Scaffolds for Soft-Tissue Repair

Qiming Jin,[1] Peter X. Ma,[2,3] and William V. Giannobile[1,3,*]

[1]Department of Periodontics and Oral Medicine, Michigan Center for Oral Health Research, School of Dentistry, University of Michigan, Ann Arbor, Michigan.
[2]Department of Biologic and Materials Sciences, School of Dentistry, University of Michigan, Ann Arbor, Michigan.
[3]Department of Biomedical Engineering, College of Engineering, University of Michigan, Ann Arbor, Michigan.

Background: Platelet-derived growth factor (PDGF) is a multifunctional growth factor that exerts its biological effects on cellular chemotaxis, proliferation, matrix synthesis, antiapoptosis, and vascularization. PDGF is clinically approved to treat neuropathic diabetic ulcers and osseous defects due to periodontal disease.
The Problem: The short half-life *in vivo* of PDGF limits the efficacy of its biological functions. Solving this problem remains a key obstacle for PDGF clinical application. Therefore, the development of an optimized controlled release delivery system offers significant potential.
Basic/Clinical Science Advances: In this article, we highlight the development of a polymeric delivery system of nanofibrous scaffolds containing PDGF-encapsulated microspheres for tissue engineering. The designed scaffolds were evaluated in a subcutaneous implantation model for tissue neogenesis, vascularization, and chemokine gene expression, as well as soft-tissue repair. PDGF was found to strongly upregulate *in vivo* gene expression of the CXC chemokine family members such as CXC chemokine ligand *CXCL1*, *CXCL2*, and *CXCL5* that are important in angiogenesis, inflammation, and wound repair.
Clinical Care Relevance: Recombinant human PDGF is approved by the Food and Drug Administration for patients afflicted with diabetic foot ulcers or compromised periodontal wounds. Challenges related to the transient biological activity of bolus PDGF administration using currently available release systems continue. Thus, it is necessary to explore new delivery systems to optimize biological activity and bioavailability of tissue growth factors.
Conclusion: The use of a controlled, "dial-able" delivery system allows for a more tightly regulated release of factors to promote repair of soft- and hard-tissue defects for clinical application.

Abbreviations and Acronyms

AAV = adeno-associated virus
CXCL = CXC chemokine ligand
HMW = high-molecular weight
LMW = low-molecular weight
MS = microsphere
NFSs = nanofibrous scaffolds
PDGF = platelet-derived growth factor
PLGA = poly(lactide-co-glycolide)
PLLA = poly(L-lactic acid)

*Correspondence: Michigan Center for Oral Health Research, School of Dentistry, University of Michigan, 1011 N. University Ave., Ann Arbor, Michigan 48109-1078 (e-mail: william.giannobile@umich.edu).

BACKGROUND

A KEY CHALLENGE for the clinical use of growth factors for wound repair is the development of an effective delivery system that integrates appropriate scaffolds and signaling molecules for tissue repair and regeneration.[1–3] Biological delivery systems for proteins and peptides can be divided mainly into two strategies: protein delivery systems and gene delivery systems.[4] For gene delivery systems, several recombinant vectors, including plasmids, adenovirus, adeno-associated virus (AAV), and retrovirus, have been developed and tested both preclinically and clinically.[5] Vector selection and dosing can be applied to control the transduction and durationof the targeted protein.[6] However, biosafety remains a consideration with viral vector–based gene delivery

Printed in U.S.A.
DOI: 10.1089/awc.2009.0170

systems.[7] In a protein delivery system, two preparation methods—surface coating and encapsulation—are commonly used. During surface coating preparation, the release rate of the proteins and peptides is primarily determined by the physicochemical interactions between protein and biomaterial. In contrast, the release rate of proteins and peptides during encapsulation preparation occurs primarily via diffusion, polymer degradation, or a combination thereof.[8] Recently, nanofibrous scaffolds (NFSs) with controlled release growth factors encapsulated in microspheres (MSs) have shown significant potential for tissue engineering applications.[9–11]

Platelet-derived growth factor (PDGF) is a member of a multifunctional growth factor family that exerts its biological effects on cellular chemotaxis, proliferation, extracellular matrix synthesis, antiapoptosis, and vascularization.[12] PDGF not only participates in embryonic development of organs such as kidney, heart, and vasculature[13] but also plays an important role in postnatal tissue repair, regeneration, and disease development.[14] The U.S. Food and Drug Administration has approved clinical use of recombinant human PDGF-BB to treat diabetic foot ulcers and periodontal osseous defects.[15,16] However, we have sought to study the feasibility of NFS/MS constructs for tissue engineering as well as the role of PDGF biological functions in tissue neogenesis and vascularization.[9]

TAKE-HOME MESSAGE FOR THE USE OF NFSS FOR GROWTH FACTOR DELIVERY

Basic science advances

- Growth factor as a major local regulator participates in tissue repair and regeneration.
- PDGF has multiple biological functions, such as cellular chemotaxis, proliferation, extracellular matrix synthesis, antiapoptosis, and vascularization.
- PDGF not only improves soft-tissue neogenesis but also enhances hard-tissue formation such as bone and cementum.
- *In vivo* biological functions of PDGF depend on the release delivery system and dosage.
- For PDGF, polymer molecular weight control release rate of PDGF and encapsulation is more effective than surface coating.
- PDGF stimulates gene expression of chemokines such as *CXCL-1*, *-2*, and *-5*, which may modulate PDGF's effects on cell chemotaxis, proliferation, and angiogenesis.

Clinical science advances

- Development of a controlled release system that allows for the administration of bioactive molecules for soft-tissue repair.
- The use of this NFS controlled release system incorporating PDGF was able to accelerate tissue invasion and tissue neogenesis, both of which are important for wound repair.
- The controlled release system can allow for the release of growth factors over days, weeks, or months, which may be of great value for specific clinical situations depending on the dosing needs to specific defects.

Relevance to clinical care

- The use of NFSs incorporating growth factor MSs may allow for the controlled release of biological factors within harsh wound-healing environments (such as the chronic wound site) that will improve bioavailability and potency of growth factor molecules for regenerative medicine applications.
- Controlled delivery systems may abrogate the need for multiple applications of growth factors in the clinical arena where it is not efficient or feasible for clinicians and patients to manage successive, inconvenient applications of exogenous growth factors.

CLINICAL PROBLEM ADDRESSED

The short duration of *in vivo* biological activity (on the order of hours or days) of proteins and peptides limits the efficacy of their function *in vivo* for tissue engineering applications. Therefore, the development of controlled release delivery systems is essential for the clinical application of growth factors. Research efforts are now focused on the "on-demand," controllable systems to promote repair of soft- and hard-tissue defects. Polymers such as poly(L-lactic acid) (PLLA) and poly(lactide-co-glycolide) (PLGA) can be processed into MSs with a desired size and can be loaded with growth factor of required concentrations for clinical applications in regenerative medicine.

RELEVANT BASIC SCIENCE CONTEXT

Biodegradable polymer degradation *in vivo* occurs mainly via hydrolysis and host phagocytosis.[10] Because these polymers possess good biocompatibility, PLLA and PLGA have been widely used for the delivery of polypeptides, proteins, and cells.[17,18] The release rate of polypeptides carried by these polymers can be controlled by adjusting the factor loading, polymer molecular weight, lactide-to-glycolide ratio within the copolymer, and formulation methods.[19,20] Compared with the traditional simple coating method in which the release rate of growth factor depends on physico-chemical interactions between the adsorbed growth factors and scaffold surfaces (that typically results in rapid release [hours or days release of factors]), the release rate of growth factor embedded in MSs is more easily controlled by the molecular weight. High-molecular weight (HMW) polymers are hydrolyzed more slowly than those with a low-molecular weight (LMW) polymers, which result in a slower release rate for polypeptides encapsulated by HMW polymers.

Recently, our group has developed novel macroporous NFSs, which are fabricated using a combination of phase separation and sugar-leaching techniques. The unique characteristic of this NFS is the nanofibrous pore walls instead of the solid pore walls, which increases the scaffold porosity to 98%, favoring diffusion of nutrients and oxygen.[10] This NFS has been shown to support bone formation induced by bone morphogenetic proteins and soft-tissue neogenesis initiated by PDGF.[10,11]

EXPERIMENTAL MODEL OR MATERIAL—ADVANTAGES AND LIMITATIONS

NFS/MS delivery system preparation

Polymer spheres, with diameters in the submicrometer to nanometer range, were fabricated using an established double emulsion technique.[21] PDGF-BB was encapsulated within the MSs with molecular weights of 65 and 6.4 kDa, respectively, and stored at −80°C until use. Macroporous NFSs were fabricated by a combination of the phase separation and sugar-leaching techniques as previously described.[22] The scaffolds were fabricated into disc shapes 7.2×2 mm in size, with a 250–425 μm pore size. PDGF-BB MS solution was added dropwise into nanofibrous disc-shape scaffolds, then divided into seven groups of specimens to investigate the effect of PDGF release rate on PDGF biological function using a rat dorsal subcutaneous implantation model. Under anesthesia, subcutaneous pockets on the dorsum of rats were surgically created, and the scaffolds were placed into the

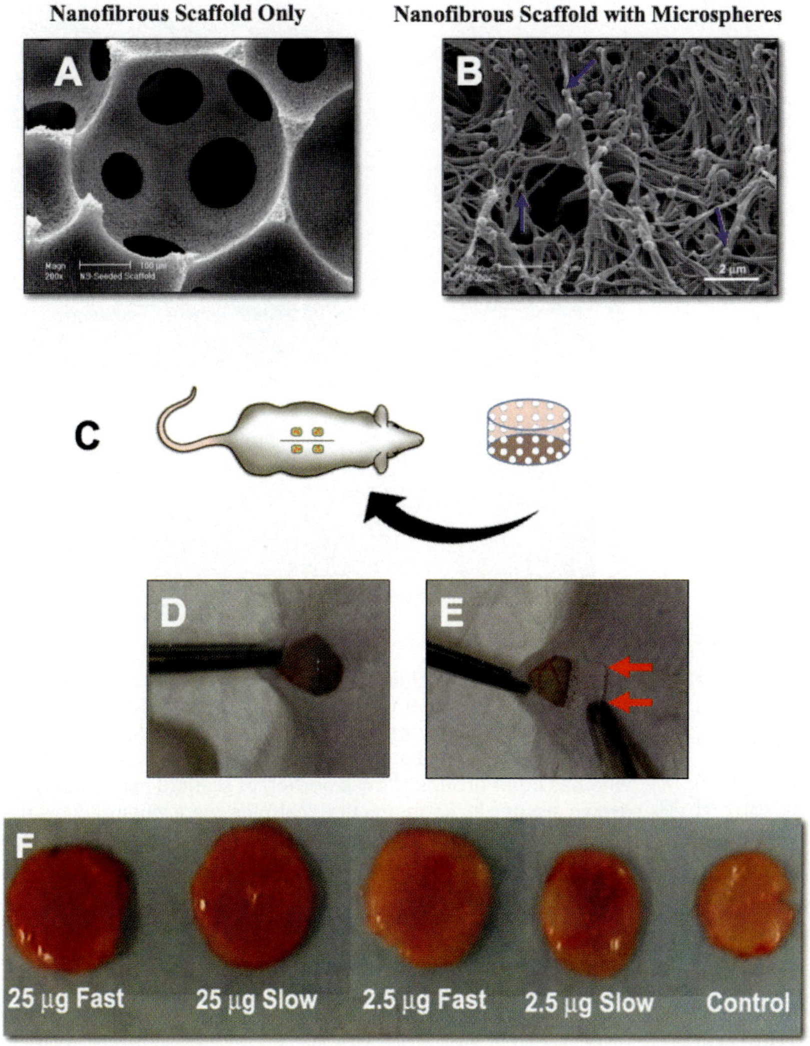

Figure 1. NFSs incorporating MSs for soft-tissue engineering. This schematic represents the application of NFS incorporating MSs that can be used for transplantation of cells or proteins (such as PDGF) for tissue regeneration applications. (**A**) NFS only, (**B**) NFS with MSs. Blue arrows in (**B**) point to MSs. Panel (**C**) demonstrates the utilization of the rodent animal model used in these studies whereby the scaffold construct is placed ectopically into the dorsa of the animals to evaluate tissue and vascular invasion into the devices (**D, E**). Red arrows in (**E**) point to scaffold placement. Panel (**F**) shows the macroscopic view of scaffolds and corresponding tissue after 7 days *in vivo*. Adapted from Jin *et al.*[9] and Wei *et al.*[10]

pockets (Fig. 1). The groups evaluated included the following: NFS alone; NFS with 2.5 μg PDGF-BB coating; NFS with 25 μg PDGF-BB coating; NFS with 6.4 kDa MSs containing 2.5 μg PDGF-BB; NFS with 6.4 kDa MSs containing 25 μg PDGF-BB; NFS with 65 kDa MSs containing 2.5 μg PDGF-BB; and NFS with 65 kDa MSs containing 25 μg PDGF-BB.[9]

RNA extraction and purification

RNA was extracted and purified according to the manufacturer's instructions (Qiagen, Valencia, CA), followed by Affymetrix GeneChip analysis. Following the identification of genes that demonstrated significant induction or repression, follow-up quantitative PCR was performed on the tissue-scaffold samples.

Statistical analyses

The differences among groups regarding tissue penetration, tissue area, blood vessel number, and real-time PCR gene expression were statistically assessed using one-way analysis of variance with Tukey multiple comparison *post hoc* test using a statistical software package Prism 4 (GraphPad, San Diego, CA). There was a minimum of three samples per group available for analysis. The level of significance was considered as $p < 0.05$. For microarray assessments, triplicate samples were pooled for gene chip analyses. Samples were displayed using an arbitrary 10-fold change cut-off for subsequent assessment with quantitative real-time PCR analysis.[9]

DISCUSSION OF FINDINGS AND RELEVANT LITERATURE

The efficiency of *in vivo* biological functions of PDGF-BB is controlled by the delivery system

For the descriptive analysis of tissue neogenesis, histological observations were carried out at 3 days after implantation, and no significant tissue in-growth into the scaffolds was found in any of the groups (data not shown). However, by 7 days, penetrating tissue occupied the entire scaffold spaces in several groups containing PDGF encapsulated in MSs, while tissue penetration was seen only in the superficial regions of scaffolds in the groups with PDGF-coating only and the groups devoid of PDGF (Figs. 2 and 3). In addition, we observed more vascularization and thicker connective tissue capsules surrounding scaffolds in the groups with PDGF encapsulation by MSs compared with groups without MSs (Fig. 3).

Concurrent with the first week histological observations, the histomorphometric measurements

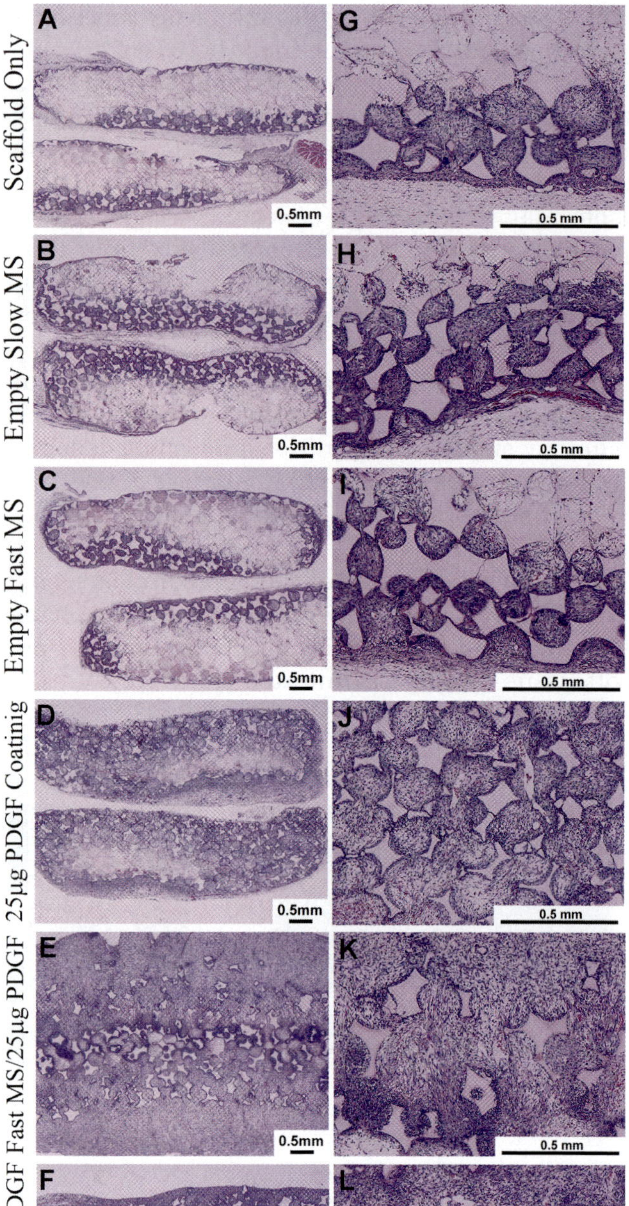

Figure 2. PDGF-containing MSs in NFSs stimulates tissue invasion *in vivo*. Left panel (A to F) at low magnification (2×) shows the tissue completely penetrated the entire NFS for the groups with PDGF encapsulated in poly(lactide-co-glycolide) MSs, whereas other groups show a portion of scaffold occupied by in-grown tissue. In addition, the scaffolds were enlarged by the penetrated tissues in the groups with high-dose PDGF encapsulated in poly(lactide-co-glycolide) MSs. Right panel (G to L) at high magnification (10×) demonstrated that most of the cells in the penetrated tissues were fibroblast-like and lymphocyte-like cells. On the scaffold pore surfaces, multiple macrophage-like cells were seen. Hematoxylin and eosin staining. Bars indicate 0.5 mm. Adapted from Jin *et al.*[9] PDGF = platelet-derived growth factor; MSs = microspheres; NFSs = nanofibrous scaffolds.

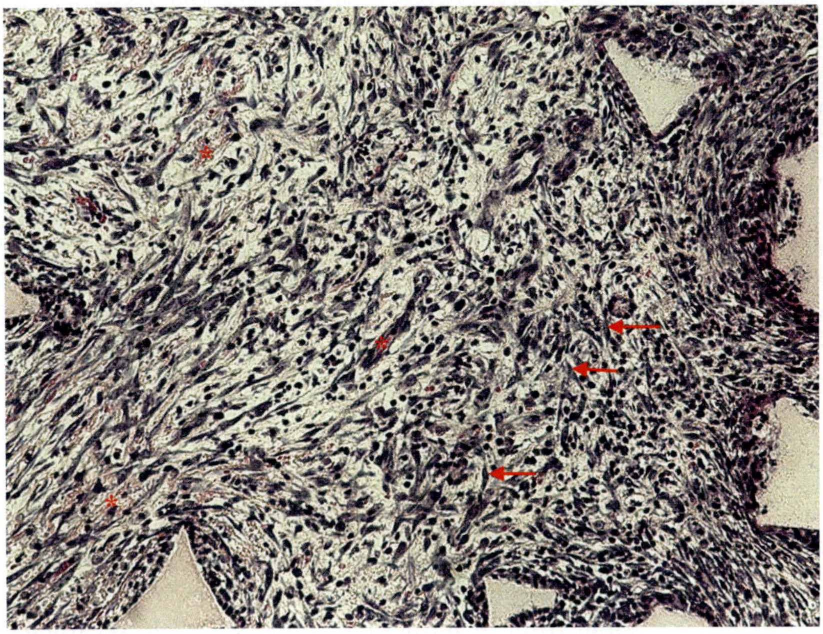

Figure 3. High magnification of histological microphotograph of the biopsies of NFS with high-molecular weight polymer MSs containing 25 μg PDGF at 1 week after implantation. Many fibroblast-like cells occupied the pore space, and a large amount of blood vessels was also formed. Red arrows indicate fibroblast-like cells. Red stars indicate mature blood vessels. Hematoxylin and eosin staining, 20×magnification.

on the 1 week specimens showed that the areas representing the specimen volume were significantly greater in the groups with NFSs containing either PDGF encapsulated in HMW MSs or high-dose PDGF encapsulated in LMW MSs compared with the other groups. With regard to the tissue penetration percentage (penetration tissue area *vs.* the whole area), tissue invasion in the groups containing PDGF encapsulated by MSs was greater than the groups with PDGF and the group with 2.5 g PDGF coating. Further, using factor VIII immunostaining to view and quantitate blood vessels using light microscopy, we observed that vascularization forming inside scaffolds was greater for the groups with PDGF encapsulated in HMW MSs, which was in accordance with the results of measurements of blood vessel number. There were significantly more blood vessels formed in the groups containing NFSs plus PDGF encapsulated in HMW MSs (data not shown).

Therefore, the above results indicate that *in vivo* PDGF-BB biological functions, such as proliferation, neogenesis, and vascularization, are mediated predominantly using a slow control release delivery system, such as NFS/HMW MSs. Molecular weight has an obvious relationship to the *in vivo* effects of PDGF encapsulated by the polymers. The groups with PDGF encapsulated within polymer MSs yielded 100% tissue penetration, whereas the groups having PDGF coated on the surface of the NFSs resulted in only 20–75% tissue penetration. Further, specimen areas were much larger for the groups with 25 g PDGF encapsulated in LMW and HMW MSs or 2.5 g PDGF encapsulated in HMW MSs when compared with other groups. These results demonstrate that tissue penetration and specimen area are dependent on the *in vivo* PDGF release rate. The results of blood vessel number and area also showed a similar correlation with the *in vivo* PDGF release rate.

The effect of PDGF-BB on the increasing gene expression of chemokines is also related to a release control delivery system

The family of chemokines is composed of low-molecular weight peptides with highly conserved cysteine motifs, which have biological functions on lymphocyte trafficking inflammation and immunity, angiogenesis, hematopoiesis, wound healing, and stem-cell chemotaxis,[23] and which may modulate PDGF biological functions on cell proliferation, chemotaxis, and vascularization. PDGF is thought to stimulate chemokine expression through the NF-kappa B (nuclear factor kappa-light-chain-enhancer of activated B cells) pathway.[24,25]

In our study, Affymetrix GeneChip analysis demonstrated that PDGF upregulated gene expression of several members of chemokine family, such as CXC chemokine ligand *CXCL-1*, *-2*, and *-5*, more than 10-fold compared with non-PDGF groups (data not shown). Using quantitative PCR to confirm the GeneChip results, PDGF was shown to induce chemokine gene expression in both a dose-dependent and duration-dependent manner.[9] The *CXCL1* gene expression induced by the 25 g PDGF encapsulated in both LMW and HMW PLGA MSs was higher than that in the scaffold-alone group, PDGF-coating group, or low-dose PDGF MS group. In contrast, *CXCL1* gene expression induced by 2.5 g PDGF encapsulated in LMW and HMW PLGA MSs showed no significant differences from either the scaffold alone or PDGF-coating groups, which indicates that upregulation of *CXCL1* gene expression stimulated by PDGF is dependent on the PDGF dose. This relationship is also seen for chemokines *CXCL-2* and *-5*. However, the gene expression of *CXCL-1*, *-2*, and *-5* induced by 25 g PDGF coated on PLLA scaffolds (not encapsulated in PLGA MSs) was not different from the empty scaffold or 2.5 g (low dose) PDGF MS groups, suggesting that the PDGF release from PDGF-coated scaffolds may be too rapid to be effective. The utilization of other gene-specific approaches and transcriptome analyses offers much potential for the evaluation of wound repair genetic regulation *in vivo*.[26] Thus, the controlled delivery of PDGF will likely be critical for clinical success (Fig. 2).

CAUTION, CRITICAL REMARKS, AND RECOMMENDATIONS

The use of polymeric delivery systems for clinical procedures has a long track record of use as implantable devices, including suture materials, scaffold matrices for soft-tissue repair, and more recently, drug delivery.[27] The use of polymeric scaffolds for regenerative medicine applications is still in the early stages of clinical development for widespread use. MS technologies have been used in a variety of clinical situations, as in drug delivery of antimicrobial molecules.[28] However, controlled human clinical trials are necessary to determine the optimal delivery strategy to promote tissue regeneration beyond that of current bolus type delivery systems for tissue repair.[29] Given that box warnings have been issued for the multiple applications of PDGF for soft-tissue ulcers (*e.g.*, up to 144 applications given), it may be of value to consider controlled delivery approaches that may expose patients to greatly reduced dosages of growth stimulatory factors.

FUTURE DEVELOPMENT

Future development in the field will include the delivery of multiple factors important for tissue repair, host defense, and antiinfective governance in the regenerative medicine field.[30–32] The consideration of on-demand and dial-able strategies for delivery of growth-promoting molecules may provide for a more finely tuned delivery system to allow for exquisite controlled delivery of tissue regenerating molecules.

ACKNOWLEDGMENT

This research was supported by NIH/NIDR DE 13397 and DE 15384.

AUTHOR DISCLOSURE STATEMENT

W.V.G. has financial interest in BioMimetic Therapeutics (Franklin, TN).

REFERENCES

1. Eming SA, Krieg T, and Davidson JM: Inflammation in wound repair: molecular and cellular mechanisms. J Invest Dermatol 2007; **127:** 514.
2. Kaigler D, Cirelli JA, and Giannobile WV: Growth factor delivery for oral and periodontal tissue engineering. Expert Opin Drug Deliv 2006; **3:** 647.
3. Langer R and Tirrell DA: Designing materials for biology and medicine. Nature 2004; **428:** 487.
4. Eming SA, Krieg T, and Davidson JM: Gene therapy and wound healing. Clin Dermatol 2007; **25:** 79.
5. Phillips JE, Gersbach CA, and Garcia AJ: Virus-based gene therapy strategies for bone regeneration. Biomaterials 2007; **28:** 211.
6. Ramseier CA, Abramson ZR, Jin Q, and Giannobile WV: Gene therapeutics for periodontal regenerative medicine. Dent Clin North Am 2006; **50:** 245, ix.
7. Chang PC, Cirelli JA, Jin Q, Seol YJ, Sugai JV, D'Silva NJ, Danciu TE, Chandler LA, Sosnowski BA, and Giannobile WV: Adenovirus encoding human platelet-derived growth factor-B delivered to alveolar bone defects exhibits safety and biodistribution profiles favorable for clinical use. Hum Gene Ther 2009; **20:** 486.
8. Faisant N, Siepmann J, and Benoit JP: PLGA-based microparticles: elucidation of mechanisms and a new, simple mathematical model quantifying drug release. Eur J Pharmacol Sci 2002; **15:** 355.
9. Jin Q, Wei G, Lin Z, Sugai JV, Lynch SE, Ma PX, and Giannobile WV: Nanofibrous scaffolds incorporating PDGF-BB microspheres induce chemokine expression and tissue neogenesis *in vivo*. PLoS ONE 2008; **3:** e1729.
10. Wei G, Jin Q, Giannobile WV, and Ma PX: Nano-fibrous scaffold for controlled delivery of recombinant human PDGF-BB. J Control Release 2006; **112:** 103.
11. Wei G, Jin Q, Giannobile WV, and Ma PX: The enhancement of osteogenesis by nano-fibrous scaffolds incorporating rhBMP-7 nanospheres. Biomaterials 2007; **28:** 2087.
12. Andrae J, Gallini R, and Betsholtz C: Role of platelet-derived growth factors in physiology and medicine. Genes Dev 2008; **22:** 1276.
13. Kaminski WE, Lindahl P, Lin NL, Broudy VC, Crosby JR, Hellstrom M, Swolin B, Bowen-Pope DF, Martin PJ, Ross R, Betsholtz C, and Raines EW: Basis of hematopoietic defects in platelet-derived growth factor (PDGF)-B and PDGF beta-receptor null mice. Blood 2001; **97:** 1990.
14. Alvarez RH, Kantarjian HM, and Cortes JE: Biology of platelet-derived growth factor and its involvement in disease. Mayo Clin Proc 2006; **81:** 1241.
15. Nevins M, Giannobile WV, McGuire MK, Kao RT, Mellonig JT, Hinrichs JE, McAllister BS, Murphy KS, McClain PK, Nevins ML, Paquette DW, Han TJ, Reddy MS, Lavin PT, Genco RJ, and Lynch SE: Platelet-derived growth factor stimulates bone fill and rate of attachment level gain: results of a large multicenter randomized controlled trial. J Periodontol 2005; **76:** 2205.

16. Steed DL: Clinical evaluation of recombinant human platelet-derived growth factor for the treatment of lower extremity ulcers. Plast Reconstr Surg 2006; **117:** 143S; discussion 150S–151S.

17. Lee KY, Peters MC, Anderson KW, and Mooney DJ: Controlled growth factor release from synthetic extracellular matrices. Nature 2000; **408:** 998.

18. Richardson TP, Peters MC, Ennett AB, and Mooney DJ: Polymeric system for dual growth factor delivery. Nat Biotechnol 2001; **19:** 1029.

19. Grayson AC, Voskerician G, Lynn A, Anderson JM, Cima MJ, and Langer R: Differential degradation rates *in vivo* and *in vitro* of biocompatible poly(lactic acid) and poly(glycolic acid) homo- and co-polymers for a polymeric drug-delivery microchip. J Biomater Sci Polym Ed 2004; **15:** 1281.

20. Lee S, Kim MS, Kim JS, Park HJ, Woo JS, Lee BC, and Hwang SJ: Controlled delivery of a hydrophilic drug from a biodegradable microsphere system by supercritical anti-solvent precipitation technique. J Microencapsul 2006; **23:** 741.

21. Wei G, Pettway GJ, McCauley LK, and Ma PX: The release profiles and bioactivity of parathyroid hormone from poly(lactic-co-glycolic acid) microspheres. Biomaterials 2004; **25:** 345.

22. Wei G and Ma PX: Macroporous and nanofibrous polymer scaffolds and polymer/bone-like apatite composite scaffolds generated by sugar spheres. J Biomed Mater Res A 2006; **78:** 306.

23. Rollins BJ: Chemokines. Blood 1997; **90:** 909.

24. Romashkova JA and Makarov SS: NF-kappaB is a target of AKT in anti-apoptotic PDGF signalling. Nature 1999; **401:** 86.

25. Wood LD, Farmer AA, and Richmond A: HMGI(Y) and Sp1 in addition to NF-kappa B regulate transcription of the MGSA/GRO alpha gene. Nucleic Acids Res 1995; **23:** 4210.

26. Roy S, Patel D, Khanna S, Gordillo GM, Biswas S, Friedman A, and Sen CK: Transcriptome-wide analysis of blood vessels laser captured from human skin and chronic wound-edge tissue. Proc Natl Acad Sci USA 2007; **104:** 14472.

27. Ma PX: Biomimetic materials for tissue engineering. Adv Drug Deliv Rev 2008; **60:** 184.

28. Williams RC, Paquette DW, Offenbacher S, Adams DF, Armitage GC, Bray K, Caton J, Cochran DL, Drisko CH, Fiorellini JP, Giannobile WV, Grossi S, Guerrero DM, Johnson GK, Lamster IB, Magnusson I, Oringer RJ, Persson GR, Van Dyke TE, Wolff LF, Santucci EA, Rodda BE, and Lessem J: Treatment of periodontitis by local administration of minocycline microspheres: a controlled trial. J Periodontol 2001; **72:** 1535.

29. Farokhzad OC and Langer R: Impact of nanotechnology on drug delivery. ACS Nano 2009; **3:** 16.

30. Hafeman AE, Li B, Yoshii T, Zienkiewicz K, Davidson JM, and Guelcher SA: Injectable biodegradable polyurethane scaffolds with release of platelet-derived growth factor for tissue repair and regeneration. Pharm Res 2008; **25:** 2387.

31. Li B, Davidson JM, and Guelcher SA: The effect of the local delivery of platelet-derived growth factor from reactive two-component polyurethane scaffolds on the healing in rat skin excisional wounds. Biomaterials 2009; **30:** 3486.

32. Liu X, Smith LA, Hu J, and Ma PX: Biomimetic nanofibrous gelatin/apatite composite scaffolds for bone tissue engineering. Biomaterials 2009; **30:** 2252.

WHS
Wound
Healing
Society

Gene Delivery to Wounds Using Allogenic Keratinocytes

Taro Koyama,[1] Pejman Aflaki,[1] Jan Jeroen Vranckx,[2] Feng Yao,[1] and Elof Eriksson[1,*]

[1]Laboratory of Tissue Repair and Gene Transfer, Division of Plastic Surgery, Brigham and Women's Hospital, Harvard Medical School, Boston, Massachusetts.
[2]Laboratory of Plastic Surgery and Tissue Engineering Research, Department of Plastic and Reconstructive Surgery, KU Leuven University Hospitals, Leuven, Belgium.

Abbreviations and Acronyms

hEGF = human epidermal growth factor

PDGF = platelet-derived growth factor

TGF-β = transforming growth factor-β

VEGF = vascular endothelial growth factor

*Correspondence: Joseph E. Murray Professor of Plastic and Reconstructive Surgery, Laboratory of Tissue Repair and Gene Transfer, Division of Plastic Surgery, Harvard Medical School, Brigham and Women's Hospital, Boston, Massachusetts 02115 (e-mail: eeriksson@partners.org).

Background: Gene therapy is a potentially attractive option in the treatment of nonhealing wounds. It aims at delivering the growth-modulating genes to the wound, enabling over or underexpression of specific molecules hence modifying the healing process. Transplantation of gene-transfected cells (*ex vivo* gene delivery) is one of the methods of delivering specific genes to the wound. Use of autologous keratinocytes as *ex vivo* gene delivery vehicles has previously been reported. In addition, successful clinical application of allogenic cultured keratinocyte as a temporary biological dressing for wounds has been described. Combining the two approaches, we evaluated the feasibility of transplantation of allogenic keratinocytes as gene delivery vehicles to accelerate wound healing.
The Problem: Prompt skin replacement is critical in the treatment of skin defects to prevent fluid loss and infection. Autografts are the most common technique; however, donor site shortage is a major limiting factor in resurfacing the extensive wounds. Despite the successful clinical application of *in vitro*–expanded autologous keratinocytes, the long process of preparation is a disadvantage of this approach.
Basic/Clinical Science Advances: Allogenic keratinocytes can function as temporary biological dressings, and in combination with gene delivery they can potentially optimize the host skin regenerative capacity before they are eventually rejected by the immune system.
Clinical Care Relevance: In a clinical context, cell cultures need to be readily available for treatment. Allogenic cell cultures can be cryopreserved, genetically modified, and used when required.
Conclusion: We demonstrated that human epidermal growth factor–transfected allogenic keratinocytes enhance re-epithelialization in porcine full-thickness wounds.

BACKGROUND

Gene therapy is a potentially attractive option in the treatment of nonhealing wounds. It aims at delivering the growth-modulating genes to the cells in the wound microenvironment, enabling overexpression or underexpression of specific molecules like cytokines and growth factors hence modifying the healing process. By providing a sustained delivery of these growth-modulating polypeptides, gene therapy has the advantage over direct application of recombinant factors, which are expensive and have a short half-life requiring frequent applications. The influence of growth factor gene delivery in wound healing, such as epidermal growth factor (EGF), keratinocyte growth factor, platelet-derived growth factor (PDGF), vascular endothelial growth factor (VEGF), transforming growth factor-β1 (TGF-β1), and insulin-like growth factor, has previously been investigated.[1–5]

Transplantation of gene-transfected cells to wounds (*ex vivo* gene

ADVANCES IN WOUND CARE, VOLUME 1

Printed in U.S.A.
DOI: 10.1089/awc.2009.0034

delivery) is one of the methods of delivering specific genes to the wound environment. The advantage of this approach over direct application of genes (*in vivo* gene delivery) is adding an extra cell source to the regenerating wound: transplanted cells serve as both regenerative seeds and carriers for specific genes to maximize the healing potential.

Use of autologous keratinocytes or fibroblasts as *ex vivo* gene delivery vehicles has previously been reported.[4,6] In addition, successful clinical application of allogenic cultured keratinocyte as a temporary biological dressing for wounds has been described.[7] Combining the two approaches, we evaluated the feasibility of transplantation of allogenic keratinocytes as efficient gene delivery vehicles to accelerate wound healing. Considering that allogenic cells can be prepared in advance, cryopreserved, and stored for later usage, such an approach aims to eliminate the lengthy process of preparation, which is a major limiting factor to the use of autologous cells in the critically ill patients often in urgent need for skin coverage.

CLINICAL PROBLEM ADDRESSED

Prompt skin replacement is critical in the treatment of skin defects to prevent fluid loss and infection. Autografts are the most commonly used technique for coverage of extensive acute burns or chronic nonhealing ulcers; however, donor site shortage is a major limiting factor in resurfacing the extensive wounds. Despite the successful clinical application of *in vitro*–expanded autologous keratinocytes as epidermal sheets,[8,9] the long process of approximately 3–4 weeks to obtain sufficient number of cells is a disadvantage of this approach.[10] Allogenic keratinocytes can function as temporary biological dressings, and in combination with gene delivery to overexpress growth factors they can potentially maximize the host skin regenerative capacity before they are eventually rejected by the immune system. They can be cryopreserved, stored in skin banks, and used when required.

RELEVANT BASIC SCIENCE CONTEXT

Wound healing is a complex biological process involving interaction of cellular and biochemical events. At the molecular level, wound healing is initiated and maintained by several cytokines and growth factors released from inflammatory cells, fibroblasts, platelets, and epithelial cells, regulating cell–cell interactions, cell migration, proliferation, and differentiation in a paracrine and autocrine fashion. Of particular importance are EGF, TGF-β, fibroblast growth factor, VEGF, and PDGF. The constant presence of these growth factors at various stages of wound healing appears to be responsible for the maintenance of the complex biological events that lead to complete skin regeneration.

Originally reported by Dr. Stanley Cohen and coworkers,[11] EGF is secreted by platelets, macrophages, keratinocytes, and fibroblasts and plays an important role in re-epithelialization by increasing keratinocyte proliferation and migration in acute wounds.[12,13] EGF binds to the EGF receptor, a tyrosine kinase transmembrane protein, resulting in dimerization of the receptor, autophosphorylation, and tyrosine phosphorylation of downstream proteins.[14] Ultimately this signaling pathway leads to the activation of a number of converging pathways promoting cell migration and proliferation.

While the topical administration of recombinant EGF and other growth factors has been reported to enhance wound healing,[15,16] their clinical application is limited due to their short half-life requiring repetitive doses, high cost, and lack of proper post-translational modifications that may impair its biological functions.[17,18] By temporary overexpression of EGF, gene therapy seems to be an effective approach to maintain a continuous EGF concentration, sustaining its presence in the wound and preventing its rapid proteolytic degradation.

EXPERIMENTAL MODEL OR MATERIAL—ADVANTAGES AND LIMITATIONS

Although a large number of studies on wound healing have used small animal models, the similarities between human and pig skin, in terms of the structure of dermis and epidermis and the cell turnover time, make the porcine model an excellent tool for studying wound healing.[19,20] We have developed and validated a unique wet wound healing model that employs a flexible, transparent polyurethane chamber developed by the senior author (Fig. 1A).[1–6,21] This unique liquid environment acts as an "*in vivo* incubator" allowing for controlling the wound microenvironment and daily analysis of the wound fluid. Wound chambers are placed over 1.5 cm × 1.5 cm full-thickness wounds created on dorsum of the Yorkshire pigs, and treatment fluid (saline with antibiotics) is injected.

Using the same model, we reported the positive effect of autologous transplantation of cell suspensions of keratinocytes (cultured and noncultured) on healing of full-thickness wounds.[21] Subsequently, we combined cell transplantation with

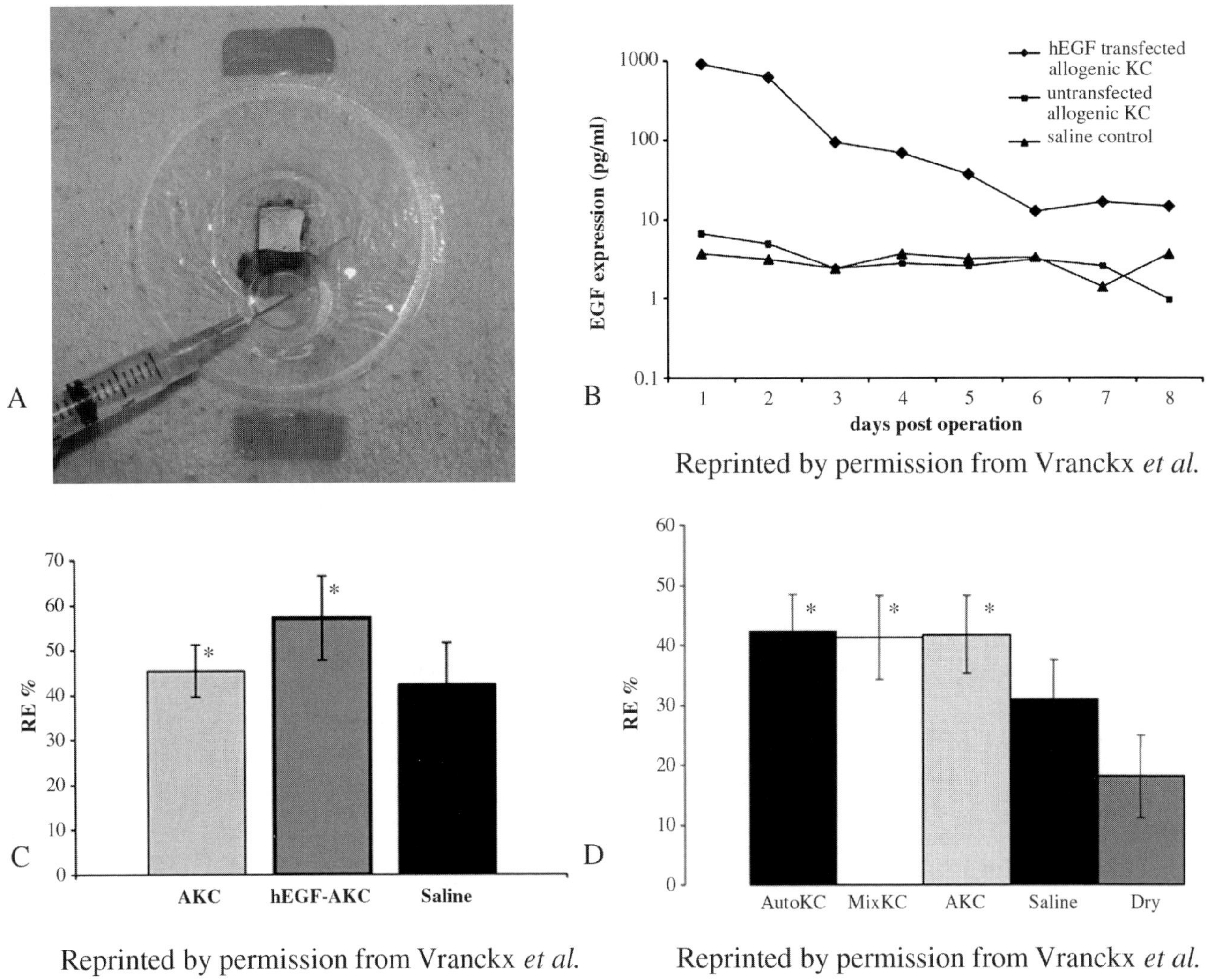

Figure 1. (**A**) Illustration of the liquid wound healing model provided by flexible, transparent polyurethane wound chambers placed over the 1.5×1.5 cm porcine full-thickness wound. The self-sealing injection pad incorporated into the chamber provides a port through which the treatment fluid (saline with antibiotics) or cell suspension cultures can be injected into the wound environment. The chamber's adhesive base has an opening corresponding to the wound size and is attached to the wound periphery. This closed liquid environment also protects against wound desiccation. (**B**) Comparison of *in vivo* human epidermal growth factor (hEGF) expression between transfected allogenic keratinocyte (KC), untransfected allogenic KC, and saline-treated wounds. hEGF expression in transfected group peaked on postoperative day 1 (920 pg/mL) with a steady decline to postoperative day 5. Overexpression remained significant until the biopsies on day 8. (**C**) Comparison of re-epithelialization between 3×10^5 hEGF-allogenic KCs (AKC), 3×10^5 untransfected AKCs, and saline-treated wounds. Mean re-epithelialization percentage (RE%) was significantly higher in hEGF-AKC transplanted compared with AKC and saline-treated wounds. No significant difference was noted between AKC and saline controls. $*p < 0.02$ versus saline control. (**D**) Comparison of RE% between full-thickness wounds treated with 5×10^5 AKCs, 5×10^5 autologous keratinocytes, 5×10^5 mixed AKC/autologous cells, saline-treated wounds, and dry wounds on day 8 reveals a significantly higher RE% in all groups of transplanted wounds compared with the saline and dry controls. No significant difference was noted between AKC, autologous, and mixed AKC/autologous groups. $*p < 0.02$ versus saline control.

gene therapy to maximize the healing potential. We achieved successful gene overexpression using autologous keratinocytes as vehicles for delivery of human growth hormone or insulin-like growth factor-1 and were able to demonstrate wound healing acceleration.[3,4]

Consecutively, six 4-month-old female Yorkshire pigs weighing 40–60 kg entered the animal facility 1 week before surgery. Under general anesthesia, full-thickness wounds measuring $1.5\,\text{cm} \times 1.5\,\text{cm}$ were created on dorsum of pigs with a depth of 1 cm, comprising a full-thickness skin layer down to the fascial plane. The current study was performed in two steps. In the first experiment, wounds were transplanted with 5×10^5 of allogenic or autologous keratinocytes. The control wounds were treated with saline alone or left dry. Next wounds were treated with 3×10^5 human EGF (hEGF)–transfected allogenic keratinocytes, 3×10^5 untransfected allogenic keratinocytes, or saline as control. Transfection of the allogenic keratinocytes was performed using hEGF-expressing plasmid with lipofectin (Invitrogen, Carlsbad, CA). The details of our keratinocytes isolation protocol and transfection protocol are described in our original paper.[22] Every 20–24 h after surgery, we collected wound fluids to evaluate hEGF expression until the experiment was terminated. Wound biopsies were performed on postoperative days 8, 11, 14, 21, and 28 to evaluate wound re-epithelialization. Long-term stability of the allogenic keratinocyte-treated wounds in terms of the wound breakdown, epidermal defects, or clinical blister formation was separately evaluated macroscopically and microscopically till postoperative day 35. Pigs were penned individually to minimize the risk of chamber disruption.

DISCUSSION OF FINDINGS AND RELEVANT LITERATURE

Various cell transplantation techniques, including fibrin suspension of cultured autologous keratinocytes or use of sheets of keratinocytes, have been described.[8,23] Our liquid environment wound model allows for transplantation of cell suspension cultures into the wound environment and is an excellent experimental tool for assessment of behavior of transplanted cells and daily analysis of gene expression.

Ex vivo gene delivery to wounds can be achieved using viral (*e.g.*, adenovirus) or nonviral vectors (*e.g.*, cationic liposomal method). Vogt *et al.* showed enhanced re-epithelialization of porcine full-thickness wounds using transplantation of autologous keratinocytes transfected with recombinant retroviral human growth hormone.[4] Svensjo *et al.* demonstrated successful gene delivery to similar wounds by transplantation of hEGF-transfected fibroblasts using nonviral vector (with lipofectin).[6] This study assessed the efficiency of allogenic keratinocytes as gene delivery vehicles to the wound environment. Specifically, using hEGF-expressing plasmid with a cationic liposomal method (lipofectin), we performed *in vitro* gene transfer to cultured allogenic keratinocytes and evaluated the effect of transplanting the gene-expressing cells on the re-epithelialization of porcine full-thickness wounds.

The efficiency of allogenic keratinocytes as gene delivery vehicles was assessed by daily analysis of wound fluid. Overall, the amount of hEGF expression was comparable with our earlier experiments with *in vivo* gene transfer to wounds using microseeding technique.[2] The hEGF allogenic keratinocytes–transplanted group revealed a peak hEGF expression of 920.8 pg/mL on postoperative day 1 with a steady decrease to 36.9 pg/mL on day 5. Overexpression of hEGF remained significant until the biopsies on day 8 (Fig. 1B). Wounds treated with hEGF-transfected allogenic keratinocytes

TAKE-HOME MESSAGE

Basic science advance

- Wound healing is a normal physiological response regulated by numerous inflammatory cytokines and growth factors. These regulatory polypeptides are secreted by a variety of cells in the wound environment and exert their influence in an autocrine and paracrine fashion. Of particular importance are EGF, TGF-β, VEGF, and PDGF secreted by keratinocytes, fibroblasts, endothelial cells, and platelets. In an attempt to accelerate the wound healing process, topical administration of recombinant growth factors has been reported. However, these approaches fail to achieve a sustained therapeutic level of the growth factors in the wound microenvironment, necessitating frequent applications. Gene therapy seems to be an attractive option in the management of nonhealing wounds. Transplantation of gene-transfected skin cells to wounds (*ex vivo* gene delivery) aims at delivering both a sustained level of growth-modulating agents and a source of regenerative cells. In this chapter, we focused on allogenic keratinocytes as the vehicles for hEGF as the growth-modulating molecule.

Clinical science advance

- Prompt skin replacement is critical in the management of extensive skin injuries or nonhealing ulcers. Autografts are commonly used procedures for wound coverage; however, they have limitations in resurfacing extensive skin defects. Despite the successful clinical application of *in vitro*–expanded autologous keratinocytes as epidermal sheets, the long process of approximately 3–4 weeks to obtain sufficient number of cells and graftable sheet production is a disadvantage of this approach. Allogenic keratinocytes can function as immediately available temporary biological dressings, and in combination with gene delivery to overexpress growth factors they can potentially optimize the host skin regenerative capacity before they are eventually rejected by the immune system. They can be cryopreserved, stored in skin bank, and used when required.

Relevance to clinical care

- We demonstrated that transfected allogenic keratinocytes enhance re-epithelialization in porcine full-thickness wounds. In a clinical context, cell cultures need to be readily available for treatment, such as in the treatment of extensively burned patient, where early excision should be immediately followed by immediate closure. Allogenic cell cultures can be cryopreserved and used when required. In addition, our results show that allogenic keratinocytes can be efficient gene delivery vehicles to wounds.

showed higher rate of re-epithelialization (56.96%) compared to untransfected allogenic keratinocytes (45.38%) or saline-treated wounds (42.01%) (Fig. 1C).

There was no statistical difference in re-epithelialization rate between wounds treated with allogenic and autologous keratinocytes, which was significantly higher in both groups compared with saline-treated or dry wounds (Fig. 1D). Transplantation of allogenic keratinocytes showed no adverse effects on epidermal thickness, size of the rete ridges, and degree of inflammation up to postoperative day 35.

Treatment of extensive nonhealing skin defects remains challenging. Skin autografts are the most widely used surgical procedures for resurfacing acute burns or chronic ulcers, but lack of adequate donor site limits their use in coverage of extensive defects. Transplantation of *in vitro*–expanded autologous keratinocytes achieved successful clinical application;[8,9] however, it requires a period of 3–4 weeks to obtain sufficient number of keratinocytes, restricting its widespread clinical application.

In the clinical setting such as in the treatment of critically ill burned patient, the vital need for immediate wound coverage necessitates that cell cultures or other skin replacement modalities be readily available. Allogenic keratinocytes can be expanded to sufficient numbers, prepared in advance, and stored frozen in the skin bank for later application. It is generally accepted that allografts are efficient biological dressings that cover the base of chronic wounds and acute burns and induce granulation and vascularization.[7] Despite the reports claiming that allogenic keratinocytes may tolerate rejection and survive permanently,[24] there is a strong evidence that rejection does occur, though the rejection process seems to be delayed for 4–5 days in comparison with transplanted split-thickness skin allografts, typically occurring 2 weeks after transplantation.[25] In our study, allogenic and autologous keratinocytes equally enhanced the wound re-epithelialization compared to control wounds. Further, we did not observe any adverse effect or increased inflammatory reaction in the allogenic-treated wounds. In addition, the rejection of allogenic cells does not seem to interfere with their role as gene delivery vehicles, as they exert their function of overexpression of growth factors before they are gradually replaced by autologous keratinocytes. Our study demonstrated that allogenic keratinocytes can serve as efficient gene delivery vehicles and accelerate the wound re-epithelialization. In addition to our study, recently Thomas-Virnig *et al.* also demonstrated the feasibility of allogenic keratinocytes as a gene delivery vehicle to wounds.[26]

CAUTION, CRITICAL REMARKS, AND RECOMMENDATIONS

We demonstrated that hEGF-transfected allogenic keratinocytes can enhance re-epithelialization in porcine full-thickness wounds. This study has some limitations. Even though the porcine skin has many similarities to human skin, further studies may be required to evaluate whether these results will also be applicable in the clinical setting. Our unique liquid environment in small wounds provided by the wound chambers is a valuable tool for studying the principles of wound healing. Whether the results are also valid in the large wound model and clinically achievable wet environment needs further studies.

FUTURE DEVELOPMENT

Wound healing is a complex biological process regulated by various cytokines and growth factors. Despite various studies into the role of growth factors and other regulatory peptides, the exact mechanism of their action and their effect on wound healing is poorly understood. There is no growth-modulating molecule that can dramatically improve the healing process. Further research on understanding the molecular basis of wound healing and effect of multiple genes is required.

Gene therapy seems to be an attractive option in the treatment of problem wounds, leading to sustained overexpression of regulatory growth factors. *Ex vivo* gene delivery has the advantage over *in vivo* techniques as it combines overexpression of growth-modulating agents and cell transplantation to maximize the healing potential. The clinical applicability of viral vectors as vehicles for gene delivery is restricted due to potential adverse effects. Therefore, further studies to develop nonviral vectors and more efficient gene delivery methods are required for future clinical application of this technique.

ACKNOWLEDGMENT

This work was supported by Public Health Grants RO1 GM51449 from the National Institutes of Health.

AUTHOR DISCLOSURE STATEMENT

No competing financial interests exist.

REFERENCES

1. Andree C, Swain WF, Page CP, *et al.*: *In vivo* transfer and expression of a human epidermal growth factor gene accelerates wound repair. Proc Natl Acad Sci USA 1994; **91:** 12188.
2. Eriksson E, Yao F, Svensjo T, *et al.*: *In vivo* gene transfer to skin and wound by microseeding. J Surg Res 1998; **78:** 85.
3. Hirsch T, Spielmann M, Velander P, *et al.*: Insulin-like growth factor-1 gene therapy and cell transplantation in diabetic wounds. J Gene Med 2008; **10:** 1247.
4. Vogt PM, Thompson S, Andree C, *et al.*: Genetically modified keratinocytes transplanted to wounds reconstitute the epidermis. Proc Natl Acad Sci USA 1994; **91:** 9307.
5. Vranckx JJ, Yao F, Petrie N, *et al.*: *In vivo* gene delivery of Ad-VEGF121 to full-thickness wounds in aged pigs results in high levels of VEGF expression but not in accelerated healing. Wound Repair Regen 2005; **13:** 51.
6. Svensjo T, Yao F, Pomahac B, Winkler T, and Eriksson E: Cultured autologous fibroblasts augment epidermal repair. Transplantation 2002; **73:** 1033.
7. Harding KG, Krieg T, Eming SA, *et al.*: Efficacy and safety of the freeze-dried cultured human keratinocyte lysate, LyphoDerm 0.9%, in the treatment of hard-to-heal venous leg ulcers. Wound Repair Regen 2005; **13:** 138.
8. Green H: The birth of therapy with cultured cells. Bioessays 2008; **30:** 897.
9. Hernon CA, Dawson RA, Freedlander E, *et al.*: Clinical experience using cultured epithelial autografts leads to an alternative methodology for transferring skin cells from the laboratory to the patient. Regen Med 2006; **1:** 809.
10. Rouabhia M: Permanent skin replacement using chimeric epithelial cultured sheets comprising xenogeneic and syngeneic keratinocytes. Transplantation 1996; **61:** 1290.
11. Cohen S and Elliott GA: The stimulation of epidermal keratinization by a protein isolated from the submaxillary gland of the mouse. J Invest Dermatol 1963; **40:** 1.
12. Tokumaru S, Higashiyama S, Endo T, *et al.*: Ectodomain shedding of epidermal growth factor receptor ligands is required for keratinocyte migration in cutaneous wound healing. J Cell Biol 2000; **151:** 209.
13. Hardwicke J, Schmaljohann D, Boyce D, and Thomas D: Epidermal growth factor therapy and wound healing—past, present and future perspectives. Surgeon 2008; **6:** 172.
14. Oda K, Matsuoka Y, Funahashi A, and Kitano H: A comprehensive pathway map of epidermal growth factor receptor signaling. Mol Syst Biol 2005; **1:** 2005 0010.
15. Hong JP, Jung HD, and Kim YW: Recombinant human epidermal growth factor (EGF) to enhance healing for diabetic foot ulcers. Ann Plast Surg 2006; **56:** 394; discussion 9–400.
16. Richard JL, Parer-Richard C, Daures JP, *et al.*: Effect of topical basic fibroblast growth factor on the healing of chronic diabetic neuropathic ulcer of the foot. A pilot, randomized, double-blind, placebo-controlled study. Diabetes Care 1995; **18:** 64.
17. Martin P: Wound healing—aiming for perfect skin regeneration. Science 1997; **276:** 75.
18. Rumalla VK and Borah GL: Cytokines, growth factors, and plastic surgery. Plast Reconstr Surg 2001; **108:** 719.
19. Sullivan TP, Eaglstein WH, Davis SC, and Mertz P: The pig as a model for human wound healing. Wound Repair Regen 2001; **9:** 66.
20. Weinstein GD: Autoradiographic studies on turnover time and protein synthesis in pig epidermis. J Invest Dermatol 1965; **44:** 413.
21. Svensjo T, Yao F, Pomahac B, and Eriksson E: Autologous keratinocyte suspensions accelerate epidermal wound healing in pigs. J Surg Res 2001; **99:** 211.
22. Vranckx JJ, Hoeller D, Velander PE, *et al.*: Cell suspension cultures of allogenic keratinocytes are efficient carriers for *ex vivo* gene transfer and accelerate the healing of full-thickness skin wounds by overexpression of human epidermal growth factor. Wound Repair Regen 2007; **15:** 657.
23. Bannasch H, Unterberg T, Fohn M, Weyand B, Horch RE, and Stark GB: Cultured keratinocytes in fibrin with decellularised dermis close porcine full-thickness wounds in a single step. Burns 2008; **34:** 1015.
24. De Luca M, Albanese E, Bondanza S, *et al.*: Multicentre experience in the treatment of burns with autologous and allogenic cultured epithelium, fresh or preserved in a frozen state. Burns 1989; **15:** 303.
25. Aubock J, Irschick E, Romani N, *et al.*: Rejection, after a slightly prolonged survival time, of Langerhans cell-free allogeneic cultured epidermis used for wound coverage in humans. Transplantation 1988; **45:** 730.
26. Thomas-Virnig CL, Centanni JM, Johnston CE, *et al.*: Inhibition of multidrug-resistant *Acinetobacter baumannii* by nonviral expression of hCAP-18 in a bioengineered human skin tissue. Mol Ther 2009; **17:** 562.

WHS
Wound
Healing
Society

Plasmid-Based Gene Transfer of Homeobox Genes and Improved Wound Healing

Kimberly A. Mace[1] and Nancy Boudreau[2,*]

[1]Faculty of Life Sciences, University of Manchester, Manchester, United Kingdom.
[2]Department of Surgery, University of California San Francisco, San Francisco, California.

Abbreviations and Acronyms

BMDC = bone marrow–derived cells

db = diabetes

Hox = homeobox

Lepr = leptin receptor

ob = obese

VEGF = vascular endothelial growth factor

*Correspondence: Department of Surgery, University of California San Francisco, Box 1302, San Francisco, California 94143-1302 (e-mail: nboudreau@sfghsurg.ucsf.edu).

Background: Repair of injured tissue is a dynamic, multifactorial process involving coordinate responses between various cell types. Delayed activation or failure to attenuate repair programs within these cell populations results in impaired, chronic, or nonhealing wounds.
The Problem: Chronic wounds in elderly and diabetic patients require costly medical intervention, or in severe cases, amputations. Current treatments, such as application of growth factors to wounds, yield only mild improvements; thus, more comprehensive approaches to coordinate the activities of the heterogeneous cell populations within the wound are needed.
Basic/Clinical Science Advances: Advances in our understanding of how cells activate and subsequently attenuate repair programs to restore tissue homeostasis have identified key pathways that could be exploited therapeutically to improve healing. Although gene therapy holds promise to achieve this goal, concerns regarding the long-term safety of these methods have impeded progress toward clinical application. Nonetheless, transient gene transfer technologies that temporally coordinate the behaviors of different cell populations required for effective repair and/or regeneration may prove more effective and safe.
Clinical Care Relevance: Patients with chronic wounds experience an impaired quality of life, significant morbidity, and increased mortality, and amputations arising from nonhealing wounds account for over 60% of all nontraumatic amputations. Thus, finding safe, cost-effective, and efficacious treatments has high clinical relevance. Plasmid-based gene transfer technologies provide a relatively safe and potentially inexpensive therapy to address these issues.
Conclusion: Herein, we describe a simple plasmid-based gene transfer method and its limitations, and summarize data from our lab using this technique.

BACKGROUND

Nonviral transfection to directly introduce genes into eukaryotic cells has been used for over 40 years,[1,2] and has utilized a variety of delivery methods from polymer- and lipid-based reagents to electroporation and gene guns. This technique has not only been essential for studying gene function but also more recently has been adapted for therapeutic application. Although viral-mediated transduction is more efficient, the main advantage of plasmid transfection over viral transduction is safety. Indeed, viral-mediated gene transfer has been plagued by safety issues due to genomic integration, and subsequent activation of oncogenes, inactivation of tumor suppressor genes, and uncontrolled immune response to viral components.[3]

Plasmid-mediated gene transfection, while transient, is particularly

ADVANCES IN WOUND CARE, VOLUME 1

Printed in U.S.A.
DOI: 10.1089/awc.2009.0182

useful in conditions in which short-term gene therapy is desirable. One prominent example is cutaneous wound healing. Skin wounds provide easy access to cells that may benefit from transient gene therapy. In addition, animal models of impaired wound healing, such as the leptin receptor–deficient ($Lepr^{db-/-}$) diabetic mouse, provide well-characterized pathologies suitable for testing gene therapy applications to improve angiogenesis, promote re-epithelialization, or attenuate sustained inflammatory responses.

The gene encoding the Lepr was identified as the diabetes (*db*) gene in mutant mice by Chen *et al.* in 1996,[4] although the use of this model to investigate complications associated with diabetes began 30 years earlier.[5] These mice develop hyperglycemia, hyperinsulinemia insulin resistance, glucose intolerance, abnormal islet morphology, and peripheral neuropathy, and are now one of the most well-established models of type 2 diabetes mellitus.[6,7] They also display poor vascularization and severely impaired wound healing,[8] similar to human patients with type 2 diabetes.[9] Analysis of wound tissue has demonstrated that diabetic wounds fail to express a variety of important factors, ranging from transcriptional regulators to secreted signaling molecules, many of which are required for efficient healing (reviewed in Brem and Tomic-Canic[10]), as well as exhibiting sustained inflammatory responses that contribute to impaired healing.[11] Moreover, pioneering studies investigating the effects of growth factor application to stimulate angiogenesis in diabetic wounds, or, conversely, blocking inflammatory mediators,[12] indeed show an improvement in both angiogenesis and overall repair.[8,13–15] Ideally then, stimulating angiogenesis while attenuating the excessive inflammatory response should further improve healing and has provided the basis for the subsequent approach described in this chapter, which focuses on coordinately regulating these responses by utilizing 'master regulator' transcription factors.

CLINICAL PROBLEM ADDRESSED

The number of people worldwide with diabetes is projected to reach 221 million by 2010,[16] and in the United States the direct medical cost of complications caused by diabetes was $116 billion in 2007.[17] Chronic wounds are the most common complication resulting from diabetes and are the leading cause of nontraumatic amputations in the developed world today.[16,18] Although treatments exist for diabetic chronic wounds, they are often not effective due to the poor understanding of the underlying mechanisms that contribute to chronic wounds. New data suggest that gene- and cell-based therapies aimed at treating multiple pathologies of the diabetic chronic wound environment simultaneously will result in a more beneficial outcome for patients with chronic wounds.[19]

RELEVANT BASIC SCIENCE CONTEXT

The homeobox (Hox) genes, encoding homeodomain transcription factors, have long been known for their highly conserved role in directing both anterior–posterior identity specification and organogenesis during development.[20] More recently, they have been shown in adult tissues to play a role in both tissue remodeling, such as mammary gland development,[21] as well as maintenance of positional identity[22] and differentiated tissue function.[23,24] Not surprisingly, misregulation of Hox genes is also associated with cancer and impaired wound healing, as these processes share many commonalities with development at both the molecular level and cellular level.[25–27] In particular, neovascularization is required for all three events, development, tumorigenesis, and wound healing, and several Hox genes have been found to regulate neovascularization in either a positive or a negative manner. The Hox-3 paralog group in particular has been shown to promote angiogenesis.[28–31] Indeed, enforced expression of *HOXA3* was as potent as vascular endothelial growth factor (*VEGF*) in inducing angiogenesis in chick chorioallantoic membrane assays,[31] whereas some central class (*e.g.*, *HOXA5*) and posterior class (*e.g.*, *HOXD10*) Hox genes function in endothelial cells to inhibit angiogenesis.[23,32] Moreover, inhibition of angiogenesis by Hox transcription factors appears to be dominant over induction. This is reminiscent of the phenomenon of posterior prevalence, in which the more posterior Hox gene function exerts phenotypic suppression over the more anterior Hox gene.[33,34] In addition to the direct effects in endothelial cells, production of Hox factors by adjacent epithelial cells also influences angiogenesis by regulating expression and secretion of key angiogenic factors, including VEGF. For example, *HOXB7* expressed in tumor cells leads to activation of adjacent cocultured endothelial cells, whereas *HOXD10* attenuates the ability of tumor epithelial cells to produce VEGF and activate angiogenesis.[35,36] Although not all of the relevant downstream target genes or mechanisms controlling Hox-mediated regulation of the angiogenic switch have been elucidated, several pathways involved in endothelial cell migration in particular have been identified by plasmid-mediated gene transfer experiments and will be discussed in more detail below.

EXPERIMENTAL MODEL OR MATERIAL—ADVANTAGES AND LIMITATIONS

We have used the *Lepr*-deficient mouse model of type 2 diabetes mellitus ($Lepr^{db-/-}$, *db/db*), which is the most widely used model of type 2 diabetes and exhibits poor granulation tissue formation, poor neovascularization, poor collagen deposition, and severely impaired wound healing.[8] Analysis of wound tissue from these mice has demonstrated that diabetic wounds fail to express a variety of key factors, ranging from transcriptional regulators to secreted signaling molecules, many of which are required for efficient healing.[13,31,37] Although these mice share many of the characteristics of human patients with type 2 diabetes, some criticisms of this model are valid. For example, chronic wounds that develop on the distal regions of the arms and legs, most often in the feet, in human patients are phenotypically different from wounds created on the dorsum of *db/db* mice in an experimental context. The chronic wounds in diabetic patients often occur as ulcerations and can often fail to heal completely, while induced wounds on *db/db* mice always heal completely, although at a much slower rate. Nonetheless, several growth factor–based therapies, first shown to be effective in the *db/db* (or *ob/ob*, the related leptin-deficient mouse model of type 2 diabetes), have successfully advanced to the clinic, and, although not quite as effective on human chronic wounds as in mouse models, do improve wound healing in a majority of patients (recently reviewed in Davidson[38]). This mouse model thus provides an opportunity to test new approaches to improve wound repair that could have real clinical relevance.

DISCUSSION OF FINDINGS AND RELEVANT LITERATURE

Transient gene transfer to full-thickness excisional wounds is performed by applying a dehydrated pellet containing 25 μg plasmid DNA in 1% methylcellulose to the wound at the time of wounding. Transient gene transfer of a Hox gene to a diabetic wound was first performed with human *HOXD3*.[27] This study was motivated by previous work identifying *HOXD3* as an angiogenic factor[28] that failed to be appropriately upregulated in response to cutaneous injury in the diabetic environment.[30] Application of 25 μg of a plasmid encoding hemagglutinin-tagged human *HOXD3* to 0.8-cm-diameter full-thickness excisional wounds in *db/db* mice at the time of wounding was found to mimic endogenous *Hoxd3* expression in wounded wild-type mice.[27] In this study, transgene expression was examined using anti-hemagglutinin antibodies and colorimetric detection in the wound tissue at several time points (up to 7 days) post transfer. Although codetection of cell-specific markers was not performed in this study, cells that expressed transgene applied with this method were identified, using cellular morphology and localization to specific proliferating cell types in the skin, including angiogenic endothelium, basal keratinocytes, and activated fibroblasts.[27] Moreover, we have observed that expression of the transgene is transient, lasting 7–10 days, does not integrate into host cell DNA, remains localized to the wound site, and does not detectably diffuse into peripheral blood.[19,31] Interestingly, we have also recently used multiplex fluorescent labeling analyses to show that leukocytes recruited to the wound site take up and transiently express the transgene as well.[19]

Gene transfer of *HOXD3* was found to result in an increase in collagen 1A1

TAKE-HOME MESSAGE

Basic science advances

- Optimization of plasmid gene transfer of Hox genes during tissue repair and regeneration.
- Identification of a gene that coordinately improves angiogenesis, directly stimulates keratinocyte migration, and attenuates excess inflammation in skin.
- Potential for transient reprogramming of progenitor cells in accessible tissue (*e.g.*, skin).

Clinical science advances

- Single application leads to a significant improvement in rate and quality of healing in diabetic wound model.
- Flexibility of gene transfer for development of transient gene therapies.
- Practical alteration of gene function for therapeutic benefit.
- Improvements in autonomous progenitor cell behavior without need for transplantation of autologous cells.

Relevance to clinical care

- Large unmet need: tens of thousands of amputations due to chronic wounds each year.
- Simple, inexpensive, noninvasive method to improve chronic wound care.
- Can be adapted for additional skin pathology treatments.

(*Col1A1*), β3 integrin (*Itgb3*), and urokinase plasminogen activator (*Plau*), all of which have been demonstrated to play a positive role in wound healing *in vivo*, by enhancing neovascularization and re-epithelialization.[27,39] Although HOXD3 directly promotes endothelial cell migration, introduction into keratinocytes impedes migration, suggesting that the enhanced re-epithelialization observed is an indirect effect of HOXD3, perhaps via increased collagen deposition, which has been shown previously to stimulate keratinocyte migration.[40]

In a complementary study, the human *HOXA3* gene was transferred to wounds of *db/db* mice, as endogenous *Hoxa3* expression is also reduced compared to wild-type mice in response to cutaneous injury. Again, enforced expression of the *HOXA3* transgene rescued a variety of the *db/db* impaired wound healing phenotypes, most notably neovascularization and re-epithelialization. However, examination of previously identified HOXD3 target genes, such as *Col1A1*, *Itgb3*, and *Plau*, revealed that they were unaffected by *HOXA3* expression. Interestingly, HOXA3 regulated target genes that were distinct from HOXD3, yet affected a similar result: collagen 6A1, integrin α3, and urokinase plasminogen activator receptor. Like the HOXD3 target genes, the products of these genes have direct roles in promoting angiogenesis via enhancing cell migration. Indeed, like *HOXD3*, overexpression of *HOXA3* in cultured endothelial cells significantly induced migration. Moreover, unlike HOXD3, HOXA3 also directly promoted keratinocyte migration[31] and thus coordinately regulates the response of both the vasculature and epidermis during the repair process.

In a follow-up study, a more detailed analysis of *HOXA3* gene transfer to diabetic wounds using bone marrow chimeras evaluated the effect of localized *HOXA3* on bone marrow–derived cell (BMDC) mobilization and recruitment.[19] BMDCs have been shown to contribute significantly to tumor-induced neovascularization.[41] Gene transfer of *HOXA3* to wounds of diabetic mice enhanced endothelial progenitor cell mobilization and recruitment to wounds, and also suppressed leukocyte recruitment. Thus, HOXA3 could promote angiogenesis while attenuating the prolonged and sustained inflammatory response that accompanies chronic nonhealing wounds. Because leukocytes at the wound site also incorporate the *HOXA3* transgene, it is possible that HOXA3 may directly attenuate their ability to further stimulate inflammatory cell recruitment. Microarray analyses of diabetic wound tissue that had received gene transfer using *HOXA3* versus control plasmid revealed extensive transcriptional changes in signaling pathways influencing leukocyte behavior. In particular, suppression of the nuclear factor-kappa B pathway was identified as one of the most likely mechanisms underlying the HOXA3-mediated suppression of the inflammatory

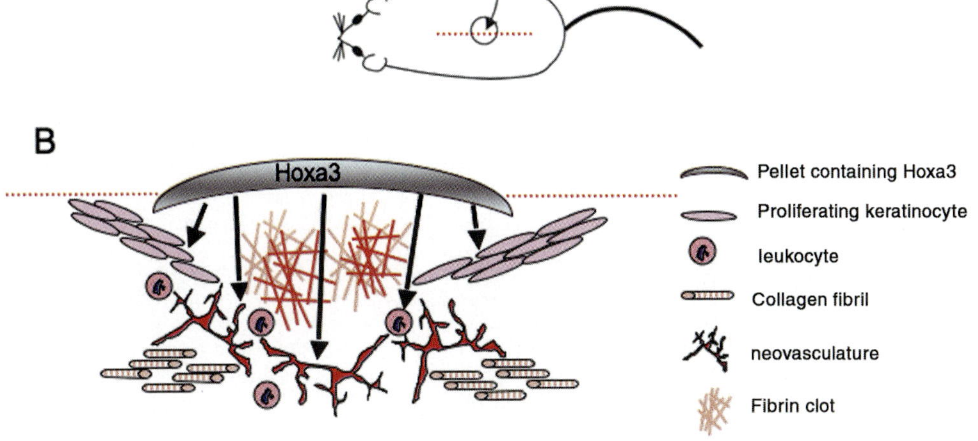

Figure 1. Gene transfer of *HOXA3* during wound healing. (**A**) Twenty-five micrograms *HOXA3* plasmid in 50 μL 1% methylcellulose is spotted in sterile Petri dishes and allowed to air-dry for 2 h. The dried pellet is then transferred to an excisional wound on the dorsum of the mouse. Dotted red line indicates the plane of view shown in cross section in (**B**). (**B**) Schematic drawing representing wound cross section that has been treated with *HOXA3* plasmid DNA pellet. *HOXA3* plasmid DNA rehydrates and is taken up and expressed predominantly by basal keratinocytes, leukocytes, and endothelial cells.

response.[19] A recent study by Milsom *et al.* suggests that HOXB4 also repressed components of the nuclear factor-kappa B pathway when overexpressed in BMDCs,[42] although via regulation of different target genes that affect BMDC behavior. Taken together, these results indicate that Hox gene transfer is capable of coordinating the behavior of endothelial cells, keratinocytes, and inflammatory cells within the diabetic wound to restore normal temporal and spatial control of tissue repair and remodeling (Fig. 1).

CAUTION, CRITICAL REMARKS, AND RECOMMENDATIONS

The use of plasmid DNA–based therapies for short-term correction or enhancement of gene expression and function in human patients has already met with some success, particularly with regard to angiogenesis in patients with critical limb ischemia.[43,44] Although transfer of naked DNA is considered the safest method of gene delivery, there still exists some potential for integration of the plasmid DNA into the host chromosome. If this event results in the activation of an oncogene, it could contribute to the development of cancer; thus, benefits must be weighed against potential risks before utilizing this approach. One viable alternative to plasmid gene transfer of Hox genes to mammalian cells is protein transfection/transduction. The third helix of Hox transcription factor homeodomains confer the ability to passively translocate through the plasma membrane, facilitating cellular uptake of this class of homeodomain proteins. However, this approach is likely to be far more costly and less effective due to high levels of proteolytic activity in the harsh chronic wound environment. Alternatively, strategies involving genetically modified autologous cells that can be applied to the wound and secrete needed factors are also likely to provide additional benefit; however, further investigation into how the chronic wound environment impacts the growth and/or differentiation state of engrafted cells will be necessary to ensure the safety of these approaches and provide important insights into therapeutically managing chronic wounds.

FUTURE DEVELOPMENT

Previous studies have focused on characterizing the global effects of delivering Hox genes to multiple cell types in the wound environment. Use of cell type–specific promoters to restrict plasmid expression to distinct cell types, or application at different stages of repair to mimic the temporally and spatially restricted patterns of endogenous Hox expression may further improve healing. For example, it may be more beneficial to direct Hoxa3 expression to inflammatory cells initially, followed by endothelial cells, and then keratinocytes, allowing for more precise orchestration of cell behaviors. Future investigations will aim to better understand the distinct effects Hox genes have on different cell types at specific time points, and how these effects mediate wound healing.

AUTHOR DISCLOSURE STATEMENT

The authors have nothing to disclose.

REFERENCES

1. McCutchan JH and Pagano JS: Enhancement of the infectivity of simian virus 40 deoxyribonucleic acid with diethylaminoethyl-dextran. J Natl Cancer Inst 1968; **41:** 351.
2. Graham FL and van der Eb AJ: Transformation of rat cells by DNA of human adenovirus 5. Virology 1973; **54:** 536.
3. Thomas CE, Ehrhardt A, and Kay MA: Progress and problems with the use of viral vectors for gene therapy. Nat Rev Genet 2003; **4:** 346.
4. Chen H, Charlat O, Tartaglia LA, Woolf EA, Weng X, Ellis SJ, *et al.*: Evidence that the diabetes gene encodes the leptin receptor: identification of a mutation in the leptin receptor gene in db/db mice. Cell 1996; **84:** 491.
5. Hummel KP, Dickie MM, and Coleman DL: Diabetes, a new mutation in the mouse. Science 1966; **153:** 1127.
6. Coleman DL: Diabetes-obesity syndromes in mice. Diabetes 1982; **31(Suppl 1 Pt 2):** 1.
7. Srinivasan K and Ramarao P: Animal models in type 2 diabetes research: an overview. Indian J Med Res 2007; **125:** 451.
8. Greenhalgh DG, Sprugel KH, Murray MJ, and Ross R: PDGF and FGF stimulate wound healing in the genetically diabetic mouse. Am J Pathol 1990; **136:** 1235.
9. Greenhalgh DG: Wound healing and diabetes mellitus. Clin Plast Surg 2003; **30:** 37.
10. Brem H and Tomic-Canic M: Cellular and molecular basis of wound healing in diabetes. J Clin Invest 2007; **117:** 1219.
11. Wetzler C, Kampfer H, Stallmeyer B, Pfeilschifter J, and Frank S: Large and sustained induction of chemokines during impaired wound healing in the genetically diabetic mouse: prolonged persistence of neutrophils and macrophages during the late phase of repair. J Invest Dermatol 2000; **115:** 245.
12. Goren I, Muller E, Schiefelbein D, Christen U, Pfeilschifter J, Muhl H, *et al.*: Systemic anti-TNFalpha treatment restores diabetes-impaired skin repair in ob/ob mice by inactivation of macrophages. J Invest Dermatol 2007; **127:** 2259.
13. Werner S, Breeden M, Hubner G, Greenhalgh DG, and Longaker MT: Induction of keratinocyte growth factor expression is reduced and delayed during wound healing in the genetically diabetic mouse. J Invest Dermatol 1994; **103:** 469.
14. Galeano M, Deodato B, Altavilla D, Cucinotta D, Arsic N, Marini H, *et al.*: Adeno-associated viral vector-mediated human vascular endothelial growth factor gene transfer stimulates angiogenesis and wound healing in the genetically diabetic mouse. Diabetologia 2003; **46:** 546.

15. Galiano RD, Tepper OM, Pelo CR, Bhatt KA, Callaghan M, Bastidas N, *et al.*: Topical vascular endothelial growth factor accelerates diabetic wound healing through increased angiogenesis and by mobilizing and recruiting bone marrow-derived cells. Am J Pathol 2004; **164:** 1935.

16. Amos AF, McCarty DJ, and Zimmet P: The rising global burden of diabetes and its complications: estimates and projections to the year 2010. Diabet Med 1997; **14 Suppl 5:** S1.

17. NIDDK: 2007 *Fact Sheet: National Diabetes Statistics*, edited by Services UDoHaH. Bethesda, MD: National Institutes of Health, 2008. http://diabetes.niddk.nih.gov/DM/PUBS/statistics.

18. Falanga V: *Cutaneous Wound Healing*. London: Martin Dunitz, 2001.

19. Mace KA, Restivo TE, Rinn JL, Paquet AC, Chang HY, Young DM, *et al.*: HOXA3 modulates injury-induced mobilization and recruitment of bone marrow-derived cells. Stem Cells 2009; **27:** 1654.

20. McGinnis W and Krumlauf R: Homeobox genes and axial patterning. Cell 1992; **68:** 283.

21. Chen F and Capecchi MR: Paralogous mouse Hox genes, Hoxa9, Hoxb9, and Hoxd9, function together to control development of the mammary gland in response to pregnancy. Proc Natl Acad Sci USA 1999; **96:** 541.

22. Rinn JL, Wang JK, Allen N, Brugmann SA, Mikels AJ, Liu H, *et al.*: A dermal HOX transcriptional program regulates site-specific epidermal fate. Genes Dev 2008; **22:** 303.

23. Myers C, Charboneau A, Cheung I, Hanks D, and Boudreau N: Sustained expression of homeobox D10 inhibits angiogenesis. Am J Pathol 2002; **161:** 2099.

24. Carrio M, Arderiu G, Myers C, and Boudreau NJ: Homeobox D10 induces phenotypic reversion of breast tumor cells in a three-dimensional culture model. Cancer Res 2005; **65:** 7177.

25. Cantile M, Pettinato G, Procino A, Feliciello I, Cindolo L, and Cillo C: *In vivo* expression of the whole HOX gene network in human breast cancer. Eur J Cancer 2003; **39:** 257.

26. Debernardi S, Lillington DM, Chaplin T, Tomlinson S, Amess J, Rohatiner A, *et al.*: Genome-wide analysis of acute myeloid leukemia with normal karyotype reveals a unique pattern of homeobox gene expression distinct from those with translocation-mediated fusion events. Genes Chromosomes Cancer 2003; **37:** 149.

27. Hansen SL, Myers CA, Charboneau A, Young DM, and Boudreau N: HoxD3 accelerates wound healing in diabetic mice. Am J Pathol 2003; **163:** 2421.

28. Boudreau N, Andrews C, Srebrow A, Ravanpay A, and Cheresh DA: Induction of the angiogenic phenotype by Hox D3. J Cell Biol 1997; **139:** 257.

29. Myers C, Charboneau A, and Boudreau N: Homeobox B3 promotes capillary morphogenesis and angiogenesis. J Cell Biol 2000; **148:** 343.

30. Uyeno LA, Newman-Keagle JA, Cheung I, Hunt TK, Young DM, and Boudreau N: Hox D3 expression in normal and impaired wound healing. J Surg Res 2001; **100:** 46.

31. Mace KA, Hansen SL, Myers C, Young DM, and Boudreau N: HOXA3 induces cell migration in endothelial and epithelial cells promoting angiogenesis and wound repair. J Cell Sci 2005; **118 (Pt 12):** 2567.

32. Rhoads K, Arderiu G, Charboneau A, Hansen SL, Hoffman W, and Boudreau N: A role for Hox A5 in regulating angiogenesis and vascular patterning. Lymphat Res Biol 2005; **3:** 240.

33. Duboule D: Patterning in the vertebrate limb. Curr Opin Genet Dev 1991; **1:** 211.

34. Duboule D and Morata G: Colinearity and functional hierarchy among genes of the homeotic complexes. Trends Genet 1994; **10:** 358.

35. Care A, Felicetti F, Meccia E, Bottero L, Parenza M, Stoppacciaro A, *et al.*: HOXB7: a key factor for tumor-associated angiogenic switch. Cancer Res 2001; **61:** 6532.

36. Chen A, Cuevas I, Kenny PA, Miyake H, Mace K, Ghajar C, *et al.*: Endothelial cell migration and vascular endothelial growth factor expression are the result of loss of breast tissue polarity. Cancer Res 2009; **69:** 6721.

37. Mace KA, Yu DH, Paydar KZ, Boudreau N, and Young DM: Sustained expression of Hif-1alpha in the diabetic environment promotes angiogenesis and cutaneous wound repair. Wound Repair Regen 2007; **15:** 636.

38. Davidson JM: First-class delivery: getting growth factors to their destination. J Invest Dermatol 2008; **128:** 1360.

39. Eming SA, Brachvogel B, Odorisio T, and Koch M: Regulation of angiogenesis: wound healing as a model. Prog Histochem Cytochem 2007; **42:** 115.

40. Guo M, Toda K, and Grinnell F: Activation of human keratinocyte migration on type I collagen and fibronectin. J Cell Sci 1990; **96 (Pt 2):** 197.

41. Lyden D, Hattori K, Dias S, Costa C, Blaikie P, Butros L, *et al.*: Impaired recruitment of bone-marrow-derived endothelial and hematopoietic precursor cells blocks tumor angiogenesis and growth. Nat Med 2001; **7:** 1194.

42. Milsom MD, Schiedlmeier B, Bailey J, Kim MO, Li D, Jansen M, *et al.*: Ectopic HOXB4 overcomes the inhibitory effect of tumor necrosis factor-{alpha} on Fanconi anemia hematopoietic stem and progenitor cells. Blood 2009; **113:** 5111.

43. Baumgartner I, Pieczek A, Manor O, Blair R, Kearney M, Walsh K, *et al.*: Constitutive expression of phVEGF165 after intramuscular gene transfer promotes collateral vessel development in patients with critical limb ischemia. Circulation 1998; **97:** 1114.

44. Baumgartner I, Chronos N, Comerota A, Henry T, Pasquet JP, Finiels F, *et al.*: Local gene transfer and expression following intramuscular administration of FGF-1 plasmid DNA in patients with critical limb ischemia. Mol Ther 2009; **17:** 914.

WHS
Wound
Healing
Society

Clinical Biomaterials for Scar-Free Healing and Localized Delivery of Cells and Growth Factors

Glenn D. Prestwich*

Departments of Medicinal Chemistry and Bioengineering, Center for Therapeutic Biomaterials, The University of Utah, Salt Lake City, Utah.

Abbreviations and Acronyms

bFGF = basic fibroblast growth factor

CMHA-S = thiolated carboxymethyl-HA

CS = chondroitin-6-sulfate

DBM = demineralized bone matrix

ECM = extracellular matrix

GMP = Good Manufacturing Practices

HA = hyaluronic acid or hyaluronan

HGF = hepatocyte growth factor

HP = heparin

MSC = mesenchymal stem cell

sECM = semisynthetic ECM

3D = three-dimensional

VEGF = vascular endothelial growth factor

*Correspondence: Departments of Medicinal Chemistry and Bioengineering, Center for Therapeutic Biomaterials, The University of Utah, 419 Wakara Way, Suite 205, Salt Lake City, Utah 84108-1257 (e-mail: gprestwich@pharm.utah.edu).

Background: Effective cell therapy will require a U.S. Food and Drug Administration–approved injectable, biocompatible material for cell placement and retention. The challenge is to replicate the complexity of the native extracellular matrix (ECM) with a minimum set of components necessary for tissue regeneration.
The Problem: Design criteria for matrices for encapsulation of cells include chemical, biological, mechanical, and rheological considerations but often ignore the critical marketing, regulatory, and financial constraints. Biocompatible materials for cell expansion and differentiation offer (i) ease of use, (ii) customizable composition and compliance, and (iii) seamless translation from *in vitro* to *in vivo* use.
Basic/Clinical Science Advances: The ECM can be deconstructed to modular components, which can be reassembled into biomimetic materials meeting the design criteria. These semisynthetic ECMs (sECMs) employ thiol-modified derivatives of hyaluronic acid that can form covalently crosslinked, biodegradable hydrogels. The sECMs are living biopolymers that can be crosslinked in the presence of cells and tissues to enable cell therapy and tissue engineering. Moreover, biological cues can be added to simulate the complexity of the ECM to control cell differentiation during tissue neogenesis.
Clinical Care Relevance: Applications of the sECM include delivery of primary or progenitor cells for repair of damage to skin, ear, nose, throat, neural, renal, ophthalmic, hepatic, bone, cartilage, and other tissues.
Conclusion: The sECM technology offers a manufacturable, highly reproducible, versatile, and U.S. Food and Drug Administration–approvable material for cell expansion and differentiation.

BACKGROUND

Hyaluronic acid (HA) or hyaluronan forms viscoelastic and lubricious solutions that can protect eye tissues during ophthalmic surgeries, provide viscosupplementation in joints, reduce postsurgical adhesions, and deliver drugs. *In vivo*, HA promotes scar-free wound healing in the fetus and maintains tissue hydration in all tissues in adults. However, the short residence time *in vivo* of HA and its poor mechanical properties led to many chemical modifications of HA. In the last two decades, HA-based medical devices and coatings have addressed clinical needs with different levels of success.[1] Chemically modified HA derivatives fall into two categories: monolithic, in which final form that cannot form new chemical bonds in the presence of cells or tissues, and living, in which the modification permits the formation of new covalent bonds in the presence of cells, tissues, or bioactive factors.

Chemical modification of HA has thus generated a number of living

Printed in U.S.A.
DOI: 10.1089/awc.2009.0124

biomaterials for reparative and regenerative medicine[2,3] that are biocompatible, bioactive, and possess physical properties optimized to specific clinical uses. One end-user-oriented strategy involves deconstruction of the extracellular matrix (ECM) to its simplest components, followed by reassembly for wound repair, tissue engineering, or growth factor delivery.[4,5] In this approach, HA is first carboxymethylated followed by introduction of crosslinkable thiol residues[4,6–8] to produce thiolated carboxymethyl-HA (CMHA-S, also known as Carbylan-S). This new HA derivative can be either rapidly crosslinked *in situ* with a thiol-reactive crosslinker such as polyethylene glycol diacrylate, or more slowly by disulfide bond formation. In addition, disulfide-containing crosslinkers can be used to make fall-apart hydrogels that permit cell recovery after expansion under mild, nonenzymatic conditions.[9] The crosslinked hydrogels can also be dried to form thin films.[10,11] Crosslinked CMHA-S films accelerate wound closure by re-epithelialization in acute full-thickness wounds in mice, and the quality of the regenerated dermis was significantly better than in untreated wounds.[5] In addition, the CMHA-S films and gels have been shown to be effective *in vivo* for the treatment of injured vocal folds,[12] for scar-free healing after endoscopic sinus surgery,[13] for preventing stenosis after tracheal injury,[14] and for preventing post-surgical adhesions after cardiac surgery,[15] abdominal surgery,[16] and tendon surgery.[17]

CLINICAL PROBLEM ADDRESSED

Many current clinical protocols involve delivery of cells, for example, autologous or allogeneic mesenchymal stem cells (MSCs), either intravenously or by direct injection into a damaged tissue. The problem is poor engraftment and low efficacy, and there are even problems caused by blood vessel occlusion by cell aggregates. Similarly, when growth factors, for example, vascular endothelial growth factor (VEGF) or platelet-derived growth factor, are delivered to cutaneous wounds or to internal damaged tissues in bolus form, rapid proteolytic degradation occurs within 5–30 min. This short half-life effectively precludes treatment with these expensive and highly active biological agents. The use of a suitable clinical biomaterial for cell or growth factory delivery would address this clinical problem.

RELEVANT BASIC SCIENCE CONTEXT

The classical paradigm of tissue engineering as used in regenerative and reparative medicine involves the delivery of cells and biological factors in a biocompatible matrix. To obtain integrated, functional, multicellular systems that recapitulate tissues and organs, the need of the true end users—physicians and patients—must dictate the key design criteria.[18] The semisynthetic ECM (sECM) technology enables tissue formation *in vivo* and also permits three-dimensional (3D) culture of cells *in vitro*. In contrast to materials that were designed for *in vitro* cell culture and then found unsuitable for clinical use, these semisynthetic HA-derived materials were specifically developed for scar-free wound healing, surgical adhesion prevention, and for delivery of cells and growth factors *in vivo*. In anticipation of the importance of stem cells in the future of cell therapy, sECMs are now being re-engineered for *in vitro* applications in research, focusing on 3D expansion and controlled differentiation of pluripotent progenitor cells. Several examples below describe uses of specific sECMs for cell delivery in preclinical models.

To solve the problem of rapid growth factor degradation *in vivo*, an sECM was developed that mimicked the chemistry and controlled release inherent in the naturally occurring heparan sulfate proteoglycans. By covalent modification of heparin (HP) with thiol groups, a co-crosslinked sECM was obtained that continuously released basic fibroblast growth factor (bFGF) over more than 1 month.[19] Dual delivery of VEGF and angiopoetin-1 both increased neovascularization indices and the number of patent microvessel beds when implanted into the ear pinnae of mice.[20] Similar results were observed with the corelease of VEGF and bFGF or the corelease of VEGF and keratinocyte growth factor; in both cases, the extent of release was enhanced by the presence of covalently bound gelatin in the matrix.[21–23] Examples of growth factor release in injury treatment are discussed below.

An interesting possibility in regenerative medicine is to enhance recruitment of endogenous progenitor cells to the site of injury, rather than adding the cells exogenously. To test this possibility, the heparan sulfate proteoglycan–like sECM known as Heprasil was loaded with hepatocyte growth factor (HGF). Migration of human bone marrow MSCs into the HGF–Heprasil mixtures was significantly enhanced relative to Heprasil or HGF alone.[24]

EXPERIMENTAL MODELS AND MATERIALS

The next two sections focus on selected papers in two areas in which the living sECMs exhibit their unique capabilities as clinically useful injectable or implantable agents in tissue repair. Specifically, examples from recent preclinical studies in cell delivery and growth factor delivery will be highlighted.

Cell delivery

Three models for cell delivery are presented. In the first, human adipose–derived stem cells were encapsulated in the injectable, crosslinkable HA–only sECM and were seeded into human placental decellular matrix.[25] The construct was implanted into a nude mouse model. In the second, autologous bone marrow–derived MSCs were encapsulated in Extracel, the cocrosslinked gelatin-HA sECM, and injected into a patellar groove defect in the femoral articular cartilage of rabbits.[26] In the third, a hybrid scaffold was created using poly (e-caprolactone)/collagen coelectrospun with gelatin into micron-sized fibers, which were then electrosprayed with the Heprasil sECM.[27] This hybrid scaffold was used to investigate the role of the hydrogel in promoting cellular infiltration into the mesh by human fetal osteoblast precursor cells.

Growth factor delivery

Two distinctly different *in vivo* models for growth delivery are discussed. First, we compared the injectable sECM Extracel and porous sponge of the same hydrogel to deliver human demineralized bone matrix (DBM) in a rat femoral defect model. The experimental design tested the importance of physical form as well as the presence or absence of a growth factor mixture in accelerating bone repair.[28] In the second model, we compared the role of the immobilized HP and bFGF released from chrondroitin sulfate–based hydrogel dressings placed on large full-thickness cutaneous defects on the backs of genetically diabetic (*db*/*db*) mice.[29]

DISCUSSION OF FINDINGS AND RELEVANT LITERATURE

Cell delivery

In the first model, the placental decellular matrix scaffolds macroscopically maintained their 3D volume and supported mature adipocyte populations *in vivo* and showed evidence of implant integration and a host contribution to the adipogenic response. Incorporating the HA-derived sECM had a positive effect on both angiogenesis and adipogenesis, suggesting that the hybrid materials provide a balance of chemical and biological cues suitable for regeneration of adipose tissue.[25]

In the rabbit osteochondral defect model, four experimental groups were (i) untreated control, (ii) autologous MSCs only, (iii) sECM only, and (iv) MSCs + sECM. At 12 weeks postsurgery, control defects were filled with fibrous tissue. In MSC-only group, hyaline-like cartilage filled the peripheral area of the defect, but the center was filled with fibrous tissue. In the sECM-only group, hyaline cartilage with zonal architecture filled the defect at 12 weeks, but a sharp interface was evident between the neocartilage and adjacent host cartilage. In the MSCs + sECM group, defects were completely filled with elastic, firm, translucent cartilage at 12 weeks, and showed superior integration of the repair tissue with the normal cartilage. The injectable sECM allowed delivery and retention of the MSCs in the defect, and facilitated the healing process involving endogenous cells.[26]

In the *in vitro* study, several electrospun scaffolds were combined with electrosprayed hydrogels to combat the common problem of poor cellular infiltration into the construct. Each of the scaffold types supported attachment and proliferation of human fetal osteoblasts, and the greatest degree of cell penetra-

TAKE-HOME MESSAGE

Basic science advances

- Modular sECMs with chemically defined, user-controlled compositions and stiffness
- Injectable hydrogels, implantable sponges, and films
- Batch-to-batch consistency
- Easy-to-use under ambient, physiological conditions
- Deliver cells and biological factors with the same biomaterial
- Seamless translation from *in vitro* to *in vivo*

Clinical science advances

- Scar-free healing of chronic and acute wounds
- Repair bone and cartilage
- Reconstruct or repair tissues and organs
- Prevent postsurgical adhesions
- Models to validate and accelerate drug development

Relevance to clinical care

- Simple compositions are the pathway to U.S. Food and Drug Administration–approvable devices for cell delivery
- Simple-to-use materials facilitate acceptance by physicians and patients
- Affordable production costs desirable for health care payer reimbursement

tion was seen in poly (e-caprolactone)/collagen microfibers, and this effect was more pronounced when the Heprasil hydrogel was present in the structure. These hybrid scaffolds suggest further opportunities for the design of cell permeable fibrous meshes for tissue engineering applications.[27]

Growth factor delivery

In the femoral defect model, injuries were either untreated or filled with Extracel hydrogel or sponges with or without 20% (w/v) DBM. The healing process was followed by radiography over the course of 8 weeks. Animals were sacrificed at week 8 postsurgery, and each femur was fixed, embedded, sectioned, and stained with Masson's trichrome. The average fractions of bone healing for each group were statistically different among all groups, and all treatment groups were significantly better than the control group. The Extracel sponge with DBM was superior to the sponge without DBM, and also healed faster than the hydrogel containing DBM. Histologically, defects treated with the Extracel sponge plus DBM were completely filled with newly generated bone tissue with a thickness comparable to native bone. From a clinical viewpoint, the most important observation was that the radiographic healing at 4 weeks was remarkably higher for the Extracel sponge containing human DBM, showing a marked acceleration of femoral repair in a young, healthy animal.[28]

Finally, we used the diabetic wound healing model to simulate a chronic wound in a compromised individual (Fig. 1). The sECM hydrogels in this model were co-crosslinked thiolated chondroitin 6-sulfate (CS) and thiolated HP, and were used to provide controlled-release delivery of bFGF at 2, 10, or 20 μg per wound to full-thickness wounds in diabetic mice. Wounds were treated with CS, CS-bFGF, or CS-HP-bFGF films that were secured with Tegaderm and an elastic bandage. At 2 weeks postinjury, both CS and CS-HP hydrogel films accelerated wound repair, even without bFGF. Addition of bFGF into CS films showed a marked dose-dependent acceleration of wound repair, but the most dramatic result was the dose-responsive effect of bFGF in the CS-HP films. Compared to 27% wound closure in 2 weeks in the controls, up to 89% wound closure was observed in the CS-HP-bFGF (20 μg) treatment. Animals were sacrificed at 4 weeks postinjury, and the thickness of newly formed epidermis and vascularized dermis was significantly improved in the CS-HP-bFGF treatments. This experiment confirms the clinical potential for topical delivery of growth factors to patients with compromised wound healing status.[29]

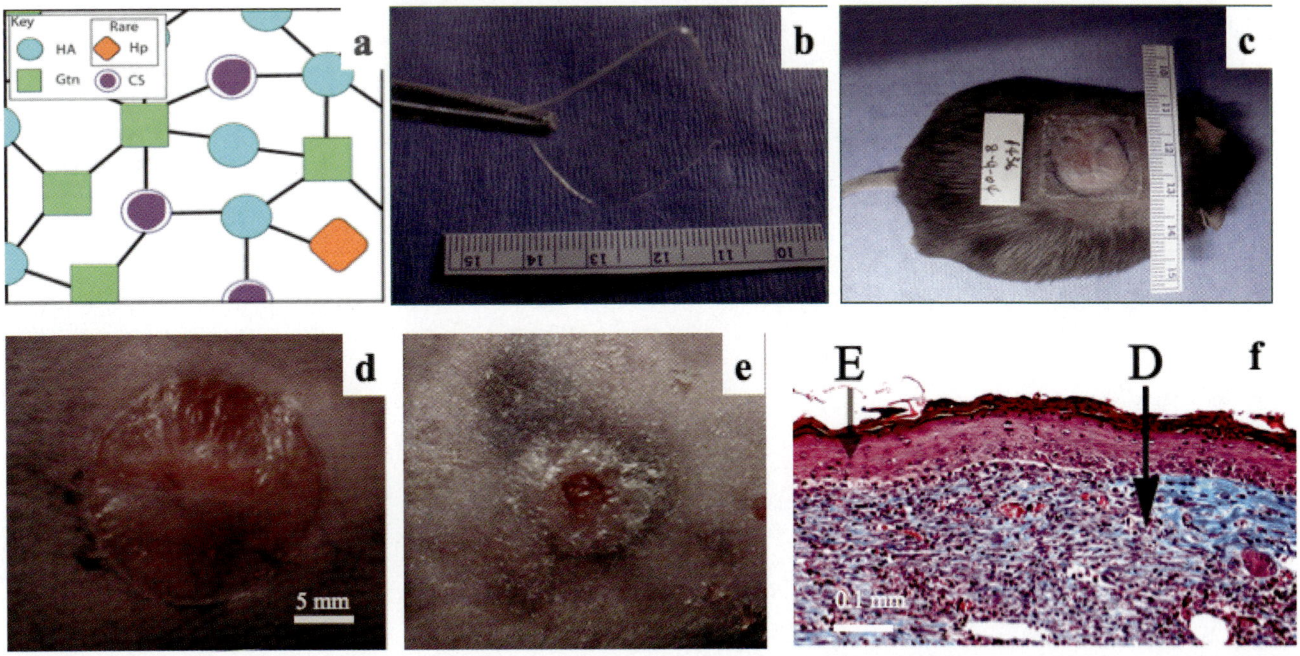

Figure 1. The modular sECM composed of crosslinked thiol-modified CS and heparin (HP) (**a**) can be formed into readily handled hydrogel films (**b**) and applied to the surface of a 1.6-cm full-thickness defect on a diabetic (*db*/*db*) mouse (**c**). After 2 weeks, the control wound is only 27% closed (**d**), but the CS-HP hydrogel containing 20 μg of basic fibroblast growth factor is 89% closed (**e**). After 4 weeks, the histology for the CS-HP-20 μg basic fibroblast growth factor treatment shows full-thickness re-epithelialization and vascularized dermal tissue (**f**). E = epidermis; D = dermis. See Liu *et al.*[29] for additional details.

CAUTION, CRITICAL REMARKS, AND RECOMMENDATIONS

The complexity of the ECM environment can be approximated in modular biomaterials that can deliver and retain cells and growth factors *in vivo*. The temptation among academic scientists—chemists, cell and molecular biologists, polymer and materials scientists, and biomedical engineers—is to create increasingly complex systems that approach ever closer to native tissues. This can lead to elegant, yet over-engineered, constructs that fail to take into account the fundamental principle of market research—make what your end user wants. To reach the clinic, we must embrace biological complexity, engineer versatility, and ultimately deliver a simple and easy-to-use product. Products by their nature need to be elegant in their simplicity, and the simplest approach to wound repair and tissue regeneration is to offer biology the basic tools to enhance and augment the natural healing and regenerative response.

FUTURE DEVELOPMENT

Nothing reaches patients unless it is commercialized, and it is important to note that products based on the sECM technology are in the marketplace already. Products for stem cell research, 3D cell culture, *in vivo* cell therapy models, and sECMs for tumor xenografts are now readily available. As cell therapy opportunities become realistic, highly purified Good Manufacturing Practices (GMP) materials will be submitted for U.S. Food and Drug Administration approval for cell delivery. Crosslinked HA derivatives are available as gels and films for surgical adhesion prevention, and gels and films for wound care for skin and eye injuries in small animals, exotics, and horses. These simple but elegant products are becoming well-accepted and well-liked clinical products in veterinary practice. Finally, selected HA-based sECMs have been granted 510 (k) status and have entered clinical trials, and phase I trial data are being accumulated. Each commercial opportunity has many hurdles, but we foresee that the sECM technology will play an important role in cell therapy strategies of the next decade.

AUTHOR DISCLOSURE STATEMENT

G.D.P is an equity holder and consultant for Glycosan BioSystems, Inc., Sentrx Animal Care, Inc., and Carbylan Biosurgery, Inc., each of which are developing or marketing products based on the sECM technology.

REFERENCES

1. Prestwich GD and Kuo J-w: Chemically-modified HA for therapy and regenerative medicine. Curr Pharm Biotech 2008; **9:** 242.
2. Liu Y, Skardal A, Shu XZ, and Prestwich GD: Prevention of peritendinous adhesions using a hyaluronan-derived hydrogel film following partial-thickness flexor tendon injury. J Orthop Res 2008; **26:** 562.
3. Allison D and Grande-Allen K: Hyaluronan: a powerful tissue engineering tool. Biomaterials 2006; **12:** 2131.
4. Liu Y, Cai S, Shu XZ, Shelby J, and Prestwich GD: Release of basic fibroblast growth factor from a crosslinked glycosaminoglycan hydrogel promotes wound healing. Wound Repair Regen 2007; **15:** 245.
5. Prestwich GD: Engineering a clinically-useful matrix for cell therapy. Organogenesis 2008; **4:** 42.
6. Shu XZ, Liu Y, Luo Y, Roberts MC, and Prestwich GD: Disulfide cross-linked hyaluronan hydrogels. Biomacromolecules 2002; **3:** 1304.
7. Shu XZ, Liu Y, Palumbo FS, Luo Y, and Prestwich GD: *In situ* crosslinkable hyaluronan hydrogels for tissue engineering. Biomaterials 2004; **25:** 1339.
8. Shu XZ, Ahmad S, Liu Y, and Prestwich GD: Synthesis and evaluation of injectable, *in situ* crosslinkable synthetic extracellular matrices for tissue engineering. J Biomed Mater Res A 2006; **79:** 902.
9. Zhang J, Skardal A, and Prestwich GD: Engineered extracellular matrices with cleavable crosslinkers for cell expansion and easy cell recovery. Biomaterials 2008; **29:** 4521.
10. Shu XZ, Liu Y, Palumbo F, and Prestwich GD: Disulfide-crosslinked hyaluronan-gelatin hydrogel films: a covalent mimic of the extracellular matrix for *in vitro* cell growth. Biomaterials 2003; **24:** 3825.
11. Liu Y, Shu XZ, and Prestwich GD: Biocompatibility and stability of disulfide-crosslinked hyaluronan films. Biomaterials 2005; **26:** 4737.
12. Duflo S, Thibeault SL, Li W, Shu XZ, and Prestwich GD: Vocal fold tissue repair *in vivo* using a synthetic extracellular matrix. Tissue Eng 2006; **12:** 2171.
13. Proctor M, Proctor K, Shu XZ, McGill LD, Prestwich GD, and Orlandi RR: Composition of hyaluronan affects wound healing in the rabbit maxillary sinus. Am J Rhinol 2006; **20:** 206.
14. Sondrup C, Liu Y, Shu XZ, Prestwich GD, and Smith ME: Cross-linked hyaluronan-coated stents in the prevention of airway stenosis. Otolaryngol.-Head Neck Surg 2006; **135:** 28.
15. Connors RC, Muir JJ, Liu Y, Reiss GR, Kouretas PC, Whitten MG, Sorenson TK, Prestwich GD, and Bull DA: Postoperative pericardial adhesion prevention using Carbylan-SX in a rabbit model. J Surg Res 2007; **140:** 237.
16. Liu Y, Shu XZ, and Prestwich GD: Reduced postoperative intra-abdominal adhesions using Carbylan-SX, a semisynthetic glycosaminoglycan hydrogel. Fertil Steril 2007; **87:** 940.
17. Liu Y, Skardal A, Shu XZ, and Prestwich GD: Prevention of peritendinous adhesions following flexor tendon injury with Carbylan™-SX, a semisynthetic glycosaminoglycan hydrogel. J Orthopedic Res 2008; **26:** 562.
18. Prestwich GD: Simplifying the extracellular matrix for 3-D cell culture and tissue engineering: a pragmatic approach. J Cell Biochem 2007; **101:** 1370.
19. Cai S, Liu Y, Shu XZ, and Prestwich GD: Injectable glycosaminoglycan hydrogels for controlled release of basic fibroblast growth factor. Biomaterials 2005; **26:** 6054.
20. Riley CM, Fuegy PW, Firpo MA, Shu XZ, Prestwich GD, and Peattie RA: Stimulation of *in vivo* an-

giogenesis using dual growth factor-loaded crosslinked glycosaminoglycan hydrogels. Biomaterials 2006; **27:** 5935.

21. Pike DB, Cai S, Pomraning KR, Firpo MA, Fisher RJ, Shu XZ, Prestwich GD, and Peattie RA: Heparin-regulated release of growth factors *in vitro* and angiogenic response *in vivo* to implanted hyaluronan hydrogels containing VEGF and bFGF. Biomaterials 2006; **27:** 5242.

22. Peattie RA, Yu B, Cai S, Pike DB, Firpo MA, Fisher RJ, Shu XZ, and Prestwich GD: Effect of gelatin on heparin regulation of cytokine release from hyaluronan-based hydrogels. Drug Deliv 2008; **15:** 363.

23. Hosack L, Firpo MA, Scott JA, Prestwich GD, and Peattie RA: Microvascular maturity elicited in tissue treated with cytokine-loaded hyaluronan-based hydrogels. Biomaterials 2008; **29:** 2336.

24. Zhao J, Zhang N, Scott JA, Prestwich GD, and Wen X: Recruitment of endogenous stem cells for tissue repair. Macromol Biosci 2008; **8:** 836.

25. Flynn L, Prestwich GD, Semple JL, and Woodhouse KA: Adipose tissue engineering *in vivo* with adipose-derived stem cells on naturally derived scaffolds. JBMR 2008; **29:** 1862.

26. Liu Y, Shu XZ, and Prestwich GD: Osteochondral defect repair with autologous bone marrow-derived mesenchymal stem cells in an injectable, *in situ*, cross-linked synthetic extracellular matrix. Tissue Eng 2006; **12:** 3405.

27. Ekapurta AK, Prestwich GD, Cool S, and Hutmacher DW: Combining electrospun scaffolds with electrosprayed hydrogels leads to three dimensional cellularization of hybrid constructs. Biomacromolecules 2008; **9:** 2097.

28. Liu Y, Ahmad S, Shu XZ, Sanders RK, Kopesec SA, and Prestwich GD: Accelerated repair of cortical bone defects using a synthetic extracellular matrix to deliver human demineralized bone matrix. J Orthoped Res 2006; **24:** 1454.

29. Liu Y, Cai S, Shu XZ, Shelby J, and Prestwich GD: Release of basic fibroblast growth factor from a crosslinked glycosaminoglycan hydrogel promotes wound healing. Wound Repair Regen 2007; **15:** 245.

WHS
Wound
Healing
Society

Matrix-Enabled Gene Delivery for Tissue Repair

Lois A. Chandler,[1] Robert Engler,[2] and Barbara K. Sosnowski[1,*]

[1]Tissue Repair Company, San Diego, California.
[2]Cardium Therapeutics, Inc., San Diego, California.

Abbreviations and Acronyms

Ad5PDGF-B = adenovirus serotype 5, E1a/b deleted, encoding PDGF-B

AdBMP2 = adenovirus serotype 5, E1a/b deleted, encoding BMP2

BMP-2 = bone morphogenetic protein-2

FGF = fibroblast growth factor

GAM = gene activated matrix

GAM501 = Ad5PDGF-B in 2.6% collagen

PDGF-BB = platelet-derived growth factor-B homodimer

*Correspondence: Tissue Repair Company, 12255 El Camino Road, Suite 250, San Diego, California 92130 (e-mail: bsosnowski@t-r-co.com).

Background: Inflammatory cells and fibroblasts orchestrate repair of hard and soft tissues by infiltrating the injured site and secreting growth factors and cytokines, stimulating tissue regeneration, progenitor cells, and laying down scar tissue. Although growth factor proteins have demonstrated efficacy in preclinical models of tissue repair, most have failed to produce significant improvements in the clinical setting.

The Problem: The limited clinical success of growth factor proteins has been attributed to poor delivery methods and short half-lives. If the gene encoding a growth factor could be transfected into cells in the tissue defect, prolonged production of growth factor could improve efficacy over protein therapy. Combining gene therapy vectors with biocompatible matrices to hold the vector for transfection and provide a scaffolding for cell migration could improve tissue repair. This approach is called gene-activated matrix (GAM).

Basic/Clinical Science Advances: Stimulation of tissue repair with GAMs has been demonstrated in preclinical models of cutaneous wound repair, nerve regeneration, ischemia, and bony defects. A phase 1/2 clinical study for the treatment of chronic diabetic neuropathic wounds utilizing the gene encoding human platelet-derived growth factor-B (Ad5PDGF-B in 2.6% collagen, GAM501) demonstrated safety and potential biological activity. A doubled-blinded, randomized, placebo-controlled phase 2b study to evaluate the safety and efficacy of a single and double application is currently underway.

Clinical Care Relevance: New treatment options are needed to provide a better daily quality of life and avoid amputations in patients having diabetic foot ulcers. Advanced products such as GAM501 with a single or double administration could offer medical practitioners and patients an important new treatment option having a potentially higher therapeutic efficacy, as well as enhancing patient compliance.

Conclusion: GAM501 is the first GAM product to progress to phase 2 development. GAMs offer promise in multiple areas of tissue regeneration and repair, including angiogenesis, bone fracture, nerve, cartilage, ligament, and surgical applications.

BACKGROUND

Gene therapy vectors formulated in biocompatible matrices, otherwise known as gene-activated matrices (GAMs), have been evaluated for the treatment of injured tissues, including skin,[1,2] bone,[3] muscle,[4] and central nervous system.[5,6] Tissue repair cells, including inflammatory cells, endothelial cells, fibroblasts, and progenitor cells, originating in the viable tissue surrounding the defect migrate into the matrix and then take up and transiently express the therapeutic transgene. Depending on the specific application, the goal can be relatively complex, such as complete regeneration of normal tissue to fill

Printed in U.S.A.
DOI: 10.1089/awc.2009.0006

a physical void[2,3] or more limited, such as induction of angiogenesis to perfuse ischemic tissue.[7] By applying GAMs directly within a tissue defect, the DNA vector as well as the transgene product (*i.e.*, the therapeutic protein) are retained within the defect site. Thus, there is an increased opportunity for achieving a maximal therapeutic response with a decreased likelihood of the DNA vector or the therapeutic protein disseminating to nontarget areas.

GAMs are versatile in that the choice of matrix and transgene can be varied based on the therapeutic target. For example, injectable, implantable, or topical formulations can be used. The matrix is considered to have at least two key beneficial functions. First, the matrix holds the DNA vector in place at the wound site until infiltrating wound repair cells arrive. Second, the matrix acts as scaffolding that promotes migration and in-growth of cells that are responsible for accumulation of *de novo* tissue, a key part of any wound healing process. Once in the matrix, cells that have been transfected by the DNA vector act as local bioreactors that produce the therapeutic transgene protein. The transgene is selected based on the desired therapeutic effect; for example, specific growth factors and cytokines that promote granulation tissue formation, angiogenesis, and bone formation. Finally, further versatility of GAMs is achieved through the use of viral or nonviral DNA vectors.

CLINICAL PROBLEM ADDRESSED

In chronic dermal wounds, such as pressure ulcers, venous stasis ulcers, and diabetic neuropathic foot ulcers, the natural process of healing is impaired for a variety of reasons, including inadequate blood flow, increased inflammatory response, impaired innervation, and a deficiency of key growth factors. In diabetic patients, the incidence of chronic lower extremity ulcers (neuropathic, ischemic, or combined etiology) is high, as is the associated morbidity. Approximately 24 million people in the United States have diabetes and 800,000 new cases are identified each year.[8,9] Fifteen percent of diabetic patients will eventually develop a lower extremity ulcer; 25% of those who develop an ulcer will have a foot amputated, and diabetics with lower-limb amputations have a 3-year survival rate of only 50%.

The current standard of care for diabetic foot ulcers (surgical debridement, daily moist dressing changes, and off-loading) results in healing incidences of only 24–31%.[10] Although growth factor proteins have demonstrated efficacy in preclinical models of tissue repair, most have failed to produce more than marginal improvements in clinical practice. The limited clinical success of growth factor proteins has been attributed to poor delivery methods and short half-lives. Becaplermin (Regranex®, Systagenix, North Yorkshire, UK), platelet-derived growth factor-B homodimer [PDGF-BB]), is the only growth factor protein approved for use in diabetic ulcers; however, the healing incidence is only 15% greater than placebo.[11] Further, Becaplermin requires daily application for up to 20 weeks. GAMs are being investigated as a therapeutic alternative (in conjunction with standardized care) for the treatment of chronic diabetic ulcers of the lower extremities. The potential ability of GAMs to achieve more sustained, localized delivery of growth factor proteins may translate into a treatment regimen requiring only one or two administrations. This is turn could lead to improved patient compliance and quality of life, and thus a better therapeutic outcome than provided by current approaches.

RELEVANT BASIC SCIENCE CONTEXT

GAMs consist of two key components, each of which can be varied to increase the versatility of this therapeutic approach. In its simplest form, a GAM consists of a gene that encodes a therapeutic protein and a biocompatible matrix. The matrix component can be customized for the target organ, for physical properties that improve local retention such as high viscosity, and for signaling or binding sequences for migrating cells such as Arginine-Glycine-Aspartic Acid-integrin, selectin, or elastin-elastin binding proteins. It can be further customized for electrostatic charge to bind plasmid DNA or viral vectors, or perhaps with viral receptors to localize the virus during the time required for cell migration into the matrix from the wound edge.

EXPERIMENTAL MODEL OR MATERIAL

Within the last decade, the evaluation of GAMs for tissue repair has progressed from preclinical to clinical studies. A GAM consisting of a replication incompetent, nonintegrating adenoviral vector encoding the human platelet-derived growth factor-B (PDGF-B) gene formulated in a 2.6% bovine type I collagen matrix (Ad5PDGF-B/Collagen) has emerged as a promising candidate therapeutic for the treatment of chronic diabetic neuropathic ulcers of the lower extremities. Adenoviral vectors are appealing for use as they can be efficiently manufactured and purified, they do not integrate into the genome of target cells, they can be genetically engineered to be nonreplicating, they efficiently transduce cells, they efficiently express therapeutic transgenes, and expression is transient and thus well suited for wound healing. Therefore, adenoviral vectors are efficient and cost effective, and have favorable safety profiles. Bovine type I collagen is favorable for use as the matrix component of GAM; it is a component of products already approved for human use, and is a natural component of healing wounds providing a scaffold for migratory repair cells. Bovine type I collagen also interacts electrostatically with adenoviral vectors, which serves to retain the vector at the site of application, a key beneficial feature of GAMs. Further, it contains Arginine-Glycine-Aspartic Acid sequences that facilitate inflammatory cell and fibroblast migration and mimic the scaffolding of normal tissue. Ad5PDGF-B/collagen has progressed from preclinical efficacy and safety evaluation to phase 2b clinical evaluation in chronic diabetic foot ulcers.

DISCUSSION OF FINDINGS AND RELEVANT LITERATURE

Stimulation of tissue repair with GAMs has been demonstrated in preclinical models of bone repair, nerve repair, ischemia, and dermal wound repair. Schreiber *et al.*[12] formulated adenoviral vectors encoding bone morphogenetic protein 2 (BMP2) with allogenic bone collagen (AdBMP2/collagen) and examined them in a rat orthotopic model. AdBMP2/collagen implants induced robust bone formation by day 14 after implantation compared to collagen implants alone. Alkaline phosphatase–specific activity, a measure of the rate of bone formation within the implants, peaked at day 14 in the AdBMP2/collagen-treated sites. In contrast, alkaline phosphatase levels were negligible through day 35 for the implants treated with collagen alone. Berry *et al.*[5] tested the efficacy of GAMs to promote survival of retinal ganglion cells after transection of axons in a rat optic nerve model. In this model, most rat ganglion cells die within the first week, with the remainder dying over a period of several months. Nonviral plasmid vectors encoding either a reporter gene or neurotrophic factors (mixtures of neurotrophin-3, fibroblast growth factor 2 (FGF2), and brain-derived neurotrophic factor plasmids) formulated in a collagen lyophile promoted sustained survival of retinal ganglion cells for over 3 months after the initial injury. The findings demonstrated that GAM-immobilized plasmid DNA implanted into the central nervous system lesion was taken up by severed axons for retrograde transport and transgene was expressed in the nucleus, thus possibly being a useful agent for neuron survival and axon regeneration. In later studies, Gonzalez *et al.*[6] demonstrated that GAMs could be used to deliver genes to axotomized dorsal root ganglion cells after spinal cord injury. One week postinjury, polymerase chain reaction analyses demonstrated that the DNA within the GAM had been retrogradely transported from the dorsal column lesion to the brain cortex and to the caudal dorsal root ganglion neurons and reverse transcriptase–polymerase chain reaction analyses demonstrated expression of the transgene. *In situ* hybridization localized the transgene DNA and RNA within fibroblasts, glial cells, endothelial cells, and inflammatory cells invading the GAM and in the dorsal root ganglion neurons. In addition, by 7 weeks the presence of the GAM also appeared to reduce secondary cavitation and scar deposition at the lesion site.

In a rodent skeletal muscle excisional model, Doukas *et al.*[4] found that the basic FGF2 gene formulated in a collagen/gelatin matrix led to increased angiogenesis, arteriogenesis, and myotube regeneration when compared with reporter gene formulations. Horvath *et al.*[7] further demonstrated in a porcine model of chronic myocardial ischemia that delivery of the FGF2/collagen-gelatin GAM led to a significant restoration of myocardial function as measured by myocardial wall thickening compared to control-treated animals. This functional improvement was confirmed by cine magnetic resonance imaging in which greater than 65% of the treated area showed improvement in wall motion compared to no improvement in the untreated area. In a follow-on study, Horvath *et al.*[13] demonstrated that adenovirus serotype 5, E1a/b-deleted, encoding FGF2/collagen-gelatin formulations in combination with CO_2 transmyocardial laser revascularization had a 105% increase in arteriolar development in treated areas compared to either treatment alone, and a 390% increase compared to saline-formulated adenovirus serotype 5, E1a/b-deleted, encoding FGF2. These data support the hypothesis that the matrix functions to hold the vector in place until repair cells arrive, take up, express, and secrete the transgene product.

The *PDGF-B* formulated in collagen matrices has been evaluated in both soft and hard tissue repair models. PDGF-BB is a known chemoattractant that can induce repair cells to migrate from the normal wound margins into the wound bed.[14] PDGF-BB is also known for its ability to stimulate repair cell proliferation, so those cells that have migrated into the wound bed and are exposed to the protein will increase in number leading to a greater amount of granulation tissue.[15,16] In addition, Keswani *et al.*[17] demonstrated that delivery of Ad5PDGF-B to several diabetic mouse models leads to the augmentation of endothelial precursor cell recruitment to the wound bed.

In a rat alveolar bone defect model, Jin *et al.*[18] demonstrated that adenoviral vector encoding PDGF-B (Ad5PDGF-B) formulated in a collagen matrix resulted in four times greater bone and six times greater cementum regeneration compared to reporter gene controls. Chang *et al.*[19] further demonstrated that Ad5PDGF-B/collagen formulations delivered to rat alveolar bone defects were well contained within the localized osseous defect and exhibited a high safety profile as measured by hematological and blood chemistry measurements. In a soft tissue model, Hijjawi *et al.*[20] described the use of nonviral plasmid DNA encoding human PDGF-B formulated in collagen to improve survival of ischemic myocutaneous flaps. Transdermal spectral imaging demonstrated an increase in patent blood vessels supporting blood flow in ischemic flaps with PDGF-B gene matrix formulations compared to controls (collagen alone).

Gu *et al.*[21] described the preclinical development of the PDGF-B gene in a replication incompetent adenovector formulated in a bovine collagen matrix (Ad5PDGF-B/bovine type I collagen [GAM501]) that has progressed to clinical evaluation for diabetic neuropathic foot ulcers. In similar preclinical studies, Doukas *et al.*[2] demonstrated that the PDGF-B gene is expressed in tissue repair cells as early as 1-day after GAM501 application and for as long as 7 days, and that Ad5PDGF-B/collagen does not lead to long-term hyperproliferative responses or scar formation. The PDGF-BB protein that is expressed in these studies contains the endogenous collagen-binding domain and thus is retained in the wound bed environment where it is needed most. As new cells migrate into the gene-containing matrix, they are exposed to the PDGF-BB protein for a 7-day period. Although the protein is only transiently synthesized and secreted by wound repair cells, the duration of its availability is substantially prolonged relative to topical protein therapy, which must be reapplied daily. The sustained presence of the PDGF-BB protein at the precise location where it can be effective is believed to lead to the acceleration of the normal wound healing response. In a full-thickness dermal wound model in rabbits,[21] multiple doses of Ad5PDGF-B/collagen were evaluated to determine if repeated treatments altered the tissue distribution, safety, immunogenicity, and efficacy of Ad5PDGF-B/col-collagen. Large ($>6\,cm^2$) full-thickness wounds were created in the backs of rabbits. Animals received either collagen alone or Ad5PDGF-B/collagen (7×10^{10} viral particle number/cm^2). Wounds were treated four times at 1-week intervals (days 0, 7, 14, and 21). On day 22 wounds were harvested and evaluated by immunohistochemistry to determine the number of proliferating cells from the wound edge to the center of the wound. Gu *et al.*[21] demonstrated that Ad5PDGF-B/collagen lead to a visible increase in granulation tissue compared to collagen controls. The quantitative assessment of proliferating cells using *in situ* hybridization and immunohistochemistry is greatest at the wound edge and slightly decreases toward the wound center for animals treated with Ad5PDGF-B/collagen (Fig. 1A). The number of proliferating cells (primarily fibroblasts, monocytes, and macrophages) was significantly higher at all wound locations assessed in the Ad5PDGF-B/collagen group compared to the animals treated with collagen alone. In addition, despite the fact that anti-adenovirus IgG responses were detected,

TAKE-HOME MESSAGE

Basic science advances

- GAMs are composed of a viral or nonviral DNA vector transgene encoding a therapeutic protein and a biocompatible matrix.
- GAMs provide an increased opportunity for achieving a maximal therapeutic response with a decreased likelihood of the DNA vector or the therapeutic protein disseminating to nontargeted tissues.

Clinical science advances

- A GAM using Ad5PDGF-B in a bovine collagen matrix (GAM501) was well tolerated and safe in a small number of patients in an open label phase ½ study and suggested a therapeutic response.
- GAM501 has progressed to a large, multicenter, double-blind, placebo-controlled study that completed enrollment in late 2009. GAM501 appeared to be safe and well-tolerated. Efficacy results are pending.

Relevance to clinical care

- There is a critical need for new therapies to enhance wound healing in a number of areas, especially in diabetic foot ulcers, which involve millions of patients. Potential patient benefits from a single administration of GAM501 could offer medical practitioners and diabetic foot ulcer patients an important new treatment option having a higher degree of therapeutic efficacy, as well as enhanced patient compliance.

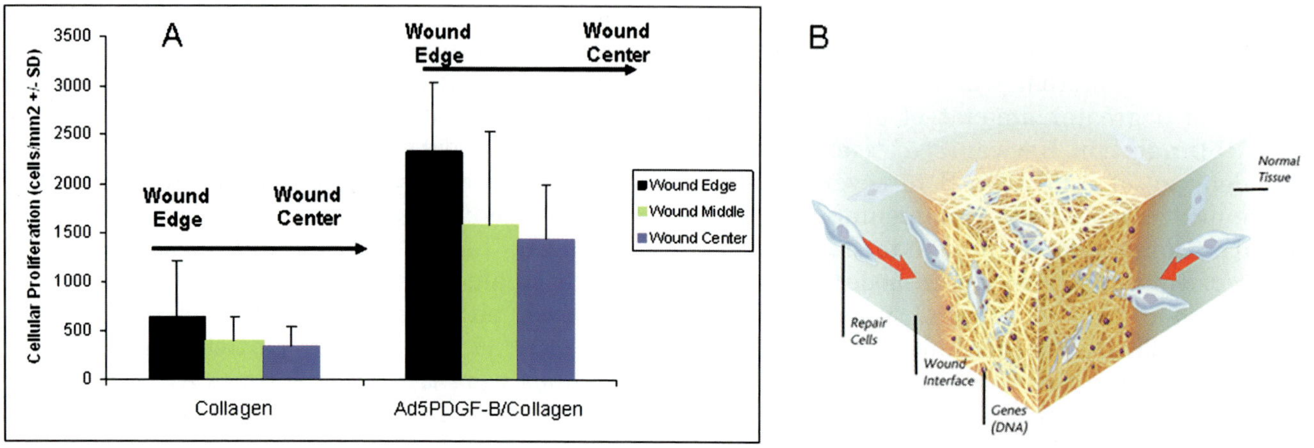

Figure 1. Ad5PDGF-B/collagen stimulates tissue repair and cell proliferation. Approximately 6 cm^2 wounds were created on the backs of rabbits on day 0. Wounds were immediately treated with either 700 μL collagen alone or 7×10^{10} viral particles of Ad5PDGF-B in an equal volume collagen matrix. Repeat treatments were given on days 7, 14, and 21. On day 22, wounds were harvested, and tissue sections were evaluated for increased cellularity using an antibody to Ki-67 (**A**). Image analysis of Ki-67-positive stains revealed an increase in the number of proliferating cells at the wound edge and slightly decreasing toward the wound center. All Ad5PDGF-B/collagen-treated animals had significantly greater number of proliferating cells for all assessed tissues compared to the animals treated with collagen alone. (**B**) Schematic of migrating cells from the viable tissue at the wound margin into the matrix.

multiple applications of Ad5PDGF-B/collagen each lead to significant increases in granulation tissue compared to saline and collagen alone controls.[21] These data support the hypothesis that cells are migrating from the viable tissue at the wound margin into the matrix and subsequently taking up and expressing the PDGF-B gene, which leads to an increase in proliferating cells (Fig. 1B).

The clinical safety and efficacy of Ad5PDGF-B/collagen (GAM501) was evaluated in a multicenter, open-label, dose-escalation phase 1/2 study. Fifteen patients with previously nonhealing foot ulcers ($\geq$6 weeks) were enrolled into this first in-man topical gene therapy study. Patients received either a single dose or four administrations of GAM501 at 1-week intervals and were then evaluated for up to 6 months. In addition to application of GAM501, patients also followed a standard of care regimen including off-loading and surgical debridement for the entire treatment and evaluation periods. Results of the phase 1/2 study indicated that GAM501 was well tolerated and there were no dose-limiting toxicity effects, including antibody responses, due to the product candidate. In addition, most of the patients (93%) had a positive response to GAM501, with 67% of the patients with small to large ulcers achieving complete wound closure (Mulder *et al.*).[22]

A phase 2b clinical study was initiated to evaluate the safety and efficacy of GAM501 for the potential treatment of nonhealing diabetic neuropathic foot ulcers. The MATRIX study is a randomized, double-blind, placebo-controlled, comparator arm clinical trial and will enroll patients found to have type I or II diabetes with a nonhealing neuropathic (but not ischemic) foot ulcer present for at least 6 weeks. The five arms of the study include standardized care, one or two applications of placebo, and one or two applications of GAM501. The study's primary endpoint is complete ulcer closure at 12 weeks or earlier. Secondary endpoints will be time to complete ulcer closure, change in ulcer area, safety, and tolerance and durability of wound closure. Enrollment is anticipated to be completed in 2009 with trial results available by the end of the year (http://clinicaltrials.gov/ct/show/NCT00493051).

CAUTION, CRITICAL REMARKS, AND RECOMMENDATIONS

The clinical development of growth factor protein therapeutics for hard and soft tissue repair and regeneration has been hampered by the inherent instability of the proteins, especially in the hostile wound environment. Consequently, frequent dosing and large quantities of protein are required for a therapeutic effect, thus making protein therapy labor intensive and expensive for both the patient and doctor. Only two recombinant human proteins, PDGF-BB and BMP2, have been approved for the treatment of diabetic ulcers and spinal fusion, respectively. The need for improved therapeutics is highly warranted.

GAM501 has not been approved by FDA and is currently in its first-blinded, placebo-controlled trial. Potential patient benefits from a single or double administration of GAM501 could one day offer medical practitioners and their diabetic foot ulcer patients an important new treatment option with a high degree of therapeutic efficacy, as well as enhanced patient compliance. Such a new treatment option could thereby provide a better daily quality of life and avoid amputations for an increasing population of patients having diabetic foot ulcers.

FUTURE DEVELOPMENT

Significant progress has been made in recent years in the development of gene therapeutics for soft and hard tissue repair. Gene therapy offers the potential for sustained local availability of the therapeutic proteins, decreased frequency of dosing, and improved therapeutic responses at reduced costs. GAM delivery provides further efficacy and cost benefits. The phase 2b MATRIX study currently in progress is evaluating the efficacy of a topically applied formulation of Ad5PDGF-B in collagen. This study represents the first of its kind topical gene therapy trial. GAMs offer promise in other areas of tissue repair and regeneration, including therapeutic angiogenesis, bone fracture repair, nerve repair, cartilage repair, ligament repair, and surgical applications.

ACKNOWLEDGMENTS

The phase 1/2 clinical study was partially supported by a grant from the National Institutes of Health/National Institute of Arthritis and Musculoskeletal and Skin Diseases (NIAMS) (5R44AR46154-03).

AUTHOR DISCLOSURE STATEMENT

L.A.C. and B.K.S. are employees of and hold stock options in Cardium Therapeutics, Inc. R.E. is a consultant to and owns stock options in Cardium Therapeutics. Cardium Therapeutics is the owner of Tissue Repair Company and of intellectual property used in the Gene Activated Matrix technology.

REFERENCES

1. Tyrone J, Mogford JE, Chandler LA, Ma C, Xia Y, Pierce GF, and Mustoe TA: Collagen-embedded platelet-derived growth factor DNA plasmid promotes wound healing in a dermal ulcer model. J Surg Res 2000; **93:** 230.
2. Doukas J, Chandler LA, Gonzalez AM, Gu DL, Hoganson DK, Ma C, Nguyen T, Printz MA, Nesbit M, Herlyn M, Crombleholme TM, Aukerman SL, Sosnowski BA, and Pierce GF: Matrix immobilization enhances the tissue repair activity of growth factor gene therapy vectors. Hum Gene Ther 2001; **12:** 783.
3. Goldstein SA: *In vivo* nonviral delivery factors to enhance bone repair. Clin Orthop 2000; **379:** S113.
4. Doukas J, Blease K, Craig D, Ma C, Chandler LA, Sosnowski BA, and Pierce GF: Delivery of FGF genes to wound repair cells enhances arteriogenesis and myogenesis in skeletal muscle. Mol Ther 2002; **5:** 517.
5. Berry M, Gonzalez AM, Clarke W, Greenlees L, Barrett L, Tsang W, Seymour L, Bonadio J, Logan A, and Baird A: Sustained effects of gene-activated matrices after CNS injury. Mol Cell Neurosci 2001; **17:** 706.
6. Gonzalez AM, Berry M, Greenlees L, Logan A, and Baird A: Matrix-mediated gene transfer to brain cortex and dorsal root ganglion neurons by retrograde axonal transport after dorsal column lesion. J Gene Med 2006; **8:** 901.
7. Horvath K, Doukas J, Lu CY, Belkind N, Greene R, Pierce GF, and Fullerton DA: Myocardial functional recovery after fibroblast growth factor 2 gene therapy as assessed by echocardiography and magnetic resonance imaging. Ann Thorac Surg 2002; **74:** 481.
8. National Diabetes Information Clearing House (NDIC). http://diabetes.niddk.nih.gov/dm/pubs/statistics/#allages.
9. Reiber GE, Vileikyte L, Boyko EJ, del Aguila M, Smith DG, Lavery LA, and Boulton AJ: Causal pathways for incident lower-extremity ulcers in patients with diabetes from two settings. Diabetes Care 1999; **22:** 157.
10. Margolis DJ, Kantor J, and Berlin JA: Healing of diabetic neuropathic foot ulcers receiving standard treatment. Diabetes Care 1999; **22:** 692.
11. Smiell JM, Wieman TJ, Steed DL, Perry BH, Sampson AR, and Schwab BH: Efficacy and safety of becaplermin (recombinant human platelet-derived growth factor-BB) in patients with nonhealing, lower extremity diabetic ulcers: a combined analysis of four randomized studies. Wound Repair Regen 1999; **7:** 335.
12. Schreiber RE, Blease K, Ambrosio A, Amburn E, Sosnowski B, and Sampath TK: Bone induction by AdBMP-2/collagen implants. J Bone Joint Surg 2005; **87:** 1059.
13. Horvath KA, Yang C, Robert E, Pierce GF, Greene R, Sosnowski BA, and Doukas J: Improvement of myocardial contractility in a porcine model of chronic ischemia using a combined transmyocardial revascularization and gene therapy approach. J Thorac Cardiovasc Surg 2004; **129:** 1071.
14. Deuel TF, Kawahara RS, Mustoe TA, and Pierce GF: Growth factors and wound healing: platelet-derived growth factor as a model cytokine. Annu Rev Med 1991; **42:** 567.
15. Pierce GF, Mustoe TA, Senior RM, Reed J, Griggin GL, Thomason A, and Deuel TF: *In vivo* incisional wound healing augmented by platelet-derived growth factor and recombinant c-sis gene homodimeric proteins. J Exp Med 1988; **167:** 974.
16. Pierce GF, Tarpley JE, Allman RM, Goode PS, Serdar CM, Morris B, Mustoe TA, and Vande Berg J: Tissue repair response in healing chronic pressure ulcers treated with recombinant platelet-derived growth factor BB. Am J Pathol 1994; **145:** 1399.
17. Keswani SG, Katz AB, Lim FY, Zoltick P, Radu A, Alaee DM, Herlyn M, and Crombleholme TM: Adenoviral mediated gene transfer of PDGF-B enhances wound healing in type I and type II diabetic wounds. Wound Repair Regen 2004; **12:** 497.
18. Jin Q, Anusaksathien O, Webb AS, Printz MA, and Giannobile WV: Engineering of tooth-supporting structures by delivery of PDGF gene therapy vectors. Mol Ther 2004; **9:** 519.
19. Chang PC, Cirelli JA, Seol Q, Sugai JV, D'Silva NJ, Danciu TE, Chandler LA, Sosnowski BA, and

Giannobile WV: Adenovirus encoding human platelet-derived growth factor-B delivered to alveolar bone defects exhibits safety and biodistribution profiles favorable for clinical use. Hum Gene Ther 2009; **20:** 486.

20. Hijjawi J, Mogford JE, Chandler LA, Cross KJ, Sosnowski BA, and Mustoe TA: Platelet-derived growth factor-B, but not fibroblast growth factor 2, plasmid DNA improves survival of ischemic myocutaneous flaps. Arch Surg 2004; **139:** 142.

21. Gu DL, Nguyen T, Gonzalez AM, Printz MA, Pierce GF, Sosnowski BA, Phillips ML, and Chandler LA: Adenovirus encoding human platelet-derived growth factor-B delivered in collagen exhibits safety, biodistribution, and immunogenicity profiles favorable for clinical use. Mol Ther 2004; **9:** 699.

22. Mulder G, Tallis AJ, Marshall VT, Mozingo D, Phillips L, Pierce GF, Chandler LA, and Sosnowski BK: Treatment of nonhealing diabetic foot ulcers with a platelet-derived growth factor gene-activated matrix (GAM501): results of a phase 1/2 trial. Wound Repair Regen 2009; **17:** 772.

Section 9

TISSUE ENGINEERING

Section Editors: Jonathan Mansbridge and Hans-Oliver Rennekampff

WHS
Wound
Healing
Society

Tissue-Engineered Skin Substitutes

Jonathan Mansbridge[1,*] and Hans-Oliver Rennekampff[2]

[1]Tecellact LLC, La Jolla, California.
[2]Department of Plastic, Hand, and Reconstructive Surgery, Burn Center, Hannover, Germany.

THE HISTORY OF TISSUE ENGINEERING as applied to skin substitutes now stretches back 30 years.[1] The industry saw explosive growth during the decade before 2002, with the appearance of three products. That high point was followed by a decline, coincident with the dot com collapse. Since then, there has been a marked resurgence, with a fourfold increase in activity over the previous peak.[2] Most of this increase has been driven by investment in stem cells. The development of skin substitutes and artificial skin has reached a plateau, and the established commercial products are growing into their market. It has been realized that only a small proportion of the sums expended annually on wound care that were hyped during the heady days can actually be addressed by tissue-engineered skin substitutes. However, the established companies in the field have focused on manufacturing their products, reducing their expectations, and are doing well. New developments on skin substitutes have been in the direction of acellular products, autologous systems, model systems, and improvements in the clinical applicability of the products.

The general rubric of tissue-engineered skin substitutes includes combinations of scaffold, cells, and growth factors. All appear in this section. Products involving cells are inevitably expensive to produce. The development, application, and future directions of cellular skin substitutes are well discussed in the article by Ronfard (page 412). Since the manufacturing of cellular products is exacting and costly,[3] there has been much interest in systems consisting of scaffolds alone. The first tissue-engineered skin substitutes were of this kind, developed by Burke *et al.*[4] and commercialized as Integra. This product was originally designed for the treatment of acute burns but has expanded into such fields as scar revision surgery. Several noncellular materials that are intended to provide a conductive substrate for migration of the host cells into the wound and to act as a template for the synthesis of a dermal-like structure have appeared in the market, including Oasis, Hyafilm, Alloderm, and others. Some of these have been used as supports for host cells, expanded and seeded.[5] Growth factors alone have received much attention but have produced few products, only Regranex platelet-derived growth factor (PDGF B chain) being available for the treatment of chronic wounds and Juvista (transforming growth factor β_3) for the prevention of scars.[6] The article by Jin and colleagues (page 375) explores an interesting direction in the sustained release of PDGF, which provides considerable benefit in terms of cellular ingrowth into a bead per microgram of PDGF supplied.

Abbreviation and Acronym

PDGF = platelet-derived growth factor

*Correspondence: Tecellact LLC, 1685 Calle Camille, La Jolla, California 92037 (e-mail: jonathanmansbridge@yahoo.com).

Printed in U.S.A.
DOI: 10.1089/awc.2009.0176

Table 1. *Examples of hypotheses for the development and maintenance of chronic wounds*

1. Transient nature of growth factor stimulation
2. Bacterial colonization and biofilm formation[9]
3. Fibroblast senescence[10–12]
4. Lactate imbalance[13]
5. Genetic defects
6. Extracellular matrix migration substrate degradation[14]
7. Oxidative damage (repetitive ishemia-reperfusion)[12]
8. Nutritional deficiency (ischemia, capillary cuffing, poor diet)[15,16]
9. Inadequate stem-cell recruitment[17]
10. Changes in the stress response[18]
11. Growth factor deficiency/proteolysis, reduced cell responsiveness[19]
12. Reduced antimicrobial peptide production[20]
13. Vitamin D deficiency[21]

This table is not intended to be exhaustive.

In systems involving cells alone, an approach of supplying large numbers of allogeneic fibroblasts to wounds to assist in healing in a clinical setting is being explored. Fibroblasts are a diverse group of cells, whose properties vary. A fibroblast population becomes dominated by one type of fibroblast or another, either through the overgrowth of a particular cell type or through a senescence process affecting each cell. This is discussed in an article by Rennekampff (page 419).

A continuing major problem in wound repair remains the mechanisms whereby some wounds become and remain chronic. A selection of mechanisms is listed in Table 1. One approach to testing and distinguishing these hypotheses is through the use of model skin equivalent. The article by Garlick (page 425) deals with a model system of wound healing that may be developed to examine the mechanisms involved in chronic wounding through the addition of microbial agents and studies that cannot be performed *in vivo*.

A question that has been raised with respect to allogeneic skin substitutes from the earliest days has been immunological rejection. Although the rejection of transplanted allogeneic organs is well established, acute rejection of allogeneic skin substitutes has never been observed in commercial products. It is conjectured that the lack of immunological response is related to the lack of antigen-presenting cells, such as dendritic or endothelial cells.[7] Nonetheless, much of the current, academic development of skin substitutes is related to autologous systems, despite the challenges presented to commercialization of the resulting systems. Some reasons for this are given in the article by Middlekoop (page 432) who also emphasizes the increasing stringency imposed by regulatory authorities on the raw materials used to make the constructs, with the complete elimination of components of animal origin. This will impose restrictions on the use, and ultimately the elimination, of bovine serum, bovine pituitary extract, bovine collagen and mouse 3T3 cells. Three approaches to autologous tissue-engineered skin substitutes can be envisaged. At one extreme is the tissue culture approach. This has been used successfully for the treatment of burns in an academic setting[8] and realized commercially (Episkin). However, the manufacture of this type of product is limited to a few centers and it requires skilled and specialized operators, who are expensive in a commercial setting. At the other extreme is the use of scaffolds, such as Integra, Oasis, etc., either alone or seeded with cells harvested during the implantation procedure. Matriderm, discussed here by Haslik and colleagues (page 438), is a good example of this approach. In this case, the patient is his own tissue culture suite, and the method is both cheap and practical. Other examples are by Bates (page 457) and Morgan (page 451). However, this approach may not meet all situations. A third approach is to use a robotic tissue culture system, which would accept a piece of tissue and provide a finished skin substitute some weeks later. The machine although expensive would be cheaper than skilled technicians, and all product-contact components (flasks, tubing, etc.) would be closed and disposable, minimizing the regulatory requirements. Such machines have been developed with a view to their use in the space program and may provide a solution to the problems of autologous tissue engineering.

As one of the simpler tissue-engineered systems, skin models have lead the way in tissue engineering, both in the development of experimental systems and in commercialization. One of the central problems in the field is the vascularization of implanted tissue. This severely limits the thickness of implants and is of particular importance in the field that deals with the organs rather than skin or cartilage. Skin substitutes are very thin, and it appears that the survival of the implanted cells is adequate under most conditions. Nonetheless, cell performance after implantation could be improved. Moreover, cellular skin implants provide an excellent test bed for the development of vascularization systems. The article by Berthod (page 445) discusses one such device, which has the potential for great impact in the general field of tissue engineering, while also pointing the way to a technique that may provide a clinical benefit in the treatment of difficult skin wounds.

The use of skin substitutes continues to fill a moderately sized but important niche in the treatment of acute and chronic wounds. In the future, we can expect refinements to be developed in the form of genetically engineered systems, sprayed cells, and improved inosculation of cellular systems. Noncellular dermal scaffolds, incorporating polymers, or an increasing range of biological molecules, will be developed that will encourage tissue repair. The movement toward autologous products is likely to be restricted to universities and nonprofit groups unless an automatic system for growing the tissues on an individual basis can be devised.

REFERENCES

1. Bell E, Ivarsson G, and Merrill C: Production of a tissue-like structure by contraction of collagen lattices by human fibroblasts of different proliferative potential *in vitro*. Proc Natl Acad Sci USA 1979; **76:** 1274.
2. Lysaght MJ, Jaklenec A, and Deweerd E: Great expectations: private sector activity in tissue engineering, regenerative medicine, and stem cell therapeutics. Tissue Eng Part A 2008; **14:** 305.
3. Mansbridge J: Commercial considerations in tissue engineering. J Anat 2006; **209:** 527.
4. Burke JF, Yannas IV, Quinby WCJ, Bondoc CC, and Yung WK: Successful use of a physiologically acceptable artificial skin in the treatment of extensive burn injury. Ann Surg 1981; **194:** 413.
5. Kalyanaraman B and Boyce ST: Wound healing on athymic mice with engineered skin substitutes fabricated with keratinocytes harvested from an automated bioreactor. J Surg Res 2009; **152:** 296.
6. Occleston NL, Laverty HG, O'Kane S, and Ferguson MW: Prevention and reduction of scarring in the skin by transforming growth factor beta 3 (TGFbeta3): from laboratory discovery to clinical pharmaceutical. J Biomater Sci Polym Ed 2008; **19:** 1047.
7. Mansbridge J: Transplantation of engineered cells and tissues. In: *Tissue Engineering Using Ceramics and Polymers*, edited by Boccaccini ARG and Gough JE. Cambridge, UK: Woodhead, 2007, p. 93.
8. Compton CC: Current concepts in pediatric burn care: the biology of cultured epithelial autografts: an eight-year study in pediatric burn patients. Eur J Pediatr Surg 1992; **2:** 216.
9. Dowd SE, Wolcott RD, Sun Y, McKeehan T, Smith E, and Rhoads D: Polymicrobial nature of chronic diabetic foot ulcer biofilm infections determined using bacterial tag encoded FLX amplicon pyrosequencing (bTEFAP). PLoS ONE 2008; **3:** e3326.
10. Stanley A and Osler T: Senescence and the healing rates of venous ulcers. J Vasc Surg 2001; **33:** 1206.
11. Harding KG, Moore K, and Phillips TJ: Wound chronicity and fibroblast senescence—implications for treatment. Int Wound J 2005; **2:** 364.
12. Wall IB, Moseley R, Baird DM, Kipling D, Giles P, Laffafian I, Price PE, Thomas DW, and Stephens P: Fibroblast dysfunction is a key factor in the non-healing of chronic venous leg ulcers. J Invest Dermatol 2008; **128:** 2526.
13. Ghani QP, Wagner S, Becker HD, Hunt TK, and Hussain MZ: Regulatory role of lactate in wound repair. Methods Enzymol 2004; **381:** 565.
14. Grinnell F and Zhu M: Fibronectin degradation in chronic wounds depends on the relative levels of elastase, alpha1-proteinase inhibitor, and alpha2-macroglobulin. J Invest Dermatol 1996; **106:** 335.
15. Pompeo M and Baxter C: Sacral and ischial pressure ulcers: evaluation, treatment, and differentiation. Ostomy Wound Manage 2000; **46:** 18.
16. Galkowska, H., Olszewsk WL, Wojewodzka U, Mijal J, and Filipiuk E: Expression of apoptosis- and cell cycle-related proteins in epidermis of venous leg and diabetic foot ulcers. Surgery 2003; **134:** 213.
17. Simka M: Delayed healing of chronic leg ulcers can result from impaired trafficking of bone marrow-derived precursors of keratinocytes to the skin. Med Hypotheses, 2007; **69:** 637.
18. Mustoe T.A., O'Shaughnessy K, and Kloeters O: Chronic wound pathogenesis and current treatment strategies: a unifying hypothesis. Plast Reconstr Surg 2006; **117:** 35S.
19. Brem H, Young J, Tomic-Canic M, Isaacs C, and Ehrlich HP: Clinical efficacy and mechanism of bilayered living human skin equivalent (HSE) in treatment of diabetic foot ulcers. Surg Technol Int 2003; **11:** 23.
20. Galkowska H, Olszewski WL, and Wojewodzka U: Expression of natural antimicrobial peptide beta-defensin-2 and Langerhans cell accumulation in epidermis from human non-healing leg ulcers. Folia Histochem Cytobiol 2005; **43:** 133.
21. Schauber J, Dorschner RA, Coda AB, Buchau AS, Liu PT, Kiken D, Helfrich YR, Kang S, Elalieh HZ, Steinmeyer A, Zugel U, Bikle DD, Modlin RL, and Gallo RL: Injury enhances TLR2 function and antimicrobial peptide expression through a vitamin D-dependent mechanism. J Clin Invest 2007; **117:** 803.

Developments in Cell-Based Therapy for Wounds

Vincent Ronfard* and Thomas Williams

Research and Development, Organogenesis, Inc., Canton, Massachusetts.

*Correspondence: Research and Development, Organogenesis, Inc., 150 Dan Road, Canton, Massachusetts 02021 (e-mail: vronfard@organo.com).

Background: Over the last 30 years, the development and use of cell-based therapy advanced from a scientific discovery to a series of commercially viable products. Several bioengineered tissues are now used in the clinic to treat venous leg ulcers (Apligraf®; Organogenesis, Canton, MA), diabetic foot ulcers (Apligraf and Dermagraft®; Advanced Biohealing, La Jolla, CA), or burns (Epicel®; Genzyme Biosurgery, Cambridge, MA). Numerous other products are in development for acute or chronic wounds.

The Problem: Currently available cell-based therapies offer good clinical outcomes for their approved indications. However, other areas of tissue repair, such as pressure ulcers, remain elusive. The ultimate goal is to regenerate skin with the complete structural and functional properties comparable to those of the wounded area before injury, regardless of the location or causation of the wound.

Basic/Clinical Science Advances: In 1988, Epicel was introduced into the burn market. In 1998, Apligraf became the first tissue-engineered product to be approved by the Food and Drug Administration for use in venous leg ulcers with duration of more than 1 month. It continues to be the only product with this approval.

Clinical Care Relevance: The existing living cell therapies offer self-modulating physiologic dosing of a full, normal range of cytokines and growth factors to induce the body to heal. The delivery methods for allogeneic living cell therapies explored thus far have included systemic injection, topical spray, and fabricated biomaterials.

Conclusion: In this chapter, the clinical development of cell-based therapy is discussed. The discussion ends with a glimpse of possible future developments in cellular therapy as a means to stimulate wound repair and regeneration.

BACKGROUND

In 2004, approximately 1.5 million tissue allografts were used for human transplantation in the United States[1] in the treatment of burns, skin loss, surgical wounds, and bullous diseases.[2] This was the culmination of many developments in tissue engineering and cell therapy over the last 30 years. Around 1980, three major advances were made. First, Rheinwald and Green were able to grow serial passage keratinocytes from a single-cell suspension of dissociated skin tissue, enabling human epidermal cells to be cultured into multiple epithelia suitable for grafting.[3] Second, Bell and colleagues produced a tissue-like structure *in vitro* by contraction of collagen lattices using human fibroblasts.[4,5] Third, Yannas *et al.* conceived a fully artificial bilayered skin made of a synthetic epidermis (semipermeable silicone layer) coupled to a collagen/glycosaminoglycan sponge acting as a template for dermal regeneration.[6] These three breakthroughs became

ADVANCES IN WOUND CARE, VOLUME 1

Printed in U.S.A.
DOI: 10.1089/awc.2009.0068

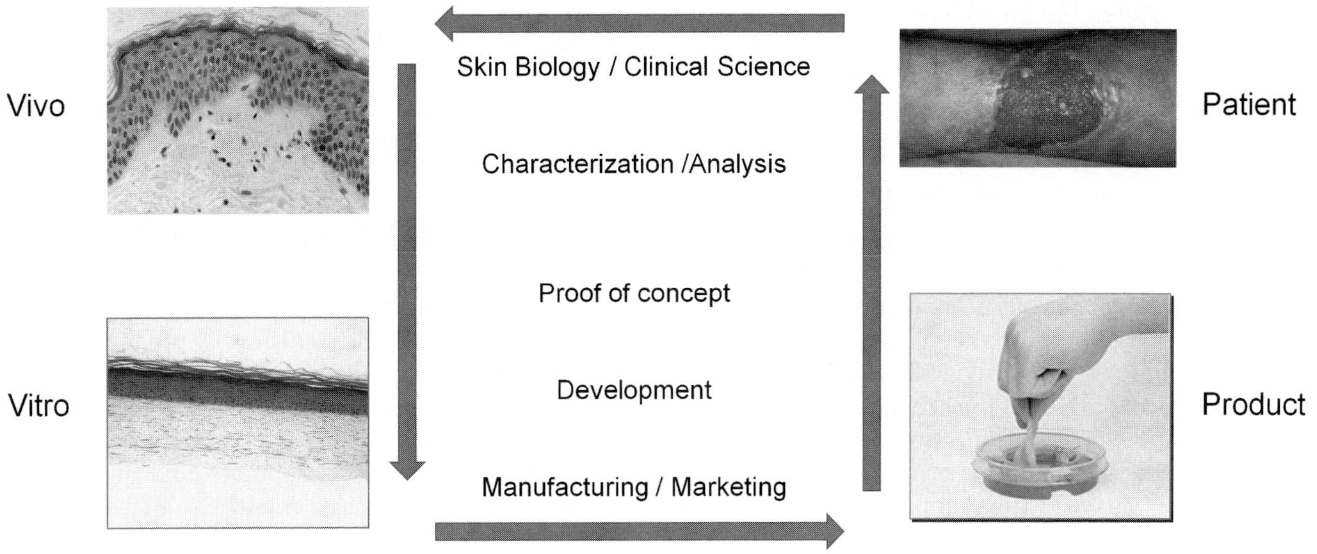

Figure 1. From cell biology to tissue engineering: a continuous cross-talk. The four pillars (*vivo, vitro,* product, and patient) must be linked during the development of a tissue engineering product. Understanding of skin development and wound healing, combined with scientific assessment of the nonhealing wound, would lead to the processing of a bioengineered tissue and its maturation into a product fulfilling the unmet clinical need. This continuous cross-talk allows safe and efficient treatment for wounds.

the opening chapter for the field of tissue engineering. More than a decade later, Langer and Vacanti[7] described tissue engineering as an interdisciplinary field that applies the principles of engineering and life science to the development of biological substitutes that restore, maintain, or improve function of the whole organ. Since that time, applied research has focused on the development of new therapeutic agents based on cellular, tissue, and growth factor therapy. From this, the novel concept of regenerative medicine has emerged. In the field of wound healing, this has led to three major approaches to product development: (1) cells, (2) biomaterials +/− cells, and (3) bioactive molecules.[8] There are still many challenges to overcome before concepts derived from scientific discoveries can be translated into viable products. All products created would ultimately have to be approved as treatments for specific conditions before they could be distributed for clinical use.

The successful large-scale production of engineered cellular products requires a source of materials and cells, and optimization of the processes needed to achieve adequate amplification of cell numbers sufficient to fabricate safe, effective, and low-cost products.[9] Additional challenges include the preservation of the product between manufacturing and application, and identification of the most effective ways to use the product[10] (Fig. 1).

CLINICAL PROBLEM ADDRESSED

Chronic ulceration of the skin is a common problem with huge impact on healthcare utilization. Of the 150 million people with diabetes worldwide, 15% suffer from foot ulceration. Many of these ulcers go on to become nonhealing chronic wounds.[11] In the United States, 82,000 limb amputations are performed on patients with diabetes mellitus each year. The majority of these amputations are in response to problems that originated from chronic ulcers in an elderly population.[12] Less than half of these amputees survive more than 5 years.[13] Venous ulcers are estimated to affect approximately 2.5 million people in the United States. Pressure ulcers afflict an additional 1.3 to 3 million people, including an estimated 10% to 18% of the patients in acute care and up to 28% of the patients in extended care facilities.[14] The American Burn Association reported that there were 500,000 burn injuries that received medical treatment in 2007.[15] Given the very high numbers of patients with skin injury, there is an obvious need for better treatment of these wounds and to ensure durable positive outcomes. In contrast, unsuccessful treatment of these wounds increases morbidity, patient suffering, physician frustration, and waste of healthcare resources.

RELEVANT BASIC SCIENCE CONTEXT

The repair of wounds is one of the most complex biological processes that occur during human life.[16] When an injury occurs, a set of complex biochemical and cellular events take place in an orderly manner to induce the cascade leading to repair. These events are divided into three major phases: inflammation, proliferation, and remodeling. If this process becomes chaotic or disrupted, the formation of scar tissue or the inability of the wound to heal itself properly (*i.e.*, to transition from an acute to a chronic wound) is increased. Yet this is not always so—fetal wound repair is essentially a regenerative process characterized by the absence of scarring and fibrosis.[17] Cell therapy using postnatal isolated fibroblasts may contain some unique features of "fetal wound repair" such as the production of transforming growth factor β_3 and high expression of glycosaminoglycan and hyaluronic acid. Better understanding of how the fetal process differs from the adult process could lead to better healing of wounds. It may be possible that the selection of fibroblast populations containing features of "fetal cells" would lead to a more perfect regeneration process.[18]

Skin breakdown may be caused by a variety of reasons including trauma, burns, arterial or venous insufficiency, diabetic neuropathy, or prolonged pressure. The pathologic processes are as varied as the causes, and the treatments utilized must be determined by the pathology. Acute wounds should show progress toward healing quickly, but some will become nonhealing, chronic wounds. These may exhibit multiple etiologic factors and cellular impairments such as inadequate angiogenesis, deficient cellular migration and proliferation, or abnormal cellular activation and differentiation. The term "chronic wound" might be more accurately phrased as "physiologically impaired wound."[19]

Some of the genes associated with inflammation, angiogenesis, response to reactive oxygen species, and regulation of extracellular matrix categories have been identified. These genes may evolve to be a valuable reference tool in the development of a better understanding of the biology of cutaneous wound healing[20] and to evaluate new treatments. The development of molecular biomarkers for wound care currently underway may complement this cellular approach by identifying an optimal time, cell type, and methodology to optimize patient response. The combined use of biomarkers and stem cells currently contained within living biomaterials may represent a more effective approach in the treatment of wounds.

EXPERIMENTAL MODEL OR MATERIAL

Multiple physiologic impairments are responsible for chronic wounds, and different loci within a chronic wound may have different physiologic factors in play. When cultured cells derived from patients with chronic wounds (venous ulcers) were tested to evaluate their response to growth factors such as granulocyte–macrophage colony-stimulating factor, the fibroblasts from the nonhealing edge were found to have almost no migration capacity, while fibroblasts originating away from the edge did. Similar studies performed with cultured fibroblasts from wounds in patients with diabetes[21] showed similar results. Cultured cells from chronic wounds have played a major role in providing a better understanding of the mechanisms of cellular wound physiology and in evaluating the effects of wound-healing stimulators *in vitro*.[19]

Three-dimensional human tissue models, referred to as "human skin equivalents," provide convenient, noninvasive experimental systems in which to study signaling pathways as well as disease processes (*e.g.*, cancer growth and wound reepithelialization).[22] The use of molecular biology tools[23] to elucidate the genetics of wound healing has opened the possibility of studying the molecular pathology of wounds.[24] This may ultimately allow a personalized approach to a patient or perhaps even their individual wounds.

Mouse models are widely used in wound-healing research because of supplier availability, easy handling, and cost. Yet this model is not optimal since many differences exist between typical mouse and human skin anatomy. Some specific animal models have been developed to overcome these limitations. The db/db mouse has been used to evaluate the synergy of age and diabetes to impair wound healing.[25] Nude mice have been used to study long-term remodeling and potency of bilayered human skin constructs.[26] Because pig skin is very similar to human skin in many ways, several models have been developed using pig skin to study wound healing,[27] hypertrophic scar formation,[28] and biomaterials.[29] The drawbacks of using pig models are expense and the special training, handling, and facilities needed for large versus small animals.

Mathematical modeling of wound healing is in the early stages of development. This approach may help to evaluate the effectiveness of specific treatments if our understanding allows enough relevant variables to be considered.[30]

DISCUSSION OF FINDINGS AND RELEVANT LITERATURE

The vast majority of chronic wounds are not treated with advanced therapies. The tendency to wait before using advanced skin substitutes is partly due to inconsistent expectations of the pace at which healing can and should occur. Advancement in care of chronic wounds will be dependent on better diagnostics to identify the reason for healing impairment, as well as the use of effective treatments to address the impairment.

The primary causes of impaired healing probably have to do with our inability to completely correct the specific pathophysiological abnormalities responsible using standard care. Gene array technologies may eventually provide a way to profile the molecular activity in a chronic wound. This may help to select the best treatment choice to overcome the specific cause for the inhibition of the wound-healing process.[31] If done quickly enough, a patient and treatment could be matched in real time, improving outcomes. Noninvasive techniques, such as optical coherence tomography, are in development to evaluate biomaterial remodeling during wound healing.[32] Modeling living products wounded *in vitro* may provide some understanding of their healing behavior when used *in vivo*.[33] These methods should provide insight into how the body responds to biomaterials and cell-based therapy, and expand our understanding of wound-healing mechanisms in general. They may also prove valuable in developing new therapies, combinations, or sequences to use in the clinic.

The mechanisms of action of bioengineered products have not been fully elucidated. They may act in several ways: (1) as an occlusive biologic dressing, promoting healing by secondary intention; (2) as a "smart material" that stimulates and reacts with the healing process; (3) as a "source" of growth factors that promote cell regulation, growth, and differentiation; (4) as a template capable of inducing revascularization; or (5) as a source of antibacterial peptides that suppress bioburden, allowing the natural healing process to continue normally. The currently available bioengineered products express and secrete numerous growth factors *in vitro*[34] and *in vivo*.[35] The production of these factors at a physiological level may explain their efficacy as compared to that seen following application of single growth factor therapy. Better understanding of these mechanisms could lead to the development of better practices for use of cell-based therapy, thus improving the clinical outcome.

The persistence of exogenous cells and the interaction of the construct with the wound needs to be evaluated further. Little is known about the

TAKE-HOME MESSAGE

Basic science advances

- Learning from wound repair to create regenerative medicine
- Explore differences between fetal versus adult wound-healing process
- Identify genes involved during cutaneous wound healing
- Characterize genes associated with inflammation, angiogenesis, reactive oxygen species, and extracellular matrix
- Clarify mechanisms and players in the molecular pathology of wounds
- Understand how cytokines and growth factors delivered by living cell therapies self-modulate
- Refine specific cellular markers and techniques to identify and select cell subpopulations
- Engineer living tissue constructs for predefined applications
- Discover the clinical applicability of stem-cell therapy to treat wounds
- Safely prolong the regenerative efficacy of allogeneic cells applied to a wound
- Evaluate the role of mesenchymal stem cells in wound healing
- Develop animal models to study wound healing

Clinical science advances

- Refining our understanding from "chronic wound" to "physiologically impaired wound"
- Develop assay using cultured cells from chronic wounds to study cellular wound physiology mechanisms
- Evaluate wound-healing stimulators using a chronic wound cell-based assay
- Clarify signaling pathways and disease processes using three-dimensional human tissue models
- Develop a personalized medicine approach to an individual patient or wound
- Mathematically model wound healing to evaluate the effectiveness of treatments
- Elucidate the mechanisms of action of currently available bioengineered products
- Evaluate the persistence of exogenous cells and the interaction between the construct and the wound

(continued)

Relevance to clinical care

- From anecdotal wound care to evidence-based medicine
- Identify molecular biomarkers for wound care to optimize patient response
- Assess delivery methods for allogeneic living cell therapies and new biomaterials
- Improve outcomes by optimizing combination therapies
- Apply currently available technologies within existing regulatory guidelines to find solutions to clinical problems
- Profile molecular activity in a chronic wound using gene array technologies to identify optimal treatment
- Develop noninvasive techniques to evaluate biomaterial remodeling during healing
- Focus on clinical benefit and ease of use to advance patient compliance
- Assess regulatory guidelines early on to facilitate the final approval of the product
- Develop product concepts and treatments that are safe, efficient, and economically viable for the industry and the society

mechanisms that would improve or degrade the persistence of allogeneic cellular products in the body. Due to its original neonatal sourcing, the allogeneic product Apligraf® does not trigger the acute rejection mediated by professional antigen-presenting cells. Allogeneic cells provided by bioengineered tissues persist for 4 to 28 weeks after grafting, depending on the wound type and method of detection. There is no evidence that chronic or delayed rejection occurs.[36] To date, more than 250,000 patients have been treated with Apligraf® with no immune activation responses reported.

The bilayered, multicellular construction of Apligraf® produces a synergy and self-regulating balance not seen in monocellular constructs. The keratinocyte stem cells present in each Apligraf® offer enhanced flexibility as compared to fully differentiated allogeneic cells. This self-modulating capability might prove to be of value in clinically unresponsive wounds. Stem cells alone or in combination with biomaterials have shown positive impact on wound healing when assessed using re-epithelialization, angiogenesis, and dermal regeneration.[37,38] Stem-cell research will need to evaluate the pros and cons of using them in humans. In addition, the regulatory environment will need to be clarified before investment can lead to commercial success. Research may be well served to focus on discovering the potential of stem-cell therapies where current treatments are lacking, such as in burns and pressure ulcers. It has been shown that autologous epidermal equivalent tissue engineered from follicular outer root sheath keratinocytes is as effective in healing recalcitrant vascular leg ulcers as split-thickness skin autografts.[39] This may be due to the presence of pluripotent epithelial stem cells residing in the outer root sheath. The use of autologous platelet concentrate combined with a skin substitute may have a positive effect on wound closure.[40]

New tissue engineering concepts such as fully human skin equivalents,[41] electrospun collagen,[42] microspheres,[43] and micronized acellular dermal matrix[44] are being developed for use in skin regeneration therapies.[45] The fully human skin equivalent made of *de novo* dermal matrix may provide suitable niches for stem cells, allowing for better soft-tissue regeneration. When electrospun collagen is used as a scaffold for engineered skin substitute, the product is of high quality and exhibits reduced contraction in an athymic mice model.

For bioengineered products to be commercially viable: (1) there must be exquisite, efficient quality control throughout the manufacturing process; (2) production scale manufacturing must be cost effective; (3) the container used in production should continue to be used as the final shipping package; and (4) automation must be implemented early in the process to improve safety, consistency, and scalability. Achieving consistency between batches is one of the most difficult challenges when working with variable biological materials. Bioequivalence assays are used to measure the functionality of the product and additional testing guarantees that all products approved for release meet stringent safety and purity requirements as required by the Food and Drug Administration and other regulatory bodies.

CAUTION, CRITICAL REMARKS, AND RECOMMENDATIONS

When advancing tissue engineering products from the bench to the clinic, three main pillars should be operating at the same time:

(1) Research. The sources of the biomaterials and/or cells needed should ensure safety, availability, and quantity. A solid scientific rationale for believing that a product will be beneficial, and extensive scientific capabilities to support the effort, must be in place before product development can begin. One of the first steps should include a proof

of concept evaluating the *in vivo* effect of the product. It is important to note that the models may need to differ based on indication, for, while successful in diabetic foot ulcers or venous ulcers, efficacy for cell therapy has been elusive in pressure ulcers.

(2) Process development and manufacturing techniques must take into account the fact that cell-based products are usually sophisticated and fragile. This makes them difficult to scale up, especially since the manufacturing process often includes manual procedures that are costly and sensitive to contamination. It is crucial to foresee these issues early in the development of a new product. Automation and closed culture systems may help reduce overall production costs, but they increase the start-up time and cost substantially. The use of animal-derived products (*e.g.*, bovine serum) and xenogenic cells in the cell banking process should be evaluated carefully from the risk/benefit perspective.

(3) Product development should be heavily guided to maximize the degree of clinical benefit and ease of use. The appropriate regulatory guidelines should be considered at every step to ensure the final approval of the product.

FUTURE DEVELOPMENTS

Autologous cell therapy is a life-saving technique for burns with high total burn surface area and has been helpful in repairing burn wounds because they take permanently. Despite their efficacy, these autologous therapies are tailor-made and thus very costly. Allogeneic cell therapy, however, can provide the molecules growth factors and coverage to induce self-regeneration. While more expensive to start up, this methodology can be expanded to treat a large population, thereby reducing the net cost to an individual. The differences between wound repair and wound regeneration are illustrated by the autologous and allogeneic approaches. Advances in allogeneic cell therapy, whether alone or housed within an engineered tissue, faces many technical challenges. Only two products are currently available "off the shelf" (Dermagraft®; and Apligraf®), and only one is multicellular (Apligraf®). Both use neonatal foreskin as a source of cells to expand into large cell banks. The use of specific proprietary cellular markers and techniques to identify and select cell subpopulations has enabled tailored tissue-engineered constructs with improved properties and clinical outcomes to be developed. The current indications of these cell therapies are limited to the treatment of diabetic foot ulcers (Dermagraft® and Apligraf®) and venous leg ulcers (Apligraf®). If allogeneic cells delivered to a pressure ulcer could survive longer without compromising safety, it might be possible to achieve similar regenerative efficacy. The use of "immune-privileged" cells, like stem cells, may eventually be shown to offer this increased efficacy while meeting safety and regulatory requirements. In the end, the key challenge will be to produce a safe and efficient product that is economically viable for the industry and the society that uses it.

AUTHOR DISCLOSURE STATEMENT

V.R. and T.W. are currently full-time employees of Organogenesis, Inc.

REFERENCES

1. Wang S, *et al.*: Infections and human tissue transplants: review of FDA MedWatch reports 2001–2004. Cell Tissue Bank 2007; **8:** 211.
2. Fimiani M, *et al.*: Other uses of homologous skin grafts and skin bank bioproducts. Clin Dermatol 2005; **23:** 396.
3. Rheinwald JG and Green H: Serial cultivation of strains of human epidermal keratinocytes: the formation of keratinizing colonies from single cells. Cell 1975; **6:** 331.
4. Bell E, Ivarsson B, and Merrill C: Production of a tissue-like structure by contraction of collagen lattices by human fibroblasts of different proliferative potential *in vitro*. Proc Natl Acad Sci USA 1979; **76:** 1274.
5. Parenteau NL, *et al.*: Epidermis generated *in vitro*: practical considerations and applications. J Cell Biochem 1991; **45:** 245.
6. Yannas IV, *et al.*: Wound tissue can utilize a polymeric template to synthesize a functional extension of skin. Science 1982; **215:** 174.
7. Langer R and Vacanti JP: Tissue engineering. Science 1993; **260:** 920.
8. Metcalfe AD and Ferguson MW: Tissue engineering of replacement skin: the crossroads of biomaterials, wound healing, embryonic development, stem cells and regeneration. J Royal Soc Interface 2007; **4:** 413.
9. Kemp P: History of regenerative medicine: looking backwards to move forwards. Regen Med 2006; **1:** 653.
10. Lysaght MJ, Jaklenec A, and Deweerd E: Great expectations: private sector activity in tissue engineering, regenerative medicine, and stem cell therapeutics. Tissue Eng Part A 2008; **14:** 305.
11. Boulton AJ, *et al.*: Diabetic neuropathies: a statement by the American Diabetes Association. Diabetes Care 2005; **28:** 956.
12. Brem H, Sheehan P, and Boulton AJ: Protocol for treatment of diabetic foot ulcers. Am J Surg 2004; **187:** 1S.
13. Reiber GE, Lipsky BA, and Gibbons GW: The burden of diabetic foot ulcers. Am J Surg 1998; **176 (Suppl 2A):** 5S.
14. Falanga V, *et al.*: Maintenance debridement in the treatment of difficult-to-heal chronic wounds.

Recommendations of an expert panel. Ostomy Wound Manag 2008; **Suppl:** 2–13 quiz 14–15.

15. American Burn Association 2005. Available at: www.ameriburn.org/resources_factsheet.php.
16. Gurtner GC, *et al.*: Wound repair and regeneration. Nature 2008; **453:** 314.
17. Ferguson MW, *et al.*: Scar formation: the spectral nature of fetal and adult wound repair. Plast Reconstr Surg 1996; **97:** 854.
18. Sorrell JM and Caplan AI: Fibroblast heterogeneity: more than skin deep. J Cell Sci 2004; **117(Pt 5):** 667.
19. Brem H, *et al.*: Primary cultured fibroblasts derived from patients with chronic wounds: a methodology to produce human cell lines and test putative growth factor therapy such as GMCSF. J Transl Med 2008; **6:** 75.
20. Roy S, *et al.*: Characterization of the acute temporal changes in excisional murine cutaneous wound inflammation by screening of the wound-edge transcriptome. Physiol Genomics 2008; **34:** 162.
21. Loot MA, *et al.*: Fibroblasts derived from chronic diabetic ulcers differ in their response to stimulation with EGF, IGF-I, bFGF and PDGF-AB compared to controls. Eur J Cell Biol 2002; **81:** 153.
22. Carlson MW, *et al.*: Three-dimensional tissue models of normal and diseased skin. Curr Protoc Cell Biol 2008; **3(Suppl 41):** 19.9.1–19.9.17.
23. Harty M, *et al.*: Regeneration or scarring: an immunologic perspective. Dev Dyn 2003; **226:** 268.
24. Stojadinovic O, *et al.*: Molecular pathogenesis of chronic wounds: the role of beta-catenin and c-myc in the inhibition of epithelialization and wound healing. Am J Pathol 2005; **167:** 59.
25. Brem H, *et al.*: The synergism of age and db/db genotype impairs wound healing. Exp Gerontol 2007; **42:** 523.
26. Guerret S, *et al.*: Long-term remodeling of a bilayered living human skin equivalent (Apligraf) grafted onto nude mice: immunolocalization of human cells and characterization of extracellular matrix. Wound Repair Regen 2003; **11:** 35.
27. Miller SJ, *et al.*: Re-epithelialization of porcine skin by the sweat apparatus. J Invest Dermatol 1998; **110:** 13.
28. Xie Y, *et al.*: The microvasculature in cutaneous wound healing in the female red Duroc pig is similar to that in human hypertrophic scars and different from that in the female Yorkshire pig. J Burn Care Res 2007; **28:** 500.
29. Navsaria HA, *et al.*: An animal model to study the significance of dermis for grafting cultured keratinocytes on full thickness wounds. Burns 1994; **20 Suppl 1:** S57.
30. Waugh HV and Sherratt JA: Modeling the effects of treating diabetic wounds with engineered skin substitutes. Wound Repair Regen 2007; **15:** 556.
31. Tomic-Canic M and Brem H: Gene array technology and pathogenesis of chronic wounds. Am J Surg 2004; **188 (1A Suppl):** 67.
32. Wang Z, *et al.*: Assessment of dermal wound repair after collagen implantation with optical coherence tomography. Tissue Eng Part C Methods 2008; **14:** 35.
33. Garlick JA: Engineering skin to study human disease—tissue models for cancer biology and wound repair. Adv Biochem Eng Biotechnol 2007; **103:** 207.
34. Milstone L, *et al.*: Growth factor expression, healing, and structural characteristics of Graftskin (Apligraf) Wounds 2000; **12(5 Suppl A):** 12A.
35. Brem H, *et al.*: Clinical efficacy and mechanism of bilayered living human skin equivalent (HSE) in treatment of diabetic foot ulcers. Surg Technol Int 2003; **11:** 23.
36. Mansbridge J: Commercial considerations in tissue engineering. J Anat 2006; **209:** 527.
37. Falanga V, *et al.*: Autologous bone marrow-derived cultured mesenchymal stem cells delivered in a fibrin spray accelerate healing in murine and human cutaneous wounds. Tissue Eng 2007; **13:** 1299.
38. Fioretti F, *et al.*: Human bone marrow-derived cells: an attractive source to populate dermal substitutes. Wound Repair Regen 2008; **16:** 87.
39. Tausche AK, *et al.*: An autologous epidermal equivalent tissue-engineered from follicular outer root sheath keratinocytes is as effective as split-thickness skin autograft in recalcitrant vascular leg ulcers. Wound Repair Regen 2003; **11:** 248.
40. Knox RL, *et al.*: Platelet-rich plasma combined with skin substitute for chronic wound healing: a case report. J Extra Corpor Technol 2006; **38:** 260.
41. El Ghalbzouri A, *et al.*: Replacement of animal-derived collagen matrix by human fibroblast-derived dermal matrix for human skin equivalent products. Biomaterials Epub 2008 Oct. 5; **30**(1): 71.
42. Powell HM, Supp DM, and Boyce ST: Influence of electrospun collagen on wound contraction of engineered skin substitutes. Biomaterials 2008; **29:** 834.
43. Chan BP, *et al.*: Self-assembled collagen-human mesenchymal stem cell microspheres for regenerative medicine. Biomaterials 2007; **28:** 4652.
44. Zhang X, *et al.*: Expansion and delivery of human fibroblasts on micronized acellular dermal matrix for skin regeneration. Biomaterials 2009; **30:** 2666.
45. MacNeil S: Biomaterials for tissue engineering of skin. Mater Today 2008; **26:** 11.

TISSUE ENGINEERING

Fibroblast Subsets for Skin Substitute Engineering

Hans-Oliver Rennekampff,[1,*] Weiguo Xu,[2] and H. Peter Rodemann[2]

[1]Department of Plastic, Hand, and Reconstructive Surgery, Medical School Hannover, Hannover, Germany.
[2]Division of Radiobiology and Environmental Molecular Biology, University of Tuebingen, Tuebingen, Germany.

Background: Enormous advances in the development of skin substitutes have occurred over the years. Acellular and fibroblast-seeded dermal substitutes have been shown to improve scarring and contraction in animal studies, the latter substitutes yielding the most favorable results. Mesenchymal-derived signals are essential for epithelial proliferation, skin morphogenesis, homeostasis, and differentiation.
The Problem: Fibroblasts at different culture conditions display different functional properties that may affect their suitability for dermal substitutes.
Basic/Clinical Science Advances: Previously we have shown that fibroblasts differentiate along a lineage from highly proliferative progenitor fibroblasts with characteristic spindle shape appearance to differentiated postmitotic polygonal fibrocytes. We demonstrated that the different subsets of fibroblasts exert significantly different patterns of cytokine release, for example, keratinocyte growth factor and transforming growth factor-β1. Coculture studies with keratinocytes revealed that postmitotic fibroblasts stimulated keratinocyte proliferation to a greater extent than progenitor fibroblasts.
Clinical Care Relevance: The design and engineering of suitable skin substitutes, for example, for the treatment of chronic wounds, will likely have to take the diversity of these fibroblasts into account.
Conclusion: Fibroblasts represent a diverse population of cells. Phenotypic differences are manifested in a variety of ways: extracellular matrix production as well as secretion of growth factors. These differences will have importance for tissue engineering of skin substitutes for *in vivo* use.

Abbreviations and Acronyms

HIF = hypoxia-inducible factor
IL = interleukin
KGF = keratinocyte growth factor
MF = progenitor fibroblast
MMP = metalloproteinase
PMF = postmitotic fibrocyte
TGF = transforming growth factor

*Correspondence: Department of Plastic, Hand, and Reconstructive Surgery, Medical School Hannover, Carl Neubergstrasse 1, 30625 Hannover, Germany (e-mail: rennekampff.oliver@mh-hannover.de).

BACKGROUND

Engineering of skin substitutes is considered to be an additional source for soft tissue coverage when autologous skin grafts are not available. The ultimate purpose for a skin substitute is to restore the normal anatomy and physiology of uninjured skin. Potentially, engineering of skin substitutes can allow for the fabrication of biological substitutes for various dermatopathologic conditions such as burns and cutaneous ulcers. The importance of dermal components and mesenchymal support for the engineering of skin substitutes is increasingly being recognized. In a variety of studies it has been demonstrated that the addition of an acellular dermal matrix can improve scar contraction when applied to full thickness wounds; however, complete restoration of a dermal architecture could never be demonstrated.

There is accumulating evidence that fibroblasts are dynamic cells occurring in functionally and morphologically heterogeneous subpopulations and that culture conditions alter fibroblast function.

Printed in U.S.A.
DOI: 10.1089/awc.2009.0132

CLINICAL PROBLEM ADDRESSED

The wound healing process involves changes in the resident dermal fibroblast population from that of quiescence to one of migration and proliferation, contraction of cells, and production of extracellular matrix. As a result of this process scar develops. None of the currently available acellular skin substitutes have been able to restore normal skin architecture and pliability. Only recently the importance of subpopulations of fibroblasts with respect to keratinocyte function and engineering of a skin substitute has been addressed.

RELEVANT BASIC SCIENCE

Recent work[1,2] has demonstrated that dermal fibroblasts from different body sites significantly differ in size and gene expression. Growth kinetics and transforming growth factor (TGF)-β1 receptor II expression as well as the ability to contract collagen lattices were found to differ with palmoplantar skin-derived fibroblasts having lower receptor levels and an increased mitotic rate. Sorrel and Caplan[3] have reviewed the differences between papillary fibroblasts that reside in the superficial dermis and reticular fibroblasts that reside in the deeper dermis, highlighting the difference in matrix molecule production in these two distinct cell populations. Versican is produced at low levels by papillary fibroblasts, whereas reticular fibroblasts produce high levels of this molecule. In contrast, decorin is produced in high levels by papillary fibroblast and in small amounts by reticular fibroblasts. Collagen types I and III production and the subsequent ratio of these two dermal collagens were not found to differ between these populations of fibroblasts.

Studies from the laboratory of the senior author also pointed toward the existence of different morphological subsets of fibroblasts within the same tissue.[4–6] Two major populations of fibroblasts have been detected in the dermis, termed mitotically active, replicative progenitor fibroblasts (MFs) and irreversible postmitotic fibrocytes (PMFs). These two subsets have been subsequently classified by cytomorphological and biochemical characteristics. According to their cytomorphology, replicative potential, and ability to synthesize specific cytokines and growth factors, such as TGF-β and keratinocyte growth factor (KGF), the MFs can be classified into the cell types MF I, MF II, and MF III.[6,7] Subcloning experiments have revealed that these cell types differentiate along the lineage MF I, MF II, and MF III, before differentiation into irreversible PMFs occurs.[8,9] The cell type MF I has the highest replicative capacity and can go through about 25–30 cell divisions before differentiating into MF II. This cell type can divide approximately 15–20 times before differentiating into the cell type MF III which has the potential for only five to eight cell division cycles before differentiating spontaneously into irreversible PMFs.[7] Based on its biochemical activity the latter cell type reflects the functional cell type of the fibroblast–fibrocyte cell system. Per cell it produces about five to eight times more total collagen when compared with MFs and provides the correct ratio of interstitial collagen types I, III, and V needed for homeostasis and maintenance of interstitial tissues.[7]

Fibroblasts are able to secrete interleukin (IL)-6, IL-8, hepatocyte growth factor, and KGF all of which are known to stimulate keratinocyte proliferation and migration. In work by Fusenig and coworker[10,11] it was demonstrated that growth-arrested x-irradiated fibroblasts and proliferating fibroblasts differ in their profiles of IL-1 alpha-stimulated cytokines and growth factor secretion. IL-1 alpha-stimulated postmitotic fibroblasts depicted lower transcriptional levels (mRNA) of KGF, IL-1 alpha, IL-8, whereas hepatocyte growth factor mRNA was dramatically increased.

As previously described, TGF-β, another important growth factor, is secreted by fibroblasts and counteracts the mitotic effect of KGF on keratinocytes. Among the three isoforms of TGF-β, TGF-β1 is the most prominent regulator. TGF-β1 was shown to downregulate epithelial growth and induce differentiation and apoptosis in keratinocytes.[12] Falanga *et al.*[13] have also reported differences in TGF-β1 mRNA and alpha 1(I) procollagen mRNA levels between clones of cultured fibroblasts. TGF-β plays an important role in the autocrine regulation of the differentiation process of MFs to functional fibrocytes through the induction of cell cycle inhibitor proteins such as p21 and p27 which mediate permanent cell cycle arrest in G_0.

At present, two major approaches have been used to generate dermal substitutes (reviewed by Boyce[14]). The first has been to fabricate a cell-free matrix for cellular ingrowth and restructuring *in vivo*. A second approach has utilized an *in vitro* cell-seeded biological matrix. There is evidence that fibroblasts play a major role in basement membrane formation either alone or in conjunction with overlying keratinocytes.[15,16] These studies have demonstrated that keratinocytes alone were either unable to or limited in the production of laminin 1, collagen IV, and laminin 5. In contrast, human fibroblasts, alone or in combination with overlying keratinocytes, showed significant production of laminin 1, collagen IV, and laminin 5. Subsequently, fibroblasts seeded into a collagen–glycosaminoglycan matrix were shown to promote basement membrane formation and epidermal homeostasis when compared with a nonseeded collagen–glycosaminoglycan. Most commercial products utilize allogeneic proliferative fibroblasts of early culture passages preferably from foreskins to construct seeded skin substitutes.

At present, none of the fibroblast-seeded substitutes has taken the different sources of fibroblasts or the phenotypic differences of fibroblasts into account. It is hypothesized that engineering of fibroblast-seeded dermal equivalents has to address these aspects to accomplish normal or even scarless healing.

EXPERIMENTAL MATERIALS

Human fibroblasts of various organs, for example, skin, lung, and kidney, have been described *in vivo* and *in vitro* to present a differentiation lineage of potentially dividing MFs and functional irreversible PMFs (Fig. 1A and B). The MFs are composed of three cell types MF I, MF II, and MF III characterized by a specific division potential (MF I: 25–30; MF II: 15–20; MF III: 5–10).[5,6] Especially, in human skin, but most likely in other organs as well, a constant ratio in the *in vivo* proportion of MFs and functional PMFs of 2:1 exists. MFs and PMFs present distinct differences in the expression of pH6-activity of β-galactosidase[17] which has also been reported to be a marker for "senescent" fibroblasts.[4,6,17]

We have also shown that nonstimulated subpopulations of dermal-derived fibroblasts constitutively secrete significantly different amounts of KGF. When compared with MFs the amount of KGFs produced per cell increases significantly in PMFs.

Hakenjos *et al.*[18] and von Pfeil *et al.*[19] from our laboratory have previously demonstrated that TGF-β1 is predominantly produced by MF III type cells and PMFs.

The senior author has shown evidence that collagen production is dependent on the subpopulation of fibroblasts, with postmitotic fibroblasts producing five to eight times more collagen types I, III, and V when compared with MFs.[7]

In further experiments in normoxic conditions on cultured composite skin substitutes composed of a collagen/elastin matrix seeded with various subsets of fibroblasts, we were able to demonstrate a distinct effect on basement membrane formation.

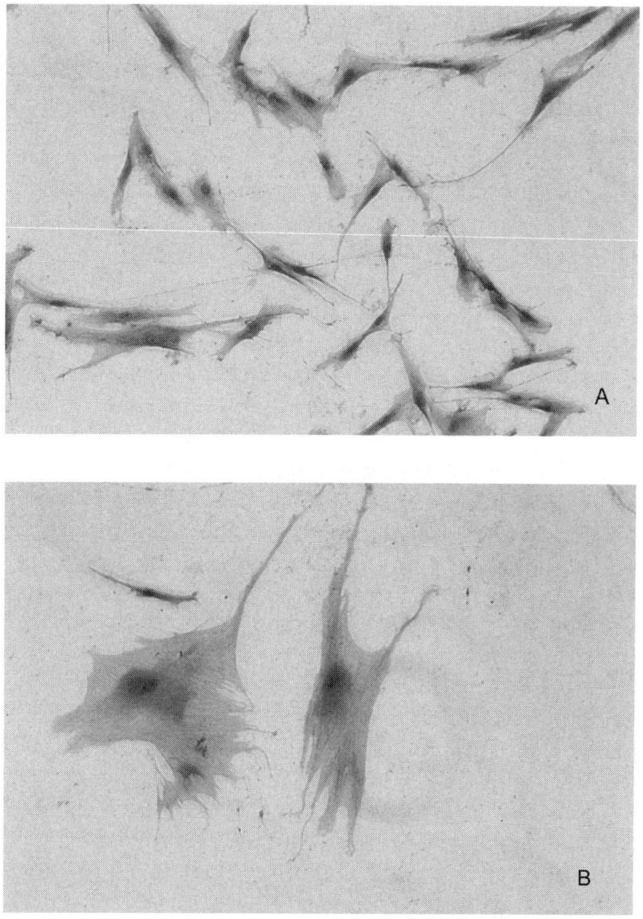

Figure 1. Cytomorphological characteristics of progenitor fibroblasts (MFs) and functional postmitotic fibrocytes (PMFs). **(A)** Mitotically active MFs of the cell type MF I display a typical spindle shape appearance; **(B)** functional PMFs appear as flattened polygonal cells.

Important in this study was the finding that postmitotic fibroblasts when cultured together with keratinocytes did not produce basement membrane proteins. In contrast, MFs in combination with keratinocytes were necessary for collagen IV and laminin 5 production.

DISCUSSION OF FINDINGS

An extensive body of literature exists on the clinical use of dermal replacements.[14,20] While a reduction in scar contracture was noticed,[21,22] true regeneration of the dermis was never achieved. While acellular dermal substitutes may be repopulated *in vivo* from day 3 onward, the addition of dermal-derived autologous fibroblasts is likely to modulate dermal tissue regeneration. Middelkoop and coworkers have shown extensive experimental evidence that an autologous fibroblast-seeded matrix improves scar contraction

TAKE-HOME MESSAGE

Basic science advances

- Dermal fibroblast phenotypes vary depending on body site
- Dermal fibroblast function varies depending on location in the dermis
- Dermal fibroblasts can be distinguished into progenitor and postmitotic fibroblasts
- Subtypes of dermal fibroblasts produce different amounts of growth factors and matrix molecules
- Fibroblast phenotype varies with time in culture and culture conditions
- Functionality of dermal fibroblasts depends on oxygenation

Clinical science advances

- Acellular matrix materials can be seeded with keratinocytes and fibroblasts
- Basement membrane formation is improved by coculture of fibroblasts with keratinocytes
- Functionality of composite grafts is improved by preseeding with fibroblasts
- Generation of fibroblast-seeded skin substitutes with particular properties may be possible using selected populations of fibroblasts

Relevance to clinical care

- Wound closure in large wounds when autologous skin grafts are not available can be facilitated with skin substitutes
- Handling characteristics are improved by matrix-derived skin substitutes over cell sheets
- Scarring is reduced with autologous fibroblast-seeded matrices
- Vulnerability may be reduced in fibroblast–keratinocyte composite skin substitutes

in a cell number-dependent fashion in porcine full-thickness wounds.[23,24] Fibroblast ingrowth from the surrounding tissue was reduced when an autologous fibroblast-seeded matrix was used in this type of acute full-thickness wound model. In these experiments proliferating dermal-derived fibroblasts were used, which do not represent the normal ratio of mitotically active and postmitotic fibroblasts in the dermis. Further *in vivo* experiments seem necessary to evaluate the function of different fibroblast subpopulations in seeded skin substitutes.

Tissue hypoxia with repetitive ischemia reperfusion injury is considered a reason for skin breakdown, skin ulceration, and chronic wound healing.[25] Hypoxia has a wide range of molecular effects on cells in the skin through hypoxia-inducible factor (HIF)1alpha-dependant as well as HIF1alpha-independent mechanisms.[26] Distler *et al.*[27] identified a significant expression of HIF1alpha in hypoxic fibroblasts. Although short-term exposure (<6 h) of fibroblasts to hypoxia has no effect on HIF1alpha stabilization,[26] prolonged hypoxia has a profound influence on extracellular matrix production. A hypoxia-induced increase of extracellular matrix proteins, for example, fibronectin and proalpha2 (I) collagen, was demonstrated on the RNA and protein levels. Interestingly, an accumulation of matrix proteins has been demonstrated in various skin ulcer types. Norman *et al.* investigated the effect of hypoxia on renal fibroblasts.[28] No difference in cell morphology was observed after 48 h of hypoxia; however, hypoxia increased the tissue inhibitor of metalloproteinase (MMP)-1 on the mRNA level as well as the protein level. Although hypoxia induces MMP1 expression,[29] no change in MMP2 expression was observed after hypoxia.[28] This may have an impact on matrix degradation and scar formation. In summary, these results indicated that it is crucial to control the levels of oxygen tension during engineering of fibroblast-seeded matrices.[30] In addition, the induction of major extracellular matrix proteins by hypoxia raises the question whether the initial hypoxia in non-perfused cell-seeded skin substitutes after transplantation *in vivo* may already determine subsequent scarring and fibrosis.

SUMMARY ILLUSTRATION

Illustration demonstrates the interaction between the two subsets of dermal-derived fibroblasts: mitotic fibroblasts and postmitotic fibroblasts on basement membrane protein expression.

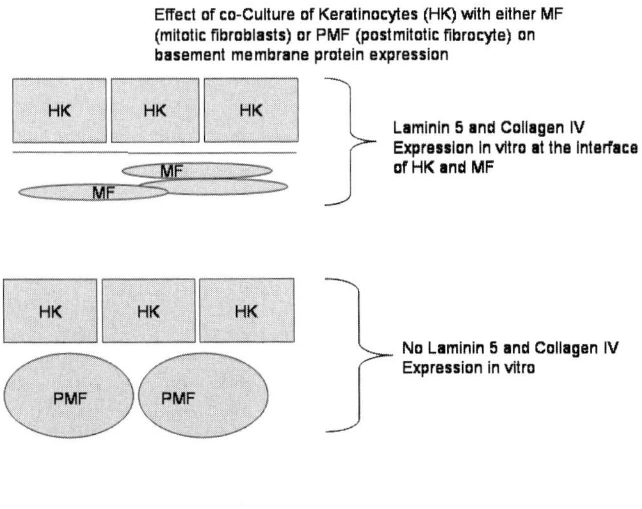

CAUTION, CRITICAL REMARKS, AND RECOMMENDATIONS

Fibroblasts represent a diverse population of cells depending on the anatomic origin and individual disease state. The fibroblast phenotype identified in ulcers from diabetic and venous insufficiency patients differs from normal nondiseased skin in these patients as well as healthy skin of volunteers. Phenotypic differences are manifested in a variety of ways: extracellular matrix production, degradation, and organization as well as secretion of growth factors. Similarly, culture conditions such as hypoxia *in vitro* and growth conditions *in vivo* alter fibroblast function. Therefore, for the development and application of dermal substitutes it may be necessary to be particularly selective about the choice of fibroblasts to be employed.

FUTURE DEVELOPMENT

The design and engineering of suitable skin substitutes for the treatment of different wound entities, for example, chronic wounds, burn wounds, and scar revision, may have to take the diversity of fibroblasts into account. Further experiments are necessary to examine the effect of subtypes of fibroblasts from different body origin on dermal regeneration *in vivo*.

ACKNOWLEDGMENT

This study was funded in part by the German Ministry of Research and Technology.

AUTHOR DICLOSURE STATEMENT

H.O.R. has presented for and received speaker honorarium from Dr. Suwelack Skin and Health Care, the producer of Matriderm Collagen/Elastin matrix. W.X. and H.P.R. declare that no competing financial interests exist. The products mentioned in this article are not all-inclusive, exclusive, or an endorsement.

REFERENCES

1. Chipev CC and Simon M: Phenotypic differences between dermal fibroblasts from different body sites determine their responses to tension and TGFβ1. BMC Dermatol 2002; **2:** 13.
2. Rinn JL, Bondre C, Gladstone HB, Brown PO, and Chang HY: Anatomic demarcation by positional variation in fibroblast gene expression programs. PloS Genet 2006; **2:** 1084.
3. Sorrell JM and Caplan AI: Fibroblast heterogeneity: more than skin deep. J Cell Sci 2004; **117:** 667.
4. Bayreuther K, Rodemann HP, Francz PI, and Maier K: Differentiation of fibroblast stem cells. J Cell Sci Suppl 1988; **10:** 115.
5. Rodemann HP: Differential degradation of intracellular proteins in human skin fibroblasts of mitotic and mitomycin C(MMC)-induced postmitotic differentiation states. Differentiation 1989; **42:** 37.
6. Herskind C, Bentzen SM, Overgaard J, Bamberg M, and Rodemann HP: Differentiation state of skin fibroblast cultures versus risk of subcutaneous fibrosis after radiotherapy. Radiother Oncol 1998; **47:** 263.
7. Rodemann HP, Bayreuther K, Francz PI, Dittmann K, and Albiez M: Selective enrichment and biochemical characterisation of seven fibroblast cell types of human skin fibroblast populations *in vitro*. Exp Cell Res 1989; **180:** 84.
8. Bayreuther K, Rodemann HP, Hommel R, Dittmann K, Albiez M, and Francz PI: Human skin fibroblasts *in vitro* differentiate along a terminal cell lineage. Proc Natl Acad Sci USA 1998; **85:** 5112.
9. Rodemann HP, Binder A, Burger A, Löffler H, and Bamberg M: The underlying cellular mechanisms of fibrosis. Kidney Int 1996; **49:** 32.
10. Fusenig NE: Epithelia-mesenchymal interactions regulate keratinocyte growth and differentiation *in vitro*. In: *The Keratinocyte Handbook*, edited by Leigh I, Lane B, and Watt F. Cambridge, MA: Cambridge University Press, 1994, pp. 71–94.
11. Maas-Szabowski N and Fusenig NE: Interleukin-1-induced growth factor expression in postmitotic and resting fibroblasts. J Invest Dermatol 1996; **107:** 849.
12. Mansbridge JN and Hanawalt PC: Role of transforming growth factor beta in the maturation of human epidermal keratinocytes. J Invest Dermatol 1988; **90:** 336.
13. Falanga V, Zhou LH, Takagi H, Murata H, Ochoa S, Martin TA, and Helfman T: Human dermal fibroblast clones derived from single cells are heterogeneous in the production of mRNAs for alpha 1(I) procollagen and transforming growth factor-beta 1. J Invest Dermatol 1995; **105:** 27.
14. Boyce ST: Design principles for the composition and performance of cultured skin substitutes. Burns 2001; **27:** 523.
15. Cooper ML, Andree C, Hansbrough JF, Zapata-Sirvent RL, and Spielvogel RI: Direct comparison of a cultured composite skin substitute containing human keratinocytes and fibroblasts to an epidermal sheet graft containing human keratinocytes on athymic mice. J Invest Dermatol 1993; **101:** 811.
16. Sahuc F, Nakazawa K, Berthod F, Collombel C, and Damour O: Mesenchymal–epithelial interactions regulate gene expression of type VII collagen and kalinin in keratinocytes and dermal–epidermal junction formation in a skin equivalent model. Wound Rep Regen 1996; **4:** 93.
17. Rodemann HP: Differential gene expression, protein synthesis, and degradation in ageing fibroblasts. In: *Cell Culture Models for Dermatological Research*, edited by Bernd A, Bereiter-Hahn J, Hevert F, and Holzmann H. Berlin-Heidelberg, New York: Springer, 1993, pp. 272–277.
18. Hakenjos L, Bamberg M, and Rodemann HP: TGF-β1-mediated alterations of rat lung fibroblast differentiation resulting in the radiation-induced fibrotic response. Int J Radiat Biol 2000; **76:** 503.
19. von Pfeil A, Hakenjos L, Herskind C, Dittmann K, Weller M, and Rodemann HP: Irradiated homozygous TGF-1 knockout fibroblasts show enhanced clonogenic survival as compared with TGF-1 wild-type fibroblasts. Int J Radiat Biol 2002; **78:** 331.
20. Kearney JN: Clinical evaluation of skin substitutes. Burns 2001; **27:** 545.
21. Sheridan RL, Choucair R, Donelan M, Lydon M, Petras L, and Tompkins R: Acellular allodermis in burn surgery: 1 year results of a pilot trial. J Burn Care Rehabil 1998; **19:** 528.
22. Van Zuijlen PPM, Vloemans JFPM, van Trier AJM, Suijker MH, van Unen E, Groenevelt F,

Kreis RW, and Middelkoop E: Dermal substitution in acute burns and reconstructive surgery: a subjective and objective long-term follow-up. Plast Reconstr Surg 2001; **108:** 1938.

23. Lamme EN, van Leeuwen RTJ, Jonker A, van Marle J, and Middelkoop E: Living skin substitutes: Survival and function of fibroblasts seeded in a dermal substitute in experimental wounds. J Invest Dermatol 1998; **111:** 989.

24. Lamme EN, van Leeuwen RTJ, Brandsma K, van Marle J, and Middelkoop E: Higher number of autologous fibroblasts in an artificial dermal substitute improve tissue regeneration and modulate scar-tissue formation. J Pathol 2000; **190:** 595.

25. Mustoe RA, O'Shaughnessy K, and Kloeters O: Chronic wound pathogenesis and current treatment strategies: a unifying hypothesis. Plast Reconstr Surg 2006; **117:** 35S.

26. Distler JH, Wenger RH, Gassmann M, Kurowska M, Hirth A, Gay S, and Distler O: Physiologic responses to hypoxia and implications for hypoxia-inducible factors in the pathogenesis of rheumatoid arthritis. Arthritis Rheum 2004; **50:** 10.

27. Distler JHW, Jüngel A, Pileckyte M, Zwerina J, Michel BA, Gay RE, Kowal-Bielecka O, Matucci-Cerinic M, Schett G, Marti HH, Gay S, and Distler O: Hypoxia induced increase in the production of extracellular matrix proteins in systemic sclerosis. Arthritis Rheum 2007; **56:** 4203.

28. Norman JT, Clark IM, and Garcia PL: Hypoxia promotes fibrogenesis in human renal fibroblasts. Kidney Int 2000; **58:** 2351.

29. Kan C, Abe M, Yamanaka M, and Ishikawa O: Hypoxia-induced increase of matrix metalloproteinase-1 synthesis is not restored by reoxygenation in a three-dimensional culture of human dermal fibroblasts. Dermatol Sci 2003; **32:** 75.

30. Tokuda Y, Crane S, Yamaguchi Y, Zhou L, and Falanga V: The levels and kinetics of oxygen tension detectable at the surface of human fibroblast cultures. J Cell Physiol 2000; **182:** 414.

TISSUE ENGINEERING

WHS
Wound
Healing
Society

Human Skin–Equivalent Platforms for the Preclinical Development and Testing of New Wound Healing Agents

Christophe Egles and Jonathan A. Garlick*

Division of Cancer Biology and Tissue Engineering, Department of Oral and Maxillofacial Pathology, Tufts University School of Dental Medicine, Boston, Massachusetts.

Background: The discovery, development, and rapid translation of new wound therapies remains dependent on the screening and testing of novel candidate compounds and wound dressings in model systems that can predict how these agents will stimulate wound repair *in vivo*.
The Problem: Potential wound healing agents are currently evaluated and developed in two-dimensional monolayer cultures and cell-based assays that do not mimic the complexity of human skin and are not predictive of *in vivo* tissue responses.
Basic/Clinical Science Advances: The development and application of tissue-engineered models that mimic the form and function of human skin, known as human skin equivalents (HSEs), provide *in vivo*–like tissues to study the biology of skin and other stratified squamous epithelia. We have adapted HSEs to study wound reepithelialization by establishing that these tissues re-establish epithelial integrity in a manner that simulates the temporal and spatial chronology of events that occur during restoration of epithelial integrity after wounding of human skin.
Clinical Care Relevance: Wounded HSEs now provide a translational platform to yield more meaningful correlations between *in vitro* and *in vivo* tissue wound responses and can now accelerate development and translation wound repair products and therapeutics for wound care.
Conclusion: We have customized wounded HSE platforms to serve as tools to screen the mechanism of action, efficacy, and safety of many types of potential wound therapeutics, including cellular therapy, topical agents that enhance wound reepithelialization, and bioengineered dressings that deliver bioactive compounds. Thus, HSEs can be modified to study the biology of specific wound environments and to screen agents tailored to them.

Abbreviations and Acronyms

2D = two-dimensional
3D = three-dimensional
ECM = extracellular matrix
HDF = human dermal fibroblasts
HSEs = human skin equivalents

*Correspondence: Division of Cancer Biology and Tissue Engineering, Department of Oral and Maxillofacial Pathology, Tufts University School of Dental Medicine, 55 Kneeland St., South Cove Building, Room 116, Boston, Massachusetts 02111 (e-mail: jonathan.garlick@tufts.edu).

BACKGROUND

A SIGNIFICANT PROBLEM facing the discovery and development of next-generation wound therapies is that candidate agents are primarily tested and screened in two-dimensional (2D) monolayer cultures and cell-based assays that do not manifest the architectural features of human skin or other stratified epithelial tissues. While these studies in 2D cultures have allowed elucidation of key cellular and molecular factors involved in cell migration and proliferation in monolayer scratch wounds,[1–5] these relatively simple culture systems lack the complexity of the wound healing microenvironment. As a result, 2D culture systems do not mimic *in vivo* wound responses and are limited in their ability to predict how potential therapeutics can enable wound repair in an *in vivo* context. It is therefore essential to move

Printed in U.S.A.
DOI: 10.1089/awc.2009.0032

wound healing science into more predictive, experimental paradigms that provide skin-like tissues with three-dimensional (3D) tissue architecture that will best advance the discovery and testing of agents targeted to improve clinical wound care. In recent years, our laboratory has adapted 3D human skin equivalents (HSEs) to serve as surrogate tissues that provide a translational platform to establish more meaningful correlations between *in vitro* and *in vivo* wound healing responses. These tools are now playing a pioneering role by enabling the evaluation of novel wound care agents in 3D *in vitro* tissue platforms that provide a focus on clinical relevance. We present an overview of how we have adapted HSEs to study or test three types of potential wound therapeutics: (1) cellular therapy by manipulating dermal fibroblast subpopulations to optimize stromal–epithelial crosstalk needed to stimulate wound reepithelialization; (2) screening efficacy of novel agents on wound reepithelialization by testing their capacity to accelerate wound reepithelialization; and (3) testing the potential of bioengineered wound dressings that incorporate bioactive agents.

CLINICAL PROBLEM ADDRESSED

As bi-directional interactions between basic and clinical wound healing scientists play an ever-increasing role in the development of new wound care strategies, the stage is set for the use of powerful new tools that can further unravel the complex regulation of wound repair processes while providing 3D tissue platforms that can predict therapeutic efficacy. To accomplish this, HSE models of wound reepithelialization now serve as surrogate tissues that enable the efficient translation of discoveries to a patent-care setting. In this light, adapting HSEs to monitor *in vivo*–like wound responses can now accelerate development and translation wound repair products and therapeutics. These 3D *in vitro* tissue technologies now more efficiently can link basic discovery in wound healing science to eventual clinical application.

BASIC SCIENCE CONTEXT

The development and application of tissue-engineered models that mimic human skin, known as HSEs, provide *in vivo*–like tissues to study epidermal biology.[6,7] These tissues are constructed by growing skin-derived keratinocytes on the surface of a type I collagen gel that is populated with dermal fibroblasts. After several days during which tissue constructs are submerged in medium, HSEs are grown at an air–liquid interface to enable tissues to fully recapitulate their *in vivo*–like morphology and patterns of gene expression that are seen in human skin *in vivo*. HSEs provide a flexible platform for the engineering of human skin and other stratified epithelial tissues due to the ability to modify their constituent cells,[8,9] extracellular matrix (ECM) proteins,[10] basement membrane,[6] and growth factors[11] incorporated into them. We have adapted HSEs to study wound reepithelialization by determining that these tissues restore epithelial integrity in a manner that simulates the temporal and spatial chronology of events that occur during reepithelialization in human skin and the oral mucosa.[8,12] Until this point, *in vitro* studies and assays of reepithelialization have been limited by their inability to simulate wound repair as it occurs in humans, as the 2D monolayer cultures widely used demonstrate limited stratification, partial differentiation, and hyperproliferative growth. Since HSEs fully mimic the complex nature of skin and other stratified epithelial tissues, we have modified them to develop a wound healing model that has been shown to mimic events linked to early wound repair, including keratinocyte proliferation,[9] migration,[11] differentiation, growth-factor response,[8,9] and protease expression[8] after an incisional wound. This wound repair model demonstrates the utility of HSEs to study phenotypic responses that are characteristic of the switch from a normal to a regenerative epithelium.[13]

EXPERIMENTAL MODEL

HSEs are constructed using skin keratinocytes and fibroblasts that are first grown in 2D, monolayer cultures in a way that optimizes their proliferative potential.[7,8] For all experiments, keratinocytes and fibroblasts are derived from the same donor to avoid any unwanted variations in keratinocyte response[14] to wounding. After 3D tissue fabrication, basal keratinocytes in HSEs demonstrate a basal rate of proliferation that is similar to skin as well as a well-differentiated, stratified epithelium.[12] HSEs are wounded with a scalpel to create an incisional wound or with a dermatological punch to create an excisional wound (Fig. 1). Wound reepithelialization then ensues in a very similar manner to that seen in full-thickness incisional wounds *in vivo* in the following discrete, temporal stages[15]: (a) Reepithelialization is initiated after a short delay (8 h) as an epithelial tongue of keratinocytes begins to migrate onto the wound bed. (b) This is followed by a transient, proliferative burst in keratinocytes at

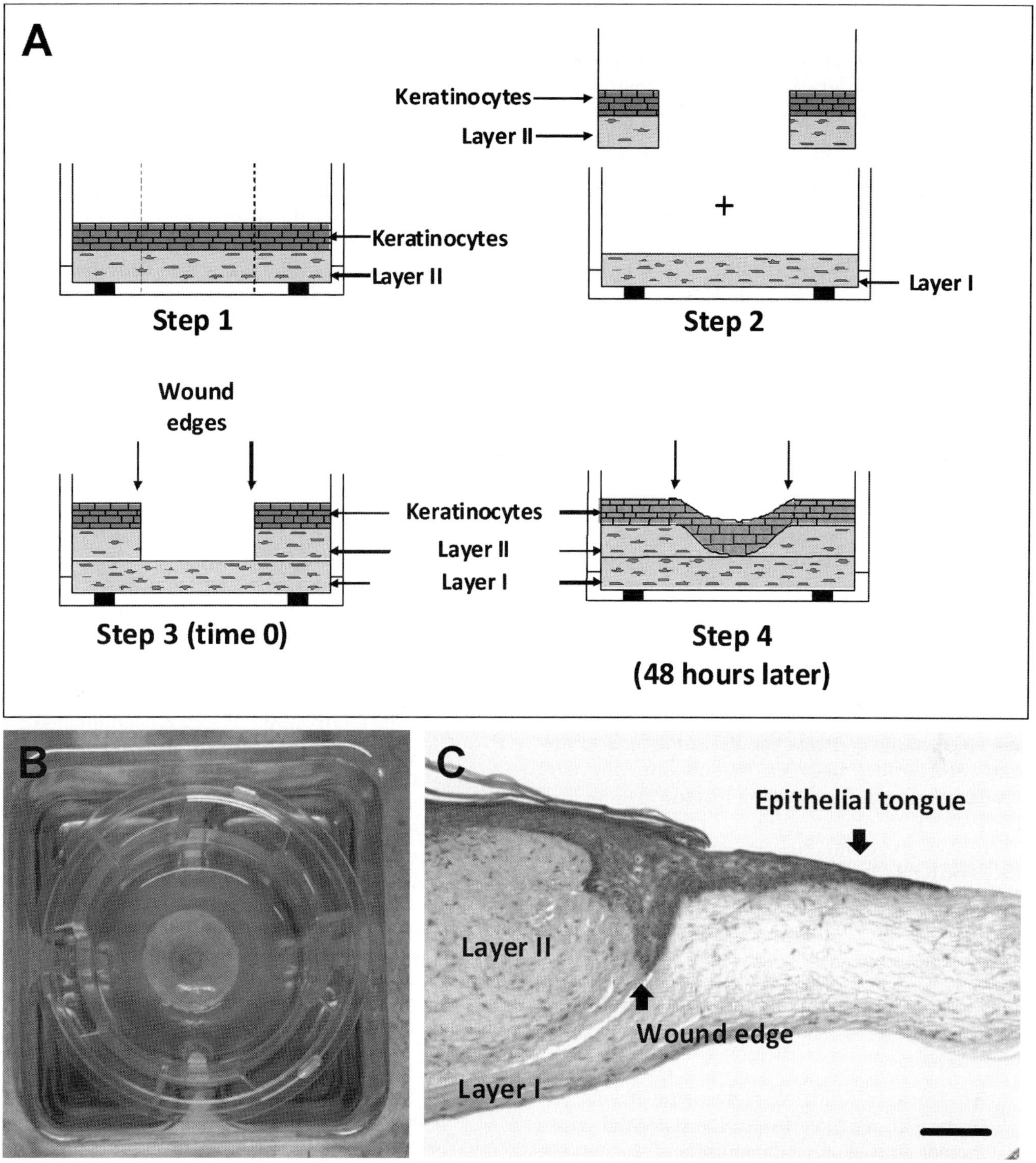

Figure 1. Construction of the wound healing model. (**A**) Schematic of stratified keratinocyte sheet growing on contracted collagen matrix containing fibroblasts (layer II). This human skin equivalent (HSE) rests on a semipermeable membrane and is nourished with medium from below and is exposed to an air–liquid interface. Step 1, a wound is formed by punching a hole into the epithelium and collagen matrix. Step 2, the wounded culture is transferred onto a second collagen matrix that has previously undergone contraction (layer I). Step 3, the resultant composite tissue consists of two layers of contracted matrix and one layer of epithelium. Wound edges are seen at the transition zone from layer I to layer II and are noted with arrows. Step 4, reepithelialization occurs as wounded keratinocytes migrate onto the collagenous wound bed in layer II and is then followed by stratification to reconstitute a fully stratified epithelium that covers the wound bed. (**B**) A characteristic wounded HSE at step 3 in the reepithelialization process. A 0.4 cm punch has been used to create a wound in the tissue that has penetrated the epithelium and the underlying collagen matrix. (**C**) Hematoxylin and eosin staining of wounded HSE showing the epithelial tongue migrating across the wound bed as it begins to close the wound. Scale bar = 100 μm.

the wound margin that occurs 24 h after wounding. (c) Production of the matrix-degrading protease, matrix metalloproteinase 1 (MMP-1), is expressed in keratinocytes migrating onto the wound bed resulting in the remodeling of ECM proteins at this interface. (d) Wound reepithelialization is complete as epithelial integrity is restored after 48–72 h. (e) Basement membrane proteins are deposited to organize and reestablish the basement membrane interface. (f) Stratification of the restored tissue then occurs to regenerate a fully differentiated, stratified squamous epithelium. Healing epithelial tissues are amenable to manipulation of medium composition,[16] modification of the ECM substrate interface on which keratinocytes are grown,[6,10] and alteration of its cellular constituents[9] to create microenvironments that mimic a variety of wound conditions in stratified epithelial tissues. For example, epithelial tissues can be constructed in the presence or absence of basement membrane proteins[10] or in the presence of various stromal cells that are incorporated into the contracted collagen gel. During tissue construction, tissues are maintained in a medium that contains low levels of serum (2%) and antibiotics. However, tissues are usually grown in the absence of serum or antibiotics during wound reepithelialization if a test compound is used, medium are changed every 2 days, and wound controls use the same medium to avoid interference between the medium ingredients and the agent or dressing tested.

DISCUSSION OF FINDINGS AND RELEVANT LITERATURE

In light of the flexibility of HSEs to create wound microenvironments that enable the development and/or testing of novel wound therapies, we present three examples in which we have used them to study and screen novel approaches to enable wound repair:

1. To assess cellular therapy using dermal fibroblasts, we have tested the potential of selected fibroblast subpopulations to enable cross-talk with the overlying epithelial cells that can stimulate wound reepithelialization.[9] In addition, this allowed us to further understand the role of epithelial–mesenchymal interactions in modulating skin repair by studying how the phenotype of human dermal fibroblasts (HDF) was linked to the healing response of wounded HSEs. We compared fibroblasts extensively cultivated in 2D monolayer culture under three distinct conditions, on denatured collagen matrix, native collagen, and tissue culture plastic before incorporation into HSEs. Our results demonstrated that extended passage of HDF on denatured collagen was able to accelerate the rate of wound healing by 38%. This increased rate of wound closure was linked to the stimulation of keratinocyte proliferation seen when HDF expanded on denatured collagen were incorporated into the collagen gels on which wound reepithelialization occurred. Therefore, modification of cells that can mediate and direct interactions with their ECM or epithelial microenvironment holds potential for novel cell therapy applications and for understanding mechanisms through which cross-talk between fibroblasts and keratinocytes may stimulate wound repair to reestablish tissue homeostasis. Use of such modified fibroblasts, which can be selected based on their interactions with specified ECM components, may provide useful therapies to identify and select cell subpopulations that may best treat patients at elevated risk for the healing of chronic wounds.
2. To screen the efficacy of potential wound healing agents that may accelerate wound reepithelialization. We have established the utility of the 3D wound HSE model to test the capacity of novel agents designed to improve tissue repair by using these tissue platforms to measure the degree of reepithelialization when wounds are exposed to a soluble test agent. To accomplish this, multiple concentrations of the agent to be tested can be added directly to the culture media or provided topically to the surface of the tissue, and the degree of reepithelialization is compared to nontreated wounds. Reepithelialization can be directly measured and the tissue phenotype monitored using immunohistochemical stains for cell proliferation (incorporation of BrdU), differentiation (keratins 1 and 10, involucrin), ECM production (laminin 5), and reestablishment of basement membrane (types IV and VII collagen). In this way, it is possible to screen large numbers of agents by testing their efficacy at various doses, thus paving the way for clinical testing of these new wound treatments.
3. Testing the release and efficacy of a bioactive wound repair agent incorporated into wound dressings. We have used wounded HSEs as a platform to test novel nanotechnology-

inspired biomaterials that can act as a bioactive wound dressing, to topically deliver compounds that may promote wound healing. As an example of this approach, we have tested two types of materials: a hydrogel made of self-assembling peptide nanofiber that can physically be placed into the wound bed[17] and silk mats made of electrospun nanoscale silk fibers that can cover over the wound bed.[18] In both cases, a potential wound stimulant (epidermal growth factor) was incorporated into these biomaterial dressings and determined that these dressings could augment wound reepithelialization by reducing the time of wound closure.[17,18] These results proved that the wound HSE platform facilitated the testing of functional biomaterial devices on human tissues to enable the development of biomaterials with properties that can be optimized for the new generation of biologically active wound dressings. In addition, this platform has the flexibility to allow the simultaneous testing of synergistic growth factors by screening the efficacy of biomaterial-mediated delivery of multiple topically acting growth factors. Other applications of this platform have been to utilize multifunctionalized biomaterials that incorporate antimicrobial molecules to deliver antibacterial factors that can provide wound protection that may stimulate wound closure.

The HSE wound model is well adapted to the use of cellular and molecular analyses for the study of signaling pathways involved in wound closure. If needed, such studies can be expanded to include ECM remodeling and revascularization by grafting HSEs to the dorsum of nude mice by our lab[19,20] or SCID mice.[21] The generation of such mouse/human chimera[21] will allow longer-term studies and can provide stromal elements, such as blood vessels, that are absent in HSEs and provide a more *in vivo*–like wound environment.

TAKE-HOME MESSAGE

Basic science advances

- HSEs are bioengineered 3D human *in vitro* tissue models constructed by growing keratinocytes on the surface of a contracted collagen gel containing HDF.
- HSEs generate a well-stratified, fully differentiated epithelium that demonstrates a basal level of keratinocyte proliferation by growing these tissues at an air–liquid interface.
- HSEs can be wounded to serve as an *in vitro* tissue model that recapitulates the temporal and spatial events that occur during wound repair of human skin and other epithelial tissues.
- Wounded HSEs closely mimic the proliferation, migration, differentiation, growth-factor response, and protease expression seen after an incisional wound *in vivo* that is characteristic of the switch from a normal to a regenerative epithelium.
- HSEs currently lack blood vessels and immune cells and need to be supplemented by *in vivo* animal studies to provide a more complete analysis of wound reepithelialization.
- The wounded HSE model enables basic science discovery into the complex interplay between multiple cell and tissue types present in the wound microenvironment in a biologically meaningful 3D tissue context.

Clinical science advances

- Wounded HSEs provide a platform for the rapid testing of lead candidate drugs and compounds that can accelerate the design and screening of drugs and compounds targeted for specific therapeutic wound care applications.
- Wounded HSEs now serve as powerful new tools that can further unravel the complex regulation of wound repair processes and provide 3D tissue platforms that can predict therapeutic efficacy in the development of new wound care strategies.
- We have illustrated the capacity of using HSEs to evaluate three types of potential wound therapeutics—cellular therapy, topically delivered wound care agents, and bioinspired wound dressings delivering bioactive agents.

Relevance to clinical care

- HSEs can monitor *in vivo*–like wound responses and have been adapted to direct the translation of new wound repair products and therapeutics to clinical application.
- Wounded HSEs are clinically relevant tissues because they provide readouts and tissue outcomes that are more predictive of *in vivo* responses than more conventional 2D monolayer cultures.
- HSE wound models can now be scaled to high-throughput formats that will enable the rapid screening of the safety and efficacy of potential wound repair agents on human skin.
- In the future, wounded HSEs can be modified to study the biology of specific wound environments, such as the chronic wounds, by screening the response to agents that are tailored to them. Further, other cell types, such as blood vessels and immune cells, should be added to the model to increase tissue complexity and to provide a closer approximation to *in vivo* models.
- Adding such complexity to existing wounded HSE platforms will create new synergies among wound care communities that will economize and streamline the pharmaceutical design and screening of new wound repair agents that will impact on patient care.

CAUTION, CRITICAL REMARKS, AND RECOMMENDATIONS

While the HSE wound model described represents an important upgrade over simple 2D monolayer culture systems, these tissues currently exist in prototypical, low-throughput formats that limit an even greater applicability as platforms for the preclinical development of new wound healing agents. The following modifications of existing HSE platforms would greatly facilitate their use throughout the wound healing community. (1) High-throughput platforms need to be developed for wounded HSEs that will further refine their utility as a screening tool by enabling the simultaneous testing of a wider number of potential wound care products and therapies. (2) Incorporation of additional cell types, such as endothelial cells or inflammatory cells, to HSEs would generate an more *in vivo*–like tissue microenvironment. For example, the use of microfluidic networks capable of providing physiological fluid flow properties is currently under development for this purpose.[22] (3) Integration of real-time imaging tools into 3D tissue platforms will allow dynamic monitoring of the sequential stages of wound healing responses. The design and development of interoperable, advanced HSE tissue platforms will impact directly on the science of wound healing and will create new synergies throughout the wound healing community that will economize and streamline the pharmaceutical design, screening, and therapeutic application of lead candidate compounds and devices targeted to the treatment of human wounds.

FUTURE DEVELOPMENTS

In their current format, the wound HSEs described are well adapted to mimic the response of normal skin after an excisional wound. However, these HSEs can be modified to study the biology of specific wound environments and to screen agents tailored to them. A future goal is to generate wound HSEs that can simulate the chronic wound environment. This could be accomplished by modifying ECM components on which cells undergo reepithelialization or by directly manipulating keratinocyte gene expression or function to impede repair. Further, incorporation of fibroblasts or keratinocytes from aged individuals would open new doors to the direct study of the relationship between wound healing and aging. This will also lead toward testing the feasibility of using patient-specific cells to develop personalized, 3D tissues that will begin to establish their utility to screen host-specific wound responses. Such patient-specific 3D tissue platforms will allow future screening and product development that will better predict responses to individualized, targeted therapies.

ACKNOWLEDGMENTS

This study was supported by the Center for Integrated Tissue Engineering at School of Dental Medicine at Tufts University, the National Institutes of Dental and Craniofacial Research, and the NIH/NIBIB via Tufts University's Tissue Engineering Resource Center. The authors thank Judith Edwards for her help in the preparation of this manuscript.

AUTHOR DISCLOSURE STATEMENT

The authors (C.E. and J.A.G.) declare no conflict of interest. There are no commercial associations that pose any such conflict of interest with the information contained in this article.

REFERENCES

1. Woodley DT, Bachmann PM, and O'Keefe EJ: Laminin inhibits human keratinocyte migration. J Cell Physiol 1988; **136:** 140.
2. Brown C, Stenn KS, Falk RJ, Woodley DT, and O'Keefe EJ: Vitronectin: effects on keratinocyte motility and inhibition of collagen-induced motility. J Invest Dermatol 1991; **96:** 724.
3. Cha D, O'Brien P, O'Toole EA, Woodley DT, and Hudson LG: Enhanced modulation of keratinocyte motility by transforming growth factor-alpha (TGF-alpha) relative to epidermal growth factor (EGF). J Invest Dermatol 1996; **106:** 590.
4. Sarret Y, Woodley DT, Grigsby K, Wynn K, and O'Keefe EJ: Human keratinocyte locomotion: the effect of selected cytokines. J Invest Dermatol 1992a; **98:** 12.
5. Sarret Y, Stamm C, Jullien D, and Schmitt D: Keratinocyte migration is partially supported by the cell-binding domain of fibronectin and is RGDS-dependent. J Invest Dermatol 1992b; **99:** 656.
6. Andriani F, Margulis A, Lin N, Griffey S, and Garlick JA: Analysis of microenvironmental factors contributing to basement membrane assembly and normalized epidermal phenotype. J Invest Dermatol 2003; **120:** 923.
7. Kolodka TM, Garlick JA, and Taichman LB: Evidence for keratinocyte stem cells *in vitro*: long term engraftment and persistence of transgene expression from retrovirus-transduced keratinocytes. Proc Natl Acad Sci USA 1998; **95:** 4356.
8. Garlick JA, Parks WC, Welgus HG, and Taichman LB: Re-epithelialization of human oral keratinocytes *in vitro*. J Dent Res 1996; **75:** 912.
9. Egles C, Shamis Y, Mauney JR, Volloch V, Kaplan DL, and Garlick JA: Denatured collagen modulates the phenotype of normal and wounded human skin equivalents. J Invest Dermatol 2008; **128:** 1830.
10. Segal N, Andriani F, Pfeiffer L, Kamath P, Lin N, Satyamurthy K, Egles C, and Garlick JA: The basement membrane microenvironment directs the normalization and survival of bioengineered human skin equivalents. Matrix Biol 2008; **27:** 163.

11. Garlick JA and Taichman LB: Effect of TGF-beta 1 on re-epithelialization of human keratinocytes *in vitro*: an organotypic model. J Invest Dermatol 1994; **103:** 554.

12. Garlick JA and Taichman LB: Fate of human keratinocytes during reepithelialization in an organotypic culture model. Lab Invest 1994; **70:** 916.

13. DePianto D and Coulombe PA: Intermediate filaments and tissue repair. Exp Cell Res 2004; **15:** 68.

14. Johnen C, Hartmann B, Steffen I, Bräutigam K, Witascheck T, Toman N, Küntscher MV, and Gerlach JC: Skin cell isolation and expansion for cell transplantation is limited in patients using tobacco, alcohol, or are exhibiting diabetes mellitus. Burns 2006; **32:** 194.

15. Winter GD: Epidermal regeneration in the domestic pig. In: *Epidermal Wound Healing*, edited by Maibach HI and Rovee DT. Chicago: Yearbook Medical, 1972, pp. 71–112.

16. Carlson MW, Alt-Holland A, Egles C, and Garlick JA: Three-dimensional tissue models of normal and diseased skin. Curr Protoc Cell Biol 2008; Chapter 19: Unit 19.9.

17. Schneider A, Garlick JA, and Egles C: Self-assembling peptide nanofiber scaffolds accelerate wound healing. PLoS ONE 2008; **9:** e1410.

18. Schneider A, Wang XY, Kaplan DL, Garlick JA, and Egles C: Biofunctionalized electrospun silk mats as a topical bioactive dressing for accelerated wound healing. Acta Biomater 2008; **32:** Issue 2, 194–200.

19. Greenberg S, Margulis A, and Garlick JA: *In vivo* transplantation of engineered human skin. Methods Mol Biol 2005; **289:** 425.

20. Greenberg S, Kamath P, Petrali J, Hamilton T, Garfield J, and Garlick JA: Characterization of the initial response of engineered human skin to sulfur mustard. Toxicol Sci 2006; **90:** 549.

21. Kalish RS, Simon M, Harrington R, Gottlieb AB, and Gilhar A: Skin equivalent and natural killer cells: a new model for psoriasis and GVHD. J Invest Dermatol 2009; **129:** 773.

22. Borenstein JT, Keegan M, Megley K, Tao S, Truong S, Demidova-Rice T, Garlick JA, Kaplan DL, and Herman IM: Innovations in 3-D Bioreactors for Wound Healing and Regenerative Medicine (TERMIS abstract, 2008).

WHS Wound Healing Society

Future Perspectives of Tissue-Engineered Skin: Xenobiotic-Free Culture Systems

Neeltje A. Coolen,[1,2] Magda M.W. Ulrich,[1,2,*] and Esther Middelkoop [1,2]

[1]Association of Dutch Burn Centres, Beverwijk, The Netherlands.
[2]Department of Plastic, Reconstructive and Hand Surgery, VU University Medical Centre, Amsterdam, The Netherlands.

Abbreviations and Acronyms

BSE = bovine spongiform encephalopathy

FCS = fetal calf serum

*Correspondence: Association of Dutch Burn Centres, P.O. Box 1015, 1940 EA Beverwijk, The Netherlands (e-mail: mulrich@burns.nl).

Background: The standard therapy for large skin defects (*e.g.*, chronic wounds or burn wounds) is unsatisfactory in terms of quality and rate of healing. Therefore, there is a high demand for tissue-engineered skin that improves wound healing. Several cellular and acellular constructs have been developed in the past years, and these substitutes accelerate wound closure and decrease length of hospital stay.

The Problem: To construct these skin equivalents, several xenobiotic (animal-derived) materials are needed. However, use of xenobiotic components is a potential risk for the patient, because of possible disease transfer (*e.g.*, prions or animal viruses). For that reason, it is likely that xenobiotic materials will be prohibited by national and international authorities in the future.

Basic/Clinical Science Advances: Several approaches have been suggested to establish xenobiotic-free skin equivalents. Some of these methods are very promising, but a complete ban of animal-derived materials is still not accomplished, and more research is necessary.

Clinical Care Relevance: Use of xenobiotic-free skin constructs is safer for the patient, because it reduces risks of infection and immune responses.

Conclusion: Tissue-engineered skin is beneficial in the treatment of deep skin wounds, but further improvements are needed to create ideal skin substitutes. Special attention should be paid to the generation of xenobiotic-free skin equivalents.

BACKGROUND

HEALING OF FULL-THICKNESS skin defects, such as chronic wounds or deep burns, is problematic. Chronic wounds (*e.g.*, leg ulcers and diabetic foot ulcers) can persist for several years. Prevalence of underlying diseases, such as diabetes mellitus or venous disease, is increasing because of changing life styles and aging of the population. Several therapies have been developed for these wounds, but some ulcers still have a low tendency to heal. Full-thickness burn wounds close faster than chronic wounds, but they heal with the formation of a hypertrophic scar. These severe scars affect appearance and cause serious restrictions on joint mobility. The standard treatment for deep burn wounds is transplantation with a meshed split skin autograft. However, healing still results in scar formation, and morbidity at the donor site may occur. In addition, insufficient donor sites may be present in patients with extensive burns because of limited availability of healthy skin. Therefore, there is a high demand for alternative therapies, particularly in the field of tissue engineering.

In recent years, both acellular and cellular tissue-engineered products

ADVANCES IN WOUND CARE, VOLUME 1

Printed in U.S.A.
DOI: 10.1089/awc.2009.0141

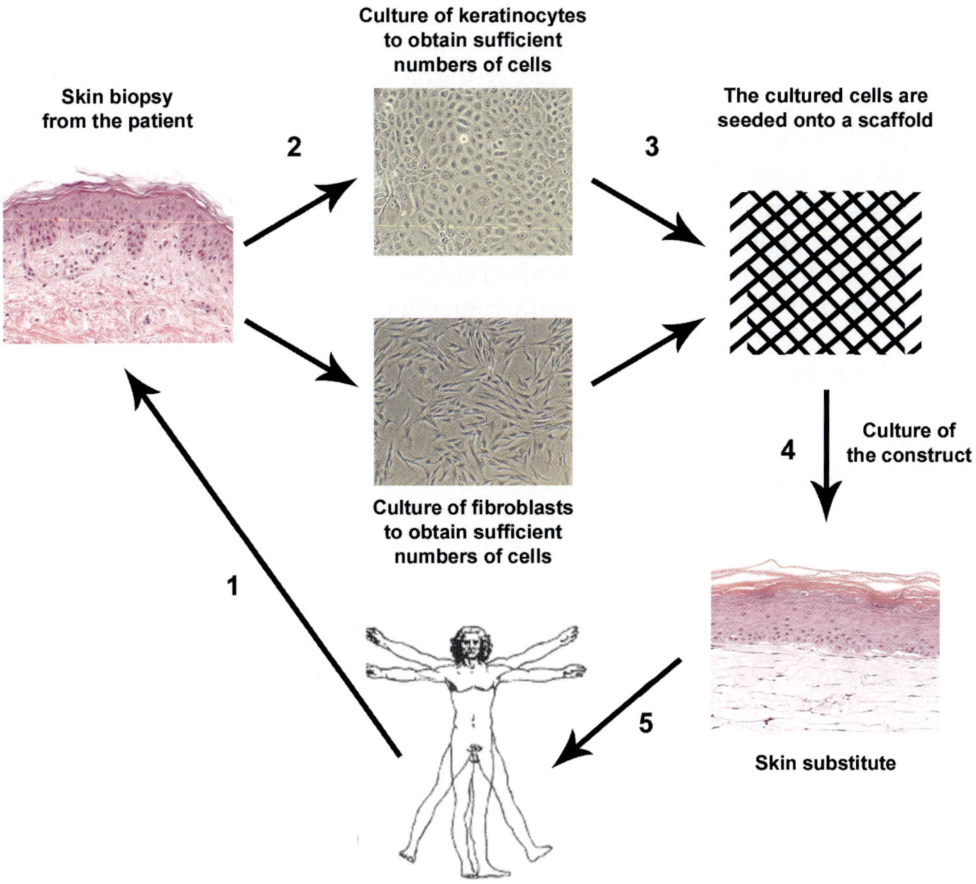

Figure 1. Overview of the generation of autologous skin substitutes. Tissue-engineered skin constructs are beneficial in the treatment of deep skin defects. To generate autologous skin equivalents, skin biopsies are obtained from the patient (1) and transferred to the laboratory. Keratinocytes are isolated from the epidermis and fibroblasts are isolated from the dermis of each biopsy (2). To acquire sufficient numbers of skin cells, the cells are expanded in the laboratory. As soon as adequate cell numbers are obtained, keratinocytes and fibroblasts are seeded onto a scaffold (a rat tail collagen type I gel) (3). Subsequently, this construct is cultured to form a skin substitute (4). When the cultured autologous skin equivalent is ready, it is transplanted to the patient (5). Conventionally, xenobiotic (animal-derived) culture ingredients are used for the expansion of skin cells and dermal scaffolds contain animal-derived proteins. Since use of xenobiotic constituents is a potential risk for the patient, xenobiotic-free skin substitutes need to be developed.

have been developed.[1,2] The acellular constructs can be used as dermal substitutes that encourage autologous cell recruitment and tissue formation. These matrices are mostly composed of animal-derived extracellular matrix molecules (*e.g.*, Integra®[3], Integra Life Sciences, Plainsboro, NJ; Matriderm®[4,5], Skin and Health Care AG, Billerbeck, Germany) or utilize allogeneic human dermis (*e.g.*, AlloDerm®[6], Lifecell Corp., Branchburg, NJ). The cellular tissue-engineered products usually consist of a synthetic or biological matrix that is populated with one or more skin cell types (Fig. 1). These constructs generally contain keratinocytes, the main epidermal cell type, and fibroblasts, the prominent dermal cell type, which produce the extracellular matrix of the dermis. The skin cells have to be expanded in the laboratory to obtain sufficient numbers of cells.

CLINICAL PROBLEM

For the manufacturing of skin substitutes, several xenobiotic (animal-derived) materials are used. Xenobiotic culture ingredients are required for the expansion of skin cells (*e.g.*, bovine serum), and extracellular matrix molecules, which are needed for the production of scaffolds, are often animal derived. The utilization of xenobiotic constituents is a potential risk for the patient, because of possible disease transfer (*e.g.*, prions or animal viruses).[7] In addition, these components may induce an immunological response in the recipient patient.[8] Therefore, the European and U.S. authorities prefer xenobiotic-free conditions for clinical applications. To construct a successful skin substitute, new strategies need to be developed to circumvent this problem. Recently, bovine serum–free media have become commercially available. However, these products (*e.g.*, EpiLife®, Cascade Biologics, Inc., Portland, OR) have not been approved for clinical use, or still contain animal components such as bovine serum albumin, bovine transferrin, or an extract from the bovine pituitary gland.

BASIC SCIENCE CONTEXT

The first cellular skin substitute was achieved by culturing autologous keratinocytes to form a confluent epithelial sheet. To obtain sufficient numbers of cells, the keratinocytes were cocultured with irradiated mouse 3T3 feeder layer cells in the presence of fetal calf serum (FCS): the Rheinwald and Green method.[9] These xenobiotic compounds supply mitogens and attachment factors for the cells. The cultured epithelial autografts can restore epidermal coverage and can be life-saving for patients suffering from extensive burns. However, the take of the sheets was variable and often poor, and there was a high chance of blistering.[10] In addition, the grafts were fragile and it took 3 to 5 weeks to culture the sheets. An alternative for the transplantation with keratinocyte sheets is transfer of preconfluent keratinocytes. These proliferating cells have a better take rate than confluent sheets and were shown to facilitate healing of both chronic ulcers and burn wounds.[11,12] In addition, the use of preconfluent keratinocytes decreased culture time and costs. Transfer of these cells to the wound bed can be accomplished by a variety of carrier systems,[13–15] which makes them easier to handle than the cultured epithelial autografts.

It is generally accepted that a dermal component is also needed in the treatment of large skin defects.[16,17] Dermal constructs might improve graft take and esthetic and functional outcome. It has been shown that it is beneficial to incorporate fibroblasts into dermal substitutes.[18] We and others found that the presence of fibroblasts in skin equivalents not only stimulated keratinocyte outgrowth and differentiation, but also improved the quality of dermal tissue regeneration.[18–20] Fibroblast-populated matrices can be used in combination with a thin-split skin autograft; however, the persisting need for large donor sites is disadvantageous. Therefore, several researchers have developed full skin equivalents consisting of a fibroblast-populated matrix and a cultured epidermis.[21,22] Some years ago, a full skin substitute (*i.e.*, Apligraf® Organogenesis, Canton, MA) was approved by the U.S. Food and Drug Administration for the treatment of venous leg ulcers and diabetic foot ulcers. However, this construct contains allogeneic skin cells and is therefore less appropriate for the permanent repair of large burn wounds.

MATERIAL—ADVANTAGES AND LIMITATIONS

As described above, use of engineered skin constructs can be beneficial in the treatment of deep skin defects. Application of these skin substitutes accelerates healing of both chronic ulcers and burn wounds and decreases length of hospital stay.[12,22–24] In addition, cultured skin substitutes can reduce requirements for split skin autografts.[21] However, there are also major disadvantages of tissue-engineered skin. An important disadvantage is that tissue-engineered products are difficult to store and transport. In addition, treatment with skin substitutes is expensive, especially with the use of autologous cells. Another significant disadvantage is that xenobiotic materials are necessary during the culture process of the current skin equivalents. Keratinocytes and fibroblasts are conventionally cultured in medium containing FCS, and keratinocyte culture techniques also require mouse feeder layer cells. These xenobiotic components may possibly contain prions (*e.g.*, bovine spongiform encephalopathy [BSE]) or animal viruses that are able to infect human cells. To reduce the risk, FCS can be obtained from countries where cow herds are free from BSE. However, if BSE spreads worldwide, serum-free culture medium will be necessary. Apart from the risk of disease transfer, patients can raise antibodies against FCS and murine cells after transplantation with tissue-engineered skin. This may lead to graft loss, anaphylaxis, and serum sickness.[7,8,25] Due to these risks, national and international legislation would favor approval of xenobiotic-free materials above xenobiotic-containing materials for clinical use. In addition, it is feasible that xenobiotic materials will be banned completely in future. Therefore, further improvements of tissue-engineered products are necessary to reduce the risk of xenotransplantation.

DISCUSSION OF FINDINGS AND RELEVANT LITERATURE

In the past few years, several approaches have been developed to establish xenobiotic-free culture systems. A first strategy is to omit FCS from the culture media. At this moment, some serum-free culture media are commercially available for the expansion of skin cells in the laboratory (*e.g.*, EpiLife or Gibco's Keratinocyte-SFM). These media have been demonstrated to support the proliferation of epidermal and dermal cells. However, cells grown using those serum-free media require plating at high cell-seeding densities, and this may not be possible or practical in a clinical setting. Further, some formulations still contain animal-derived proteins, such as bovine pituitary extract or bovine serum albumin, which carries the risk of BSE transmission. Even when serum-free media do not contain xenobiotic components, manufacturers do not fully disclose the composition of the medium. Consequently, none of these culture media are currently approved for clinical use. Since commercial media have several limitations, it is important to search for other serum-free culture methods. Smola *et al.* showed that FCS can also be replaced by autologous patient serum in keratinocyte cultures.[26] Experiments show that patient serum was equally or even better suited than FCS to stimulate keratinocyte proliferation. However, murine feeder layer cells were still necessary in the culture process. In addition, it is undesirable to draw blood from patients with large burn wounds, because these patients already have a fluid shortage and blood cell shortage. A second approach to avoid xenobiotic constituents was shown by MacNeil's group. They reported that murine feeder layer cells can be replaced by human dermal fibroblasts under serum-free conditions.[27–29] Keratinocytes were able to attach and proliferate well on a chemically defined plasma polymer surface in combination with human feeder cells. However, it took some weeks before sufficient numbers of the fibroblasts were cultured and the cells could be used as a feeder layer. Another possible solution is the replacement of mice feeder layer cells by extracellular matrix molecules.[30–32] We found that keratinocytes can be cultured on collagen type IV, derived from human placenta, without the need of mouse feeder cells and FCS, and that these cells were still able to create a fully differentiated epidermis.[30] Several investigators have reported that keratinocyte stem cells adhere more rapidly to human placental collagen type IV than transient amplifying keratinocytes.[33,34] For this reason, human collagen type IV may support the growth of keratinocytes. Besides collagen type IV, other extracellular matrix proteins can replace mouse feeder layer cells. Keratinocytes were able to attach and grow on bovine collagen type I membranes without feeder layers under serum-free conditions.[31] These keratinocytes could form a fully differentiated epidermis after transplantation to a nude mice model. However, more research is necessary to replace the bovine-derived collagen type I by human-derived collagen. Mannosides, present in the basement membrane, can also be used as a substitute for mice feeder layer cells.[32] Attachment and proliferation of keratinocytes was better on a chemically synthesized mannose-rich matrix than on feeder cells; however, FCS was still necessary in this culture system. A final strategy to avoid xenobiotic components is the use of a dermal scaffold that is completely composed of human-derived materials. To generate such a construct, human dermal fibroblast can be stimulated to produce a protein-rich matrix.[35] This cell-derived matrix had a high mechanical strength and is therefore probably suitable for transplantation. Next to a cell-derived construct, clotted human plasma can be used as a dermal scaffold.[36] Both keratinocytes and fibroblasts proliferate well on this matrix and it was successfully transplanted to burn patients. To avoid risks, this construct can be generated from autologous plasma.

In conclusion, some of these strategies are very promising in establishing xenobiotic-free cultures.

TAKE-HOME MESSAGE

Basic sciences

- The current skin substitutes consist of both cellular and acellular skin substitutes. Acellular matrices are fabricated from animal-derived extracellular matrix molecules (*e.g.*, Integra®) or utilize allogeneic human dermis (*e.g.*, AlloDerm®). Cellular constructs are composed of a synthetic or biological matrix that is populated with keratinocytes and/or fibroblasts.
- In the past few years, several efforts have been made to develop xenobiotic-free skin substitutes. We and others showed that it is possible to replace bovine serum and mouse cells, needed for the expansion of skin cells, by animal-free alternatives. In addition, dermal substitutes can be constructed from human-derived materials.
- In addition to safety aspects, the current skin substitutes have other disadvantages. Treatment with these constructs is very expensive at this moment, and these tissue-engineered products are difficult to store and transport.
- Further improvements are needed to create ideal skin substitutes that are in agreement with national and international legislation.

Clinical sciences

- Tissue-engineered skin is beneficial in the treatment of deep skin defects. Application of these skin substitutes accelerates healing of both chronic ulcers and burn wounds and decreases length of hospital stay.
- More *in vivo* studies are necessary to prove the clinical efficacy of the developed xenobiotic-free skin constructs.
- National and international authorities would favor approval of xenobiotic-free skin substitutes above xenobiotic-containing constructs for clinical use, because of the possible risks.

Relevance to clinical care

- Since the standard treatments of large skin wounds are inadequate, there is a high demand for tissue-engineered skin.
- Currently, several xenobiotic (animal-derived) materials are used during the manufacturing process of skin substitutes. However, use of xenobiotic components is a potential risk for the patient, because of possible disease transfer (*e.g.*, prions or animal viruses) and the possible immunological response in the patient. Due to these risks, development of animal-free constructs should be promoted.

However, extensive *in vivo* studies have to be performed to test the efficacy of these methods in patients.

CAUTION, CRITICAL REMARKS, AND RECOMMENDATIONS

For the development of tissue-engineered skin, it is important that this construct is in accordance with national and international legislation. Recently, the European Union has adopted a regulation on advanced therapy medicinal products, which includes tissue-engineered products.[37] To safeguard public health, clinical studies on advanced therapy medicinal products should be conducted in accordance with the principles and guidelines for good clinical practice, as laid down in Directive 2001/20/EC. In addition, the manufacture of these products should be in compliance with the principles of good manufacturing practice, as set out in Commission Directive 2003/94/EC. However, the European Commission still has to draw up detailed guidelines on good clinical practice and good manufacturing practice specific to advanced therapy medicinal products. During the production process, the European authority tolerates use of animal cells, but very detailed information has to be provided about many aspects of the involved animals. Similar to the European authority, the American U.S. Food and Drug Administration approves xenotransplantation. However, extensive safety tests have to be performed and many data have to be supplied about health and husbandry of the source animal.

A framework for the regulations of tissue-engineered constructs is just beginning to evolve. Clear international laws and regulatory controls are needed to make commercialization of these products possible. Prompt development of such legislation is crucial for the success of tissue-engineered constructs.

FUTURE DEVELOPMENT

Further improvements are needed to develop an ideal tissue-engineered skin. The perfect skin equivalent should be safe, clinically effective, and commercially viable. To generate safe skin substitutes, xenobiotic-free skin equivalents should be developed. Besides safety, the clinical efficacy of skin constructs should be optimized. Current skin constructs improve healing of deep wounds, but they do not restore complete tissue function or prevent scar formation. Finally, production costs need to be contained to generate commercially viable tissue-engineered constructs. For this reason, culture techniques have to be less labor intensive, and user-friendly products must be created that do not need specialist expertise. To reduce the risk of commercial failure, it is essential that cost-effectiveness studies are conducted before product development is considered.

In the past decades, tissue-engineered skin has shown a proof of concept in being beneficial for the treatment of deep skin defects. It has a tremendous therapeutic potential that is just beginning to be realized.

AUTHOR DISCLOSURE STATEMENT

No conflict of interest disclosed.

REFERENCES

1. Kearney JN: Clinical evaluation of skin substitutes. Burns 2001; **27:** 545.
2. Metcalfe AD and Ferguson MW: Bioengineering skin using mechanisms of regeneration and repair. Biomaterials 2007; **28:** 5100.
3. Burke JF, Yannas IV, Quinby WC, Jr., Bondoc CC, and Jung WK: Successful use of a physiologically acceptable artificial skin in the treatment of extensive burn injury. Ann Surg 1981; **194:** 413.
4. Haslik W, Kamolz LP, Nathschlager G, Andel H, Meissl G, and Frey M: First experiences with the collagen-elastin matrix Matriderm as a dermal substitute in severe burn injuries of the hand. Burns 2007; **33:** 364.
5. van Zuijlen PP, Vloemans JF, van Trier AJ, Suijker MH, van Unen E, Groenevelt F, Kreis RW, and Middelkoop E: Dermal substitution in acute burns and reconstructive surgery: a subjective and objective long-term follow-up. Plast Reconstr Surg 2001; **108:** 1938.
6. Wainwright DJ: Use of an acellular allograft dermal matrix (AlloDerm) in the management of full-thickness burns. Burns 1995; **21:** 243.
7. MacNeil S: Progress and opportunities for tissue-engineered skin. Nature 2007; **445:** 874.
8. Meyer AA, Manktelow A, Johnson M, deSerres S, Herzog S, and Peterson HD: Antibody response to xenogeneic proteins in burned patients receiving cultured keratinocyte grafts. J Trauma 1988; **28:** 1054.
9. Rheinwald JG and Green H: Serial cultivation of strains of human epidermal keratinocytes: the formation of keratinizing colonies from single cells. Cell 1975; **6:** 331.
10. Desai MH, Mlakar JM, McCauley RL, Abdullah KM, Rutan RL, Waymack JP, Robson MC, and Herndon DN: Lack of long-term durability of cultured keratinocyte burn-wound coverage: a case report. J Burn Care Rehabil 1991; **12:** 540.
11. Harris PA, Leigh IM, and Navsaria HA: Pre-confluent keratinocyte grafting: the future for cultured skin replacements? Burns 1998; **24:** 591.
12. Zhu N, Warner RM, Simpson C, Glover M, Hernon CA, Kelly J, Fraser S, Brotherston TM, Ralston DR, and MacNeil S: Treatment of burns and chronic wounds using a new cell transfer dressing for delivery of autologous keratinocytes. Eur J Plast Surg 2005; **28:** 319.
13. Pellegrini G, Ranno R, Stracuzzi G, Bondanza S, Guerra L, Zambruno G, Micali G, and De Luca M: The control of epidermal stem cells (holoclones) in the treatment of massive full-thickness burns

with autologous keratinocytes cultured on fibrin. Transplantation 1999; **68:** 868.

14. van den Bogaerdt AJ, Ulrich MM, van Galen MJ, Reijnen L, Verkerk M, Pieper J, Lamme EN, and Middelkoop E: Upside-down transfer of porcine keratinocytes from a porous, synthetic dressing to experimental full-thickness wounds. Wound Repair Regen 2004; **12:** 225.
15. Navarro FA, Stoner ML, Park CS, Huertas JC, Lee HB, Wood FM, and Orgill DP: Sprayed keratinocyte suspensions accelerate epidermal coverage in a porcine microwound model. J Burn Care Rehabil 2000; **21:** 513.
16. Cooper ML, Hansbrough JF, Spielvogel RL, Cohen R, Bartel RL, and Naughton G: *In vivo* optimization of a living dermal substitute employing cultured human fibroblasts on a biodegradable polyglycolic acid or polyglactin mesh. Biomaterials 1991; **12:** 243.
17. Cuono C, Langdon R, and McGuire J: Use of cultured epidermal autografts and dermal allografts as skin replacement after burn injury. Lancet 1986; **1:** 1123.
18. Marks MG, Doillon C, and Silver FH: Effects of fibroblasts and basic fibroblast growth factor on facilitation of dermal wound healing by type I collagen matrices. J Biomed Mater Res 1991; **25:** 683.
19. Lamme EN, Van Leeuwen RT, Brandsma K, Van Marle J, and Middelkoop E: Higher numbers of autologous fibroblasts in an artificial dermal substitute improve tissue regeneration and modulate scar tissue formation. J Pathol 2000; **190:** 595.
20. Cooper ML, Andree C, Hansbrough JF, Zapata-Sirvent RL, and Spielvogel RL: Direct comparison of a cultured composite skin substitute containing human keratinocytes and fibroblasts to an epidermal sheet graft containing human keratinocytes on athymic mice. J Invest Dermatol 1993; **101:** 811.
21. Boyce ST, Kagan RJ, Greenhalgh DG, Warner P, Yakuboff KP, Palmieri T, and Warden GD: Cultured skin substitutes reduce requirements for harvesting of skin autograft for closure of excised, full-thickness burns. J Trauma 2006; **60:** 821.
22. Gibbs S, van den Hoogenband HM, Kirtschig G, Richters CD, Spiekstra SW, Breetveld M, Scheper RJ, and de Boer EM: Autologous full-thickness skin substitute for healing chronic wounds. Br J Dermatol 2006; **155:** 267.
23. Gore DC: Utility of acellular allograft dermis in the care of elderly burn patients. J Surg Res 2005; **125:** 37.
24. Ryan CM, Schoenfeld DA, Malloy M, Schulz JT, 3rd, Sheridan RL, and Tompkins RG: Use of Integra artificial skin is associated with decreased length of stay for severely injured adult burn survivors. J Burn Care Rehabil 2002; **23:** 311.
25. Cairns BA, deSerres S, Brady LA, Hultman CS, and Meyer AA: Xenogeneic mouse fibroblasts persist in human cultured epidermal grafts: a possible mechanism of graft loss. J Trauma 1995; **39:** 75; discussion 79.
26. Smola H, Reinke M, Shephard P, Krieg T, and Hess S: Autologous patient serum for the culture of keratinocyte transplants reduces risk of transmittable disease. Lancet 1999; **353:** 641.
27. Bullock AJ, Higham MC, and MacNeil S: Use of human fibroblasts in the development of a xenobiotic-free culture and delivery system for human keratinocytes. Tissue Eng 2006; **12:** 245.
28. Higham MC, Dawson R, Szabo M, Short R, Haddow DB, and MacNeil S: Development of a stable chemically defined surface for the culture of human keratinocytes under serum-free conditions for clinical use. Tissue Eng 2003; **9:** 919.
29. Sun T, Higham M, Layton C, Haycock J, Short R, and MacNeil S: Developments in xenobiotic-free culture of human keratinocytes for clinical use. Wound Repair Regen 2004; **12:** 626.
30. Coolen NA, Verkerk M, Reijnen L, Vlig M, van den Bogaerdt AJ, Breetveld M, Gibbs S, Middelkoop E, and Ulrich MM: Culture of keratinocytes for transplantation without the need of feeder layer cells. Cell Transplant 2007; **16:** 649.
31. Horch RE, Debus M, Wagner G, and Stark GB: Cultured human keratinocytes on type I collagen membranes to reconstitute the epidermis. Tissue Eng 2000; **6:** 53.
32. Labsky J, Dvorankova B, Smetana K, Holikova Z, Jr., Broz L, and Gabius HJ: Mannosides as crucial part of bioactive supports for cultivation of human epidermal keratinocytes without feeder cells. Biomaterials 2003; **24:** 863.
33. Jones PH and Watt FM: Separation of human epidermal stem cells from transit amplifying cells on the basis of differences in integrin function and expression. Cell 1993; **73:** 713.
34. Jones PH, Harper S, and Watt FM: Stem cell patterning and fate in human epidermis. Cell 1995; **80:** 83.
35. Throm AM, Liu WC, Lock CH, and Billiar KL: Development of a cell-derived matrix: Effects of epidermal growth factor in chemically defined culture. J Biomed Mater Res A 2009; Epub ahead of print, DOI: 10.1002/Jbm.a.32369.
36. Llames SG, Del Rio M, Larcher F, Garcia E, Garcia M, Escamez MJ, Jorcano JL, Holguin P, and Meana A: Human plasma as a dermal scaffold for the generation of a completely autologous bioengineered skin. Transplantation 2004; **77:** 350.
37. Regulation (EC) No 1394/2007 of the European Parliament and of the Council of 13 November 2007 on advanced therapy medicinal products and amending Directive 2001/83/EC and Regulation (EC) No 726/2004. Off J Eur Union 2007; **L324:** 121.

WHS
Wound
Healing
Society

The Use of a Collagen–Elastin Matrix as Dermal Regeneration Template for the Treatment of Full-Thickness Skin Defects

Werner Haslik, David B. Lumenta, Lars Peter Kamolz,* and Manfred Frey

Division of Plastic and Reconstructive Surgery, Department of Surgery, Medical University of Vienna, Vienna, Austria.

Abbreviation and Acronym

VSS = Vancouver Scar Scale

*Correspondence: Division of Plastic and Reconstructive Surgery, Department of Surgery, Vienna Burn Centre, Medical University of Vienna, Waehringer Guertel 18-20, A-1090 Vienna, Austria (e-mail: lars-peter.kamolz@meduniwien.ac.at).

Background: The gold standard for coverage of full-thickness skin defects is skin grafting. However, since not all layers of skin are replaced adequately by split-thickness skin grafts alone, poor skin quality and scar contractures represent common problems in grafted regions.

The Problem: Dermal substitutes are used to improve the quality of skin-grafted areas, but due to the increased distance between the skin graft and its wound bed, most materials require a two-step procedure to overcome the problem of diminished take-rate of skin grafts.

Basic/Clinical Science Advances: The dermal substitute Matriderm® (Dr. Otto Suwelack Skin & Health Care AG, Billerbeck, Germany) is composed of native structurally intact collagen fibrils coated with elastin for supporting dermal regeneration. The collagen of the three-dimensional matrix is obtained from bovine dermis and contains collagen type I, III, and V. Elastin is obtained from bovine nuchal ligament by hydrolysis. The thickness of the matrix is 1 or 2 mm; it is sterilized with γ-irradiation and can be stored at room temperature.

Clinical Care Relevance: Matriderm is a matrix that allows for a simultaneous application of the dermal substitute combined with immediate skin grafting in a one-stage procedure.

Conclusion: This simultaneous application of this collagen–elastin matrix with skin grafts represents a viable alternative to other types of defect coverage like pedicled or free flaps, which should be considered in the treatment of full-thickness skin injuries.

BACKGROUND

THE LOSS OF SKIN and soft tissue in the upper extremity due to burn, trauma, or after-surgical procedures represents a major impairment for each patient. Traditionally, autologous skin grafting alone is used for coverage of full-thickness skin defects without exposure of bone or vessels. Since split-thickness skin grafts contain epidermis and only a small layer of dermis, the resulting skin quality is often poor, and the developing scar contractures can lead to functional impairment, for example, reduced range of movement. Consequently, in areas of functional importance, it is essential to reestablish as close as possible properties of healthy skin to reach full functional recovery.

The reconstruction of the dermal component with a dermal substitute represents one possibility to optimize results for the grafted area.[1–9] Great efforts have been made for developing appropriate dermal substitutes[10] to overcome poor skin quality. Several main goals for the improvement of skin graft quality can be postulated:

- application in a one-stage procedure
- reduced incidence of scar contractures

Printed in U.S.A.
DOI: 10.1089/awc.2009.0140

- improved skin pliability and elasticity
- pleasant aesthetic appearance
- off the shelf availability
- fully resorbable

CLINICAL PROBLEM ADDRESSED

The interposition of a dermal substitute between the wound bed and the split-thickness skin graft results in an increased distance to be overcome for capillary in-growth (angiogenesis) and diffusion of nutrients. This can diminish the take-rate of the skin graft. As a result, the majority of dermal substitutes were used in a two-stage procedure, where in a first operation the substitute is applied on a well-perfused wound bed. After a distinct period of time with sufficient vascularization of the scaffold reached, which may depend on the type of dermal substitute used, the split-thickness skin graft is finally applied on top of it.

While in severely burned patients with the omnipresent lack of donor sites a two-stage procedure can be useful to delay further split-skin graft harvests, there is no doubt that a one-stage procedure with skin substitutes offers several advantages.[11]

First, the number of operations is reduced. Second, the overall time for wound healing is shortened due to the omission of the period allowed for vascularization of the substitute alone, before actual skin grafting takes place as performed in two-stage procedures. Third, the incidence of infections is reduced as a result of the shorter healing period and the omission of a temporary coverage (usually silicone) frequently used for two-stage templates, which requires an intensified wound care management. Fourth, due to the above-mentioned points, physiotherapy and scar prevention strategies can be initiated earlier to prevent the development of contractures. Last, but not least, it should be taken into account that wound-healing periods beyond a period of 14 to 21 days are often associated with the development of hypertrophic scarring.[12]

RELEVANT BASIC SCIENCE CONTEXT

The dermal substitute Matriderm® (Dr. Otto Suwelack Skin & Health Care AG, Billerbeck, Germany) is composed of native structurally intact collagen fibrils coated with elastin for supporting dermal regeneration. The collagen of this three-dimensional matrix is obtained from bovine dermis and contains the dermal collagen type I, III, and V. The elastin is obtained from bovine nuchal ligament by hydrolysis. The product is according to the annex II, section 4 of the Council Directive 93/42 EEC concerning Medical Devices and Commission Directive 2003/32 EC. The thickness of the matrix is 1 or 2 mm; it is sterilized with γ-irradiation and can be stored at room temperature. The collagen–elastin matrix Matriderm offers the possibility to perform dermal substitution and split-thickness skin grafting in a one-stage procedure without diminished take-rate of the skin (Table 1).

EXPERIMENTAL MODEL OR MATERIAL—ADVANTAGES AND LIMITATIONS

To minimize bacterial colonization, acute burn wounds were scrubbed with chlorhexidine (Octenisept®; S&M, Norderstedt, Germany) or other antiseptics. An early radical debridement was performed in all patients to minimize the rate of infections. In case of scar revisions or other clean surgical wounds, single-shot antibiotics were employed. After accurate hemostasis, the matrix is prepared. Since the wound bed allows in most cases for a sufficient moisturization of the matrix with blood and wound fluid, easing access of wound-healing factors to the matrix, immersion of the matrix in normal saline, is rarely necessary. However, if the matrix remains dry after application to the wound, we prefer to immerse the matrix with normal saline. After the matrix is placed onto the wound bed, a thin unmeshed split-thickness skin graft, harvested with the Zimmer® (Freiburg, Germany) dermatome, is placed on top of the matrix

Table 1. *Different kind of templates*

Material	bovine collagen-based dermal component with glycosaminoglycan (chondroitin-6-sulphate) temporary epidermal silicone sheet	dermal collagen types I, III and V with elastin component	bioabsorbable polyglactin mesh seeded with allogeneic neonatal fibroblasts	acellular dermis processed from human cadaver skin	bilayered living skin equivalent composed of type I bovine collagen, allogeneic keratinocytes and fibroblasts from neonatal foreskin	porous collagen sponge with co-cultured allogeneic donor epidermal keratinocytes and dermal fibroblasts from neonatal foreskin
Product name	Integra™	Matriderm®	Dermagraft™	Alloderm®	Apligraf®	OrCel®
Producer	Integra LifeScience, Plainsborough, NJ, USA	Dr. Suwelack Skin & Health Care AG, Billerbeck, Germany	Advanced Tissue Sciences, LaJolla, CA, USA	Lifecell Corporation, Branchberg, NJ, USA	Organogenesis, Canton, MA, USA	Forticell Bioscience, New York, NY, USA

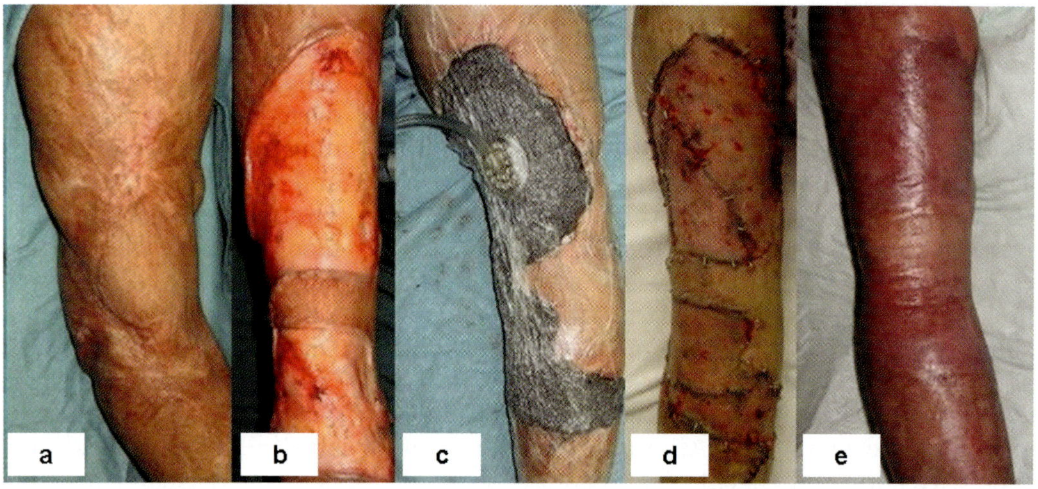

Figure 1. (**a**) Scars and scar contractures after deep burns to the right arm; (**b**) after deep excision of the contracted and scarred areas. Wound bed (subcutaneous tissue and facia) already covered with Matriderm (1 mm); (**c**) immobilization of the grafted areas (Matriderm and unmeshed skin graft in the single step procedure) by use of the V.A.C.® (Vienna, Austria) (**d**) Early result after removal of the V.A.C.—100% take-rate. (**e**) Later result 2 months after the operation: full range of motion and good aesthetic result.

(Fig. 1a–e). The grafts are fixed by the use of sutures or staples. For dressings we used paraffin gauzes (Bactigras®, Smith and Nephew Medical Limited, Hull, England) and gauze swabs (Gazin®, Lohmann&Rauscher International, Rengsdorf, Germany). To allow for undisturbed wound healing, we prescribed immobilization of the hands concerned for 5 days before the first deep dressing change.

All admissions were treated as in-patients until sufficient wound closure was achieved. This time-point also marks the beginning of physiotherapy and application of compression garments, which were worn for at least 1 year postoperatively according to our clinical protocol.

DISCUSSION OF FINDINGS AND RELEVANT LITERATURE

The first clinical reports on the dermal substitute Matriderm were published by van Zuijlen *et al.*, in which the authors examined its application in acute burns and for scar revision surgery.[13] The results of the matrix with skin grafts were intra-individually compared to the contralateral side, where just split-thickness skin grafts were used. While the take-rate was reported to be equal in both collectives (without the need for regrafting), in burn patients, where Matriderm was used, the resulting take-rate was reported to be 9% lower. For assessment of scar quality after surgery, the authors used the Vancouver Scar Scale (VSS) and cutometry (Courage and Khazaka Electronic, Cologne, Germany) after 3 and 12 months. The parameters of reconstructed scars with the dermal substitute demonstrated in cutometry measures a significantly increased pliability, elasticity, extension, and reduced retraction as compared to skin grafted–only wounds. There were no significant differences observed after 3 months in burn wounds or after 12 months in either group. As a clinical note, the chosen time-point for debridement of burn wounds in the above study at 3 weeks was rather late, and it is a known phenomenon, if wound healing has not occurred by that time, that the development of hypertrophic scarring is very likely to occur.[12] This can possibly explain the early results after 3 months in the above series.

In a study of 10 patients, Haslik *et al*[14] observed a 97% take-rate of unmeshed split-thickness skin grafts in combination with Matriderm. The VSS revealed in conjunction with other reports a good aesthetic result after 3 months. In another report by the same group,[15] analyzing patients receiving in one operative procedure the dermal matrix and unmeshed split-thickness skin grafts for soft-tissue defects of the hand and wrist region after burns or radial forearm flap harvest sites, favorable aesthetic for VSS and functional outcome for Disability of Arm Shoulder Hand score (assessing activities of daily living on a 5-scale item list with 30 questions) were observed in the long-term after 12 months postoperatively. In addition to that Ryssel *et al*[16] did not observe a reduced take-rate, when applying split-thickness skin grafts on Matriderm in a one-stage procedure. After 3 months a statistically significantly improved pliability as compared to the control group (split-thickness skin graft only) was observed; however, no long-term data beyond this period exist. Kolokythas *et al*[17] consistently found a comparable take-rate in 14 patients after the one-stage procedure with Matriderm, so that in sum, it can be concluded that if early debridement was performed, the use of the dermal matrix can be regarded as a safe method without compromising the take-rate. All the above-mentioned reports have used a 1 mm thick matrix.

The dermal matrix also turned out to be feasible for use in intensive care unit patients in a one-stage procedure, as it has been applied in a considerable percentage of severely burned patients in the previously mentioned study by Haslik *et al*[15] and has successfully been integrated for special indications in a whole-treatment concept of severely burned patients.[18] As most of the intensive care unit patients require low-dose catecholamine support, it is interesting to note that the use of peripheral acting vasoconstrictors did not affect the take-rate of the split-thickness skin grafts in combination with the dermal matrix. The combination of vacuum-assisted closure (negative pressure wound therapy), split-thickness skin grafts, and the matrix is discussed controversially. Although it seems that this composite application can be beneficial for the overall take-rate, there is a lack of studies currently supporting their combined use. The difference of 1 or 2 mm thick matrices on the final impact of skin properties has not been described in the current literature.

Whether the indication of the dermal template is restricted to the use in combination with skin grafts can be challenged by the finding of Keck *et al.*,[19] who have successfully applied the matrix alone subcutaneously under the atrophic skin adhering to the tendons after paravasation injury with a cytostatic drug in a case report.

Future therapeutic approaches will reveal if the potential indications for Matriderm are restricted to superficial soft-tissue defects or can be extended to deeper structures requiring comparable constructs or even applied for soft-tissue augmentations.

There are numerous reports and studies on different skin substitutes for burns, but the level of evidence for most of them is characterized by generally poor reporting of methodological detail and small sample sizes.[20] Another problem is that most reports focus on different entities of indications for the use of skin grafts. Consequently, it is difficult to be confident to establish a state-of-the-art comparison from the literature available.

Other skin substitutes, which can be used for full-thickness wound coverage, include Integra,

TAKE-HOME MESSAGE

Basic science advances

- Skin grafts are used to cover surface defects of the body.
- Split-thickness skin grafts are used, if larger areas need to be grafted and the morbidity caused by full-thickness skin grafts to the donor region outweighs its overall benefits.
- Split-thickness skin-grafted areas do not have the same properties as healthy (full-thickness) skin due to the partial lack of the dermal layer.
- In split-thickness skin-grafted areas scar contractions can occur and may result in functional and aesthetic limitations.

Clinical science advances

- The use of dermal substitutes is a possibility to improve the properties of areas receiving split-thickness skin grafts.
- The interposition of a dermal substitute between the wound bed and a skin graft results in an increased distance to overcome for capillary ingrowth and diffusion of nutrients. This can diminish the take-rate of skin grafts, and as a result, the majority of the dermal substitutes are used in a two-stage procedure to allow for sufficient vascularization of the dermal template before skin grafting.
- The dermal collagen–elastin matrix Matriderm has shown to be suitable for a one-step procedure without affecting the actual take-rate of split-thickness skin grafts.
- Current reports support a favorable outcome in terms of skin pliability after 3 months postoperatively.
- Numerous reports and studies on different skin substitutes for burns have a low level of evidence due to generally poor reporting of methodological detail and small sample sizes. Consequently, it is difficult to establish a state-of-the-art comparison from the literature available.

Relevance to clinical care

- The number of operations in a one-stage procedure is reduced.
- The overall time for wound healing is reduced due to the omission of the period allowed for vascularization of the substitute alone, before actual skin grafting takes place as performed in two-stage procedures.
- The rate of infections is reduced as a result of the shorter healing period, and the omission of a temporary coverage frequently used for two-stage templates, which requires an intensified wound care management.
- Due to the shorter healing period, physiotherapy and scar prevention strategies can be initiated earlier to prevail the development of contractures.
- Wound-healing periods beyond a period of 14 to 21 days are often associated with the development of hypertrophic scarring.

Dermagraft, Alloderm, Apligraf, and OrCel (Table 1). Both not primarily intended for the use in burns, Dermagraft[21,22] and Apligraf[23] are mainly used for small size areas, for example, lower extremity defects, and are not regarded as suitable for coverage of larger wound surfaces.

Alloderm is classified as banked human tissue and even if the dermal cells are removed, precautions to the use of human donor skin apply. The product comes in different thicknesses of up to 3.3 mm (0.13 inch), yet only the thinnest variants of less than 0.5 mm (0.02 inch) are recommended for skin grafting.

While Alloderm provides the structure of human dermis and should therefore be a suitable dermal substitute, the majority of the literature focuses on hernia repair[24,25] and breast augmentation rather than skin reconstruction. This reflects a rather low utilization of Alloderm for dermal reconstruction at least in the European medical community. About OrCell[26] there are only a few reports available in the literature. Apligraft has been thoroughly tested in multicentre trials for application in diabetic foot ulcers.[27,28] Following Dermagraft, Transcyte was developed by Advanced Tissue Sciences as burn product (subsequently Smith and Nephew), with the main indication for the coverage of partial-thickness burn wounds.[29–32]

Most clinical experience for the use in full-thickness burns to date exists on the dermal matrix Integra, which consists of a bovine collagen-based dermal component with glycosaminoglycan (chondroitin-6-sulphate) and a temporary epidermal silicone sheet: a two-step procedure is recommended with removal of the silicone layer after sufficient healing of the neodermis, before definite closure can be achieved upon application of a split-thickness skin graft.

As an emergency treatment for life-threatening burns, the outer silicone layer was intended to decrease fluid loss and to act as a bacterial barrier. Aiming for sufficient persistence after implantation, the collagen–glycosaminoglycan matrix was chemically cross linked, increasing the time to full disintegration substantially. The product requires about 3 weeks after implantation for vascularization of the dermal matrix. Only thereafter, in an obligatory second operation the wound could be finally closed with a split-skin transplant.

In a multicentre postapproval clinical trial, Integra was found to be safe with a reliable take-rate and low infection rates in the presence of burn wounds.[33] Only few studies on Integra with regard to scar quality exist, which have compared the final results with an adequate control group.[34] The major challenges were infections in the closed wound chamber requiring wound revision and regrafting, instigating growing need for a less demanding product with more reliable results.

A silicone-free variation of Integra was recently cleared by the Food and Drug Administration as a wound dressing, but the critical element for one-stage dermal regeneration is much more than the plain absence of a silicone cover. Immediate "overgrafting" with skin graft requires rapid integration of the dermal matrix into cellularized and vascularized tissue to ensure sufficient nutrition, while porosity will be the key element in the first few days only.

Finally the matrix needs to last long enough to provide a guiding structure for tissue reorganization without becoming a foreign element in the healing tissue for many months. The first publications on Matriderm, which involves bovine collagen and elastin, date back to the year 2006.

How can rapid integration be accomplished in Matriderm? Natural, native collagen features well-defined binding sites for fibroblasts, enabling them to grow along the fibers, immediately followed by endothelial cells. A dermal matrix needs to present the same native structure, otherwise in-growth will be delayed. For Matriderm, vascular structures have been demonstrated as early as day 5 after implantation.[17] At the same time the matrix was fully colonized by fibroblasts.

Denatured collagen—or even worse, chemically cross-linked collagen, like in Integra—does not present the native structure and lacks on binding sites. Cellular in-growth into such matrices is known to last for about 3 to 4 weeks, way too long for a skin graft to survive on top. One potential solution may be to mesh such matrices,[35] but yet there is no clinical evidence proving the long-term benefit for the skin quality based on a meshed dermal matrix. Free permeability for nutrients is the key for early skin graft survival on any given matrix. The term "porosity" evokes associations with holes in a solid material, poorly describing the three-dimensional fibers Matriderm reveals in a micro-computed tomography analysis (Fig. 2).

Durability of the scaffold during wound healing and tissue reorganization is an ambivalent goal. On the one hand the matrix structures need to stay in place long enough to enable neodermis formation instead of plain repair tissue, on the other hand the material shall be integrated and finally metabolized without causing foreign body reaction. During the matrix development for Matriderm, combinations of a number of different components of extracellular matrix in collagen were tested. The

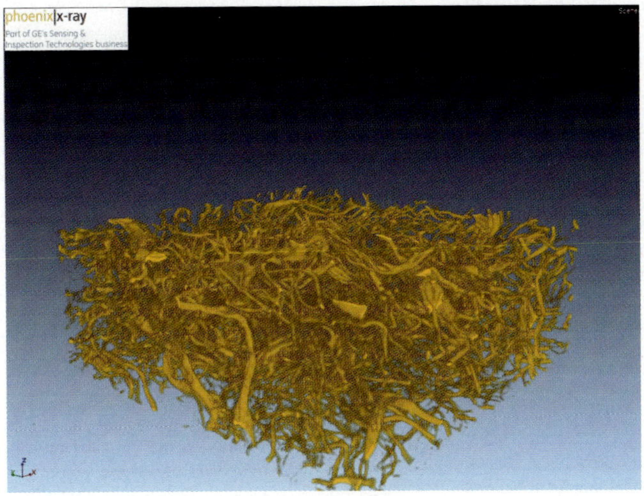

Figure 2. Micro-computed tomography scan of Matriderm. The architecture of the collagen matrix seems to provide a nearly unimpaired fluid exchange between wound bed and graft, enabling an early and complete take of the skin graft in a one-step procedure.

addition of partially hydrolyzed elastin resulted in significantly reduced wound contraction.[36] At the same time this combination proved to be a viable basis for the one-stage grafting procedure with split-skin autograft, and the resulting skin elasticity was significantly improved.[13]

So far, except for the difference associated with the surgical technique (one- *vs.* two-step procedure), where a two-step procedure translates in a prolonged length-of-stay and the need for a second operation, there is no evidence in the literature to be found on the superiority of one of the matrices.

CAUTION, CRITICAL REMARKS, AND RECOMMENDATIONS

The dermal matrix Matriderm has so far delivered reliable results in the one-stage treatment of full-thickness skin defects. The use of the template with split-thickness skin grafts in a one-stage procedure reduces the number of operations, length-of-hospital stay, and time allowed for recovery and reintegration in daily and work life. However, there are some restrictions applying to the use of Matriderm. Its use is only recommended in clean surgical or freshly debrided wounds with no signs of infection. In case of burn injuries, it should be used only after early debridement to result in a similar take-rate of split-thickness skin grafting alone. In the presence of clinical signs of infection its application is not recommended. The use of meshed split-thickness skin grafts in combination with the matrix seems to deliver inferior results in comparison to unmeshed split-thickness skin grafts. Although there are a number of papers in the literature dealing with Matriderm, there is a lack of randomized blinded studies proving its benefit against skin grafting alone or in combination with other dermal substitutes.

FUTURE DEVELOPMENT

With this matrix, an important step in the ladder of developing an ideal skin substitute has been made. The dream of artificial skin off-the-shelf, with all desired layers of subcutis, dermis, and epidermis, integrated seamlessly into a given host organism, however, is still afar. The need for further research and development of skin substitutes is undeniable. Thereby, the technique of tissue engineering will play an important role to reconstruct a skin-like equivalent with similar off-the-shelf properties to a reasonable financial expense.

As economic on a producers' as well as scientific considerations on treating physicians' and surgeons' side come into play, only large multicentric studies will provide a sufficient statistically based power to render results for a health authority–approved broad range of applications for skin-like constructs.

AUTHOR DISCLOSURE STATEMENT

No competing financial interests exist.

REFERENCES

1. Atiyeh BS, Gunn SW, and Hayek SN: State of the art in burn treatment. World J Surg 2005; **29:** 131.
2. Dantzer E and Braye FM: Reconstructive surgery using an artificial dermis (Integra): results with 39 grafts. Br J Plast Surg 2001; **54:** 659.
3. Dantzer E, Queruel P, Salinier L, Palmier B, and Quinot JF: Dermal regeneration template for deep hand burns: clinical utility for both early grafting and reconstructive surgery. Br J Plast Surg 2003; **56:** 764.
4. Heimbach D, Luterman A, Burke J, Cram A, Herndon D, Hunt J, Jordon M, McManus W, Solem L, Warden G, and Zawacki B: Artificial dermis for major burns. A multi-center randomized clinical trial. Ann Surg 1988; **208:** 313.
5. Heitland A, Piatkowski A, Noah EM, and Pallua N: Update on the use of collagen/glycosaminoglycate skin substitute—six years of experiences with artificial skin in 15 German burn centers. Burns 2004; **30:** 471.
6. Jones I, Currie L, and Martin R: A guide to biological skin substitutes. Br J Plast Surg 2002; **55:** 185.

7. Shakespeare P: Burn wound healing and skin substitutes. Burns 2001; **27:** 517.

8. Yannas IV and Burke JF: Design of an artificial skin. I. Basic design principles. J Biomed Mater Res 1980; **14:** 65.

9. Yannas IV, Burke JF, and Gordon PL: Design of an artificial skin. II. Control of chemical composition. J Biomed Mater Res 1980; **14:** 107.

10. Kamolz LP, Kitzinger HB, Karle B, and Frey M: The treatment of hand burns. Burns 2008; **9:** 327.

11. Behr B, Megerle KO, Germann G, and Kloeters O: New concepts in local burn wound therapy. Handchir Mikrochir Plast Chir 2008; **40:** 361.

12. van der Veer WM, Bloemen MC, Ulrich MM, Molema G, van Zuijlen PP, Middelkoop E, and Niessen FB: Potential cellular and molecular causes of hypertrophic scar formation. Burns 2009; **35:** 15.

13. van Zuijlen PP, van Trier AJ, Vloemans JF, Groenevelt F, Kreis RW, and Middelkoop E: Graft survival and effectiveness of dermal substitution in burns and reconstructive surgery in a one-stage grafting model. Plast reconstr Surg 2000; **106:** 615.

14. Haslik W, Kamolz LP, Nathschlager G, Andel H, Meissl G, and Frey M: First experiences with the collagen-elastin matrix Matriderm as a dermal substitute in severe burn injuries of the hand. Burns 2007; **33:** 364.

15. Haslik W, Kamolz LP, Manna F, Hladik M, Rath T, and Frey M: Management of full-thickness skin defects in the hand and wrist region: first long-term experiences with the dermal matrix Matriderm®. J Plast Reconstr Aesthet Surg 2008.

16. Ryssel H, Gazyakan E, Germann G, and Ohlbauer M: The use of MatriDerm in early excision and simultaneous autologous skin grafting in burns—a pilot study. Burns 2008; **34:** 93.

17. Kolokythas P, Aust MC, Vogt PM, and Paulsen F: Dermal subsitute with the collagen-elastin matrix Matriderm in burn injuries: a comprehensive review. Handchir Mikrochir Plast Chir 2008; **40:** 367.

18. Lumenta DB, Kamolz LP, and M.Frey: Adult burn patients with more than 60%TBSA involved—Meek and other techniques to overcome restricted skin harvest availability—the Viennese concept. J Burn Care Res 2009; **30:** 231.

19. Keck M and Ueberreiter K: Successful correction of an adherent scar on the dorsal hand with Matriderm. Handchir Mikrochir Plast Chir 2008; **40:** 197.

20. Pham C, Greenwood J, Cleland H, Woodruff P, and Maddern G: Bioengineered skin substitutes for the management of burns: a systematic review. Burns 2007; **33:** 946.

21. Omar AA, Mavor AI, Jones AM, and Homer-Vanniasinkam S: Treatment of venous leg ulcers with Dermagraft. Eur J Vasc Endovasc Surg 2004; **27:** 666.

22. Marston WA: Dermagraft, a bioengineered human dermal equivalent for the treatment of chronic nonhealing diabetic foot ulcer. Expert Rev Med Devices 2004; **1:** 21.

23. Edmonds M: Apligraf in the treatment of neuropathic diabetic foot ulcers. Int J lower extrem wounds 2009; **8:** 11.

24. Vertrees A, Greer L, Pickett C, Nelson J, Wakefield M, Stojadinovic A and Shriver C: Modern management of complex open abdominal wounds of war: a 5-year experience. J Am Coll Surg 2008; **207:** 801.

25. Awad SS, Rao RK, Berger DH, Albo D, and Bellows CF: Microbiology of infected acellular dermal matrix (AlloDerm) in patients requiring complex abdominal closure after emergency surgery. Surg Infect 2009; **10:** 79.

26. Still J, Glat P, Silverstein P, Griswold J, and Mozingo D: The use of a collagen sponge/living cell composite material to treat donor sites in burn patients. Burns 2003; **29:** 837.

27. Falanga VJ: Tissue engineering in wound repair. Adv Skin Wound Care 2000; **13(2 Suppl):** 15.

28. Veves A, Falanga V, Armstrong DG, and Sabolinski ML: Graftskin, a human skin equivalent, is effective in the management of noninfected neuropathic diabetic foot ulcers: a prospective randomized multicenter clinical trial. Diabetes Care 2001; **24:** 290.

29. Tenenhaus M, Bhavsar D, and Rennekampff HO: Treatment of deep partial thickness and indeterminate depth facial burn wounds with water-jet debridement and a biosynthetic dressing. Injury 2007; **38 Suppl 5:** S39.

30. Amani H, Dougherty WR, and Blome-Eberwein S: Use of Transcyte and dermabrasion to treat burns reduces length of stay in burns of all size and etiology. Burns 2006; **32:** 828.

31. Kumar RJ, Kimble RM, Boots R, and Pegg SP: Treatment of partial-thickness burns: a prospective, randomized trial using Transcyte. ANZ J Surg 2004; **74:** 622.

32. Pape SA and Byrne PO: Safety and efficacy of TransCyte for the treatment of partial-thickness burns. J Burn Care Rehabil 2000; **21:** 390.

33. Heimbach DM, Warden GD, Luterman A, Jordan MH, Ozobia N, Ryan CM, Voight DW, Hickerson WL, Saffle JR, De Clement FA, Sheridan RL and Dimick AR: Multicenter postapproval clinical trial of Integra dermal regeneration template for burn treatment. J Burn Care Rehabil 2003; **24:** 42.

34. Jeng JC, Fidler PE, Sokolich JC, Jaskille AD, Khan S, White PM, Street JH, Light TD, and Jordan MH: Seven years' experience with Integra as a reconstructive tool. J Burn Care Res **2007;** 28: 120.

35. Chu CS, McManus AT, Matylevich NP, Goodwin CW, and Pruitt BA, Jr.: Integra as a dermal replacement in a meshed composite skin graft in a rat model: a one-step operative procedure. J Trauma 2002; **52:** 122.

36. De Vries HJ, Zeegelaar JE, Middelkoop E, Gijsbers G, Van Marle J, Wildevuur CH, and Westerhof W: Reduced wound contraction and scar formation in punch biopsy wounds. Native collagen dermal substitutes. A clinical study. Br J Dermatol 1995; **132:** 690.

How to Achieve Early Vascularization of Tissue-Engineered Skin Substitutes

François Berthod,[1,2,*] Lucie Germain,[1,2] Roxane Pouliot,[1,3] and François A. Auger[1,2]

[1]Laboratoire d'Organogénèse Expérimentale (LOEX), Centre de recherche FRSQ du CHA universitaire de Québec, Hôpital du Saint-Sacrement, Québec, Canada.
[2]Département de chirurgie, Faculté de médecine, Université Laval, Québec, Canada.
[3]Faculté de Pharmacie, Université Laval, Québec, Canada.

Background: The coverage of deep and extensive burns with autologous tissue-engineered skin is a promising strategy to improve the cosmetic aspect and functionality of the skin, compared to the transplantation of simple epithelial sheets. Indeed, a dermal compartment could markedly help to prevent hypertrophic scar formation and to strengthen the dermal–epidermal junction while increasing skin suppleness and pliability.
The Problem: The thickness of the dermis could be a limitation to the survival of the tissue after transplantation, since its vascularization can take up to 2 weeks to occur through neovascularization. This delay could lead to graft necrosis.
Basic/Clinical Science Advances: To overcome this problem, the reconstruction of a preformed network of branching capillaries in the dermis before grafting has proven to be an efficient solution in connecting to the host's vasculature in less than 4 days after grafting. The formation of this capillary-like network is achieved by the coculture of human fibroblasts and endothelial cells in a collagen sponge for a 1-month *in vitro* maturation period. The successful inosculation process between human capillaries and the host's vasculature was demonstrated after grafting onto nude mice.
Clinical Care Relevance: In addition to autologous epithelial sheets and split-thickness autografts, this endothelialized reconstructed skin made of the patient's own cells could be a valuable additional strategy to permanently cover deep wounds.
Conclusion: The reconstruction in tissue-engineered organs of a capillary-like network made of the patient's own cells before grafting is a promising approach to promote their early vascularization.

Abbreviations and Acronyms

CLT = capillary-like tube
ECM = extracellular matrix
VEGF = vascular endothelial growth factor

*Correspondence: Laboratoire d'Organogénèse Expérimentale (LOEX), Centre de recherche FRSQ du CHA universitaire de Québec, Hôpital du Saint-Sacrement, 1050 chemin Sainte-Foy, Québec G1S 4L8, Canada (e-mail: francois.berthod@chg.ulaval.ca).

BACKGROUND

THE COVERAGE OF deep and extensive burns using autologous epithelial sheets has already proven its efficiency as a life-saving treatment. It can considerably decrease the patient's stay in the intensive care burn unit, but the esthetical outcome remains still not optimal. Thus, patients may benefit from the transplantation of an autologous full-thickness tissue-engineered skin, instead of only the epidermis, since the dermis is expected to prevent hypertrophic scar formation and to improve skin elasticity and strength of the dermal–epidermal junction. However, a major drawback is hidden behind this advantage; the quick vascularization of a thicker tissue (over 2-mm thick) remains a challenge. Indeed, the grafted tissue will need to be colonized by new blood vessels through the process of

Printed in U.S.A.
DOI: 10.1089/awc.2009.0084

angiogenesis that will take more time with thicker tissues. Hence, the complete vascularization of a reconstructed skin made of a 2-mm thick dermis was shown to be achieved 2 weeks after transplantation on the nude mouse.[1,2] During this delay, the tissue only survived through diffusion of oxygen and nutrients from the wound bed, and this passive process of diffusion is theoretically limited to a distance of 100 μm (Fig. 1).[3] Thus, this slow vascularization may lead to at least a partial necrosis of the graft, inducing important contraction of the tissue and potential loss of the entire epidermis.

A strategy to overcome this limitation was to impregnate dressings protecting the graft with culture medium during the first week. This procedure works but needs a highly qualified nursing team, is time consuming, and increases the risks of infection.[4]

In addition to the necessary autologous nature of the reconstructed skin (as a permanent coverage), its survival during the first 2 weeks after transplantation still remains a challenge.

CLINICAL PROBLEM ADDRESSED

The best example of a fast vascularization in the treatment of deep and extensive burns is the grafting of cadaver skin as a temporary coverage of the wound bed. This tissue is rapidly and fully revascularized after grafting, as attested by its pink appearance. The fast revascularization of cadaver skin was demonstrated to be mediated through the

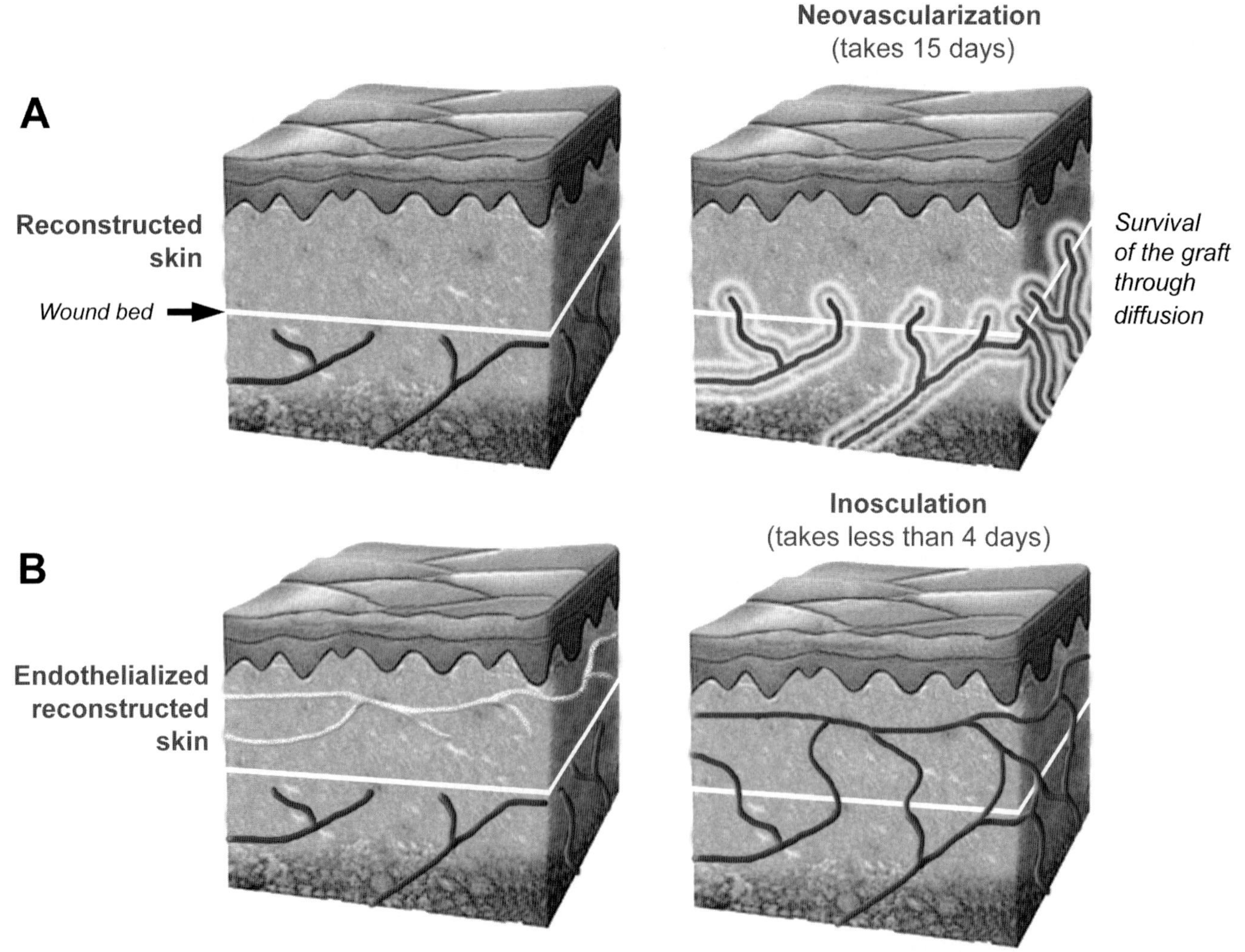

Figure 1. (**A**) When a conventional tissue-engineered reconstructed skin is transplanted on a wound, the graft vascularization is promoted through the process of neovascularization, which needs 2 weeks to be completed. During that period, the graft is nourished through the diffusion of oxygen and nutrients from the blood vessels of the wound. (**B**) When an endothelialized reconstructed skin is transplanted on a wound, the preformed capillary network connects spontaneously with the host's vasculature through the inosculation process. The graft can be fully vascularized in less than 4 days.

process of inosculation, namely, the spontaneous reconnection of the capillaries from the grafted skin with the host's vasculature.[5] This spontaneous anastomosis between capillaries allows a complete vascularization of the whole graft in a matter of hours, instead of weeks through angiogenesis.

RELEVANT BASIC SCIENCE CONTEXT

The best way to achieve a fast vascularization of a reconstructed skin after transplantation should be to speed up angiogenesis to promote a fast growth of new blood vessels in the graft or to build a preformed vascular network inside the reconstructed skin before transplantation.[6] Recombinant growth factors with angiogenic properties are used in the clinic to enhance wound healing.[7] These molecules can be applied on open wounds using ointments, but are much more complex to add in the context of a reconstructed skin that is impermeable after grafting. Since the vascular endothelial growth factor (VEGF) is one of the most potent angiogenic factors, it has been used to promote vascularization in tissue-engineered skin models. A reconstructed skin made of keratinocytes overexpressing VEGF was shown to induce less contraction but did not demonstrate a significant effect 1 week after grafting.[8,9] Moreover, permanent overexpression of VEGF, as well as any angiogenic factor, could be detrimental over time since uncontrolled angiogenesis is implicated in cancer growth, and retroviral transfection could also be a concern.

Since the cells themselves produce growth factors, the addition of endothelial cells instead of molecules was attempted. Endothelial cells are expected at least, to secrete angiogenic factors, and at best, to actively participate in the formation of new capillaries. The incorporation of human endothelial cells into mixed collagen/fibrin gels promoted cord formation within 24 h, but then went into apoptosis.[10] Apoptosis was prevented by transfection of these cells using retroviral-mediated overexpression of a caspase-resistant Bcl-2 protein. These Bcl-2–transduced endothelial cells formed structures resembling microvessels after grafting in mice and enhanced neovascular formation 2 weeks after transplantation.[10,11] Similar works were performed using human endothelial cells or endothelial progenitor cells without Bcl-2 transduction and showed that these cells formed new capillaries after transplantation.[3,8,12,13] However, since endothelial cells were seeded in the reconstructed tissue just before grafting, neovessels were detected in the constructs only after 2 weeks, and thus with such a delay did not provide a significant advantage to these models.

THE ENDOTHELIALIZED HUMAN RECONSTRUCTED SKIN: ADVANTAGES AND LIMITATIONS

To achieve a fast vascularization (within hours) of a tissue-engineered reconstructed skin, capillaries need to be established inside the tissue before grafting. This means that an *in vitro* maturation period of the reconstructed skin is necessary to allow for capillary-like structure formation and organization into a network. Since neovessels need about 2 weeks to form into the entire thickness of a reconstructed skin after transplantation, a similar delay is foreseeable *in vitro* in physiological conditions. To prevent human endothelial cell apoptosis and the use of large amounts of growth factors or tumor-derived molecules such as phorbol myristate acetate or Matrigel™, the coculture of these cells with naturally occurring partners in connective tissues (*e.g.*, fibroblasts) was used in our reconstructed skin model. The key elements to promote capillary-like formation with human endothelial cells are the presence of an extracellular matrix (ECM) on which cells can attach and a source of angiogenic growth factors, such as VEGF. Fibroblasts can provide both components to endothelial cells. A porous scaffold is a good mean to promote ECM production by fibroblasts in a three-dimensional architecture. Since these cells are usually embedded in ECM, they secrete high amounts of collagen and proteins until they fill with ECM the empty pores in which they spread.[14,15] This will allow the deposition of a highly physiological ECM made of human proteins that contains highly specialized molecules such as type XII and XIV collagens as previously described.[16] Another alternative could also be the so-called self-assembly method, that is, the long-term culture of fibroblasts in monolayer on plastic in the presence of ascorbic acid, which promotes ECM deposition around cells. After 28 days of maturation, fibroblasts produce a manipulable cellular sheet made of a very physiological ECM.[17–21] The production of stable capillary-like tubes (CLTs) can also be induced in this model.[22,23]

DISCUSSION

We used a collagen–chitosan sponge scaffold to promote ECM deposition by the coculture of human endothelial cells and fibroblasts, because this model is easy to handle and allows a suitable modulation of the final size of the reconstructed tissue. We demonstrated that ECM produced by fibroblasts is an ideal environment that promotes capillary-like formation. In the presence of fibroblasts, but in conditions that prevent ECM deposition, only very few capillaries were detected.[24] However, ECM alone in the absence of living fibroblasts was not sufficient to promote capillary-like formation. In addition, fibroblasts need to be closely associated with the endothelial cells to trigger capillary-like formation, mainly through the local release of VEGF.[24]

Then, after 31 days of *in vitro* maturation, a three-dimensional network of capillary-like structures is formed in the reconstructed tissue.[25] These capillaries present an internal lumen in which no ECM was observed, indicating that it is a closed structure. They are made of endothelial cells, as demonstrated by the presence of Weibel Palade bodies in their cytoplasm (using transmission electron microscopy) and closely associated through tight junctions.[26] This CLT formation was shown to be sensitive to angiogenic and angiostatic drugs. This is a powerful model to study human angiogenesis *in vitro*.[27]

But the fundamental question to address was to determine whether these CLTs composed of a preformed network of capillaries in a reconstructed skin could connect to the host's vasculature after transplantation on wounds, and if they could speed up the vascularization of the graft.

The human endothelialized reconstructed skin was transplanted on immunodeficient mice for 2 weeks, and the graft vascularization was followed. In the nonendothelialized reconstructed skin used as negative controls, no blood was detected underneath the epidermis before 2 weeks, and this late vascularization was achieved through neovascularization as assessed by the staining of mouse endothelial cells.[1] In contrast, we demonstrated that some human capillaries (detected by their expression of both, the human leukocyte antigen and the von Willebrand factor) containing mouse blood (stained by a specific mouse red blood cells antibody) were observed underneath the endothelialized reconstructed skin epidermis at 4 days after transplantation.[1] This showed that (1) the human capillaries can connect through inosculation to the mouse vasculature, (2) this connection occurred very early after transplantation, and (3) vascularization occurred throughout the whole thickness of the graft and up to the epidermis, which shows that the CLT network was well distributed and that these capillaries communicate to each other (Fig. 1). After 2 weeks, some chimeric blood vessels

TAKE-HOME MESSAGE

Basic science advances

- The endothelialized reconstructed skin is a powerful *in vitro* model to study angiogenesis and to determine the angiogenic or angiostatic potential of various molecules or drugs. Indeed, this model allows the spontaneous formation of a network of CLTs in absence of extraphysiological amounts of growth factors or tumor-derived molecules.
- This enables the detection of a subtle angiogenic effect of a molecule.
- The model can be cultured for over 40 days *in vitro*, which allows the analysis of the long-term effect of drugs on angiogenesis.
- Molecules can be supplemented in the culture medium for 1 week at an early stage (*i.e.*, during CLT formation) or a late stage (after CLT stabilization). Their effect can be followed for 1 or 2 weeks after removal to assess whether it is reversible.
- An effect of general toxicity can also be monitored.[27]
- Such long-term effect assessment of the angiostatic potential of drugs is essential in the perspective of the evaluation of an anticancer therapy.

Clinical science advances

- The development of an autologous endothelialized reconstructed skin is a major breakthrough in the coverage of deep and extensive burns.
- It allows the reconstruction of a 2-mm thick dermis, which is known to achieve a much better healing quality compared to autologous epithelial sheets and efficiently prevents hypertrophic scar formation.
- The preformed capillary network in this thick reconstructed skin promotes a fast vascularization of the graft in less than 4 days that enhances its survival and prevents contraction.
- The efficacy of this tissue-engineered skin to cover burns should be equivalent to split-thickness skin grafts while being available in large surface without the need to harvest skin on donor sites.

Relevance to clinical care

- Based on our practice with autologous epithelial sheet transplantation, handling and grafting of endothelialized reconstructed skin on wounds may be even simpler than epidermal sheets since these constructs are much less fragile and are easier to manipulate.
- Because this autologous reconstructed skin accomplishes a permanent coverage of the wound, it should considerably decrease the length of stay of the patient in the burn unit, and thus decrease the risk of infection for the patient and the cost of the treatment while achieving a functionally better and more cosmetically pleasing skin.

made of the human and mouse endothelial cells in a branching pattern were observed.[1]

This work provides the first demonstration of an inosculation process between human reconstructed capillaries and the mouse vasculature in a tissue-engineered skin.

This result shows that the reconstruction of a CLT network in a tissue-engineered organ before its transplantation could be a valuable strategy to achieve a very fast vascularization of the tissue after grafting. Theoretically, if a CLT network is homogeneously distributed throughout the whole tissue, vascularization of thick tissues may no longer be a limitation.

Nevertheless, this strategy implies that we have access to fibroblasts, keratinocytes, and endothelial cells from the patient by isolation from a single small skin biopsy. Such triple cell extraction is feasible (Marie-Hélène Rochon, unpublished observation, and Ref.[28]), though difficult to perform, especially if it needs to be done rapidly and to generate large amounts of cells. In addition, the preformed CLT network needs at least 3 weeks of *in vitro* maturation to be properly organized.

For clinical applications, the preparation of an autologous endothelialized reconstructed skin will need highly qualified personnel and infrastructures to be applied in the clinic. However, the example of the commercialization of autologous epithelial sheets by Genzyme Corporation™ (Cambridge, MA) is a proof of concept that it is feasible. The cost of this product may be very high, but it will be a permanent coverage that could save the life of severely burnt patients. Also, it might notably decrease the length of the patient's stay at the burn unit. Thus, it would be cost efficient.

CAUTION, CRITICAL REMARKS, AND RECOMMENDATIONS

As experienced in the clinic with the coverage of wounds using autologous epithelial sheets, this approach of harvesting and growing patient's cells *in vitro*, followed by engineered tissue reconstruction, is very efficient to treat deep and extensive burns. As with epithelial sheets, the primary aim is to save patients' lives, but with endothelialized reconstructed skin, a secondary goal will be to greatly improve the healing quality and cosmetic results. However, this new skin will still lack melanocytes, hair, and sweat and sebaceous glands. Moreover, the preparation of the tissue will take at least 1 month before being able to perform the first transplantation. Thus, a combination of techniques should be the best way to treat the severely burnt patients. Conventional split-thickness autografts in the initial weeks will still be the gold standard for burn treatment. However, autograft harvesting will generate additional donor sites that could be covered with autologous epithelial sheets, known by clinicians to be an excellent strategy for a much faster and better healing of these secondary wounds. After 1 month, endothelialized reconstructed skin will be available for transplantation on the remaining wounds. Moreover, the subsequent esthetical surgery procedures can be performed using reconstructed skin engineered from previously developed cell banks from each patient, which in turn avoids additional and painful patient skin harvesting. As discussed above, the production of these living tissue-engineered substitutes requires good infrastructures and quality control to ascertain the quality of the reconstruction methods and cell populations. For example, the preservation of stem cells during the epithelial cell culture *in vitro* is essential to insure long-term regeneration of the epidermis.[29]

FUTURE DEVELOPMENTS

Vascularization of tissue-engineered organs is essential to achieve lasting survival after transplantation. However, incorporation of melanocytes and sweat and sebaceous glands into a reconstructed skin could be a set of important next steps. The recovery of pain, temperature, and sensory perception of skin is also of major importance. Incorporation of molecules in the tissue-engineered skin that enhance nerve regeneration after grafting has been shown as a powerful strategy to promote sensory perception recovery.[30] The integration of hair follicles and Schwann cells could also be beneficial.

Finally, the enrichment of the tissue-engineered skin with the patient's own stem cells could be a valuable strategy to speed up its reconstruction and in the development of tissues that will retain a strong potential for autorepair after grafting.[29,31]

ACKNOWLEDGMENTS

This research was supported by the Canadian Institutes of Health Research grant MOP-14364. The authors thank Todd Galbraith for his skilled revision of the manuscript.

AUTHOR DISCLOSURE STATEMENT

No competing financial interests exist.

REFERENCES

1. Tremblay PL, Hudon V, Berthod F, Germain L, and Auger FA: Inosculation of tissue-engineered capillaries with the host's vasculature in a reconstructed skin transplanted on mice. Am J Transplant 2005; **5:** 1002.
2. Berthod F, Germain L, Li H, Xu W, Damour O, and Auger FA: Collagen fibril network and elastic system remodeling in a reconstructed skin transplanted on nude mice. Matrix Biol 2001; **20:** 463.
3. Kannan RY, Salacinski HJ, Sales K, Butler P, and Seifalian AM: The roles of tissue engineering and vascularisation in the development of microvascular networks: a review. Biomaterials 2005; **26:** 1857.
4. Boyce ST, Supp AP, Harriger DM, Greenhalgh DG, and Warden GD: Topical nutrients promote engraftment and inhibit wound contraction of cultured skin substitutes in athymic mice. J Invest Dermatol 1995; **104:** 345.
5. Young DM, Greulich KM, and Weier HG: Species-specific *in situ* hybridization with fluorochrome-labeled DNA probes to study vascularization of human skin grafts on athymic mice. J Burn Care Rehabil 1996; **17:** 305.
6. Sahota PS, Burn JL, Brown NJ, and MacNeil S: Approaches to improve angiogenesis in tissue-engineered skin. Wound Repair Regen 2004; **12:** 635.
7. Li WW, Talcott KE, Zhai AW, Kruger EA, and Li VW: The role of therapeutic angiogenesis in tissue repair and regeneration. Adv Skin Wound Care 2005; **18:** 491.
8. Supp DM, Wilson-Landy K, and Boyce ST: Human dermal microvascular endothelial cells form vascular analogs in cultured skin substitutes after grafting to athymic mice. FASEB J 2002; **16:** 797.
9. Dickens S, Vermeulen P, Hendrickx B, Van den Berge S, and Vranckx JJ: Regulable vascular endothelial growth factor165 overexpression by *ex vivo* expanded keratinocyte cultures promotes matrix formation, angiogenesis, and healing in porcine full-thickness wounds. Tissue Eng Part A 2008; **14:** 19.
10. Schechner JS, Nath AK, Zheng L, Kluger MS, Hughes CC, Sierra-Honigmann MR, *et al.*: *In vivo* formation of complex microvessels lined by human endothelial cells in an immunodeficient mouse. Proc Natl Acad Sci USA 2000; **97:** 9191.
11. Schechner JS, Crane SK, Wang F, Szeglin AM, Tellides G, Lorber MI, *et al.*: Engraftment of a vascularized human skin equivalent. FASEB J 2003; **17:** 2250.
12. Nor JE, Peters MC, Christensen JB, Sutorik MM, Linn S, Khan MK, *et al.*: Engineering and characterization of functional human microvessels in immunodeficient mice. Lab Invest 2001; **81:** 453.
13. Shepherd BR, Enis DR, Wang F, Suarez Y, Pober JS, and Schechner JS: Vascularization and engraftment of a human skin substitute using circulating progenitor cell-derived endothelial cells. FASEB J 2006; **20:** 1739.
14. Berthod F, Hayek D, Damour O, and Collombel C: Collagen synthesis by fibroblasts cultured within a collagen sponge. Biomaterials 1993; **14:** 749.
15. Berthod F, Sahuc F, Hayek D, Damour O, and Collombel C: Deposition of collagen fibril bundles by long-term culture of fibroblasts in a collagen sponge. J Biomed Mater Res 1996; **32:** 87.
16. Berthod F, Germain L, Guignard R, Lethias C, Garrone R, Damour O, *et al.*: Differential expression of collagen XII and XIV in human skin and in reconstructed skin. J Invest Dermatol 1997; **108:** 737.
17. Laplante AF, Germain L, Auger FA, and Moulin V: Mechanisms of wound reepithelialization: hints from a tissue-engineered reconstructed skin to long-standing questions. FASEB J 2001; **15:** 2377.
18. Grenier G, Remy-Zolghadri M, Larouche D, Gauvin R, Baker K, Bergeron F, *et al.*: Tissue reorganization in response to mechanical load increases functionality. Tissue Eng 2005; **11:** 90.
19. Laflamme K, Roberge CJ, Pouliot S, D'Orleans-Juste P, Auger FA, and Germain L: Tissue-engineered human vascular media produced *in vitro* by the self-assembly approach present functional properties similar to those of their native blood vessels. Tissue Eng 2006; **12:** 2275.
20. Larouche D, Paquet C, Fradette J, Carrier P, Auger FA, and Germain L: Regeneration of skin and cornea by tissue engineering. Methods Mol Biol 2009; **482:** 233.
21. Jean J, Lapointe M, Soucy J, and Pouliot R: Development of an *in vitro* psoriatic skin model by tissue engineering. J Dermatol Sci 2009; **53:** 19.
22. Rochon M-H, Fradette J, Fortin V, Tomasetig F, Roberge C-J, Baker K, *et al.*: Normal human epithelial cells regulate the size and morphology of tissue-engineered capillaries. Tissue Eng 2010; Under revision.
23. Sorrell JM, Baber MA, and Caplan AI: A self-assembled fibroblast-endothelial cell co-culture system that supports *in vitro* vasculogenesis by both human umbilical vein endothelial cells and human dermal microvascular endothelial cells. Cells Tissues Organs 2007; **186:** 157.
24. Berthod F, Germain L, Tremblay N, and Auger FA: Extracellular matrix deposition by fibroblasts is necessary to promote capillary-like tube formation *in vitro*. J Cell Physiol 2006; **207:** 491.
25. Hudon V, Berthod F, Black AF, Damour O, Germain L, and Auger FA: A tissue-engineered endothelialized dermis to study the modulation of angiogenic and angiostatic molecules on capillary-like tube formation *in vitro*. Br J Dermatol 2003; **148:** 1094.
26. Black A, Berthod F, L'Heureux N, Germain L, and Auger FA: *In vitro* reconstruction of a human capillary-like network in a tissue-engineered skin equivalent. FASEB J 1998; **12:** 1331.
27. Tremblay PL, Berthod F, Germain L, and Auger FA: *In vitro* evaluation of the angiostatic potential of drugs using an endothelialized tissue-engineered connective tissue. J Pharmacol Exp Ther 2005; **315:** 510.
28. Magnan M, Berthod F, Champigny M-F, Soucy F, and Bolduc S: *In vitro* reconstruction of a tissue-engineered endothelialized bladder from a single porcine biopsy. J Pediatr Urol 2006; **2:** 261.
29. Larouche D, Tong X, Fradette J, Coulombe PA, and Germain L: Vibrissa hair bulge houses two populations of skin epithelial stem cells distinct by their keratin profile. FASEB J 2008; **22:** 1404.
30. Caissie R, Gingras M, Champigny MF, and Berthod F: *In vivo* enhancement of sensory perception recovery in a tissue-engineered skin enriched with laminin. Biomaterials 2006; **27:** 2988.
31. Trottier V, Marceau-Fortier G, Germain L, Vincent C, and Fradette J: IFATS collection: using human adipose-derived stem/stromal cells for the production of new skin substitutes. Stem Cells 2008; **26:** 2713.

WHS
Wound
Healing
Society

Self-Assembled Scaffold-Free Three-Dimensional Micro-Tissues for Tissue Repair

Jacquelyn Youssef and Jeffrey R. Morgan*

Department of Molecular Pharmacology, Physiology, and Biotechnology, Brown University, Providence, Rhode Island.

Background: The growth of cells *in vitro* is of great importance to basic and applied research in all areas of biomedical research, including wound healing.
The Problem: For years, the two-dimensional culture of cells on rigid plastic dishes has been the method of choice; however, it is increasingly recognized that three-dimensional (3D) models more closely mimic *in vivo* tissue architecture and function. Most 3D models combine a small number of cells with a large amount of scaffold (natural or synthetic), maximizing cell-to-scaffold interactions, but in most *in vivo* tissues, cell-to-cell interactions are the most important.
Basic/Clinical Science Advances: We have developed a new, straightforward, scaffold-free method to culture cells in 3D, which thus maximizes cell-to-cell interactions. Monodispersed cells are added to micro-molded agarose and they self-assemble into 3D micro-tissues. Size is easy to control, and we have shown that cells will self-assemble complex branching structures such as a honeycomb. When a mix of two different cell types is added, the cells will self-assemble and often self-sort with one cell type forming the core, and the other the outer coating. Such structures more closely mimic the heterotypic cell-to-cell interactions of *in vivo* tissues.
Relevance to Clinical Care: 3D micro-tissues will be useful for understanding disease processes, drug discovery, and toxicity testing and may be useful as tissue transplants.
Conclusion: A new 3D cell culture method that maximizes cell-to-cell interactions has been developed with a wide range of basic and translational applications.

Abbreviations and Acronyms

2D = two-dimensional
3D = three-dimensional
ECM = extracellular matrix
NHF = normal human fibroblast
PDMS = polydimethylsiloxane

*Correspondence: Department of Molecular Pharmacology, Physiology, and Biotechnology, Brown University, 34 Olive St., Providence, Rhode Island 02912 (e-mail: jeffrey_morgan@brown.edu).

BACKGROUND

THE CHALLENGE OF DEVELOPING *in vitro* culture conditions that more closely mimic the *in vivo* environment is ever present. Current two-dimensional (2D) models, such as the rigid plastic Petri dish, are inadequate at emulating the complex mechanical and biochemical surroundings of the body.[1] Culturing cells on flat surfaces results in the loss of important cell-to-cell and cell-to-extracellular matrix (ECM) interactions critical for cellular phenotype.[2] As a result, new three-dimensional (3D) models are being developed.

Many approaches have been developed to culture cells in 3D using scaffolds, sponges, and gels. In these methods, cells are combined with either a natural (*e.g.*, collagen) or a synthetic [*e.g.*, poly(lactic-co-glycolic acid)] biomaterial to form a 3D construct where cell-to-ECM interactions are maximized. Research in the field of wound healing led to the development of one of the first and most successful 3D models—the

Printed in U.S.A.
DOI: 10.1089/awc.2009.0130

fibroblast-populated collagen lattice.[3] In this 3D model, a relatively small number of fibroblasts is gelled within a collagen lattice to create a mimic of the dermis, a tissue where cell density is low and ECM is abundant. The fibroblasts contract and remodel the collagen gel, and this model has been widely used in wound healing research. These sorts of scaffolds have been proposed for both *in vitro* research and *in vivo* transplantation.[4–6] A limitation, however, is that cell-to-ECM interactions are maximized while cell-to-cell interactions are minimized, as the percentage of scaffold greatly outnumbers the percentage of cells. Although these environments are a step closer to the *in vivo* environment, they are inadequate for tissue environments in which cell-to-cell interactions dominate such as epithelial, hepatic, and many other organ types in which the ECM is a small fraction of the tissue's composition. These models also do not emulate processes such as embryogenesis, morphogenesis, tumorigenesis, and tissue fusion, all of which are thought to rely highly on cell-to-cell interactions.[7–9] Necessary for *in vitro* research are 3D cellular constructs that maximize cell-to-cell interactions.

CLINICAL PROBLEM ADDRESSED

The culture of cells *in vitro* is a process of fundamental importance to a wide range of clinical problems. Often, cells from patients or animal models are cultured *in vitro* in an attempt to mimic the disease process and to seek an understanding of the molecular basis of disease for basic science studies. Cultured cells are also used in the drug discovery process to find new therapeutics and to test for toxicity. With breakthroughs in stem cell research and the emerging field of tissue engineering, cultured cells are increasingly being considered as transplants to replace or repair diseased tissues.

RELEVANT BASIC SCIENCE CONTEXT

Self-assembly is the process by which monodispersed cells will aggregate via cell-to-cell adhesions, thus forming a 3D cellular micro-tissue. In self-assembled micro-tissues, the only ECM present is that which is produced by the cells. Because cell-to-cell interactions are maximized, self-assembled micro-tissues are thought to more closely emulate processes driven by cell-to-cell contacts that are hard to model in traditional 3D culture.[7–9] Moreover, micro-tissues exhibit properties closer to that of native tissues, including micro-tissues of myocardial cells that beat with a human-like rhythm, hepatocyte micro-tissues that have superior detoxifying function, cartilage micro-tissues that maintain their differentiated phenotype, dorsal root ganglion cells extending projections into fibroblast micro-tissues, and human endothelial cells vascularizing fibroblast micro-tissues.[10–13]

Prior methods (liquid overlay, spinner culture, and hanging drop) have associated limitations (Table 1). In liquid overlay, cells are seeded onto a flat nonadhesive material such as agarose.[14] With small amounts of shaking, the cells aggregate and form spherical micro-tissues (spheroids). However, there is a large and heterogeneous distribution in the sizes of the spheroids and also a small yield of micro-tissues. The spinner culture and rotating wall vessel methods prevent cells from settling, and as they collide with one another, they form spheroids.[15–17] Although these methods can form large numbers of micro-tissues, it is difficult to control size, and therefore sizes vary. In the hanging drop method, a small volume of cell suspension is pipetted onto the surface of a Petri dish lid, which is inverted causing the cells to settle to the bottom of the drop where they form spheroids. Spheroid size is less variable, but the method is labor intensive and it is difficult to change

Table 1. *Techniques for the self-assembly of micro-tissues with associated benefits*

	Hanging Drop	Liquid Overlay	Rotating Wall Vessel	Spinner Culture	Micro-Molded Hydrogels
Good size control	+				+
Low shear stresses	+	+			+
High yield			+	+	+
Good control of heterotypic cell-to-cell ratio	+				+
Minimal labor			+	+	+
Easy-to-handle micro-tissues			+	+	+
Possibility of complex shapes					+
Observe by microscopy	+	+			+
Cell-type independent	+	+			+
Ubiquitous	+	+		+	

medium or harvest spheroids. None of these methods can self-assemble micro-tissues with complex shapes.

EXPERIMENTAL MODEL AND MATERIALS

Many of the limitations of the past methods were overcome when our lab developed a new method based on micro-molded nonadhesive hydrogels for the self-assembly of 3D micro-tissues.[18,19] This versatile technology starts with computer-aided design software and uses rapid prototyping and replica molding to make a polydimethylsiloxane (PDMS) rubber mold for casting agarose gels. In one design, the PDMS mold has an array of 820 cylindrical pegs, which are 800 μm tall, each with a hemispherical cap. These pegs are situated on a rectangular stage. Molten agarose is added to the PDMS mold, and after the agarose solidifies it is separated from the PDMS mold. The resulting agarose gel has a seeding chamber with 820 small recesses that are molded into the surface of the gel. The gels are then equilibrated in cell culture medium for at least 12 h; when a cell suspension is added to the seeding chamber, the cells settle and aggregate on the bottom of the small recesses. Because the agarose environment is nonadhesive, the cells attach to one another and form a single spherical micro-tissue at the bottom of each recess. In a single pipetting step it is possible to form 820 micro-tissues. The hydrogel technology has the high throughput and ease of handling of the spinner culture method combined with the size consistency of the hanging drop method. The method has been used with a variety of cell types derived from many tissues, including the skin, brain, liver, heart, artery, breast, and ovary. To date, over 20 different cell types have been tested. Because the gels are transparent, the process of self-assembly can be monitored by microscopy.

DISCUSSION OF FINDINGS AND RELEVANT LITERATURE

In addition to forming large numbers of uniform-sized micro-tissues in a single step, the micro-molded gels have several other practical advantages. First, micro-tissue size can be easily controlled by adjusting the number of cells seeded. Fewer cells form smaller micro-tissues. Second, micro-tissues with two or more cell types can be formed by seeding a mixture of cells. The ratio of cells in the micro-tissue is controlled by the ratio of cells in the mixture. Lastly, changing the medium or adding growth factors or even a second batch of cells is easy to do because the micro-tissues are at the bottom of the recesses.

TAKE-HOME MESSAGE

New *in vitro* 3D cell culture models are needed to better mimic tissue architecture, function, and disease processes. These 3D models can bridge the gap between *in vitro* and *in vivo* studies and serve to provide more clinically relevant data. Such models can provide important basic information about disease processes, and serve as platforms for drug discovery and toxicity testing. Moreover, some 3D culture models are being transplanted and used for tissue regeneration and repair.

We have developed a new and straightforward method for 3D cell culture that maximizes cell-to-cell interactions that may be useful for bridging this difficult gap between *in vitro* and *in vivo* research. The technology relies on the ability of cells to aggregate and self-assemble a 3D micro-tissue, and the method provides straightforward ways for monitoring the process of self-assembly for a variety of cell types. It also presents the option of examining how cells self-assemble and what mechanisms are directing the process. Novel assays based on shapes such as rods, toroids, and loop-ended dogbones present simple models of phenomena that occur in the body such as tissue fusion, tissue contraction, cell elongation, and morphogenesis.

Using the micro-molded hydrogel technology, there are new potential methods to engineer tissues with a variety of structures. Past methods of self-assembly only could create spherical micro-tissues. With this new method, micro-tissues with complex shapes can be easily created. The technology also presents the option of creating living building blocks that can be fused to form even larger more complex structures and to control the position of different cell types within those structures. By being able to control cell position, the possibility of making epithelialized or vascularized tissues is now feasible. Moreover, having the ability to control cell location and tissue shape has the potential of overcoming past limitations associated with using self-assembled micro-tissues as viable tissue replacements. Unlike many engineered tissue replacements, which are simplified as cells randomly distributed within a scaffold, these micro-tissues mimic natural tissues that are conglomerates of multiple cell types located in distinct regions within a complex architecture. Also toward more natural tissue models and tissue replacements, complex-shaped micro-tissues may provide more flexibility in terms of size. Spherical micro-tissues are constrained in size by the diffusion limits of nutrients and waste products. However, shapes such as the toroid and honeycomb have open lumens that could result in much larger micro-tissues that could accommodate for nutrient diffusion. In comparison to many current tissue replacements, these micro-tissues are a scaffold-free tissue. This eliminates any adverse reactions to the scaffold (synthetic or natural), and these micro-tissues may more closely emulate tissues with low ECM content. All of these benefits render self-assembled micro-tissues as a feasible and attractive addition to the current tissue replacement and *in vitro* models.

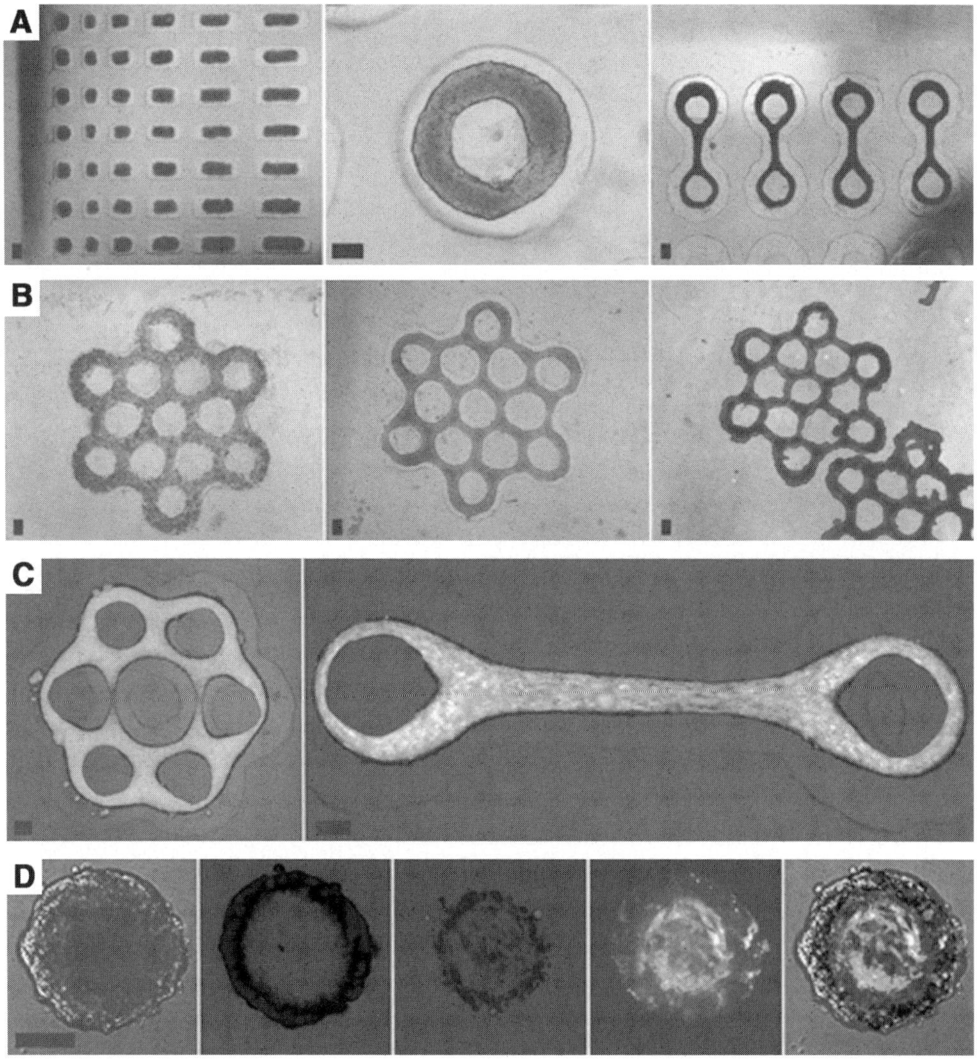

Figure 1. Micro-molded hydrogels can be used to direct the self-assembly of a number of shapes, including rods, toroids, loop-ended dogbones, and honeycombs. (**A**) H35 rods (left), MCF-7 (a breast cancers cell torid) (middle), and H35 loop-ended dogbone (right). (**B**) MCF-7 seeded in honeycomb recesses (left), MCF-7s honeycomb compacts slightly 1 day after seeding (middle), and MCF-7s maintain patent lumens of branched structure up to 3 days postremoval from gels (right). (**C**) Heterotypic honeycomb (left) and loop-ended dogbone (right) micro-tissues composed of normal human fibroblasts and H35s (right). (**D**) Self-sorting of 2-day tritypic spheroid from left to right: differential interference contrast microscopy; H35s; normal human fibroblasts; human umbilical vein endothelial cells; and the composite image. Scale bars are 200 μm in (**A–C**) and 100 μm in (**D**).[19] © 2007 BioTechniques. Used by permission.

A key advance uncovered with the micro-molded hydrogel technology is the observation that self-assembly is not limited to spherical structures; that is, cells can be directed to self-assemble complex-shaped structures such as a honeycomb[18–20] (Fig. 1). Past methods were not able to form complex shapes. In fact, it was thought that cells could only self-assemble a spheroid, because that structure minimized surface free energy. Micro-molded hydrogels can also be used for the assembly of rod-shaped, toroid-shaped, loop-ended dogbone-shaped, and honeycomb-shaped micro-tissues by changing the design of the recess features.[19]

Another key finding was that different cell types differ in their ability to form and maintain these complex shaped micro-tissues.[19,20] Specifically, we compared the self-assembly of two distinct cell types—normal human fibroblast (NHF), derived from neonatal foreskin, and H35 cells, a rat hepatocyte cell line.[20] By seeding NHFs and H35s into trough-like recesses, it was demonstrated that NHFs assembled into micro-tissues rapidly ($<$12 h) and did not maintain elongated structures, but rather contracted to spherical micro-tissues. In contrast, H35s self-assembled much slower (1–2 days), and maintained complex shapes such as a rod, a toroid, and a honeycomb.[20]

We have used micro-tissues with complex shapes to understand the fundamental processes controlling cell-to-cell adhesion and self-assembly. For example, we used molds with trough-shaped recesses to show that cytoskeletal-mediated tension is important in self-assembly.[21] Inhibitors of cytoskeletal-mediated tension, such as blebbistatin and Y-27632, slowed the rate of self-assembly and also stabilized micro-tissues with complex shapes, such as a toroids and loop-ended dogbones.[21,22] Moreover, these inhibitors were shown to influence the self-sorting of cells in 3D.[21] Before these studies, it was thought that self-assembly was driven predominately by the action of surface adhesion molecules such as cadherins.[8,23,24] The processes of cell-to-cell adhesion and cytoskeletal-mediated tension are of fundamental importance to wound healing, where cells need to exert adhesive and traction forces to move into or cover areas in need of repair. Likewise, cellular mechanical forces are highly active in areas of repair and fibrosis. In our loop-ended dogbone molds, NHFs exerted strong forces that caused the dramatic elongation of cells and ultimately the rupture of the 3D micro-tissue. Such 3D micro-tissues can be used to investigate these forces.

With an eye toward tissue engineering, we have used molds with honeycomb-shaped recesses showing that one or more cell types can be used to form honeycombs with patent lumens. Such complex-shaped micro-tissues could be used in a number of applications, including bioreactor development and the engineering of tissue equivalents with endothelialized lumens.[20] We have also shown that 3D micro-tissues can be used as building blocks to make even larger structures.[25] Spheroids formed in micro-molded agarose were cultured for different times, harvested, and added to a second mold with trough-shaped recesses, where these living building blocks underwent tissue fusion. An important finding was that tissue fusion could be controlled by preculture time. Longer preculture time resulted in less and more controllable tissue fusion. This finding was extended to show that it could be used to control cell position in 3D when fusing heterotypic building blocks containing two different cell types. Previously, it was thought that cell position in heterotypic spheroids was solely determined by cohesive and adhesive surface interactions of the cell types involved. Using this straightforward approach, it was possible to generate a number of archetypal 3D structures that mimic complex *in vivo* tissue architectures.

CAUTION, CRITICAL REMARKS, AND RECOMMENDATIONS

Although there are advantages to 3D micro-tissues compared to 2D culture, there are still a number of limitations that must be overcome. Micro-tissues are several cell layers thick and depend on diffusion for gas and nutrient exchange, and the size of the aggregate has to be carefully controlled to avoid necrotic cores. It is not clear if this size constraint is the same for all cells, as cell types may differ on their requirements for oxygen and nutrients. Size constraints could be overcome with the development of vascularized or lumen containing micro-tissues that can be perfused and there is exciting progress in this area.[26,27] Also as a caution, nearly all cell culture medium has been optimized for cell growth and differentiation in conventional 2D culture dishes. To account for differences in cell phenotype, migration, and proliferation, medium needs be optimized for 3D. When compared to cells grown on flat dishes, 3D micro-tissues are considerably thicker and not as amenable to high magnification microscopy techniques. Currently, there are a number of automated assays and culture techniques that have been developed for 2D culture, and these methods need to be developed for 3D micro-tissues. As well, for these tissues to be a viable tissue replacement, limitations associated with size, transplantability, mechanical strength, and biological function need to be further investigated.

FUTURE DEVELOPMENTS

As a platform technology, future work with self-assembled 3D micro-tissues can proceed in a number of directions. As a basic science tool, the technology can be used to develop new and more realistic models of normal and diseased tissues for basic and applied studies. The method is especially useful in cases such as fibrotic diseases where cellular mechanics contribute to the progression of disease. Our lab is using the method to understand the self-assembly process by quantifying the role of cell-to-cell adhesion, cytoskeletal-mediated tension, and the contribution of specific molecules. Understanding the rules of self-assembly and how to control them will provide insight into biological processes of fundamental importance to wound healing, cancer, and developmental biology. This information and an understanding of tissue fusion will enable us to build ever more complex structures and to test these structures as tissue replacements and substitutes.

AUTHOR DISCLOSURE STATEMENT

The authors do not have commercial associations that might create or pose a conflict of interest in connection with this chapter.

REFERENCES

1. Pampaloni F, Reynaud EG, and Stelzer EH: The third dimension bridges the gap between cell culture and live tissue. Nat Rev Mol Cell Biol 2007; **8:** 839.
2. Kleinman HK, Philp D, and Hoffman MP: Role of the extracellular matrix in morphogenesis. Curr Opin Biotechnol 2003; **14:** 526.
3. Bell E, Ehrlich HP, Buttle DJ, and Nakatsuji T: Living tissue formed *in vitro* and accepted as skin-equivalent tissue of full thickness. Science 1981; **211:** 1052.
4. Griffith LG and Naughton G: Tissue engineering—current challenges and expanding opportunities. Science 2002; **295:** 1009.
5. Ingber DE and Levin M: What lies at the interface of regenerative medicine and developmental biology? Development 2007; **134:** 2541.
6. Langer R and Vacanti JP: Tissue engineering. Science 1993; **260:** 920.
7. Duguay D, Foty RA, and Steinberg MS: Cadherin-mediated cell adhesion and tissue segregation: qualitative and quantitative determinants. Dev Biol 2003; **253:** 309.
8. Foty RA, Pfleger CM, Forgacs G, and Steinberg MS: Surface tensions of embryonic tissues predict their mutual envelopment behavior. Development 1996; **122:** 1611.
9. Moscona A and Moscona H: The dissociation and aggregation of cells from organ rudiments of the early chick embryo. J Anat 1952; **86:** 287.
10. Fukuda J and Nakazawa K: Orderly arrangement of hepatocyte spheroids on a microfabricated chip. Tissue Eng 2005; **11:** 1254.
11. Kelm JM and Fussenegger M: Microscale tissue engineering using gravity-enforced cell assembly. Trends Biotechnol 2004; **22:** 195.
12. Kelm JM, Ittner LM, Born W, Djonov V, and Fussenegger M: Self-assembly of sensory neurons into ganglia-like microtissues. J Biotechnol 2006; **121:** 86.
13. Kunz-Schughart LA, Schroeder JA, Wondrak M, van Rey F, Lehle K, Hofstaedter F, and Wheatley DN: Potential of fibroblasts to regulate the formation of three-dimensional vessel-like structures from endothelial cells *in vitro*. Am J Physiol Cell Physiol 2006; **290:** C1385.
14. Enmon RM Jr., O'Connor KC, Lacks DJ, Schwartz DK, and Dotson RS: Dynamics of spheroid self-assembly in liquid-overlay culture of DU 145 human prostate cancer cells. Biotechnol Bioeng 2001; **72:** 579.
15. Castaneda F and Kinne RK: Short exposure to millimolar concentrations of ethanol induces apoptotic cell death in multicellular HepG2 spheroids. J Cancer Res Clin Oncol 2000; **126:** 305.
16. Foty RA and Steinberg MS: The differential adhesion hypothesis: a direct evaluation. Dev Biol 2005; **278:** 255.
17. Manley P and Lelkes PI: A novel real-time system to monitor cell aggregation and trajectories in rotating wall vessel bioreactors. J Biotechnol 2006; **125:** 416.
18. Napolitano AP, Chai P, Dean DM, and Morgan JR: Dynamics of the self-assembly of complex cellular aggregates on micromolded nonadhesive hydrogels. Tissue Eng 2007; **13:** 2087.
19. Napolitano AP, Dean DM, Man AJ, Youssef J, Ho DN, Rago AP, Lech MP, and Morgan JR: Scaffold-free three-dimensional cell culture utilizing micromolded nonadhesive hydrogels. Biotechniques 2007; **43:** 494, 496.
20. Dean DM, Napolitano AP, Youssef J, and Morgan JR: Rods, tori, and honeycombs: the directed self-assembly of microtissues with prescribed microscale geometries. FASEB J 2007; **21:** 4005.
21. Dean DM and Morgan JR: Cytoskeletal-mediated tension modulates the directed self-assembly of microtissues. Tissue Eng A 2008; **14:** 1989.
22. Dean DM, Rago AP, and Morgan JR: Fibroblast elongation and dendritic extensions in constrained versus unconstrained microtissues. Cell Motil Cytoskelet 2009; **66:** 129.
23. Foty RA and Steinberg MS: Cadherin-mediated cell-cell adhesion and tissue segregation in relation to malignancy. Int J Dev Biol 2004; **48:** 397.
24. Steinberg MS: Mechanism of tissue reconstruction by dissociated cells. II. Time-course of events. Science 1962; **137:** 762.
25. Rago AP, Dean DM, and Morgan JR: Controlling cell position in complex heterotypic 3D microtissues by tissue fusion. Biotechnol Bioeng 2009; **102:** 1231.
26. Khademhosseini A and Langer R: Microengineered hydrogels for tissue engineering. Biomaterials 2007; **28:** 5087.
27. McGuigan AP and Sefton MV: Modular tissue engineering: fabrication of a gelatin-based construct. J Tissue Eng Regen Med 2007; **1:** 136.

WHS
Wound
Healing
Society

An Inductive Approach to Wound Repair and Regeneration Using a Tissue-Engineered Product

Damien Bates* and Stephen Farrell

Organogenesis, Inc., Canton, Massachusetts.

Background: While allogeneic tissue-based products can be engineered, they do not themselves have to replace missing host tissue to provide significant clinical efficacy. In this case, the role of the tissue-engineered product is to induce a healing response.
The Clinical Problem: A better understanding of a tissue-engineered product's mechanism of action and determining in which clinical settings it should be used is necessary if wound care is to be improved.
The Clinical Solution (Product): Given the Level 1 evidence available, tissue-engineered products should be considered in the treatment of wounds where primary intention strategies are not appropriate.
Market—History, Current, and Prospects: Traditional approaches to wound care have focused on wound management. Tissue-engineered products approved for the treatment of wounds are now growing at a rate faster than the general wound care market.
Business Challenges—Policies, Practices, Legal, and Geographical: Products designed for wound management can still get approval by the relatively straightforward 510(k) process. Products seeking specific wound treatment indications require Premarket Approval, Biologic License Application, or New Drug Application approval.
Public–Private Partnership SWOT Analysis: Academia and industry must continue to partner to translate scientific breakthroughs into safe and effective treatment for patients. Opportunities for partnership occur throughout the lifecycle of the product.
Conclusion: Allogeneic tissue-engineered products are safe and effective means for treating wounds by improving secondary intention healing. Better wound care will continue to depend on public–private partnerships that increase our understanding of how tissue-engineered approaches to wound care work, and by doing so provide opportunities for further product improvement.

Abbreviations and Acronyms

DFU = diabetic foot ulcer
FDA = Food and Drug Administration
VLU = venous leg ulcer

*Correspondence: Organogenesis, Inc., 150 Dan Road, Canton, Massachusetts 02021 (e-mail: dbates@organo.com).

BACKGROUND

Tissue engineering combines the principles of engineering and cell biology to unite the three traditional elements of cells, scaffolds, and growth factors to generate new three-dimensional tissues.[1] Organogenesis has been involved in the evolution of tissue-engineered approaches to wound care over the last 30 years. Formed in 1985, Organogenesis aimed to improve upon the skin tissue engineering technology first described by Dr. Eugene Bell and coworkers from Massachusetts Institute of Technology.[2] Organogenesis' initial goal was to produce a tissue *in vitro* which when grafted would help establish normal functional skin as quickly and effectively as possible.[3] These efforts culminated in the development and mass production of

Printed in U.S.A.
DOI: 10.1089/awc.2009.0090

Apligraf® (Organogenesis Inc., Canton, MA), a bilayered tissue structure consisting of a well-differentiated, cornified human epithelial layer and a collagenous layer containing allogeneic human keratinocytes and fibroblasts. Historically the goal of tissue engineering was to produce living structures that would mimic as closely as possible the anatomical tissue that was missing or needing to be replaced.[3] Conceptually this tissue-engineered product would serve as either a permanent or temporary replacement for the missing tissue. Limitations to this strategy are both blood supply and biocompatibility.[1] Since that time there has been a gradual realization that while allogeneic tissue-based products can be engineered, they do not necessarily themselves have to replace missing host tissue to provide significant clinical efficacy.[4–6] Rather than filling a defect or acting as a scaffold for tissue ingrowth, the role of the tissue-engineered product is to induce a healing response.

THE CLINICAL PROBLEM

Wounds are characterized by loss or disruption of anatomical integrity or continuity that may impair function of the part.[7] It is estimated that, in 1992, there were 35.2 million cases of significant skin loss (U.S. data) that required major therapeutic intervention.[8] Of the total number of skin loss cases described above, approximately 7 million wounds become chronic.[8] For demographic reasons, cost, and the limitation of standard surgical approaches (*e.g.*, primary intention healing), tissue-engineered approaches to wound care have focused on chronic wounds.

Delays in understanding how tissue-engineered products actually work have unfortunately led to inappropriate clinical usage and disappointment.[9] In the case of Apligraf, the initial understanding that this was a skin substitute led to its early use as an alternative to a skin autograft.[10,11] The clinical problems facing tissue-engineered approaches to wound care are reaching a better understanding of the product's mechanism of action and determining in which clinical settings they should be used. To be successful from the clinical perspective, tissue-engineered products need to be able to demonstrate clinical safety and efficacy in a consistent and predictable manner, be cost effective, and be easy to use.[9,12]

THE CLINICAL SOLUTION (PRODUCT)

Apligraf is Food and Drug Administration (FDA) approved for the treatment of both venous leg ulcer (VLU)[4,5] and diabetic foot ulcer (DFU)[6] and has now been used safely in the treatment of over 250,000 patients during the last 11 years. It is delivered fresh to clinics with a usable in-clinic shelf life of at least 10 days and is fully reimbursed by Medicare. This product does not function as a skin autograft[13–15] but improves the rate and quality of healing of both acute and chronic wounds by secondary intention.[4–6,10,11,16] Apligraf is a bilayered cellularized tissue construct that utilizes a systems biology approach to wound healing by elaborating a network of growth factors and cytokines,[17,18] which interact with underlying host tissue. This property of tissue-engineered products stands in sharp contrast to the historical reductionist or single supraphysiological growth factor approaches to wound care.[19]

The challenge then for the physician, acknowledging that improved outcomes with secondary intention healing are now within grasp, is which wounds to treat by primary intention and which ones to treat by secondary intention. Wounds that are treated by primary intention require the following: sufficient tissue elasticity, tissue integrity, vascularity, available donor tissue, ability to immobilize or splint the affected part, adequate hemostasis, and freedom from infection. Especially in the case of chronic wounds, these prerequisites are often absent necessitating a secondary intention healing approach. In this case, given the Level 1 evidence available for improved outcomes using Apligraf, this tissue-engineered approach to wound care should be seriously considered. In the case of acute wounds, some primary intention surgical strategies such as grafting give inferior cosmesis as the graft retains the characteristics of the tissue of origin and not the recipient site.[20] We are now faced with the exciting and revolutionary prospect of preferentially choosing modified secondary intention healing with Apligraf over primary intention healing to achieve improved wound-healing outcomes. The goal is to use tissue-engineered products to push wound healing away from repair with scar toward regeneration. This concept is now supported with Level 1 data showing site appropriate tissue regeneration in terms of color and texture in the oral cavity.[16]

MARKET—HISTORY, CURRENT, AND PROSPECTS

The total cost of acute and chronic wound care is estimated to be approximately $25–35 billion in the United States.[21] This includes the use of therapies, supplies, as well as the cost of medical personnel involved in the treatment of these wounds. Chronic wounds account for nearly two-thirds of this total. The magnitude of the clinical challenge is huge: of the 21 million individuals in the United States with diabetes, the lifetime risk of developing foot ulceration has been estimated at 25%[22] resulting in approximately 82,000 lower extremity amputations annually[9]; VLU affect 0.18% to 1.35% of the population equating to approximately 600,000 such wounds in the United States[9]; another 1.4 million people in the United States have pressure ulcers.[9] With challenges in record keeping and even sometimes diagnosis, these numbers are likely to be understated.

Traditional approaches to wound care have focused on wound covering and providing an environment in which healing can occur. Today, a large part of the wound care market still consists of these dressings, which have become increasingly sophisticated, yet still fall short of promoting healing. Collagen-based dressings were introduced in the late 1990s and early 2000s. These products, while still not approved by the FDA for healing, did aim at providing a more biological approach to managing wounds. In 1997, a growth factor therapy formulated with platelet-derived growth factor was introduced to the market for the treatment of DFU. It was supported by randomized controlled trial evidence of superior efficacy over standard care. Subsequent efforts on single growth factor therapy persist to this day. Tissue-engineered approaches to wound care began in the 1990s and resulted in the development and commercialization of two therapies approved by the FDA, Apligraf and Dermagraft. Tissue-engineered products continue to grow at a rate faster than the general wound care market, but still represent a fraction of the overall treatments for VLU and DFU. There is no tissue-engineered product approved for the treatment of pressure ulcers.

BUSINESS CHALLENGES—POLICIES, PRACTICES, LEGAL, AND GEOGRAPHICAL

With the increasing incidence of diabetes in a generally aging population, chronic ulcers are on the incline and represent an evergrowing portion of overall medical costs. In some instances, the government is employing punitive measures for the development of chronic wounds, such as pressure ulcers, during hospitalization. Chronic wounds also represent a significant factor impacting quality of life, mobility, and mortality of the aging population. With the increasing costs come the increased need for therapies that conclusively and practically resolve these wounds.

While products designed for wound management can still get approval by the relatively straightforward 510(k) process, products seeking specific healing indications require Premarket Approval, Biologic License Application, or New Drug Application approval in the United States. These efforts require many more years of research and study, along with millions of dollars in investment. Depending on the nature of the product, various sections of the FDA may be involved including Center for Devices and Radiological Health, Center for Biologics Evaluation and Research, or Center for Drug Evaluation and Research. Products marketed on a global basis face particular challenge as European Medicines Agency and FDA do not have completely harmonized views of advanced products, especially cell-based therapies.

The production of advanced therapies for chronic wounds can be quite costly and complex as most involve some form of cell culture, either employing cells to produce growth factors or using the cells themselves as the therapy.

PUBLIC–PRIVATE PARTNERSHIP—SWOT ANALYSIS

The challenges for public–private partnerships in tissue engineering are similar to those in other fields. Academia brings a great deal of expertise often in narrow areas of specialization. This may be extremely relevant in the understanding of the molecular basis of regeneration and how that may be recapitulated through tissue-engineered approaches to wound care. Industry brings a vast experience in product development (*e.g.*, process development and validation, manufacturing, quality control and assurance, regulatory, and clinical operations), which is essential if breakthroughs in scientific understanding (which often arise in academia) are ever to be translated into a product that ultimately benefits patients. This focus on product approval has a beneficial effect (in terms of patient care) by forcing the research activities in the public realm to be more pragmatic and less theoretical (Fig. 1).

Balanced with these positives is the need for both parties to realize where the expertise actually lies. While the public partner may have experience as a principal investigator in a clinical trial or participation in an advisory board, this is a far cry

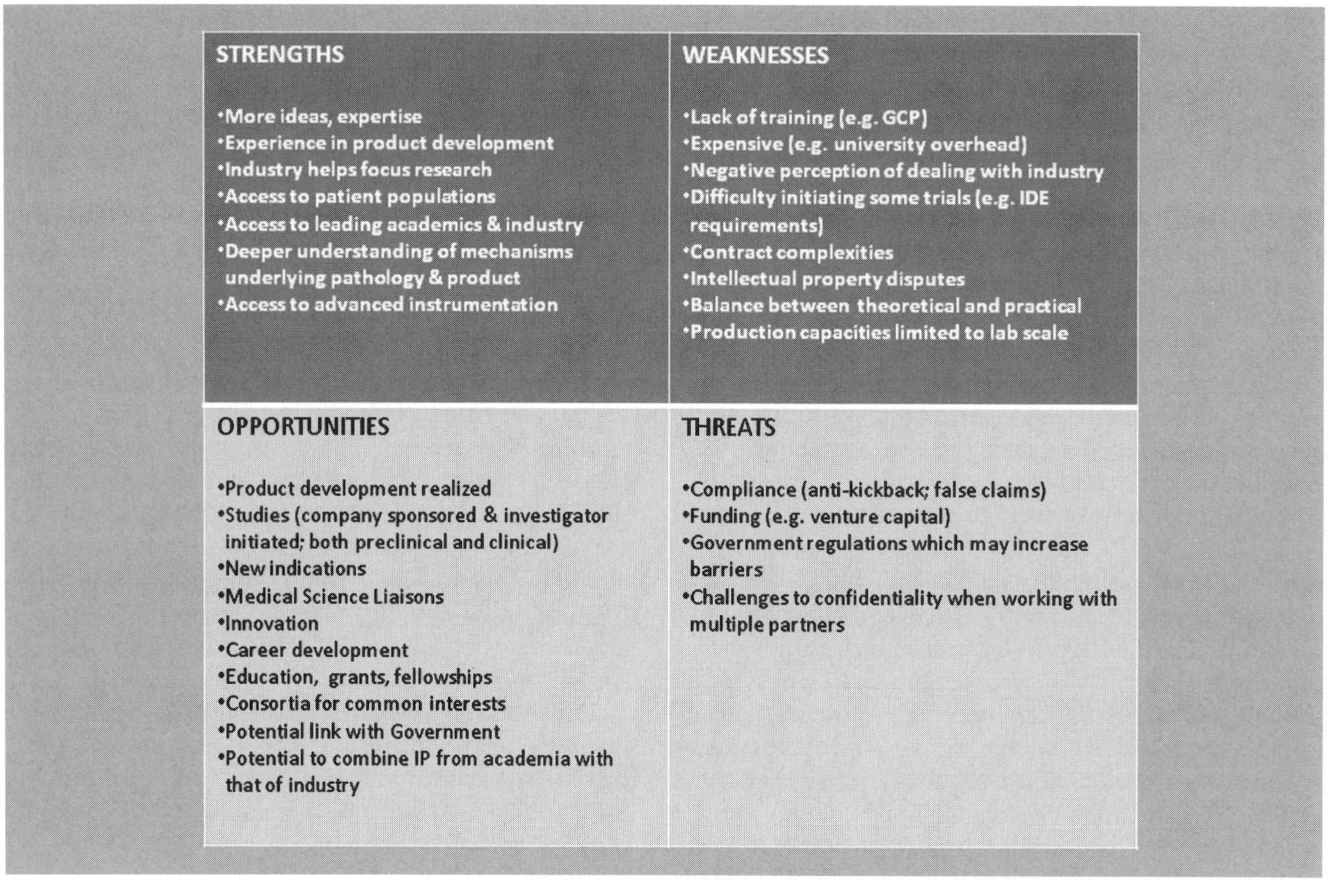

Figure 1. Strengths and weaknesses (Internal) and opportunities and threats (External) (SWOT analysis) of public-private partnerships.

from the actual operational implementation of a multicenter clinical trial with adherence to all the Good Clinical Practice and regulatory guidelines. Likewise the manufacturing capability of the public institution may be inadequate from an industry and product development point of view as their production capacities are limited to laboratory scale.

Some clinical trials may be overly burdensome to the investigator. In the case of tissue-engineered products, many of which are currently regulated as devices, there is a need to file an Investigational Device Exemption before running a clinical trial that is outside of the product's FDA-approved label. Similarly, university rules and regulations have the potential to add significant cost to research funded by industry (*e.g.*, departmental overheads). Intellectual property and contract disputes may further undermine the realization of a fruitful collaboration.

When it does occur, public–private partnerships can be very productive. Research collaboration, for example, can either be in the form of a company-sponsored clinical trial or an investigator-initiated study (preclinical or clinical). The latter study is often facilitated by a Medical Science Liaison who operates between the public and private partners: bringing product education and opportunity to the investigator and bringing innovation and research opportunities to the company. These relationships can be enormously beneficial both to the company in the form of hypothesis-generating studies that may ultimately lead to a new indication for their product and to the physician in terms of helping establish their academic career and bringing additional funding opportunities for education (*e.g.*, grants and fellowships). By virtue of their collaboration, new funding opportunities may be applied for (*e.g.*, National Institutes of Health, Small Business Innovation Research Program, Small Business Technology Transfer Program) that may not have been possible without such collaboration. Academia also brings potential opportunities for diffusion of company innovation to the peers of a physician who is a leader in their field. It is useful to remember that if public–private partnerships are guided by scientific merit, fair balance, evidence-based medicine, and ultimately for patient benefit, this will militate against the negative stereotype of collaborating with industry.

Potential barriers or threats to this partnership are in the form of excessive government regulation of industry–physician interaction (*e.g.*, new compliance measures) that, although designed to protect patient safety and welfare and limit wasteful spending of public money through potential conflicts of interest, may actually stifle innovation and medical progress. The other potential threat includes lack of funding both on the front end of product development (*e.g.*, venture capital funding) and the back end (*e.g.*, no product reimbursement). Both scenarios ultimately undermine the ability to generate the money that underpins public–private partnerships.

CONCLUSION

Over the last 30 years there has been an evolution in the way tissue-engineered products are being developed, perceived, and used in wound care. Tissue-engineered wound care products began with matrices and growth factors alone and now the more sophisticated approaches combine these important elements together with cells. For these three-dimensional tissues, there has been a transition from a paradigm of tissue replacement to one of tissue induction. The broad swath of high-level data supporting the use of Apligraf to improve the rate and quality of healing by secondary intention now allows the physician to focus on the appropriate surgical approach to the patient rather than deciding which product to use in which specific wound state or indication. If the physician decides that secondary intention healing is the preferable approach to heal a wound, then a tissue-engineered product such as Apligraf should be seriously considered for reasons of safety, efficacy, and cost effectiveness.

Despite this new understanding, significant challenges remain. Wounds of all types remain an enormous public health burden and the ultimate challenge is how to provide the safest and most clinically effective treatments to patients in a fiscally responsible manner. This goal demands a better understanding of wound pathophysiology, tissue repair, and regeneration. The regulatory landscape is in flux and manufacturing challenges abound. However, there are many opportunities for public–private partnerships to further this exciting field of tissue engineering and continue to push it toward regenerative medicine in the literal sense.

CRITICAL REMARKS AND RECOMMENDATIONS

- Tissue engineering combines cells, extracellular matrices, and signaling molecules.
- Allogeneic tissue-based products such as Apligraf do not replace tissue but induce a healing response.
- The induced healing response is manifested clinically as an improved rate and quality of healing by secondary intention.
- Clinicians need to be strategic with respect to wound care: is primary intention or secondary intention more appropriate?
- The potential to improve the rate and quality of healing by secondary intention now exists.
- By improving the quality of healing by secondary intention, Apligraf has provided a window into the possibility of inducing site appropriate tissue regeneration.
- Traditional approaches to wound care have focused on wound management rather than wound treatment.
- Tissue-engineered products provide a systems biology approach rather than a reductionist single growth factor approach to wound care.
- There is a significant regulatory burden for tissue-engineered product approval.
- Tissue-engineered products have a higher level of evidence to support their use than wound management products approved through the 510(k) pathway.
- Academia and industry must continue to partner to translate scientific breakthroughs into safe and effective treatment for patients.

AUTHOR DISCLOSURE STATEMENT

Both authors of this manuscript are full-time employees of Organogenesis, Inc.

REFERENCES

1. Morrison WA: Progress in tissue engineering of soft tissue and organs. Surgery 2009; **145:** 127.
2. Bell E, Ehrlich HP, Buttle DJ, and Nakatsuji T: Living tissue formed *in vitro* and accepted as skin-equivalent tissue of full thickness. Science 1981; **211:** 1052.
3. Wilkins LM, Watson SR, Prosky SJ, Meunier SF, and Parenteau NL: Development of a bilayered living skin construct for clinical applications. Biotechnol Bioeng 1994; **43:** 747.
4. Falanga V, Margolis D, Alvarez O, Auletta M, Maggiacomo F, Altman M, Jensen J, Sabolinski M, and Hardin-Young J: Rapid healing of venous ulcers and lack of clinical rejection with an allogeneic cultured human skin equivalent. Human Skin Equivalent Investigators Group. Arch Dermatol 1998; **134:** 293.
5. Falanga V and Sabolinski M: A bilayered living skin construct (APLIGRAF) accelerates complete closure of hard-to-heal venous ulcers. Wound Repair Regen 1999; **7:** 201.
6. Veves A, Falanga V, Armstrong DG, and Sabolinski ML: Graftskin, a human skin equivalent, is effective in the management of noninfected neuropathic diabetic foot ulcers: a prospective randomized multicenter clinical trial. Diabetes Care 2001; **24:** 290.
7. Lazarus GS, Cooper DM, Knighton DR, Percoraro RE, Rodeheaver G, and Robson MC: Definitions and guidelines for assessment of wounds and evaluation of healing. Wound Repair Regen 1994; **2:** 165.
8. Clark RA, Ghosh K, and Tonnesen MG: Tissue engineering for cutaneous wounds. J Invest Dermatol 2007; **127:** 1018.
9. Ehrenreich M and Ruszczak Z: Update on tissue-engineered biological dressings. Tissue Eng 2006; **12:** 2407.
10. Muhart M, McFalls S, Kirsner RS, Elgart GW, Kerdel F, Sabolinski ML, Hardin-Young J, and Eaglstein WH: Behavior of tissue-engineered skin: a comparison of a living skin equivalent, autograft, and occlusive dressing in human donor sites. Arch Dermatol 1999; **135:** 913.
11. Waymack P, Duff RG, and Sabolinski M: The effect of a tissue engineered bilayered living skin analog, over meshed split-thickness autografts on the healing of excised burn wounds. The Apligraf Burn Study Group. Burns 2000; **26:** 609.
12. Metcalfe AD and Ferguson MW: Bioengineering skin using mechanisms of regeneration and repair. Biomaterials 2007; **28:** 5100.
13. Badiavas EV, Paquette D, Carson P, and Falanga V: Human chronic wounds treated with bioengineered skin: histologic evidence of host-graft interactions. J Am Acad Dermatol 2002; **46:** 524.
14. Gohari S, Gambla C, Healey M, Spaulding G, Gordon KB, Swan J, Cook B, West DP, and Lapiere JC: Evaluation of tissue-engineered skin (human skin substitute) and secondary intention healing in the treatment of full thickness wounds after Mohs micrographic or excisional surgery. Dermatol Surg 2002; **28:** 1107; discussion 1114.
15. Griffiths M, Ojeh N, Livingstone R, Price R, and Navsaria H: Survival of Apligraf in acute human wounds. Tissue Eng 2004; **10:** 1180.
16. McGuire MK, Scheyer ET, Nunn ME, and Lavin PT: A pilot study to evaluate a tissue-engineered bilayered cell therapy as an alternative to tissue from the palate. J Periodontol 2008; **79:** 1847.
17. Brem H, Young J, Tomic-Canic M, Isaacs C, and Ehrlich HP: Clinical efficacy and mechanism of bilayered living human skin equivalent (HSE) in treatment of diabetic foot ulcers. Surg Technol Int 2003; **11:** 23.
18. Milstone LM, Asgari MM, Schwartz PM, and Hardin-Young J: Growth factor expression, healing, and structural characteristics of graftskin (Apligraf). Wounds 2000; **12:** 12A.
19. Steed DL: Clinical evaluation of recombinant human platelet-derived growth factor for the treatment of lower extremity diabetic ulcers. Diabetic Ulcer Study Group. J Vasc Surg 1995; **21:** 71; discussion 79–81.
20. Karring T, Ostergaard E, and Loe H: Conservation of tissue specificity after heterotopic transplantation of gingiva and alveolar mucosa. J Periodontal Res 1971; **6:** 282.
21. Landers, SJ. New Approaches Aimed at Healing Wounds. American Medical News, Jan. 14, 2008. http://www.ama-assn.org/amednews/2008/01/14/hlsc0114.htm.
22. Singh N, Armstrong DG, and Lipsky BA: Preventing foot ulcers in patients with diabetes. JAMA 2005; **293:** 217.

Section 10

Stem and Progenitor Cells

Section Editors: Timothy M. Crombleholme and Kenneth W. Liechty

STEM AND PROGENITOR CELLS

WHS
Wound
Healing
Society

Mesenchymal Stem Cells and Wound Repair

Charles Bellows[1] and Donald G. Phinney[2,*]

[1]Department of Surgery, Tulane University Health Sciences Center, New Orleans, Louisiana.
[2]Department of Molecular Therapeutics, The Scripps Research Institute, Jupiter, FL.

Background: The wounding of healthy tissues invokes a physiologic response involving initially inflammation, followed by formation of granulation tissue and subsequently neovascularization and re-epithelialization. This process, which involves the concerted action of various cell types, soluble factors, and extracellular matrix components, is rapid and efficient in most healthy individuals.

The Problem: Imbalances resulting from sickness, disease, and injury can impair the wound-healing process resulting in the formation of chronic, nonhealing wounds. Although a number of treatment options exist for managing chronic wounds, a large percentage of such wounds fail to heal.

Basic/Clinical Science Advances: In the past decade, cell-based therapies have been explored as a means to augment the healing of chronic wounds. Specifically, mesenchymal stem cells (MSCs) derived from bone marrow have proven efficacious in healing cutaneous wounds, diabetic skin ulcers, and burns in various animal models and human patients. MSC-induced healing appears to occur through a variety of mechanisms, most of which involve paracrine signaling.

Clinical Care Relevance: It is estimated that 5.7 million people in the United States suffer from some form of chronic wound. Moreover, there is little evidence that standardized treatments are effective in promoting the healing of such wounds. Therefore, chronic wounds continue to represent a significant cause of disability for patients, and new treatment regimens are desperately needed.

Conclusion: MSC-based therapies are effective in augmenting the healing of chronic wounds. However, further research is needed to delineate their mechanism of action and optimize their methods of procurement and delivery so that their therapeutic benefit can be maximized.

Abbreviations and Acronyms

CCL21 = chemokine, CC motif, ligand 21
CCR7 = chemokine, CC motif, receptor 7
CXC = cysteine-x-cysteine
EGF = epidermal growth factor
FPR1 = formyl peptide receptor 1
GFP = green fluorescent protein
HGF = hepatocyte growth factor
KGF = keratinocyte growth factor
MSCs = mesenchymal stem cells
PDGF = platelet-derived growth factor
TACR1 = tachykinin receptor 1
TGF-β = transforming growth factor beta
TNF-α = tumor necrosis factor alpha
VEGF = vascular endothelial growth factor

*Correspondence: The Scripps Research Institute, Department of Molecular Therapeutics, A213, 130 Scripps Way, Jupiter, Florida 33458 (e-mail: dphinney@scripps.edu).

BACKGROUND

Wound healing occurs in all tissues and organs of the body and is orchestrated by a highly integrated and ordered series of molecular, cellular, and biochemical events. However, various conditions, including infection, venous or arterial disease, and diabetes, can disrupt the process at different phases, leading to the formation of chronic nonhealing wounds. To effectively manage these wounds, one must understand the normal healing process, which is categorized into separate phases: inflammatory, proliferative, and remodeling. The inflammatory phase begins immediately after wounding and is characterized by hemostasis and inflammation. Cytokines (tumor necrosis factor alpha [TNF-α], transforming growth factor beta [TGF-β], and interleukin 1), chemokines (thromboxane A2 and prostaglandins), and growth factors

Printed in U.S.A.
DOI: 10.1089/awc.2009.0139

(epidermal growth factor [EGF], platelet-derived growth factor [PDGF], fibroblast growth factor 2, and keratinocyte growth factor [KGF]) released in response to injury orchestrate subsequent phases of the healing process by recruiting other cell types to the injured tissue and promoting their growth and differentiation.[1]

The proliferative phase is characterized by angiogenesis, collagen deposition, granulation tissue formation, and epithelialization. Fibroblasts recruited to the site of injury produce collagen, glycoproteins, and other matrix proteins that replace the provision fibrin-based matrix produced by clotting. Angiogenesis, which is stimulated by TNF-α, is also critical for proper wound healing, as new capillaries deliver nutrients to the wound and help maintain the granulation tissue bed. Keratinocytes and endothelial cells also proliferate during this time, eventually producing autocrine growth factors that sustain the healing process. Keratinocytes also migrate across the granulation tissue to close the wound. Although many cytokines and growth factors are expressed early in the wound-healing process, others such as chemokine, cysteine-x-cysteine (CXC) motif, ligand 10 (CXCL 10) and chemokine, CXC motif, ligand 11 (CXCL 11) appear later and may induce a transition to the remodeling phase.[2] Herein, collagen type III is degraded and replaced by collagen type 1, which is reorganized and cross-linked to increase the tensile strength of the healing tissue. Cells no longer needed in the wound repair process are also eliminated by apoptosis.

CLINICAL PROBLEM ADDRESSED

Chronic wounds arise because of a number of underlying physiological conditions. In the United States they are estimated to affect some 5.7 million patients at a cost of 20 billion dollars annually.[3] Economic analyses may under estimate the total cost of chronic wound care due to incomplete reporting and ineffectiveness of treatment regimens. The most common chronic wounds encountered in Western medical practice result from diabetes. Up to 15% of the 20 million diabetics in the United States are at risk of developing chronic wounds, many of whom will require limb amputations. Infection is also a common problem in chronic wounds, resulting in increased patient morbidity and mortality. Molecular studies have shown that chronic wounds contain diverse microbial communities, which form biofilms that protect them against killing by systemic antibiotics, topical antiseptics, and the host defenses.[4] Lack of oxygen at the wound site because of compromised blood flow and/or bacterial respiration also impairs the normal healing process.[5]

BASIC SCIENCE CONTEXT

Although cell-based therapies are well established in clinical medicine, for example, bone marrow transplantation, the past few decades have seen major advances in the field of stem cell research. These include the discovery that most adult tissues in the body harbor some type of stem and/or progenitor cells that play a role in tissue homeostasis. For example, the identification of neural stem cells disproved the notion that the adult central nervous system lacks any regenerative capacity, and neural stem cells are now being employed in clinical trials to treat a variety of neurological disorders. Similarly, adult bone marrow is now thought to harbor three phenotypically and functionally distinct stem cell populations: hematopoietic, mesenchymal, and endothelial.[6] These stem cells and their progeny possess unique properties that make them well suited for use in wound healing, such as the capacity to induce angiogenesis, secrete growth factors and extracellular matrix proteins, and modulate immune cell function. However, elucidating which marrow-derived subpopulations are best suited to augment wound healing, and determining how such cells may be recruited from marrow to sites of tissue injury remain important challenges for developing effective cell-based therapies.

EXPERIMENTAL MODEL OR MATERIAL—ADVANTAGES AND LIMITATIONS

Mesenchymal stem cells (MSCs) were initially identified in bone marrow as fibroblastoid-like cells with the capacity to generate a heterotopic osseous tissue when transplanted *in vivo*.[7] Based on these findings, the cells were exploited as feeder layers to establish long-term bone marrow cultures and shown to express a variety of cytokines, growth factors, and adhesion molecules that regulate aspects of hematopoiesis.[6] Subsequently, the stem cell nature of the cells was inferred from studies showing that clonally derived populations retained the capacity to differentiate into adipocytes, chondrocytes, and osteoblasts *in vitro*.[8] Based on these early findings, MSCs were used in human clinical trials to treat osteogenesis imperfecta.[9]

More recently, MSCs have gained traction as cell-based vectors for treating ischemic, inflammatory, neurologic, and immune-related disorders. The broad therapeutic efficacy of MSCs was initially attributed to their ability to differentiate into nonhematopoietic cell types in a context-dependent manner *in vivo*, thereby contributing directly to tissue regeneration.[10] More recently, their capacity to alter the tissue microenvironment via paracrine signaling is thought to be the principle mechanism by which MSCs affect tissue repair. Paracrine signaling has been shown to modulate inflammatory responses, immune cell function, angiogenesis, and the growth and survival of host cells at sites of injury and disease.[11,12] These attributes, together with the fact that the cells are readily available, amenable to genetic engineering, can be expanded to large numbers *in vitro*, and have a good safety record in clinical trials, has fueled tremendous growth in their popularity as vectors to treat nonhematological diseases.

DISCUSSION OF FINDINGS AND RELEVANT LITERATURE

Various groups have reported that topical, intradermal, or systemic administration of MSCs augments the healing of thermal,[13] radiation,[14] and chemical-induced burns,[15] diabetic skin ulcers,[16] and full-thickness cutaneous wounds.[17–20] Early work in the field indicated that MSCs acted by participating directly in the regeneration of wounded tissue. For example, several groups reported that MSCs expressing green fluorescent protein (GFP) or labeled with 5-bromo-2-deoxyuridine and administered to wounded animals[13,17,19,20] localized within skin structures and coexpressed cytokeratin. However, in one study a much higher percentage of GFP^+ cells in the wound were shown to coexpress the endothelial (13.2%) or pericyte (33%) markers CD31 or alpha smooth muscle actin, respectively.[17] Moreover, fluorescence-activated cell sorting analysis of dissociated wound tissue revealed a precipitous decline in number of GFP^+ MSCs engrafted within the wound, which ranged from 10.1% at day 7 to 1.8% by day 28 postinjury.[19] Although the reason for the decline was not investigated, these results are similar to that seen after MSC administration to infarcted myocardial tissue.[21] Other studies have demonstrated that MSCs accelerate wound healing in normal and diabetic mice in the absence of transdifferentiation,[16] and Francois *et al.*[14] reported that human MSCs delivered intravenously to immunodeficient mice with radiation-induced skin lesions could not be detected using a sensitive PCR assay in the wound by

TAKE-HOME MESSAGE

Basic science advances

- MSCs express receptor proteins that bind to factors released into the circulation in response to tissue injury, such as HGF, N-formyl peptides, and substance P.
- MSCs recruited to sites of tissue injury localize around blood vessels and within skin structures, including the dermis, hair follicles, and sebaceous glands. Transdifferentiation into epithelial cell fates appears to occur at a low frequency, but does not result from cell fusion. The majority of MSCs engrafted in wounds adopt characteristics of endothelial cells and pericytes.
- MSCs appear to be cleared from wounds during the healing process and do not contribute long term to the structure of the healed tissue.
- Paracrine signaling appears to be the principal mechanisms by which MSCs accelerate wound healing. MSCs secrete growth factors, angiogenins, and inflammatory mediators that contribute to various phases of the wound-healing process, including formation of granulation tissue, neovascularization, and re-epithelialization.

Clinical science advances

- Many of the cellular and molecular events that contribute to the different phases of wound healing have been well described, thereby providing insight into the mechanisms by which cell-based therapies augment the healing process.
- MSC-based therapies were evaluated in various experimental animal models and were found to be efficacious for treating a number of different wound types.
- Preliminary studies indicate that MSC-based therapies also accelerate healing of deep skin burns, cutaneous wounds, and diabetic ulcers in human patients.
- Owing to their ready availability, ease of isolation, unique molecular attributes, and good safety record in clinical trials, MSCs appear well suited for treating chronic, nonhealing wounds.

Relevance to clinical care

- The number of patients suffering from chronic wounds attributable to diseases such as diabetes mellitus and peripheral vascular disease is on the rise, imposing a large burden on the nation's healthcare industry.
- There is very little evidence for the efficacy of current wound care treatment strategies to reduce the burden of chronic wounds.
- MSC-based therapies represent a promising new treatment option for patients with chronic wounds.
- MSC populations are heterogeneous, so screening would be desirable to ensure that cells applied to wounds produce copious amounts of the proper factors to accelerate the healing process.
- Chronic wounds have underlying causes that must be addressed for the wound to heal properly. Therefore, cell-based therapy alone may be insufficient to promote permanent healing of a wound.

8 weeks postinjury, although a significant enhancement in wound healing was observed. Therefore, while these studies indicate that MSCs are recruited to sites of injury, sometimes in large numbers, and augment the healing process, their direct contribution to new dermal tissue appears modest and short lived.

Recently, several groups have identified receptors on MSCs that may recruit the cells to sites of tissue injury. These include the c-met receptor,[22] which binds to hepatocyte growth factor (HGF), as well as the N-formyl peptide receptor.[23] HGF and N-formyl peptides are released in response to tissue injury and function in recruitment of immune cells and fibroblasts to stimulate tissue repair. Both receptors were shown to be functional in MSCs and promote chemotaxis in response to their cognate ligands, suggesting a role in homing *in vivo*. MSCs have also been shown to express receptors for the neuro-peptide substance P.[24] More recently, Hong *et al.*[25] reported that levels of substance P are rapidly elevated in peripheral blood after tissue injury and induce mobilization of $CD29^{+}$ cells, which are phenotypically and functionally similar to MSCs, into the circulation. This response was shown to positively correlate with accelerated wound healing. Similarly, intradermal injection of chemokine, CC motif, ligand 21 into the periphery of wounded skin also increased MSC recruitment to the wound and accelerated its closure.[17] Therefore, MSCs appear to employ several sensing mechanisms to respond to tissue injury (Fig. 1). This conclusion is consistent with that of studies by Mansilla *et al.*,[26] who showed that the proportion of circulating MSCs was on average 21-fold higher in human patients with severe burns than in healthy controls, and the number correlated with the size and severity of the burn.

Once recruited to a wound, MSCs appear to augment healing by paracrine signaling. For example, Liu *et al.*[27] showed that rat MSCs constitutively expressed a number of growth factors

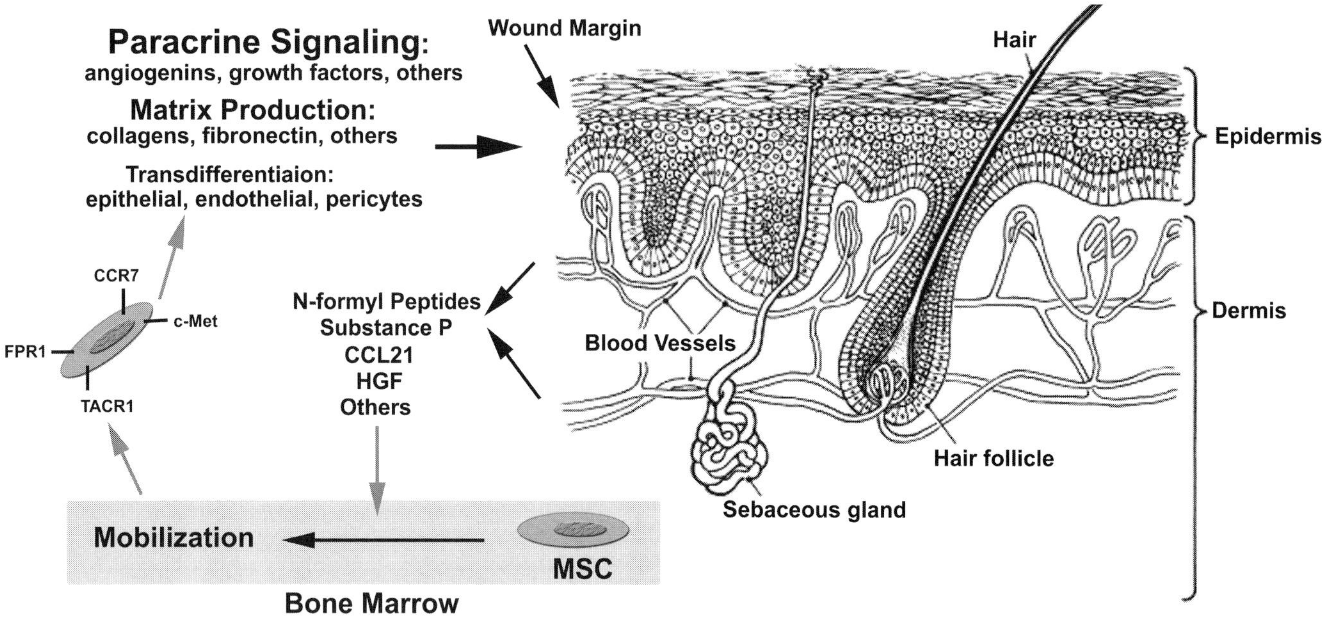

Figure 1. MSCs promote wound healing by various mechanisms. After tissue injury, a variety of substances are released locally and systemically that function to recruit cells to the wound to initiate healing. Recent studies indicate that HGF, N-formyl peptides, substance P (tachykinin 1), and CCL21 are among these factors. Moreover, these proteins have been shown to bind specific receptors (c-Met, TACR1, CCR7, and FPR1) expressed on the surface of MSCs, inducing mobilization from marrow and chemotaxis to the site of tissue injury. Subsequently, MSCs engrafted within the wound augment healing by several distinct mechanisms. Paracrine signaling via release of angiogenins (vascular endothelial growth factor, erythropoietin, cysteine-rich, and angiogenic inducer 61), growth factors (epidermal growth factor, fibroblast growth factor 2, insulin-like growth factor 1, keratinocyte growth factor, platelet-derived growth factor, and transforming growth factor beta), and other soluble factors promotes angiogenesis, keratinocyte proliferation and migration, and may also modulate the activity of inflammatory cells. MSCs are also known to secrete a large array of extracellular matrix molecules, including collagens, fibronectin, and various matrix metalloproteinases. Therefore, MSCs may directly contribute to tissue repair by functioning akin to fibroblasts. Alternatively, MSCs may trans-differentiate into epithelial or vascular cell types although this process occurs at a low frequency, and therefore its contribution to wound healing may be minimal. MSCs = mesenchymal stem cells; HGF = hepatocyte growth factor; CCL21 = chemokine, CC motif, ligand 21; TACR1 = tachykinin receptor 1; CCR7 = chemokine, CC motif, receptor 7; FPR1 = formyl peptide receptor 1.

important in wound healing, including PDGF, epidermal growth factor (EGF), TGF-β, vascular endothelial growth factor (VEGF), KGF, fibroblast growth factor 2, and HGF, and that expression of PDGF, EGF, KGF, and HGF was significantly elevated when cells were exposed to lipopolysaccharide or interleukin 1. Similarly, treatment of MSCs with superfusates from wounded abdominal tissue was shown to upregulate expression of TGF-β, EGF, and VEGF. Human MSCs and adipose-derived cells were also reported to secrete appreciable levels of insulin-like growth factor 1, VEGF, and HGF, the latter two of which were upregulated by exposure to TNF-α.[28] Therefore, exposure to the wound microenvironment appears to induce expression in MSCs of various angiogenins and mitogens that normally participate in the wound-healing process (Fig. 1). MSCs have also been reported to secrete significantly higher levels of angiopoietin 1, KGF, insulin-like growth factor 1, PDGF, and erythropoietin than compared to dermal fibroblasts,[18,19] which may explain their superior healing capacity.[19] MSCs have also been shown to secrete high levels of cysteine-rich angiogenic inducer 61, and depletion of this protein from the MSC-conditioned medium abolished the angiogenic activity of the cells.[29] This is consistent with studies showing that the MSC-conditioned medium also stimulates wound healing.[18]

CAUTION, CRITICAL REMARKS, AND RECOMMENDATIONS

The aforementioned studies indicate that MSCs are recruited via receptor-mediated processes to sites of tissue injury and accelerate wound healing principally via paracrine-mediating signaling. However, caution is urged in generalizing these findings. For example, MSC populations are known to be functionally heterogeneous with respect to their differentiation potential, and our own studies have shown that many paracrine factors expressed by MSCs are restricted to specific subpopulations.[12] This heterogeneity likely reflects the functional complexity of bone marrow stroma and may account for the broad therapeutic effects of MSCs. However, because of the lack of standardized methods to isolate, culture-expand, and characterize these populations, their cellular composition may vary significantly. Therefore, the low frequency of transdifferentiation to epithelial cells may reflect the lack of bona fide stem/progenitors within populations administered to wounds. Also, few studies have quantified the proportion of MSCs that secrete wound-healing–promoting factors or have demonstrated if these factors are coexpressed with receptor proteins that mediate homing to sites of injury *in vivo*. Also, MSCs may also secrete factors that may antagonize the wound-healing process, such as inflammatory cytokines. To address these potential confounds, we recommend future studies to more accurately quantify the number of stem/progenitors within MSC populations applied to wounds, demonstrate dose-related responses in wound healing, and perform fractionation studies to determine the contribution of different MSC subpopulations to the wound-healing process. Finally, recent studies have shown that MSCs also have a propensity to home to sites of tumor formation *in vivo*, and confer upon cancer cells more invasive and metastatic properties in part through secretion of angiogenins, cytokines, and chemokines.[30] Consequently, caution must be taken when administering MSCs to treat chronic wounds to ensure that cells remain within the wound bed and do not home to other ectopic sites *in vivo*, such as micrometastasis.

FUTURE DEVELOPMENTS

Recent advances that have shed light on the mechanism of action of MSCs in accelerating wound healing offer promise for the development of improved treatment strategies for chronic wound care. Specifically, areas of future research include development of improved fractionation methods to enrich for cell populations that express the appropriate surface receptors to enhance homing *in vivo*, secrete high levels of paracrine factors to accelerate wound healing, or exhibit more robust transdifferentiation toward epithelial or endothelial cell lineages. Genetic approaches also offer the potential to engineer improved cell-based vectors that combine some or all of the aforementioned properties, and could also be used to increase resistance to hypoxia or other adverse environmental conditions within wounds, thereby enhancing their potency. Finally, advances in scaffold development may yield materials that can be colonized by cells for improved topical administration, or that can also regulate the growth, differentiation, or secretory functions of cellular vectors *in vivo*.

AUTHOR DISCLOSURE STATEMENT

The authors (D.G.P. and C.B.) certify that no competing financial interests exist with regard to the work cited in this chapter.

REFERENCES

1. Barrientos S, Stojadinovic O, Golinko MS, Brem H, and Tomic-Canic M: Growth factors and cytokines in wound healing. Wound Repair Regen 2008; **16:** 585.

2. Yates CC, Whaley D, Y-Chen A, Kulescekaran P, Hebda PA, and Wells A: ELR-negative CXC chemokines CXCL11 (IP-9/I-TAC) facilitates dermal and epidermal maturation during wound repair. Am J Pathol 2008; **173:** 643.

3. Branski LK, Gauglitz GG, Herndon DN, and Jeschke MG: A review of gene and stem cell therapy in cutaneous wound healing. Burns 2009; **35:** 171.

4. Bjarnsholt T, Kirketerp-Møller K, Jensen PØ, Madsen KG, Phipps R, Krogfelt K, Høiby N, and Givskov M: Why chronic wounds will not heal: a novel hypothesis. Wound Repair Regen 2008; **16:** 2.

5. Gordillo GM, Schlanger R, Wallace WA, Bergdall V, Bartlett R, and Sen CK: Protocols for topical and systemic oxygen treatments in wound healing. Methods Enzymol 2004; **381:** 575.

6. Phinney DG: Marrow stem cells. In: *Advances in Tissue Engineering*, edited by Polak J, Mantalaris S, and Harding S. London: Imperial College Press, 2008, pp. 95–122.

7. Phinney DG: Building a consensus regarding the nature and origin of mesenchymal stem cells. J Cell Biochem 2002; **S38:** 7.

8. Pittenger MF, MacKay AM, Beck SC, Jaiswal RK, Douglas R, Mosca JD, Moorman MA, Simonetti DW, Craig S, and Marshak DR: Multilineage potential of adult human mesenchymal stem cells. Science 1999; **284:** 143.

9. Horwitz EM, Gordon PL, Koo WK, Marx JC, Neel MD, McNall RY, Muul L, and Hofmann T: Isolated allogeneic bone marrow-derived mesenchymal cells engraft and stimulate growth in children with osteogenesis imperfecta: implications for cell therapy of bone. Proc Natl Acad Sci USA 2002; **99:** 8932.

10. Grove JE, Bruscia E, and Krause DS: Plasticity of bone marrow-derived stem cells. Stem Cells 2004; **22:** 487.

11. Kinnaird T, Stabile E, Burnett MS, and Epstein SE: Bone-marrow-derived cells for enhancing collateral development: mechanisms, animal data, and initial clinical experiences. Circ Res 2004; **95:** 354.

12. Phinney DG and Prockop DJ: The state of transdifferentiation and modes of tissue repair: current views. Stem Cells 2007; **25:** 2896.

13. Fu X, Fang L, Li X, Cheng B, and Sheng Z: Enhanced wound healing quality with bone marrow mesenchymal stem cells autografting after skin injury. Wound Repair Regen 2006; **14:** 325.

14. Francois S, Mouiseddine M, Mathieu N, Semont A, Monti P, Dudoignon N, Sache A, Boutarfa A, Thierry D, Gourmelon P, and Chapel A: Human mesenchymal stem cells favor healing of the cutaneous radiation syndrome in xenogenic transplant model. Ann Hematol 2007; **86:** 1.

15. Oh JY, Kim MK, Shin MS, Lee HJ, Ko JH, Wee WR, and Lee JH: The anti-inflammatory and anti-angiogenic role of mesenchymal stem cells in corneal wound healing following chemical injury. Stem Cells 2008; **26:** 1047.

16. Javazon EH, Keswani SG, Badillo AT, Crombleholme TM, Zoltick PW, Radu AP, Kozin ED, Beggs K, Malik AA, and Flake AW: Enhanced epithelial gap closure and increased angiogenesis in wounds of diabetic mice treated with adult murine bone marrow stromal progenitors. Wound Repair Regen 2007; **15:** 350.

17. Sasaki M, Abe R, Fujita Y, Ando S, Inokuma D, and Shimizu H: Mesenchymal stem cells are recruited into wounded skin and contribute to wound repair by transdifferentiation into multiple skin cell types. J Immunol 2008; **180:** 2581.

18. Chen L, Tredget EE, Wu PYG, and Wu Y: Paracrine factors of mesenchymal stem cells recruit macrophages and endothelial lineage cells and enhance wound healing. PLoS ONE 2008; **4:** e1886.

19. Wu Y, Chen L, Scott PG, and Tredget EE: Mesenchymal stem cells enhance wound healing through differentiation and angiogenesis. Stem Cells 2007; **25:** 2648.

20. Li H, Fu X, Ouyang Y, Cai C, Wang J, and Sun T: Adult bone marrow-derived mesenchymal stem cells contribute to wound healing of skin appendages. Cell Tissue Res 2006; **326:** 725.

21. Noiseux N, Gnecchi M, Lopez-Ilasaca M, Zhang L, Solomon SD, Deb A, Dzau VJ, and Pratt RE: Mesenchymal stem cells over expressing Akt dramatically repair infarcted myocardium and improve cardiac function despite infrequent cellular fusion or differentiation. Mol Ther 2006; **14:** 840.

22. Neuss S, Becher E, Woltje M, Tietze L, and Jahnen-Dechent W: Functional expression of HGF and HGF receptor/c-met in adult human mesenchymal stem cells suggests a role in cell mobilization, tissue repair, and wound healing. Stem Cells 2004; **22:** 405.

23. Viswanathan A, Painter RG, Lanson NA Jr., and Wang G: Functional expression of N-formyl peptide receptors in human bone marrow-derived mesenchymal stem cells. Stem Cells 2007; **25:** 1263.

24. Rameshwar P and Gascón P: Substance P (SP) mediates production of stem cell factor and interleukin-1 in bone marrow stroma: potential auto-regulatory role for these cytokines in SP receptor expression and induction. Blood 1995; **86:** 482.

25. Hong HS, Lee J, Lee E, Kwon YS, Lee E, Ahn W, Jiang MH, Kim JC, and Son Y: A new role for substance P as an injury-inducible messenger for mobilization of CD29+ stromal-like cells. Nat Med 2009; **15:** 425.

26. Mansilla E, Marin GH, Drage H, Sturla F, Salas E, Gardiner C, Bossi S, Lamonega R, Guzman A, Nunez A, Gil MA, Piccinelli G, Ibar R, and Soratti C: Bloodstream cells phenotypically identical to mesenchymal bone marrow stem cells circulate in large amounts under the influence of acute large skin damage: new evidence for their use in regenerative medicine. Transplant Proc 2006; **38:** 967.

27. Liu Y, Dulchavsky DS, Xiaohua G, Kwon D, Chopp M, Dulchavsky S, and Gautam SC: Wound repair by bone marrow stromal cells through growth factor production. J Surg Res 2006; **136:** 336.

28. Wang M, Crisostomo PR, Herring C, Meldrum KK, and Meldrum DR: Human progenitor cells from bone marrow or adipose tissue produce VEGF, HGF, and IGF-1 in response to TNF by a p38 MAPK-dependent mechanism. Am J Physiol Regul Integr Comp Physiol 2006; **291:** R880.

29. Estrada R, Li N, Sarojini H, An J, Lee M-J, and Wang E: Secretome from mesenchymal stem cells induces angiogenesis via Cyr61. J Cell Physiol 2009; **219:** 563.

30. Kidd S, Spaeth E, Klopp A, Andreeff M, Hall B, and Marini FC: The (in) auspicious role of mesenchymal stromal cells in cancer: be it friend or foe. Cytotherapy 2008; **10:** 657.

Mesenchymal Stem Cells in Ischemic Wound Healing

Susan W. Volk*

Department of Clinical Studies, University of Pennsylvania School of Veterinary Medicine, Philadelphia, Pennsylvania.

Background: Regenerative medical strategies using adult stem cells promise to revolutionize the treatment of a variety of diseases and conditions for which effective therapies are currently lacking. Recent advancements in the field of regenerative medicine have highlighted the potential of mesenchymal stem cells (MSCs) as a potential source of cells capable of differentiating and mediating repair of a variety of tissues, including the skin.
The Problem: Despite an increasing awareness of the pathophysiologic events that occur in the development of chronic wounds of various underlying etiologies, chronic wounds remain a burdensome problem for more than 5 million patients and the healthcare providers who treat them in the United States each year. The impact of ischemia on the process of dermal healing is profound and has been considered one of the most significant contributing factors in the development of chronic wounds.
Basic/Clinical Science Advances: Regenerative medicine was in its infancy almost two decades ago when MSCs were targeted to improve orthopedic repair in a variety of preclinical models. Continued advances in our understanding of the importance of the stem cell niche, mechanisms by which MSCs mediate tissue repair, and optimization of their cellular delivery have further contributed to the expansion of their use in regenerative therapies for many tissues. Most recently, MSC-based therapies have been shown to improve healing of chronic cutaneous wounds, including ischemic ulcers.
Clinical Care Relevance: The ability of MSC-based therapy to overcome the detrimental effects of ischemia in the wound-healing process may provide innovative approaches to chronic wounds secondary to a variety of underlying etiologies.
Conclusion: Cellular-based therapies using MSCs offer significant promise as a novel approach to restore healing to chronic wounds and deservedly are the focus of intensive research efforts in the field of wound bioscience.

Abbreviations and Acronyms

bFGF = basic fibroblast growth factor

ECM = extracellular matrix

MSCs = mesenchymal stem cells

*Correspondence: Department of Clinical Studies, University of Pennsylvania School of Veterinary Medicine, 3800 Spruce St., Philadelphia, Pennsylvania 19104 (e-mail: swvolk@vet.upenn.edu).

BACKGROUND

For wounds to heal progressively, inflammatory, vascular, mesenchymal, and epithelial cells must coordinate production of a variety of growth factors, cytokines, extracellular matrix (ECM), and the enzymes necessary to modify this ECM. Ischemia induces a loss of the balanced activities of these cellular components and leads to chronic, impaired wound healing.[1] Although it has been known for more than 30 years that oxygen tension is a key regulator in wound repair,[2] ischemic wounds remain a burdensome challenge to the healthcare industry. Ischemia, a major factor of which is tissue hypoxia, has been shown to decrease granulation tissue formation, impair epithelialization, and diminish biomechanical strength parameters in wounds.[3,4] Decreased tissue oxygen tension has been shown

Printed in U.S.A.
DOI: 10.1089/awc.2009.0020

to diminish collagen production in wounds, increase matrix metalloproteinase activity, and cause aberrant expression of a variety of growth factors and cytokines within the wound.[2,5–7] These quantitative and qualitative differences in growth factors and ECM components further contribute to diminished proliferative and migratory capacity of key cellular components (fibroblasts, endothelial cells, and keratinocytes) within and recruitment into the wound.[8–10] Unless sufficient cell numbers can be generated within the wound from existing precursors or progenitors enter the wound from distant sites, these wounds will remain unhealed. Therefore, chronic wounds appear to be appropriate targets for regenerative medical strategies that seek to heal the body either by stimulation of endogenous cells to repair damaged tissues or through transplantation of cells or engineered tissues to replace injured or diseased ones. Regenerative medicine is an emerging field of wound biomedicine that promises to provide new and exciting therapeutic modalities.

CLINICAL PROBLEM ADDRESSED

Chronic wounds are a formidable clinical challenge that is associated with significant social and economic consequences. Ischemia has been implicated as one of the most serious contributing factors leading to the development of chronic wounds.[11] Chronic nonhealing wounds, including ischemic ulcers, plague more than 5 million Americans each year with an estimated financial burden of more than $20 billion.[12] Despite the enormous impact on both individuals and society, there remains a significant need for effective therapies for ischemic and other chronic nonhealing wounds.

BASIC SCIENCE CONTEXT

Cellular therapy is an emerging therapeutic strategy for cutaneous wounds. In addition to skin-derived cells (fibroblasts and keratinocytes), the bone marrow provides another source of cells that contribute to normal wound repair. Although bone marrow–derived inflammatory cells have long been recognized to play a critical role in wound repair, the mesenchymal stem cell (also referred to as marrow stromal cells or MSCs) is another component of the bone marrow that has exceptional potential to improve healing of chronic wounds, particularly those with an ischemic component. Recent investigations have begun to elucidate the role of MSCs in response to dermal injury. Bone marrow–derived MSCs are capable of homing to sites of injury, including cutaneous wounds,[13,14] and are thought to contribute to healing through a variety of mechanisms. MSCs may participate directly in wound closure through progenitor cell proliferation and differentiation, as well as production of an ECM by these cells.[14–16] Alternatively, MSCs may indirectly participate in the healing process through the production of paracrine growth factors that would result in proliferation and improved function of resident cell populations, that is, fibroblasts, endothelial, or epithelial cells. The effect of paracrine factors may go beyond the wound to recruit additional regulatory cell populations such as monocytes and macrophages from distant sites. Wound tissue may be particularly suitable for MSC-based therapeutic strategies, as the granulation tissue bed is produced within a defect, unlike other damaged tissues that may require repopulation of existing tissues with MSCs. Collectively, these results suggest that although current knowledge about vulnerary effects of MSCs for chronic wound therapy is just beginning to be understood, MSCs may be particularly suited to promote repair of nonhealing wounds through a variety of mechanisms that target many of the cellular and growth factor alterations present within the chronic wound.

EXPERIMENTAL MODEL

Although there is currently no ideal model of the chronic wound, the rabbit ischemic ear model developed by the Mustoe laboratory[3] has been considered the gold standard in the investigation of ischemic wounds for many reasons. This model, in which two of the three major arteries to the ear are ligated and divided, provides significant and prolonged ischemia to the ear (at least 14 days). Second, healing occurs with minimal contraction because of the adherence of soft tissues to underlying auricular cartilage, thus more closely approximating distal extremity wounds in people where chronic wounds tend to occur. Last, the size of the rabbit allows for multiple wounds to be created on the same ear (ischemic or nonischemic), creating intraanimal controls and therefore increasing statistical power of studies. To address the relative lack of molecular tools available in the rabbit, several rodent models have been developed. Both a modified ischemic ear and a dorsal pedal model have been described in the rat, as well as several other models in which ischemia is created on the dorsum of the animal using implants to prevent neovascularization and/or contraction.[6,17–19] Although rodent models allow for a more efficient mechanistic dissection of therapies for ischemic wounds and are less costly, the smaller size limits both size and number of wounds possible on each individual, which does diminish their usefulness in the assessment of therapeutic strategies for ischemic wounds. Delivery of MSCs to cutaneous wounds created in other animal wound models has been by injection into the wound periphery or application onto the wound bed in a simple cellular suspension or within a variety of matrices or biosynthetic materials.[15,20–22] The latter approach may help retain cells within the wound and influence their fate within the wound.

DISCUSSION OF FINDINGS AND RELEVANT LITERATURE

MSCs have received tremendous attention regarding their clinical potential in regenerative medicine, particularly for orthopedic and ischemic myocardial diseases, but also in neurologic, renal, and hepatic diseases.[23–26] They have been shown to accelerate dermal repair not only in acute wounds but also when applied to chronic wounds in both animal models and human patients.[15,16,20,22,27] The ability of MSCs to treat ischemic wounds has been assessed using allogeneic MSCs in the rabbit ischemic ear model.[15] In this study, topically applied bone marrow–derived MSCs were capable of reversing the detrimental effects of ischemia on wound repair by promoting both an increase in granulation tissue formation as well as reepithelialization. Mechanistic dissection suggested that the ability of MSCs to improve dermal healing in the face of ischemia is multifactorial, including both direct and indirect mechanisms. Applied MSCs were found to persist in the granulation tissue of the wound bed, contributing to the increase in granulation tissue of ischemic wounds compared to vehicle-treated or bone marrow mononuclear cell–treated ischemic wounds. Additional data support that these cells may assume a myofibroblast phenotype in granulation tissue based upon their expression of the myofibroblast marker α-smooth muscle actin and their constitutive expression of type I and III collagens in culture. The production

TAKE-HOME MESSAGE

Basic science advances

- MSCs are attractive candidates for cell-based therapies because of their relative ease of isolation, broad differentiation potential, and ability to be expanded *in vitro.*
- Bone marrow–derived MSCs are capable of homing to sites of injury, including cutaneous wounds, and participating in dermal repair.
- Application of MSCs to ischemic wounds led to improved reepithelialization and increased granulation tissue formation.
- Implanted MSCs provide cellular precursors that are capable of engrafting and directly contributing to dermal repair.
- The production of a rich ECM by transplanted MSCs may contribute to wound repair by improving mechanical properties of the wound as well as modulating activity of other cells within the wound through cellular–matrix interactions.
- The expression of trophic factors and chemokines by MSCs is an important mechanism by which cutaneous wound repair is enhanced in MSC-based therapies.
- The robust expression of various angiogenic factors by MSCs is thought to be the primary mechanism by which MSCs increase neovascularization of damaged tissues. This property of MSCs makes them highly attractive candidates for repair of ischemic tissues, including ischemic dermal wounds.

Clinical science advances

- Therapeutic application of MSCs to ischemic wounds has been shown to reverse the detrimental effects of ischemia on wound-healing parameters in the ischemic rabbit ear model.
- MSC-based therapeutic strategies have been shown to be effective in improving dermal healing in several animal models of chronic wounds as well as in several studies examining their efficacy in treating chronic wounds in human patients.
- Delivery of MSCs for wound therapy may be by direct application to the wound bed, injection into the periphery of the wound, or within a variety of matrices or biosynthetic materials, the latter of which may assist in cellular retention as well as direct differentiation capacity within the wound.

Relevance to clinical care

- At present, MSC-based therapies have shown tremendous promise for the treatment of chronic cutaneous wounds in multiple animal models and in several small studies in human patients. Their therapeutic success in the treatment of ischemic wounds in the rabbit ear model is particularly promising as it provides proof in principle that MSCs are able to overcome the detrimental effects of ischemia, a major contributing factor to the development of many types of chronic cutaneous wounds.

of a rich ECM by MSCs is likely to contribute to wound repair by improving mechanical properties of the wound as well as modulating activity of other cells within the wound through cellular–matrix interactions.

Although other studies have suggested that MSCs are capable of differentiating into epithelial and/or vascular endothelial cells,[16,28,29] there was no evidence for these events within the ischemic wounds.[15] This discrepancy could be explained by differences in wound microenvironments, as both lactate and oxygen levels have been shown to regulate MSC properties and may potentially limit differentiation potential.[30,31] Rather than transdifferentiation, the positive effects of applied MSCs on both reepithelialization and neovascularization in the ischemic wounds appear to be through the production of multiple paracrine mediators. To explain the observation that MSC application to ischemic wounds was able to increase vascular density within the newly formed granulation tissue sixfold compared to control wounds without directly contributing to vascular progenitors, an examination of soluble mediators of angiogenesis by MSCs was performed. MSCs were found to express several important angiogenic cytokines, particularly basic fibroblast growth factor (bFGF) and vascular endothelial growth factor, as well as platelet-derived growth factor and connective tissue growth factor, which have been shown to promote endothelial cell recruitment and modulate vascular remodeling. The powerful ability of MSCs to improve angiogenesis within ischemic tissues through the production of soluble factors is consistent with results of other studies examining MSC-based therapeutic strategies for ischemic myocardial disease, as well as renal and neurologic injury.[24,26,32]

Similarly, several growth factors important to keratinocyte proliferation and migration, such as heparin-binding epidermal-like growth factor, transforming growth factor-α, epidermal growth factor, keratinocyte growth factor, and bFGF, were found to be expressed by MSCs and provide a mechanism by which MSCs improve reepithelialization in the absence of their epithelial transdifferentiation in ischemic wounds. The ability of conditioned media from MSC cultures to promote keratinocyte proliferation and outgrowth from epidermal explants supported this hypothesis of indirect participation by MSCs on reepithelialization of the ischemic wounds. MSCs were also found to express connective tissue growth factor, bFGF, and platelet-derived growth factor-B, which may function in both an autocrine or a paracrine role within the wound to positively regulate ECM production, as well as proliferation and chemotaxis of other mesenchymal progenitors within the wound. These combined observations in this preclinical model support the further development of MSC-based therapeutic strategies for ischemic wounds and elucidate several mechanisms by which MSCs may be able to initiate healing in these problematic wounds (Fig. 1).

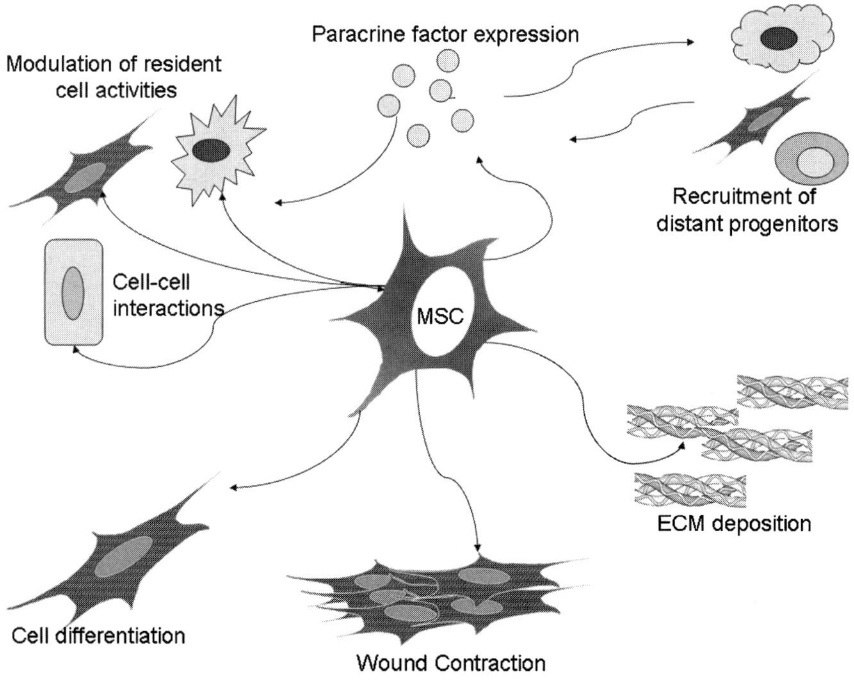

Figure 1. Mesenchymal stem cells (MSCs) may improve ischemic wound healing by a variety of mechanisms. MSCs may directly improve wound healing by providing progenitor cells that engraft and differentiate into fibroblasts/myofibroblasts (potentially additional cell types in other chronic wounds). These cells may elaborate a rich extracellular matrix and participate in wound contraction. Activities of resident cells in the wound may be influenced by direct contact with the MSCs or their differentiated cell types as well as through the effects of paracrine growth factors secreted by the MSCs. Expression of chemokines by MSCs may also be responsible for the recruitment of distant progenitors to or migration of local cells within the wound bed.

CAUTION, CRITICAL REMARKS, AND RECOMMENDATIONS

Although MSC treatment has been shown to positively influence healing of chronic wounds due to a variety of underlying etiologies, it should be remembered that the particular microenvironment of an individual wound may influence both the differentiation potential of delivered MSCs as well as their activity within the wound (proliferative capacity, migration, apoptosis, and secretion of paracrine factors). Therefore, the response to MSC therapy may vary in wounds of differing etiologies as well as with the chronicity of individual wounds. It is also important to note that MSC application and systemic administration for regenerative therapies in rodent models has revealed MSC differentiation to undesirable phenotypes, including dystrophic mineralization associated with osteogenic differentiation within cutaneous wounds[33] and malignant transformation.[34,35] Evolution of our understanding of both the cues required by MSCs, as well as the responses elicited in MSCs, to facilitate cutaneous wound repair will improve our ability to harness the potential of these cells and avoid complications associated with therapies.

FUTURE DEVELOPMENT

Regenerative medicine and tissue engineering strategies that seek to harness the potential of MSCs for treatment of chronic cutaneous wounds are still in development; however, initial basic and clinical studies have shown that they offer tremendous promise for a clinical problem in desperate need of effective therapy. To reap their clinical benefits will require an improved understanding of the biology of these cells as well as the development of technologies for delivery or endogenous recruitment of MSCs to sites of repair.

ACKNOWLEDGMENT

Wound-healing research in the author's laboratory was funded by NIH Award K08AR53945.

AUTHOR DISCLOSURE STATEMENT

No conflict of interest disclosed.

REFERENCES

1. Bennett NT and Schultz GC: Growth factors in wound healing: part II. Role in normal and chronic wound healing. Am J Surg 1993; **166:** 74.
2. Hunt TK and Pai MP: The effect of varying ambient oxygen tensions on wound metabolism and collagen synthesis. Surg Gynecol Obstet 1972; **135:** 561.
3. Ahn ST and Mustoe TA: Effects of ischemia on ulcer wound healing: a new model in the rabbit ear. Ann Plast Surg 1990; **24:** 17.
4. Stephens EO and Hunt TK: Effect of changes in inspired oxygen and carbon dioxide tension on wound tensile strength. An experimental study. Ann Surg 1971; **173:** 515.
5. Beckert S, Hierlemann H, Muschenborn N, Witte M, Ranke M, and Coerper S: Experimental ischemic wounds: correlation of cell proliferation and insulin-like growth factor 1 expression and its modification by different local IGF-1 release systems. Wound Repair Regen 2005; **13:** 278.
6. Mogford JE, Sisco M, Bonomo SR, Robinson AM, and Mustoe TA: Impact of aging on gene expression in a rat model of ischemic cutaneous wound healing. J Surg Res 2004; **118:** 190.
7. Shukla A, Dubey MP, Srivastava R, and Srivastava BS: Differential expression of proteins during healing of cutaneous wounds in experimental normal and chronic models. Biochem Biophys Res Commun 1998; **244:** 434.
8. Seah CC, Phillips TJ, Howard CE, Panova IP, Hayes CM, Assandra AS, and Park HY: Chronic wound fluid suppresses proliferation of dermal fibroblasts through a Ras-mediated signaling pathway. J Invest Dermatol 2005; **124:** 466.
9. Falanga V: Growth factors and chronic wounds: the need to understand the microenvironment. J Dermatol 1992; **19:** 667.
10. Badiavas EV: The potential of bone marrow cells to orchestrate homeostasis and healing in skin. Blood Cells Mol Dis 2004; **32:** 21.
11. Schäffer M, Witte M, and Horst-Dieter B: Models to study ischemia in chronic wounds. Int J Low Extrem Wounds 2002; **1:** 104.
12. Attinger CE, Hoang H, Steinberg J, Couch K, Hubley K, Winger L, and Kugler M: How to make a hospital-based wound center financially viable: the Georgetown University Hospital model. Gyn Oncol 2008; **111:** S92.
13. Liechty KW, MacKenzie TC, Shaaban AF, Radu A, Moseley AB, Deans R, Marshak DR, and Flake AW: Human mesenchymal stem cells engraft and demonstrate site-specific differentiation after *in utero* transplantation in sheep. Nat Med 2000; **6:** 1282.
14. Fathke C, Wilson L, Hutter J, Kapoor V, Smith A, Hocking A, and Isik F: Contribution of bone marrow-derived cells to skin: collagen deposition and wound repair. Stem Cells 2004; **22:** 812.
15. Volk SW, Radu A, Zhang L, and Liechty KW: Stromal progenitor cell therapy corrects the wound healing defect in the ischemic rabbit ear model of chronic wound repair. Wound Repair Regen 2007; **15:** 736.
16. Wu Y, Chen L, Scott PG, and Tredget EE: Mesenchymal stem cells enhance wound healing through differentiation and angiogenesis. Stem Cells 2007; **25:** 2648.
17. Harder Y, Amon M, Erni D, and Menger MD: Evolution of ischemic tissue injury in a random pattern flap: a new mouse model using intravital microscopy. J Surg Res 2004; **121:** 197.
18. Schwarz DA, Lindblad WJ, and Rees RS: Altered collagen metabolism and delayed healing in a novel model of ischemic wounds. Wound Repair Regen 1995; **3:** 204.
19. Alizadeh N, Pepper MS, Modarressi A, Alfo K, Schlaudraff K, Montandon D, Gabbiani G, Bochaton-Piallat M-L, and Pittet B: Persistent ischemia impairs myofibroblast development in wound granulation tissue: a new model of delayed wound healing. Wound Repair Regen 2007; **15:** 809.
20. Badillo AT, Redden RA, Zhang L, Doolin EJ, and Liechty KW: Treatment of diabetic wounds with fetal murine mesenchymal stromal cells enhances wound closure. Cell Tissue Res 2007; **329:** 301.
21. Kim SS, Song CK, Shon SK, Lee KY, Kim CH, Lee MJ, and Wang LW: Effects of human amniotic membrane grafts combined with marrow mesenchymal stem cells on healing of full-thickness skin defects in rabbits. Cell Tissue Res 2009 (Epub ahead of print).
22. Falanga V, Iwamoto S, Chartier M, Yufit T, Butmarc J, Kouttab N, Shrayer D, and Carson P: Autologous bone marrow-derived cultured

mesenchymal stem cells delivered in a fibrin spray accelerate healing in murine and human cutaneous wounds. Tissue Eng 2007; **13:** 1299.

23. Young RG, Butler DL, Weber W, Caplan AI, Gordon SL, and Fink DJ: Use of mesenchymal stem cells in a collagen matrix for Achilles tendon repair. J Orthop Res 1998; **16:** 406.

24. Togel F, Hu Z, Weiss K, Isaac J, Lange C, and Westenfelder C: Administered mesenchymal stem cells protect against ischemic acute renal failure through differentiation-independent mechanisms. Am J Physiol 2005; **289:** 31.

25. Sato Y, Araki H, Kato J, Nakamura K, Kawano Y, Kobune M, Sato T, Miyanishi K, Tekayama T, Takahashi M, Takimoto R, Iyama S, Matsunaga T, Ohtani S, Matsuura A, Hamada H, and Niitsu Y: Human mesenchymal stem cells xenografted directly to rat liver are differentiated into human hepatocytes without fusion. Blood 2005; **106:** 756.

26. Shi E, Kazui T, Jiang X, Washiyama N, Yamashita K, Terada H, and Bashar AH: Therapeutic benefit of intrathecal injection of marrow stromal cells on ischemia-injured spinal cord. Ann Thorac Surg 2007; **83:** 1484.

27. Yoshikawa T, Mitsuno H, Nonaka I, Sen Y, Kawanishi K, Inada Y, Takakura Y, Okuchi K, and Nonomura A: Wound therapy by marrow mesenchymal cell transplanted. Plast Reconstr Surg 2008; **121:** 860.

28. Sasaki M, Abe R, Fujita Y, Ando S, Inokuma D, and Shimizu H: Mesenchymal stem cells are recruited into wounded skin and contribute to wound repair by transdifferentiation into multiple skin cell types. J Immunol 2008; **180:** 2581.

29. Li H, Fu X, Ouyang Y, Cai C, Wang J, and Sun T: Adult bone marrow-derived mesenchymal stem cells contribute to wound healing of skin appendages. Cell Tissue Res 2006; **326:** 725.

30. Zieker D, Schafer R, Glatzle J, Nieselt K, Coerper S, Northoff H, Konlgsrainer A, Hunt H, Konlgsrainer A, Hunt TK, and Beckert S: Lactate modulates gene expression in human mesenchymal stem cells. Langenbecks Arch Surg 2008; **393:** 297.

31. Ohnishi S, Yasuda T, Kitamura S, and Nagaya N: Effect of hypoxia on gene expression of bone marrow-derived mesenchymal stem cells and mononuclear cells. Stem Cells 2007; **25:** 1166.

32. Kinnaird T, Stabile E, Burnett MS, Lee CW, Barr S, Fuchs S, and Epstein SE: Marrow-derived stromal cells express genes encoding a broad spectrum of arteriogenic cytokines and promote *in vitro* and *in vivo* arteriogenesis through paracrine mechanisms. Circ Res 2004; **94:** 678.

33. Javazon EH, Keswani SG, Badillo AT, Crombleholme TM, Zoltick PW, Radu AP, Kozin ED, Beggs K, Malik AT, and Flake AW: Enhanced epithelial gap closure and increased angiogenesis in wounds of diabetic mice treated with adult murine bone marrow stromal progenitor cells. Wound Repair Regen 2007; **15:** 350.

34. Tolar J, Nauta AJ, Osborn MJ, Mortari AP, McElmurry RT, Bell S, Xia L, Zhou N, Riddle M, Schroeder TM, Westendorf JJ, McIvor RS, Hofendoom PCW, Szuhai K, Oseth L, Hirsch B, Yant SR, Kay MA, Peister A, Prockop DJ, Fibbe E, and Blazar BR: Sarcoma derived from cultured mesenchymal stem cells. Stem Cells 2007; **25:** 371.

35. Miura M, Miura Y, Padilla-Nash HM, Molinolo AA, Fu B, Patel V, Seo B-M, Sonoyama W, Zheng JJ, Baker CC, Chen W, Reid T, and Shi S: Accumulated chromosomal instability in murine bone marrow mesenchymal stem cells leads to malignant transformation. Stem Cells 2005; **24:** 1095.

Mesenchymal Stem Cells in Diabetic Wound Healing

Dustin M. Bermudez[1,2] and Kenneth W. Liechty[1,2,3,*]

[1]Department of Surgery, University of Pennsylvania School of Medicine, Philadelphia, Pennsylvania.
[2]Center for Fetal Research, Children's Hospital of Philadelphia, Philadelphia, Pennsylvania.
[3]The University of Mississippi Medical Center, Jackson, Mississippi

Background: Diabetic wounds are slow to heal and are the source of considerable health care expenditures. The etiology of the wound-healing defect of diabetes is myriad: a more proteolytic extracellular matrix, decreased levels of growth factors and cytokines, poor macrophage function, and a depressed immune system. Mesenchymal stem cells (MSCs) offer a novel cellular approach to correct the multitude of causes of the diabetic wound-healing defect.
The Problem: The incidence of diabetic wounds and lower extremity ulcers is rapidly increasing; currently, 22 million Americans suffer from diabetes and by 2030 this number is expected to double. An effective therapy to treat chronic ulcers of the diabetic is still lacking.
Basic/Clinical Science Advances: MSCs appear to correct the wound-healing defect of diabetes in a diabetic murine model. Application of autologous MSCs in one human study demonstrated improved wound healing.
Clinical Care Relevance: The application of allogeneic MSCs to chronic ulcers of diabetics may be an effective and cost-efficient strategy. Given that a lower extremity ulcer precedes most amputations, treatment of these wounds will significantly impact morbidity and mortality among diabetics (estimated to be responsible for up to $58 billion of annual health care costs in the United States alone in 2007).
Conclusion: MSCs may offer a novel and cost-effective therapy to treat diabetic ulcers. Randomized controlled trials assessing safety and effectiveness in human subjects are still lacking.

Abbreviations And Acronyms

BM = bone marrow
DFU = diabetic foot ulcer
ECM = extracellular matrix
EPC = endothelial progenitor cell
FGF = fibroblast growth factor
HBOT = hyperbaric oxygen therapy
HLA = human leukocyte factor
MSC = mesenchymal stem cell
PDGF = platelet-derived growth factor
PIGF = placental growth factor
SDF-1α = stromal-derived factor 1 alpha
TGF-β = transforming growth factor beta
VEGF = vascular endothelial growth factor

*Correspondence: Department of Surgery, University of Mississippi Medical Center, 2500 North State St., Jackson, Mississippi 39216 (e-mail: kliechty@surgery.umsmed.edu).

BACKGROUND

Dermal injury sets into motion a complex cascade of molecular events that orchestrate hemostasis, cell migration, and scar deposition that ultimately lead to a well-healed wound. Alteration of this normal physiology can lead to either a chronic ulcer that fails to heal or a keloid scar that heals with profound fibrosis. Effective treatment for either of these extremes is still lacking. Further elucidation of the precise mechanism by which wounds heal as well as novel therapies that address the myriad defects that likely occur in these aberrations are necessary.

Diabetes is a common scenario in which the wound-healing process is significantly impaired. This is of particular concern to the health care establishment as a whole (as well as the American economy) as approximately $58 billion was spent in the United States alone in 2007 on the treatment of diabetic wounds and their resultant complications.[1] There are approximately 22 million people in the United States alone who now suffer from diabetes. Over the next 15 years this number is expected to double.[2,3]

As the prevalence of diabetes rises drastically, so do its resultant

Printed in U.S.A.
DOI: 10.1089/awc.2009.0064

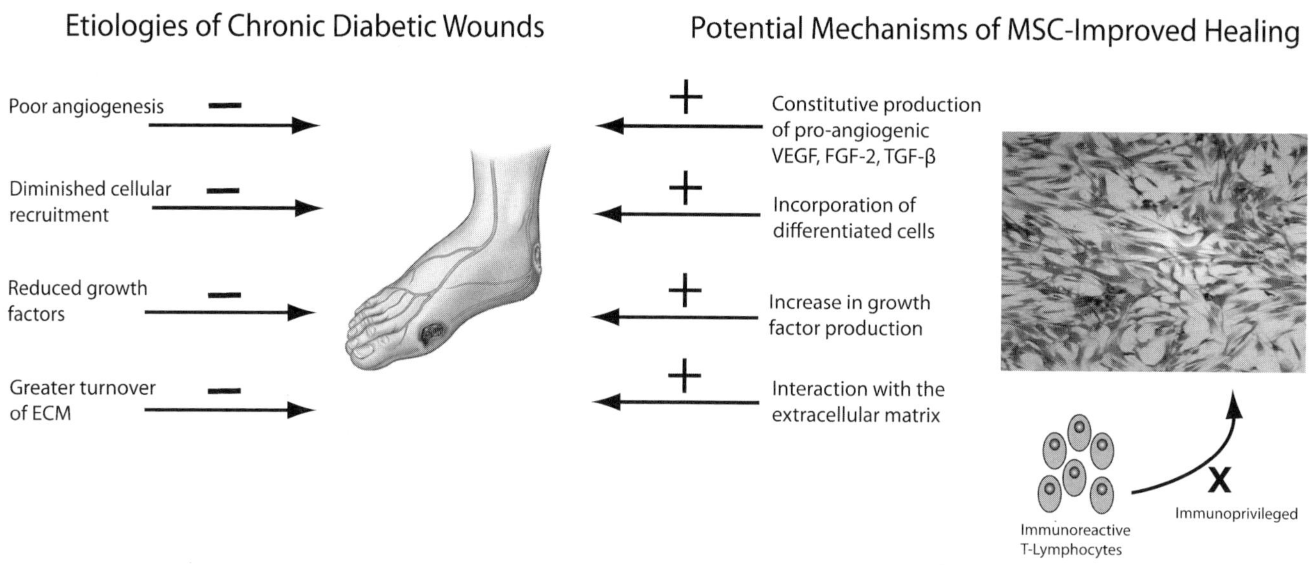

Figure 1. Chronic diabetic wounds arise from a multitude of factors relating to angiogenesis, cellular recruitment, growth factor production, and ECM turnover. MSCs have the potential to play a significant role in the treatment of these wounds due to a variety of unique properties. Additionally, it is believed that MSCs are immunoprivileged; in the setting of an allogeneic, HLA-nonmatched MSC treatment, the recipient will be unlikely to mount a profound inflammatory response. ECM = extracellular matrix; HLA = human leukocyte antigen; MSC = mesenchymal stem cell.

complications—chief among which are diabetic foot ulcers (DFUs). DFUs generally occur when an insensate lower extremity, already deficient in arterial inflow, is subjected to an incidental traumatic cut or scrape that never heals and becomes a chronic ulcer. When paired with an already compromised immune system, there is a significant risk of amputation. Lower extremity foot ulcers are the number one cause of inpatient admissions in diabetic patients in the United States.[4,5] Approximately 84% of patients who undergo amputation have a DFU as the primary cause.[1,4]

Despite the great increase in incidence and prevalence of DFUs, novel therapies are lacking. Attempts have been made at improving wound healing through basic wound care, empiric antibiotic therapy, and hyperbaric oxygen therapy (HBOT). Unfortunately, these therapies have not had a major impact on the propensity for diabetic lower extremity ulcers to heal. Application of dermal grafts, recombinant growth factors, and HBOT have been investigated as alternative approaches to improve wound healing.[6–8]

Cellular therapy, however, may hold great promise for the treatment of DFUs. Specifically, mesenchymal stem cells (MSCs) are currently being investigated as a method to treat diabetic wounds given their multiple unique and advantageous properties.[9–16] We propose that MSCs should be further investigated as a novel therapy that may change the way chronic diabetic wounds are treated (Fig. 1).

CLINICAL PROBLEM ADDRESSED

The wound-healing defects known to exist in diabetic patients are myriad. They include fewer endothelial progenitor cells (EPCs); diminished macrophage function; lower levels of the chemokine stromal-derived factor 1 alpha (SDF-1α) and growth factors, fibroblast growth factor (FGF), epithelial growth factor, and platelet-derived growth factor (PDGF); decreased levels of endothelial nitric oxide synthase synthesis; reduced collagen deposition; greater proteolysis in the extracellular matrix (ECM); less angiogenesis; and diminished keratinocyte and fibroblast migration and proliferation.[4,17,18] With this multitude of alterations in the physiology of diabetic wounds, an effective treatment strategy must address multiple aspects of this wound-healing impairment simultaneously.

Basic wound care, HBOT, and prophylactic antibiotics, while unlikely to be cost prohibitive, have been met with minimal success at improving wound closure rates in diabetics. A recent Cochrane Review examined five trials from 1992 to 2003 that assessed the impact that HBOT had on outcomes. They found little evidence that HBOT improved wound healing and limited evidence that it decreased the frequency of major amputations.[8]

Newer therapies, such as recombinant PDGF or the use of dermal grafts, have been met with some success. Regranex, a recombinant form of PDGF-BB, that is deficient in diabetic wounds, demonstrated a 14% improvement in wound closure when used clinically.[6,19] Although PDGF is an important growth factor in wound healing, it is not the only one affected by diabetic physiology.

Apligraf is a biologic dressing approved for use in diabetic and chronic wounds. It is composed of an epidermal layer formed from human keratinocytes on one side and a dermal layer composed of human fibroblasts in a bovine type I collagen matrix on the other. Dermagraft, another biologic dressing, is composed of human foreskin fibroblasts cultured onto an absorbable scaffold and is approved for use in full-thickness DFUs. These biologic dressings have demonstrated some improvement in wound healing.[7]

Many of the initial studies directed at assessment of cytotherapy in the context of diabetes utilized whole bone marrow (BM).[20–23] Most cells, however, derived from BM do not have a regenerative capacity, like that of EPCs and MSCs. Numerous studies have utilized whole BM, through direct injection, collagen matrix, or a fibrin spray, and demonstrated an improvement in wound healing in lower extremity ulcers and radiation burn injuries.[20–23] While none of these were randomized controlled trials, many enrolled patients had chronic wounds for over a year, refractory to current therapy, and found their wounds healed after BM application.

RELEVANT BASIC SCIENCE CONTEXT

Myriad aspects of the molecular physiology of the wound-healing process are deranged in the diabetic—leading to a delay in healing and chronic inflammatory states. These include a more proteolytic ECM, a deficiency of growth factors, inadequate collagen deposition, and deficient tensile strength. The ECM of a wound is integral for deposition of collagen (leading to increased tensile strength), migration of inflammatory cells into the wound, regulation of the proteolytic state of a tissue, and serving as a scaffold for cellular development.

Growth factors play an essential part of the wound-healing process. They can influence cell migration and homing, cellular proliferation, angiogenesis, and metalloproteinase activity. Transforming growth factor beta 1 (TGF-β1), insulin-like growth factor-1, vascular endothelial growth factor (VEGF), basic FGF, keratinocyte growth factor, and interleukin 6 all play a role in angiogenesis.[18] When decreased, as is the case in diabetes, less angiogenesis takes place.

Initial studies investigated the effect of whole BM on wound healing. The appeal of whole BM was that it could be derived from autologous sources, and along with numerous other inflammatory and progenitor cells, it carries with it MSCs. Preliminary studies suggested that application of BM progenitor cells might improve wound closure.[11,20,21,23]

MSCs have the unique capacity of exhibiting pluripotency, or the ability to differentiate into a variety of tissues, as well as remaining self-renewing. They can also be isolated from adult tissue.[24–26] MSCs are a heterogeneous group of cells, mesodermal in origin, that can differentiate into a multitude of cell lines: adipocytes, chondrocytes, osteocytes, and myocytes.[24–26] Moreover, MSCs can be induced to transform into cells of ectodermal (neurons) and endodermal (hepatocytes) origin as well.[13] These cells have the unique capacity to constitutively produce growth factors integral to the wound-healing process and to differentiate into cells necessary for wound contraction and the healing process as a whole, and can interact with the ECM.[14,24–26] Specifically, MSCs have been found to constitutively produce VEGF, FGF, and TGF-β—all of which promote angiogenesis.[27]

EXPERIMENTAL MODEL

MSCs, by definition, are self-renewing and multipotent as well as clonogenic. However, culture of these cells *in vitro* may alter the phenotype such that these cells no longer represent the parent cell.[14,26] MSCs are usually isolated in humans based on several markers, including CD73, CD90, and CD105, and lack of CD45. It has also been suggested that expression of Stro-1 and VCAM-1 could also be used to preferentially enrich for MSCs.[10] There is still debate, however, whether isolating MSCs with these cell-surface markers results in a pure MSC population.

A number of different mouse models exist that serve to replicate the pathophysiology of diabetes. The nonobese diabetic mouse is a spontaneous animal model of type I diabetes. This mouse, however, was generated through inbreeding of hyperglycemic mice that may enrich for genes not relevant to the human phenotype. Streptozotocin and alloxan induce a diabetic state through mediating pancreatic islet cell destruction. These rodents develop a hyperglycemic, hypoinsulinemic state. This is in contrast to the monogenic model of leptin resistance.[28] These mice, known as db/db mice, are obese, hyperglycemic, and hyperinsulinemic. In contrast to the streptozocin-induced diabetic state that most closely resembles type I diabetes, these db/db mice more closely resemble the pathophysiology of type II diabetes. Direct applicability to type II diabetes in humans, however, is still unclear. Human diabetes is more likely a product of numerous genetic and epigenetic factors.

Integral to the safety of allogeneic MSCs for therapeutic use in humans is ensuring their relatively immunoprivileged status. Although some data have suggested that MSCs are immunoprivileged, this has been supported in only one clinical study thus far.[25,29]

TAKE-HOME MESSAGE

Basic science advances

- Badillo *et al.*[9] found that the wound-healing defect of genetically diabetic mice (db/db) can be corrected with the application of 1×10^6 fetal MSCs. Mice that received the treatment also demonstrated elevated levels of SDF-1α, VEGF, TGF-β1, epithelial growth factor, PDGF-BB, placental growth factor (PIGF), murine inhibitory peptide-2, and interleukin 6.
- Wu *et al.*[15] found that application of MSCs in a dermal graft model will significantly improve healing in a dermal splint model specifically increasing angiogenesis, wound closure, and epithelialization.
- MSCs can be used not only in the setting of diabetic wounds but they may also be used for treatment of other injured tissue.[10,14,30,31]

Clinical science advances

- Yoshikawa *et al.*[16] have demonstrated that use of a collagen sponge impregnated with autologous BM-derived MSCs will promote closure in chronic wounds of multiple etiologies.
- Falanga *et al.*[11] show that application of increasing levels of autologous BM-derived MSCs will hasten the wound-healing process of chronic lower extremity ulcers as well as acute surgical ulcers.
- MSCs possess immunosuppressive properties that likely occur through T-cell suppression.[29] Additionally, MSCs can be transplanted across the major histocompatibility complex barrier without the need for immunosuppression.

Relevance to clinical care

- Cellular therapy has the advantage of exploiting a cell's machinery to produce various cytokines, growth factors, ECM components, and other products, all of which contribute to the impaired healing found in diabetics. MSCs are a potentially ideal cell to treat a chronic diabetic ulcer. They are self-renewable and may thus be expanded in culture *ex vivo*. They are immunoprivileged and are thus theoretically able to be extracted from a healthy, unrelated donor; expanded *ex vivo*; and then transplanted into major histocompatibility complex–unmatched recipients without any need for immunosuppression. Finally, they have been proven in animal models to correct the diabetic wound-healing defect.

DISCUSSION OF FINDINGS AND RELEVANT LITERATURE

It has recently been demonstrated that in the db/db mouse model of diabetes, application of MSCs reverses the wound-healing defect found at baseline.[9] Application of MSCs to injured tissue has not been limited to dermis alone. Implantation of BM-derived MSCs to sphingomyelinase-deficient mice delays neurologic impairment, and injection of MSCs into swine myocardium after infarction reduced pathologic scarring and minimized ventricular contractile dysfunction.[14,30] Additionally, injection of MSCs into rats after stroke demonstrated smaller infarct size, and improved axonal growth.[31] One clinical study has suggested that application of MSCs can augment the rate of wound closure with chronic wounds.[16]

Growth factors, however, have been tested more thoroughly than cellular therapy. Regranex, a recombinant form of PDGF, has been approved by the Food and Drug Administration for use in DFUs since 1998. Randomized clinical trials suggested an impact on wound healing—one clinical trial demonstrated a significant difference in likelihood to heal (34% vs. 26%) and propensity for amputation (4.9% vs. 6.4%). The benefit demonstrated with these newer therapies is mitigated by their prohibitive cost.[32]

The ECM, in particular, may be a key factor in the etiology of chronic, diabetic wounds. Ladwig *et al.* demonstrated that the matrix metalloproteinase and tissue inhibitor metalloproteinase composition of the ECM contribute to chronic wounds' failure to heal.[33] Studies have demonstrated that diabetic chronic wounds possess higher levels of the proteolytic matrix metalloproteinases and lower levels of their inhibitors, tissue inhibitor metalloproteinases.[18,33] MSCs possess the ability to interact with the ECM—thus potentially addressing this imbalance.[34]

Cellular migration may also be addressed by MSC therapy. EPCs are recruited to the site of injury via SDF-1α secretion.[4] Decreased expression of SDF-1α results in fewer EPCs migrating to the site of injury. Diabetic wounds demonstrate both lower levels of EPCs and SDF-1α.[4,9,17,18] MSC application can lead to improved SDF-1α levels, recruited macrophages, and cells of endothelial lineage.[22]

It has been demonstrated that MSCs preferentially home to sites of injury. Ortiz *et al.* showed that MSCs preferentially engraft in murine lung parenchyma with bleomycin exposure (leading to pulmonary fibrosis), and Mouisseddine *et al.* demonstrated greater migration of MSCs in the setting of multiorgan injury from radiation exposure.[35,36] Wu *et al.* found that application of allogeneic MSCs will improve angiogenesis, hasten wound closure, and enhance re-epithelialization in diabetic mice.[15] Direct injection of MSCs into dermal wounds also corrects the diabetic defect.[9] Thus far, only one clinical study has employed MSCs to heal a chronic wound (none have been directed at diabetic wounds specifically).[16]

CAUTION, CRITICAL REMARKS, AND RECOMMENDATIONS

Cellular therapy has tremendous potential to treat chronic diabetic wounds. Unlike targeted therapies that may address a single aspect of a deficiency in diabetic wounds, cellular therapy can address a multitude of deficiencies simultaneously. Enthusiasm for this approach, however, should be tempered by a dearth of thorough investigations performed thus far. There is a lack of randomized controlled trials that address MSC application in patients with diabetes. Although a number of studies have attempted to assess this with BM progenitor cells, there was neither sufficient power nor were there adequate controls to deduce whether these were effective therapies. A phase 1 study to demonstrate safety of use would be worthwhile. Additionally, insufficient data exist as to the method of delivery. Application of allogeneic BM-derived MSCs can be injected intradermally, applied topically, or adhered with a biologic matrix.

Data have suggested that CD45 cells (common leukocyte antigen) alone may also have some action on levels of growth factors, cytokines, and ECM proteins.[9] The distinct characteristics that make an MSC effective at improving the wound-healing process are still unclear.

Further, the immunoprivileged status that MSCs are afforded has yet to be thoroughly studied in human subjects in a controlled fashion. While it is assumed that the use of allogeneic MSCs will not incite an immune response, this has not been accurately studied to date.

Finally, Javazon *et al.*[27] found that with application of adult-derived MSCs to diabetic mice, a notable increase in dystrophic calcification was encountered with a suggestion that teratomas may develop. This risk must be studied further to ensure that this is not encountered in human subjects.

FUTURE DEVELOPMENT

An effective and cost-efficient treatment for chronic diabetic wounds is sorely needed. As the prevalence of diabetes increases and as health care costs in the United States skyrocket, the need for such a therapy becomes even more critical. MSCs may offer hope to provide a safe, effective, and cost-efficient therapy to treat these wounds. To begin to consider its implementation in clinical practice, randomized clinical trials are necessary to demonstrate its purported safety and efficacy. Further, animal studies addressing the most effective mode of delivery (injection, topical application, and synthetic graft) must also be pursued. Once safety, efficacy, and efficiency have been addressed with the use of MSCs on chronic wounds, they may be applied to a variety of other clinical scenarios, including fistulas in Crohn's patients, myocardium following infarction, and brain parenchyma following stroke.

ACKNOWLEDGMENTS

Wound-healing research conducted in the senior author's laboratory has been funded by NIH Grants #R56DK080672-01A1 and DP2DK083085-01.

AUTHOR DISCLOSURE STATEMENT

No conflict of interest disclosed.

REFERENCES

1. Health, United States, 2007. Center for Disease Control and Prevention. U.S. Department of Health and Human Services.

2. Boulton AJ, Vileikyte L, Ragnarson-Tennvall G, and Apleqvist J: The global burden of diabetic foot disease. Lancet 2005; **366:** 1719.

3. Wild S, Roglic G, Green A, Sicree R, and King H: Global prevalence of diabetes: estimates for the year 2000 and projections for 2030. Diabetes Care 2004; **27:** 1047.

4. Brem H and Tomic-Canic M: Cellular and molecular basis of wound healing in diabetes. J Clin Invest 2007; **117:** 1219.

5. National Diabetes Information Clearinghouse: National Diabetes Statistics fact sheet. http://diabetes.niddk.nih.gov/dm/pubs/satistics/index.htm.

6. Bennett SP, Griffiths GD, Schor AM, Leese GP, and Schor SL: Growth factors in the treatment of diabetic foot ulcers. Br J Surg 2003; **90:** 133.

7. Veves A, Falanga V, Armstrong DG, and Sabolinski ML: Graftskin, a human skin equivalent, is effective in the management of noninfected neuropathic diabetic foot ulcers: a prospective randomized multicenter clinical trial. Diabetes Care 2001; **24:** 290.

8. Kranke P, Bennett MH, Debus SE, Roeckl-Wiedmann I, and Schnabel A: Hyperbaric oxygen therapy for chronic wounds. Cochrane Database Syst Rev 2004, Issue 1. Art. No.: CD004123.

9. Badillo AT, Redden RA, Zhang L, Doolin EJ, and Liechty KW: Treatment of diabetic wounds with fetal murine mesenchymal stromal cells enhances wound closure. Cell Tissue Res 2007; **329:** 301.

10. Brooke G, Cook M, Blair C, Han R, Heazlewood C, Jones B, Kambouris M, Kollar K, McTaggart S, Pelekanos R, Rice A, Rossetti T, and Atkinson K: Therapeutic applications of mesenchymal stromal cells. Semin Cell Dev Biol 2007; **18:** 846.

11. Falanga V, Iwamoto S, Chartier M, Yufit T, Butmarc J, Kouttab N, Shrayer D, and Carson P: Autologous bone marrow-derived cultured mesenchymal stem cells delivered in a fibrin spray accelerate healing in murine and human cutaneous wounds. Tissue Eng 2007; **13:** 1299.

12. Lataillade JJ, Doucet C, Bey E, Carsin H, Huet C, Clairand I, Bottollier-Depois JF, Chapel A, Ernou I, Gourven M, Boutin L, Hayden A, Carcamo C, Buglova E, Joussemet M, de Revel T, and Gourmelon P: New approach to radiation burn treatment by dosimetry-guided surgery combined with autologous mesenchymal stem cell therapy. Regen Med 2007; **2:** 785.

13. Phinney DG and Prockop DJ: Concise review: mesenchymal stem/multipotent stromal cells: the state of transdifferentiation and modes of tissue repair–current views. Stem Cells 2007; **25:** 2896.

14. Psaltis PJ, Zannettino AC, Worthley SG, and Gronthos S: Concise review: mesenchymal stromal cells: potential for cardiovascular repair. Stem Cells 2008; **26:** 2201.

15. Wu Y, Chen L, Scott PG, and Tredget EE: Mesenchymal stem cells enhance wound healing through differentiation and angiogenesis. Stem Cells 2007; **25:** 2648.

16. Yoshikawa T, Mitsuno H, and Nonaka I: Wound therapy by mesenchymal cell transplantation. Plast Reconstr Surg 2008; **121:** 860.

17. Badillo AT, Chung S, Zhang L, Zoltick P, and Liechty KW: Lentiviral gene transfer of SDF-1α to wounds improves diabetic wound healing. J Surg Res 2007; **143:** 35.

18. Blakytny R and Jude E: The molecular biology of chronic wounds and delayed healing in diabetes. Diabet Med 2006; **23:** 594.

19. Steed DL: Clinical evaluation of recombinant human platelet-derived growth factor for the treatment of lower extremity ulcers. Plast Reconstr Surg 2006; **117:** 143S.

20. Badiavas EV and Falanga V: Treatment of chronic wounds with bone marrow-derived cells. Arch Dermatol 2003; **139:** 510.

21. Badiavas EV, Ford D, Liu P, Kouttab N, Morgan J, Richards A, and Maizel A: Long-term bone marrow culture and its clinical potential in chronic wound healing. Wound Repair Regen 2007; **15:** 856.

22. Chen L, Tredget EE, Wu PY, and Wu Y: Paracrine factors of mesenchymal stem cells recruit macrophages and endothelial lineage cells and enhance wound healing. PLoS ONE 2008; **3:** 1886.

23. Ichioka S, Kouraba S, Sekiya N, Ohura N, and Nakatsuka T: Bone marrow-impregnated collagen matrix for wound healing: experimental evaluation in a microcirculatory model of angiogenesis, and clinical experience. Br J Plast Surg 2005; **58:** 1124.

24. Herdrich BJ, Lind RC, and Liechty KW: Multipotent adult progenitor cells: their role in wound healing and the treatment of dermal wounds. Cytotherapy 2008; **10:** 543.

25. Keating A: Mesenchymal stromal cells. Curr Opin Hematol 2006; **13:** 419.

26. Pittenger MF, Mackay AM, Beck SC, Jaiswal RK, Douglas R, Mosca JD, Moorman MA, Simonetti DW, Craig S, and Marshak DR: Multilineage potential of adult human mesenchymal stem cells. Science 1999; **284:** 143.

27. Javazon EH, Keswani SG, Badillo AT, Crombleholme TM, Zoltick PW, Radu AP, Kozin ED, Beggs K, Malik AA, and Flake AW: Enhanced epithelial gap closure and increased angiogenesis in wounds of diabetic mice treated with adult murine bone marrow stromal progenitor cells. Wound Repair Regen 2007; **15:** 350.

28. Rees DA and Alcolado JC: Animal models of diabetes mellitus. Diabet Med 2005; **22:** 359.

29. Aggarwal S and Pittenger MF: Human mesenchymal stem cells modulate allogeneic immune cell responses. Blood 2005; **105:** 1815.

30. Jin HK, Carter JE, Huntley GW, and Schuchman EH: Intracerebral transplantation of mesenchymal stem cells into acid sphingomyelinase-deficient mice delays the onset of neurological abnormalities and extends their life span. J Clin Invest 2002; **209:** 1183.

31. Yoo SW, Kim SS, Lee SY, Lee HS, Kim HS, Lee YD, and Suh-Kim H: Mesenchymal stem cells promote proliferation of endogenous neural stem cells and survival of newborn cells in a rat stroke model. Exp Mol Med 2008; **40:** 387.

32. Chow I, Lemos EV, and Einarson TR: Management and prevention of diabetic foot ulcers and infections: a health economic review. Pharmacoeconomics 2008; **26:** 1019.

33. Ladwig GP, Robson MC, Liu R, Kuhn MA, Muir DF, and Schultz GS: Ratios of activated matrix metalloproteinase-9 to tissue inhibitor of matrix metalloproteinase-1 in wound fluids are inversely correlated with healing of pressure ulcers. Wound Repair Regen 2002; **10:** 26.

34. Xu X, Xu Z, Xu Y, and Cui G: Effects of mesenchymal stem cell transplantation on extracellular matrix after myocardial infarction in rats. Coron Artery Dis 2005; **16:** 245.

35. Mouisseddine M, Francois S, Semont A, Sache A, Allenet B, Mathieu N, Frick J, Thierry D, and Chapel A: Human mesenchymal stem cells home specifically to radiation-injured tissues in a non-obese diabetes/severe combined immunodeficiency mouse model. Br J Radiol 2007; **80:** 49.

36. Ortiz LA, Gambelli F, McBride C, Gaupp D, Baddoo M, Kaminski N, and Phinney DG: Mesenchymal stem cell engraftment in lung is enhanced in response to bleomycin exposure and ameliorates its fibrotic effects. Proc Natl Acad Sci USA 2003; **100:** 8407.

The Systems Biology of Diabetic Wound Healing: Insights from Transcriptomic and Functional Genomics Analyses

Arturo R. Maldonado,[1,2,*] Bruce J. Aronow,[3,4] and Timothy M. Crombleholme,[1,2,5]

[1]Division of Pediatric General and Thoracic Surgery, The Center for Molecular Fetal Therapy, Cincinnati, Ohio.
[2]Molecular & Developmental Biology Graduate Program, The University of Cincinnati College of Medicine, Cincinnati, Ohio.
[3]Divisions of Biomedical Informatics & Computational Medicine Center, Department of Pediatrics, Cincinnati Children's Hospital Medical Center, Cincinnati, Ohio.
[4]Departments of Pediatrics, Cancer & Cell Biology and [5]Surgery, The University of Cincinnati College of Medicine, Cincinnati, Ohio.

Background: Diabetes is associated with significant morbidity, mortality, and cost to society. Despite improvements in our understanding and therapeutics, diabetes remains a leading cause of chronic nonhealing wounds and amputations.
The Problem: Diabetes is associated with abnormal healing, and multiple studies have shown that the disease leads to altered signaling and function of multiple wound components. We have shown perturbed cellular function and impaired healing conferred by diabetic versus normal endothelial progenitor cells (EPCs). However, because the basis for diabetic effects on EPC and other wound cell types appears complex, genome-wide identification of EPC perturbations represents an unbiased examination.
Basic/Clinical Science Advances: Transcriptional profiling reveals a multiplicity of wound field responses. Coupled with siRNA gene knockdown screens, a wealth of novel insights into genes and pathways required for wound healing can be obtained. To date, comparing EPCs from diabetic to normal in two type I diabetic models has allowed us to identify 270 genes differentially expressed, many of which play critical roles in angiogenesis. Their analysis using systems biological network and pathway approaches implicates a critical role for altered Chemokine, CXC motif, ligand 12(CXCL12)–Chemokine, CXC motif, receptor 4(CXCR4) signaling in diabetic bone marrow–derived EPC wound healing function.
Clinical Care Relevance: Improved understanding of diabetes-altered regulatory pathways, identification of novel biomarkers, and pathway-targeted therapies may allow us to overcome diabetes-impaired wound healing and to decrease severe outcomes such as amputation.
Conclusions: Gene expression profiling and siRNA-based gene function screens represent important tools to elucidate the impact of diabetes on wound healing and EPC function. Their use for further evaluation of pathophysiologic and therapeutic implications is critically needed.

Abbreviations and Acronyms

AGE = advanced glycation end products

CXCL12 = Chemokine, CXC motif, ligand 12; also SDF-1

CXCR4 = Chemokine, CXC motif, receptor 4

EPC = endothelial progenitor cell

*Correspondence: Timothy M. Crombleholme MD, 3333 Burnet Ave, MLC 11025, Cincinnati, OH 45231 (e-mail: timothy.crombleholme@cchmc.org).

BACKGROUND

The complex biology of normal wound healing has made understanding of diabetes-impaired wound healing a great challenge. While early systems biology approaches focused on this complex molecular biology, modern systems biology addresses this complexity with the additional goals of creating bridges from the bench to the bedside. The toll of diabetes on society continues to mount, and there is an urgent need to understand the pathogenesis of this disease.

Several studies have shown that normal wound healing requires neovascularization or new blood vessel

Printed in U.S.A.
DOI: 10.1089/awc.2009.0050

formation from angiogenesis, the branching of preexisting blood vessels, and vasculogenesis, *de novo* blood vessel formation. Early wound healing studies done in animals transplanted with bone marrow expressing reporter genes have shown that bone marrow–derived cells incorporate into blood vessels in the wounds. Asahara *et al.* were the first to infer the bone marrow origin of cells that differentiated into mature endothelial cells incorporated into blood vessels in wounds.[1] These endothelial progenitor cell, (EPC), display undifferentiation markers similar to stem cells such as CD133, Sca-1, and c-Kit. Unlike mesenchymal stem cells, the EPCs express vascular lineage markers such as Tie-2 and Flk1 and are Brachyury negative. However, Flk-1 and Tie-2 are also expressed in hematopoietic stem cells and endothelial cells.[2,3] Because there are no EPC-specific markers, cells isolated using these markers contain a diverse population of progenitors and are considered cell populations enriched for EPC.

Because of the complex nature and the multiorgan involvement of EPCs, their function has been divided into three categories: mobilization, the entry of EPCs into circulation from the bone marrow; recruitment, the targeting and invasion of EPC from peripheral blood into damaged or ischemic tissue such as provisional wound matrix; and local function, the effects of EPC on the cells and extracellular matrix in the wound environment.

CLINICAL PROBLEM ADDRESSED

In the United States, direct economic costs from diabetes reached 174 billion dollars in 2007.[4] This disease causes a great amount of morbidity such as chronic, nonhealing wounds. The problem is accentuated by a greater risk of limb amputations compared to nondiabetics. Diabetics have increased mortality through multiple organ dysfunction, and half of diabetic amputees die by the third year after the amputation.[5] Through systems biology approaches, we hope to gain new insights into the complex molecular pathways underlying normal wound healing that are impaired in diabetes. To achieve this goal, scientists have employed a number of tools, including transcriptomics, functional genomics, and regulatory network analysis.

RELEVANT BASIC SCIENCE CONTEXT

Since normal wound healing is a complex process, the underlying mechanisms involved in the pathophysiology of impaired healing have been elusive. Biologists have recently made attempts to characterize normal cellular functions using siRNA loss of function screens *in vitro* and transcriptional profiling of normal acute wounds *in vivo*.[6,7]

Our laboratory and others have shown that diabetic wounds are characterized by impaired angiogenesis.[8,9] The molecular mechanisms that underlie altered angiogenesis are complex and are reflected in the large number of altered wound growth factors and cytokines. Multiple studies have examined the proteome of diabetic wounds and identified decreased pleiotropic growth factors such as insulin growth factor 1, transforming growth factor beta 1, and platelet-derived growth factor.[10] Alteration in these proteins results in far-reaching effects not only in endothelial proliferation and function, but also on keratinocytes, fibroblasts, and infiltrating leukocytes in wound provisional matrix.[10] Vasculogenesis is also altered in diabetes, and there are data that EPC mobilization, recruitment, and function are abnormal.[9,11,12] In addition to various wound effects, response to ischemia is altered in diabetes.[13]

Many human and animal studies have shown that diabetics have an abnormal response to ischemia. Ischemic tissues in diabetics have worsening edema, fibrosis, and necrosis compared to nondiabetics. *In vitro* and *in vivo* evaluations of the abnormal responses show that an altered EPC response is associated with this phenomenon.[13] Mobilization and recruitment of EPC from the bone marrow to ischemic tissue are decreased in a similar fashion as occurs in diabetic cutaneous wounds.

Since diabetes-impaired healing is associated with abnormal angiogenesis in wounds and response to ischemia, we have focused on the bone marrow EPC and its role in the abnormal wound healing process.[9] Although it has been shown that EPC function is altered in both type I and type II diabetes, we decided to analyze the transcriptome of EPC in two models of type I diabetes to better understand the perturbations in genetic and molecular regulation.

Although systems biology traditionally generates hypotheses from a complex model to be tested using reductionist experimental designs, we have taken a "bottom up approach" by focusing on a specific cell type, the EPC, under diabetic conditions in the bone marrow, and applying a transcriptomic analysis to evaluate complex gene perturbations from diabetes.

EXPERIMENTAL MODEL AND LIMITATIONS

Mouse models and induction of diabetes

The nonobese (*i.e.*, NOD/LtjNOD) mice develop insulin-dependent diabetes from insulitis-related β islet destruction resulting in a hyperglycemic hypoinsulinemic state similar to human type I diabetes. One limitation of this model is the amount of time and variability to onset of hyperglycemia and fragility of the hyperglycemic animals. Another type I diabetes model can be produced by injecting control mice, usually C57BL/6 (C57), with streptozotocin, a glucosamine-nitrosourea alkylating agent that has β islet specificity.

For type II diabetes, one can use leptin receptor defective mice (db/db). When homozygous, these mice become obese at 3 to 4 weeks of age and hyperglycemic and hyperinsulinemic between 4 to 8 weeks of age similar to human type II diabetes.

Systems biology approaches to wounds and EPCs

For wound transcriptomics, total RNA is harvested from the wound at serial time points or from individual cell types in the wound.[7] A limitation of whole-wound samples is the averaging of transcripts among different cell types. To help analyze the effectiveness of wound therapies, another systems approach is to evaluate the transcriptomics of various wound therapies as was done by Derrick *et al.* for vacuum-assisted closure, wet to moist gauze therapy, and gauze under suction.[14]

In functional genomics analysis of wound healing, individual wound cell types are cultured and high-throughput loss of function screens are performed, such as with an siRNA library.[6] After identifying altering siRNA, further analysis is needed to determine gain of functionality and functional rescue in those cells *in vitro* and *in vivo*.

EPCs can be isolated from whole bone marrow by immunostaining with either magnetic bead isolation or fluorescence-activated cell sorting. After RNA quality assessment by an Agilent Bioanalyzer, RNA is processed through an Affymetrix gene chip and transcriptomics obtained.

Transcriptomics, gene ontology, hierarchical gene clusters, and regulatory network analysis can be performed using GeneSpring (Agilent Technologies, Santa Clara, CA), ToppGene Suite (Cincinnati Children's Research Foundation, Cincinnati, OH), and Ingenuity Pathway Analysis software (Ingenuity Systems, Mountain View, CA). Database cross-integration, mathematical model creation of complex biological processes, and regulatory model isomorphism are widely used in systems biology.

DISCUSSION OF FINDINGS AND RELEVANT LITERATURE

To unveil complex regulatory processes in normal wound healing, Roy *et al.* analyzed early wound edge transcriptomics.[7] At serial time points from 0 to 96 h after flank wounding, wound edge tissue was harvested and expression analysis performed. RNA was analyzed for significant expression changes at the various time points and further classified by functional category and wound-specific cell-type category. As one would anticipate, the wound transcriptome is very dynamic and significant changes can be identified even at short time intervals. This serves as a good starting point to identify early candidate genes and generate testable hypotheses of their function in the first 96 h of normal wound healing.

A systems biology approach to network nodal testing has been recently performed on endothelial cells, their migration individually and as a sheet, and their response to bFGF. For loss of function, an siRNA functional screen was conducted using a 2,400 protein-diced siRNA library transfected into human umbilical vein cells to examine the role of potential regulatory proteins in endothelial cell motility, directed migration, cell–cell coordination, and cell density.[6] For sheet migration kinetics analysis, endothelial cells were cultured in monolayers and stained with a fluorophore, and the monolayer was then scraped to create an acellular wound and then photographed after 15 min and 15 h. Live cell tracking was then performed by staining human umbilical vein cells with nuclear dye and taking serial images. Velocity of wound closure, velocity of cell movement, directionality, proliferation, and cell–cell coordination were digitally analyzed and correlated to individual siRNA effects. One of the novel conclusions from these studies is that the majority of proteins knocked down resulted in single category perturbations. This is in contrast to the belief that most of these proteins behave in a pleiotropic manner and affect multiple functional categories. However, these results need to be validated *in vivo*. In addition, this approach would be useful for the study of EPCs and may prove that EPCs have similar analogous migration mechanisms, at least *in vitro*.

Our laboratory has focused on the isolation of EPCs from type I diabetic mice to perform genomic expression analysis on this important cell in neovascularization and wound healing (Fig. 1). Of the top 270 most perturbed genes in diabetic EPC, CXCL12 is most upregulated (5.4-fold, $p < 0.01$). Not only is it upregulated, but it also belonged to

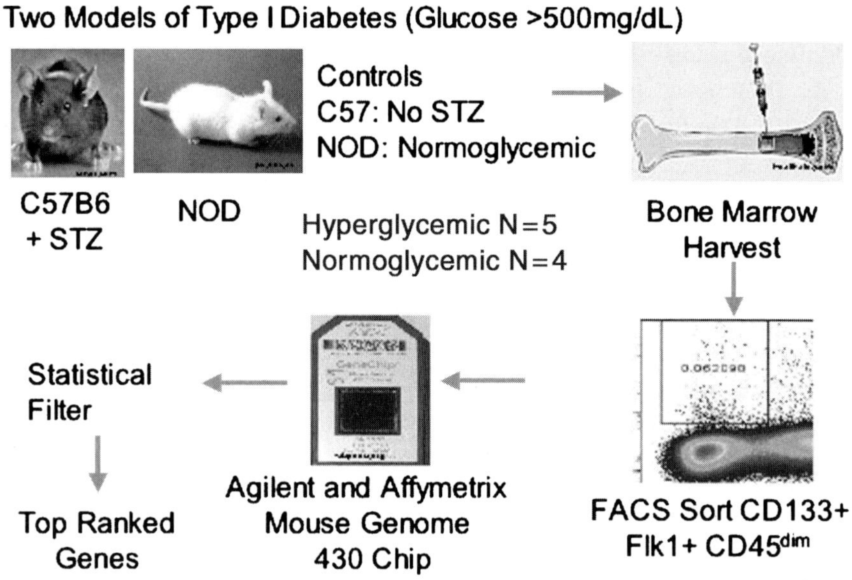

Figure 1. Transcriptional profiling of disease-perturbed cells. Transcriptomics of diabetic endothelial progenitor cell was performed with the following experimental design. Endothelial progenitor cells from two different models of type I diabetes were harvested from hyperglycemic mice and from normoglycemic controls. Fluorescence-activated cell sorting was performed to isolate CD133+ Flk1+ $CD45^{dim}$ cells and RNA extracted. RNA quality was determined followed by Affymetrix chip processing. Raw data were filtered through a statistical filter and top ranked genes obtained. Functional gene categories were analyzed followed by regulatory network clustering analysis to obtain gene signatures.

the top seven of eight functional gene categories with the angiogenesis genes being among the largest group of perturbed genes in the diabetic EPC transcriptome. These data suggest that the EPC transcriptome is significantly altered under diabetic conditions and lend support to the hypothesis that diabetic EPC are dysfunctional.[15]

Although our analysis was performed in models of both type I diabetes, others have evaluated CXCL12 and found expression changes in both type I models (streptozotocin), and type II models (db/db) in wounds and bone marrow.[16–18] It is likely that the diabetic EPC acts as a window into a systemic perturbation in CXCL12 regulation. While evidence exists that CXCL12 expression is increased in various bone marrow cell types, wound provisional matrix cells in multiple mouse models of diabetes show decreased CXCL12 expression. The significance of this reversal in CXCL12 expression pattern and gradient is noteworthy considering that the CXCL12-CXCR4 axis is an important mechanism for bone marrow–derived cell homing and targeting to injured tissue and sites of neovascularization. The CXCL12–CXCR4 axis as an impaired molecular mechanism in diabetic EPCs is supported by results from experiments using topical CXCL12 protein or lentiviral-mediated gene transfer of CXCL12 in which there is an improvement in wound healing parameters, including increased speed of epithelial gap closure, angiogenesis, and accelerated wound closure rates.[16,17] In addition, supplementing hyperbaric oxygen treatment to exogenous CXCL12 synergistically increased wound EPC number and wound closure. This synergism was ablated by simultaneous addition of a nitric oxide synthase inhibitor, suggesting that hyperbaric oxygen therapy acts through a nitric oxide synthase–dependent pathway.[17]

The verteporfin injury model was used to study the effect of advanced glycation end products (AGE) on the repair function of EPC on injured endothelial cells. On injuring a portion of the endothelial monolayer, the labeled EPC could be seen migrating to the injury site and formed tight junctions with the endothelial cells at the site of injury. EPC-mediated recovery of the denuded culture section and transendothelial electric resistance were used as measures of repair, and these variables were adversely inhibited by AGE.[19] These *in vitro* findings suggest that the diabetic hyperglycemic glycosylation effects on wound provisional matrix could adversely alter integrin-dependent EPC functions. These findings need to be investigated *in vivo*.

CAUTION, CRITICAL REMARKS, AND RECOMMENDATIONS

Systems biology, transcriptomics, regulatory network analysis, and functional genomic approaches are great tools to help us understand complex regulatory networks. However, these methodologies and their interpretation must be combined with translational experiments that bridge the process of validating hypotheses of gene network structure and function to improving experimental models and identifying critical interventions. Unlike static pathway diagrams, the promise of systems biology is the opportunity to better understand dynamic processes that are closer to the critical pathophysiology being studied.

There is still much that we do not understand about the pathophysiology of impaired wound healing in diabetes. We have not identified any single EPC-specific marker. The population that contains cells we call EPC is undifferentiated, arises from the bone marrow, is released into the circulation in response to a set of signals, circulates to and navigates through target tissue, and assists in wound repair and neovascularization. It is possible that these cells represent a heterogeneous population of cells that maximally exert their effects in concert.

The inability to perpetuate EPC in culture without differentiation after they are extracted from mice creates many challenges. Many advances in the field may be possible if we can learn to culture mouse EPC and create great numbers that can then be used not only for *in vitro* assays, but also for genetic manipulation, bone marrow transplantation, and wound cell therapy.

Future Development

Since EPC transcriptomic analyses show significant perturbations in type I models of diabetes, it is important to also study the EPC in type II models. Because there is decreased CXCL12 expression in mouse diabetic wounds, human wounds should also be examined for perturbed CXCL12 expression. In addition, the effects of ECM glycosylation and AGE on EPC function should also be examined, which may also represent potential therapeutic targets.

Bioinformatic approaches like temporal transcriptomics of wound edge and granulation tissue should be repeated in impaired wound healing models and performed on individual wound cell types under normal and abnormal wound healing conditions. Further, siRNA functional genomic screens of EPC and other wound matrix cells will help elucidate their molecular functions, regulation, and roles in wound healing biology. Finally, a comprehensive approach to studying the complexities of wound healing under normal and abnormal conditions will hopefully provide new insights and paradigms for the treatment of patients with significant morbidity and mortality related to impaired wound healing.

GLOSSARY OF TERMS

Advanced Glycation End Product: Products of the Milliard Reaction, a nonenzymatic glycation oxidation process that occurs in chronic hyperglycemia. Advanced products are irreversibly glycated as opposed to intermediate glycation products that are reversible, but promote further glycation. These products are implicated in the molecular pathophysiology of multiple diseases.[20]

Angiogenesis: The formation of new blood vessels from branching of preexisting blood vessels.

Biomarker: A molecule indicating the past or present state of a biological process.

Functional Genomics: The molecular study of dynamic gene regulation and gene product interaction effects on cellular function.

Gene Ontology: A structured vocabulary describing gene and gene product function using biological, molecular, and cellular concepts that are generally accepted among multidisciplinary biologists.[21]

Gene Regulatory Network: Interaction relationships among genes, RNAs, and proteins associated with the transcriptional, translational, modification, and other mechanisms regulating their activation and function.

Glycation: The nonenzymatic bonding of sugar molecules to proteins, lipids, and other molecules that often leads to impaired molecular function.

Glycosylation: Glycan production from carbohydrate enzymatic processing that can be free or attached to proteins, lipids, or other molecules.

TAKE-HOME MESSAGE

Basic science advances

- Wound edge transcriptomics show dynamic changes in gene expression at short time intervals within the first 96 h of normal wound healing.[7]
- Functional genomic siRNA screen of endothelial cell function elucidates many migration regulatory proteins and a similar analysis should be done with normal and diabetic EPCs.[6]
- EPC show 270 differentially expressed genes consistently altered in two different type I diabetic models.[15]
- Most altered genes in the EPC play a role in angiogenesis.[15]
- CXCL12 expression is increased in diabetic EPC.[15]

Clinical science advances

- EPC mobilization, recruitment, and function appear to be abnormal in humans with diabetes.

Relevance to clinical care

- EPC-targeted therapies may improve diabetic wound healing in humans.
- Better understanding of wound provisional matrix gene expression dynamics may present therapeutic targets for impaired healing states.

This process is important for the molecular function of many molecules.

Hierarchical Gene Clusters: Gene expression pattern analyses used to distinguish groups of genes that exhibit similar regulation across a series of independent samples. Gene clusters that exhibit coordinated regulation are then analyzed for the enrichments in shared gene functions based on ontologic features.

Knockdown: A partial reduction in gene expression sometimes done by hybridization of an oligonucleotide to the gene transcript of interest.

Mobilization: The movement of bone marrow cells from the marrow to the systemic circulation.

Model Isomorphism: The application of models developed for one biological process that can be used to predict outcomes of another biological process based on similar components.

Neovascularization: The development of new blood vessels either by angiogenesis or vasculogenesis.

Progenitor Cells: Lineage-fated cells that are partially undifferentiated and are committed to a specialized type or subtype of cell population. These cells arise from stem cells that partially mature or from rapidly dividing progenitor cells.

Recruitment: The homing of bone marrow–derived cells to sites of disease that requires mobilization and traversing from systemic circulation through endothelium to the target tissue.

Reductionism: The study of a complex process by examining the fundamental parts of the process.

siRNA: Small interfering RNA are short RNA oligonucleotides that are used to knockdown gene expression by hybridizing with messenger RNA. The double-stranded RNA molecule can lead to RNA degradation.

Stem Cells: Undifferentiated or immature cells that are pluripotent; that is, they can self-renew or form a wide variety of mature cell types.

Systems Biology: The systematic study of complex biology using various bioinformatics tools to identify novel molecular pathways and therapeutic targets not identified by reductionist science.

Transcriptome/Transcriptomics: The genome-wide study of gene expression using high-throughput methods such as gene microarrays.

Undifferentiation: An immature state characteristic of stem cells and progenitor cells.

Vasculogenesis: The process of forming new blood vessels *de novo* and not from branching angiogenesis.

Verteporfin: A derivative of benzoporphyrin that is used to damage endothelium by production of oxygen radicals when exposed to 680–695 nm wavelength light.

ACKNOWLEDGMENT

Supported in part by grants RO1s DK072446 and DK074055 (T.M.C.).

AUTHOR DISCLOSURE STATEMENT

A.R.M., B.J.A., and T.M.C. do not have any commercial associations that may pose a conflict of interest in connection with this article.

REFERENCES

1. Asahara T, Murohara T, Sullivan A, Silver M, van der Zee R, Li T, Witzenbichler B, Schatteman G, and Isner JM: Isolation of putative progenitor endothelial cells for angiogenesis. Science 1997; **275:** 964.
2. TL, Huber V, Kouskoff H, Joerg Fehling J, Palis and G: Keller haemangioblast commitment is initiated in the primitive streak of the mouse embryo. Nature 2004; **432:** 625.
3. Shalaby F, Ho J, Stanford WL, Fischer K-D, Schuh AC, Schwartz L, Bernstein A, and Rossant J: A requirement for Flk1 in primitive and definitive hematopoiesis and vasculogenesis. Cell 1997; **89:** 981.
4. Economic costs of diabetes in the U.S. in 2007. Diabetes Care 2008; **31:** 596.
5. Miyajima S, Shirai A, Yamamoto S, Okada N, and Matsushita T: Risk factors for major limb amputations in diabetic foot gangrene patients. Diabetes Res Clin Pract 2006; **71:** 272.
6. Vitorino P and Meyer T: Modular control of endothelial sheet migration. Genes Dev 2008; **22:** 3268.
7. Roy S, Khanna S, Rink C, Biswas S, and Sen CK: Characterization of the acute temporal changes in excisional murine cutaneous wound inflammation by screening of the wound-edge transcriptome. Physiol genomics 2008; **34:** 162.
8. Ferguson MW, Herrick SE, Spencer MJ, Shaw JE, Boulton AJ, and Sloan P: The histology of diabetic foot ulcers. Diabet Med 1996; **13 Suppl 1:** S30.
9. Keswani SG, Katz AB, Lim FY, Zoltick P, Radu A, Alaee D, Herlyn M, and Crombleholme TM: Adenoviral mediated gene transfer of PDGF-B enhances wound healing in type I and type II diabetic wounds. Wound Repair Regen 2004; **12:** 497.
10. Blakytny R and Jude E: The molecular biology of chronic wounds and delayed healing in diabetes. Diabet Med 2006; **23:** 594.
11. Tepper OM, Galiano RD, Capla JM, Kalka C, Gagne PJ, Jacobowitz GR, Levine JP, and Gurtner GC: Human endothelial progenitor cells from type II diabetics exhibit impaired proliferation, adhesion, and incorporation into vascular structures. Circulation 2002; **106:** 2781.
12. Loomans CJ, de Koning EJ, Staal FJ, Rookmaaker MB, Verseyden C, de Boer HC, Verhaar MC, Braam B, Rabelink TJ, and van Zonneveld AJ: Endothelial progenitor cell dysfunction: a novel concept in the pathogenesis of vascular complications of type 1 diabetes. Diabetes 2004; **53:** 195.
13. Fadini GP, Sartore S, Schiavon M, Albiero M, Baesso I, Cabrelle A, Agostini C, and Avogaro A: Diabetes impairs progenitor cell mobilisation after hindlimb ischaemia-reperfusion injury in rats. Diabetologia 2006; **49:** 3075.
14. Derrick KL, Norbury K, Kieswetter K, Skaf J, and McNulty AK: Comparative analysis of global gene

expression profiles between diabetic rat wounds treated with vacuum-assisted closure therapy, moist wound healing or gauze under suction. Int Wound J 2008; **5:** 615.

15. Maldonado AR, Aronow BJ, Uzvolgyi E, Cohen RM, Parvadia JK, Morris LM, Vulentin-Solis JF, Lim FY, and Crombleholme TM: Identification of altered genomic signatures in diabetic endothelial progenitor cells through a computational systems biology approach. Wound Repair Regen 2008; **16:** A10. Abstract no. 11.

16. Badillo AT, Chung S, Zhang L, Zoltick P, and Liechty KW: Lentiviral gene transfer of SDF-1alpha to wounds improves diabetic wound healing. J Surg Res 2007; **143:** 35.

17. Gallagher KA, Liu ZJ, Xiao M, Chen H, Goldstein LJ, Buerk DG, Nedeau A, Thom SR, and Velazquez OC: Diabetic impairments in NO-mediated endothelial progenitor cell mobilization and homing are reversed by hyperoxia and SDF-1 alpha. J Clin Invest 2007; **117:** 1249.

18. Leng Q, Nie Y, Zou Y, and Chen J: Elevated CXCL12 expression in the bone marrow of NOD mice is associated with altered T cell and stem cell trafficking and diabetes development. BMC Immunol 2008; **9:** 51.

19. Bhatwadekar AD, Glenn JV, Li G, Curtis TM, Gardiner TA, and Stitt AW: Advanced glycation of fibronectin impairs vascular repair by endothelial progenitor cells: implications for vasodegeneration in diabetic retinopathy. Invest Ophthalmol Vis Sci 2008; **49:** 1232.

20. Huijberts MS, Schaper NC, and Schalkwijk CG: Advanced glycation end products and diabetic foot disease. Diabetes Metab Res Rev 2008; **24 Suppl 1:** S19.

21. Ashburner M, Ball CA, Blake JA, Botstein D, Butler H, Cherry JM, Davis AP, Dolinski K, Dwight SS, Eppig JT, Harris MA, Hill DP, Issel-Tarver L, Kasarskis A, Lewis S, Matese JC, Richardson JE, Ringwald M, Rubin GM, and Sherlock G: Gene ontology: tool for the unification of biology. The Gene Ontology Consortium. Nat Genet 2000; **25:** 25.

WHS Wound Healing Society

Bone Marrow Adult Stem and Progenitor Cells in the Treatment of Chronic Wounds

John Kowalczyk and Evangelos Badiavas*

Department of Dermatology, Interdisciplinary Stem Cell Institute, University of Miami Miller School of Medicine, Miami, Florida.

Abbreviations and Acronyms

ESCs = embryonic stem cells

HSCs = hematopoietic stem cells

MSCs = mesenchymal stem cells

*Correspondence: Department of Dermatology, Interdisciplinary Stem Cell Institute, University of Miami Miller School of Medicine, 1600 NW 10th Ave., RMSB 2023A, Miami, Florida 33136 (e-mail: ebadiavas@med.miami.edu).

Background: A variety of stem cells have captured the attention of the scientific community and lay press. Collectively, these cells have great potential for the repair and regeneration of a variety of tissues. Wound healing has been a primary focus for many recent studies.
The Problem: Chronic wounds represent a failure of the normal mechanisms involved in healing. Even when wounds do heal, the healed area has significant alteration of the normal anatomy predisposing the area to rewounding.
Basic/Clinical Science Advances: Stem and progenitor cells have been shown to reside locally within the skin and traffic to the skin from distant sites, particularly in response to injury. Recent studies have attempted to identify the function of these cells and how they participate in the healing process.
Clinical Care Relevance: The use of bone marrow–derived stem and progenitor cells has shown promise in laboratory wound models and in the treatment of recalcitrant chronic wounds in patients.
Conclusion: Adult stem and progenitor cells derived from skin, bone marrow, and other tissues hold great promise for wound healing and tissue regeneration with return of normal function.

BACKGROUND

All of us are the product of a unique single stem cell, the fertilized egg. As one develops, new stem cells are formed that ultimately give rise to all the tissues of the body. Stem cells are, however, important throughout development and into adult life for critical functions such as growth, repair, and tissue regeneration after injury. As such, these cells have been a major topic of research in the area of cutaneous wound healing with particular attention paid to chronic wounds. Much emphasis has been placed on two distinct classes of stem cells for the treatment of wounds: embryonic and adult stem cells. Although embryonic stem cells (ESCs) have the greatest potential for self-renewal and the ability to form tissues derived from all germ layers, their potential for clinical use is currently limited due to ethical and safety concerns. ESCs also cannot (without genetic manipulation) be obtained from an autologous source. Adult stem cells do not have these difficulties but may be more restricted (without genetic manipulation) in their ability to form multiple tissues. Different types of adult stem cells are currently being studied with respect to wound healing. A few such stem cells are epidermal stem cells, hematopoietic stem cells (HSC), and mesenchymal stem cells (MSC). Epidermal stem cells have been found in the bulge region of the hair follicle, interfollicular epidermis, and sebaceous glands.[1,2] HSC and their progenitors have been classically described in the bone marrow, but more recent evidence has identified rich

ADVANCES IN WOUND CARE, VOLUME 1

Printed in U.S.A
DOI: 10.1089/awc.2009.0067

sources of these stem cells in umbilical cord blood. Low levels of HSC normally circulate in the blood stream; however, their number in circulation can be greatly enhanced by administration of hematopoietic hormones such as granulocyte colony–stimulating hormone.[3] MSC were also initially described in the bone marrow; however, similar (if not identical) stem cells can also be found in other sources such as adipose tissue.[4] Likely due to their regenerative capability, adult stem cells and their progenitors have the capacity to "home," or migrate, to areas of tissue injury.[5–11] These cells residing in normal skin and distant organs are therefore likely to play an important role in normal wound healing. The apparent lack of stem and progenitor cells at the site of injury could precipitate the formation of a chronic wound. It is believed that by replacing these stem and progenitor cells, dermal rebuilding and closure of nonhealing chronic wounds may occur.[12] Although the exact mechanism of stem cell participation (or lack of participation) in chronic wounds is not yet fully understood, current research shows promise that stem cells may potentially play a pivotal role in their treatment.

CLINICAL PROBLEM ADDRESSED

The management of chronic wounds remains a challenge for clinicians as almost 50% of the wounds that are present for more than 1 year remain resistant to current treatment modalities.[13] We believe that stem cells play a crucial role in normal wound healing and that a lack of stem cells or inability of these cells to home to sites of cutaneous injury can hinder wounds from healing spontaneously. Several hypotheses are being examined to determine why these cells are unable to reach the site of tissue injury. It has been proposed that the body's capacity to signal the proper cells in response to injury may be weakened.[14] It could also be that once the appropriate stem cells are signaled, they may encounter a physical and/or physiological barrier making them unable to infiltrate the wound.[5,15] A prime example of this type of barrier could be the fibrin cuff formation observed in patients suffering from chronic venous ulcers and other chronic wounds.[16] Recent data have indicated that there may not be a sufficient number of stem cells available at the wound site.[17] By harvesting stem cells and then applying them more directly to chronic wounds, researchers are able to potentially bypass many problems these cells may face on their own such as their ability to be signaled and home to the wound site.[6,7,15] Obtaining a

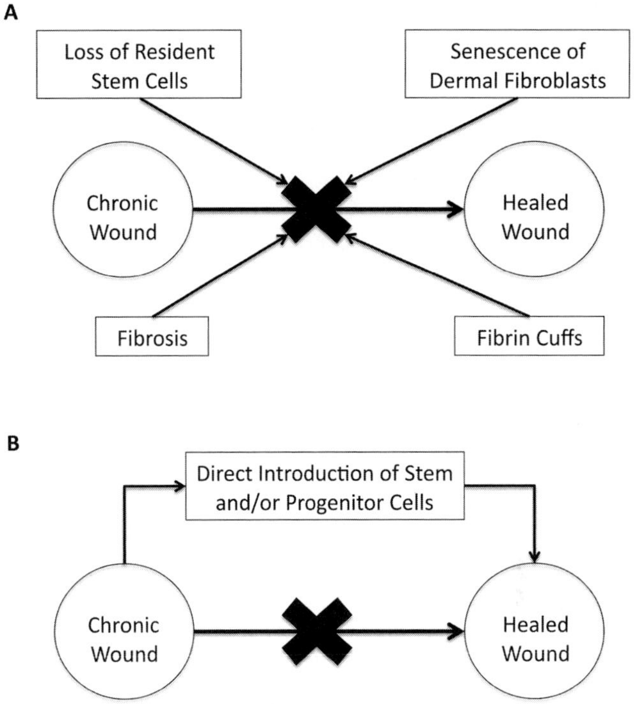

Figure 1. A. Chronic wounds may fail to heal due to the loss of resident stem cells and the loss of function or senescence of cells in the wound. There are also likely impediments to the repopulation of stem and progenitor cells from distant sites. Fibrin cuffs may stop circulating stem/progenitor cells from migrating out of blood vessels and the fibrosis associated with chronic wounds could also limit cell migration to the wound site. B. Applying stem and/or progenitor cells directly to wounds circumvents the inhibition of cell migration to the wound site and may provide a means for repopulating a chronic wound with stem/progenitor cells leading to healing.

durable closure in chronic wounds is often difficult.[18,19] Histologically, even when healing does occur, there is scarring with loss of adnexal structures, elastic, and reticulin fibers. The lack of proper dermal rebuilding can lead to loss of function and propensity for reinjury. Through the introduction of these cells at the site of cutaneous injury, it is believed that dermal rebuilding in chronic wounds can be achieved. Several researchers have already demonstrated dermal rebuilding and at least partial closure of chronic wounds through the application of adult stem cells or whole bone marrow (Fig. 1).[6,7,13,20]

RELEVANT BASIC SCIENCE CONTEXT

The advances made in stem cells and regenerative medicine have been both exciting and controversial. The most pluripotent stem cells have been derived from the early embryos of both humans and animals. As these cells may be derived from different stages of gestation, location in the embryo and species of origin, variations in their growth requirements, gene expression, and potential for differentiation exist.[21,22] More recent work has shown that pluripotent cells, induced pluripotent cells, can be derived from even mature cells by genetic manipulation.[23,24] The use of ESCs and induced pluripotent cells is, however, hampered for clinical use by their propensity to form tumors.[25] While adult stem cells may be recruited by tumors,[26] they have not been demonstrated to produce tumors on administration to animals or patients. Clinical studies have therefore been focused on adult stem cells.

EXPERIMENTAL MODEL OR MATERIAL—ADVANTAGES AND LIMITATIONS

Since animal models for chronic wounds are often lacking, several trials thus far have been conducted on human patients. To best provide evidence that this type of treatment modality is effective, patients chosen for these trials will often have prolonged, recalcitrant, chronic wounds that have failed standard and advanced treatments. Most experimental therapies have focused on the use of autologous bone marrow. Whole marrow, cultured marrow cells, and MSC have been used. The cells are typically harvested from the patient's bone marrow through an aspirate of the posterior iliac crest. The bone marrow–derived cells are directly applied to patient's wounds in a variety of ways, such as direct injection, topical application, in combination with bioengineered or autologous skin substitutes, or as part of a fibrin spray,[27] among others. The patient's wounds are monitored over time and depending on the wound's response to treatment, the patient may require more aspirations and applications of these autologous cells. Bone marrow cells are often chosen also due to their ability to be maintained in culture. Some cells, such as MSC's, can be expanded to provide an almost limitless supply of material that can be studied. Although these cells are proliferative in culture, not all cell cultures grow the same. It has been shown that bone marrow cultures from patients with chronic wounds may not grow as well as cultures from normal patients,[7] which may yield a less than optimal number of cells for treatment. This has lead to the search for modifications to the culture systems[7] to improve growth.

TAKE-HOME MESSAGE

Basic science advances

- Various types of multipotential stem cells exist.
- Early stem cells are hampered by their ability to form tumors on *in vivo* administration.

Clinical science advances

- Stem cells and other bone marrow–derived cells have been shown to play a role in normal wound healing. These cells have been shown to make up components of normal skin and it is possible that a deficiency of these cells at the site of cutaneous injury may lead to the formation of chronic wounds.
- Experiments have illustrated that bone marrow–derived stem and progenitor cells have the ability to home to the site of cutaneous wound injury. The inability of these cells to home to the site of tissue injury can potentially lead to the formation of chronic wounds. One possible obstacle for these cells may be the presence of fibrin cuffs around blood vessels seen in various forms of chronic ulceration.
- Stem cells and other bone marrow–derived cells have displayed the ability to differentiate into multiple cell types that form different structures of the skin. It is still not yet fully understood how these cells differentiate or what the extent of their differentiation potential is.
- Further study is required to optimize the use of adult stem cells for therapy and to fully evaluate their safety.

Relevance to clinical care

- Nearly 50% of all wounds present at least 1 year remain resistant to conventional and advanced therapies.
- When applied to chronic cutaneous wounds, bone marrow cells have thus far proven to be useful for inducing dermal rebuilding and wound closure.

DISCUSSION OF FINDINGS AND RELEVANT LITERATURE

Adult stem cells have been shown to aid in wound repair of many tissues including blood vessels, myocardium, cardiac valves, bone, skin, cartilage, tendon, meniscus, and more.[12] Although the exact mechanism by which these stem cells aid in cutaneous wound healing is not yet fully understood, studies have shown significant benefit from their use in chronic wounds. It is known that epidermal stem cells play a role in normal wound regeneration, and it has recently been discovered that certain types of chronic wounds are lacking epidermal stem cells.[17] Research, however, has focused on the use of MSCs, HSCs, and whole bone marrow aspirates for the treatment of chronic wounds.

MSCs are multipotent cells compromising 0.001–0.01% of all nucleated bone marrow cells.[4,28,29] They are proliferative in culture and have been shown to differentiate into osteoblasts, chrondocytes, astrocytes, pneumocytes, hepatocytes, neurons, and cardiac myocytes.[12] In an experiment using intravenously injected fluorescent-labeled sex-mismatched murine MSCs, it has been shown that MSC can differentiate into keratinocytes, endothelial cells, pericytes, and monocytes at the site of a cutaneous wound.[30] Autologous, human MSCs were also combined with an artificial dermis made of a collagen sponge and applied to the wounds of 20 patients with intractable dermopathies.[31] The investigators reported that 18 of the 20 patients' wounds treated were "mostly closed" with the remaining 2 patients having died of causes unrelated to the experiment.[31] These studies highlight the potential of MSCs to home to sites of injury, differentiate into skin cells and aid in wound repair.

HSCs are mulitpotent cells originating in the bone marrow that give rise to blood cells. Just as with the MSCs mentioned above, HSCs have also been shown to have the potential to home to the skin and differentiate into skin cells. Krause *et al.* showed that HSCs reintroduced into mice home to the bone marrow and can be seen differentiating into epithelial cells of the liver, lung, GI tract, and skin.[32] Although there have been no clinical trials that use only HSCs to aid in wound healing, Chan *et al.* successfully used a side population of bone marrow–derived HSCs to promote wound healing in diabetic mice when applied topically to the wound.[33] As with the MSCs, it is unknown how HSCs differentiate into skin cells, but it may be possible for stem cells that are committed to differentiate along a particular pathway to differentiate along a different pathway in the presence of certain signals.

Whole bone marrow contains not only MSCs and HSCs as mentioned above, but also progenitor cells, scavenger cells, and inflammatory cells. Some of these nonstem cell components of bone marrow have been demonstrated to aid in wound healing, such as the endothelial progenitor cell's ability to repair vascular structures within the skin.[34] The importance of bone marrow cells in wound healing has been seen in leukemia patients with malfunctioning bone marrow, as their wounds have been shown to have markedly impaired healing.[33] Bone marrow cells play a role in cutaneous wound healing, which can be seen through the production of type 3 collagen. Uninjured skin normally possesses a 4:1 ratio of collagen type 1 to type 3; during wound healing, however, this ratio changes to 2:1 due to an increase in collagen type 3 which is a unique product of bone marrow–derived cells.[35] When patients with wounds present for at least 1 year (having failed both conventional and advanced therapies) were given autologous fresh bone marrow aspirate and/or cultured bone cells, all patients showed at least some degree of dermal rebuilding.[6,7] Bone marrow has shown its ability to home, differentiate to, and create skin structures in response to wounding; how to incorporate this into a common therapy is being examined.

These and other studies show the great potential of adult stem cells and other bone marrow–derived cells to participate in wound healing and form skin structures. Although these cells have shown the capacity to differentiate into skin cells, it is still not understood exactly how this takes place or how functional these new cells are. More clinical trials are needed to optimize the use of these cells, determine the best course of therapy, and to examine any possible adverse effects.

CAUTION, CRITICAL REMARKS, AND RECOMMENDATIONS

Although experimental findings appear promising, more studies are needed to validate the ability of stem cells to aid in the healing of chronic cutaneous wounds. Multiple animal and *in vitro* studies support that stem and other bone marrow–derived cells can form structures in the skin, but future clinical studies will be needed to confirm these findings and prove that these newly formed structures are functional. Randomized clinical trials comparing the different stem cell regimens are also needed to determine which cells or combination of cells will be the most efficient to induce dermal rebuilding and wound closure.

The use of adult stem and other bone marrow–derived cells have thus far shown no significant adverse effects. Earlier stem cells derived from embryos have been shown to produce tumor formation when administered *in vivo* to animals,[25,36] and there has been a recent report of tumor formation in a clinical trial using fetal cells.[37] Future studies will be required to better evaluate the safety and effectiveness for different stem cell populations.

FUTURE DEVELOPMENT

Through ongoing studies we hope to better understand the physiology of how stem cells aid in cutaneous wound healing. With a more thorough understanding, treatments can be tailored toward using not only the correct cells but also the proper amount. It is possible that different stem cells, such as follicular or epidermal stem cells, may be more efficient for the treatment of chronic wounds. While it appears that bone marrow stem cells are important in dermal repair, research indicates that follicular stem cells have great potential for reepithelialization.[2,38] It is, however, too early to know which cells or combination of cells will be most efficient.

There is also need for improvement of current culture systems as cultures derived from patients with chronic wounds are sometimes difficult to grow.[7] With more efficient culture systems, it may be possible to greatly expand cells for therapy and reduce the frequency of cell harvests from patients.

AUTHOR DISCLOSURE STATEMENT

The authors, John Kowalczyk and Evangelos Badiavas, have no commercial associations or conflicts of interest to disclose. No competing financial interests exist. The National Institute on Aging supported the authors' work discussed within (R01AG027874). The National Institute on Aging is a component of the National Institutes of Health (NIH).

REFERENCES

1. Ambler CA and Maatta A: Epidermal stem cells: location, potential and contribution to cancer. J Pathol 2009; **217:** 206.
2. Blanpain C and Fuchs E: Epidermal homeostasis: a balancing act of stem cells in the skin. Nat Rev Mol Cell Biol 2009; **10:** 207.
3. Pusic I and DiPersio JF: The use of growth factors in hematopoietic stem cell transplantation. Curr Pharm Des 2008; **14:** 1950.
4. Phinney DG and Prockop DJ: Concise review: mesenchymal stem/multipotent stromal cells: the state of transdifferentiation and modes of tissue repair current views. Stem Cells 2007; **25:** 2896.
5. Badiavas EV: The potential of bone marrow cells to orchestrate homeostasis and healing in skin. Blood Cells Mol Dis 2004; **32:** 21.
6. Badiavas EV and Falanga V: Treatment of chronic wounds with bone marrow-derived cells. Arch Dermatol 2003; **139:** 510.
7. Badiavas EV, Ford D, Liu P, Kouttab N, Morgan J, Richards A, and Maizel A: Long-term bone marrow culture and its clinical potential in chronic wound healing. Wound Repair Regen 2007; **15:** 856.
8. Chamberlain G, Fox J, Ashton B, and Middleton J: Concise review: mesenchymal stem cells: their phenotype, differentiation capacity, immunological features, and potential for homing. Stem Cells 2007; **25:** 2739.
9. Fu X, Fang L, Li X, Cheng B, and Sheng Z: Enhanced wound-healing quality with bone marrow mesenchymal stem cells autografting after skin injury. Wound Repair Regen 2006; **14:** 325.
10. Rea S, Giles NL, Webb S, Adcroft KF, Evill LM, Strickland DH, Wood FM, and Fear MW: Bone marrow-derived cells in the healing burn wound—more than just inflammation. Burns 2009; **35:** 356.
11. Fox JM, Chamberlain G, Ashton BA, and Middleton J: Recent advances into the understanding of mesenchymal stem cell trafficking. Br J Haematol 2007; **137:** 491.
12. Wu Y, Wang J, Scott PG, and Tredget EE: Bone marrow-derived stem cells in wound healing: a review. Wound Repair Regen 2007; **15 Suppl 1:** S18.
13. Falanga V, and Sabolinski M: A bilayered living skin construct (APLIGRAF) accelerates complete closure of hard-to-heal venous ulcers. Wound Repair Regen 1999; **7:** 201.
14. Simka M: Delayed healing of chronic leg ulcers can result from impaired trafficking of bone marrow-derived precursors of keratinocytes to the skin. Med Hypotheses 2007; **69:** 637.
15. Lin CD, Allori AC, Macklin JE, Sailon AM, Tanaka R, Levine JP, Saadeh PB, and Warren SM: Topical lineage-negative progenitor-cell therapy for diabetic wounds. Plast Reconstr Surg 2008; **122:** 1341.
16. Joshi A and Sloan P: Role of "fibrin" cuffs in chronic nonspecific oral ulceration. Wound Repair Regen 2004; **12:** 18.
17. Morasso MI and Tomic-Canic M: Epidermal stem cells: the cradle of epidermal determination, differentiation and wound healing. Biol Cell 2005; **97:** 173.
18. Finlayson K, Edwards H, and Courtney M: Factors associated with recurrence of venous leg ulcers: a survey and retrospective chart review. Int J Nurs Stud 2009; **46:** 1071.
19. Herschthal J and Kirsner RS: Current management of venous ulcers: an evidence-based review. Surg Technol Int 2008; **17:** 77.
20. Rogers LC, Bevilacqua NJ, and Armstrong DG: The use of marrow-derived stem cells to accelerate healing in chronic wounds. Int Wound J 2008; **5:** 20.
21. Rossant J: Stem cells and early lineage development. Cell 2008; **132:** 527.
22. Silva J and Smith A: Capturing pluripotency. Cell 2008; **132:** 532.
23. Takahashi K and Yamanaka S: Induction of pluripotent stem cells from mouse embryonic and adult fibroblast cultures by defined factors. Cell 2006; **126:** 663.
24. Takahashi K, Tanabe K, Ohnuki M, Narita M, Ichisaka T, Tomoda K, and Yamanaka S: Induction of pluripotent stem cells from adult human fibroblasts by defined factors. Cell 2007; **131:** 861.
25. Yu J and Thomson JA: Pluripotent stem cell lines. Genes Dev 2008; **22:** 1987.
26. Stagg J: Mesenchymal stem cells in cancer. Stem Cell Rev 2008; **4:**119.
27. Falanga V, Iwamoto S, Chartier M, Yufit T, Butmarc J, Kouttab N, Shrayer D, and Carson P: Autologous bone marrow-derived cultured mesenchymal stem cells delivered in a fibrin spray accelerate healing in murine and human cutaneous wounds. Tissue Eng 2007; **13:** 1299.
28. Uccelli A, Moretta L, and Pistoia V: Mesenchymal stem cells in health and disease. Nat Rev Immunol 2008; **8:** 726.
29. Pittenger MF, Mackay AM, Beck SC, Jaiswal RK, Douglas R, Mosca JD, Moorman MA, Simonetti DW, Craig S, and Marshak DR: Multilineage potential of adult human mesenchymal stem cells. Science 1999; **284:** 143.
30. Sasaki M, Abe R, Fujita Y, Ando S, Inokuma D, and Shimizu H: Mesenchymal stem cells are recruited into wounded skin and contribute to wound repair by transdifferentiation into multiple skin cell type. J Immunol 2008; **180:** 2581.
31. Yoshikawa T, Mitsuno H, Nonaka I, Sen Y, Kawanishi K, Inada Y, Takakura Y, Okuchi K, and Nonomura A: Wound therapy by marrow mesenchymal cell transplantation. Plast Reconstr Surg 2008; **121:** 860.
32. Krause DS, Theise ND, Collector MI, Henegariu O, Hwang S, Gardner R, Neutzel S, and Sharkis SJ: Multi-organ, multi-lineage engraftment by a single bone marrow-derived stem cell. Cell 2001; **105:** 369.
33. Chan RK, Garfein E, Gigante PR, Liu P, Agha RA, Mulligan R, and Orgill DP: Side population hematopoietic stem cells promote wound healing in diabetic mice. Plast Reconstr Surg 2007; **120:** 407; discussion 12–3.
34. Asahara T, Masuda H, Takahashi T, Kalka C, Pastore C, Silver M, Kearne M, Magner M, and Isner JM: Bone marrow origin of endothelial progenitor cells responsible for postnatal vasculogenesis in physiological and pathological neovascularization. Circ Res 1999; **85:** 221.
35. Fathke C, Wilson L, Hutter J, Kapoor V, Smith A, Hocking A, and Isik F: Contribution of bone marrow-derived cells to skin: collagen deposition and wound repair. Stem Cells 2004; **22:** 812.
36. Blum B and Benvenisty N: The tumorigenicity of human embryonic stem cells. Adv Cancer Res 2008; **100:** 133.
37. Amariglio N, Hirshberg A, Scheithauer BW, Cohen Y, Loewenthal R, Trakhtenbrot L, Paz N, Koren-Michowitz M, Waldman D, Leider-Trejo L, Toren A, Constantini S, and Rechavi G: Donor-derived brain tumor following neural stem cell transplantation in an Ataxia Telangiectasia patient. PLoS Med 2009; **6:** e29.
38. Taylor G, Lehrer MS, Jensen PJ, Sun TT, and Lavker RM: Involvement of follicular stem cells in forming not only the follicle but also the epidermis. Cell 2000; **102:** 451.

STEM AND PROGENITOR CELLS

A Review of the Therapeutic Potential of Adipose-Derived Stem Cells

Liam C. Macleod, Aaron W. James, Antoine L. Carre, Michael T. Longaker, and Hermann P. Lorenz*

Department of Surgery, Lucile Packard Children's Hospital, Stanford University School of Medicine, Stanford, California.

Background: Stem cell treatment for wound defects is a promising new therapy. Stem cell types that are being investigated include human embryonic pluripotent stem cells, induced pluripotent stem cells, and bone marrow–derived stem cells. Recently, adipose-derived stem cells (ASCs) have emerged as a leading therapy for wound repair among regenerative cells. ASCs are acquired with little morbidity, are multipotent, and have a high yield of primary cells.
The Problem: Each stem cell considered for therapy has unique disadvantages. Bone marrow–derived stem cells have a low yield and require a painful procedure for harvest. Embryonic pluripotent stem cells are mired in ethical debate, and induced pluripotent stem cells cannot be efficiently induced to stem-cell-like states without viral or plasmid vectors used in transfection of genes. The use of transfection incurs unknown long-term risks. Because ASCs are autologous, postnatal, and readily available, they have important advantages over other types of stem cells.
Basic Clinical/Science Advances: In the early 2000s, the byproducts of liposuction (commonly referred to as lipoaspirate) were shown to contain ASCs, which are isolated by relatively simple methodology. Chondrocyte, osteoblast, myocyte, endothelial, epithelial, neuron, and other lineages can be differentiated from ASCs. Many of these observations were verified morphologically and by functional assays. Increasingly, the ability of ASC grafts to enhance tissue repair and function postinjury is becoming the benchmark for successful differentiation and incorporation of stem cell–based therapy.
Clinical Care Relevance: ASC-based therapy has improved closure of calvarial bone defects; generated transplantable cartilage when implanted on a scaffold; improved cardiac, skeletal, and smooth muscle function; aided in skin healing; and played a supportive role in neuronal convalescence in a stroke model.
Conclusion: The ASC is a promising stem cell with potential for repairing bone, cartilage, muscle, endothelial tissue, skin, and possibly neurons. However, mechanistic understanding of lineage differentiation, appropriate scaffolds, and standardization of clinical trials are currently lacking.

Abbreviations and Acronyms

ASCs = adipose-derived stem cells

BMP = bone morphogenic protein

BMSCs = bone marrow–derived stem cells

HEKs = human epidermal keratinocytes

IFATS = International Fat Applied Technology Society

MI = myocardial infarction

TGFβ1 = transforming growth factor β1

UVB = ultraviolet B light

VEGF = vascular endothelial growth factor

*Correspondence: Department of Surgery, Lucile Packard Children's Hospital, Stanford University School of Medicine, 770 Welch Road, Suite 440, Stanford, California 94305 (e-mail: plorenz@stanford.edu).

BACKGROUND

RESEARCH ON CELL SOURCES for therapeutic interventions, such as tissue defect healing or hematopoietic transplantation, has accelerated since the late 20th century. Stem cell types considered for cell-based therapy include human embryonic pluripotent stem cells, induced pluripotent stem cells, bone marrow mesenchymal stem cells, and bone marrow–derived stem cells (BMSCs). Each of these cell types has advantages and problems. Acquisition of human embryonic

Printed in U.S.A.
DOI: 10.1089/awc.2009.0110

pluripotent stem cells is surrounded by ethical debate, and a well-evidenced tendency for tumorigenesis with teratoma formation. Similarly, efficient induction of induced pluripotent stem cells is still being elucidated.[1] While bone marrow mesenchymal stem cells have shown promise in being inducible down a variety of lineages and BMSCs have met with clinical success in hematopoietic transplants, severe donor-site pain and low stem cell yield upon harvest are nontrivial obstacles for their wider use.

Another stem cell worthy of attention is the adipose-derived stem cell (ASC). ASCs are acquired from a discarded product (lipoaspirate) obtained with liposuction. ASCs isolated from lipoaspirate are multipotent and are easy to expand in culture. ASC isolation yields many cells. ASCs are described by several names elsewhere in the literature, including adipose stem cells, processed lipoaspirate cells, adipose-derived adult stromal cells, human multipotent ASCs, and adipose mesenchymal cells. To minimize confusion, the International Fat Applied Technology Society (IFATS) reached a consensus on the name ASCs, hence its use in this review.

CLINICAL PROBLEM ADDRESSED

ASCs are easily harvested by liposuction, a common, well-tolerated procedure. In the United States, over 400,000 liposuction operations are performed per year, and aspirated material (roughly 3 L) is often discarded.[2] However, this lipoaspirate contains a variety of cell types, including ASCs, which have multilineage potential and ability to self-renew in culture. Therefore, a critical question remains as to which therapies ASCs are most suited and whether they can be safely harvested, expanded, and distributed.

RELEVANT BASIC SCIENCE CONTEXT

In 2003, the Hedrick group showed that the primary harvest yield and proliferative capacity of ASCs was greater than BMSCs.[3] However, despite the different tissue source and yield, the biology of the two cell types was similar in terms of multipotent potential and cell markers. Both cell types express CD105, SH3, Stro-1, CD90, and CD44. However, ASCs do not express CD45 or CD31, hallmark hematopoietic and endothelial markers, respectively. Research demonstrates that ASCs can differentiate toward a number of distinct lineages, including adipo-, chondro-, osteo-, myo- (cardiac, smooth, and skeletal), endothelial-, epithelial-, and neuro- (with less evidence). The evidence is strongest for mesodermal fates. In this review, differentiation techniques, lineage confirmatory methods, and therapeutic models are emphasized. Due to its direct relevance for skin wound healing, recent research on epithelial differentiation is discussed in greatest detail.

EXPERIMENTAL MODEL OR MATERIAL

Since the early 2000s, a number of research teams isolated and induced ASCs to differentiate along osteo-, chondro-, myo-, endothelial-, epithelial-, and neuro-cell lineages (Fig. 1). Most relevant to skin wound healing is the epithelial differentiation pathway.[4] ASC isolation involves a liposuction procedure, washing the liposuction products, lysis of red blood cells, incubation with collagenase, and centrifugation.[5] These manipulations result in a pellet called the stromal vascular fraction, which contains a variety of cells from blood, endothelium, and a sizeable population of ASCs. ASCs are isolated from the many cells comprising the stromal vascular fraction by plastic adherence. Finally, ASCs are expanded in culture. Early attempts to differentiate specific cell lineages from ASCs borrowed methods used in research with BMSCs. However, differentiation methods are continually being refined for specific use with ASCs. In most cases, differentiation of ASCs toward a given lineage was assessed by functional assays and markers specific to each desired cell type. Finally, models ranging from mouse, rabbit, and pig, to human have sought to show functional improvement post-ASC injection in a number of organ systems. ASCs have found limited early clinical application and harbor future promise. In an often-cited case report, autologous ASCs were implanted into a congenital calvarial defect in a 7-year-old girl, and the surprising achievement of near closure was verified 3 months postoperatively.[6]

DISCUSSION OF FINDINGS AND RELEVANT LITERATURE

Bone

ASCs become osteoblast-like when cultured with ascorbic acid, β-glycerophosphate, dexamethasone, and vitamin D.[7] ASC-derived bone cells have osteoblast-like morphology and marker expression (cbfa-1, alkaline phosphatase, and others).[2,8] ASCs were implanted on an apatite-coated resorbing scaffold into a 4-mm murine calvarial defect.[7] Complete bone healing is impossible in a defect this size. Our laboratory demonstrated that over

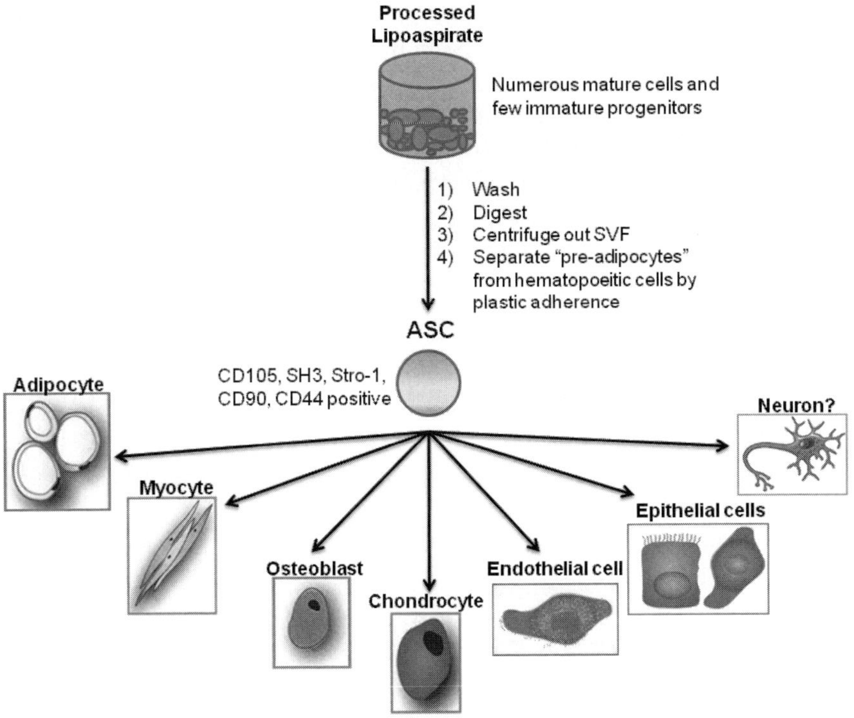

Figure 1. Schematic showing adipose-derived stem cell isolation and established lineages of adipose-derived stem cell differentiation.

3 months, 90% closure and density were achieved. The ASC origin of the new bone was verified with Y chromosome detection in sex mismatching of donor-recipient pairs.[7] One mechanism of osteogenic differentiation in ASCs exposed to retinoic acid and bone morphogenic protein 2 (BMP-2) is upregulation of the BMP receptor 1B.[9] When this receptor is blocked by RNAi, osteogenesis is impaired, showing that the 1B receptor is a necessary pathway for induction. Despite such details, much work remains to be completed in elucidating the mechanisms by which ASCs adopt the morphology and function of various lineages.

Cartilage

ASCs have been induced to form chondrocytes.[2] Chondrocyte differentiation occurs in a high-cell-density microenvironment with exposure to transforming growth factor β1 (TGFβ1).[8] Chondrocyte markers for differentiation include cartilage extracellular matrix molecules such as collagen II and IV, and proteoglycans.[2,10] ASCs have been shown to have therapeutic value in a rabbit cartilage injury model. ASC injection into the femoral condyle cartilage in this model resulted in significant functional improvement compared to controls. Improvement was based on resistance to biomechanical stress and histological grading.[11] The exact mechanism of the cartilage repair is not well understood. Another group implanted a subcutaneous, ASC-seeded, poly-lactide-co-glycolide scaffold in mice. At 8 weeks, these TGFβ-treated ASCs displayed cartilage-like phenotype, determined by mRNA expression and histological staining for collagens.[12]

Muscle

Much work addresses the repair and differentiation of ASCs toward skeletal, smooth, and cardiac muscle.[10] Skeletal muscle lineage differentiation is shown by expression of MyoD1, myosin, myf5, myf6, and myogenin.[10] Myo-induction involves treatment with dexamethasone, hydrocortisone, and sometimes azacytidine.[13] *In vivo*, *LacZ*-transduced ASCs were observed incorporating into muscle fibers of cardiotoxin-mediated rabbit tibialis anterior injuries at 2 weeks postinjection.[14] Additionally, ASC-treated tibialis anterior muscles demonstrated greater mass and contractile function than cardiotoxin-injured controls that were not treated with ASCs. The muscle regenerative ability of ASCs was tested in the Duchenne muscular dystrophy mouse.[15] The tibialis anterior muscle was damaged with cardiotoxin before intravenous injection of human ASCs. Human flk-1+ ASCs trafficked to the damaged murine muscle and reconstituted dystrophin expression. Further, flk-1+ human cells, along with murine cells, were viable long term in the muscle satellite compartment, which becomes depleted in muscular dystrophies. Human cell markers were also observed in nascent endothelial cells, suggesting that ASCs contributed to muscle repair partly through stimulation of angiogenesis.

ASCs can become smooth muscle–like when cultured in media with MCDB131 and heparin, on plates coated with laminin or collagen.[16] Smooth muscle identity was assessed by protein and gene expression of smooth muscle–specific proteins (α-actin, calponin, caldesmon, SM22, myosin heavy chain, and smoothelin). *In vivo*, human ASCs were injected into the bladders and urethras of mice and dispersed stably (up to 12 weeks) throughout mouse bladder smooth muscle, which suggests a potential for an ASC role in repair.[17]

ASCs differentiate into cardiomyocytes *in vivo, in vitro*, and clinically.[18,19] Planat-Benard confirmed cardiomyocyte identity morphologically and with markers such as Nkx2.5, troponin I, and myosin heavy chain. In a murine myocardial infarction (MI) model, Mazo *et al.* demonstrated superior improvement in cardiac function post-MI with ASC engraftment versus either BMSC grafts and cell-free control groups.[20] Improvement was based on percent tissue viability at the infarct site and left ventricular ejection fraction.

Endothelial

Vascular endothelial growth factor (VEGF)–supplemented and insulin-like growth factor 1–supplemented medium induces an endothelial cell phenotype in cultured ASCs.[21] In a mouse model of hindlimb ischemia, gross improvement in blood flow and capillary density after intravenous ASC injection was observed although the exact role of ASCs in this process was not described.[21]

Skin

Application of ASCs to cutaneous wounds can improve epithelial migration, vasculogenesis, scar cosmetics, and healing rate. One study cultured ASCs with human epidermal keratinocytes (HEKs) and observed more rapid HEK migration in coculture than controls.[22] Another study examined the medium of cultured of ASCs and found that the cells secreted platelet-derived growth factor, fibroblast growth factor 2, keratinocyte growth factor, TGFβ1, hepatocyte growth factor, VEGF, collagen I, and fibronectin.[23] These factors all have stimulatory effects on wound repair. A third research group suspended autologous ASCs in an atelocollagen matrix with a silicone membrane and implanted the scaffold into full-thickness cutaneous wounds in diabetic mice.[24] Histologic examination demonstrated significantly advanced granulation, capillary formation, and epithelialization in ASC-treated mice versus mice treated with the silicone membrane alone.

TAKE-HOME MESSAGE

Basic science advances

- ASC isolation methods are well established, and differentiation along numerous lineages is possible.
- Efforts aim to improve efficiency of differentiation and explore other inducible cell types.
- Osteogenic conditions include ascorbic acid, β-glycerophosphate, dexamethasone, vitamin D, all-trans retinoic acid, and BMP-2.
- Chondrogenic differentiation conditions include high cell density and TGFβ1.
- Myogenic differentiation conditions include corticosteroids and azacytidine (skeletal), MCDB131, and heparin on laminin- or collagen-coated plates (smooth), and DNA demethylating chemical 5-azacytidine or coculture (cardiac).
- Endothelial differentiation is achieved by exposing ASCs to insulin-like growth factor 1 and VEGF.
- Neurogenic differentiation remains controversial.
- Transdifferentiation is typically assessed by gene and protein expression.
- ASCs secrete numerous cytokines relevant to repair, including platelet-derived growth factor, fibroblast growth factor 2, VEGF, and TGFβ.

Clinical science advances

- A stable cartilaginous identity is observed among TGFβ-treated ASCs seeded on a poly-lactide-co-glycolide scaffold in a mouse model—this is promising for therapies involving cartilage transplant.
- In a Duchenne muscular dystrophy mouse model, ASC-injected tibialis anterior injuries had greater contractile function, mass, and dystrophin reconstitution.
- Injection of human pretreated ASCs into mouse bladders resulted in stable incorporation of human smooth muscle cells. ASCs should be considered for therapy in a variety of systems that rely on smooth muscle such as the gastrointestinal tract and urogenital tracts.
- Postmyocardial infarction, ASC-injected mice have greater left ventricular ejection fraction and infarct site tissue viability than controls.
- ASCs accelerate HEK migration, reduce wrinkles, and are well suited to use with scaffolds in epithelial wound healing.
- ASCs provide UVB protection to fibroblasts in coculture.
- ASC-mediated repair poststroke may be attributable to ASC release of growth factors rather than neuronal transdifferentiation.
- ASCs seeded on a collagen matrix and implanted in a mouse wound improved repair.

Relevance to clinical care

- To date, most therapeutic effects of ASCs have been observed in animal models. Diseases and procedures most likely to benefit from ASC therapy, based on completed animal research include defects of bone (congenital abnormalities and trauma), defects of joints (arthritides and trauma), and procedures requiring cartilage (*e.g.*, rhinoplasty), Duchenne muscular dystrophy, myocardial infarction, cutaneous scar treatment, skin wound healing, and various vascular disorders.
- ASC osteogenesis has been used to close murine calvarial defects, and in one case, a human calvarial defect.
- IFATS and several biotechnology companies are dedicated to developing ASC-based therapies. A few clinical trials have taken place, but no products are currently widely available.
- Work remains in understanding the mechanisms by which ASCs differentiate and repair tissues as well as appropriate scaffolds, microenvironments and host side effects.

ASCs have been combined with various scaffolds, and the constructs' capacity to improve repair has been demonstrated. Altman seeded ASCs on silk suture material and used it to close a 6-mm full-thickness skin defect in mice.[25] Wound closure was significantly enhanced in the group that received ASC-coated sutures compared to the control group. Researchers compared six topical treatments that combined ASCs (vs. saline) with plasma (platelet poor or rich), and fibrin gels.[26] ASCs did not significantly increase the rate of closure in full-thickness porcine skin wounds, but each of the study treatments containing ASCs, whether with or without fibrin or platelets, resulted in better cosmetic results (based on gross appearance of the scar) and increased microvessel density. The topical treatment that most increased microvessel density was ASCs carried in a fibrin gel with platelet-rich plasma. These results suggest that each tested component may contribute to wound closure in an additive manner.

Finally, ASCs have also been successfully used to reduce photo-induced wrinkles in mice based on gross observation and *in vitro* experiments.[27] Decreased skin wrinkles occurred after 8 weeks of ultraviolet B light (UVB) exposure in mice injected subcutaneously with ASCs. To investigate possible mechanisms, ASCs were cocultured with human dermal fibroblasts, and exposed to UVB. UVB exposure decreased fibroblast proliferation in the control culture dishes, but not in the ASC–fibroblast coculture. These results suggest a paracrine effect in which factors released from ASCs provided UVB protection to fibroblasts. This, in turn, may provide benefit in preventing solar elastosis, which occurs in chronic UVB exposure. Thus, ASCs have been shown to have potential therapeutic benefit for skin healing.

Neurons

ASCs treated with β-mercaptoethanol develop a neuron-like morphology and express neuronal markers such as nestin, neuron-specific enolase, and neuron-specific nuclear protein.[8] The possibility that cell toxicity drove a disordered morphology and gene expression resulted in criticism of these differentiation techniques. Thus, milder neuronal differentiation methods have been studied, such as, exposure to insulin, indomethacin, and isobutylmethylxanthine,[8] or brain-derived neurotrophic factor and all-trans retinoic acid.[28] However, neuronal differentiation has yet to be validated conclusively by recapitulation of neuronal function, such as forming synapses or transmitting action potentials. Many believe that the reported improvements in stroke models after ASC treatment are mediated by vasculogenesis or ASC release of regenerative growth factors. No clean evidence of ASC transdifferentiation has been shown.[8]

CAUTION, CRITICAL REMARKS, AND RECOMMENDATIONS

There are several notable knowledge gaps in the induction, modulation mechanisms, duration of viability, and appropriate scaffolds for ASCs. For example, BMSC culture methods often serve as a model for selecting specific lineages in ASCs. Yet, this transfer of methods from one type of cell to another does not always function as well as intended. For example, hypoxia and BMP-6 are better inducers of chondrogenesis in ASCs than the methods used to differentiate cartilage from BMSCs.[29,30] Regarding modulation of ASCs, a problem with osteo-induction using retinoic acid is that this stimulates osteoclastogenesis that resorbs some of the ASC-derived bone.[31] This cross-stimulation requires predictable modulation before ASCs can be used in bone repair. ASC multipotency does not endure indefinitely, and ideal microenvironments maintaining a multipotent state are not well understood. For example, ASCs' ability to differentiate into skeletal muscle attenuates when cultured longer than 7 days. Neuronal cell fate is an unexpected outcome for ASCs, and skepticism is prudent. Yet, ASC-based therapies in neurological disease remain possible, given ASCs' potential to mediate neuronal repair through supportive mechanisms such as vasculogenesis.

FUTURE DEVELOPMENT

Current research on ASC multipotency demonstrates promising therapeutic potential. To translate basic work to a clinical therapy, further elucidation of the mechanisms involved in ASC lineage selection and tissue repair is needed. IFATS is an organization devoted to pooling information regarding ASCs in an effort to accelerate the many potential therapies that ASCs represent. Further, there are several biotechnology companies devoted to the development of these cells. Ultimately, in addition to mechanistic understanding, a number of other challenges must be considered. ASCs are undergoing clinical trials, and strategies to coordinate these trials would be useful in evaluating their success. Many preclinical animal trials are still needed. For example, should cells be pretreated to encourage specific differentiation? What is the best site, dose, and delivery method of cells destined for each organ system or disease? What influence will the host tissue microenvironment have on ASCs? Are ASCs competent to respond to host signals in a predictable, reproducible manner? Are there any unforeseen safety issues such as ectopic tissue or tumor potential? What is the ideal cell–scaffold–environment combination for each desired tissue type? As ASCs make their way from basic research laboratories to clinical applications, sound initial engineering that addresses these questions can help ensure rapid, safe, and efficacious implementation.

AUTHOR DISCLOSURE STATEMENT

No competing financial interests exist.

REFERENCES

1. Okita K, Nakagawa M, Hyenjong H, Ichisaka T, and Yamanaka S: Generation of mouse induced pluripotent stem cells without viral vectors. Science 2008; **322:** 949.
2. Zuk PA, Zhu M, Mizuno H, Huang J, Futrell JW, Katz AJ, *et al.*: Multilineage cells from human adipose tissue: implications for cell-based therapies. Tissue Eng 2001; **7:** 211.
3. De Ugarte DA, Morizono K, Elbarbary A, Alfonso Z, Zuk PA, Zhu M, *et al.*: Comparison of multilineage cells from human adipose tissue and bone marrow. Cells Tissues Organs 2003; **174:** 101.
4. Branski LK, Gauglitz GG, Herndon DN, and Jeschke MG: A review of gene and stem cell therapy in cutaneous wound healing. Burns 2009; **35:** 171.
5. Bunnell BA, Estes BT, Guilak F, and Gimble JM: Differentiation of adipose stem cells. Methods Mol Biol 2008; **456:** 155.
6. Lendeckel S, Jodicke A, Christophis P, Heidinger K, Wolff J, Fraser JK, *et al.*: Autologous stem cells (adipose) and fibrin glue used to treat widespread traumatic calvarial defects: case report. J Craniomaxillofac Surg 2004; **32:** 370.
7. Cowan CM, Shi YY, Aalami OO, Chou YF, Mari C, Thomas R, *et al.*: Adipose-derived adult stromal cells heal critical-size mouse calvarial defects. Nat Biotechnol 2004; **22:** 560.
8. Fraser JK, Wulur I, Alfonso Z, and Hedrick MH: Fat tissue: an underappreciated source of stem cells for biotechnology. Trends Biotechnol 2006; **24:** 150.
9. Wan DC, Shi YY, Nacamuli RP, Quarto N, Lyons KM, and Longaker MT: Osteogenic differentiation of mouse adipose-derived adult stromal cells requires retinoic acid and bone morphogenetic protein receptor type IB signaling. Proc Natl Acad Sci USA 2006; **103:** 12335.
10. Zuk PA, Zhu M, Ashjian P, De Ugarte DA, Huang JI, Mizuno H, *et al.*: Human adipose tissue is a source of multipotent stem cells. Mol Biol Cell 2002; **13:** 4279.
11. Nathan S, Das De S, Thambyah A, Fen C, Goh J, and Lee EH: Cell-based therapy in the repair of osteochondral defects: a novel use for adipose tissue. Tissue Eng 2003; **9:** 733.
12. Mehlhorn AT, Zwingmann J, Finkenzeller G, Niemeyer P, Dauner M, Stark B, *et al.*: Chondrogenesis of adipose-derived adult stem cells in a polylactide-co-glycolide scaffold. Tissue Eng A 2009; **15:** 1159.
13. Strem BM, Hicok KC, Zhu M, Wulur I, Alfonso Z, Schreiber RE, *et al.*: Multipotential differentiation of adipose tissue-derived stem cells. Keio J Med 2005; **54:** 132.
14. Bacou F, el Andalousi RB, Daussin PA, Micallef JP, Levin JM, Chammas M, *et al.*: Transplantation of adipose tissue-derived stromal cells increases mass and functional capacity of damaged skeletal muscle. Cell Transplant 2004; **13:** 103.
15. Liu Y, Yan X, Sun Z, Chen B, Han Q, Li J, *et al.*: Flk-1+ adipose-derived mesenchymal stem cells differentiate into skeletal muscle satellite cells and ameliorate muscular dystrophy in mdx mice. Stem Cells Dev 2007; **16:** 695.
16. Rodriguez LV, Alfonso Z, Zhang R, Leung J, Wu B, and Ignarro LJ: Clonogenic multipotent stem cells in human adipose tissue differentiate into functional smooth muscle cells. Proc Natl Acad Sci USA 2006; **103:** 12167.
17. Jack GS, Almeida FG, Zhang R, Alfonso ZC, Zuk PA, and Rodriguez LV: Processed lipoaspirate cells for tissue engineering of the lower urinary tract: implications for the treatment of stress urinary incontinence and bladder reconstruction. J Urol 2005; **174:** 2041.
18. Planat-Benard V, Menard C, Andre M, Puceat M, Perez A, Garcia-Verdugo JM, *et al.*: Spontaneous cardiomyocyte differentiation from adipose tissue stroma cells. Circ Res 2004; **94:** 223.
19. Rangappa S, Fen C, Lee EH, Bongso A, and Sim EK: Transformation of adult mesenchymal stem cells isolated from the fatty tissue into cardiomyocytes. Ann Thorac Surg 2003; **75:** 775.
20. Mazo M, Planat-Benard V, Abizanda G, Pelacho B, Leobon B, Gavira JJ, *et al.*: Transplantation of adipose derived stromal cells is associated with functional improvement in a rat model of chronic myocardial infarction. Eur J Heart Fail 2008; **10:** 454.
21. Miranville A, Heeschen C, Sengenes C, Curat CA, Busse R, and Bouloumie A: Improvement of postnatal neovascularization by human adipose tissue-derived stem cells. Circulation 2004; **110:** 349.
22. Yuan F, Lei YH, Fu XB, Sheng ZY, Cai S, and Sun TZ: Promotive effect of adipose-derived stem cells on the wound model of human epidermal keratinocytes *in vitro*. Zhonghua Wai Ke Za Zhi 2008; **46:** 1575.
23. Park BS, Jang KA, Sung JH, Park JS, Kwon YH, Kim KJ, *et al.*: Adipose-derived stem cells and their secretory factors as a promising therapy for skin aging. Dermatol Surg 2008; **34:** 1323.
24. Nambu M, Kishimoto S, Nakamura S, Mizuno H, Yanagibayashi S, Yamamoto N, *et al.*: Accelerated

wound healing in healing-impaired db/db mice by autologous adipose tissue-derived stromal cells combined with atelocollagen matrix. Ann Plast Surg 2009; **62:** 317.

25. Altman AM, Yan Y, Matthias N, Bai X, Rios C, Mathur AB, *et al.*: IFATS series: Human adipose-derived stem cells seeded on a silk fibroin-chitosan scaffold enhance wound repair in a murine soft tissue injury model. Stem Cells 2009; **27:** 250.

26. Blanton MW, Hadad I, Johnstone BH, Mund JA, Rogers PI, Eppley BL, *et al.*: Adipose stromal cells and platelet-rich plasma therapies synergistically increase revascularization during wound healing. Plast Reconstr Surg 2009; **123(Suppl 2):** 56S.

27. Kim WS, Park BS, Park SH, Kim HK, and Sung JH: Antiwrinkle effect of adipose-derived stem cell: activation of dermal fibroblast by secretory factors. J Dermatol Sci 2009; **53:** 96.

28. Anghileri E, Marconi S, Pignatelli A, Cifelli P, Galie M, Sbarbati A, *et al.*: Neuronal differentiation potential of human adipose-derived mesenchymal stem cells. Stem Cells Dev 2008; **17:** 909.

29. Xu Y, Malladi P, Chiou M, Bekerman E, Giaccia AJ, and Longaker MT: *In vitro* expansion of adipose-derived adult stromal cells in hypoxia enhances early chondrogenesis. Tissue Eng 2007; **13:** 2981.

30. Hennig T, Lorenz H, Thiel A, Goetzke K, Dickhut A, Geiger F, *et al.*: Reduced chondrogenic potential of adipose tissue derived stromal cells correlates with an altered TGFbeta receptor and BMP profile and is overcome by BMP-6. J Cell Physiol 2007; **211:** 682.

31. Wan DC, Siedhoff MT, Kwan MD, Nacamuli RP, Wu BM, and Longaker MT: Refining retinoic acid stimulation for osteogenic differentiation of murine adipose-derived adult stromal cells. Tissue Eng 2007; **13:** 1623.

WHS
Wound
Healing
Society

Endothelial Progenitor Cell's Contribution to Wound Healing and Skin Graft Neovascularization

Michael G. Galvez, Edward I. Chang, and Geoffrey C. Gurtner*

Division of Plastic and Reconstructive Surgery, Department of Surgery, Stanford University School of Medicine, Stanford, California.

Abbreviations and Acronyms

eNOS = endothelial nitric oxide synthase

EPC = endothelial progenitor cell

HIF-1α = hypoxia-inducible factor-1 alpha

HMG-CoA = hydroxymethyl-glutaryl coenzyme-A

ICAM-1 = intercellular adhesion molecule 1

MMP = matrix metallo-proteinase

NO = nitric oxide

PHD = prolyl hydroxylase

SDF-1α = stromal cell–derived factor-1 alpha

VEGF = vascular endothelial growth factor

*Correspondence: Division of Plastic and Reconstructive Surgery, Department of Surgery, Stanford University School of Medicine, 257 Campus Drive West, Hagey Building GK-201, Stanford, California 94305-5148 (e-mail: ggurtner@stanford.edu).

Background: Neovascularization, comprised of angiogenesis and vasculogenesis, is essential for wound healing and skin graft revascularization. Although the relative importance of vasculogenesis remains unclear, it is certain that this process requires bone marrow–derived endothelial progenitor cells (EPCs) to respond rapidly to hypoxic stimuli, mobilize into the circulation, home to sites of ischemia, and mature into new vessels.

The Problem: To maximize EPC therapeutic potential in the treatment of ischemic wounds in the elderly or diabetic population, the underlying mechanisms governing the mobilization and targeting of EPCs must be elucidated.

Basic/Clinical Science Advances: In the past year, impairments in the ability of EPCs to home to sites of ischemia in aging were linked to decreased hypoxia-inducible factor-1 alpha (HIF-1α) stabilization. Hyperglycemia as occurs in diabetes was also linked to hypoxia-inducible factor-1 alpha dysfunction and impaired nitric oxide–mediated EPC mobilization, which was corrected by both hyperoxia and the chemokine, stromal cell–derived factor-1 (SDF-1). The combination of a statin with SDF-1 improved EPC mobilization and function. Activated Akt, a downstream effector of SDF-1, increased EPC trafficking. A novel graft model for determining revascularization and novel EPC delivery strategies were also developed.

Clinical Care Relevance: EPC-based therapeutics for wound healing has great potential for the revascularization and regeneration of tissue in aging and diabetes.

Conclusion: Understanding the mechanisms underlying normal EPC function and developing novel EPC-based strategies for improving wound healing and skin graft neovascularization can have a profound impact on the management and treatment of wounds in a clinical setting.

BACKGROUND

Neovascularization, or the formation of new blood vessels, is critical for granulation tissue formation and tissue regeneration in wound healing.[1] During the proliferative phase, neovascularization provides efficient delivery of nutrients and maintenance of oxygen homeostasis allowing cellular proliferation and tissue regeneration. Neovascularization occurs by two distinct processes: angiogenesis and vasculogenesis, both of which are mediated by the transcription factor hypoxia-inducible factor-1 alpha (HIF-1α). Tissue injury and subsequent hypoxia initiate the release of cytokines and a cascade of growth factors that stimulate resident endothelial cells to proliferate and sprout new blood vessels (angiogenesis).

In addition, these growth factors also mobilize and recruit endothelial

Printed in U.S.A.
DOI: 10.1089/awc.2009.0113

progenitor cells (EPCs) to sites of injury where they contribute to neovessel formation (vasculogenesis).[2] EPCs, thought to be related to embryonic hemangioblasts, are mobilized from the bone marrow and selectively home to areas of ischemia.[3–6] Trafficking of EPCs is contingent on appropriate environment-specific signals and the response of normally functioning stem and progenitor cells.[7,8] Vasculogenesis represents a significant contribution to neovascularization in wound healing and occurs in the most ischemic tissue during skin graft revascularization.[9]

Any tissue transferred without its blood supply from one part of the body to another in reconstructive surgery, such as a skin graft, immediately becomes ischemic and slowly revascularizes through the wound bed.[10] Initially nourished by imbibition, or diffusion through wound surface contact, the skin graft then undergoes inosculation, where capillary buds from the wound bed join the microvasculature of the skin graft to restore blood flow through preexisting channels. Ultimately, *de novo* blood vessels grow into the skin graft and revascularize the skin graft through a combination of angiogenesis and vasculogenesis. Proper skin graft revascularization and wound healing requires intact EPC function and trafficking.

CLINICAL PROBLEM ADDRESSED

Neovascularization is an essential component for granulation tissue formation, nutrient delivery, and proper wound healing. This process is also vital for skin graft revascularization, an important component for soft tissue coverage in reconstructive surgery. Impairments in neovascularization are a major cause for the development of chronic wounds.[11] Aging and diabetes result in poor neovascularization and wound healing due to an impaired ischemic response linked to HIF-1α dysfunction[12–14] (Fig. 1).

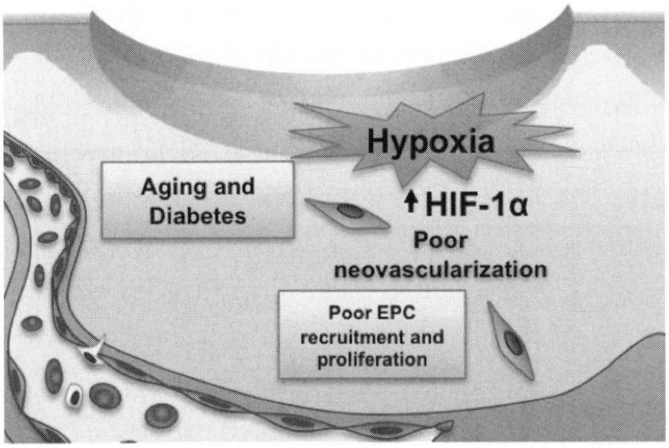

Figure 1. In the setting of aging and diabetes, neovascularization results in hypoxia-inducible factor-1 alpha (HIF-1α) dysfunction with subsequent poor neovascularization and deficient endothelial progenitor cell (EPC) recruitment and proliferation.

RELEVANT BASIC SCIENCE CONTEXT

The neovascularization process in wound healing is mediated by HIF-1α. This transcription factor is constitutively expressed intracellularly and is posttranslationally regulated through a complex mechanism involving prolyl hydroxylases (PHDs). In the presence of oxygen and iron, PHDs hydroxylate HIF-1α and target it for proteosomal degradation. However, in the absence of oxygen (hypoxia), PHDs are unable to hydroxylate HIF-1α, leading to increased HIF-1α accumulation. Insufficient blood flow to provide adequate oxygenation of tissue (ischemia) leads to increased HIF-1α as a result of hypoxia and followed by the formation of a heterodimer transcriptional complex with HIF-1β. This HIF heterodimer is capable of binding hypoxia response element sequences, which initiate the transcription of multiple genes involved in the response to ischemic injury.[15] Binding increases transcription of stromal cell–derived factor-1 (SDF-1), a known chemokine stimulator of vasculogenesis, and vascular endothelial growth factor (VEGF), a potent proneovascular cytokine that can augment both angiogenesis and vasculogenesis. Signals released by injured tissue mediate the recruitment and retention of mobilized stem cells in tissues requiring repair or regeneration. Receptor/ligand interactions either at the level of the blood vessel endothelium or within the injured tissue itself are likely responsible for the targeted homing of stem cells to injured tissues. CXCR4/SDF-1 and c-kit/stem cell factor have been identified as receptor/ligand pairs involved in the trafficking of stem cells.[16–21] Specifically, CXCR4/SDF-1 is a critical mediator in the mobilization and homing of EPCs from the bone marrow niche to regions of injury or ischemia.[9,22] Further, EPC recruitment from the bone marrow is enhanced by VEGF, matrix metalloproteinases (MMPs), endothelial nitric oxide synthase (eNOS), and estrogen.

EXPERIMENTAL MODEL OR MATERIAL—ADVANTAGES AND LIMITATIONS

This past year, several key studies have attempted to determine neovascularization deficiencies in the setting of aging and diabetes, elucidate the mechanism for EPC mobilization and homing, and describe novel therapeutic EPC delivery methods. A combination of molecular techniques, and *in vitro* and *in vivo* studies were utilized to make these advances.

EPC deficiencies in aged mice and humans were linked to HIF-1α dysfunction,[13,23] and reduced EPC levels was noted in adult human life compared with childhood.[24] Further, hyperglycemia was linked to HIF-1α dysfunction,[12] and diabetes was shown to have impaired nitric oxide (NO)–mediated EPC mobilization, reversed by both hyperoxia and SDF-1 in a murine ischemic hindlimb model.[25] Combining low-dose statin and SDF-1 improved neovascularization through improved EPC mobilization and proliferation, leading to enhanced incorporation into neovessels.[26] Activated Akt, a key downstream effector of SDF-1, was shown to increase EPC survival, NO production, and increased EPC localization to sites of ischemia.[27] Recently, a novel murine model was created allowing *in vivo* analysis of the microcirculation during skin graft healing.[28] Promising techniques for enhancing EPC therapy efficiency by taking advantage of paracrine effects[29] and novel EPC delivery utilizing implanted scaffolds were also assessed.[30] However, limited studies involving translational approaches and therapies utilizing human EPCs for wound healing and graft revascularization were undertaken.

TAKE-HOME MESSAGE

Basic science advances

- Decreased HIF-1α levels in aging murine tissue resulted in poor vasculogenesis and angiogenesis. This age-related decline in HIF-1α stabilization was linked to increased PHD-mediated degradation in peripheral tissue.
- Hyperglycemia impaired NO-mediated EPC mobilization through decreased phosphorylation of eNOS. The stimulation of eNOS by hyperoxia and local SDF-1 improved EPC trafficking and neovascularization in diabetic wounds.
- Direct modification of HIF-1α by the glyoxalase 1 substrate methylglyoxal, in the setting of hyperglycemia, resulted in poor HIF-1α activity.
- The combination of low-dose statin and SDF-1 improved neovascularization through increased EPC mobilization and proliferation, leading to enhanced incorporation.
- The activation of the Akt/NOS pathway by SDF-1 increased EPC proliferation, reduced apoptosis, and increased ICAM-1 resulting in increased EPC incorporation at ischemic sites and improved transendothelial migration.
- A novel murine model allowed *in vivo* analysis of the microcirculation during skin graft revascularization.
- Attributed to paracrine effects, EPCs and smooth muscle cells increased vessel density and perfusion more than each cell type alone.
- EPC delivery method of incorporating a microenvironment of arginine–glycine–aspartic acid peptides and VEGF onto a scaffold was a reliable method for consistent delivery of EPCs *in vivo*.

Clinical science advances

- Human EPC baseline levels in adult life are reduced compared with childhood.

Relevance to clinical care

- Aging and diabetes are known risk factors for delayed wound healing, chronic wound, and pressure ulcer development.
- Understanding the mechanisms of appropriate EPC function and developing new EPC-based strategies for improving wound healing and graft neovascularization are promising areas for providing better wound care, revascularization, and regeneration of tissue.

DISCUSSION OF FINDINGS AND RELEVANT LITERATURE

Aging and diabetes are known risk factors for delayed wound healing due to an inability to mount an appropriate neovascular response following an ischemic insult. Analysis of the prevalence of circulating EPCs in adult patients demonstrated reduced baseline levels compared with childhood levels,[24] suggesting that the observed impairments in the vascular regenerative potential in adults may be a reflection of reduced EPC levels. Decreased HIF-1α levels were also seen in aged ischemic muscle and skin tissue in murine models, resulting in poor vasculogenesis and angiogenesis.[13,23] The underlying mechanism for the age-related decline in HIF-1α stabilization was due to increased PHD expression in peripheral tissue and subsequent PHD-mediated HIF-1α degradation. Thus in aging, the combination of an impaired hypoxic response and potentially low EPC levels represent targets for future therapeutic interventions.

NO, synthesized by eNOS, is essential in the bone marrow microenvironment and in EPC mobilization. Hyperglycemia in a diabetic wound-healing murine model was shown to have impaired NO-mediated EPC mobilization due to decreased phosphorylation of eNOS.[25]

However, NO levels can be increased via hyperbaric oxygen, which stimulates eNOS activity. Although hyperoxia increased EPC mobilization, EPC trafficking to ischemic diabetic wounds was only achieved when SDF-1 was applied concurrently with hyperbaric oxygen therapy, which resulted in improved neovascularization and wound healing. Hyperglycemia also results in increased intercellular reactive oxygen species, which was shown to cause HIF-1α dysfunction.[12] This decreased function was shown to be due to direct modification of HIF-1α by the glyoxalase 1 substrate methylglyoxal, resulting in reduced heterodimer formation and thus poor HIF-1α binding to hypoxia response elements. The paradox of the ability of hyperoxia to stimulate NO production as well as the association with increased reactive oxygen species production has yet to be clarified. However, despite this contradiction, it is clear that effective EPC trafficking and the correction of HIF-1α function in diabetes is promising for directing future therapeutics.

Statins, or hydroxymethylglutaryl coenzyme-A (HMG-CoA) reductase inhibitors, competitively inhibit the rate-limiting step in cholesterol biosynthesis. Clinically they are primarily used to lower cholesterol in the circulation for primary and secondary prevention of coronary artery disease, but have also been shown to stimulate angiogenesis and protect against ischemic injury of the heart. Although the mechanism of statin action on EPCs is unclear, it is certain that they result in improved EPC function, mobilization, and subsequent incorporation into new blood vessels. In the murine ischemic hindlimb model, the combination of low-dose statin and SDF-1 was shown to improve neovascularization through increased EPC mobilization, proliferation, and reduced apoptosis, leading to enhanced neovessel incorporation.[26] The improvement in EPC mobilization by statin therapy was attributed to the upregulation of MMP-2 and MMP-9, which are both involved in the degradation of extracellular matrix and in facilitating EPC release from the bone marrow. Increased proliferation and reduced apoptosis of EPCs were attributed to the activation of the Akt/NOS pathway by SDF-1. These observations demonstrated that induced release of EPCs combined with improved homing and proliferation with SDF-1 results in improved neovascularization.

A separate study further confirmed the role of Akt, a key downstream effector of SDF-1, to increase EPC survival, NO production, and the adhesion molecule, intercellular adhesion molecule 1 (ICAM-1), when activated by phosphorylation.[27] Activated Akt enhanced ICAM-1 expression on endothelial cells, resulting in increased EPC incorporation into blood vessels at ischemic sites and improved transendothelial migration. Akt gene transfer to a murine ischemic hindlimb model led to significantly increased homing of systemically administered EPCs, resulting in neovessel formation, restoration of blood flow, and tissue healing. Together these studies demonstrate the importance of understanding the mechanisms behind the many downstream effectors of drugs and cytokines important for EPC trafficking to sites of ischemia.

Quantifying skin graft healing and revascularization is limited to studies utilizing only histological means. Thus, a novel murine model was created allowing *in vivo* analysis of the microcirculation during skin graft revascularization.[28] This animal model has promising implications for designing studies to better understand the underlying mechanisms for angiogenesis, inosculation, and subsequent vasculogenesis in skin graft revascularization.

In addition to the advances in analyzing the underlying mechanisms for vasculogenesis, a number of studies have also developed some promising techniques to enhance graft revascularization utilizing EPCs. In a murine hindlimb ischemia model, the combination of EPCs and smooth muscle cells was shown to increase vessel density and perfusion more than each cell type alone,[29] suggesting that the paracrine interaction between endothelial cells and smooth muscle cells is critical for the maturation and remodeling of neovessels into functional vasculature and may represent another potential target to enhance graft revascularization. As previous studies have demonstrated, direct injection of EPCs is an inefficient means of stem cell delivery due to poor targeting and rapid clearance from the host circulation. However, novel trafficking techniques using arginine–glycine–aspartic acid amino acid sequences and VEGF-embedded scaffolds have demonstrated promising results in reliable delivery of EPCs *in vivo*.[30] This scaffold was able to enhance EPC survival and resulted in sustained release and repopulation of the surrounding tissue.

CAUTION, CRITICAL REMARKS, AND RECOMMENDATIONS

Questions still persist regarding EPC lineage and the precise panel of cell surface markers that define

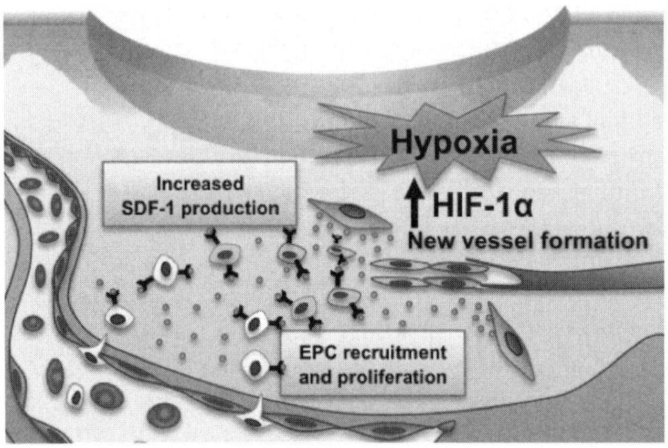

Figure 2. Strategies for rapid delivery of EPCs and increasing recruitment and proliferation have powerful implications for improving neovascularization in poor wound healing and ischemic tissue.

this cell population, especially considering the inconsistency in the literature. Are circulating progenitor/stem cells identical to bone marrow resident progenitor/stem cells? Is one progenitor/stem cell type or many different cell types involved in ischemic homing and neovascularization? Although well described in murine models, the full functional characteristics for human EPCs in wound healing and graft revascularization have only been partially described.

FUTURE DEVELOPMENTS

Human response to injury can either be classified as tissue regeneration or repair with scar. The field of regenerative medicine for wound healing requires a thorough understanding of the mechanisms that govern EPC dynamics and the ability to exploit that knowledge to enhance neovascularization in healing wounds. Thus, developing new strategies utilizing stem cell–based therapies, adjuvant growth factors, and tissue engineering approaches have promising implications on the future treatment and management of complex wounds in the diabetic and elderly population (Fig. 2).

AUTHOR DISCLOSURE STATEMENT

No competing financial interests exist.

REFERENCES

1. Gurtner GC, Werner S, Barrandon Y, and Longaker MT: Wound repair and regeneration. Nature 2008; **453:** 314.
2. Patan S: Vasculogenesis and angiogenesis as mechanisms of vascular network formation, growth and remodeling. J Neurooncol 2000; **50:** 1.
3. Shi Q, *et al.*: Evidence for circulating bone marrow-derived endothelial cells. Blood 1998; **92:** 362.
4. Asahara T, *et al.*: Bone marrow origin of endothelial progenitor cells responsible for postnatal vasculogenesis in physiological and pathological neovascularization. Circ Res 1999; **85:** 221.
5. Pelosi E, *et al.*: Identification of the hemangioblast in postnatal life. Blood 2002; **100:** 3203.
6. Reyes M, *et al.*: Origin of endothelial progenitors in human postnatal bone marrow. J Clin Investig 2002; **109:** 337.
7. Hattori K, *et al.*: Plasma elevation of stromal cell-derived factor-1 induces mobilization of mature and immature hematopoietic progenitor and stem cells. Blood 2001; **97:** 3354.
8. Gill M, *et al.*: Vascular trauma induces rapid but transient mobilization of VEGFR2(+)AC133(+) endothelial precursor cells. Circ Res 2001; **88:** 167.
9. Tepper OM, *et al.*: Adult vasculogenesis occurs through *in situ* recruitment, proliferation, and tubulization of circulating bone marrow-derived cells. Blood 2005; **105:** 1068.
10. Capla JM, *et al.*: Skin graft vascularization involves precisely regulated regression and replacement of endothelial cells through both angiogenesis and vasculogenesis. Plast Reconstr Surg 2006; **117:** 836.
11. Bauer SM, Bauer RJ, and Velazquez OC: Angiogenesis, vasculogenesis, and induction of healing in chronic wounds. Vasc Endovasc Surg 2005; **39:** 293.
12. Ceradini DJ, *et al.*: Decreasing intracellular superoxide corrects defective ischemia-induced new vessel formation in diabetic mice. J Biol Chem 2008; **283:** 10930.
13. Chang EI, *et al.*: Age decreases endothelial progenitor cell recruitment through decreases in hypoxia-inducible factor 1 alpha stabilization during ischemia. Circulation 2007; **116:** 2818.
14. Capla JM, *et al.*: Diabetes impairs endothelial progenitor cell-mediated blood vessel formation in response to hypoxia. Plast Reconstr Surg 2007; **119:** 59.
15. Safran M and Kaelin WG Jr.: HIF hydroxylation and the mammalian oxygen-sensing pathway. J Clin Investig 2003; **111:** 779.
16. Matsui Y, Zsebo KM, and Hogan BL: Embryonic expression of a haematopoietic growth factor encoded by the SI locus and the ligand for c-kit. Nature 1990; **347:** 667.
17. Heissig B, *et al.*: Recruitment of stem and progenitor cells from the bone marrow niche requires MMP-9 mediated release of kit-ligand. Cell 2002; **109:** 625.
18. Pillarisetti K and Gupta SK: Cloning and relative expression analysis of rat stromal cell derived factor-1 (SDF-1)1: SDF-1 alpha mRNA is selectively induced in rat model of myocardial infarction. Inflammation 2001; **25:** 293.
19. Salvucci O, *et al.*: Regulation of endothelial cell branching morphogenesis by endogenous chemokine stromal-derived factor-1. Blood 2002; **99:** 2703.
20. Youn BS, Mantel C, and Broxmeyer HE: Chemokines, chemokine receptors and hematopoiesis. Immunol Rev 2000; **177:** 150.
21. Lapidot T: Mechanism of human stem cell migration and repopulation of NOD/SCID and B2mnull NOD/SCID mice. The role of SDF-1/CXCR4 interactions. Ann NY Acad Sci 2001; **938:** 83.
22. Ceradini DJ, *et al.*: Progenitor cell trafficking is regulated by hypoxic gradients through HIF-1 induction of SDF-1. Nat Med 2004; **10:** 858.
23. Bosch-Marce M, *et al.*: Effects of aging and hypoxia-inducible factor-1 activity on angiogenic cell mobilization and recovery of perfusion after limb ischemia. Circ Res 2007; **101:** 1310.
24. Jie KE, Goossens MH, van Oostrom O, Lilien MR, and Verhaar MC: Circulating endothelial progenitor cell levels are higher during childhood than in adult life. Atherosclerosis 2009; **202:** 345.

25. Gallagher KA, *et al.*: Diabetic impairments in NO-mediated endothelial progenitor cell mobilization and homing are reversed by hyperoxia and SDF-1 alpha. J Clin Investig 2007; **117:** 1249.

26. Shao H, *et al.*: Statin and stromal cell-derived factor-1 additively promote angiogenesis by enhancement of progenitor cells incorporation into new vessels. Stem Cells 2008; **26:** 1376.

27. Hur J, *et al.*: Akt is a key modulator of endothelial progenitor cell trafficking in ischemic muscle. Stem Cells 2007; **25:** 1769.

28. Lindenblatt N, *et al.*: A new model for studying the revascularization of skin grafts *in vivo*: the role of angiogenesis. Plast Reconstr Surg 2008; **122:** 1669.

29. Foubert P, *et al.*: Coadministration of endothelial and smooth muscle progenitor cells enhances the efficiency of proangiogenic cell-based therapy. Circ Res 2008; **103:** 751.

30. Silva EA, Kim ES, Kong HJ, and Mooney DJ: Material-based deployment enhances efficacy of endothelial progenitor cells. Proc Natl Acad Sci USA 2008; **105:** 14347.

The Role of Bone Marrow–Derived Endothelial Progenitor Cells in Neovascularization of Engineered Skin Substitute

Lee M. Morris and Timothy M. Crombleholme*

Division of General, Thoracic, and Fetal Surgery, Center for Molecular Fetal Therapy, Cincinnati Children's Hospital Medical Center, Cincinnati, Ohio.

Abbreviations and Acronyms

EC = endothelial cell

EPC = endothelial progenitor cell

ESS = engineered skin substitute

VEGF = vascular endothelial growth factor

*Correspondence: Timothy M. Crombleholme, Division of General, Thoracic, and Fetal Surgery, Center for Molecular Fetal Therapy, Cincinnati Children's Hospital Medical Center, 3333 Burnet Ave., MLC 11025, Cincinnati, Ohio 45229-3039 (e-mail: timothy.crombleholme@cchmc.org).

Background: Ischemic tissue requires an adequate neovascularization response for proper healing to occur. Neovascularization may occur through both angiogenesis and vasculogenesis. Vasculogenesis is mediated through bone marrow–derived endothelial progenitor cells (EPCs) and has been shown to play an important role in many injury models.

The Problem: Many types of skin injuries including severe burns and chronic nonhealing ulcers may prove problematic due to prolonged healing times with associated complications. Autologous grafting of skin is the usual treatment for these types of wounds; however, the amount of skin that can be harvested is limited. Further, new epidermal damage is created at the donor site, increasing scarring and discomfort.

Basic/Clinical Science Advances: Engineered skin substitute (ESS) has offered a valuable treatment modality in these particular types of wounds. These bilayered human skin equivalents have been shown to improve healing of severe wounds while reducing wound contracture and infection. One mechanism thought to be important in this healing process is the recruitment of EPCs.

Clinical Care Relevance: Increasing evidence suggests that circulating EPCs play a major role in the neovascularization of ESS, and the availability or function of these cells may be a rate-limiting step in successful engraftment. Future developments in optimizing the vasculogenic capacity of EPCs through increased mobilization or isolation and coculturing with ESS may increase the clinical success rates of these grafts.

Conclusion: ESS offers an important treatment modality in cases of severe burns and other chronic nonhealing wounds. EPCs show promise in accelerating neovascularization of these avascular grafts and potentially enhancing engraftment.

BACKGROUND

Injured or ischemic tissue requires an appropriate vascular response to supply the regenerating tissue with adequate amounts of oxygen and nutrients for proper healing. This process of new vessel formation is termed neovascularization and, until recently, was thought to occur solely through angiogenesis or the sprouting of new vessels from preexisting ones. More recently, however, vasculogenesis, or the *de novo* formation of new blood vessels from the differentiation of stem cells known as endothelial progenitor cells (EPCs), is known to contribute to postnatal neovascularization.[1] These cells are thought to arise from the hemangioblasts, a common precursor cell for both hematopoietic stem cells and EPCs.[2] The phenotype of these cells is not completely described, but the cells are enriched within populations

ADVANCES IN WOUND CARE, VOLUME 1

Printed in U.S.A.
DOI: 10.1089/awc.2009.0036

that express both CD133 and vascular endothelial growth factor (VEGF) receptor 2.[3]

Vasculogenesis has been shown to play a role in the neovascularization of many types of ischemia and injury models including cardiac ischemia, wound healing, and tumor growth.[3] Moreover, multiple studies have found disease states such as diabetes and coronary artery disease to be associated with dysfunctional and lower numbers of circulating EPCs.[4,5] Additionally, many investigators have found both in the laboratory and now in human clinical trials that exogenously administered EPCs or pharmacologically mobilized EPCs improve neovascularization and tissue repair.[6]

The vasculogenic potential of these cells has attracted the attention of the growing field of tissue engineering. Many new therapies will come from advances in tissue engineering, but currently the biggest limiting factor for survival of these avascular three-dimensional tissue constructs is adequate neovascularization. Here we focus on the contribution of EPCs to a particular type of tissue-engineered skin construct called engineered skin substitute (ESS).

CLINICAL PROBLEM ADDRESSED

Many types of skin injuries including severe burns, chronic nonhealing ulcers, and other surgical wounds, as well as a variety of blistering and desquamating dermatological conditions, may represent significant morbidity due to prolonged healing times and associated complications such as infection and contraction. In the United States alone, chronic wounds are estimated to affect more than 2 million people with total treatment costs as high as $1 billion annually.[7] Additionally, severe burn wounds account for 50,000 hospitalizations each year with 20,000 of these patients having at least a 25% total body surface area burn.[8] Burn-related infections account for up to 10,000 deaths every year in the United States, which is the main cause of death from massive burns.[9] Rapid skin closure remains the limiting factor for reducing infection and increasing the probability of survival from extensive burn injuries.

RELEVANT BASIC SCIENCE CONTEXT

Skin performs a wide range of functions, but its role in providing a protective barrier is most critical for survival. Following injury, the skin's normal healing process originates from proliferating epidermal cells in the appendages of the deep dermal layer, such as hair follicles. Wound healing without a dermal layer results in contracture. As a result, healing of severe burn wounds and other large chronic nonhealing ulcers where the skin's appendages have been obliterated are of particular concern.

The development of skin substitutes has offered a valuable treatment modality in these particular types of wounds. They have been shown to improve the healing of severe wounds while reducing complications such as wound contracture.[10] Although autologous grafting of skin from other areas of the body is the usual treatment for burn wounds and other types of skin ulcers refractory to conventional wound therapy, the amount of skin and number of donor sites that can be harvested are limited. Further, new epidermal damage is created at the donor site, which increases scarring and discomfort. ESS has also been shown to heal with less of a meshed pattern of scarring that is seen in autografted skin[9] and may actually provide improved healing rates in chronic wounds compared to skin autograft.[11]

The mechanism of action has been shown to be multifactorial with positive effects attributed to the protection of the underlying tissue, but more importantly, through the secretion of multiple growth factors and extracellular matrix components.[11] These secreted growth factors are thought to promote neovascularization through local cellular effects as well as through recruitment of bone marrow–derived EPCs.

EPCs have been shown to contribute to neovascularization after being mobilized from the bone marrow and recruited to sites of ischemia by signals initiated from the injured tissue. Although mobilization and recruitment of EPCs are incompletely understood, specific cytokines have been implicated in this process and include stromal-derived factor-1α (CXCL12),[3] angiopoietin-1,[12] and VEGF.[3]

EXPERIMENTAL MODEL OR MATERIAL—ADVANTAGES AND LIMITATIONS

Starting from the first report of cultured human epidermis in 1975[13] by Rheinwald and Green, tissue engineering technology quickly evolved to include both dermal and epidermal components.[9,14] A bilayered skin substitute, or ESS, can promote better wound healing than a single-layered substitute due to the protective effects from external shearing provided by the epidermis and prevention of wound contraction by the dermal component.[15] ESS has been created using several techniques, but the main components are cultured keratinocytes,

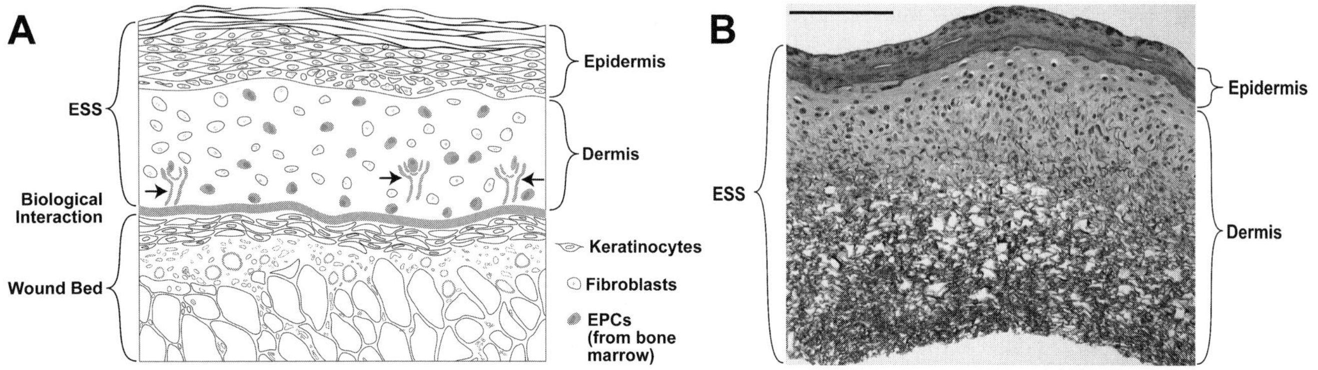

Figure 1. (**A**) Diagram of the components of engineered skin substitute (ESS) and mechanisms of action on the underlying wound bed. ESS secrete multiple growth factors and cytokines into the wound bed that assists in neovascularization through recruitment of both local endothelial cells (angiogenesis) as well as bone marrow–derived endothelial progenitor cells (EPCs) (vasculogenesis). These EPCs migrate into the ESS approaching the dermal–epidermal junction and differentiate into blood vessels (arrows). This *de novo* blood vessel formation then inosculates with the systemic mouse vasculature to perfuse the tissue. (**B**) Representative histologic section from an ESS showing the dermis and epidermis. Scale bar = 150 μm.

fibroblasts, and a matrix scaffold to support these cells. The combination of these two cell types adds to the benefit of the bilayered ESS by allowing cross-talk between the fibroblasts and keratinocytes. This cross-talk facilitates proper growth factor and cytokine release, important for the therapeutic effects and the neovascularization of the ESS.[16] Although reports have been made of coculturing microvascular endothelial cells (ECs) into ESS while *in vitro*,[17] virtually all available skin equivalents are devoid of any dermal microvasculature. These avascular skin substitutes require host EC invasion to allow for the adequate delivery of oxygen and nutrients (Fig. 1).

This lack of dermal microvasculature has proven advantageous to investigators studying neovascularization. When ESS grafts are transplanted onto mouse hosts, investigators are able to easily differentiate the newly formed vessels from the preexisting ones. Additionally, when the mouse host has been bone marrow transplanted with bone marrow from a transgenic donor expressing a reporter protein, the investigator may accurately quantify the contribution of bone marrow–derived cells to the neovasculature. These points become rather important when the experimental endpoint involves the determination of the relative contributions of angiogenesis and vasculogenesis to neovascularization. Thus, the engraftment of ESS using mice transplanted with transgenically labeled bone marrow is an ideal, *in vivo* model for determining the effects of angiogenic and vasculogenic inhibitors or stimulators.

While this model has many advantages, some limitations do exist. The process of culturing the cells and creating a mature graft takes approximately 4 weeks to complete. When these grafts are used in combination with bone marrow transplantation, this makes rapid experimentation rather difficult. Moreover, due to the human cell lines incorporated into the ESS, immunodeficient mice are required to prevent xenograft rejection.

DISCUSSION OF FINDINGS AND RELEVANT LITERATURE

EPCs have been isolated and applied to many different injury and ischemia models where they have been shown to enhance neovascularization.[3] Additionally, many tumor models have relied on recruitment of EPCs for vascular supply.[3] Although the precise contribution of EPCs to neovessel formation has not been well characterized, various studies have found a range of results. One study using bone marrow–transplanted mice found that in wound capillary bed formation, it was estimated that EPCs form 0.2% to 1.4% of the mature endothelium.[18] They also found a much higher percentage of bone marrow–derived ECs within polyvinyl alcohol sponge–induced granulation tissue, in which EPCs accounted for 8.3% to 11.2% of the vasculature. Another study using a Matrigel plug assay and corneal micropocket assay found that up to 26% of the neovasculature was derived from the bone marrow.[19]

Given these observations, investigators have looked at how EPCs may enhance the neovascularization of tissue-engineered biological substitutes. Due to the fact that cells need to be within 150–200 μm of blood supply for adequate oxygen and nutrient supply and removal of waste products,[20] tissue-engineered biological substitutes thicker than these measurements may fail *in vivo*. In particular, ESS may be dependent on imbibition or nourished through plasma secreted by the underlying tissue for up to 2 weeks following transplant, which can reduce successful engraftment.[21] To combat this problem, experiments have been conducted where EPCs were used to enhance the survival and function of a number of tissue-engineered constructs including ESS.[22]

Kung *et al.* found that after *ex vivo* expansion of human EPCs and seeding onto ESS before transplantation onto mouse hosts, these cells greatly improved the neovascularization of ESS.[22] They found that after 2 weeks *in vivo*, ESS seeded with EPCs contained microvessels extending into the mid dermis, whereas this degree of vessel formation was not seen in ESS without EPCs. Moreover, they were able to show that these vessels were of human origin and were not infiltrating mouse vessels from the wound bed. These microvessels within the ESS demonstrated functionality by 2 weeks through inosculation or connection with the recipient circulation from the bed of the wound.

Similarly, Wu *et al.* found that seeding human EPCs onto an acellular biodegradable polyglycolic acid-poly-L-lactic acid scaffold with the addition of human smooth muscle cells also produced microvessels within the scaffold.[23] As well, Vermeulen *et al.* showed using a plasma gel biomatrix placed onto full-thickness porcine skin wounds that the addition of EPCs resulted in a dramatic increase in vascular structures.[24]

Shepherd *et al.* reported the utilization of EPCs to promote neovascularization of a skin substitute formed from decellularized human dermis and human keratinocytes.[25] Isolated human EPCs were allowed to differentiate *in vitro* into ECs where they were then seeded onto skin substitutes before transplant onto immunodeficient mice. Not only were these ECs derived from EPCs able to form human vascular structures within the skin substitutes but also they were able to enhance mouse angiogenesis within the grafts.

In our laboratory, we demonstrated that after engraftment of ESS onto the bone marrow–transplanted nude mice, the bone marrow contributed to 23% at day 7 and 26% at day 14 of the microvasculature within the ESS.[26] We also observed that singular CD133+ cells (a marker for EPCs) had migrated to the superficial dermal layer

TAKE-HOME MESSAGE

Basic science advances

- EPCs have been used to enhance the survival and function of a number of tissue-engineered constructs including ESS.[22]
- Kung *et al.* found that after *ex vivo* expansion of human EPCs and seeding onto ESS before transplantation onto mouse hosts, these cells greatly improved the neovascularization of ESS.[22]
- Wu *et al.* found that seeding human EPCs onto an acellular biodegradable polyglycolic acid-poly-L-lactic acid scaffold with the addition of human smooth muscle cells also produced microvessels within the scaffold.[23] As well, Vermmeulen *et al.* showed using a plasma gel biomatrix placed onto full-thickness porcine skin wounds that the addition of EPCs resulted in a dramatic increase in vascular structures.[24] Shepherd *et al.* reported the utilization of ECs derived from EPCs promoted neovascularization of a skin substitute formed from decellularized human dermis and human keratinocytes.[25]
- Our laboratory was able to demonstrate that after engraftment of ESS onto bone marrow–transplanted nude mice, the bone marrow contributed to 23% at day 7 and 26% at day 14 of the microvasculature within the ESS.[26]

Clinical science advances

- EPCs within human peripheral blood are relatively rare and obtaining a sufficient number of these cells for experimental use has proven problematic. Clinical advances have increased EPC availability for potential use in such areas as tissue engineering.
- Clinical trials using mobilizing agents such as granulocyte colony–stimulating factor and AMD3100 have been used and resulted in rapid and potent mobilization of EPCs. With the assistance of these kinds of pharmacological agents, obtaining and storing large numbers of EPCs for use in tissue-engineered constructs may be much more feasible than previously thought.[28]

Relevance to clinical care

- ESS require more time to neovascularize than skin autografts. The delay in neovascularization is mainly due to the absence of any native microvasculature within the ESS.
- The additional time required for restoration of blood flow may cause increased cell death due to inadequate nutrient and oxygen supply. Reducing the time required for the neovascularization of ESS will likely increase clinical success rates.
- Increasing evidence suggests that circulating EPCs play a major role in the neovascularization of ESS, and the availability or function of these cells may be a rate-limiting step in successful engraftment.
- Future developments in optimizing the vasculogenic capacity of EPCs through increased mobilization or isolation and coculturing with ESS may increase the clinical success rates of these grafts.

of the ESS before the formation of the microvasculature at this level. These observations suggest that EPCs may also promote neovasculariation by releasing factors that act in a paracrine manner to support local angiogenesis and/or improve host cell survival, thereby creating a permissive environment that enables more rapid neovascularization.

To translate these results in humans, and attempt to seed ESS grafts with autologous EPCs before transplant, large numbers of EPCs will need to be isolated from peripheral blood. Due to low numbers of circulating EPCs within human blood, obtaining sufficient numbers of these cells for experimental use has proven problematic. More recently, clinical advances have been made to increase EPC availability for potential use in such areas as tissue engineering. Clinical trials using mobilizing agents such as granulocyte colony–stimulating factor and AMD3100 have been used and resulted in rapid and potent mobilization of EPCs. Additionally, progress has been made in the *ex vivo* expansion of EPCs for use *in vivo*.[27] With the assistance of these kinds of pharmacological agents or expansion *ex vivo*, obtaining and storing large numbers of EPCs for use in tissue-engineered constructs may be much more feasible than previously thought.[28]

CAUTION, CRITICAL REMARKS, AND RECOMMENDATIONS

Though tissue-engineered constructs, and in particular ESS, have generated much excitement in the medical, scientific, and biotechnology communities, enthusiasm for these products has been tempered by the variable clinical results mixed with high cost. In the future it is hoped that less expensive and more clinically effective ESS will be developed. Increasing evidence suggests that circulating EPCs play a major role in the neovascularization of these grafts, and the availability or function of these cells may be a rate-limiting step in the success rates seen clinically. Although the number of EPCs in adult blood is extremely low under normal conditions,[28] these may be increased pharmacologically or isolated and expanded *ex vivo* to assist in graft neovascularization.

The studies conducted so far using EPCs show improved neovascularization of ESS either *in vitro* or in the initial posttransplant periods. Further studies are necessary, however, to demonstrate that these results translate into improved graft survival in the long term.

FUTURE DEVELOPMENT

The largest restraint on advances in tissue engineering is arguably the current difficulty in neovascularizing these avascular constructs. To increase clinical utility of these grafts in normal and vascular compromised wounds, future developments will have to address this dilemma. In an attempt to overcome this, researchers have looked at a few avenues to improve neovascularization. One method as discussed previously is improving culturing techniques to incorporate vasculogenic cells such as EPCs into these constructs and begin the vessel formation while these constructs are still *in vitro*.

Another technique that is being studied is the genetic modification of cells within the ESS to overproduce specific growth factors known to enhance angiogenesis and vasculogenesis. Candidate factors are many but should include stromal cell–derived factor-1α (CXCL12),[29] VEGF,[12] and platelet-derived growth factor,[30] among others. Recent studies have shown that genetically modified keratinocyte-overexpressing VEGF induces a more rapid neovascularization *in vivo*.[31] Caution remains, however, as the long-term effects of these therapeutic neovascularization treatments remain unknown, and time-controlled expression of these growth factors will need to be optimized.

AUTHOR DISCLOSURE STATEMENT

L.M.M. and T.M.C. have no real or perceived conflicts of interest in connection with this manuscript and no competing financial interests exist.

REFERENCES

1. Rafii S, *et al.*: Contribution of marrow-derived progenitors to vascular and cardiac regeneration. Semin Cell Dev Biol 2002; **13:** 61.
2. Park C, Ma YD, and Choi K: Evidence for the hemangioblast. Exp Hematol 2005; **33:** 965.
3. Liu ZJ and Velazquez OC: Hyperoxia, endothelial progenitor cell mobilization, and diabetic wound healing. Antioxid Redox Signal 2008; **10:** 1869.
4. Loomans CJ, *et al.*: Endothelial progenitor cell dysfunction: a novel concept in the pathogenesis of vascular complications of type 1 diabetes. Diabetes 2004; **53:** 195.
5. Fadini GP, *et al.*: Circulating endothelial progenitor cells are reduced in peripheral vascular complications of type 2 diabetes mellitus. J Am Coll Cardiol 2005; **45:** 1449.
6. Kawamoto A and Losordo DW: Endothelial progenitor cells for cardiovascular regeneration. Trends Cardiovasc Med 2008; **18:** 33.
7. Supp DM and Boyce ST: Engineered skin substitutes: practices and potentials. Clin Dermatol 2005; **23:** 403.

8. Burn Incidence Fact Sheet: American Burn Associations, 2002. www.ameriburn.org/resources_factsheet.php.

9. Boyce ST, *et al.*: Cultured skin substitutes reduce donor skin harvesting for closure of excised, full-thickness burns. Ann Surg 2002; **235:** 269.

10. Boyce ST, Glafkides MC, Foreman TJ, and Hansbrough JF: Reduced wound contraction after grafting of full-thickness burns with a collagen and chondroitin-6-sulfate (GAG) dermal skin substitute and coverage with Biobrane. J Burn Care Rehabil 1988; **9:** 364.

11. Spiekstra SW, Breetveld M, Rustemeyer T, Scheper RJ, and Gibbs S: Wound-healing factors secreted by epidermal keratinocytes and dermal fibroblasts in skin substitutes. Wound Repair Regen 2007; **15:** 708.

12. Moore MA, *et al.*: Mobilization of endothelial and hematopoietic stem and progenitor cells by adenovector-mediated elevation of serum levels of SDF-1, VEGF, and angiopoietin-1. Ann NY Acad Sci 2001; **938:** 36–45; discussion 45.

13. Rheinwald JG and Green H: Serial cultivation of strains of human epidermal keratinocytes: the formation of keratinizing colonies from single cells. Cell 1975; **6:** 331.

14. Bell E, Ehrlich HP, Buttle DJ, and Nakatsuji T: Living tissue formed *in vitro* and accepted as skin-equivalent tissue of full thickness. Science 1981; **211:** 1052.

15. Medalie DA, *et al.*: Evaluation of human skin reconstituted from composite grafts of cultured keratinocytes and human acellular dermis transplanted to athymic mice. J Invest Dermatol 1996; **107:** 121.

16. Jimenez PA and Jimenez SE: Tissue and cellular approaches to wound repair. Am J Surg 2004; **187:** 56S.

17. Vincenzo V, Barbara Z, Giovanni A, Silvio A, Carolin T, Roberta C, and Brunio A: *In vitro* reconstruction of a micro-vascularized skin substitute. Burns 2007; **33:** S118.

18. Crosby JR, *et al.*: Endothelial cells of hematopoietic origin make a significant contribution to adult blood vessel formation. Circ Res 2000; **87:** 728.

19. Murayama T, *et al.*: Determination of bone marrow-derived endothelial progenitor cell significance in angiogenic growth factor-induced neovascularization *in vivo*. Exp Hematol 2002; **30:** 967.

20. Folkman J and Hochberg M: Self-regulation of growth in three dimensions. J Exp Med 1973; **138:** 745.

21. Tremblay PL, Hudon V, Berthod F, Germain L, and Auger FA: Inosculation of tissue-engineered capillaries with the host's vasculature in a reconstructed skin transplanted on mice. Am J Transplant 2005; **5:** 1002.

22. Kung EF, Wang F, and Schechner JS: *In vivo* perfusion of human skin substitutes with microvessels formed by adult circulating endothelial progenitor cells. Dermatol Surg 2008; **34:** 137.

23. Wu X, *et al.*: Tissue-engineered microvessels on three-dimensional biodegradable scaffolds using human endothelial progenitor cells. Am J Physiol Heart Circ Physiol 2004; **287:** H480.

24. Vermeulen P, *et al.*: A plasma-based biomatrix mixed with endothelial progenitor cells and keratinocytes promotes matrix formation, angiogenesis, and reepithelialization in full-thickness wounds. Tissue Eng Part A 2009; **15:** 1533.

25. Shepherd BR, *et al.*: Vascularization and engraftment of a human skin substitute using circulating progenitor cell-derived endothelial cells. FASEB J 2006; **20:** 1739.

26. Vaikunth SS, *et al.*: Cultured skin substitutes (CSS): an ideal model for the study of angiogenesis and vasculogenesis. Wound Repair Regen 2007; **15:** A22.

27. Kalka C, *et al.*: Transplantation of *ex vivo* expanded endothelial progenitor cells for therapeutic neovascularization. Proc Natl Acad Sci USA 2000; **97:** 3422.

28. Shepherd RM, *et al.*: Angiogenic cells can be rapidly mobilized and efficiently harvested from the blood following treatment with AMD3100. Blood 2006; **108:** 3662.

29. Yamaguchi J, *et al.*: Stromal cell-derived factor-1 effects on *ex vivo* expanded endothelial progenitor cell recruitment for ischemic neovascularization. Circulation 2003; **107:** 1322.

30. Keswani SG, *et al.*: Adenoviral mediated gene transfer of PDGF-B enhances wound healing in type I and type II diabetic wounds. Wound Repair Regen 2004; **12:** 497.

31. Supp DM, Supp AP, Bell SM, and Boyce ST: Enhanced vascularization of cultured skin substitutes genetically modified to overexpress vascular endothelial growth factor. J Invest Dermatol 2000; **114:** 5.

WHS Wound Healing Society

In Vitro Assays for Wound-Healing Properties of Stem Cells

Edward J. Doolin*

Department of General and Thoracic Surgery, Children's Hospital of Philadelphia, and Department of Clinical Surgery, University of Pennsylvania, Philadelphia, Pennsylvania.

*Correspondence: Department of General and Thoracic Surgery, Children's Hospital of Philadelphia, 34th and Civic Center Blvd., Philadelphia, Pennsylvania 19104 (e-mail: doolin@email.chop.edu).

Background: The plasticity of the stem cell has made it appealing for clinical medicine. Cellular therapy has become a method to (1) make genetic interventions, (2) create tissue grafts, (3) form cells with unique functions such as islet cells, and (4) create cells that have chemical and mechanical properties that will treat a specific clinical problem.

The Problem: When an injury occurs, a series of events are required to maintain homeostasis. The wound must be sealed, there must be restoration of tensile strength, and missing tissue must regenerate. A stem cell is a building block with plasticity and proliferation characteristics that make it an inviting tool for the enhancement of wound repair.

Basic/Clinical Science Advances: Many *in vitro* techniques exist that can be designed to manipulate cells creating the functional phenotype needed for a given wound or host. The use of growth factors, different oxygen levels, genetic transfection, and even changes in physical force can all be used to enhance the stem cells' role in wound healing.

Clinical Care Relevance: When there is an injury, the environment of the wound will contribute to the rate and success of healing. Mesenchymal stem cells can provide contraction properties to close a wound, growth factor secretion to aid in healing, and cell differentiation for tissue replacement.

Conclusion: Wounds need directed therapies dictated by the mechanism of injury, size of injury, type of tissue injured, and the health of the patient. Mesenchymal stem cells, with their growth and plasticity, provide the framework for uniquely tailored therapies.

BACKGROUND

Early after an injury the activation of adhesion molecules as well as other elements respond to control the extent of the damage. During this process circulating cells appear in the wound. These have many functions, including protection of the exposed tissue, scavenging debris, and creating a structure for repair.[1] Some of these cells are constantly in circulation so that when an injury occurs they are seen in the wound quickly.

These cells have many functions in the task of protecting and healing a wound. Their adhesive properties allow them to dress the wound by preventing blood and fluid loss and creating an environment conducive to repair. Some of these cells scavenge bacteria and debris, creating a sterile healthy environment. Finally, they contribute to a scaffold that will allow regeneration (Fig. 1).

Wounds heal poorly for many reasons. With respect to the circulating cell, inadequate numbers, poor adhesion, or poor function of these cells all contribute to a failed wound. Since these mesenchymal stem cells can be manipulated they are a potential tool

ADVANCES IN WOUND CARE, VOLUME 1

Printed in U.S.A.
DOI: 10.1089/awc.2009.0100

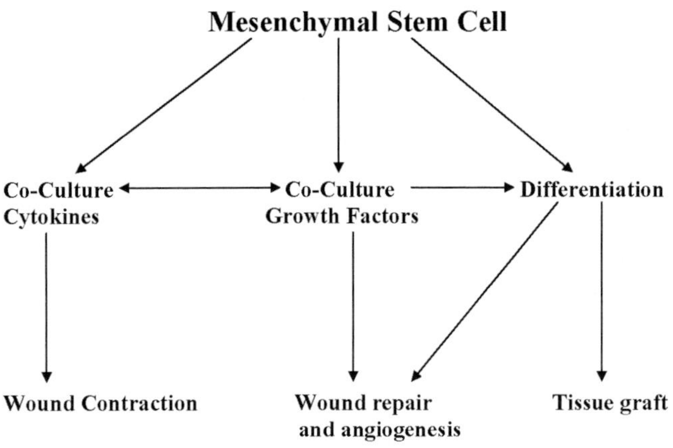

Figure 1. Mesenchymal stem cells are termed pluripotential. Their plasticity broadens the spectrum of methodology in studying or manipulating these cells. As such, their activities are intertwined. As seen here, three different methods can be used to modify or evaluate the cell. The cells' influence is not restricted, however. By inducing the cell to secrete a certain growth factor, it may also differentiate. Conversely, when cells are differentiated they will enhance the healing of similar tissues. The combinations of options are limitless.

for therapeutics interventions that can enhance wound care.[2] Several different types of cells provide these functions, including fibroblasts, circulating stem cells, platelets, endothelial cells, and *in situ* injured cells. The stem cell is the most attractive to investigate since the ability to modify their varied potential phenotypes makes them useful for many wounds, even complex ones where more than one tissue type is involved[3] (Fig. 1).

CLINICAL PROBLEM ADDRESSED

The healing wound has a complex dynamic. Studying an individual component is difficult and identifying interventions *in vivo* that are effective is elusive. *In vitro* studies have the advantage of isolating the mechanism being studied. In addition, different properties of the individual cell type can be observed, allowing the investigator to develop approaches to therapy specific to a certain wound or tissue. Adhesion, migration, proliferation, contraction, and differentiation are all characteristics of the stem cell that can be investigated and manipulated *in vitro*.

RELEVANT BASIC SCIENCE CONTEXT

The cells being considered for therapeutics can be assessed for how they respond to factors found in the wound. Cytokines are one stimulus. Compounds such as interleukin 1 and tumor necrosis factor can induce circulating stem cells to target a wound and adhere. Growth factors such as insulin growth factor, platelet-derived growth factor-AB, and stromal-derived growth factor also have such an effect.[4–6] Finally, a variety of immunologic mechanisms as well as chemokines (CXCR2 and CCR2) can contribute to stem cell migration and function. Stromal-derived growth factor has been found to be particularly useful in targeting stem cells, especially as they pertain to wound healing.[7]

The ability of the cell to contract is critical in its early effect on the wound. The cytoskeleton is responsible for early wound contraction because it occurs quickly, well before healing proteins are synthesized and before differentiation and regeneration are seen. Later, the contracture of wound occurs due to the excessive deposition of collagen III. This can be deforming and interfere with normal tissue regeneration.[6]

It is useful to observe the activity of a single cell. The extent of the contraction and the force generated can be measured as a function of the change in the size of the cell on a measuring device.[8,9] The cell's behavior in a wound-like milieu is also useful. By measuring contraction in collagen the superior mechanics of the mesenchymal stem cell can be seen compared to normal and diseased fibroblasts. The concentration of cells can also be altered giving insight into the cell–cell and cell–milieu interaction.[10]

The *in vitro* proliferation of the mesenchymal stem cell autograft can be tailored to target the type of wound that is being treated. By modifying the culture technique the mesenchymal stem cell can be partially or completely differentiated.[11,12] One method to modify the stem cells is to provide these growth factors in a more sustained fashion at a higher concentration. Further, stem cells can be modified to differentiate into endothelial-like cells, which may provide a template for neovascularization.[13]

EXPERIMENTAL METHODS

Having stem cells target the wound is the first step. Migration assays can demonstrate what factors will influence a stem cell. Here the stem cell is suspended in a matrix where a gradient of different substances is applied. The rate and distance the cell migrates is a measure of the effect of that compound on the cell.[7,14]

An appealing characteristic of the mesenchymal stem cell is its ability to reduce the size of a wound rapidly.[15] This can be seen from the first few days and up to a week in a treated wound. To understand the cell's effective contraction, a mechanical property due to a strong cytoskeleton must be studied. A common reproducible technique is the cell-populated collagen gel. Using this approach the extent and rate of contraction are measurable. The influence of cell density and the collagen concentration on contraction can also be measured.[6,10,15]

The ability to isolate a single cell and study its mechanical strengths is ideal. This allows the investigator to understand the mechanical properties of the cell without the confounding effect of matrix or other cells. Using a fabricated, deformable template of fibers, a single cell can be observed. The extent the cell deforms the fibers will measure its force of contraction.[8]

Finally, using the *in vitro* environment the cell can differentiate into whatever cell type is needed.[16,17] A myocyte-like cell, fibroblast-like cell, and osteoblast-like cell can all be fashioned with the use of correct growth and differentiation factors. This can be done in a collagen suspension, using a fabricated scaffold or in a dynamic environment such as a bioreactor.

DISCUSSION OF FINDINGS AND RELEVANT LITERATURE

Cells that participate in the repair of an injury clearly need to have the ability to find and attach to the wound. The mesenchymal stem cell has the property of differentiating into reparative tissues such as fibrous tissue, cartilage, bone, endothelium, and muscle. If these cells are to be delivered therapeutically then their interaction with the wound must be understood and they must adhere to the wound and become active.

Many chemotactic receptors have been identified.[17–19] In addition, methods to enhance the responsiveness of the cell can also be studied. Using similar migration assays it was found that the preincubation of the stem cells with cytokines improved their responsiveness to such agents.[17]

Many different proteins are helpful in the healing of a wound. Fibronectin, fibrin, and collagen (all types) contribute to the development and strength of the scar. In addition, the ability to overpopulate the wound with healing cells allows for the creation of an optimal cell/matrix ratio for the healing of the wound. It has been demonstrated that the contraction of the wound is accelerated with a high concentration of stem cells. If a more rapid contraction is provided, then a less deforming contracture is encountered because less collagen will be deposited. In other areas like healing bone, muscle, or cartilage, contraction is not desirable and regenerative proteins will be needed. This can be engineered both by developing regenerative cells and by using scaffolds to induce a specific tissue construct. Stem cells can be modified to improve osteoblastic activity or chondroitin-secreting activity.[20] Skin regeneration can also be programmed using *in vitro* stem cell modification.[21]

The mesenchymal stem cell can contribute to the closure of the wound. Some of these events can be manipulated, but a valuable asset of the mesenchymal stem

TAKE-HOME MESSAGE

Basic science advances

- Mesenchymal stem cells can be isolated from a variety of tissue and other sources. These include bone marrow, fat, amniotic fluid, and solid organs.
- Mesenchymal stem cells can be manipulated *in vitro*. Manipulations can include adjuncts to proliferation, differentiation, motility, and adhesion.
- Mesenchymal stem cells can be in heterogeneous populations. *In vitro* techniques can be used to refine these cell sources to provide the specific cell type desired.
- Mesenchymal stem cells' technologic advances continue to provide new tools that enhance our ability to control these cells, chemically, physically, and genetically.

Clinical science advance

- Mesenchymal stem cells are useful adjuncts to wound healing. They can be manipulated to target the stage of wound healing desired such as contraction or regeneration.
- Mesenchymal stem cells can be manipulated *in vitro* to overcome patient deficiencies such as hypoxia, diabetes, malnutrition, and poor circulating inflammatory cells.

Relevance to clinical care

- Wound healing is a final common pathway to all injury.
- Key cell types are important to this mechanism.
- Mesenchymal stem cells can be a source for all natural as well as uniquely effective healing cells.
- *In vitro* manipulation will be able to prepare these cells to perform specific tasks and target specific defects in the wound healing of a patient.

cell is the ability to program it to make a desirable protein and inhibit the secretion of an undesirable protein. Once the stem cell adheres to the wound, the cells will generate a force to help close and splint the wound. Later, at about day 3, there is a secondary contracture of the scar. This is a function of the protein secretion of the cell and can be eliminated with a collagen cross-linking blocker.[22,23] This stepwise effect on the wound is fundamental to many aspects of the wound healing.

Wounds are rarely ideal physiologic environments, and the ability to study the specific impact of these factors in a controlled setting can be useful. Using the collagen gel method, stem cells have been demonstrated to have a powerful ability to create a mechanical contraction. These cells are more effective than normal fibroblasts and much more effective than dermal fibroblasts coming from a compromised host such as the elderly or diabetic.[24]

If stem cell therapeutics is going to be feasible, *in vitro* expansion is critical. Mesenchymal stem cells are a small subset of any cell isolation. The need for a particular cell depends on the site of injury, mechanism, and stage of healing. Many factors can influence the effectiveness of the cellular phase of healing. Multipotential cells are a therapeutic option. The main advantage is the ability to expand the cells in their undifferentiated form when the doubling times are short, and later modifying them to the desired cell type.

As different wounds are encountered, different healing cells can be used. Fibroblasts, stromal cells, chondrocytes or osteocytes, and even epithelium all have advantages in different situations. For closure of a wound, rapidly contracting cells such as myocytes or fibroblasts are effective.

Certain wounds would be better served with a tissue graft. In these cases the stem cell can be modified *in vitro* to not only secrete the desired matrix but also actually form a small autograft, which will serve to immediately reconstruct the wound.

A vascular network is required to support a living cell structure 200 μm or greater depending on the tissue type. If the wound is to be served in a timely way the vascular network has to be available as the cells proliferate and differentiate.[25] Natural mechanisms provide this by the response of the host tissue to the growth factors such as vascular endothelial growth factor and fibroblast growth factor at the wound edge. The use of a mesenchymal stem cell autograft in the wound can enhance this.

CAUTION, CRITICAL REMARKS, AND RECOMMENDATIONS

The *in vitro* environment offers many tools to the investigator and the clinician. When trying to understand mechanism of action the ability to isolate a variable is a powerful approach. As such we have discovered what compounds have an effect on stem cells. We have been able to isolate and expand stem cells. Finally, the ability to modify a stem cell or even construct a tissue type lends an important insight into the mesenchymal stem cell as a tool. When these techniques and principles are applied clinically, it is often difficult to be certain what mechanisms are in play. Cytokine-conditioned stem cells improve adhesion. It is hard to know if this is a change in stem cell behavior or just a higher concentration of the cytokine. A higher concentration results in a more rapid wound contraction. It is not certain whether the mechanism is a change in a cell–cell interaction, a loss of matrix, or an actual change in the mechanism of the cell. The tools presented here will advance the field of wound care a great deal. Although a great understanding comes from *in vitro* observation, the translation to clinical practice must be implemented with additional studies to assure the outcome desired.

FUTURE DEVELOPMENT

In vitro cell engineering and manipulation offers a great deal of promise. In wound repair there are two obstacles: deficiencies of the host and loss of tissue. The use of stem cell engineering can provide the number of cells needed, the type of cell needed, and even tissue replacement. There will come a time when problematic wounds are characterized in a more refined way. They will be profiled by the distribution of cytokine present, the oxygen tension of the wound, the tissue type needed, and the inflammatory cells present. Using *in vitro* manipulation of mesenchymal stem cells the specific deficiency of the wound can be targeted. The healing mechanisms can be enhanced and tissue can be replaced.

AUTHOR DISCLOSURE STATEMENT

There is no conflict of interest.

REFERENCES

1. Schultz GS: The physiology of wound bed preparation. In: *Surgical Wound Healing and Management*, edited by Granick MS and Gamelli RL. New York, NY: Informa Healthcare, 2007, pp. 1–16.
2. Fu X and Li H: Mesenchymal stem cells and skin wound repair and regeneration: possibilities and questions. Cell Tissue Res 2009; **335:** 317.
3. Chamberlain G, Fox J, Ashton B, and Middleton J: Concise review: mesenchymal stem cells: their phenotype, differentiation capacity, immunological features and potential for homing. Stem Cells 2007; **25:** 2739.
4. Ponte AL, Marais E, Gallay N, Langonne A, Delorme B, Herault O, Charbord B, and Domench J: The *in vitro* migration capacity of human bone marrow mesenchymal stem cells: comparison of chemokine and growth factor chemotactic activities. Stem Cells 2007; **25:** 1737.
5. Ringe J, Strassburg S, Neumann K, Endres M, Notter M, Burmester G, Kaps C, and Sittinger M: Towards *in situ* tissue repair: human mesenchymal stem cells express chemokine receptors CXCR1, CXCR2, and CCR2, and migrate upon stimulation with CXCL8 but not CCL2. J Cell Biochem 2007; **101:** 135.
6. Redden RA and Doolin EJ: Complementary roles of microtubules and microfilaments in the lung fibroblast-mediated contraction of collagen gels: dynamics and the influence of cell density. In Vitro Cell Dev Biol Anim 2006; **42:** 70.
7. Badillo AT, Zhang L, and Liechty KW: Stromal progenitor cells promote leukocyte migration through production of stromal-derived growth factor 1 alpha: a potential mechanism for stromal progenitor cell-mediated enhancement of cellular recruitment to wounds. J Pediatr Surg 2008; **43:** 1128.
8. Sniadecki NJ and Chen CS: Microfabricated silicone elastomeric post arrays for measuring traction forces of adherent cells. In: *Methods in Cell Biology*, Vol. 83, edited by Wang YL and Discher DE. San Diego, CA: Academic Press, 2007, pp. 313–328.
9. Ji L, Loerke D, Gardel M, and Danuser G: Probing intracellular force distributions by high-resolution live cell imaging and inverse dynamics. In: *Methods in Cell Biology, Volume 83, Cell Mechanics*, edited by Wang YL and Discher DE. San Diego, CA: Academic Press, 2007, pp. 200–231.
10. Redden RA and Doolin EJ: Collagen crosslinking and cell density have distinct effects on fibroblast-mediated contraction of collagen gels. Skin Res Technol 2003; **9:** 290.
11. Zhou DH, Huang SL, Wu YF, Wei J, Chen G, Li Y, and Bao R: The expansion and biological characteristics of human mesenchymal stem cells. Zhonghua Er Ke Za Zhi 2003; **41:** 607.
12. Baksh D and Davies JE: Culture of mesenchymal stem/progenitor cells in adhesion-independent conditions. In: *Methods in Cell Biology, Volume 86, Stem Cell Culture*, edited by Mather J. San Diego, CA: Academic Press, 2008, pp. 280–292.
13. Sen KS: Tiny new genes called microRNAs regulate blood vessel formation. In: *Gene and Protein Based Therapies WHS Yearbook*, Vol. 1, pp. 2–18.
14. Herdrich BJ, Lind RC, and Liechty KW: Multipotent adult progenitor cells: their role in wound healing and the treatment of dermal wounds. Cytotherapy 2008; **10:** 543.
15. Yang Z, Jeen-Shang L, Jianxin C, and Wang JH-C: Determining substrate displacement and cell traction fields—a new approach. J Theor Biol 2006; **242:** 607.
16. Lorenz K, Sicker M, Schmelzer E, Rupf T, Salvetter J, Schultz-Siegmund M, and Bader A: Multilineage differentiation potential of human dermal skin-derived fibroblasts. Exp Dermatol 2008; **17:** 925.
17. Liechty KW, MacKenzie TC, Shaaban AF, Radu A, Moseley AB, Deans R, Marchak DR, and Flake AW: Human mesenchymal stem cells engraft and demonstrate site-specific differentiation after *in utero* transplantation in sheep. Nat Med 2000; **6:** 1282.
18. Bhakta S, Hong P, and Koc O: The surface adhesion molecule CXCR4 stimulates mesenchymal stem cell migration to stromal cell-derived factor-1 *in vitro* but does not decrease apoptosis under serum deprivation. Cardiovasc Revasc Med 2006; **7:** 19.
19. Li M, James D, Firth E, and Putnins E: An *in vitro* analysis of mechanical wounding-induced ligand-independent KGFR activation. J Dermatol Sci 2008; doi:10.1016/j.jdermsci.2008.10.008.
20. Juncosa-Melvin N, Boivin GP, Galloway MT, Gooch C, West JR, and Butler DL: Effects of cell-to-collagen ratio in stem cell-seeded constructs for achilles tendon repair. Tissue Eng 2006; **12:** 681.
21. Salem H, Ciba P, Rapoport DH, Egana JT, Reithmayer K, Kadry M, Machens HG, and Kruse C: The influence of pancreas-derived stem cells on scaffold based skin regeneration. Biomaterials 2009; **30:** 789.
22. Richards WO, Doolin EJ, Miginsky MP, and Moulton AL: Pharmacologic inhibition of scar contracture of intracardiac prosthetic patches. Annual Meeting of the Association for Academic Surgery, Syracuse, New York, 1984. J Surg Res **37:** 33.
23. Brown RA, Talas G, Porter RA, McGrouther DA, and Eastwood M: Balanced mechanical forces and microtubule contribution to fibroblast contraction. J Cell Physiol 1996; **169:** 439.
24. Badillo AT, Redden RA, Liping Z, Doolin EJ, and Liechty KW: Treatment of diabetic wounds with fetal murine mesenchymal stromal cells enhances wound closure. Cell Tissue Res 2007; **329:** 301.
25. Wang XH, Chen SF, Jin HM, and Hu RM: Differential analyses of angiogenesis and expressions of growth factors in micro- and macrovascular endothelial cells of type 2 diabetic rats. Life Sci 2009; doi:10.1016/j.lfs.2008.12.010.

WHS
Wound
Healing
Society

Progenitor Cells for the Treatment of Acute Myocardial Infarction

Benjamin J. Herdrich[1,2,*] and Robert C. Gorman[1]

[1]The University of Pennsylvania School of Medicine, Philadelphia, Pennsylvania.
[2]The Center for Fetal Research at The Children's Hospital of Philadelphia, Philadelphia, Pennsylvania.

Background: Left ventricular remodeling after myocardial infarction (MI) results in ventricular dilation, fibroplasia, and decline in cardiac function. There is significant morbidity and mortality associated with this process, often leading to heart failure despite medical management. New therapies aimed at altering ventricular remodeling after MI are needed, and cytotherapy utilizing progenitor cells is a current area of investigation.

The Problem: Many variables need to be considered to maximize the therapeutic benefit of cytotherapy, including the cell type, the method of delivery, the timing, and patient selection. Investigation into progenitor cell biology will continue to identify novel treatment strategies that then must be tested clinically to demonstrate safety, feasibility, and ultimately therapeutic benefit.

Basic/Clinical Science Advances: Although progenitor cells have the potential to affect ventricular remodeling through multiple mechanisms, their major effect is likely due to actions of secreted factors. Hepatocyte growth factor, stromal-derived growth factor-1 alpha, and stem cell factor affect the mobilization of progenitor cells, which makes it possible to develop treatment strategies based on recruitment of endogenous progenitor cells.

Clinical Care Relevance: There have been a number of randomized controlled trials demonstrating modest improvements in cardiac function using progenitor cell therapies after MI. In addition, clinical trials have used granulocyte-colony-stimulating factor as a treatment aimed at increasing progenitor cell mobilization.

Conclusion: Progenitor cell therapy after MI has been shown to be safe and feasible with some improvements in cardiac function and clinical outcomes. Further investigation is needed to better understand the biology of progenitor cells and the effects of progenitor cell–based therapies.

Abbreviations and Acronyms

BMC = bone marrow cells
EDV = end-diastolic volume
EF = ejection fraction
ESV = end-systolic volume
G-CSF = granulocyte-colony-stimulating factor
LV = left ventricle or left ventricular
MI = myocardial infarction
RCT = randomized controlled trials
SDF-1α = stromal-derived growth factor-1 alpha

*Correspondence: The Hospital of the University of Pennsylvania, 4 Maloney, 3400 Spruce St., Philadelphia, Pennsylvania 19104 (e-mail: benjamin.herdrich@uphs.upenn.edu).

BACKGROUND

Acute myocardial infarction (MI) affects over 1 million Americans each year.[1] Even with modern reperfusion therapy and optimized medical treatment, the overall prognosis after MI remains poor.[2] Soon after the ischemic insult, leukocytes migrate to the infarct and initiate the inflammatory response.[3] There is upregulation of proinflammatory cytokines and degradation of the extracellular matrix by collagenases and matrix metalloproteinases.[4] After MI, left ventricular (LV) remodeling occurs over a period of weeks, and depending on factors such as infarct size, LV remodeling can lead to progressive ventricular dilation, myocyte hypertrophy, fibrosis, and decline in function ultimately resulting in heart failure.[3] Once heart failure symptoms develop, the 5-year survival is approximately 50%, which is largely unchanged over the last 50 years.[5] Therefore, there is a need for the

Printed in U.S.A.
DOI: 10.1089/awc.2009.0121

development of new therapies aimed at preventing the decline in cardiac function associated with post-MI LV remodeling.

Cytotherapy has been an active area of research for the treatment of many diseases, including MI. Multipotent adult progenitor cell populations can be isolated from a number of different tissues, and while the therapeutic potential and mechanisms of action likely vary between progenitor cell populations, progenitor cell therapy can improve healing through a variety of mechanisms. Cell differentiation, cell fusion, production of the extracellular matrix, production of cytokines and growth factors, and modulation of the immune system are all mechanisms by which cytotherapy can potentially promote neovascularization, cardiac regeneration, recruitment of progenitor cells, and inhibition of apoptosis with an end result of cardiac repair and improved function.[6] However, there are many obstacles that need to be overcome to realize this potential. To date, cytotherapy has only produced modest results in clinical trials. A metaanalysis including 18 studies and 999 patients showed a 3.66% increase in mean ejection fraction (EF), a 5.49% reduction in infarct size, and a 4.80 mL reduction in LV end-systolic volume (ESV) in patients treated with bone marrow–derived cells compared with controls.[7] These results are encouraging as they demonstrate cytotherapy to be safe and feasible in the treatment of MI. However, there is clearly much work to be done in understanding the biology of cytotherapy and applying that knowledge to maximize the benefit of therapeutic treatment strategies.

There is a more robust human experience using progenitor cells to treat MI than has been done with some other disease processes. Many of the same cellular mechanisms controlling progenitor cell migration and function in the heart also take place elsewhere throughout the body, and understanding how to maximize cytotherapy in the heart may also help us in designing cytotherapy protocols used in dermal wounds and other organs. It should also be recognized that there are differences between organ systems that need to be considered when drawing parallels between cytotherapy strategies in different parts of the body. Nonetheless, the animal and human experiences utilizing progenitor cell therapies in the treatment of MI should be critically evaluated beyond the scope of the cardiovascular system as this may help to advance our understanding of cytotherapy with regards to other diseases.

CLINICAL PROBLEM ADDRESSED

The goal of cytotherapy after MI is to prevent the progressive decline in cardiac function associated with LV remodeling and thus impact morbidity and mortality. There are many factors affecting LV remodeling after MI, including infiltration of inflammatory cells, upregulation of proinflammatory cytokines, activation of matrix metalloproteinases, infarct size and distribution, changes in the LV strain and stress distribution, and increases in wall stress.[4,8–11] Cytotherapy has multiple mechanisms of action and therefore holds the potential to target multiple processes driving pathologic LV remodeling. To maximize the success of cytotherapy in the treatment of MI, the cell population, the time and place of delivery, the delivery mechanism, and the appropriate patient population all need to be carefully considered (Fig. 1).

RELEVANT BASIC SCIENCE CONTEXT

Bone marrow has been the most popular cell source for cytotherapy after MI; however, peripheral blood, skeletal muscle, adipose tissue, placental cord blood, skeletal myoblasts, and embryonic stem cells have all been proposed sources.[6] Bone marrow is a readily available source of progenitor cell populations, and bone marrow–derived cells have been shown to lead to myocardial regeneration after MI in experimental models.[12] Enriching bone marrow for progenitor cell populations has been done by different methods, including density gradient, plastic adherence, and cell surface markers.[12–14] It is not clear which cell population and isolation method are best, and the majority of the effects seen with bone marrow–derived progenitor cell therapy are likely not caused by cell differentiation and myocardial regeneration but rather a paracrine mechanism stimulating angiogenesis, affecting LV remodeling, and promoting endogenous cell function and tissue repair.

Cytokines and growth factors, such as stromal-derived growth factor-1 alpha (SDF-1α), hepatocyte growth factor, and stem cell factor, can affect mobilization and migration of bone marrow–derived progenitor cells.[14–16] Cell therapy using bone marrow stromal cells after MI in rabbits was shown to generate an SDF-1α gradient from the bone marrow to the heart and thus promote recruitment of endogenous progenitor cells to the heart.[17] Recruitment of endogenous progenitor cells is a therapeutic strategy that has been used and is the basis for trials using granulocyte-colony-stimulating factor (G-CSF) after MI.[18,19] Endogenous pro-

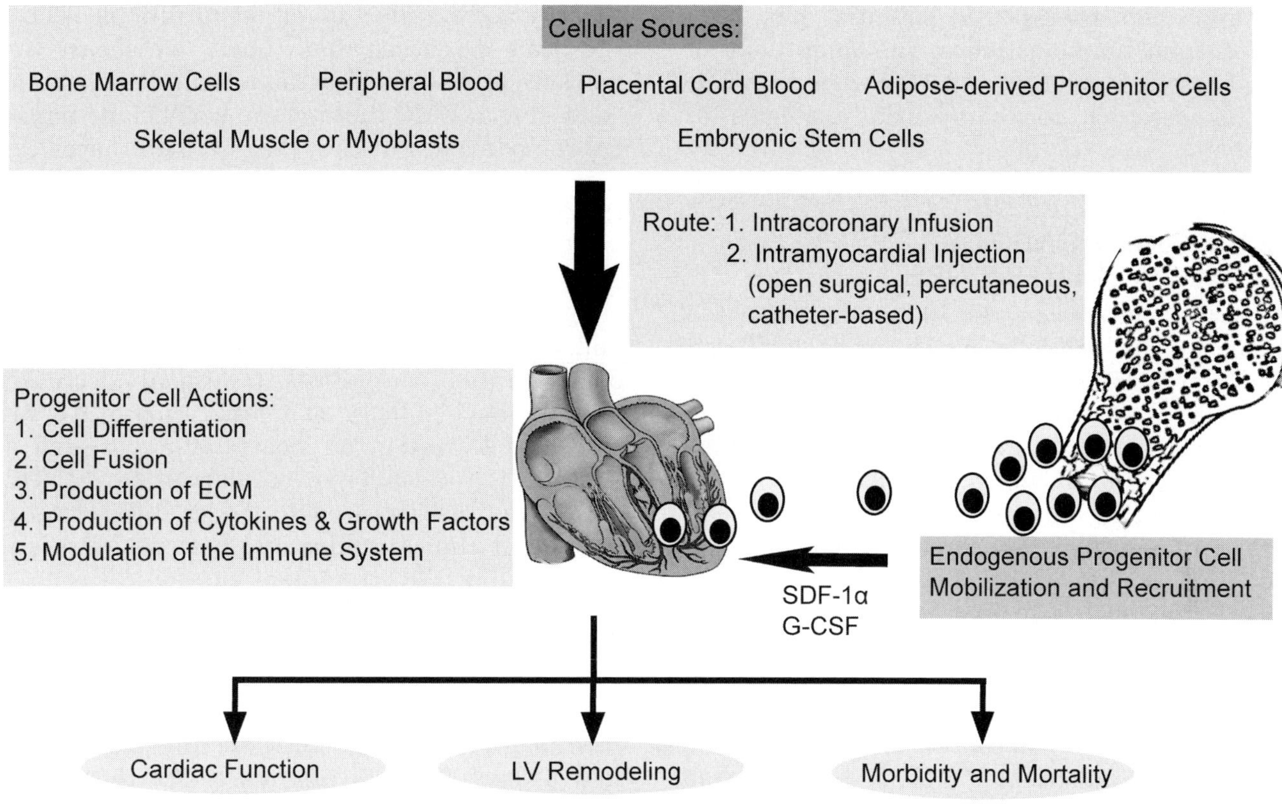

Figure 1. Overview of cellular therapy to promote cardiac healing after myocardial infarction (MI). Multiple cell sources have been proposed for use in cellular therapy after MI with bone marrow being the most utilized. Cells can be delivered to the heart via intracoronary infusion or intramyocardial injection. Progenitor cells have several different potential mechanisms by which they can act to promote myocardial healing and regeneration. Endogenous cells are mobilized into the circulation and migrate to the heart. Stromal-derived growth factor-1 alpha (SDF-1α) has been shown to be important to progenitor cell mobilization, and granulocyte-colony-stimulating factor (G-CSF) has been used clinically to mobilize progenitor cells into the circulation after MI. The goal of these therapies is to improve cardiac function, impact left ventricular remodeling, and improve morbidity and mortality after MI.

genitor cell recruitment strategies are advantageous, as they eliminate the need for cell harvest and isolation protocols. However, this strategy has challenges to overcome, including how to recruit the right cell population to the heart in numbers sufficient to affect LV remodeling. The biologic signals controlling progenitor cell homing from the bone marrow to injured myocardium are not fully understood. As these signals are better elucidated, we will better be able to design therapeutic strategies targeted at recruitment of endogenous progenitor cell populations.

EXPERIMENTAL MODEL OR MATERIAL—ADVANTAGES AND LIMITATIONS

The biology of cellular therapy utilizing bone marrow–derived progenitor cell populations continues to be an active area of research. Once therapeutic strategies are developed and validated in animal models, and the techniques are shown to be safe and feasible in human studies, they should be rigorously tested in randomized controlled trials (RCT) as was done in the STEMMI trial, REPAIR-AMI, BOOST, MYSTAR, and REGENT trials.[18–28] Only through RCT looking at end points measuring cardiac function, LV remodeling, and clinical events will the therapeutic benefit be defined as it pertains to patient selection, cell type, administration route, timing of treatment, and adverse events.

Human studies addressing cytotherapy for MI are complicated by the number of variables that may affect the outcome. Preclinical studies have addressed variables such as the type of cell, the route of administration, and the timing of treatment, but translating this to effective therapies in human trials has had only limited success.[6] Further, some complications identified in animal models have not been shown to be clinically relevant in human studies of cellular therapy for MI.[7,29] While much of our understanding of stem cells and their therapeutic potential has been learned from animal studies, the limitations of animal research must be respected when translating this research to therapeutic strategies in humans.

DISCUSSION OF FINDINGS AND RELEVANT LITERATURE

To date there have been over 1000 patients treated in clinical trials with cellular therapy after MI, and it has been shown to be safe and feasible with some success in improving EF and positively impacting LV remodeling.[7,30] Both the BOOST and REPAIR-AMI trials are RCT, which have looked at EF in patients suffering MI and treated with reperfusion therapy plus either intracoronary bone marrow cells (BMC) or best medical therapy alone. Both trials demonstrate a modest improvement in EF for BMC treatment versus the placebo at 4–6 months (BOOST: $0.7 \pm 8.1\%$ in placebo vs. $6.7 \pm 6.5\%$ in the BMC group at 6 months; REPAIR-AMI: $3.0 \pm 6.5\%$ in placebo vs. $5.5 \pm 7.3\%$ in the BMC group at 4 months).[20,23] However, there was no statistical difference in EF between the BMC and placebo groups at 12 months (REPAIR-AMI trial) or 18 month (BOOST trial).[21,25] BMC therapy improved the speed of EF recovery but did not impact EF over the long term. When comparing patients in the REPAIR-AMI trial with baseline EF $\leq 48.9\%$, there was a statistically significant improvement in EF in the BMC group, suggesting that BMC therapy may be more beneficial to patients with depressed cardiac function at baseline.[25]

EF does not tell the whole story, and both the BOOST and the REPAIR-AMI trials also looked at markers of LV remodeling. The REPAIR-AMI trial demonstrated no change in ESV in the BCM group from baseline at 4 months compared with an increase in the placebo group. End-diastolic volume (EDV) increased in both groups over 4 months.[23] Once again, subgroup analysis demonstrated that BMC therapy prevented progressive increases in EDV and ESV in patients with EF $\leq 48.9\%$ compared with placebo. In addition, BMC treatment lead to increased systolic wall thickening in the infarct segment at 12 months compared to baseline.[25] The BOOST trial demonstrated improved systolic wall motion in the borderzone at 6 months in the BMC group but not in the placebo group.[20] Markers of diastolic dysfunction, including transmitral flow velocities (E/A ratio) and diastolic myocardial velocities (Ea/Aa ratio), were improved with BMC therapy at 18 months. However, BMC therapy had no effect on either isovolumic relaxation time or deceleration time,[22] which are also markers of diastolic function. In all, these studies suggest that BMC therapy can beneficially impact LV remodeling. Further, patients with lower cardiac function will likely benefit the most from BMC therapy.

While markers of cardiac function and LV remodeling are important, the ultimate question is whether cytotherapy can impact on the morbidity and mortality after MI. The REPAIR-AMI trial demonstrated that BMC treatment decreased the combined endpoint of death, recurrence of MI, or rehospitalization for heart failure as well as death, MI, or need for revascularization.[23,24] This study was not powered to detect differences in individual clinical endpoints; however, this still suggest that BMC treatment has clinical benefits that go beyond improvements in measured cardiac function.

The timing and delivery method of BMC therapy is also important to consider. The REPAIR-AMI trial suggests that early BMC treatment within the first 4 days after MI attenuates the therapeutic effect; however, it does not look at late BMC treatment.[23] The MYSTAR trial is addressing both time (early: 21–42 days after MI vs. late: 3 months after MI) and delivery method (intracoronary vs. combined intracoronary and percutaneous intramyocardial injection).[26] Comparing combined therapy in patients with EF $< 45\%$, both early and late treatment produced similar modest decreases in infarct size (early: $-3.9 \pm 6.3\%$, late: $-3.2 \pm 6.0\%$) and increases in EF (early: $4.3 \pm 6.6\%$, late: $4.0 \pm 7.5\%$) 9–12 months after MI.[27] This demonstrated that a combined delivery method is safe and feasible. While both early and late treatment times produced similar results, it is not clear how that should be interpreted given that most RCT have used solely an intracoronary delivery method.

Both the BOOST and REPAIR-AMI trials used BMC, which were progenitor cells enriched using different methods of density gradient separation; however, it is unclear what the ideal source for cellular therapy is.[20,23] The REGENT trial compared a selected bone marrow–derived CD34+ CXCR4+ population with BMC enriched by density gradient alone. The REGENT trial did not show a difference in the selected versus the unselected BMC populations. Both cell populations demonstrated trends toward improvement in EF especially in patients with depressed EF at baseline.[28] This demonstrates safety and feasibility of both cell populations, but the ideal cell type remains unknown.

Another method of cellular therapy is to promote mobilization and recruitment of endogenous bone marrow–derived progenitor cells. There have been a number of studies investigating G-CSF, including the STEMMI trial. The STEMMI trial failed to show a difference in EF with G-CSF treatment compared with placebo; however, it showed that G-CSF was safe, produced different patterns of mobilization of CD34+ cells and MSC, and did not increase in-stent neo-intimal hyperplasia.[18,19] A metaanalysis including 8 studies and 385 patients failed to show an overall benefit of G-CSF treatment for MI; however, subgroup analysis showed a statistically significant improvement in EF in patients with depressed baseline cardiac function and also with therapy initiated $\leq$37 h after MI.[30] This suggests that G-CSF may be beneficial in the right patient population and with appropriate timing.

CAUTION, CRITICAL REMARKS, AND RECOMMENDATIONS

Cellular therapy for MI has shown some promise in RCT. The optimal cell type, method of delivery, timing, and patient population are still not fully known. However, this continues to be an active area of research, and with time and the appropriate trials, these questions should be answered. While the modest improvements in cardiac function seen with cellular therapy have been somewhat disappointing, safety and feasibility have clearly been demonstrated. Further research is warranted to better understand the biology of cellular therapy and optimize the procedures for selecting patients, isolating cells, and delivering cells to patients suffering MI.

FUTURE DEVELOPMENTS

As we continue to improve our understanding of progenitor cell homing, differentiation, interactions with the extracellular matrix, paracrine effects, and modulation of the immune response, we will better be able to devise treatment strategies that maximize cellular function and improve clinical outcome. Promoting regeneration of infarcted myocardium after MI would be the ideal result of a cellular-based therapy, but significant myocardial regeneration has not been demonstrated in postnatal humans. Clinical trials will continue to refine the therapies that have been developed, and the ongoing investigation into regenerative healing

TAKE-HOME MESSAGE

Basic science advances

- Bone marrow–derived progenitor cells have been shown to contribute to cardiac regeneration in animal models after MI.
- In addition to bone marrow, peripheral blood, skeletal muscle, adipose tissue, placental cord blood, skeletal myoblasts, and embryonic stem cells have all been proposed cell sources for cytotherapy aimed at treating MI.
- Cytotherapy has the potential to promote cardiac healing and affect LV remodeling through multiple mechanisms, including cell differentiation, cell fusion, production of the extracellular matrix, production of cytokines and growth factors, and modulation of the immune system. Paracrine actions are likely the dominant mechanism through which administered cells have their effects.
- Growth factors and cytokines, such as SDF-1α, hepatocyte growth factor, stem cell factor, and G-CSF, can affect mobilization and migration of bone marrow–derived progenitor cells to infarcted myocardium. Cellular therapy has been shown to promote progenitor cell recruitment to the heart by creating an SDF-1α gradient.

Clinical science advances

- RCT are needed to demonstrate the efficacy of emerging cellular therapies and answer questions regarding patient selection, cell type, timing of cell therapy, and delivery method.
- The BOOST and REPAIR-AMI trial both demonstrated modest improvements in cardiac function and LV remodeling in patients suffering MI and treated with BMC administered via intracoronary infusion.
- The REPAIR-AMI trial suggests that patients with impaired cardiac function at baseline derive the most benefit from BMC therapy after MI.
- Most clinical trials have utilized an intracoronary injection route; however, the MYSTAR trial has demonstrated safety and feasibility of a combined approach using both intracoronary injection and percutaneous myocardial injection.
- Cytotherapy within the first 4 days after MI does not appear to be as effective as delayed therapy, but the optimal timing is not known.
- G-CSF therapy after MI does have effects on progenitor cell mobilization, but it has not been shown to be superior to placebo.

Relevance to clinical care

- Cellular therapy after MI has repeatedly been shown to be safe and feasible.
- The REPAIR-AMI trial demonstrated that BMC therapy after MI decreased the combined clinical endpoints of (1) death, recurrence of MI, or rehospitalization for heart failure, and (2) death, MI, or need for revascularization.
- More studies are needed to define the effects of cellular therapy on morbidity and mortality after MI.

holds the promise of restoring function to an injured heart.

ACKNOWLEDGEMENTS

Cardiovascular research in the senior author's laboratory is funded by National Institutes of Health Grants HL63954, HL71137, and HL76560 (Bethesda, MD) and individual Established Investigator Awards from the American Heart Association (Dallas, TX) to J. Gorman and R. Gorman.

AUTHOR DISCLOSURE STATEMENT

The authors have no conflicts of interest to disclose.

REFERENCES

1. Rosamond W, Flegal K, Furie K, Go A, Greenlund K, Haase N, Hailpern SM, Ho M, Howard V, Kissela B, Kittner S, Lloyd-Jones D, McDermott M, Meigs J, Moy C, Nichol G, O'Donnell C, Roger V, Sorlie P, Steinberger J, Thom T, Wilson M, and Hong Y: Heart disease and stroke statistics 2008 update: a report from the American Heart Association statistics committee and stroke statistics subcommittee. Circulation 2008; **117:** e25.
2. Kaul P, Armstrong PW, Chang WC, Naylor CD, Granger CB, Lee KL, Peterson ED, Califf RM, Topol EJ, and Mark DB: Long-term mortality of patients with acute myocardial infarction in the United States and Canada. Comparison of the patients enrolled in global utilization of streptokinase and tPA for occluded arteries - Gusto-1. Circulation 2004; **110:** 1754.
3. St. John Sutton M and Sharpe N: Left ventricular remodeling after infarction: pathophysiology and therapy. Circulation 2000; **101:** 2981.
4. Cleutjens JPM, Kandala JC, Guarda E, Guntaka RV, and Weber KT: Regulation of collagen degradation in the rat myocardium after infarction. J Mol Cell Cardiol 1995; **27:** 1281.
5. Levy D, Kenchaiah S, Larson MG, Benjamin EJ, Kupka MJ, Ho KK, Murabito JM, and Vasan RS: Longterm trends in the incidence of and survival with heart failure. N Engl J Med 2002; **347:** 1397.
6. Dimmeler S, Zieher AM, and Schneider MD: Unchain my heart: the scientific foundations of cardiac repair. J Clin Invest 2005; **115:** 572.
7. Abdel-Latif A, Bolli R, Tleyjeh IM, Montori VM, Perin EC, Hornung CA, Zuba-Surma EK, Al-Mallah M, and Dawn B: Adult bone marrow-derived cells for cardiac repair: a systemic review and meta-analysis. Arch Intern Med 2007; **167:** 989.
8. Jackson BM, Gorman JH 3rd, Salgo IS, Moainie SL, Plappert T, St John-Sutton M., Edmunds LH Jr., and Gorman RC: Borderzone geometry increases wall stress after myocardial infarction: contrast echocardiographic assessment. Am J Physiol Heart Circ Physiol 2003; **284:** H475.
9. Gallagher G, Menzie S, Huang Y, Jackson C, and Hunyor SN: Regional cardiac dysfunction is associated with specific alterations in inflammatory cytokines and matrix metalloproteinases after acute myocardial infarction in sheep. Basic Res Cardiol 2006; **102:** 63.
10. Vandervelde S, van Luyn MJA, Rozenbaum MH, Petersen AH, Tio RA, and Harmsen MC: Stem cell-related cardiac gene expression early after murine myocardial infarction. Cardiovasc Res 2007; **73:** 783.
11. Jackson BM, Gorman III JH, Moainie S, Guy TS, Narula N, Narula J, St. John Sutton M, Edmunds LH Jr., and Gorman RC: Extension of borderzone myocardium in postinfarction dilated cardiomyopathy. J Am Coll Cardiol 2002; **40:** 1160.
12. Orlic D, Kajstura J, Chimenti S, Jakoniuk I, Anderson SM, Li B, Pickel J, McKay R, Nadal-Ginard B, Bodine DM, Leri A, and Anversa P: Bone marrow cells regenerate infarcted myocardium. Nature 2001; **410:** 701.
13. Leor J, Guetta E, Feinberg MS, Galski H, Bar I, Holbova R, Miller L, Zarin P, Castel D, Barbash IM, and Nagler A: Human umbilical cord blood-derived CD133+ cells enhance function and repair of the infracted myocardium. Stem Cells 2006; **24:** 772.
14. Ceradini DJ, Kulkarni AR, Callaghan MJ, Tepper OM, Bastidas N, Kleinman ME, Capla JM, Galiano RD, Levine JP, and Gurtner GC: Progenitor cell trafficking is regulated by hypoxic gradients through HIF-1 induction of SDF-1. Nat Med 2004; **10:** 858.
15. Yang ZJ, Xu SL, Chen B, Zhang SL, Zhang YL, Wei W, Ma DC, Wang LS, Zhu TB, Li CJ, Wang H, Cao KJ, Gao W, Huang J, Ma WZ, and Wu ZZ: Hepatocyte growth factor plays a critical role in the regulation of cytokine production and induction of endothelial progenitor cell mobilization: a pilot gene therapy study in patients with coronary heart disease. Clin Exp Pharmacol Physiol 2009; **36:** 790.
16. Higuchi K, Ayach B, Sato T, Chen M, Devine SP, Rasaiah VI, Dawood F, Yanagisawa T, Tei C, Takenaka T, Liu PP, and Medin JA: Direct injection of kit ligand-2 lentivirus improves cardiac repair and rescues mice post-myocardial infarction. Mol Ther 2009; **17:** 262.
17. Lee BC, Hsu HC, Tseng WY, Chen CY, Lin HJ, Ho YL, Su MJ, and Chen MF: Cell therapy generates a favourable chemokine gradient for stem cell recruitment into the infarcted heart in rabbits. Eur J Heart Fail 2009; **11:** 238.
18. Ripa RS, Jorgensen E, Wang Y, Thune JJ, Nilsson JC, Sondergaard L, Johnsen HE, Kober L, Grande P, and Kastrup J: Stem cell mobilization induced by subcutaneous granulocyte-colony stimulating factor to improve cardiac regeneration after acute ST-elevation myocardial infarction: results of the double blind, randomized, placebo-controlled Stem Cells in Myocardial Infarction (STEMMI) trial. Circulation 2006; **113:** 1983.
19. Jorgensen E, Baldazzi F, Ripa RS, Friis T, Wang Y, Helqvist S, and Kastrup J: Instent neointimal hyperplasia after percutaneous intervention for ST-elevation myocardial infarction and treatment with granulocyte-colony stimulating factor. Results from the stem cells in myocardial infarction (STEMMI) trial. Int J Cardiol Epub 2008 Dec 2.
20. Wollert KC, Meyer GP, Lotz J, Ringes-Lichtenberg S, Lippolt P, Breidenbach C, Fichtner S, Korte T, Hornig B, Messinger D, Arseniev L, Hertenstein B, Ganser A, and Drexler H: Intracoronary autologous bone-marrow cell transfer after myocardial infarction: the BOOST randomized controlled clinical trial. Lancet 2004; **364:** 141.
21. Meyer GP, Wollert KC, Lotz J, Steffens J, Lippolt P, Fichtner S, Hecker H, Schaefer A, Arseniev L, Hertenstein B, Ganser A, and Drexler H: Intracoronary bone marrow cell transfer after myocardial infarction: eighteen months' follow-up data from the randomized, controlled BOOST (Bone marrow transfer to enhance ST-elevation infarct regeneration) trial. Circulation 2006; **113:** 1287.
22. Schaefer A, Meyer GP, Fuchs M, Klein G, Kaplan M, Wollert KC, and Drexler H: Impact of intracoronary bone marrow cell transfer on diastolic function in patients after acute myocardial infarction: results from the BOOST trial Eur Heart J 2006; **27:** 929.
23. Schächinger V, Erbs S, Elsässer A, Haberbosch W, Hambrecht R, Hölschermann H, Yu J, Corti R, Mathey DG, Hamm CW, Süselbeck T, Assmus B, Tonn T, Dimmeler S, and Zeiher AM: Intracoronary bone marrow-derived progenitor cells in acute myocardial infarction. N Engl J Med 2006; **355:** 1210.
24. Schächinger V, Erbs S, Elsässer A, Haberbosch W, Hambrecht R, Hölschermann H, Yu J, Corti R, Mathey DG, Hamm CW, Süselbeck T, Werner N, Haase J, Neuzner J, Germing A, and Zeiher AM; REPAIR-AMI Investigators: Improved clinical outcome after intracoronary administration of bone-marrow-derived progenitor cells in acute myocardial infarction: final 1-year results of the REPAIR-AMI trial. Eur Heart J 2006; **27:** 2775.
25. Dill T, Schächinger V, Rolf A, Möllmann S, Thiele H, Tillmanns H, Assmus B, Dimmeler S, Zeiher AM, and Hamm C: Intracoronary administration of

bone marrow-derived progenitor cells improves left ventricular function in patients at risk for adverse remodeling after acute ST-segment elevation myocardial infarction: results of the Reinfusion of Enriched Progenitor cells and Infarct Remodeling in Acute Myocardial Infarction study (REPAIR-AMI) cardiac magnetic resonance imaging substudy. Am Heart J 2009; **157:** 541.

26. Nyolczas N, Gyöngyosi M, Beran G, Dettke M, Graf S, Sochor H, Christ G, Édes I, Balogh L, Krause KT, Jaquet K, Kuck KH, Benedek I, Hintea T, Kiss R, Préda I, Kotevski V, Pejkov H, Dudek D, Heba G, Sylven C, Charwat S, Jacob R, Maurer G, Lang I, and Glogar D: Design and rationale for the Myocardial Stem Cell Administration After Acute Myocardial Infarction (MYSTAR) Study: a multicenter, prospective, randomized, single-blind trial comparing early and late intracoronary or combined (percutaneous intramyocardial and intracoronary) administration of nonselected autologous bone marrow cells to patients after acute myocardial infarction. Am Heart J 2007; **153:** 212.e1.

27. Gyöngyosi M, Lang I, Dettke M, Beran G, Graf S, Sochor H, Nyolczas N, Charwat S, Hemetsberger R, Christ G, Édes I, Balogh L, Krause KT, Jaquet K, Kuck KH, Benedek I, Hintea T, Kiss R, Préda I, Kotevski V, Pejkov H, Zamini S, Khorsand A, Sodeck G, Kaider A, Maurer G, and Glogar D: Combined delivery approach of bone marrow mononuclear stem cells early and late after myocardial infarction: the MYSTAR prospective, randomized study. Nat Clin Pract Cardiovasc Med 2009; **6:** 70.

28. Tendera M, Wojakowski W, Ruzytto W, Chojnowska L, Kepka C, Tracz W, Musiatek P, Piwowarska W, Nessler J, Buszman P, Grajek S, Breborowicz P, Majka M, Ratajczak MZ, and for the REGENT Investigators (the REGENT investigators are listed in the Appendix): Intracoronary infusion of bone marrow-derived selected CD34+ CXCR4+ cells and non-selected mononuclear cells in patients with acute STEMI and reduced left ventricular ejection fraction: results of randomized, multicentre Myocardial Regeneration by Intracoronary Infusion of Selected Population of Stem Cells in Acute Myocardial Infarction (REGENT) Trial. Eur Heart J 2009; **30:** 1313.

29. Moelker AD, Baks T, Wever KMAM, Spitskovsky D, Wielopolski PA, van Beusekom HM, van Geuns RJ, Wnendt S, Duncker DJ, and van der Giessen WJ: Intracoronary delivery of umbilical cord blood derived unrestricted somatic stem cells is not suitable to improve LV function after myocardial infarction in swine. J Mol Cell Cardiol 2007; **42:** 735.

30. Abdel-Latif A, Bolli R, Zuba-Surma EK, Tleyjeh IM, Hornung CA, and Dawn B: Granulocyte colony-stimulating factor therapy for cardiac repair after acute myocardial infarction: a systemic review and meta-analysis of randomized controlled trials. Am Heart J 2008; **156:** 216–226.e9.

WHS Wound Healing Society

Stem Cells in Hepatic Regeneration After Injury

Unsal Kuscuoglu,[1] Katherine Bianco,[2] and Karl G. Sylvester[1,*]

[1]Hagey Laboratory for Regenerative Medicine, Department of Surgery, Stanford University School of Medicine, Stanford, California.
[2]Department of Obstetrics, Gynecology, and Reproductive Sciences, UCSF School of Medicine, University of California, San Francisco, California.

Abbreviations and Acronyms

ESCs = embryonic stem cells

FAH = fumarylacetoacetate hydrolase

iPSCs = induced pluripotent stem cells

TNF = tumor necrosis factor

*Correspondence: Hagey Laboratory for Regenerative Medicine, Department of Surgery, Stanford University School of Medicine, 257 Campus Drive, Stanford, California 94305-5148 (e-mail: sylvester@stanford.edu).

Background: Despite overall cellular quiescence during homeostasis, the liver is one of the few solid organs that maintains near-complete regenerative capacity. In contradistinction to continuously renewing organ systems like the gut, skin, and hematopoietic systems that rely on a well-ordered stem cell hierarchy, in the liver, the fully mature hepatocyte is primarily responsible for maintaining the hepatic parenchyma and its restoration after acute injury.
The Problem: A common feature to nearly all forms (congenital-metabolic, acquired-infectious, toxic, and neoplastic) of liver disease is chronic hepatocellular injury that results in an eventual deficit in hepatic regenerative capacity along with increasing inflammation and fibrosis. Currently, the only successful treatment for end-stage liver disease is whole-organ transplantation. Given the severe shortage of suitable organs for transplantation, viable alternatives to liver transplantation are critically needed. Cell-based therapies are promising yet suffer from the lack of a sufficient cell source.
Basic/Clinical Science Advances: Recent advances in our basic understanding of hepatic developmental and regenerative biology may lead to novel sources of competent cells for hepatic cell therapy to supplant current whole-organ replacement strategies. Numerous sources, including endogenous facultative hepatic progenitor cells and possible exogenous fetal and embryonic sources of liver stem and progenitor cells, are being enthusiastically pursued.
Clinical Care Relevance: To date, a limited number of successful mature hepatocyte transplantation therapies have been achieved for a select number of metabolic diseases. This experience has provided the necessary proof of principle on which to base future hepatocellular therapeutic strategies.
Conclusion: In addition to the possibility of utilizing hepatic cells for cellular therapies, the knowledge gained in the study of hepatic regeneration may also lead to novel strategies to prevent hepatocellular exhaustion and thereby ameliorate progressive hepatocellular injury, thus lessening or obviating replacement therapies.

BACKGROUND

Numerous investigative and clinical observations have provided comprehensive evidence for the singular potency of hepatic regenerative capacity among solid organs. Unlike most other regenerating epithelia (*i.e.*, skin and gut), the liver does not rely upon stem or progenitor cells as a primary participant in the injury response. Rather, the hepatocellular response is defined contextually by the nature of the injury or stimuli. In response to acute injury, fully differentiated hepatocytes and cholangiocytes reenter the cell cycle and restore hepatic parenchyma through proliferation and hypertrophy (Fig. 1A).[1,2] While mature hepatocytes are not themselves stem cells, as defined by pluripotency and self-renewal capacity, they do possess certain stem-like replicative

ADVANCES IN WOUND CARE, VOLUME 1

Printed in U.S.A.
DOI: 10.1089/awc.2009.0101

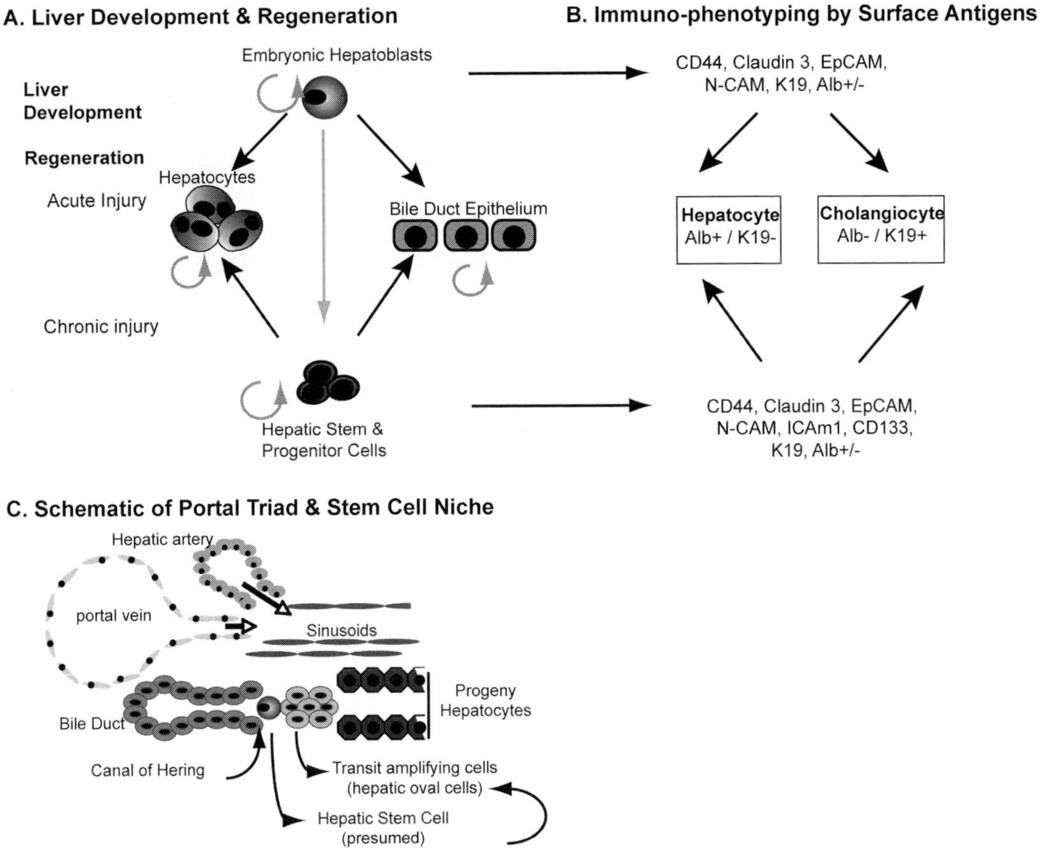

Figure 1. (**A**) Schematic of similarities in the cell biology of liver development and regeneration. During development, hepatoblasts (liver stem cells) self-renew and give rise to both hepatocytes and cholangiocytes (bile duct epithelium). In response to acute injury, hepatocytes and cholangiocytes proliferate to restore parenchyma. During overwhelming acute or chronic injury, postnatal hepatic stem and progenitor cells proliferate to restore injured parenchyma. (**B**) Immunophenotyping by surface antigen expression of the liver progenitor and progeny cells and their relationships to each other (these data are summarized from numerous sources cited in the text). (**C**) Schematic of the portal triad and the presumed niche (Canal of Hering) for the postnatal liver stem cell and the transiently amplifying hepatic oval cells or ductular reactions.

capabilities, including an ability to undergo serial transplantation. However, the morbidity of most liver diseases and liver failure result from repetitive injury stimuli that impart cumulative damage to the hepatocellular compartment. The net result of chronic injury is hepatocyte senescence that defines the earliest phase of progressive liver failure. In response to hepatocyte mitotic inhibition, a facultative and transiently amplifying hepatic progenitor population of cells proliferates to maintain liver parenchyma[1] (Fig. 1A). These cells, which have been variously called "oval cells," "ductular reactions," or "intermediate hepatobiliary cells," are thought to possess bipotent differentiation potential for both hepatocyte and cholangiocyte.[3,4] Oval cell proliferation has been observed in numerous rodent models of liver injury and in the majority of chronic human liver diseases. In both human and rodent, the oval cell response appears to vary with the severity of the disease or injury.[5] Most current theories hold that the emergence of oval cells during chronic injury occurs as a precursor cell to nascent hepatocyte progeny (hepatoblasts) to maintain liver parenchymal volume (Fig. 1A). Despite these tenets of the hepatocellular response during liver regeneration, current knowledge of the precise origin of adult liver progenitors, lineage tracing of oval cells to a precursor or stem cell, and the signaling pathways that govern these responses in postnatal liver remains incomplete.

CLINICAL PROBLEM

Given its unique physiologic role in nutrient and xenobiotic metabolism, the liver is subject to a variety of injury stimuli (*e.g.*, toxin, lipid, and viral) with cumulative effects. Taken together, each of these injury stimuli manifests a response from the cellular compartment of the liver in an attempt to maintain, repair, or restore liver form and function. During overwhelming acute injury–induced liver failure (*e.g.*, acetaminophen intoxication) or at the extremes of chronic liver disease (*e.g.*, cirrhosis [late stage viral hepatitis] or carcinoma), both the hepatocyte and facultative progenitor cell responses are insufficient. Thus, there exists an unmet need for whole-organ replacement or regeneration. Aside from supportive measures, liver transplantation remains the only replacement strategy for many hepatopathies. The limited success with hepatocyte transplantation to date, while encouraging, suffers from an inability to obtain mature hepatocytes in sufficient quantities suitable for transplantation.

RELEVANT BASIC SCIENCE CONTEXT

The endogenous two-tiered hepatocellular response (hepatocytes and oval cells) to injury and regeneration has been the most extensively studied to date (Fig. 1).[1,2] The regenerative capacity of hepatocytes has been determined in a number of rodent models that facilitate liver regeneration or repopulation based upon physical, chemical, or genetic selection advantages to engrafting hepatocytes. In addition, much has been learned about the recapitulation in adult liver of specific cellular and genetic programs employed during liver development (Fig. 1A, B).[6] However, the inability to maintain robust differentiation and proliferation of mature hepatocytes *in vitro* has limited further progress in the field as it relates to developing strategies for cellular therapies. Thus, there is currently a significant interest in generating hepatocytes from expandable precursors. This has lead to an increasing effort devoted to primarily three sources from which to derive expandable hepatocytes. Recent progress has been made with committed human fetal and adult sources of both elusive hepatic stem cells and hepatoblasts.[7,8] More recently, exogenous pluripotent sources like embryonic stem cells (ESCs) and most recently induced pluripotent stem cells (iPSCs) are perhaps the most attractive sources of a potentially unlimited number of precursors cells.[9–11] Successful strategies utilizing a pluripotent cell source to provide cells for regenerative applications would overcome the principle barriers to clinical application of deriving a sufficient quantity of healthy cells that are immune compatible with the potential host. The molecular mechanisms for hepatic induction and commitment learned from embryonic studies of liver development are being utilized to pursue the derivation of hepatocytes from these pluripotent undifferentiated sources. Despite recent progress, evidence that hepatocyte-like cells from pluripotent sources can achieve a fully mature and functional phenotype sufficient for organ repopulation is currently lacking.

EXPERIMENTAL MODEL

Rodent models have been extensively developed and utilized to study the cell and molecular biology of hepatic regeneration given their approximation of the human response to hepatic injury. In general, most rodent injury models attempt to recapitulate the acute and/or chronic nature of the pathologic causes of human liver injury. The models of acute injury that are most commonly utilized include either partial hepatectomy or treatment with carbon tetra-chloride.[1,2] In both of these models the liver parenchymal volume is fully restored within days largely due to a robust hepatocyte proliferative response. To study the second tier or oval cell contribution to liver regeneration, the proliferative capacity of hepatocytes has to be inhibited. Numerous toxins that exert a strong and persistent block of native hepatocyte proliferation have been utilized either alone or in combination with an acute stimulus-like partial hepatectomy to elicit a robust oval cell response.[1,2] To definitively examine the progenitor cell characteristics of a cell population under study, model systems that stimulate *in vivo* organ replacement or repopulation are required. As an alternative to toxin-mediated hepatocyte injury models, genetic mouse models that result in hepatocyte injury caused by the accumulation of toxic metabolites have revealed that engrafting cells can be selected for expansion if there is a survival benefit conferred by the wild-type allele (genotype). A prototypical example is the genetic mouse model of familial tyrosinemia, in which mice deficient for the enzyme fumarylacetoacetate hydrolase (FAH) develop progressive hepatic failure in the absence of the rescue metabolite 2-(2-nitro-4-trifluoro methylbenzoyl)-1,3-cyclohexanedione.[12–14] Using this model, previous authors have demonstrated that, given a powerful positive (genetic) selection for survival, it is possible to achieve complete liver repopulation by engrafting hepatocytes harboring intact FAH.[13–16] The establishment of the FAH mice on an immune-deficient background has further extended this model's utility to a number of different allogeneic and xenogeneic (human) cell transplant assays for determining a candidate cell's liver repopulating capabilities.[17]

DISCUSSION OF FINDINGS AND RELEVANT RECENT LITERATURE

Hepatic regeneration by hepatocytes

Hepatic regeneration is characterized by a tiered cellular response (Fig. 1A). In the primary response, the mature, fully differentiated hepatocyte reenters the cell cycle upon a regenerative stimulus. Despite decades of research describing the proliferative potential of hepatocytes, this is not always a typical response of cell cycle progression and the completion of mitosis with resultant two daughter cells. Hepatocytes possess the unique capacity to undergo endo-reduplication and cellular hypertrophy.[18,19] Stated differently, mature hepatocytes undergo genetic duplication without cytokinesis. This results in hepatocytes that are both multinucleate and polyploid. Despite this, polyploid hepatocytes are capable of serial transplantation and numerous population doublings.[20] Replicative senescence can and does however occur *in vivo* with serial injury or cumulative cell damage. Moreover, replicative senescence and dedifferentiation are the hallmarks of primary hepatocyte culture.

Hepatic regeneration by endogenous progenitors

When hepatocyte proliferation is impaired as occurs in chronic human liver diseases or during acute overwhelming necrosis, a population of facultative transiently amplifying progenitor cells proliferates from the portal tracts (Fig. 1C). This ductular response is the second-tier response that results in a more primitive intermediary hepatic cell for eventual parenchymal replacement. Thus, the proliferation, migration, and differentiation of the transiently amplifying oval cell appear to recapitulate the critical aspects of liver morphogenesis accomplished by the hepatic stem cell and hepatoblast during liver development (Fig. 1A). Emerging studies have found that the niche for the postnatal stem cell appears to be primarily the Canal of Hering at the terminal bile ductule in the portal triad (Fig. 1C), but also suggest that intralobular ductal or periductal cells are also competent.[6,21] Few studies to date have examined the molecular pathways regulating postnatal liver stem cell proliferation and differentiation. One of the major limitations to the study of the progenitor cell response is the absence of a uniform and consistent panel of phenotypic markers that can be utilized across species for their prospective isolation. However, very recent studies in both rodents and humans have made progress in this area (Fig. 1B).[6,22,23] Many previous studies of postnatal liver progenitor cells have utilized a variety of cell surface antigens that have also been identified during hepatic development, including alpha fetal protein, CD133, cytokeratin 19, cytokeratin 18, neural cell adhesion molecule, CD44, epithelial cell adhesion molecule (EpCAM), and the M2-isozyme of pyruvate kinase.[5,24,25] One uncharacterized epitope that has been consistently utilized by many investigators in identifying mouse ductular reactions is the A6 antigen.[4,26] However, this antigen has no known biologic role and the anti-A6 antibody seems to also recognize bile duct epithelium. More recently, several signaling pathways such as Notch/Delta/Jagged, NF-kappaβ, somatostatin, and members of the tumor necrosis factor (TNF) pathway (TWEAK/Fn14) have been described as critical molecular regulators of hepatic oval cell biology.[27–30] Similar to published evidence for the morphogen Wnt pathway involvement during liver development for growth and differentiation, there have been several recent studies describing the Wnt pathway's role in regulating hepatic oval cell directed liver regeneration in response to chronic injury.[31,32]

Hepatic regeneration from bone marrow

A possible third tier of cellular response to liver injury has been described from bone marrow–derived cells. Circulating myeloid cells have been observed to traffic to the liver in response to injury. The overall relevance of the myeloid cell contribution remains unclear; however, most evidence seems to indicate that this is largely a stochastic event with little meaningful result outside specific experimental models.[15,16] The described mechanism involves cell fusion between the engrafting myeloid cell and the resident hepatocyte resulting in myeloid cell reprogramming toward a hepatic lineage. Although this is unlikely to represent a substantial mechanism of physiologic liver regeneration, it is conceivable that this phenomenon could be exploited in a cell–gene therapy approach to liver therapies.

Derivation of exogenous hepatic stem cells

Since hepatocytes are neither pluripotent and do not undergo endless duplication through asymmetric cell division either *in vivo* or *in vitro*, they cannot be considered a true stem cell despite their other stem-like properties. Moreover, the tools for the prospective isolation and expansion of endogenous pre- and postnatal liver stem and progenitor cells are still being developed (Fig. 1B). Therefore, given these disadvantages, the utility of hepatocytes and known liver stem cells for typical stem cell applications like cell therapy remains limited. Thus, there is a recent robust interest in pluripotent iPSCs and ESCs that may allow for the derivation of an expandable and immune-compatible source of exogenous hepatic stem cells. Numerous groups have now demonstrated an ability to partially differentiate ESCs toward a hepatic fate.[33–35] This requires as an initial step the derivation of definitive endoderm by induction of ESCs by activin A.[36] Subsequent commitment to the hepatic lineage specifically has been accomplished with the use of various morphogen combinations with most involving bone morphogenetic protein-4 (BMP-4) and basic fibroblast growth factor (bFGF). The characterization of resultant hepatocyte-like cells by marker gene/protein analysis are promising, yet the lack of evidence that these cells can become mature hepatocytes *in vivo* and contribute to end-organ function remains to be determined in genetic mouse models of metabolic disease similar to those described above.[36]

CAUTION, CRITICAL REMARKS, AND RECOMMENDATIONS

Taken together, the early success with hepatocyte transplantation and recent advances in our understanding of hepatic progenitor cell biology have combined to bolster enthusiasm for the prospect of utilizing hepatic progenitor cells for liver repair and regeneration. The excitement provided by the findings with induced pluripotent cells has further broadened the interest in possible cell therapies for a variety of liver diseases. The biology of several hepatic diseases and the realization that limited replacement of the hepatic parenchyma by competent, corrected cells could have a profound impact on altering a disease phenotype (*e.g.*, hemophilia) have positioned the prospect for hepatic cell therapy as a priority among many researchers. Still, much work remains to be done so that these promising therapies can be implemented in a safe and regulated manner. Complementary studies using both available human specimens and cell sources as well as rodent models of liver injury and repopulation are needed. A great deal of basic investigation is yet to be accomplished so that the controlled proliferation and differentiation of competent cells is enacted as desired and untoward effects of cell transplantation are avoided (tumorigenesis).

TAKE-HOME MESSAGE

Basic science advances

- The endogenous hepatocellular regenerative response can be conceptualized as a two-tiered cellular response that includes the hepatocyte and the facultative hepatic progenitor cells and their precursors.
- Although hepatocytes themselves are not true "stem cells" in biologic terms, they do represent the primary cell source for hepatic regeneration.
- The postnatal hepatic stem and progenitor cell response is less well characterized, but emerging evidence does suggest that a precursor–progeny relationship exits and resembles a typical ordered stem cell hierarchy.
- Many of the same stem progenitor cell relationships and signaling pathways governing hepatic development are evident during postnatal liver repair, including the persistence of a rare pluripotent stem cell.
- Exogenous sources of cells for hepatic regeneration have included bone marrow–derived myelomonocytic cells, committed fetal hepatoblasts, and uncommitted pluripotent sources of stem cells that could potentially be expanded and derived from the host and therefore rendered immune compatible.
- The continued recognition and understanding of symmetry between hepatic development and regeneration will facilitate our ability to derive novel therapies in support of the liver injury response.

Clinical science advances

- Human hepatocyte transplantation has been successfully used to treat a limited number of hepatopathies.
- It is likely that if liver-directed cell therapies are going to succeed, then more potent, proliferative cell sources will be required.
- Conceptually, ESCs and iPSCs may represent an ideal source for the derivation of liver repopulating cells since they are pluripotent, highly proliferative, and can be derived in an immune-compatible manner with the designated host.
- Many basic biologic questions need to be addressed before the safe application of purified, well-characterized progenitor and stem cell sources can be utilized clinically.

FUTURE DEVELOPMENT

With continued study of the basic cellular and molecular mechanisms of liver regeneration, novel applications of the knowledge gained may lead to advanced cell therapies for a variety of hepatic disease states. Overall, by understanding the hierarchical role of stem cells in hepatic regeneration, broader insight to the cellular response to other organ injuries like the dermis may also be gained. Further, a deeper understanding of the signaling mechanisms by which the hepatocellular compartments respond to liver injury may also lead to non-cell-based molecular treatments to augment endogenous tissue repair and regenerative response.

ACKNOWLEDGMENTS

This work was supported in part by the Oak Foundation, The National Institutes of Health (NIH) (DK56339), The Stanford Cancer Center (Development Research Award, Transplant and Tissue Engineering Center of Excellence), and Packard Children's Hospital (all to K.G.S.).

AUTHOR DISCLOSURE STATEMENT

None of the authors have anything to disclose related to the material contained within this manuscript.

REFERENCES

1. Fausto N, Campbell JS, and Riehle KJ: Liver regeneration. Hepatology 2006; **43:** S45.

2. Fausto N: Liver regeneration and repair: hepatocytes, progenitor cells, and stem cells. Hepatology 2004; **39:** 1477.

3. Braun KM and Sandgren EP: Cellular origin of regenerating parenchyma in a mouse model of severe hepatic injury. Am J Pathol 2000; **157:** 561.

4. Wang X, Foster M, Al-Dhalimy M, Lagasse E, Finegold M, and Grompe M: The origin and liver repopulating capacity of murine oval cells. Proc Natl Acad Sci USA 2003; **100 Suppl 1:** 11881.

5. Lowes KN, Brennan BA, Yeoh GC, and Olynyk JK: Oval cell numbers in human chronic liver diseases are directly related to disease severity. Am J Pathol 1999; **154:** 537.

6. Zhang L, Theise N, Chua M, and Reid LM: The stem cell niche of human livers: symmetry between development and regeneration. Hepatology 2008; 4**8:** 1598.

7. Cheng N, Wauthier E, and Reid LM: Mature human hepatocytes from *ex vivo* differentiation of alginate-encapsulated hepatoblasts. Tissue Eng Part A 2008; **14:** 1–7.

8. Schmelzer E, Zhang L, Bruce A, Wauthier E, Ludlow J, Yao HL, Moss N, Melhem A, McClelland R, Turner W, Kulik M, Sherwood S, Tallheden T, Cheng N, Furth ME, and Reid LM: Human hepatic stem cells from fetal and postnatal donors. J Exp Med 2007; **204:** 1973.

9. Basma H, Soto-Gutierrez A, Yannam GR, Liu L, Ito R, Yamamoto T, Ellis E, Carson SD, Sato S, Chen Y, Muirhead D, Navarro-Alvarez N, Wong RJ, Roy-Chowdhury J, Platt JL, Mercer DF, Miller JD, Strom SC, Kobayashi N, and Fox IJ: Differentiation and transplantation of human embryonic stem cell-derived hepatocytes. Gastroenterology 2009; **136:** 990.

10. Safinia N and Minger SL: Generation of hepatocytes from human embryonic stem cells. Methods Mol Biol 2009; **481:** 169.

11. Stadtfeld M, Nagaya M, Utikal J, Weir G, and Hochedlinger K: Induced pluripotent stem cells generated without viral integration. Science 2008; **322:** 945.

12. Grompe M: Complete hepatic regeneration after somatic deletion of an albumin-plasminogen activator transgene, 1991. J Hepatol 2002; **37:** 422.

13. Overturf K, Al-Dhalimy M, Finegold M, and Grompe M: The repopulation potential of hepatocyte populations differing in size and prior mitotic expansion. Am J Pathol 1999; **155:** 2135.

14. Overturf K, Al-Dhalimy M, Tanguay R, Brantly M, Ou CN, Finegold M, and Grompe M: Hepatocytes corrected by gene therapy are selected *in vivo* in a murine model of hereditary tyrosinaemia type I. Nat Genet 1996; **12:** 266.

15. Lagasse E, Connors H, Al-Dhalimy M, Reitsma M, Dohse M, Osborne L, Wang X, Finegold M, Weissman IL, and Grompe M: Purified hematopoietic stem cells can differentiate into hepatocytes *in vivo.* Nat Med 2000; **6:** 1229.

16. Willenbring H, Bailey AS, Foster M, Akkari Y, Dorrell C, Olson S, Finegold M, Fleming WH, and Grompe M: Myelomonocytic cells are sufficient for therapeutic cell fusion in liver. Nat Med 2004; **10:** 744.

17. Azuma H, Paulk N, Ranade A, Dorrell C, Al-Dhalimy M, Ellis E, Strom S, Kay MA, Finegold M, and Grompe M: Robust expansion of human hepatocytes in Fah-/-/Rag2-/-/Il2rg-/- mice. Nat Biotechnol 2007; **25:** 903.

18. Lazzerini Denchi E, Celli G, and de Lange T: Hepatocytes with extensive telomere deprotection and fusion remain viable and regenerate liver mass through endoreduplication. Genes Dev 2006; **20:** 2648.

19. Duncan AW, Hickey RD, Paulk NK, Culberson AJ, Olson SB, Finegold MJ, and Grompe M: Ploidy reductions in murine fusion-derived hepatocytes. PLoS Genet 2009; **5:** e1000385.

20. Fausto N: Hepatocytes break the rules of senescence in serial transplantation studies. Is there a limit to their replicative capacity? Am J Pathol 1997; **151:** 1187.

21. Kuwahara R, Kofman AV, Landis CS, Swenson ES, Barendswaard E, and Theise ND: The hepatic stem cell niche: identification by label-retaining cell assay. Hepatology 2008; **47:** 1994.

22. Dorrell C, Erker L, Lanxon-Cookson KM, Abraham SL, Victoroff T, Ro S, Canaday PS, Streeter PR, and Grompe M: Surface markers for the murine oval cell response. Hepatology 2008; **48:** 1282.

23. Wauthier E, Schmelzer E, Turner W, Zhang L, LeCluyse E, Ruiz J, Turner R, Furth ME, Kubota H, Lozoya O, Barbier C, McClelland R, Yao HL, Moss N, Bruce A, Ludlow J, and Reid LM: Hepatic stem cells and hepatoblasts: identification, isolation, and *ex vivo* maintenance. Methods Cell Biol 2008; **86:** 137.

24. Turner WS, Schmelzer E, McClelland R, Wauthier E, Chen W, and Reid LM: Human hepatoblast phenotype maintained by hyaluronan hydrogels. J Biomed Mater Res B Appl Biomater 2007; **82:** 156.

25. Kon J, Ooe H, Oshima H, Kikkawa Y, and Mitaka T: Expression of CD44 in rat hepatic progenitor cells. J Hepatol 2006; **45:** 90.

26. Factor VM, Radaeva SA, and Thorgeirsson SS: Origin and fate of oval cells in dipin-induced hepatocarcinogenesis in the mouse. Am J Pathol 1994; **145:** 409.

27. Jung Y, Oh SH, Zheng D, Shupe TD, Witek RP, and Petersen BE: A potential role of somatostatin and its receptor SSTR4 in the migration of hepatic oval cells. Lab Investig 2006; **86:** 477.

28. Jakubowski A, Ambrose C, Parr M, Lincecum JM, Wang MZ, Zheng TS, Browning B, Michaelson JS, Baetscher M, Wang B, Bissell DM, and Burkly LC: TWEAK induces liver progenitor cell proliferation. J Clin Investig 2005; **115:** 2330.

29. Sanchez A, Factor VM, Schroeder IS, Nagy P, and Thorgeirsson SS: Activation of NF-kappaB and STAT3 in rat oval cells during 2-acetylaminofluorene/partial hepatectomy-induced liver regeneration. Hepatology 2004; **39:** 376.

30. Jensen CH, Jauho EI, Santoni-Rugiu E, Holmskov U, Teisner B, Tygstrup N, and Bisgaard HC: Transit-amplifying ductular (oval) cells and their hepatocytic progeny are characterized by a novel and distinctive expression of delta-like protein/preadipocyte factor 1/fetal antigen 1. Am J Pathol 2004; **164:** 1347.

31. Hu M, Kurobe M, Jeong YJ, Fuerer C, Ghole S, Nusse R, and Sylvester KG: Wnt/beta-catenin signaling in murine hepatic transit amplifying progenitor cells. Gastroenterology 2007; **133:** 1579.

32. Tan X, Yuan Y, Zeng G, Apte U, Thompson MD, Cieply B, Stolz DB, Michalopoulos GK, Kaestner KH, and Monga SP: Beta-catenin deletion in hepatoblasts disrupts hepatic morphogenesis and survival during mouse development. Hepatology 2008; **47:** 1667.

33. Agarwal S, Holton KL, and Lanza R: Efficient differentiation of functional hepatocytes from human embryonic stem cells. Stem Cells 2008; **26:** 1117.

34. Cai J, Zhao Y, Liu Y, Ye F, Song Z, Qin H, Meng S, Chen Y, Zhou R, Song X, Guo Y, Ding M, and Deng H: Directed differentiation of human embryonic stem cells into functional hepatic cells. Hepatology 2007; **45:** 1229.

35. Hay DC, Zhao D, Fletcher J, Hewitt ZA, McLean D, Urruticoechea-Uriguen A, Black JR, Elcombe C, Ross JA, Wolf R, and Cui W: Efficient differentiation of hepatocytes from human embryonic stem cells exhibiting markers recapitulating liver development *in vivo.* Stem Cells 2008; **26:** 894.

36. Chiao E, Elazar M, Xing Y, Xiong A, Kmet M, Millan MT, Glenn JS, Wong WH, and Baker J: Isolation and transcriptional profiling of purified hepatic cells derived from human embryonic stem cells. Stem Cells 2008; **26:** 2032.

Section 11

DEVICES

Section Editors: Paul Y. Liu and Lisa Gould

What Is New in Debridement?

Stephen C. Davis* and Aron G. Nusbaum

Department of Dermatology and Cutaneous Surgery, University of Miami Miller School of Medicine, Miami, Florida.

Background: The rationale for debridement is based on the fact that the chronic wound bed is known to contain factors that inhibit the natural healing cascade. For wound closure to occur spontaneously or via administration of novel therapies such as topically applied growth factors, physical, molecular, and cellular barriers to healing must be removed.

The Problem: Incidence of wound closure in chronic wounds is low, with estimates ranging from 25% to 50% in venous and diabetic ulcers despite 20 weeks of treatment (Falanga et al. Ostomy Wound Manage 2008; **Suppl:** 2; quiz 14). Necrotic tissue not only impedes reepithelialization and prolongs inflammation but also provides a fertile environment for bacteria, with evidence indicating that colonization of $>10^5$ colony-forming units (CFU)/g tissue delays wound healing (Schultz et al. Wound Repair Regen 2003; **11 Suppl 1:** S1).

Basic/Clinical Science Advances: Gene expression profiling has been utilized to differentiate between senescent cells from the nonhealing edge of chronic wounds and viable cells from adjacent skin (Brem et al. Mol Med 2007; **13:** 30). Future assays may be developed based on this technology to outline the optimal margins for debridement (Tomic-Canic et al. Adv Skin Wound Care 2008; **21:** 487; quiz 493). Although numerous techniques for debridement are available, all have particular shortcomings in certain situations. More recently, coblation technology has shown the ability to selectively break molecular bonds within necrotic tissue (Mancini. Aesthetic Plast Surg 2001; **25:** 372), causing minimal thermal injury to surrounding skin. Preliminary evidence shows effectiveness in removing surface debris and bacteria from partial-thickness wounds.

Clinical Care Relevance: It is estimated that 2.5 million Americans are affected by venous ulcers, 1.3–3 million suffer from pressure ulcers, and 1 million diabetics are at risk for developing neuropathic ulcers over any 3-year period (Falanga et al. Ostomy Wound Manage 2008; **Suppl:** 2; quiz 14). The inability of these wounds to heal ultimately results in long-term hospitalizations and creates an ongoing challenge for physicians.

Conclusion: Better understanding of the many techniques available for debridement is required, with respect to their effectiveness and shortcomings in different clinical situations. New technologies for debridement along with novel assays to assess the status of the wound bed should improve treatment outcomes in this complex clinical scenario.

Abbreviations and Acronyms

CT = coblation technology

ECM = extracellular matrix

MDT = maggot debridement therapy

MMPs = matrix metalloproteases

*Correspondence: Department of Dermatology and Cutaneous Surgery, University of Miami Miller School of Medicine, 1600 NW 10th Ave., Room 2089, Miami, Florida 33136 (e-mail: sdavis@med.miami.edu).

BACKGROUND

Removal of necrotic tissue has been routinely used for a variety of wound types, including chronic, acute, and burns. Devitalized tissue has been shown to not only delay the healing process but also provide a fertile environment for bacteria.[1–3] Topical growth factor delivery has been shown to be more effective after proper debridement.[4] Wound bed preparation by removing nonviable

Printed in U.S.A.
DOI: 10.1089/awc.2009.0166

Table 1. *Considerations when selecting an appropriate debridement method*

Method	Advantages	Disadvantages
Surgical (sharp)	• Wounds with large amount of necrotic tissue or eschar • Exposes undermined tissue, hidden abscesses, or sinus tracts • Removes callus in diabetic foot ulcers • Highly selective • Immediate results	• Blood loss • Very painful unless patient has neuropathy • May require operating room and general anesthesia Contraindications: • Vascular disease or ischemic wounds • Autoimmune disorders (pyoderma gangrenosum)
Mechanical	• Nonsurgical candidates • Exudative wounds with necrotic material • Faster than enzymatic and autolytic	Wet-to-dry dressings: • Nonselective • Painful • Frequent dressings changes Irrigation-pulsed lavage: • Nonselective • Forceful penetration of bacteria into wound Ultrasound: • Clinician requires protective gear because of aerosolization • Should be performed in a closed environment to prevent microbial spread • May be painful Hydrosurgery: • Requires a suction canister and an operating room setting • High risk of cross contamination due to aerosolized bacteria
Enzymatic	• Selective depending on agent • Bedside use	• Eschar must be cross-hatched prior to application • Irritation of surrounding skin and slightly painful stinging sensation • Slow process • Availability
Biological	• Selective • Possible antimicrobial effects • Bedside use	• Bleeding • Proper disposal of larvae-filled dressings • Conflicting reports regarding pain level • Psychological distress
Autolytic	• Wounds with minimal debris • Selective • Painless • Bedside use	• Exudate must be constantly monitored • Slow process
Coblation technology	• Immediate results • Can remove bacteria from wounds	• May be painful on sensate patients • May require operating room and general anesthesia

tissue and by controlling bacterial load and inflammation is an important concept that helps correct specific abnormalities found in chronic wounds, *i.e.*, high proinflammatory cytokine levels, elevated matrix metalloprotease (MMP) levels, low growth factor activities, abnormal matrix, and senescent wound cells.[5] By removing molecular,[6] physical,[2] and microbiologic[7] barriers to healing, debridement not only facilitates endogenous healing but also may render the wound amenable to a variety of novel therapeutic modalities. Although few new debridement methods are available, we recently studied the use of a novel coblation technology (CT) for debridement. In the future, molecular markers might be utilized to help differentiate between impaired and nonimpaired tissue, making surgical debridement more accurate and more efficacious.[8]

CLINICAL PROBLEM ADDRESSED

The treatment of chronic wounds significantly impacts the health-care system with U.S.$25 billion spent annually.[6,8] Wounds, especially chronic, and burns are usually characterized with an accumulation of nonviable tissue which includes cellular debris and eschar or crust. Mostly this devitalized tissue gets colonized and eventually infected with bacteria. The removal of this tissue is critical for wounds to heal. A variety of debridement methods exist and additional controlled studies are needed. One of the most important concepts in current practice is that of wound bed preparation with the goal of restoring the altered chronic wound environment to that of an acute wound.[1,5] Proper wound debridement is an essential part of wound bed preparation (Table 1).

BASIC SCIENCE CONTEXT

The cellular and molecular environment in an acute wound is capable of supporting a synchronized cascade of events leading to complete healing.[1] In chronic wounds, however, this stepwise process is interrupted by a variety of factors, resulting in an absence of healthy granulation tissue and failure of reepithelialization. Defective remodeling of the extracellular matrix (ECM) in chronic wounds is characterized by excessive concentrations of MMPs which degrade the matrix material. Macromolecules produced by matrix degradation along with extravasated fibrinogen and fibrin sequester endogenous growth factors and render them unavailable to wound-healing cells.[1] In addition, cultured fibroblasts isolated from chronic wounds show unresponsiveness to platelet-derived growth factor beta[9] and transforming growth factor beta.[10] Failure to reepithelialize is associated with epidermal hyperproliferation at the nonhealing wound edge which is postulated to occur because of lack of apoptosis in keratinocytes and fibroblasts.[1] Increased levels of β-catenin and c-myc hyperexpression may be operative in preventing cell differentiation and migration.[11] Overall, many "defective" cells and matrix material can be found in chronic wounds and elimination of this material is needed for an optimal healing environment. Removal of necrotic tissue and slough may liberate sequestered growth factors and accelerate healing.[12] In a prospective multicenter study of 118 patients with diabetic foot ulcers treated with recombinant human platelet derived growth factor, a higher rate of healing was observed with more frequent debridement.[13]

Studies have suggested that chronic ulcers contain distinct subpopulations of fibroblasts and keratinocytes at the nonhealing wound edge when compared with adjacent skin. The cells from these two locations exhibit different capacities to heal and therefore molecular markers can be used to help differentiate them. These markers might be utilized to determine the optimal margins for surgical debridement.[8]

These studies demonstrated the role of growth factors in chronic wound healing and indicated that debridement creates a wound environment where growth factors and their receptors are available for binding. In addition, debridement might restore normal reepithelialization by removing senescent cells from the wound margin.[1,2,12]

EXPERIMENTAL MODELS OR MATERIALS

Animal models of debridement consist predominantly of porcine and rodent species. Porcine models offer significant advantages for wound healing studies because of its many similarities to humans.[14] Surgical debridement has been shown to accelerate epithelialization of second-degree burns in a porcine model,[15] with excision of burns 24 h after injury being more effective than that after 96 h. Studies evaluating enzymatic debridement have been performed predominantly in porcine burn wounds,[16–19] with one model recreating a compartment syndrome using a circumferential leg burn.[16] Rat necrotic flap models have also been used to assess the ability of enzymatic debridement to penetrate full-thickness eschars.[20] Pulsed lavage methods for removing necrotic tissue have been generally studied with respect to its effects on bacterial burden and healing in deep wounds by using various contaminated animal models, including rat crushed muscle wounds,[21] goat musculoskeletal wounds,[22] and rabbit open facture model.[23]

Although animal models are helpful, well-controlled clinical randomized trials are needed to determine optimal debridement methods and parameters.

DISCUSSION OF FINDINGS AND RELEVANT LITERATURE

Various debridement methods have been studied and used clinically, including surgical, mechanical, enzymatic, biological, and autolytic. Although all show evidence of efficacy, some of the supporting literature has design limitations. No single debridement method has been shown to be ideal for all clinical situations, suggesting that there is room for further research and new advances in this field. More recently, CT has been developed for debridement and our recent work with this modality (unpublished data) will be presented.

Surgical debridement

Surgical debridement is the gold standard therapy for rapid removal of necrotic, infected tissue from a wound and can immediately expose undermined tissue, hidden abscesses, or sinus tracts. Callus formation, typically seen at the edges of diabetic foot ulcers, exerts physical traction preventing wound closure[13] and is only amenable to surgical debridement. Neuropathic foot ulcers responded with a higher rate of wound closure in centers that performed more frequent debridements.[4,13] The benefit of surgical debridement has also been demonstrated in chronic venous leg ulcers.[24]

Mechanical debridement

Mechanical debridement methods physically remove debris from the wound bed and include wet-to-dry dressings, irrigation-pulsed lavage, ultrasonic mist, and the more recently introduced is Versajet™ hydrosurgery.

Wet-to-dry dressings consist of applying saline-soaked gauze to the wound, and upon removal of the gauze, the embedded tissue and debris are removed with it. Technically, this is the simplest method of mechanical debridement but requires frequent dressing changes, is extremely painful to the patient, and can remove viable tissue.

Irrigation therapy involves directing a stream of water under low or high pressure toward the wound bed with the purpose of removing bacteria, necrotic tissue, and exudate. The main concerns with using pulsed lavage are destruction of viable tissue and forceful penetration of bacteria into the wound. In a contaminated goat musculoskeletal wound model, pulsed lavage was effective in removing bacteria immediately after irrigation; however, after 48 h, bacterial counts were elevated, implying that pressure irrigation may promote later infection.[22] Conversely, in a contaminated rat dorsal wound model, pulsed lavage resulted in lower bacterial counts for up to 10 days.[21]

Ultrasonic mist debridement removes necrotic debris and promotes wound healing using acoustic energy derived from sound waves at varying frequencies delivered by a saline mist. An unblinded study of 70 patients with ischemic leg ulcers showed a significant difference in the likelihood to achieve 50% closure at 12 weeks when ultrasonic mist was used, compared with standard wound care.[25] Nevertheless, a systematic review of online databases concluded that insufficient evidence is available to determine whether ultrasonic mist is effective in debriding devitalized tissue in nonhealing wounds.[26]

Low-frequency ultrasound without mist has been evaluated as an adjunct to the treatment of nonhealing venous ulcers in a regimen consisting of 10 min of foot bathing with application of continuous ultrasound three times per week. Studies showed a statistically significant decrease in ulcer area after 8 and 12 weeks of treatment when compared with conventional therapy alone.[27,28]

More recently, the Versajet device has been utilized for hydrosurgical debridement of chronic wounds of various etiologies.[29] This device was found to be faster and more precise than a hand-held dermatome for performing escharectomy in patients with burns,[30] although no significant difference in healing was seen. Most of the evidence for efficacy of hydrosurgery is based on expert opinion lacking control groups.[31] An increase in aerosolized bacteria was measured for up to 1 h postdebridement, implying that a risk for cross contamination exists when using this modality.[32]

Enzymatic debridement

Enzymatic debridement is the method by which the application of naturally occurring proteolytic enzymes degrades necrotic tissue. This technique can be used in the setting of either yellow slough or black eschar and has been shown to be beneficial in the treatment of leg ulcers,[33] pressure ulcers,[34] and burns.[35] Although collagenase and papain/urea have been the agents most frequently used, the Food and Drug Administration has recently removed all topical papain products from the market.

TAKE-HOME MESSAGE

Basic science advances

- The cellular and molecular environment in a chronic wound bed presents multiple barriers which inhibit wound closure and delay healing.
- Chronic wounds contain excessive concentrations of MMPs which degrade the matrix, resulting in defective remodeling of the ECM.
- Macromolecules produced by matrix degradation along with host fibrinogen and fibrin sequester growth factors and render them ineffective.
- Epidermal hyperproliferation at the nonhealing wound edge is associated with impaired migration and subsequent failure of reepithelialization.
- Debridement may influence ECM homeostasis and formation of normal granulation tissue by removal of senescent fibroblasts and MMPs from the wound base.

Clinical science advances

- The study by Steed *et al.*[13] in patients with diabetic foot ulcers treated with recombinant human platelet-derived growth factor provides evidence that more frequent debridement results in increased wound closure rates. This study not only demonstrated the effectiveness of growth factor therapy in the healing of chronic wounds, but also suggested that debridement may create a wound environment where both exogenous and endogenous growth factors can effectively bind to their receptors.
- Necrotic tissue not only presents a physical barrier to healing, but also contains bacteria and proinflammatory toxic material. To better assess efficacy, future clinical trials should use standardized endpoints such as the "healing rate" which has been shown to be 80% sensitive and specific for predicting ultimate wound closure in venous and diabetic ulcers at 4 weeks of therapy.[7]

Relevance to clinical care

- The clinician must select the appropriate method of debridement based on multiple factors such as wound characteristics, vascular status, general medical condition, and available resources.[2]
- The molecular, cellular, and bacteriologic abnormalities that impair chronic wound healing must be corrected on an ongoing basis for healing to occur.

Although several studies have shown enzymatic debridement to be efficacious in the treatment of burn wounds,[18,19,35,36] it has been previously reported that the use of this modality in wounds with $>10^5$ CFU/g tissue is unsafe unless used with topical antimicrobials.[37] These reports stated that enzymatic treatment of burn wounds may facilitate the proliferation and invasion of microorganisms, leading to sepsis.[38] More recently, a study evaluating the microbiologic effects of both collagenase and papain/urea in an infected rodent burn model showed the ability of these agents to reduce bacterial load to below 10^5 and accelerate wound closure.[37] This result refutes the notion that enzymatic debridement agents are unsafe if not used with concomitant antimicrobials.

Biological debridement

Maggot debridement therapy (MDT) is effective in degrading necrotic tissue because of larval release of proteolytic enzymes. Secretion of antimicrobial substances by these organisms has also been reported.[39]

This modality is being used more frequently in Europe[7] and mild pain occurs commonly. Bleeding has been reported with its use and MDT may be contraindicated adjacent to a major vessel.[39] Only two studies[40,41] assessed wound closure rates and the results were conflicting. The largest study comparing MDT to conventional therapy showed no benefit in reducing bacterial load,[41] whereas a limited number of small studies suggested that MDT may have some antimicrobial properties.[39]

Autolytic debridement

Autolytic debridement utilizes endogenous proteolytic enzymes derived from neutrophils (*e.g.*, elastase, collagenase, lysozyme, and myeloperoxidase) to liquefy slough or eschar.[1] Although this form of autolysis can be slow, it can be accelerated with the use of occlusive dressings which promote a moist wound environment that enhances proteolytic activity and growth factor-mediated healing.[42] When using these dressings, exudate must be constantly monitored as the accumulation of chronic wound fluid may cause degradation of ECM proteins and inhibition of cell proliferation, resulting in delayed wound healing.[43]

More studies are needed to evaluate the use of combination dressings as they may prove to be a better alternative with fewer complications than traditional wound dressings.

Coblation technology

CT, when employed using a saline medium, creates a plasma consisting of an excited electron field which causes tissue to be ablated or coagulated, depending on the voltage applied. At high voltages, a bipolar plasma field is generated at the tip of the device between active and return electrodes, which allows for devitalized tissue to be vaporized at low temperatures (40–70°C).[44,45] The ability of this device to effectively remove surface debris without causing thermal injury to surrounding tissues has resulted in its increasingly widespread use in the medical field. CT can also be used at lower voltages to coagulate small vessels, achieving a bloodless surgical field.[46]

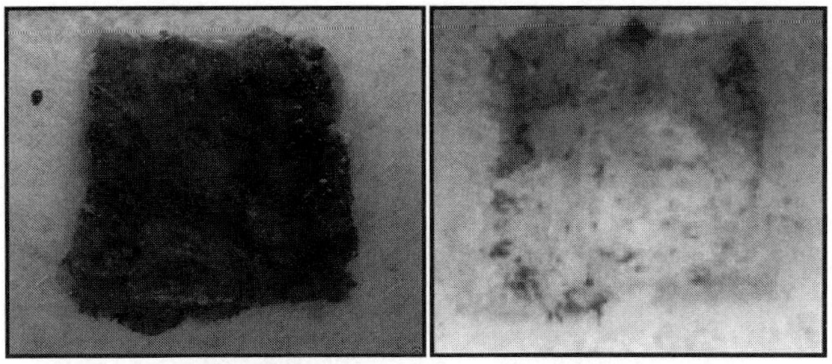

Figure 1. Photographs of dye removal with coblation.

Using a porcine model we examined the capability of CT (PROcise XP; ArthroCare, Austin, TX) to remove nonviable tissue in wound debridement as well as its effectiveness in reducing wound bacterial load. To determine wound debridement performance, we measured the effectiveness of CT to remove a black dye from partial-thickness wound sites. Pre- and posttreatment photographs were obtained and compared visually as well as by digital image analysis. Only 6.27% of the dye remained after treatment (Fig. 1), suggesting that CT could remove nonviable tissue from the wound surface. To determine the microbiologic effects, partial-thickness wounds were treated at 20 min and 24 h after inoculation. Compared with untreated controls, CT treatment resulted in a statistically significant reduction ($p < 0.05$) of planktonic and biofilm-associated bacteria (Fig. 2). These results suggest potential clinical implications for the use of this new treatment modality of wound debridement of chronic and burn wounds. Additional, well-controlled clinical trials are warranted.

CAUTION, CRITICAL REMARKS, AND RECOMMENDATIONS

Although it is widely accepted that removal of necrotic tissue from chronic wounds is beneficial, there are clinical situations in which debridement may be contraindicated. Necrotic wounds without

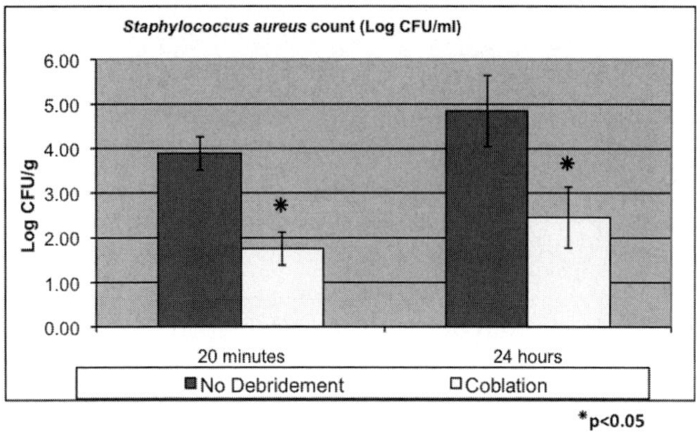

Figure 2. Staphylococcus aureus counts (log CFU/mL).

adequate blood supply, such as black eschars on ischemic toes, should not be debrided, as dry gangrenous toes could be converted to wet gangrene with subsequent infection.[2] When vascularity is adequate but general medical conditions exist which will impede healing despite debridement efforts, the underlying factors must be resolved for healing to progress.[2] If advancing necrosis or a source of infection is present, surgical debridement is the treatment of choice.[47] Conversely, when a slower approach is acceptable, enzymatic or autolytic debridement can be considered, especially when surgery or anesthesia is contraindicated. Pain must be considered when selecting a method of debridement.[3] As mechanical or surgical debridement can be very painful and requires the use of anesthetics, methods such as autolytic debridement with occlusive dressings or negative pressure wound therapy can be more comfortable for the patient. Guidelines for implementing a specific modality in a particular clinical situation are generally based on expert opinion rather than on evidence-based medicine.[2,7]

FUTURE DEVELOPMENTS

New debridement methods and assessments are being developed to help in the removal of nonviable tissue. One such method is the CT discussed earlier, which uses a focused plasma to remove necrotic tissue and bacteria at lower temperatures than previously used cautery devices.[48] Further evaluations of the value of CT in wound management, including well-controlled clinical trials, are needed.

Although, currently, clinical parameters such as the wound bed score and the debridement performance index are available to guide the clinician regarding the need for debridement as well as its effectiveness,[7] the study by Brem *et al.*,[8] using gene expression profiling to differentiate senescent from viable wound cells, provides the foreground for development of an assay to guide the margins of debridement based on molecular markers.

ACKNOWLEDGMENT

This coblation study was supported by Arthrocare, Inc.

AUTHOR DISCLOSURE STATEMENT

No competing financial interests exist.

REFERENCES

1. Schultz GS, Sibbald RG, Falanga V, Ayello E, Dowsett C, Harding K, Romanelli M, Stacey M, Teot L, and Vanscheid W: Wound bed preparation: a systematic approach to wound management. Wound Repair Regen 2003; **11 (Suppl 1):** S1.

2. Kirshen C, Woo K, Ayello EA, and Sibbald RG: Debridement: a vital component of wound bed preparation. Adv Skin Wound Care 2006; **19:** 506; quiz 517.

3. Sieggreen MY and Maklebust J: Debridement: choices and challenges. Adv Wound Care 1997; **10:** 32.

4. Steed DL: Clinical evaluation of recombinant human platelet-derived growth factor for the treatment of lower extremity ulcers. Plast Reconstr Surg 2006; **117 (Suppl 7):** 143S; discussion 150S.

5. Schultz GS, Barillo DJ, Mozingo DW, and Chin GA: Wound bed preparation and a brief history of TIME. Int Wound J 2004; **1:** 19.

6. Tomic-Canic M, Ayello EA, Stojadinovic O, Golinko MS, and Brem H: Using gene transcription patterns (bar coding scans) to guide wound debridement and healing. Adv Skin Wound Care 2008; **21:** 487; quiz 493.

7. Falanga V, Brem H, Ennis WJ, Wolcott R, Gould LJ, and Ayello EA: Maintenance debridement in the treatment of difficult-to-heal chronic wounds: recommendations of an expert panel. Ostomy Wound Manage 2008; **Suppl 2;** quiz 14.

8. Brem H, Stojadinovic O, Diegelmann RF, Entero H, Lee B, Pastar I, Golinko M, Rosenberg H, and Tomic-Canic M: Molecular markers in patients with chronic wounds to guide surgical debridement. Mol Med 2007; **13:** 30.

9. Agren MS, Steenfos HH, Dabelsteen S, Hansen JB, and Dabelsteen E: Proliferation and mitogenic response to PDGF-BB of fibroblasts isolated from chronic venous leg ulcers is ulcer-age dependent. J Invest Dermatol 1999; **112:** 463.

10. Hasan A, Murata H, Falabella A, Ochoa S, Zhou L, Badiavas E, and Falanga V: Dermal fibroblasts from venous ulcers are unresponsive to the action of transforming growth factor-beta 1. J Dermatol Sci 1997; **16:** 59.

11. Stojadinovic O, Brem H, Vouthounis C, Lee B, Fallon J, Stallcup M, Merchant A, Galiano R, and Tomic-Canic M: Molecular pathogenesis of chronic wounds: the role of beta-catenin and c-myc in the inhibition of epithelialization and wound healing. Am J Pathol 2005; **167:** 59.

12. Kirsner R: Wound bed preparation. Ostomy Wound Manage 2003; **49 (Suppl 2)**.

13. Steed DL, Donohoe D, Webster MW, and Lindsley L: Effect of extensive debridement and treatment on the healing of diabetic foot ulcers. Diabetic Ulcer Study Group. J Am Coll Surg 1996; **183:** 61.

14. Sullivan TP, Eaglstein WH, Davis SC, and Mertz P: The pig as a model for human wound healing. Wound Repair Regen 2001; **9:** 66.

15. Davis SC, Mertz PM, Bilevich ED, Cazzaniga AL, and Eaglstein WH: Early debridement of second-degree burn wounds enhances the rate of epithelization—an animal model to evaluate burn wound therapies. J Burn Care Rehabil 1996; **17(6, Pt 1):** 558.

16. Krieger Y, Rosenberg L, Lapid O, Glesinger R, Bogdanov-Berezovsky A, Silberstein E, Sagi A, and Judkins K: Escharotomy using an enzymatic debridement agent for treating experimental burn-induced compartment syndrome in an animal model. J Trauma 2005; **58:** 1259.

17. Mekkes JR, Le Poole IC, Das PK, Bos JD, and Westerhof W: Efficient debridement of necrotic wounds using proteolytic enzymes derived from Antarctic krill: a double-blind, placebo-controlled study in a standardized animal wound model. Wound Repair Regen 1998; **6:** 50.

18. Bott R, Crissman J, Kollar C, Saldajeno M, Ganshaw G, Thomas X, Lane T, Klykken P, Davidson J, and Nanney L: A silicone-based controlled-release device for accelerated proteolytic debridement of wounds. Wound Repair Regen 2007; **15:** 227.

19. Orgill DP, Liu PY, Ritterbush LS, Skrabut EM, Samuels JA, and Shames SL: Debridement of porcine burns with a highly purified, ananain-based cysteine protease preparation. J Burn Care Rehabil 1996; **17:** 311.

20. Gurfinkel R, Lavon I, Cagnano E, Volgin K, Shaltiel L, Grossman N, Kost J, Singer A and Rosenberg L: Combined ultrasonic and enzymatic debridement of necrotic eschars in an animal model. J Burn Care Res 2009; **30:** 505.

21. Brown LL, Shelton HT, Bornside GH, and Cohn I, Jr.: Evaluation of wound irrigation by pulsatile jet and conventional methods. Ann Surg 1978; **187:** 170.

22. Owens BD, White DW, and Wenke JC: Comparison of irrigation solutions and devices in a contaminated musculoskeletal wound survival model. J Bone Joint Surg Am 2009; **91:** 92.

23. Caprise PA, Jr., Miclau T, Dahners LE, and Dirschl DR: High-pressure pulsatile lavage irrigation of contaminated fractures: effects on fracture healing. J Orthop Res 2002; **20:** 1205.

24. Williams D, Enoch S, Miller D, Harris K, Price P, and Harding KG: Effect of sharp debridement using curette on recalcitrant nonhealing venous leg ulcers: a concurrently controlled, prospective cohort study. Wound Repair Regen 2005; **13:** 131.

25. Kavros SJ, Miller JL, and Hanna SW: Treatment of ischemic wounds with noncontact, low-frequency ultrasound: the Mayo Clinic experience, 2004–2006. Adv Skin Wound Care 2007; **20:** 221.

26. Ramundo J and Gray M: Is ultrasonic mist therapy effective for debriding chronic wounds? J Wound Ostomy Continence Nurs 2008; **35:** 579.

27. Mohr P, Stegmann W, and Breitbart EW: Low-frequency ultrasound treatment of chronic venous ulcers. Wound Repair Regen 1997; **5:** 18.

28. Peschen M, Weichenthal M, Schopf E, and Vanscheidt W: Low-frequency ultrasound treatment of chronic venous leg ulcers in an outpatient therapy. Acta Derm Venereol 1997; **77:** 311.

29. Gurunluoglu R: Experiences with waterjet hydrosurgery system in wound debridement. World J Emerg Surg 2007; **2:** 10.

30. Gravante G, Delogu D, Esposito G, and Montone A: Versajet hydrosurgery versus classic escharectomy for burn debridment: a prospective randomized trial. J Burn Care Res 2007; **28:** 720.

31. Sainsbury DC: Evaluation of the quality and cost-effectiveness of Versajet hydrosurgery. Int Wound J 2009; **6:** 24.

32. Bowling FL, Stickings DS, Edwards-Jones V, Armstrong DG, and Boulton AJ: Hydrodebridement of wounds: effectiveness in reducing wound bacterial contamination and potential for air bacterial contamination. J Foot Ankle Res 2009; **2:** 13.

33. Ramundo J and Gray M: Enzymatic wound debridement. J Wound Ostomy Continence Nurs 2008; **35:** 273.

34. Alvarez O, Fernandez-Obregon A, Rogers RS, Bergamo L, Masso J, Black M: A prospective randomized comparative study of collagenase and papain-urea for pressure ulcer debridement. Wounds 2002; **14:** 293.

35. Rosenberg L, Lapid O, Bogdanov-Berezovsky A, Glesinger R, Krieger Y, Silberstein E, Sagi A, Judkins K, and Singer A: Safety and efficacy of a proteolytic enzyme for enzymatic burn debridement: a preliminary report. Burns 2004; **30:** 843.

36. Soroff HS and Sasvary DH: Collagenase ointment and polymyxin B sulfate/bacitracin spray versus silver sulfadiazine cream in partial-thickness burns: a pilot study. J Burn Care Rehabil 1994; **15:** 13.

37. Payne WG, Salas RE, Ko F, Naidu DK, Donate G, Wright TE, and Robson MC: Enzymatic debriding agents are safe in wounds with high bacterial bioburdens and stimulate healing. Eplasty 2008; **8:** e17.

38. Hummel RP, Kautz PD, MacMillan BG, and Altemeier WA: The continuing problem of sepsis following enzymatic debridement of burns. J Trauma 1974; **14:** 572.

39. Gray M: Is larval (maggot) debridement effective for removal of necrotic tissue from chronic wounds? J Wound Ostomy Continence Nurs 2008; **35:** 378.

40. Armstrong DG, Salas P, Short B, Martin BR, Kimbriel H, Nixon B, and Boulton A: Maggot therapy in "lower-extremity hospice" wound care: fewer amputations and more antibiotic-free days. J Am Podiatr Med Assoc 2005; **95:** 254.

41. Dumville JC, Worthy G, Bland JM, Cullum N, Dowson C, Iglesias C, Mitchell J, Nelson E, Soares M, and Torgerson D: Larval therapy for leg ulcers (VenUS II): randomised controlled trial. BMJ 2009; **338:** b773.

42. Chen WY, Rogers AA, and Lydon MJ: Characterization of biologic properties of wound fluid collected during early stages of wound healing. J Invest Dermatol 1992; **99:** 559.

43. Bucalo B, Eaglstein WH, and Falanga V: Inhibition of cell proliferation by chronic wound fluid. Wound Repair Regen 1993; **1:** 181.

44. Woloszko J, Stalder K, and Brown I: Plasma characteristics of repetitively-pulsed electrical discharges in saline solutions used for surgical procedures. IEEE Trans Plasma Sci 2002; **30:** 1376.

45. Stalder K, Woloszko J, Brown I, and Smith C: Repetitive plasma discharges in saline solutions. Appl Phys Lett 2001; **79:** 4503.

46. Mancini PF: Coblation: a new technology and technique for skin resurfacing and other aesthetic surgical procedures. Aesthetic Plast Surg 2001; **25:** 372.

47. Schiffman J, Golinko MS, Yan A, Flattau A, Tomic-Canic M, and Brem H: Operative debridement of pressure ulcers. World J Surg 2009; **33:** 1396.

48. Shah UK and Dunham B: Coblation for tonsillectomy: an evidence-based review. ORL J Otorhinolaryngol Relat Spec 2007; **69:** 349.

Debridement in Surgical Wounds

Luc Téot*

Burns and Plastic Unit, Lapeyronie Hospital, Montpellier, France.

Abbreviations and Acronyms

EUSOL = Edinburgh University Solution of Lime

RCTs = randomized controlled trials

SD = standard deviation

*Correspondence: Burns and Plastic Unit, Hôpital Lapeyronie, 371 Ave. Doyen Giraud 34295 Montpellier cedex, Montpellier, France (e-mail: lteot@aol.com).

Background: A systematic review published in 1999 indicated that there were no studies comparing nondebridement with debridement. A guidance document on the use of debriding agents for difficult-to-heal surgical wounds highlighted the absence of randomized controlled trials to support any particular method of debridement.

The Problem: Surgical debridement may be achieved by the aggressive excision of all devitalized tissues using surgical techniques. Disadvantages associated with this method are the requirement for hospital admission, the administration of an anesthetic, and time taken in the operating theatre. Autolytic debridement is a natural tendency to remove sloughy tissues and is promoted by the maintenance of a moist environment by the judicious use of dressings and topical agents.

Basic/Clinical Science Advances: Dryburgh and colleagues had developed an extensive review to determine the effect of different methods of debridement on the rate of debridement and healing of surgical wounds. Five trials were selected and analyzed.

Clinical Care Relevance: The common outcome was the time to a clean wound bed for infected postsurgical wounds. A limited range of treatments was identified with dextranomer beads or paste and different comparisons used in each trial; therefore, it was not possible to pool the results. The enzymatic agent (streptokinase/streptodornase) demonstrated a statistically significant reduction in the time to a clean wound bed when compared with saline-soaked dressings.

Conclusion: The trials included in this review were of poor quality. Trials reflecting the wider range of debridement methods and agents for surgical wounds were not identified.

INTRODUCTION

Postoperative infection and dehiscence rate vary depending on the length of the surgical procedure, the type of surgery, and the organ involved (2.4% for skin surgery). These wounds present variable amounts of devitalized tissues, with different aspects such as necrosis, fibrous tissues, or green, thick purulent odorous exudate. This accumulation of nonviable elements will impede wound healing.

Even if surgical debridement is a natural strategy for a surgeon who allegates some responsibilities in the immediate pejorative evolution of the operative wound, no significant statistical data exist to find this attitude. Smell *et al.*,[1] in a study analyzing the interest of a becaplermin, showed a positive effect of surgical debridement as secondary outcome. A list of new debriding agents was recently proposed, which focused on the whirlpools and hydrojets, with

ADVANCES IN WOUND CARE, VOLUME 1

Printed in U.S.A.
DOI: 10.1089/awc.2009.0180

immediate removal of sloughy tissues and a peroperative obtention of a clean wound bed.[2] These purely visual arguments have not yet been considered as conclusive on the long-term capacity of expedite wound healing using these techniques.

Milder approaches have been developed, defined as the mechanical or sharp debridement. Repetitive mild excisions of devitalized tissues are often performed. This nurse-based technique is commonly realized in the nonsurgical settings (rehabilitation center or the community), where a patient has been sent from the surgical ward.

Other nonsurgical techniques have been described, like biosurgery using living maggots. *Lucilia sericata* produces enzymes like collagenases that degrade undesired tissues and swallow them. This technique became popular in the articles that were published during 1999–2003, issuing to the intensive use of these helpers, more in diabetic foot debridement and in acute trauma setting management.

Autolytic debridement is based on the natural tendency of the body to eliminate spontaneously dead tissues, and it has been extensively used since Winter demonstrated the interest of moist wound healing over situations when a limited amount of deleterious items is present. The principle of these techniques is to hydrate and moisten the wound bed, transforming the hard fibrous tissues into liquid, more easy to remove during the next dressing change.

Dextranomer (beads and paste) presented as a candidate for this purpose, until the production was stopped in 2007 (except in South Africa).

The wet to dry debridement was a method where saline-soaked gauze dressing was regularly applied over a wound. The dry eschar was softened by the wet ambiance, and once the gauze is drying, the necrotic and sloughy tissues attached to the gauze, and were removed during the next dressing. The intense provoked pain and damages to the healthy tissues were the cause for cessation of this technique.

A scoring debridement system has been proposed by Margolis and colleagues for leg ulcers,[3] but no parallel has yet been detailed concerning surgical wounds.

The Cochrane Review realized by Dryburgh and colleagues in 2009[4] gives a focus on the numerous methods available, noting that no consensus exists on which one is most effective. The result of this analysis reports that debridement for surgical wounds has not been demonstrated as getting a sufficient level of evidence, whatever be the proposed technique.

MATERIAL

Nonviable tissues not only inhibit the growth of the epithelial tissues but also increase the production of exudate, impair assessment of the wound bed, and make it more difficult to achieve wound closure, thus having an adverse effect on the quality of life.[5] Although Baharestani (6) details a number of reasons for the removal of the dead tissues (as detailed above), these reasons do not appear to be supported by the robust, scientific evidence. Debridement is the process whereby foreign material and dead or damaged tissue and debris are removed from a wound.[6] The extent of the field of debridement must be related to the large number of possible situations, ranging from prevention of accumulation of small amounts of undesired tissues to the need for life salvage in surgical debridement of extensive Fournier gangrene, a rare postoperative complication encountered after perineal surgical procedures. Usually, surgeons will tend to reapproximate the wound after a second debridement and closure of the postoperative infected wound, strongly believing that primary closure is more adapted than secondary closure, which needs more time to be completed.

There is a considerable debate on the appropriateness and efficacy of debridement methods.[7] A systematic review published in 1999 indicated that there were no studies comparing nondebridement with debridement, and therefore, the benefits of debridement on wound healing were unclear.[8] A guidance document on the use of debriding agents for difficult-to-heal surgical wounds highlighted the lack of sufficient evidence and the corresponding absence of randomized controlled trials (RCTs) to support any particular method of debridement. Edwards and Killen[9] found suggestive evidence in a higher rate of healing when using hydrogels compared with gauze in diabetic foot. This, however, did not mention infected diabetic ulcers.

Surgical debridement

Surgical debridement may be achieved by the aggressive excision of all devitalized tissues using surgical techniques.[10–12] Disadvantages associated with this method are the requirement for hospital admission, the administration of an anesthetic with associated complications, and time in the operating theatre. It is also associated with pain, bleeding and excision of healthy tissues and, as such, is not suitable or desirable for all patients. However, for both surgical and sharp procedures, issues of patient consent, training and skill of the clinician must be considered.[13]

Biosurgical/biological debridement

In biosurgical or biological debridement, sterile larvae (maggots) of the *Lucilia sericata* species of greenbottle fly were applied to a sloughy wound. There the larvae are capable of producing powerful proteolytic enzymes that destroy the dead tissues by liquifying and ingesting it.

Healthy tissues in the wound bed are not damaged; although there are aesthetic considerations, larvae are increasingly being used for wound debridement.[5,14–16]

Autolytic debridement

Over time, naturally occurring enzymes will eventually breakdown and dissolve dead or sloughy tissues in wounds. This natural process is promoted by the maintenance of a moist environment by the judicious use of dressings and topical agents (*e.g.*, hydrogels, semiocclusive, and occlusive wound dressings). Many of these dressings hydrate and remove black, necrotic tissues, and slough.[5,6,14] Dextranomer is an example of a hydroscopic dressing that has a high absorptive capacity, capable of removing bacteria, debris, and absorbing wound exudate, thereby facilitating autolytic debridement. However, worldwide production of dextranomer beads and paste was discontinued in 2007, with the exception of the paste that is still available in South Africa.

Mechanical debridement

Mechanical methods of debridement are nonselective, operator dependent, and may result in damage to healthy tissues.[5] The nurse will have a tendency to focus her debridement in the depth of 1.5 cm at the surface of the wound, when a specialized nurse will be trained to perform a deeper debridement. The techniques are essentially based on the two principles of no pain and no bleeding, preventing with an appropriate training to be aggressive to the normal healthy tissues. On the other hand, sharp debridement involves the excision of small quantities of dead tissues by a clinician using scissors or a scalpel.[16] This procedure may be performed in a community or hospital setting.[17]

Wet to dry debridement

The wet to dry method of debridement has been abandoned because of the high provoked pain this technique induced. It is based on the application of a saline-soaked gauze dressing to a wound. The moist dressing induces separation of the devitalized tissues, and once dried, the dressing is removed, together with the slough and necrotic tissues. This process is continued until all the devitalized tissues are removed. This is reported to be a painful procedure and may damage healthy tissues; fibers may be left in the wound, and the dressing does not provide a barrier to bacterial contamination.[5,15,16]

Wound cleansing debridement

Irrigating a wound with a continuous or intermittent flow of fluid delivered under mild pressure (between 8 and 12 pounds psi) is sufficient to remove devitalized tissues and wound bacteria.[5] Newer devices using higher pressures were recently proposed,[18] with a positive effect on granulation tissue formation.

Some whirlpool systems use highly pressurized saline delivered via a nozzle between 12,800 and 15,000 psi.[19] Whirlpool debridement is used for large wounds where sticky materials have to be detached from the bed wall; these devices allow harvest successive slices of tissues that are immediately extracted from the wound bed using an appropriate aspirating ending incorporated into the extremity, preventing contamination of the surrounding normal tissues.

Some authors, mainly in Central Europe and Germany, combine whirlpool and active solutions such as Lavasept or Prontosan. Composed partly of biguanides (derived from chlorhexidine solutions), they include a low concentration of antimicrobial (0.1%) solutions. The recent possibility to irrigate postoperative wounds using a modified negative pressure therapy unit has to be confirmed in terms of interest in reducing the numbers of germs and issuing to wound closure.

Chemical debridement

A range of chemical agents, including hypochlorites such as Edinburgh University Solution of Lime (EUSOL), Dakin's solution (sodium hypochlorite), hydrogen peroxide, and iodine, have been used to promote debridement of wounds. The use of chemical agents remains a controversial area, in which any benefits need to be judged against any detrimental effects on the process of healing.[5,20,21]

Enzymatic debridement

Topical enzymatic preparations are applied to moist (or moistened) devitalized tissues. Such preparations include streptokinase/streptodornase,[14,15] collagenase,[17] papain/urea, and a combination of fibrinolysin and deoxyribonuclease.[17]

This method has a number of disadvantages, including a requirement for frequent dressing changes and a slow rate of debridement. Worldwide production of the enzymatic preparation of streptokinase/streptodornase has now been discontinued.

CLINICAL PROBLEM ADDRESSED

Postoperative infections may have different potential origins, depending on the anatomical site where the infection develops. Infection can be localized at the skin level, on the surgical incision deeper along the track, or at the level of the operated organ itself.

Most of the time the surgeon, in charge of the postoperative period, will try to understand where the problem is localized and how he can fix it.

His preferred strategy will be to propose a re-operation to clean the wound and remove debris and infected tissues. Surgeons are not likely to develop RCTs, and in particular case no strong evidence can be withdrawn from the literature concerning the accuracy of these strategies.

Dryburgh and colleagues[4] had developed an extensive review to determine the effect of different methods of debridement on the rate of debridement and healing of surgical wounds. They developed a search strategy to search the following electronic databases: Wounds Group Specialised Trials Register (searched 3/3/08), Cochrane Central Register of Controlled Trials (CENTRAL) (the Cochrane Library, 2008, issue 1), MEDLINE (1950 to February Week 3 2008), EMBASE (1980 to 2008 Week 09), and CINHAL (1982 to February Week 4 2008). They checked the citations within obtained studies to identify additional articles and also relevant conference proceedings. They contacted manufactures of wound debridement agents to ascertain the existence of published, unpublished, and ongoing trials. Their search was not limited by language or publication status.

They included relevant RCTs with outcomes including at least one of the following: time to complete debridement or time to complete healing.

Two authors independently reviewed the abstracts and titles obtained from the search, two extracted data independently using a standardized extraction sheet, and two independently assessed the methodological quality. One author was involved in all stages of the data collection and extraction process, thus ensuring continuity.

Five RCTs were eligible for inclusion; all compared treatments for infected surgical wounds and reported the time required to achieve a clean wound bed (complete debridement). One trial compared an enzymatic agent (streptokinase/streptodornase) with saline-soaked dressings and reported the time to complete debridement. Four of the trials compared the effectiveness of dextranomer beads or paste with other products (different comparator in each trial) to achieve complete debridement. Meta-analysis was not possible because of the unique comparisons within each trial. One trial reported that dextranomer achieved a clean wound bed significantly more quickly than EUSOL, and one trial comparing enzymatic debridement with saline-soaked dressings reported that the enzyme-treated wounds were cleaned more quickly. However, the methodological quality was poor in these two trials.

The authors' conclude that there is a lack of large, high-quality published RCTs evaluating debridement *per se* or comparing different methods of debridement for surgical wounds, to guide clinical decision making.

BASIC SCIENCE CONTEXT

During a surgical procedure, many factors occur at the wound bed site to favor complications. Well-reported factors are the length of the procedure, the accessibility of the operated organ, the pressure exerted by retractors on the skin, the general health condition of the patient, and the septic ambiance. The resistance to closure of the wound may also be influenced by mechanical forces exerted on the wound edges, an unadapted drainage, or the presence of intense inflammation over the edges of the wounds.

Several visible complications can be observed, like damaged fat presence under a closing skin, leakage coming from an opened organ, or accumulation of pus around the operated organ, linked to poor local vascularization, or problems of ischemia and reperfusion. Collagenases and metalloproteases accumulate into the wound, turning the initially considered acute wound into a cascade of event comparable to what is usually observed in chronic wounds.

If this is well accepted that surgeons will come back to revisit their field of operation around the organs they previously operated, a few data have gone to consensus concerning the most adapted strategy to follow on a superficial dehiscence of the wound.

DISCUSSION OF FINDINGS AND RELEVANT LITERATURE

The objectives of Dryburgh *et al.*[4] were to determine the effects of different debriding methods on the rate of debridement and healing of surgical wounds.

Their methods considered the criteria for analyzing the type studies for this review, and they included all RCTs evaluating debridement in the management of surgical wounds.

Table 1.

Types of interventions, any method of debridement was accepted
Primary outcomes
Time to complete debridement
The proportion of wounds completely debrided during the trial period
The rate of reduction in wound size expressed in either absolute or relative terms
The proportion of wounds completely healed during the trial period
Time to complete healing
Secondary outcomes
When reported, we recorded the following secondary outcomes:
Patient satisfaction (*e.g.*, pain associated with treatment as recorded using a recognized pain scale)
Rate of infection
Quality of life
Length of hospital stay
Cost-effectiveness (*e.g.*, as presented in a cost-effectiveness analysis, which may include nursing time, time taken to change dressing, number of dressing changes required, cost of dressing materials)
Serious adverse events (life threatening or those leading to hospitalization)
Other adverse events (those leading to discontinuation of treatment)
Assessment of risk of bias in included studies was realized by two authors working independently on quality criteria, adequacy of the randomization process, adequacy of allocation concealment, assessment of heterogenicity, and data synthesis

The authors recruited studies on people of any age, in any care setting, with a surgical wound that required debridement, but excluded studies of wounds that were not caused by surgery (*i.e.*, trauma, wounds, burns, abscesses or sinuses, pressure ulcers, leg ulcers, diabetic foot ulcers, fungating tumors) and wounds caused by the removal of serious adverse events (life threatening or those leading to hospitalization) and other adverse events (those leading to discontinuation of treatment) (Table 1).

RESULTS OF COMPARABLE TRIALS

Trial 1: dextranomer beads compared with EUSOL gauze (1 RCT, 20 participants)

Goode *et al.*[22] compared dextranomer beads (an autolytic debridement agent) with EUSOL-soaked ribbon gauze in 20 patients with infected surgical wounds, following appendectomy or bowel surgery (Table 2).

Goode *et al.*[22] commented on the higher cost of dextranomer (£3.40 per twice-daily dressing), but the shorter hospital stay in the treatment group compensated for this. This claim was not supported by any data.

Although they demonstrated methodological adequacy in allocation concealment and blinding of outcome assessment, an unclear randomization process, a small sample size, and insufficient data mean it is difficult to place much weight on these results.

Table 2. *Outcomes of Trial 1*

Primary outcomes
Outcome 1—time to a clean wound bed and secondary wound closure
Resolution of erythema and edema, absence of pus or slough, and the formation of granulation tissue were used as the criteria to determine a clean wound bed. Mean time to a clean wound bed was significantly shorter with dextranomer; 8.1 days compared with 11.6 days for EUSOL ($p < 0.05$, Mann–Whitney *U*-test).
Outcome 2—time to complete healing
The time to complete healing was not reported though the trialists report that one wound in each group healed without secondary closure.
Secondary outcomes
Outcome 1—patient satisfaction: not reported
Outcome 2—rate of infection: not reported
Outcome 3—quality of life: not reported
Outcome 4—length of hospital stay
Patients in the dextranomer group were described as having a shorter stay by a median of 2.2 days than the EUSOL group; however, no data for the control group were reported.
Outcome 5—cost-effectiveness: not reported

EUSOL = Edinburgh University Solution of Lime.

Further the comparator (EUSOL) is rarely used due to fears of harmful effects on healthy tissues.[23]

Trial 2: dextranomer paste compared with 10% aqueous polyvinylpyrrolidone (1 RCT, 40 participants)

Michiels and Christiaens[24] compared dextranomer paste with gauze dressings soaked in 10% aqueous polyvinylpyrrolidone (an iodine-based chemical debridement agent), in people with infected surgical

Table 3. *Outcomes of Trial 2*

Primary outcomes
Outcome 1—time to clean wound bed
The disappearance or resolution of erythema, pus and debris, edema, necrotic tissue, and the presence of granulation tissue were used as the criteria to determine a clean wound bed. The results for each variable were assessed subjectively and presented individually. The development, validity, and reliability of the assessment systems used were not reported, but the trialists did acknowledge that the evaluation was an approximation. The trial reported no significant difference between the treatment and control groups for the resolution of erythema, edema, necrotic tissue, and the development of granulation tissue. The handling and reporting of the data for the pus and debris criteria was unclear and subjective, and the groups were not comparable at baseline with respect to the amount of pus and debris. Michiels and Christiaens[24] report that dextranomer significantly reduced the time taken to clean the wound bed compared with polyvinylpyrrolidone. A *p*-value < 0.05 was reported (Student's *t*-test); however, no data were provided, and the subjective assessment of the outcome increases the risk of bias.
Outcome 2—time to complete healing
The duration of the trial was 12 days, and treatment was discontinued when the wound was clean and had new granulation tissue.
Time to complete healing was not reported.
Secondary outcomes
No secondary outcomes were reported in this trial.

Table 4. *Outcomes of Trial 3*

Primary outcomes:
Outcome 1—time to clean wound bed
The trial reported the number of days required for a clean wound bed and secondary suture. Statistical analysis of the data demonstrated that the time to a clean wound bed or secondary suture was significantly shorter for the streptokinase/streptodornase group (mean 5 days [SD 2.16]) compared with the saline-soaked dressings group (mean 13.45 days [SD 6.77] $p < 0.05$ by both Student's *t*-test and Mann–Whitney *U*-test). The time to clean wound bed was analyzed using the Student's *t*-test and Mann–Whitney *U*-test. Time to debridement or discharge of the patient is the time to event outcomes and so the treatment effect should have been expressed as a hazard ratio.
Outcome 2—time to complete healing not reported

Secondary outcomes
Outcome 1—patient satisfaction: not reported
Outcome 2—rate of infection: not reported
Outcome 3—quality of life
The trial reported that no patients in either group complained of significant discomfort from the wound.
Outcome 4—length of hospital stay
Patients in the streptokinase/streptodornase group were described as having a shorter stay by 8.5 days than the saline-soaked dressings group; however, no data or statistics were included in the trial report.
Outcome 5—cost-effectiveness: not reported

SD = standard deviation.

wounds after osteosynthesis, microsurgery, and reconstructive procedures (Table 3).

The methodological quality of this trial was poor, with only the completeness of follow-up being adequate. The validity of the results is questionable.

Trial 3: streptokinase/streptodornase compared with saline-soaked dressing (1 RCT, 21 participants)

One small randomized trial compared enzymatic debridement with streptokinase/streptodornase with saline-soaked dressings. Poulson *et al* developed a trial[25] in people with infected abdominal surgical wounds after a range of operations (Table 4).

Methodological adequacy is reported in the randomization process, allocation concealment, blinded outcome assessment, and completeness of follow-up. However, poor handling and analysis of the data and a small sample size are the drawbacks of this trial. The validity of the results is therefore questionable.

Trial 4: dextranomer beads compared with 0.1% chloramine-soaked dressings (1 RCT, 28 participants)

Sondergaard and Galatius[26] randomized 28 patients with infected, open surgical wounds, to dextranomer or 0.1% chloramine group (Table 5).

Methodological quality is poor, and none of the adequacy criteria was met by this trial.

Table 5. *Outcomes of Trial 4*

Primary outcomes:
Outcome 1—time to clean wound bed
The number of days until the wounds were clinically clean were reported as a median of 6 days with dextranomer and 5 days with chloramine-soaked dressings (described as no significant difference; however, no data were provided). The criteria used to determine when the wound was clinically clean were not reported.
Outcome 2—time from the start of the treatment till the patient was assessed as ready for outpatient treatment
This was reported as a median of 9 days for dextranomer and 7 days for chloramines; the difference between the two groups was reported as not significant. However, no variance data were reported.
Outcome 3—time to complete healing
The time to complete healing was reported as a median of 27 days for the dextranomer group and 20 days for the chloramine group (no variance data provided). This was described by the trialists as no significant difference between the groups.

Secondary outcomes:
Outcome 1—patient satisfaction
The trialists reported that the dextranomer dressing was less painful as it was easier to remove. However, no data were included.
Outcome 2—rate of infection: not reported
Outcome 3—quality of life: not reported
Outcome 4—length of hospital stay: not reported
Outcome 5—cost-effectiveness
The average cost per change of dressing for the dextranomer group was 123 Danish Kroner compared with approximately 1.50 Danish Kroner for the chloramine group; however, no further cost analysis was reported.

Trial 5: dextranomer beads compared with elastomer foam (1 RCT, 50 participants)

Young and Wheeler[27] randomized 50 people with infected, open surgical wounds between treatment with dextranomer beads and a foam elastomer dressing (Table 6).

Table 6. *Outcomes of Trial 5*

Primary outcomes:
Outcome 1—time to clean wound bed: not reported
Outcome 2—time to complete healing
There was no statistically significant difference in the mean time to healing (40.92 days [SD = 3.98] with dextranomer compared with 36.90 days [SD = 3.18] for elastomer foam). The time to clean wound bed was analyzed as continuous data, using the Student's *t*-test ($p > 0.05$). The time to a clean wound bed is a time to event outcome and so the treatment effect should have been expressed as a hazard ratio.

Secondary outcomes
Outcome 1—patient satisfaction
The trialists reported that comfort of the dressing was assessed by questioning the patient. Pain of the wound was graded, and the mean time to a pain-free wound was reduced with dextranomer at 5.32 days (SD = 0.55) compared with 5.64 days (SD = 0.45) for foam. Once again the analysis of the data of time to a pain-free wound should have been expressed as a hazard ratio.
Outcome 2—rate of infection: not reported
Outcome 3—quality of life: not reported
Outcome 4—length of hospital stay: not reported
Outcome 5—cost-effectiveness
Young and Wheeler[27] discussed the cost of the dressings reporting that dextranomer was markedly less cost-effective than elastomer foam. However, no cost analysis data were included, and only approximate costings from another dextranomer trial by Goode *et al.*[22] were quoted.

CONCLUDING REMARKS

Although only five RCTs conducted before 1990 met the inclusion criteria for this review, a range of more recent research articles were identified, but following closer scrutiny were all excluded. It is apparent from these excluded studies that a range of debridement methods are being used in clinical practice including surgical debridement (Zeitani *et al.*)[28]; mechanical debridement (Allie *et al.*[29]; Granick *et al.*)[19]; however, these studies are not RCTs, and therefore are highly susceptible to selection bias. It is disappointing that recently published studies are not employing more rigorous research methods that aim to minimize bias and therefore increase the confidence with which we can view the findings. The cost of conducting an RCT may be one consideration.

Manufacturers of existing and new wound debridement products appear to use controlled trials, retrospective analysis of patient case notes, and case studies as evidence of effectiveness.

The common outcome for the five included trials was the time to a clean wound bed for infected postsurgical wounds. Three out of the four trials comparing dextranomer with other products reported shorter time to a clean wound bed for dextranomer. The trial comparing streptokinase/streptodornase with saline dressings reported a shorter time to a clean wound bed with streptokinase/streptodornase.

However, a number of trial deficiencies reduce the confidence by which we can draw any conclusions to inform practice. These deficiencies include:

1. Poor quality of the trials;
2. Small sample sizes;
3. Limited range of treatments;
4. Different control groups for each trial;
5. Lack of replication studies;
6. Inappropriate statistical analysis (time to event data not being analyzed as such).

The methodological quality of the trials was variable, with small sample sizes, method of randomization not always being clear, and inadequate allocation concealment. Data and statistical information were incomplete in three of the five trials. Blinding of the independent assessors would have been possible, but this was only clearly demonstrated in two studies.[22,25]

A limited range of treatments was identified with dextranomer beads or paste and different comparisons used in each trial; therefore, it was not possible to pool the results. The rationale for choosing dextranomer for the treatment groups was not clear, apart from Young and Wheeler,[27] who identified this as a new dressing, the trial being supported financially by the manufacturer. Dextranomer was significantly better than the EUSOL-soaked dressings,[22] but this result must be viewed with caution, as there were insufficient statistical data included in the small trial and methodological flaws in the trial. As worldwide production of dextranomer products has been discontinued, except for dextranomer paste that is currently only available in South Africa, the impact on clinical practice of findings is extremely limited.

The enzymatic agent (streptokinase/streptodornase) demonstrated a statistically significant reduction in the time to a clean wound bed when compared with saline-soaked dressings. Poor handling and analysis of the data was a limitation of this trial, and it should be noted that this enzyme is no longer available worldwide.

There is a complete absence of adequately powered, methodologically robust RCTs evaluating contemporary debridement interventions for surgical wounds. The trials included in this review investigate treatments that are no longer available, and the trials were of poor quality. Trials reflecting the wider range of surgical, biosurgical, mechanical, chemical, and autolytic debridement methods and agents for surgical wounds were not identified.

This analysis reflects the poor quality of the randomized trials developed until now. Even if surgeons are still convinced of the efficacy of an aggressive approach of debridement in surgical wounds, strong

TAKE-HOME MESSAGE

Basic science advance

- Most of the knowledge on the mechanisms of dehiscence has to be defined, with respect to the mechanical forces on the edges of the wound, the role of trauma on the subcutaneous tissues, the extent of infection, the risk of hematomas and underlying localized hyperpressure, etc. Acute postoperative wounds are still lacking scientific data on the respective role of biological agents, leading to necrosis, dehiscence, and nonhealing.

Clinical science advance

- No strong evidence has yet been given either to leave a wound opened after surgical dehiscence or on the fact that surgeons should ban the second cleaning surgical procedure and reclose the wound.

methodological trials issuing to statistical significant differences are still to be done.

AUTHOR DISCLOSURE STATEMENT

No competing financial interests exist.

REFERENCES

1. Smiell JM, Wieman TJ, Steed DL, Perry BH, Sampson AR, and Schwab BH: Efficacy and safety of becaplermin (recombinant human platelet-derived growth factor-BB) in patients with nonhealing, lower extremity diabetic ulcers: a combined analysis of four randomized studies. Wound Repair Regen 1999; **7:** 335.
2. Téot L: Surgical debridement. In: *Surgical Wound Healing and Management*, edited by Granick MS and Gamelli RL. London: Informa Healthcare Pub NY, 2007, pp. 91–102.
3. Margolis DJ, Allen-Taylor L, Hoffstad O, and Berlin JA: Diabetic neuropathic foot ulcers: predicting which ones will not heal. Am J Med 2003; **115:** 627.
4. Dryburgh N, Smith F, Donaldson J, and Mitchell M: Debridement for surgical wounds. Cochrane Database Syst Rev July 16 2008; CD006214.
5. Baharestani M: The clinical relevance of debridement. In: *The Clinical Relevance of Debridement*, edited by Baharestani M, Gottrup F, Holstein P, and Vanscheidt W. Berlin, Germany: Springer-Verlag, 1999, pp. 1–15.
6. Vowden K and Vowden P: Wound debridement, part 1: non-sharp techniques. J Wound Care 1999; **8:** 237.
7. Ashworth J: Conservative sharp debridement: the professional and legal issues. Prof Nurse 2002; **17:** 585.
8. Bradley M, Cullum N, and Sheldon T: The debridement of chronic wounds: a systematic review. Health Technol Assess 1999; **3 (17 Pt 1):** iii–iv, 1–78.
9. Edwards RH and Killen DA: Comparison of two methods of management of clean surgical wounds. JAMA 1967; **201:** 137.
10. Thomas AML and Moore K: The structure and composition of chronic wound eschar. J Wound Care 1999; **8:** 285.
11. Sibbald RG, Williamson D, Orsted HL, Campbell K, Keast D, Krasner D, Sibbald D: Preparing the wound bed debridement, bacterial balance and moisture balance. Ostomy Wound Manage 2000; **46:** 14.
12. Schultz GS, Sibbald RG, Falanga V, Ayello EA, Dowsett C, Harding K, Romanelli M, Stacey MC, Teot L, and Vanscheidt W: Wound bed preparation: a systematic approach to wound management. Wound Repair Regen 2003; **11 (Suppl):** S1.
13. Lewis R, Whiting P, ter Reit G, O'Meara S, and Glanville J: *A Rapid Systematic Review of the Clinical Effectiveness and Cost Effectiveness of Debriding Agents in Treating Surgical Wounds Healing by Secondary Intention*. York, UK: NHS Centre for Reviews and Dissemination, 2000.
14. O'Brien M: Exploring methods of wound debridement. Br J Commun Nurs 2002; **7 (Suppl):** 10, 12, 14, 16–18.
15. Poston 1996 Ramundo J, and Wells J: Wound debridement. In: *Acute and Chronic Wounds: Nursing Management*, 2nd edition, edited by Bryant RA. St. Louis, MO: Mosby, 2000, pp. 157–178.
16. Van der Plas MJ, Jukema GN, Wai SW, Dogterom-Ballering HC, Lagendijk EL, van Gulpen C, van Dissel JT, Bloemberg GV, and Nibbering PH: Maggot excretions/secretions are differentially effective against biofilms of *Staphylococcus aureus* and *Pseudomonas aeruginosa*. J Antimicrob Chemother 2008; **61:** 117.
17. Stotts NA: Wound infection: diagnosis and management. In: *Acute and Chronic Wounds: Nursing Management*, 2nd edition, edited by Bryant RA. St. Louis, MO: Mosby, 2000, pp. 179–188.
18. Dijoux C, Ribal E, and Téot L: Use of a moderate-pressure irrigation system to effect debridement in the home setting. J Wound Care 2008; **17:** 134–136, 138.
19. Granick MS, Posnett J, Jacoby M, Noruthun S, Ganchi PA, and Datiashvili RO: Efficacy and cost-effectiveness of a high-powered parallel waterjet for wound debridement. Wound Repair Regen 2006; **14:** 394.
20. Brennan SS and Leaper DJ: The effect of antiseptics on the healing wound: a study using the rabbit ear chamber. Br J Surg 1985; **72:** 780.
21. Hofman D: Debridement—a nursing issue? www.etrs.org/bulletin9_3/section5.html (accessed November 17, 2005).
22. Goode AW, Glazer G, and Ellis BW: The cost effectiveness of dextranomer and Eusol in the treatment of infected surgical wounds. Br J Clin Pract 1979; **33:** 325.
23. Morgan DA: Chlorinated solutions—an update. J Tissue Viability 1991; **2:** 31.
24. Michiels I and Christiaens MR: Dextranomer (Debrisan) paste in postoperative wounds: a controlled study. Clin Trials J 1990; **27:** 283.
25. Poulson J, Kristensen VN, Brygger HE, and Delikaris P: Treatment of infected surgical wounds with Varidase. Acta Chir Scand 1983; **149:** 245.
26. Sondergaard JO and Galatius H: Debrisan compared with chloramine packs in the treatment of postoperative infected wounds [Debrisan versus kloramin—mecheved postoperative inficerede cikatricer]. Ugeskrift for Laeger 1982; **144:** 1523.
27. Young HL and Wheeler MH: Report of the prospective trial of dextranomer beads (Debrisan) and silicone foam elastomer (silastic dressings in surgical wounds). Br J Surg 1982; **69:** 33.
28. Zeitani J, Bertoldo F, Bassano C, Penta de Peppo A, Pellegrino AP, El Fakhri FM, and Chiariello L: Superficial wound dehiscence after median sternotomy: surgical treatment versus secondary wound healing. Ann Thorac Surg 2004; **77:** 672.
29. Allie DE, Herbert CJ, Lirtzman MD, Wyatt CH, Keller VA, Souther SM, Allie, AA, Mitran EV, and Walker CM: Novel treatment strategy for leg and sternal wound complications after coronary graft surgery: bioengineered Apligraf. Ann Thorac Surg 2004; **78:** 673.

WHS
Wound
Healing
Society

Recent Advances in the Use of Ultrasound in Wound Care

Vickie R. Driver* and Matteo Fabbi

Foot Care, Vascular, and Endovascular Specialists, Boston Medical Center, Boston University School of Medicine, Boston, Massachusetts.

Abbreviations and Acronyms

ERK = extracellular signal regulated protein kinase

JNK = Jun N-terminal kinase

KGF = keratinocyte growth factor

kHz = kilohertz

MHz = megahertz

MRSA = methicillin resistant staphylococcus aureus

NO = nitric oxide

NOS = nitric oxide synthase

RCT = randomized control trials

TGF-β1 = transforming growth factor-β1

US = ultrasound

*Correspondence: Foot Care, Vascular, and Endovascular Specialists, Boston Medical Center, Boston University School of Medicine, Preston Building, 732 Harrison Ave., Boston, Massachusetts 20018 (e-mail: vickie.driver@bmc.org).

Background: The effects of ultrasound (US) on wound healing have been extensively studied over the past 50 years. In recent years the widespread use of low-frequency US for wound care has been paired by a growing body of literature showing promising preclinical and clinical data.

The Problem: The progressive increase in the utilization of low-frequency, low-intensity US devices in wound care raises the question of what are the most appropriate indications for these treatments.

Basic/Clinical Science Advances: The first application of US to wound care employed devices working with high-frequency US, and the results of metaanalyses of randomized controlled trials regarding their effectiveness are controversial. Recently, a growing number of experimental studies have provided insights into the molecular mechanism of US action, particularly regarding wound healing, angiogenesis, and bacterial load.

Clinical Care Relevance: Two distinct types of low-frequency US devices are available for clinical use: contact US devices are debriders, particularly effective for the treatment of eschar or inflammatory tissue as well as for the debridement of painful ulcers; noncontact US devices have shown to clinically affect the healing process at various phases, particularly on neuropathic diabetic foot ulcers and to a certain extent on ischemic leg ulcers. Preliminary data on other types of lower extremity ulcers show promising future developments for this treatment.

Conclusion: Low-frequency US can be useful in the management of painful ulcers, on diabetic foot ulcers, and, to a certain extent, on ischemic leg ulcers.

BACKGROUND

ONE OF THE MOST RELEVANT FEATURES of ultrasound (US) to exert a biologic effect is frequency. It affects the intensity of US delivery since absorption, which is frequency dependent, is the major cause of intensity attenuation. By increasing the frequency, the wavelength shortens and absorption increases. Low-frequency US has the potential of delivering energy with less attenuation than high-frequency US. In 1982, the World Health Organization fixed a safety standard of 3.0 W/cm^2 as the highest level of intensity to be used without inducing significant harm. Low-frequency US shows a deeper tissue penetration then high-frequency US. It displays its effect via thermal and nonthermal mechanisms. The thermal component of low-frequency US is not a major concern.

Early studies employed high-frequency US in the megahertz (MHz) range, and data from metaanalyses of randomized controlled trials (RCT) are controversial. It is suggested that US treatment in the MHz range (1–3 MHz) may be useful in the management of venous leg ulcers.[1] Conversely, an effect on pressure ulcers of MHz US has not yet been convincingly demonstrated.[2]

In recent years low-frequency, kilohertz (kHz), US devices have been

Printed in U.S.A.
DOI: 10.1089/awc.2009.0018

increasingly used for wound healing, serving as debriders or as healing promoters. Preclinical studies on both cellular and animal models have provided promising results. In particular, they have demonstrated a direct US effect on several stages of the healing process, including a beneficial action on bacterial load that could be helpful in the treatment of chronic ulcers. RCTs of low-frequency, noncontact US treatment suggest an effect on neuropathic, superficial diabetic foot ulcers,[3] with some evidence of benefit on ischemic ulcers.[4]

CLINICAL PROBLEM ADDRESSED

The growing incidence of nonhealing ulcers worldwide urges researchers to test and introduce into the clinical practice novel and effective therapeutic strategies. Since US may be one of the most promising tools for the treatment of skin ulcers, a careful review of the data available in the literature appears compulsory.

BASIC SCIENCE CONTEXT

US appears to modulate fibroblast activity,[5,6] the inflammatory response,[7] and cytokine production.[7] It appears that therapeutic US treatment may promote a clinically relevant response to injury leading to the formation of a qualitatively different tissue. Although an effect on healing time has not been confirmed in experimental models, US may enhance the formation of a stronger granulation tissue.[8] Low-frequency US treatment also may be helpful in the clinical management of ischemic wounds by promoting vasodilation and angiogenesis.[9,10] Further, US may be useful in the alteration of the bacterial load during the treatment of chronic wounds.[11] US in the kHz range shows a good tissue penetration, which is an important factor in the management of contamination/infection, since most biofilms tend to localize deeper in the wound tissue. The experimental models showing the molecular effects of US treatment are reviewed in detail in the following section.

EXPERIMENTAL MODEL OR MATERIAL

Effects on the wound healing process

The effects of low-frequency, low-intensity, pulsed US (in the kHz range) on human foreskin fibroblasts have been investigated in a recent study.[5] In this model treatment with US induced fibroblast DNA synthesis and proliferation. The mechanism by which US elicits cellular proliferation appears to be mediated by the mechanosensor integrin $\beta 1$, which activates a downstream-specific signal transduction pathway (Rho/rho-associated kinase) leading to cellular proliferation via extracellular signal–regulated protein kinase phosphorylation. The activation of the Rho/rho-associated kinase pathway is also responsible for the organization of intracellular stress fiber and focal adhesion capacity. As a morphological confirmation of this, Lai and Pittelkow[6] have shown a post-US increase in vacuolization, a marker of intracellular remodeling. Further, they evaluated the effects of 40 kHz, low-intensity, noncontact, pulsed US on either normal or scrape-wounded cultured fibroblasts. Acceleration of the molecular cascade promoted by wound healing has been observed in US-treated fibroblasts (Table 1).

Table 1. *Molecular effects of ultrasound on fibroblasts*[6]

	US-Treated Fibroblasts	Wounded Fibroblasts
KGF	↑ Early ↓ Late	↓ Early ↑ Late
TGF-$\beta 1$	↑	↓
ERK/JNK	↑↑ during day 1	↑ after day 1

US = ultrasound; KGF = keratinocyte growth factor; TGF-$\beta 1$ = transforming growth factor-$\beta 1$; ERK = extracellular signal–regulated protein kinase; JNK = Jun Jun N-terminal kinase.

US treatment led to an increase in mast cell degranulation, collagen deposition, and tensile strength in an animal model of incisional, full-thickness, and partial-thickness wounds.[7] Another group[8] observed a significantly higher amount of collagen and blood vessels in the granulation tissue of treated animals as compared with sham-treated control group.

Effects on angiogenesis

US treatment in both the MHz and the kHz range can elicit the production of angiogenic factors such as vascular endothelial growth factor and interleukin-8 in osteoblasts, fibroblasts, and circulating mononuclear cells at given intensity thresholds.[9] In an ischemic limb model, contact, low-frequency, low-intensity US determined an improvement of perfusion and a reversal of the acidotic state in the gracilis muscle of rabbits after ligation of the femoral artery.[12] This effect was blunted by the administration of a nitric oxide synthase (NOS) inhibitor. A confirmation of the post-US NO release is provided by an *in vitro* study on endothelial cells from human umbilical cord and aortic bovine endothelial cells.[10] A reversible, rapid, and transient (1 min) upregulation of endothelial NOS was noted. This resulted in increased NO production, a response comparable with that

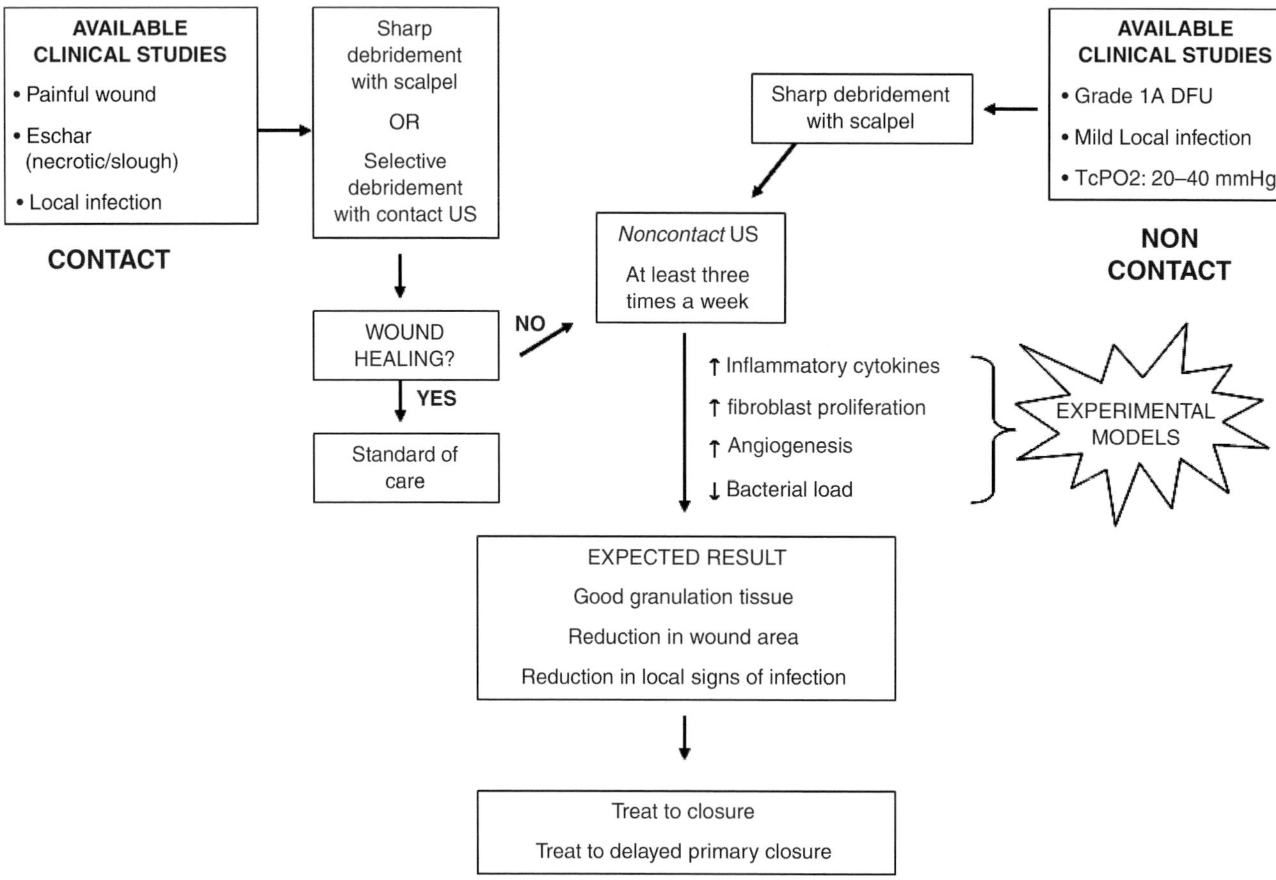

Figure 1. Ultrasound (US) treatment in wound care can be useful by providing selective painless debridement of eschar tissue or of local infection tissue especially if traditional debridement with a scalpel proves to be too painful. This goal can be achieved with contact devices. Noncontact devices can be a helpful adjunct to sharp debridement in restarting the healing process. The molecular basis for this action has been demonstrated in animal studies, but a confirmation of these findings in humans is needed. US treatment can be useful in achieving a good granulation tissue, which also could be more suitable for a delayed primary closure (*e.g.*, skin graft). The illustration presents a proposed algorithm for the integration of contact and noncontact devices into clinical practice.

obtained after administration of a known endothelial NOS inducer[10] (Fig 1).

Bactericidal effect

In a preliminary study, Serena *et al*[11] showed a bactericidal effect of noncontact low-frequency US *in vitro*. This effect was more prevalent on Pseudomonas, *Escherichia coli*, and *Enterococcus faecalis* strains, but was almost absent on methicillin resistant staphylococcus aureus (MRSA) or *Staphylococcus aureus*. A morphologic analysis showed bacterial cell wall alteration to be the basis for the bactericidal effect of US. The same group confirmed the *in vitro* observation in a clinical study on 11 patients with pressure ulcers. In this study a 2-week treatment with noncontact, low-frequency US resulted in a significant reduction of the bacterial load. A 26% decrease of the wound area was noted, and this could be at least partly attributable to the bactericidal effect of US treatment.

DISCUSSION OF FINDINGS AND RELEVANT LITERATURE

Debridement (contact devices)

In the past US debriders have been widely used for the debridement of necrotic and infected tissue in the operative room. Low-frequency, contact devices are designed and employed as debriders. They are nonsurgical devices that work through the transmission of US frequency to an edge that vibrates and is responsible for the debridement effects. Saline is used for the control of the heating effect and for cleansing of the ulcer. The available devices are Soring Sonoca 180, which employs a 25-kHz frequency; Misonix Sonic One, which employs a 22.5-kHz frequency; and Arobella Qoustic, which employs a 35-kHz frequency.

The advantage of these devices is that they are not surgical devices and can be used also in the clinical setting. Sterile saline is used for the reduction of the thermal effect on tissues, for a better transduction of the US, and for wound cleansing.

Preliminary data with contact, low-frequency US debriders on a series of 17 patients[13] showed an effective debridement of necrotic tissue, and a reduction of wound area after treatment. The wound bed quality was good enough to allow revisional surgery for some of these ulcers after US debridement. Of note, no adverse events (*e.g.*, heating effect) have been observed. Another study on 19 mainly venous, chronic leg ulcers[14] treated with 25-kHz US debrider, showed a significant reduction in ulcer pain. It appears that wound healing has to be expected in at least one-third of patients after five sessions of treatment. Even if the hypothesis of some effects of contact debriders on the wound healing process has been advocated, to date no convincing evidence of these actions has been provided. Contact US devices should therefore be considered only when debridement of necrotic or infected tissue without significant pain is desired.

Wound healing (noncontact devices)

In addition to contact US debriders, the introduction of low-frequency, noncontact devices that also can be used in a nonsurgical clinical setting has promoted new encouraging research in this field.

In an RCT of diabetic foot ulcers, Ennis *et al*[3] evaluated the effects of low-frequency, noncontact US treatment for full-thickness neuropathic diabetic foot grade 1A ulcers. The treatment scheme was a 4-min application of noncontact US three times a week. In this trial, 55 subjects were randomized to US treatment or sham placebo. After an initial surgical debridement, the rate of ulcers healed in the treatment group was significantly higher as compared to sham-treated group (40.7% vs. 14.3%). Of interest, ulcer characteristics between the two groups were significantly different in regard to exudate characteristics with the treatment group showing a smaller amount of exudate compared with controls. A safety analysis did not show any significant difference in the rate of adverse events between the two groups.

The same group evaluated the effects on the rate of healing over an 8-month period of 29 ulcers of several etiologies.[15] Patients were treated three times a week, with single treatment duration ranging from 3 to 12 min depending on wound area. In this single-center observational study, 69% of the ulcers treated with US alone or with a combination of US and advanced wound care dressings healed.

Another observational study on 51 patients with lower extremity wounds of various etiology[16] con-

TAKE-HOME MESSAGE

Basic science advances

- US therapy has been proven to act on the various phases of the healing process.
- Through a combination effect on the inflammatory phase, angiogenesis, and the bacterial load, US may be useful to obtain a more viable and strong granulation tissue.
- Delayed primary healing could be performed earlier if the granulation tissue is more viable.

Grading of clinical recommendations

Clinical recommendations are graded according to the strength of available studies[21] as

- Grade A (high quality): very unlikely that future research will change our confidence in the estimate of the effect (evidence from metaanalyses or large, well-conducted RCT).
- Grade B (moderate quality): further research is likely to have an important impact on our confidence in the estimate of the effect (evidence from prospective trials, cohort studies, and case–control studies).
- Grade C (low quality): further research is very likely to have an important effect on our confidence in the estimate of the effect (case series, retrospective studies).
- Grade D (very low quality): any estimate of the effect is very uncertain (case reports).

Clinical science advances

- The clinical debridement of necrotic and infected tissue with nonsurgical, low-frequency, contact US devices is selective and as effective as debridement with a scalpel (grade B).
- Debridement with contact, low-frequency devices allows a good wound bed preparation (grade B).
- US therapy has been shown to accelerate the healing of chronic venous ulcers (grade A).
- Noncontact, low-frequency devices, which deliver the US energy through a saline mist medium, proved to be useful in accelerating the healing of full-thickness grade 1A neuropathic diabetic foot ulcers as well as ischemic ulcers (grade B).
- The effects may be mediated by a direct mechanical effect or by the influence of some steps of the healing process as well as the management of the bacterial load (grade C).

Relevance to clinical care

- US debriders can be useful when nonpainful, selective debridement is required, particularly in a nonsurgical setting (grade B).
- Noncontact US can be useful as an adjunct to sharp debridement to improve the characteristics of the granulation tissue and allow a more rapid wound closure or delayed primary closure (grade C).

firmed a reduction in wound area in US-treated ulcers. In this study, treatment frequency ranged from three to five times a week. A prospective, open-label, parallel-group controlled trial compared the effects of low-frequency, noncontact US treatment for ischemic ulcers versus standard of care.[4] A reduction of wound area greater than 50% was achieved in 63% of US-treated ulcers as compared with 29% of standard of care-treated ulcers. The important finding of this study is the effect of US treatment in patients with transcutaneous oxygen tension values between 20 and 40 mm Hg. This is a gray zone in which the decision of whether to perform a revascularization procedure or to adopt a wait-and-see approach may be challenging, and usually the clinical course of the ulcer is the major determinant. Low-frequency US may represent an important adjunct tool for treating patients who fall in this category with ischemic. A limitation of this study is the use of the surrogate marker of 50% wound area reduction, which is only a predictor of healing.

Pain management

Few articles have addressed the issue of the effect of US treatment on ulcer pain.

In a case series of five patients with burns, Waldrop and Serfass[17] showed a significant reduction of ulcer pain during the cycle of noncontact US therapy. A retrospective chart review of 15 patients treated with noncontact US therapy showed a significant reduction of wound pain in all treated subjects.[18] Contact US therapy is also associated with a reduction in wound pain[14] and use of pain medication after six treatment sessions.[19]

Whether US treatment influences ulcer pain directly or by improving the healing process has to be ascertained.

Table 2. *Summary of indications and available devices for low-frequency ultrasound therapy in wound care (modified by Sussman and Dyson[20])*

	Contact	Noncontact
Frequency	22.5-25-35 kHz*	40 kHz
Therapeutic range (intensity)	0.1–2.0 W/cm^2	0.1–0.5 W/cm^2
Mode	Continuous/pulsed	Continuous
Fluid delivery mode	Stream/mist/spray	Mist
Duration of treatment	No standard Depends on: patient tolerance Tissue quality Size of the ulcer	No standard Depends on: Wound size
Wound bed contact	Yes Exerts both mechanical (edge) and acoustic (US) effects	No 1–1.5 cm distance
Selective debridement	Yes	No
Pain with treatment	Sometimes	No
Observation of result	Immediate	Over time Usually requires multiple applications
Thermal effect	Yes Dissipated by saline Soring Sonoca 180 Misonix Sonic One Arobella Quoustic	No
Indications	Debridement of: Painful ulcers Eschar tissue Necrotic tissue	As adjunct to sharp debridement for (1) Promoting healing of: Grade 1A diabetic foot ulcers
	Infected tissue from Venous ulcers/painful ulcers	Ischemic ulcers (2) Control bacterial load in chronic ulcers with mild local signs of infection

*(according to device type)

CAUTION, CRITICAL REMARKS, AND RECOMMENDATIONS

US treatment for wound care is a safe and potentially effective treatment that may be integrated to standard of care in the management of chronic ulcers. Table 2 summarizes the main differences between contact and noncontact US devices. Preclinical data suggest that the therapeutic effect of US may be due to a modulation of the healing process combined with the stimulation of angiogenesis and the control of the bacterial load. These effects have not yet been demonstrated in human studies. Moreover, the various preclinical and clinical studies have employed different treatment schemes, and at present it is not clear which treatment dose is likely to have the greater benefit. The small sample size of available studies and the use of surrogate markers of healing in some of them warrant caution in the widespread use of US on all kind of wounds.

Further studies are needed to address the issue of ulcer pain control, to confirm the preliminary data on chronic ulcers, and to provide a dose range for the most effective treatment.

FUTURE DEVELOPMENTS

Further research is needed to demonstrate therapeutic effects of contact US treatment other than debridement. Additional noncontact US studies are required to better understand the appropriate treatment dose as well as the angiogenic therapeutic effect. Future research may take into account the combination effects of US therapy with skin grafts, skin equivalents, and other advanced modalities.

AUTHOR DISCLOSURE STATEMENT

V.R.D. discloses no conflict of interest.
M.F. discloses no conflict of interest.

REFERENCES

1. Al-Kurdi D, Bell-Syer SEM, and Flemming K: Therapeutic ultrasound for venous leg ulcers. Cochrane Database Syst Rev 2008, Issue 1. Art n:CD001180.DOI:10.1002/14651858.CD001180.pub2.
2. Baba-Akbari Sari A, Flemming K, Cullum NA, and Wollina U: Therapeutic ultrasound for pressure ulcers. Cochrane Database Syst Rev 2006, Issue 3. Art n: CD001275.DOI:10.1002/14651858.CD001275.pub2.
3. Ennis WJ, Formann P, Mozen N, Massey J, Conner-Kerr T, Meneses P, and the MIST Ultrasound Diabetic Foot Study Group: Ultrasound therapy for recalcitrant diabetic foot ulcers: results of a randomized, double-blind, controlled, multicenter study. Ostomy Wound Manage 2005; **51:** 24.
4. Kavros SJ, Miller JL, and Hanna SW: Treatment of ischemic wounds with noncontact, low-frequency ultrasound: the Mayo Clinic experience 2004–2006. Adv Skin Wound Care 2007; **20:** 221.
5. Zhou S, Schmelz A, Seufferlein T, Yiping L, Jinshun Z, and Bachem MG: Molecular mechanisms of low intensity pulsed ultrasound in human skin fibroblasts. J Biol Chem 2004; 279, 52: 54463-9.
6. Lai J and Pittelkow MR: Physiological effects of ultrasound mist on fibroblasts. Int J Dermatol 2007; **46:** 587.
7. Byl NN, McKenzie AL, West JM, Whitney JD, Hunt TK, and Scheuenstuhl HA: Low-dose ultrasound effects on wound healing: a controlled study with Yucatan pigs. Arch Phys Med Rehabil 1993; **73:** 333.
8. Thawer HA and Houghton PE: Effects of ultrasound delivered through a mist of saline to wounds in mice with diabetes mellitus. J Wound Care 2004; **13:** 1.
9. Reher P, Doan N, Bradnock B, Meghji S, and Harris M: Effect of ultrasound on the production of IL-8, basic FGF and VEGF. Cytokine 1999; **11:** 416.
10. Altand OD, Dalecki D, Suchkova VN, and Francis CW: Low-intensity ultrasound increases endothelial cell nitric oxide synthase activity and nitric oxide synthesis. J Thromb Haemost 2003; **2:** 637.
11. Serena T, Lee K, Lam K, Attar P, Meneses P, and Ennis W: The impact of noncontact, nonthermal, low-frequency ultrasound on bacterial counts in experimental and chronic wounds. Ostomy Wound Manage 2009; **55:** 22.
12. Suchkova VA, Baggs RB, Sahni SK, and Francis CW: Ultrasound improves tissue perfusion in ischemic tissue through a nitric oxide dependent mechanism. Thromb Haemost 2002; **88:** 865.
13. Breuing KH, Bayer L, Neuwalder J, and Orgill DP: Early experience using low-frequency ultrasound in chronic wounds. Ann Plast Surg 2005; **55:** 183.
14. Tan J, Abisi S, and Burnand KG: A painless method of ultrasonically assisted debridement of chronic leg ulcers: a pilot study. Eur J Vasc Endovasc Surg 2007; **33:** 234.
15. Ennis WJ, Valdes W, Gainer M, and Meneses P: Evaluation of clinical effectiveness of MIST ultrasound therapy for the healing of chronic wounds. Adv Skin Wound Care 2006; **19:** 437.
16. Kavros SJ and Schenck EC: Use of noncontact low-frequency ultrasound in the treatment of chronic foot and leg ulcerations. A 51 patient analysis. J Am Podiatr Med Assoc 2007; **97:** 95.
17. Waldrop K and Serfass A: Clinical effectiveness of noncontact, low frequency, nonthermal ultrasound in burn care. Ostomy Wound Manage 2008; **45:** 66.
18. Gehling ML and Samies JH: The effect of noncontact, low-intensity, low frequency therapeutic ultrasound on lower extremity chronic wound pain: a retrospective chart review. Ostomy Wound Manage 2007; **53:** 44.
19. Schulze CH, Hulskamp T, Schikorski M, and Thies E: Effective, gentle, low pain wound debridement with low frequency ultrasound applied using mobile equipment. http://wundbehandlung.net/opencms/opencms/wundbehandlung/dokumente/Effectivexgentle_low-pain_wound_debridement_with_low-frequency_ultrasound_applied_using_mobile_equipment.pdf.
20. Sussman C and Dyson M: Therapeutic and diagnostic ultrasound. In: *Wound Care, a Collaborative Practice Manual for Health Professionals*, edited by Sussman C and Bates-Jensen B. Lippincott Williams & Wilkins, 2006; **25:** 617.
21. Guyatt G, Oxman AD, Vist GE, Kunz R, Falck-Ytter Y, Alonso-Coello P, and Schunemann JH, for the GRADE Working Group: GRADE: an emerging consensus on rating quality of evidence and strength of recommendations. BMJ 2008; **336:** 924.

Topical Negative Pressure Therapy for Acute and Chronic Wounds

Zena Elizabeth Helen Moore*

Faculty of Nursing and Midwifery, Royal College of Surgeons in Ireland, Dublin, Ireland.

Abbreviations and Acronyms

CI = confidence interval

EBM = evidence based medicine

RCT = randomized controlled trial

SD = standard deviation

TNP = topical negative pressure

VAC® = Vacuum-Assisted Closure

*Correspondence: Faculty of Nursing and Midwifery, Royal College of Surgeons in Ireland, 123 St. Stephens Green, Dublin D2, Ireland (e-mail: zmoore@rcsi.ie).

Background: Topical negative pressure (TNP) therapy is becoming increasingly popular for all kinds of wounds, with the best-known option being the Vacuum Assisted Closure (VAC®) system (KCI, San Antonio, TX).
The Problem: The aim of this systematic review was to summarize the evidence relating to the effectiveness of TNP on acute and chronic wound healing.
Basic/Clinical Science Advances: Principally the therapy works by removing excess exudate and edema, thereby stimulating angiogenesis and cell proliferation
Clinical Care Relevance: Evidence from studies has shown some positive effects for healing in a variety of wounds (mixed acute and chronic, diabetic wounds, skin grafts, and acute diabetic postamputation foot wounds) treated with TNP.
Conclusion: There appears to be a substantial amount of randomized controlled trial evidence that has explored TNP therapy within the clinical setting. However, interpretation of these data should have cognizance of the methodological quality of the studies

BACKGROUND

Topical negative pressure (TNP) therapy is becoming increasingly popular for all kinds of wounds,[1] with the best-known option being the Vacuum-Assisted Closure (VAC®) system (KCI, San Antonio, TX).[2] Prior to the publication of this review, a number of other reviews have been published. However, Ubbink *et al.*[1] argued that there were limitations in those reviews, for example, inclusion of studies other than randomized controlled trials (RCTs) outdated search strategies, as several trials have appeared since and limitations in wound type were included. Therefore, an updated review of the evidence was felt to be necessary. This article provides a review and critique of the systematic review.

CLINICAL PROBLEM ADDRESSED

The aim of this review[1] was to summarize the evidence relating to the effectiveness of TNP in acute and chronic wound healing. The review was based only on RCTs. The primary outcome of interest was wound healing expressed as time to complete healing, change in wound surface area, proportion of wounds healed within the trial period, survival rate of split-thickness skin grafts, or wound condition ready for surgery or skin grafting. Secondary outcomes were infection, pain, quality of life, edema, microcirculation, bacterial load, adverse events, and duration of hospital stay.

RELEVANT BASIC SCIENCE CONTEXT

TNP therapy is an interesting development in wound management which works by applying a controlled negative pressure to the surface of a wound. Although the concept of using suction in wound management is not new, the application of a negative

ADVANCES IN WOUND CARE, VOLUME 1

Printed in U.S.A.
DOI: 10.1089/awc.2009.0173

pressure at the surface of the wound is novel. TNP creates a controlled, local subatmospheric pressure in the wound.[3] The technique uses a foam dressing connected to a vacuum device. The device delivers a controlled negative pressure of −50 to −125 mmHg, which can be applied constantly or intermittently.[1] Principally the therapy works by removing excess exudate and edema, thereby stimulating angiogenesis and cell proliferation.[3] As it is a closed system it also has the advantage of helping to maintain the principles of infection control.

It is suggested that TNP works by utilizing many different mechanisms of action.[4] One such mechanism is mechanical stress, which is postulated to increase cellular activity, accelerate cell proliferation, accelerate DNA synthesis, and increase fibrogenesis.[4] A second mechanism is the growth of granulated tissue within the wound bed.[4] Indeed, granulated tissue production has been noted in wounds treated with both continuous and intermittent suctions. A further important mechanism of action is the removal of excess fluid and edema from the wound. Importantly, this fluid consists of proinflammatory cytokines and matrix metalloproteinases, which are known to impair wound healing in chronic wounds.[4] Therefore, TNP helps to create an environment at the wound surface that is conducive to more orderly wound repair.

EXPERIMENTAL MODELS OR MATERIALS—ADVANTAGES AND LIMITATIONS

RCTs that evaluated the use and effectiveness of TNP in patients aged 18 years and over, with all kinds of wounds and in all settings reporting the primary outcome of interest, were included. Fifteen reports of 13 trials matched the inclusion criteria. Of these, three described the same set of patients and reported on bacterial load, costs of the TNP technique, and treatment efficacy. Seven trials involved chronic (venous, arterial, diabetic, or pressure) wounds, two involved a mixture of chronic and acute wounds, and four dealt with acute wounds, of which three were on split skin grafts.

Mixed acute and chronic wounds

Two studies reported a faster mean time to complete wound healing using VAC therapy: 16 days for VAC group (95% confidence interval [CI]: 9–23) versus 20 days for control group (95% CI: 16–24) ($p = 0.32$)[5]; 29 days for VAC group (95% CI: 25.5–32.5) versus 45 days for control group (95% CI: 36.2–53.8) ($p = 0.001$).[6]

Two studies described greater reduction in wound surface area using VAC therapy; median reduction in wound surface area of 0.3 cm^2/day for VAC versus −0.1 cm^2/day for control group ($p = 0.83$),[5] and mean (standard deviation [SD]) reduction in wound surface area was 3.8% (0.5) per day for VAC and 1.7% (0.6) per day for gauze-treated group (mean difference was 2.10% [95% CI: 1.69–2.51]).[7]

Two studies described a faster time to being ready for surgery using VAC therapy; median time of 7 days for VAC (95% CI: 5.7–8.3) versus 17 days for control group (95% CI: 10–24),[6] and median time of 6 days for VAC versus 7 days for gauze-treated group ($p = 0.19$).[7]

Three studies reported on costs, of which one found that there was no statistical difference in costs between VAC and gauze.[7] Another study found a statistically significant difference for VAC versus the conventional group ($p = 0.09$).[5] The final study calculated the average total costs to be U.S.$5452 for conventional and U.S.$3381 for VAC treatment.[6]

Diabetic wounds

Three studies that explored the effect of TNP on diabetic foot wounds were included. The first study found a faster rate of healing in TNP versus control (mean difference was −20.00 days [95% CI: −52.31 to 12.31]).[8] The second study reported a faster reduction in wound size with VAC versus gauze (mean difference was 20.4 cm^2 for VAC; mean difference was 9.5 cm^2 for gauze group).[9] The same study also reported a faster time to become ready for surgery in the VAC group (mean difference was −4.45 [95% CI: −7.87 to −1.03]).[9] The final study reported a faster mean reduction in depth after VAC treatment versus moist dressing (mean difference was 43.10 [95% CI: 2.66–83.54]).[10]

Pressure ulcers

Two studies reported on pressure ulcers. The first study[11] found a similar number of patients healed in both groups (VAC versus a Healthpoint system). However, there was a faster reduction in wound volume in the VAC group (mean reduction in wound volume of 51.8% in VAC group versus 42.1% in Healthpoint group; $p = 0.46$).[11] Similarly, Wanner *et al.*[12] found a faster time to reach 50% of the initial wound volume with VAC (mean [SD] = 27 days [10] for VAC versus 28 days [7] for control group; $p = 0.9$) (mean difference was −1.00 [95% CI: −8.21 to 6.21]).

Skin grafts

Three studies were included relating to patients with skin grafts. The first study[13] reported a greater take rate for Integra with VAC versus conventional therapy alone (mean difference was 20% [95% CI: 13.40–26.60%]). The second study[14] found a faster rate of graft healing in TNP versus control (mean difference was −3.23 days [95% CI: −4.88 to −1.58]). The authors[14] also found that there was less graft loss with TNP versus control (mean difference was −7.62 cm^2 [95% CI: −12.06 to −3.18]) as well as less loss percentage of grafted area for TNP versus the control group (mean difference was −16.44% [95% CI: −26.03 to −6.85]). The number of patients who needed revisional skin transplantations was less in the TNP group (5 of 30 who had TNP versus 12 of 30 controls). The final study[15] found no difference on graft take rate between TNP and control (mean [SD] graft take rate was 86 [12.5] in wounds treated with TNP versus 87 [18.2] in control wounds).

Acute wounds

One study investigated acute wounds (diabetic foot amputations).[16] In this study, more patients healed over a 16-week period in the VAC group compared with controls (43 of 77 VAC-treated patients versus 33 of 85 controls). However, 13 of 77 patients in the VAC group and 5 of 85 controls developed a wound infection (risk difference was 0.11 [95% CI: 0.01–0.21]).

Authors' conclusion

Ubbink *et al.*[1] concluded that at present there is no worthwhile evidence to support the use of TNP in the treatment of various wounds. Further, a far more rigorous evaluation is needed, largely in the form of RCTs. Until this has been completed, the use of TNP should not become routine or be reimbursed for local wound care.

DISCUSSION OF FINDINGS AND RELEVANT LITERATURE

The authors'[1] conclusion appears contradictory to the evidence presented within the review. The conclusion was derived from an appraisal of the methodological quality of the studies reviewed. The authors[1] presented that the overall trial quality was moderate with true randomization (such as computer-aided) used in only three studies and allocation concealment could not be guaranteed in over half the trials. Similar findings have been noted in a recently updated Cochrane systematic review of support surfaces for pressure ulcer prevention,[17] where only 50% of the 52 studies included an adequate description of allocation concealment. The concern here is that there is a tendency for studies without adequate allocation concealment to report larger estimates of effect when compared with those who described adequate allocation concealment.[18]

The nature of the intervention in this review[1] made blinding of patients and healthcare workers impossible; thus, as expected, blinding the outcome assessor occurred in only four trials. Lack of blinding is not unique to just studies of TNP. Indeed, in a study by Fergusson *et al.*,[19] only 2% of 191 trials reported in the medical literature from 1998 to 2001 provided evidence of the success of blinding. It is well alluded that blinding is not always possible in clinical trials.[18–22] As such, Schulz[18] argued that blinding is not the most important criteria to consider; indeed, the effect of nonblinding is less than that of poor allocation concealment. Thus, as many trials cannot be blinded, other criteria are needed to assess the quality of those studies.[18]

To meet the challenge of reporting clinical trials in published literature, a group of experts met to discuss the problem. Following this meeting the Consolidated Standards of Reporting Trials (CONSORT) statement was developed and was first published in 1996.[23] Further meetings of the group took place following this inaugural meeting, and the CONSORT statement was revised and subsequently published in 2001.[24] In this instance, Ubbink *et al.*[1] have demonstrated that there is a large body of knowledge available. However, the methodological quality of some of the studies is not always in accordance with that of the CONSORT statement. Once again, this problem is not unique to studies of TNP. Indeed, a study has been conducted of RCTs published between July 2002 and June 2003 in five leading general medicine journals, to determine the quality of reporting since the CONSORT statement.[25] In 253 trials assessed, the compliance with CONSORT was found to be high in some areas, for example, sequence generation was reported in 80% (95% CI: 75–80%) of the trials. Conversely, blinding of participants was reported in 40% (34–46%) of trials, for healthcare providers in 17% (95% CI: 13–22%) of trials, for outcome assessors in 47% (95% CI: 41–53%) of trials, and for data analysts in 15% (10–19%) of trials. The authors argued that there remain inconsistencies in the application of CONSORT and these need to be addressed to improve the overall quality of reporting.[25] Of course it is possible that blinding was hard to achieve in the trials reviewed and this is the reason for failure to report, rather than it being an omission on the part of the researchers.

The authors[1] suggested that an inability to conduct meta-analysis was a problem in determining the direction of the effect of TNP. Meta-analysis involves quantitatively combining the results from individual trials that have explored a similar research question.[26] Undertaking a systematic review does not automatically imply that a meta-analysis will be conducted. Meta-analysis should only be carried out when it is appropriate.[27] The underlying premise is that the studies must be exploring a set of related research hypotheses. The purpose is to allow for greater accuracy in data analysis when using a group of studies rather than relying on the results of an individual study.[27] It is contended that the inability to conduct a meta-analysis in this instance[1] arises not primarily because of the quality of the trials, rather because of the challenges in defining clear outcome parameters that are universally accepted across all wound healing studies.[28] It is apparent that this problem is not unique to TNP studies as it is evidenced across the wide domain of wound healing literature.[29]

The authors[1] suggested that there is no aggregate evidence of more rapid complete wound healing for any wound type. However, it is not clear how this conclusion was arrived at, seeing as how no meta-analysis was conducted. Therefore, it is also reasonable to suggest that, as no meta-analysis has been conducted, there is no aggregate evidence to suggest that TNP does or does not result in more rapid complete wound healing. However, evidence from single studies has shown some positive effects on healing in a variety of wounds (mixed acute and chronic, diabetic wounds, skin grafts, and acute diabetic post amputation foot wounds) treated with TNP.

One of the major criticisms of systematic reviews is that they tend to have a narrow inclusion criterion, and thus, often, little evidence is found.[30] The rationale for this narrow focus is to reduce the margin for bias, thereby increasing the confidence which one may have in the conclusion of the review.[30] For example, a Cochrane systematic review by Moore and Cowman[31] of wound cleansing for pressure ulcers found overall that there was no good trial evidence to support use of any particular wound cleansing solution or technique for pressure ulcers. A further systematic review of silver-based wound dressings and topical agents for treating diabetic foot ulcers by Bergin and Wraight[32] found no studies that met the inclusion criteria. Similar findings have been noted in a review of repositioning for the treatment of pressure ulcers, where no trials at all were located.[33] It is evident that a lack of RCT evidence is an issue in wound management. However, in this case,[1] 15 reports of 13 trials were identified, all of which demonstrated some positive effects of TNP in a variety of acute and chronic wounds. It appears, therefore, that the authors' conclusions are not entirely justified. Even if one allows for the potential for bias, there appears to be a substantial amount of RCT evidence that has explored TNP therapy within the clinical setting. However, interpretation of these data should have cognizance of the methodological quality of the studies.

The authors[1] reported that four previous reviews have been conducted exploring the use of TNP. They rejected the findings of two of the

TAKE-HOME MESSAGE

Basic science advances

- TNP creates a controlled, local subatmospheric pressure in the wound.
- The technique uses a foam dressing connected to a vacuum device. The device delivers a controlled negative pressure of −50 to −125 mmHg, which can be applied constantly or intermittently.
- Principally the therapy works by removing excess exudate and edema, thereby stimulating angiogenesis and cell proliferation.
- As it is a closed system it also has the advantage of helping to maintain the principles of infection control.

Clinical science advances

- Fifteen reports of 13 trials matched the inclusion criteria.
- Three described the same set of patients and reported on bacterial load, costs of the TNP technique, and treatment efficacy.
- Seven trials involved chronic (venous, arterial, diabetic, or pressure) wounds, two involved a mixture of chronic and acute wounds, and four dealt with acute wounds, of which three were on split skin grafts.
- Fifteen reports of 13 trials demonstrated some positive effects of TNP in a variety of acute and chronic wounds.

Relevance to clinical care

- As no meta-analysis has been conducted, there is no aggregate evidence to suggest that TNP does or does not result in more rapid complete wound healing.
- Evidence from studies has shown some positive effects on healing in a variety wounds (mixed acute and chronic, diabetic wounds, skin grafts, and acute diabetic post amputation foot wounds) treated with TNP.
- There appears to be a substantial amount of RCT evidence that has explored TNP therapy within the clinical setting. However, interpretation of this data should have cognizance of the methodological quality of the studies.
- Restriction of evidence to only those included in RCTs may limit the applicability and value of all the available evidence and this should be borne in mind when reading the review of Ubbink *et al.*

reviews[34,35] because they included nonrandomized trials and case series, which they say may yield erroneously positive results. Further, they argued that inclusion of subjective outcomes may impact on the quality of the data yielded from the reviews.[1] The underlying feature of evidence-based medicine (EBM) is "The conscientious explicit and judicious use of current best evidence in making decisions about the care of individual patients . . ." (Ref.[36]: p. 71). In essence, clinical decision making should, on the one hand, have cognizance of the specific evidence and experience to support practice, but conversely should also bear in mind the uniqueness of each patient and their individual responses to particular treatments. It is clear that the patient's experiences, often assessed using subjective measures, are important and impact enormously on the acceptability of the given treatment. EBM is, in essence, not limited to randomized trials and meta-analyses; it incorporates clinical expertise and the best available external evidence and we cannot have one without the other.[37] Indeed, even well-conducted studies may be inapplicable or inappropriate for an individual patient and this will be determined by clinical experience. Conversely, without knowledge of what constitutes current best evidence, clinical practice may become rapidly out of date, and thus evidence and experience are two sides of the same coin.[37] If very limited criteria, such as overwhelming conclusive level I evidence, are used as the bright line for use and/or reimbursement of a technology, while ignoring all other types of evidence, the treatment of patients may end up being suboptimal. In other words, restriction of evidence to only those included in RCTs may limit the applicability and value of all the available evidence and this should be borne in mind when reading the review of Ubbink *et al.*[1]

CAUTION, CRITICAL REMARKS, AND RECOMMENDATIONS

Ubbink *et al.*[1] have completed a systematic review exploring TNP therapy for acute and chronic wounds. They concluded that at present there is no worthwhile evidence to support the use of TNP in the treatment of various wounds. Further, a far more rigorous evaluation is needed, largely in the form of RCTs. It is contended, however, that the review has presented data from 13 RCTs and the evidence from these studies has shown that TNP has some positive effects across a variety of wound types. However, it is acknowledged that there are methodological issues arising from these studies which should be borne in mind when reviewing the evidence. These methodological issues are not unique to studies of TNP, and they appear to be problems in many instances of clinical research in wound healing.[29] One should be aware that RCT is only one form of evidence and in reality the practice of EBM beholds the clinician to consider all of the available evidence. As such the review by Ubbink *et al.*[1] is a summary of part of the evidence and is not the entirety of what is known about TNP. Indeed, there are a number of papers not included in this review,[38,39] probably because of publication dates, and consideration should be given to the implications of this for the conclusions of the review and more importantly for clinical practice.

FUTURE DEVELOPMENTS

TNP therapy is widely used as an intervention in wound healing and a large body of scientific literature has explored its use within the clinical setting. The range of TNP devices has increased and the clinician needs to be aware of the evidences that support the use of the newer models. One should be aware that RCT is only one form of evidence and in reality the practice of EBM beholds the clinician to consider all of the available evidences. Future studies should distinguish between the different TNP devices, and outcome measures chosen should be those that are most clinically applicable.

AUTHOR DISCLOSURE STATEMENT

No competing financial interests exist.

REFERENCES

1. Ubbink DT, *et al.*: A systematic review of topical negative pressure therapy for acute and chronic wounds. Br J Surg 2008; **95:** 685.
2. Argenta LC and Morykwas MJ: Vacuum-assisted closure: a new method for wound control and treatment: clinical experience. Ann Plast Surg 1997; **38:** 563.
3. Shirakawa M and Isseroff RR: Topical negative pressure devices: use for enhancement of healing chronic wounds. Arch Dermatol 2005; **141:** 1449.
4. Jones SM, Banwell PE, and Shakespeare PG: Advances in wound healing: topical negative pressure therapy. Postgrad Med J 2005; **81:** 353.
5. Braakenburg A, *et al.*: The clinical efficacy and cost effectiveness of the vacuum-assisted closure technique in the management of acute and chronic wounds: a randomized controlled trial. Plast Reconstr Surg 2006; **118:** 390.
6. Vuerstaek JD, *et al.*: State of the art treatment of chronic leg ulcers: a randomized controlled trial

comparing vacuum-assisted closure (V.A.C.) with modern wound dressings. J Vasc Surg 2006; **44:** 1029.

7. Mouës CM, *et al.*: Bacterial load in relation to vacuum-assisted closure wound therapy: a prospective randomized trial. Wound Repair Regen 2004; **12:** 11.
8. McCallon SK, *et al.*: Vacuum-assisted closure versus saline-moistened gauze in the healing of postoperative diabetic foot wounds. Ostomy Wound Manage 2000; **46:** 28.
9. Etöz A, Özgenel Y, and Özcan M: The use of negative pressure wound therapy on diabetic foot ulcers: a preliminary controlled trial. Wounds 2004; **16:** 264.
10. Eginton M, *et al.*: A prospective randomized evaluation of negative-pressure wound dressing for diabetic foot wounds. Ann Vasc Surg 2003; **17:** 645.
11. Ford CN, *et al.*: Interim analysis of a prospective, randomized trial of vacuum-assisted closure versus the Healthpoint system in the management of pressure ulcers. Ann Plast Surg 2002; **49:** 55.
12. Wanner MB, *et al.*: Vacuum-assisted wound closure for cheaper and more comfortable healing of pressure sores: a prospective study. Scand J Plast Reconstr Surg Hand Surg 2003; **37:** 28.
13. Jeschke MG, *et al.*: Development of new reconstructive techniques: use of Integra in combination with fibrin glue and negative-pressure therapy for reconstruction of acute and chronic wounds. Plast Reconstr Surg 2004; **113:** 525.
14. Llanos S, *et al.*: Effectiveness of negative pressure closure in the integration of split thickness skin grafts. Ann Surg 2006; **244:** 700.
15. Moisidis E, *et al.*: A prospective, blinded, randomized, controlled clinical trial of topical negative pressure use in skin grafting. Plast Reconstr Surg 2004; **114:** 917.
16. Armstrong DG and Lavery LA: Negative pressure wound therapy after partial diabetic foot amputation: a multicentre, randomised controlled trial. Lancet 2005; **366:** 1704.
17. McInnes E, *et al.*: Support surfaces for pressure ulcer prevention. Cochrane Database of Systematic Reviews, 2008 (4. art. no.: CD001735. DOI: 10.1002/14651858.CD001735.pub3.).
18. Schulz KF: Assessing allocation concealment and blinding in randomised controlled trials: why bother? Evid Based Med 2000; **5:** 36.
19. Fergusson D, *et al.*: Turning a blind eye: the success of blinding reported in a random sample of randomised, placebo controlled trials. BMJ 2004; **328:** 432.
20. Pocock SJ: Blinding and placebos. In: *Clinical Trials: A Practical Approach*. Chichester: John Wiley & Sons, 1983, pp. 90–105.
21. Devereaux PJ, *et al.*: Double blind, you are the weakest link—goodbye! Evid Based Nurs 2002; **5:** 36.
22. Bang H, Ni L, and Davis CE: Assessment of blinding in clinical trials. Controlled Clin Trials 2004; **25:** 143.
23. Begg C, *et al.*: Improving the quality of reporting of randomized controlled trials. The CONSORT statement. JAMA 1996; **276:** 637.
24. Moher D, Schulz KF, and Altman D: The CONSORT statement: revised recommendations for improving the quality of reports of parallel-group randomized trials. CONSORT Group. J Am Med Assoc 2001; **285:** 1987.
25. Mills EJ, *et al.*: The quality of randomized trial reporting in leading medical journals since the revised CONSORT statement. Contemp Clin Trials 2005; **26:** 480.
26. Naylor D: Meta-analysis and the meta-epidemiology of clinical research. BMJ 1997; **315:** 617.
27. Greener J and Grimshaw J: Using meta-analysis to summarise evidence within systematic reviews. Nurse Res 1996; **4:** 27.
28. Gottrup F: Evidence is a challenge in wound care. Int J Lower Extrem Wounds 2006; **5:** 74.
29. Clark M and Price P: Evidence-based practice: sound in theory, weaker in practice? ETRS Bull 2005; **12:** 5.
30. Moore Z and Cowman S: The Cochrane Collaboration, systematic reviews and meta analysis. In: *Nursing Research: Designs and Methods*, edited by Watson R. London: Churchill Livingstone, 2008, pp. 101–111.
31. Moore ZEH and Cowman S: Wound cleansing for pressure ulcers. In: *Cochrane Database of Systematic Reviews*. Wiley and Sons, 2005.
32. Bergin S and Wraight P: Silver based wound dressings and topical agents for treating diabetic foot ulcers. In: *Cochrane Database of Systematic Reviews*. Wiley, 2006.
33. Moore ZEH and Cowman S: Repositioning for treating pressure ulcers. In: *Cochrane Database of Systematic Reviews*. Wiley, 2009.
34. Mendonca D, Papini R, and Price PE: Negative-pressure wound therapy: a snapshot of evidence. Int Wound J 2006; **3:** 261.
35. Pham CT, Middleton PF, and Maddern GJ: The safety and efficacy of topical negative pressure in non-healing wounds: a systematic review. J Wound Care 2006; **15:** 240.
36. Sackett DL, *et al.*: *Evidence-Based Medicine: How to Practice and Teach EBM*. New York: Churchill Livingstone, 1997.
37. Sackett DL, *et al.*: Evidence-based medicine: what it is and what it isn't. BMJ 1996; **312:** 71.
38. Apelqvist J, *et al.*: Resource utilization and economic costs of care based on a randomized trial of vacuum-assisted closure therapy in the treatment of diabetic foot wounds. Am J Surg 2008; **195:** 782.
39. Blume PA, *et al.*: Comparison of negative pressure wound therapy using vacuum-assisted closure with advanced moist wound therapy in the treatment of diabetic foot ulcers: a multicenter randomized controlled trial. Diabetes Care 2008; **31:** 631.

WHS
Wound
Healing
Society

Tangential Hydrosurgery—A New Tool for Wound Debridement

Mark J. Ferretti and Paul Y. Liu*

Department of Surgery, Roger Williams Medical School, Boston University School of Medicine, Providence, Rhode Island.

*Correspondence: Department of Surgery, Roger Williams Medical School, Boston University School of Medicine, 825 Chalkstone Ave., Providence, Rhode Island 02908 (e-mail: pliu@rwmc.org).

Most wounds, whether created by a surgeon's scalpel, or the product of trauma to the integument, heal without more than routine methods of cleansing and reapproximation. But dirty wounds, as well as chronically contaminated wounds such as pressure sores, venous, and arterial ulcers, may need more radical debridement to produce a clean bed. Traditional sharp methods of debridement, relying on sharp implements such as scalpels and curettes, cause significant bloodletting and are imprecise in the amount of tissue removed. This chapter introduces a fairly recent device useful for debriding acute and chronic wounds, the Versajet®. The principles behind this device will be discussed, as well as an overview of other methods of wound debridement. Tangential hydrosurgery, as the technique employed by the Versajet is known, employs a hair-thin high-pressure stream of saline directed orthogonal to the wound surface. This creates a vacuum and cutting effect that slices off fractions of millimeters of tissue with each pass. We believe that this novel device is a significant addition to the armamentarium available in the treatment of wounds. It is rapid, safe (after a learning curve), and precise, with an adjustable power setting. This allows the operator to remove only the targeted tissue, one thin layer at a time, and has yielded superior results in burn wound debridements in areas such as eyelids and hands where sparing tissue is of paramount importance.

BACKGROUND

It is estimated that more than 6.5 million Americans suffer from chronic wounds.[1] One of the factors leading to nonhealing is the presence of bacteria and the associated biofilm in the wound bed which prevent the normal events leading to a closed, healed wound.[2] This biofilm consists of a tough, impermeable layer of glycocalyx which is extremely difficult to remove (dental plaque is perhaps the best-known example of a biofilm in daily evidence). Rapid and efficient methods of removing bacteria and biofilms are thought to be a "best practice" in getting chronic wounds to heal.[3] Traditional methods of removing bacteria and biofilm include dressing changes, topical antimicrobials, sharp debridement, and nonsurgical wound debridement. The efficacy of such methods is highly variable.[4,5]

In acute wounds such as burns or motor-vehicle accidents involving road rash, nonviable tissue and debris need to be removed before the wound can be grafted or healed by secondary intention. The mainstay of clinical burn care is timely eschar removal (deep second- and third-degree burns) before these areas become infected, and immediate split-thickness grafting.[6,7] In large burns involving a significant percentage of the burn victim's total body surface area, this debridement is limited by blood loss, which in turn is a function of both speed of eschar removal and depth of

ADVANCES IN WOUND CARE, VOLUME 1

Printed in U.S.A.
DOI: 10.1089/awc.2009.0177

tissue removal. Dermatomes and Weck or Goulian knives are the mainstay tools of such debriding sessions,[7] and because they rely on pressure on the tissue bed to determine the depth of debridement, they can be imprecise and excessive amount of tissue may be removed. In this arena of wound care, a rapid and more precise method of necrotic tissue removal could also be of benefit.

CLINICAL PROBLEM ADDRESSED

Debridement of the wound bed is the basis of modern wound care. Clinicians have many methods for removing nonviable tissue, slough, and debris from the base and edges of wounds, ranging from wet to dry dressing changes, to using scalpels and curettes to cut and scoop away tissue. These latter tools can cause extreme pain to the patient and may require local anesthetics to be injected around the edges and into the wound bed before beginning the debridement. Surgeons have the option of employing monitored or general anesthesia care to minimize patient discomfort, but this adds considerable expense and recovery time to every operative wound debridement. Other practitioners have relied on other, sometimes less effective means of debridement to minimize pain and expense. Centers for Medicare and Medicaid Services, the parent governmental department overseeing Medicare, has recently targeted the potentially fraudulent practices of some clinicians billing for "partial-thickness wound debridements" consisting of nothing more than saline irrigation and rubbing the wound surface with gauze.[8]

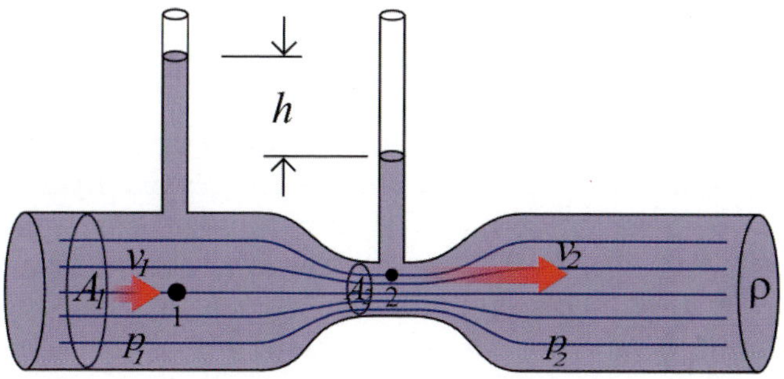

Figure 1. The Venturi effect—fluid velocity speeds up from point 1 to point 2 as a function of the narrowing of the tube diameter. This results in lowered pressure, h, at point 2. This vacuum effect draws the tissue into the path of the saline stream.

RELEVANT BASIC SCIENCE CONTEXT

The physical principles underlying the process of tangential hydrosurgery are fascinating. The vacuum responsible for lifting tissue into the path of the cutting saline stream occurs because of the Venturi effect, which describes the increase in fluid velocity across a narrowing of the stream path, as illustrated in Fig. 1.[9]

Decreased pressure is a side effect of this increased fluid stream velocity, which draws material toward or into the stream. Figure 2 demonstrates how this occurs with the Versajet® device and also shows the tip of the device. As an aside, birds sucked into the intake of jet engines is a modern and hazardous example of the manifestation of the Venturi effect.

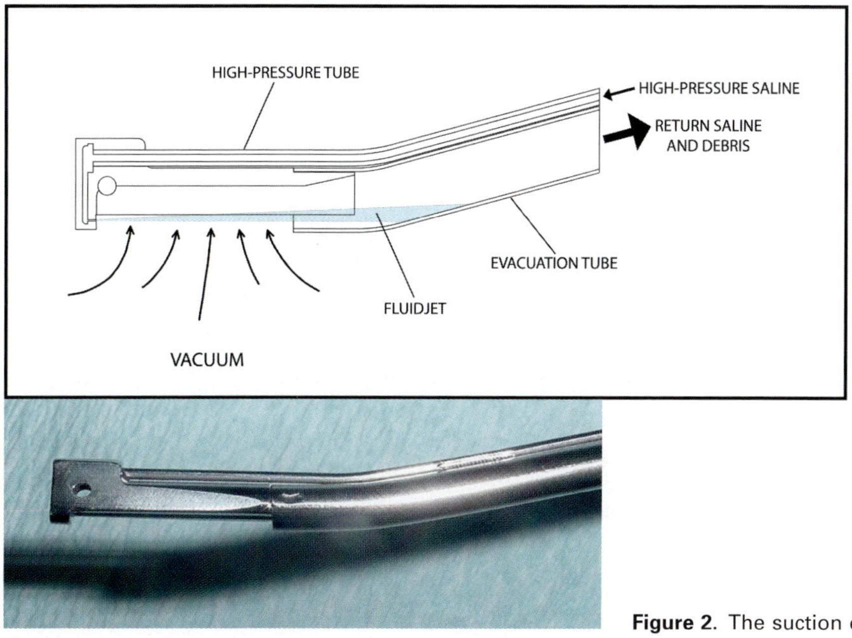

Figure 2. The suction effect at the tip of the Versajet®.

DISCUSSION OF RESULTS/RELEVANT LITERATURE

Several centers in the United States and Europe have already begun to employ tangential hydrosurgery as a method of removing burn eschar and creating a graftable bed.[10–12] In one study, areas traditionally difficult to excise, such as eyelids and hand webspaces, were successfully debrided and grafted with 100% graft take in all 44 patients studied.[10] The thin layers of tissue removed using tangential hydrosurgery leaves delicate viable tissue behind, a situation distinct from using a Goulian-Weck dermatome or Humby knife, where the thickness of eschar removed is both a function of the thickness of a shim placed inside a frame containing a straight edge razor blade, and the amount of pressure exerted by the burn surgeon. An earlier report utilizing these methods for debriding hand burns reported complete take in 93% of patients, so there may be a slight advantage accruing to the use of the Versajet with respect to attaining a graftable bed.[13]

Gravante and colleagues, in a prospective, randomized trial conducted in Belgium, assigned 87 consecutive burned patients in a 1-year time period to eschar debridement using either conventional means or the Versajet.[12] They found that tangential hydrosurgery was significantly faster (and could translate into less blood loss) and was more accurate in finding the correct plane between viable and nonviable dermal remnant.

In a recent study on the debridement of 155 chronic and subacute wounds, Vanwijck and colleagues found that the use of Versajet produced a graftable bed 95% of the time.[14] They concluded that tangential hydrosurgery was a useful technique and a "more highly selective" method of debridement compared with conventional techniques. There has been one published, prospective, randomized trial comparing the Versajet to standard debridement techniques on lower extremity ulcers, performed by Caputo *et al.*[15] They reported that in 41 patients (22 treated with Versajet, 19 treated with scalpel debridement and pulsed lavage), no differences in wound healing rates were recorded, but the Versajet was 39% faster in accomplishing the debridement.

One study looked at the potential role of tangential hydrosurgery in reducing the bacterial bioburden in the wound. Bowling and colleagues used the Versajet on foot ulcers, and then cultured the wounds after the session.[16] They found no statistically significant reduction in the semiquantitative bacterial counts taken from the wound surfaces. This may point to the need to refine techniques to ensure that sufficient tissue is planed off and the biofilm and entrapped bacteria are removed, or to repeat the experiments after controlling for the effects of aerosolized bacteria.

TAKE-HOME MESSAGE

The options for wound debridement vary depending on the tissue and clinical scenario. A synopsis (not meant to be exhaustive) is provided in a tabular form below:

Methods of Debridement	Indications	Caveats
Scalpel	Wound edges, burn eschar, connective tissue	Painful, bloody, imprecise, requires anesthetized area/patient
Curette	Granulation tissue, necrotic bone	Not sharp enough for skin, connective tissue, or intact bone
Enzymatic	Less pain	Slow, may encourage tissue sepsis[16]; animal data show decreased infection[22]
Hydrotherapy	Crust and scale	Bulky apparatus; sterile whirlpools not commonly available
Dressings (occlusive, wet-to-dry)	Less pain, minimal necrotic tissue, eschar	Ineffective or at best slow
Biological (*e.g.*, maggots)	Third-world locale, large volume of necrotic tissue	Blowflies everywhere, "yech" factor
Tangential hydrosurgery	Large surface areas, thinner skin/cosmetically or functionally sensitive areas where tissue sparing is important	Learning curve, expense, usually requires anesthesia, may spread infection via aerosolization,[23] operator risk

SUMMARY ILLUSTRATION

Part of the expense of the Versajet device (between $300 and $400 at our hospital) is the fact that the tubing and handpiece have to be strong enough to withstand the enormous pressures generated by the pump. The tubing, for example, is constructed of Kevlar® (Dupont, Wilmington, DE), the same material used in bulletproof vests by law enforcement personnel. It is also a single-use device, to maintain sterility and prevent cross-contamination.

Accumulating evidence from experimental models and analyses of real wounds is pointing to the importance of biofilm in perpetuating a state of inflammation, rather than substrate replenishment in chronic wounds.[17,18] Mechanical removal of biofilm may be critical as an adjunct to successful wound closure. However, even though the link between biofilm and wound chronicity has not been definitively established, effective wound debridement does help wounds to heal.[19–22] Multicenter trials, such as the recombinant platelet-derived growth factor (Regranex®, Ortho-McNeil Pharmaceutical, Titusville, NJ) study, showed much better healing rates at sites where frequent and aggressive debridement accompanied study visits (Greg Schultz, pers. comm.).

CAUTION AND RECOMMENDATIONS

There are now two forms of the Versajet (Smith & Nephew, Hull, UK): the original handpiece, with about 12,000 lbs/inch^2 of water pressure, called the Versajet Exact®; and a new handpiece, called the Versajet Plus®, which is capable of delivering a couple of thousand additional pounds per square inch of saline jet pressure tangential to the wound surface. This latter device is quite powerful and is much more difficult to plane smoothly over tissue at the highest settings. Bone is not debrided by either device (though marrow spaces are), and the stringy nature of tendon lends itself better to scissor debridement than tangential hydrosurgery. In our experience, composite tissues incorporating hyperkeratotic plantar skin (*e.g.*, surrounding a diabetic plantar foot ulcer) represent the only common wound material requiring the additional expense of the Versajet Plus. Skin paddle deepithelialization, a common technique in plastic surgical procedures where burying a skin/muscle flap is called for, seems to progress more quickly when the Versajet Exact is employed, with a middling power setting between 5 and 7 (Ferretti and Liu, unpublished data).

One additional caution is when the saline stream encounters tissue such as bone or leathery eschar, rather than slice it, there is a splash effect. Operators should therefore wear protective eyewear such as a mask with a clear eyeshield, or goggles with side shields. One group found that bacteria aerosolized from contaminated wounds by the action of the Versajet could be cultured in Petri dishes placed some distance from the operating room table.[16]

FUTURE DEVELOPMENT

There are 23.6 million diabetics in the United States, with 60–70% of them living with some degree of peripheral neuropathy.[23] Though numbness in hands and feet is a significant issue in itself, it sometimes obviates the need for anesthesia before wound debridement. In these cases, the Versajet may be employed without the need for anesthesia. This may make it suitable for use in outpatient wound centers, where the bulk of wound care is carried out. (The senior author served as a nonpaid consultant to the company that invented the Versajet [Hydrocision, Burlington, MA] and discussed the development of a disposable sterile tip, which could be changed between patients.) There are significant engineering issues to overcome, such as the possibility of a dislodged tip being propelled at 12,000 psi across the room or into a patient, but the vast increase in potential numbers of wounds treated in the clinic as opposed to operating room venue might make such a development economically feasible.

AUTHOR DISCLOSURE STATEMENT

The senior author (P.Y.L.) is a compensated speaker for Smith and Nephew (Largo, FL), which owns the rights to the Versajet.

REFERENCES

1. Singer AJ and Clark RA: Cutaneous wound healing. N Engl J Med 1999; **341:** 738.
2. James GA, Swogger E, Wolcott R, Pulcini E, Secor P, Sestrich J, Costerton JW, and Stewart PS: Biofilms in chronic wounds. Wound Repair Regen 2008; **16:** 37.
3. WHS Guidelines for Management of Chronic Wounds.
4. Bowler PG. Wound pathophysiology, infection and therapeutic options. Ann Med 2002; **34:** 419.
5. Akiyama H, Oono T, Saito M, and Iwatsuki K: Assessment of cadexomer iodine against *Staphylococcus aureus* biofilm *in vivo* and *in vitro* using confocal laser scanning microscopy. J Dermatol 2004; **31:** 529.
6. Jeffery SL: Device related tangential excision in burns. Injury 2007; **38(Suppl 5):** S35.
7. Heimbach DM: Early burn excision and grafting. Surg Clin North Am 1987; **67:** 93.
8. In: Proceedings of the *2008 Payment Policy Committee of the American Society of Plastic Surgeons*, Chicago, IL, October 31, 2008.
9. Public domain illustration. www.wikipedia.org.
10. Klein MB, Hunter S, Heimbach DM, Engrav LH, Honari S, Gallery E, Kiriluk DM, and Gibran NS: The Versajet water dissector: a new tool for tangential excision. J Burn Care Rehabil 2005; **26:** 483.
11. Rennekampff HO, Schaller HE, Wisser D, and Tenenhaus M: Debridement of burn wounds with a water jet surgical tool. Burns 2006; **32:** 64.
12. Gravante G, Delogu D, Esposito G, and Montone A: Versajet hydrosurgery versus classic escharectomy for burn débridment: a prospective randomized trial. J Burn Care Res 2007; **28:** 720.
13. Hunt JL, Sato R, and Baxter CR: Early tangential excision and immediate mesh autografting of deep dermal hand burns. Ann Surg 1979; **189:** 147.
14. Vanwijck R, Kaba L, Boland S, Gonzales Y, Azero M, Delange A, and Tourbach S: Immediate skin grafting of sub-acute and chronic wounds debrided by hydrosurgery. J Plast Reconstr Aesthet Surg 2009, February 3.
15. Caputo WJ, Beggs DJ, DeFede JL, Simm L, and Dharma H: A prospective randomised controlled clinical trial comparing hydrosurgery debridement

with conventional surgical debridement in lower extremity ulcers. Int Wound J 2008; **5:** 288.

16. Bowling FL, Stickings DS, Edwards-Jones V, Armstrong DG, and Boulton AJ: Hydrodebridement of wounds: effectiveness in reducing wound bacterial contamination and potential for air bacterial contamination. J Foot Ankle Res 2009; **2:** 13.
17. Rhoads DD, Wolcott RD, and Percival SL: Biofilms in wounds: management strategies. J Wound Care 2008; **17:** 502.
18. Hurlow J and Bowler PG: Clinical experience with wound biofilm and management: a case series. Ostomy Wound Manage 2009; **55:** 38.
19. Granick M, Boykin J, Gamelli R, Schultz G, and Tenenhaus M: Toward a common language: surgical wound bed preparation and debridement. Wound Repair Regen 2006; **14(Suppl 1):** S1.
20. Steed DL, Donohoe D, Webster MW, Lindsley L, and the Diabetic Ulcer Study Group: Effect of extensive debridement on the healing of diabetic foot ulcers. J Am Coll Surg 1996; **183:** 61.
21. Saap LJ and Falanga V: Debridement performance index and its correlation with complete closure of diabetic foot ulcers. Wound Rep Reg 2002; **10:** 354.
22. Payne WG, Salas RE, Ko F, Naidu DK, Donate G, Wright TE, and Robson MC: Enzymatic debriding agents are safe in wounds with high bacterial bioburdens and stimulate healing. Eplasty 2008; **8:** e17.
23. American Diabetes Association www.diabetes.org.

WHS Wound Healing Society

Electrical Activation of Wound-Healing Pathways

Min Zhao,[1,3]* Josef Penninger,[2] and Roslyn Rivkah Isseroff[1,4]

[1] Department of Dermatology, School of Medicine, University of California Davis, Davis, California.
[2] Institute of Molecular Biotechnology of the Austrian Academy of Sciences, Vienna, Austria.
[3] Department of Ophthalmology, University of California Davis, Davis, California
[4] Wound Clinic, VA Medical Center, Mather, California

Background: Effective wound healing has been a lasting and challenging topic in health care. Various strategies have been used to accelerate and perfect the healing process. One such strategy has involved the application of an exogenous electrical stimulus to chronic wounds with the aim of stimulating healing responses.

The Problem: The biology of electric stimulation to instigate healing, however, is very poorly understood. How does electric stimulation induce healing responses?

Basic/Clinical Science Advances: Recent research shows that the electric fields (EFs) activate multiple signaling pathways that are critical for wound healing. Importantly, the EFs provide a powerful, sometimes an overriding, directional signal for cell migration in wound healing. Unlike other stimuli, EFs have the intrinsic property of being directional. The EF-directed cell migration (electrotaxis/galvanotaxis) appears to be a consequence of EF-induced polarized signaling of epidermal growth factor receptors, integrins, and phosphoinositide 3 kinase/Pten, and may be mediated by protein kinase C, intracellular Ca^{2+}, and cyclic adenosine monophosphate (cAMP). Because directional cell migration is a key component in wound healing, galvanotaxis may represent an important mechanism of wound healing.

Clinical Care Relevance: With the constantly enlarging diabetic and aging population, chronic or nonhealing wounds pose increasing health and economic problems, and currently there is no effective therapy available. Electric stimulation activates important intracellular signaling pathways that are polarized in the EF direction, resulting in enhanced and stimulated directional cell migration. Electric stimulation offers a novel approach to achieve better and accelerated wound healing.

Conclusion: Experimental evidence suggests a significant role of endogenous EFs in cell migration in wound healing. Most importantly, EFs are a very powerful signal to direct cell migration. Electric stimulation therefore may represent a promising and unique strategy to induce cell and tissue growth in a directional manner, to enhance wound healing, and to achieve better wound healing.

BACKGROUND

Injury elicits multiple signaling pathways.[1–3] To restore tissue integrity and homeostasis effectively, those signaling pathways have to be well coordinated. Impairment of signaling orchestration may lead to defective healing, and chronic and nonhealing wounds.[4] Many strategies have been used in an attempt to accelerate the healing response. One strategy is application of an exoge-

Abbreviations and Acronyms

AC = alternating current

Akt = a downstream effecter of PI3 kinase. Akt is activated as a result of PI3 kinase activity

cAMP = cyclic adenosine monophosphate (cyclic AMP or 3′-5′-cyclic adenosine monophosphate) is a second messenger that is important in many biological processes

chemoattractant = inorganic or organic substances possessing chemotaxis inducer effect in motile cells

chemotaxis = the phenomenon in which cells direct their movements according to certain chemicals in their environment

contact inhibition = a natural process of arresting cell growth and movement when two or more cells come into contact with each other

DC EFs = direct current electric fields

ECM = extracellular matrix

EF(s) = electric field(s)

EGFR = epidermal growth factor receptor

ERK1/2 = extracellular-signaling regulated kinase 1/2

FAD = Food and Drug Administration

galvanotaxis/electrotaxis = directional cell migration in an electric field

(continued)

Printed in U.S.A.
DOI: 10.1089/awc.2009.0021

(continued from page 567)

integrins = cell surface receptors that interact with the ECM and mediate various intracellular signals. They define cellular shape, mobility, and regulate the cell cycle

pAkt = activated form of Akt

PI3 kinase = phosphoinositide 3-kinases (PI 3-kinases or PI3Ks) are a family of related enzymes that are capable of phosphorylating the 3 position hydroxyl group of the inositol ring of phosphatidylinositol (PtdIns). They are also known as phosphatidylinositol-3-kinases

PKC = protein kinase C

population pressure = growth of adjacent cells form a pressure to push cells to move into a wound

Pten = short of phosphatase and tensin homolog is a protein that acts as a tumor suppressor gene through the action of its phosphatase protein product. This phosphatase is involved in the regulation of the cell cycle, preventing cells from growing and dividing too rapidly

Rac = subfamily of the Rho family of GTPases, small (~21 kDa) signaling G proteins (more specifically a GTPases)

transepithelial potential difference = electric potential difference between the basal side and apical side of epithelial layers

VEGF = vascular endothelial growth factor

VEGFR = vascular endothelial growth factor receptor

*Correspondence: Department of Dermatology, School of Medicine, University of California Davis, 1515 Newton Court, Davis, California 95618-4859 (e-mail: minzhao@ucdavis.edu).

nous electrical stimulus to activate healing.[5–8] Despite encouraging results being reported and approval of Medicare and other insurance policies for use of electric stimulation in some types of chronic and nonhealing wounds, the advancement in using electric stimulation to achieve effective wound healing is limited.[9] Yet, recent research has provided significant insights into electrical stimulation of wound healing.

Endogenous wound electric fields (EFs) are present at human skin wounds, generated immediately upon wounding. Application of EFs, in dose ranges of those generated naturally, activates signaling molecules critical for wound healing in many types of exposed cells, including epidermal growth factor receptors (EGFRs), integrins, and phosphoinositide 3 (PI3) kinases and Pten (phosphatase and tensin homolog).[8,10–13] Significantly, these signaling molecules are activated in a directional manner, often on the side of the cell facing the cathodal pole of the EF. This provides a unique prohealing advantage to application of EF as a therapeutic modality, since the directional cueing of the repair response is maintained as long as the EF is present—unlike the topical application of growth factors or other stimulatory compounds, which normally are difficult to maintain as a stable gradient to sustain directional migratory or proliferative responses. Importantly, the electric signaling appears to be a predominant signaling mechanism in guiding cell migration in epithelial wound healing.[11]

Clinically, both direct current (DC) stimulation and alternating current (AC) stimulation have been tested for wound healing. The stimulation schemes include constant DCs, DC pulses, and ACs. The electric stimulation comes with a huge number of choices of different amplitudes, frequencies (AC and pulsed DC), duty cycles, durations, current strengths, and so on. Current is usually very small for DC stimulation (hundreds of μA–mA). Low-voltage pulsed currents are pulses with durations up to 1 s and voltages up to 150 V. Monophasic and biphasic pulsed currents can be low voltage and high voltage up to several hundred volts with short duration (μs).[7,14–17] For example, a recent clinical study in Germany used Dermapulse® (Gerromed, Hamburg, Germany) with varied polarity, a pulse frequency of 128 Hz, and an average current strength of 300 μA. This double-blinded, placebo-controlled clinical study demonstrated pain relief, improved perfusion, and a tendency of improved healing in chronic venous leg ulcers.[18] Because there are many modalities of using pulsed DC and AC, understanding the effects of those modalities on wound-healing signaling pathways will offer better choice of those many parameters.

In addition to wound healing, electric stimulation has been used in orthopedics, sports medicine, and neurology.[19–22] For bone and cartilage cells, a specific, defined capacitively coupled electrical signal can result in significant upregulation of cartilage matrix protein production, and nitric oxide–dependent chondrocyte proliferation.[14,19]

This short perspective focuses on activation of signaling pathways by DC EFs. Because cells are responsive to DC EFs, exogenously applied electric stimulation is likely to affect cells through same or similar mechanisms. Those responses are likely to be cell-type specific, and stimulation parameter dependent.

CLINICAL PROBLEM ADDRESSED

The clinical problems presented by chronic, nonhealing wounds are familiar to the readers of this review. While acute wounds normally heal without many complications, the comorbidities of diabetes, mal-

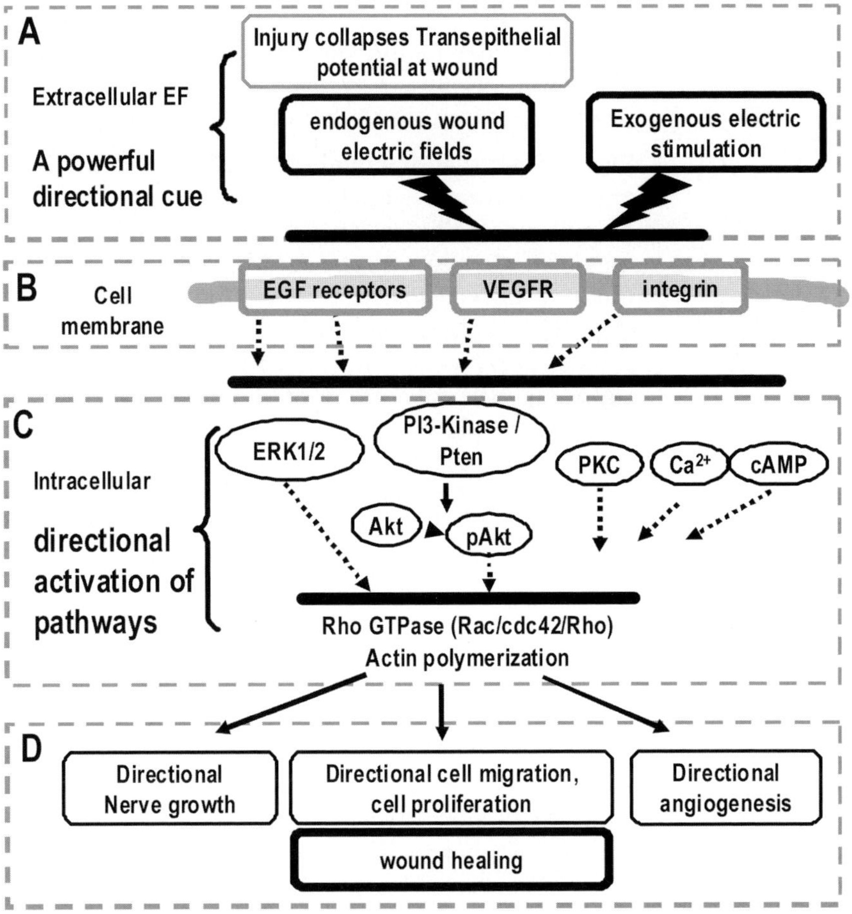

Figure 1. Electrical activation of wound-healing pathways. Schematic diagram shows the generation of the endogenous wound electric signals and the electrical activation of some important signaling pathways for cell migration and wound healing. (**A**) Injury breaks the epithelial barrier and induces endogenous wound electric fields (EFs). Electric stimulation can also be exogenously applied; (**B**) extracellular EFs may activate epidermal growth factor receptors (EGFRs), vascular endothelial growth factor receptors (VEGFRs), and integrins; (**C**) polarized activation of membrane receptors induces asymmetric intracellular signaling, notably extracellular-signaling regulated kinase 1/2 (ERK1/2), phosphoinositide 3 (PI3) kinase/Akt, Rac, and protein kinase C (PKC) to induce downstream cascades; (**D**) the orchestration of the polarized intracellular signaling results in directional cell migration and proliferation, and perhaps directional nerve growth and new blood vessel formation. These effects may lead to improved wound-healing response.

nutrition, pressure, infection, chronic inflammation, and aging can create a scenario that leads to nonhealing wounds. The biologic impediments that prevent healing are poorly understood.[23] Chronic wounds generate significant economic burden to our health care system.[4,24] Even with the best standard of care, up to 30% of venous leg ulcers and 65% of diabetic foot ulcers fail to heal[25] and few therapeutic advances have significantly altered these figures. Thus, new treatment paradigms are needed to address this burgeoning problem.

RELEVANT BASIC SCIENCE CONTEXT

Du-Bois Reymond, a founder of electrophysiology, detected wound EFs on a cut in his fingertip 160 years ago.[26] The existence of endogenous wound EFs has been confirmed in all wounds that have been measured using various modern techniques. When guinea pig skin is wounded, a large and steady EF arises, measuring $\sim 140\,\mathrm{mV/mm}$.[12,27,28] The vibrating probe technique has allowed noninvasive measurements with great temporal and spatial resolution of endogenous electric currents.[11,29,30] The electric currents (flow of positive charge) are oriented toward the wound and, therefore, are well positioned to guide and stimulate the migration and other healing responses of cells at wounds (Fig. 1A).

Impaired cell migration into wounds is characteristic of chronic wounds in the elderly, pressure ulcers, and venous stasis ulcers of the skin.[2,24,31] To heal a wound effectively, cells must not only become motile, but also migrate in the correct direction. Many types of cells migrate directionally in an EF, a phenomenon called electrotaxis or galvanotaxis.[32] Because the cells have to migrate directionally to heal a wound, and because endogenous EFs naturally occur at wounds and cells migrate directionally in EFs, it has long been postulated that the wound EFs might have a role in wound healing in directing cell and tissue growth.[33–35]

EXPERIMENTAL MODEL OR MATERIAL—ADVANTAGES AND LIMITATIONS

We have used a vibrating probe system to measure the endogenous wound electric currents at epithelial wounds of skin and cornea. While not a chronic wound, the acute wound offers the advantage of being easier to manipulate. Using the vibrating probe system requires specialized instrument and special expertise, which limits the use of this technique in the clinical situation. A noninvasive device currently being developed may offer opportunities to measure EFs in patients and determine to what extent the changes in wound EFs correlate to impaired wound healing.[28] This may lead to diagnostic and prognostic application of measuring EFs and indicate manipulation of wound EFs to achieve better wound healing.

We use digital video microscopy to observe EF-induced cellular responses, for example, cell migration, division, and signaling mechanisms. This allows us to mimic the effects of endogenous EFs on the cells. Our results show that keratinocytes, corneal epithelial cells, fibroblasts, endothelial cells, and neutrophils—when cultured in an EF—all migrate directionally. The advantages of this approach include precise control of the experimental conditions, the stimulating parameters, and direct evaluation of the cellular response and signaling mechanisms. We have identified some important signaling mechanisms that are activated by EFs. Most importantly, the electric signaling gives cells a sense of direction by activating EGFR, extracellular-signaling regulated kinase 1/2 (ERK1/2), and PI3 kinase in a polarized manner. The directionality of EFs when combined with promising therapies of using biochemical stimulators such as growth factors may achieve better wound healing, especially in chronic, nonhealing wounds. However, the extrapolation and translation of the results to clinical application are still a major challenge.

With further understanding of the molecular and cellular mechanisms, and development in techniques of application of EFs, electric stimulation may lead to effective therapies.

DISCUSSION OF FINDINGS AND RELEVANT LITERATURE

Newly developed tools such as microneedle arrays and a bioelectric imager have confirmed and greatly extended our understanding of the existence of wound EFs. A shallow slit wound ($\sim$1 mm in depth and $\sim$1–2 mm in length) on human finger tip produces an electric current of 8–10 μA/cm^2.[29] The microneedle arrays and bioelectric imager have measured very similar wound EFs (100–177 mV/mm) on human skin immediately upon wounding.[27,28] EFs of similar strength activate multiple signaling pathways important to wound healing (Fig. 1).

EFs relocalize and activate EGFRs and downstream signaling pathways

EFs induce polarization and activation of EGFRs in keratinocytes and corneal epithelial cells. We have observed cathodal redistribution of EGFRs (Fig. 1B) on keratinocytes and corneal epithelial cells as early as 10 min in an EF. The downstream signaling–dua-phosphorylated ERK1/2 and actin filament are also polarized to the cathodal side.[8,12,41] Long-time exposure in combination with extracellular matrix (ECM) upregulates expression of EGFRs in corneal epithelial cells in culture.[36]

TAKE-HOME MESSAGE

Basic science advances

- Injury induces naturally occurring, endogenous wound EFs, which measure $\sim$100–200 mV/mm at skin and corneal wounds.
- EFs redistribute and activate important membrane receptors for wound healing—EGFRs, VEGFRs, and integrins.
- Importantly, EF-induced activation of the signaling pathways is directional. EFs activate mitogen-activated kinase ERK1/2, PI3 kinase/Akt at the cathodal side in which direction cells migrate.
- EFs of physiological strength stimulate directional cell migration and cell proliferation.
- EFs of physiological strength override other directional cues and are able to guide cell migration against other directional cues in wound healing.
- EFs stimulate endothelial cells to produce VEGF, and direct alignment, migration, and elongation of endothelial cells.
- EFs stimulate and direct nerve sprouting into the wounds and in culture.
- Exogenously applied electrical stimulation mimics the effects of the endogenous wound EFs, and is likely to stimulate and guide cell migration, thus enhances wound healing.
- Pharmacological manipulation of ion transportation at the wound may be an effective way of enhancing the endogenous EFs and achieve better wound healing.

Clinical sciences

- EF-based therapies may represent a powerful approach and a direction of future wound management. With the convincing demonstration of the effect of EFs in directing cell migration, medical bioengineering companies are developing and improving devices for electrical stimulation of wound healing.
- Alternatively, pharmacological manipulation of the endogenous wound EFs may offer novel and effective approaches to develop wound-healing therapies, circumventing concerns of exogenous EF application—variable tissue resistance resulting in uneven distribution of EFs and EF effects to nontargeted tissues.

Relevance to clinical care

- The Center for Medicare and Medicaid Services as well as third-party payers have approved coverage for electric stimulation to treat stage III and stage IV pressure ulcers, arterial ulcers, diabetic ulcers, and venous stasis ulcers. Chronic ulcers are defined as ulcers that have not healed in 30 days.
- Considerable off-label use of electrical stimulatory devices, approved by Food and Drug Administration (FDA) for indications such as bone healing and deep brain stimulation, has been the practice until now (HCPCS code G0281). Currently, several companies are developing devices or bandages using EF-based concept specifically for wound-healing indications. One such bandage has FDA 510(k) premarketing approval (Prosit adhesive bandage; Vomaris (Chandler, AZ); www.accessdatafda.gov/cdrh_docs/pdf8/K081977.pdf).
- Numerous reports suggest efficacy of these devices, but a Cochrane Review protocol reviewing the evidence[40] now underway has still not come to any conclusions. Randomized clinical trials will be needed.
- Pharmacological manipulation of ion transport of the epithelial cells may represent a promising new approach to achieve better wound healing based on the concept of EF-directed cell and tissue growth.
- Use of diuretics, such as furosemide, may interfere with ion transport mechanisms in epithelial cells. Because ion transport is the basis of the endogenous wound EFs, which plays a significant role in wound healing, attention should be paid to diabetic patients who use diuretics and have nonhealing wounds or refractory wounds. Alternative medicine may minimize possible detrimental side effects on wound healing.

EGFR signaling is a ubiquitous signaling mechanism following wounding, and its activation results in many important prohealing responses, such as enhanced directional cell motility and proliferation. Activation of EGFRs also has antiapoptotic effects.

EFs have the intrinsic property of being directional, and do not easily dissipate like soluble chemicals. EFs thus provide a persistent directional signal through activation of intracellular pathways in a polarized manner, different from activation of intracellular signaling by diffusible molecules. This gives the therapeutic approach of electrical stimulation an advantage over conventional approaches with diffusing agents.

Signaling through integrins—Rac

EFs redistribute integrins in fibroblasts.[37] Integrins are cell surface receptors that cells use to bind and respond to the ECM. Integrins have diverse functions. They regulate cell adhesion to ECM and to neighbor cells. They also contribute to the control of cell proliferation, shape, and motility. Integrins also mediate many important signal pathways. Knockout of $\beta 4$ integrin abrogated the electrotaxis of keratinocytes in the absence of EGF, which can be recovered by transfection and expression of $\beta 4$ integrin.[13] Two distinct but synergistic signaling pathways—EGFR and integrin $\beta 4$—coordinate galvanotaxis and are required for the activation of Rac that was essential for directional migration of keratinocytes in response to an EF (Fig. 1B,C).

PI3 kinase and Pten are key molecules that mediate electrotaxis

PI3 kinase/Akt and Pten are compass molecules in directional sensing and migration of cells in response to chemical gradients. EFs activate PI3 kinase/Akt signaling pathway in neutrophils and keratinocytes that are cultured in serum-free medium. The activation of PI3 kinase/Akt and several other kinases in keratinocytes is rapid and specific.[11] Most strikingly, the activation of those signaling pathways is polarized in the direction of cell migration. When the polarity of EF is reversed, PI3 kinase signaling is activated at the new cathode-facing side, membrane protrusion, and directional migration in the new direction ensue.[10,11] Genetic disruption or pharmacological inhibition of PI3 kinase abrogated electrotaxis of corneal epithelial cells and keratinocytes in wound healing in monolayer and organ cultures. Those results suggest that the EF-induced directional activation of PI3 kinase underlies the directional cell migration (Fig. 1C).

EFs are an overriding guidance cue directing cell migration in wound healing

It is generally accepted that the following cues give cells a sense of direction and the cells migrate and grow directionally: (i) injury stimulation *per se*; (ii) gradients of chemoattractants; (iii) contact inhibition release; (iv) wound void; (v) population pressure—growth of adjacent cells; and (vi) changes in mechanical force after injury.[1–3,38] However, when an EF of physiological strength is applied in the opposite direction of those cues, cell migration simply follows the direction of EF,[11] suggesting that EFs are able to override other cues in directing cell migration.

EFs induce and direct proangiogenic responses and nerve growth

In addition to guiding epithelial cells, EFs may direct angiogenesis and nerve growth.[39] An EF upregulates the expression of vascular endothelial growth factor (VEGF). EFs as low as 75–100 mV/mm direct the reorientation, elongation, and migration of endothelial cells in culture. These proangiogenic responses require VEGF receptor (VEGFR) activation and are mediated through PI3 kinase-Akt and the small GTPase Rho kinase (ROCK) signaling pathways, resulting in reorganization of the actin cytoskeleton. Thus, the endogenous EFs might play a role in angiogenesis *in vivo* by stimulating the VEGFR signaling pathway, to induce angiogenic responses. Nerve sprouting at corneal wounds increases in number and grows more directionally when the endogenous would EFs are increased.[12]

Manipulation of endogenous EFs

As the endogenous wound EFs are generated because of transport of ions by ion channels and pumps, we have used pharmacological agents to increase wound EFs, which indeed significantly enhanced wound healing and nerve growth.[11,30]

CAUTION, CRITICAL REMARKS, AND RECOMMENDATIONS

Currently, electric stimulation is being used in certain refractory and nonhealing wounds. While there are reports with encouraging outcomes, there is no FDA-approved device specifically for the indication of skin wound healing. Great discrepancy exists in the reported clinical protocols that claim to have achieved improved wound healing using electric stimulation. Well-controlled, randomized clinical trials and standardization of the device and protocols for electric stimulation are needed.

Practical application of electrical stimulation itself may need to be carefully considered and designed. The endogenous EFs are generated at the leading edge, very focally because of tightly regulated ion transport at the breach to skin electrical resistant barrier. Experimentally applied EFs in culture dish can be precisely controlled. Exogenously applied electric stimulation at wounds in patients, however, can generate highly uneven current density, path, and voltage distribution. Those are significantly confounding factors in electric stimulation for wound healing in patients. These confounding factors may explain the discrepant results reported in some of the clinical trials.

At the same time, electric stimulation for wound healing requires thorough understanding of the underlying mechanisms before therapeutic applications may be more successful, reliable, and consistent. Because electric stimulation may have numerous signaling and cellular targets, appropriate tests are needed to ensure that any beneficial outcome of electric stimulation targeting one type of cell or some particular signaling pathway is not counteracted by other effects on different types of cells and signaling pathways. Understanding how EFs may affect cellular behaviors and signaling pathways in tissues and their functional consequences should bring a new tool to manage chronic wounds.

FUTURE DEVELOPMENT

Despite the remarkable guidance effects of EF on many types of cells, it is still not known how the cells sense the EFs. This type of basic scientific understanding is fundamental to develop effective therapies. It would be important to delineate the signaling pathways and mechanisms of EF-induced cellular responses and the effects on the biology of wound healing.

It is highly important that devices and practice be standardized for wound care clinical trials. From a therapeutic standpoint, the development of safe, effective, and reliable stimulators to specifically manipulate cellular and tissue response *in vitro* as well as *in vivo* could have tremendous impact in this field. We are developing pharmacological approaches to affect the endogenous wound EFs through manipulation of ion transport in epithelial cells. This may represent a practical and easier way to standardize for manipulation of local EFs rather than by application of physical electrodes.

ACKNOWLEDGMENT

Wound healing research in the authors' laboratory is supported by the Wellcome Trust, UC Davis Dermatology Development Fund (to M.Z.) and NIH R01-AR44518 (to R.R.I.). The project described was also supported by Award Number R01EY019101 from the National Eye Institute. The content is solely the responsibility of the authors and does not necessarily represent the official views of the National Eye Institute or the National Institutes of Health.

AUTHOR DISCLOSURE STATEMENT

No competing financial interests exist.

REFERENCES

1. Martin P: Wound healing—aiming for perfect skin regeneration. Science 1997; **276:** 75.
2. Singer AJ and Clark RA: Cutaneous wound healing. N Engl J Med 1999; **341:** 738.
3. Gurtner GC, Werner S, Barrandon Y, and Longaker MT: Wound repair and regeneration. Nature 2008; **453:** 314.
4. Falanga V: Wound healing and its impairment in the diabetic foot. Lancet 2005; **366:** 1736.
5. Stewart S, Rojas-Muñoz A, and Belmonte JCI: Bioelectricity and epimorphic regeneration. Bioessays 2007; **29:** 1133.
6. Olyaee Manesh A, Flemming K, Cullum NA, and Ravaghi H: Electromagnetic therapy for treating pressure ulcers. Cochrane Database Syst Rev 2006; CD002930. DOI: 10.1002/14651858.CD002930.pub3.
7. Kloth LC: Electrical stimulation for wound healing: a review of evidence from *in vitro* studies, animal experiments, and clinical trials. Int J Low Extrem Wounds 2005; **4:** 23.
8. Ojingwa JC and Isseroff RR: Electrical stimulation of wound healing. J Invest Dermatol 2003; **121:** 1.
9. Schaum KD: Decision on national coverage of electromagnetic therapy for wounds. Adv Skin Wound Care 2004; **17:** 316.
10. Huttenlocher A and Horwitz AR: Wound healing with electric potential. N Engl J Med 2007; **356:** 303.
11. Zhao M, Song B, Pu J, Wada T, Reid B, Tai G, Wang F, Guo A, Walczysko P, Gu Y, Sasaki T, Suzuki A, Forrester JV, Bourne HR, Devreotes PN, McCaig CD, and Penninger JM: Electrical signals control wound healing through phosphatidylinositol-3-OH kinase-gamma and PTEN. Nature 2006; **442:** 457.
12. McCaig CD, Rajnicek AM, Song B, and Zhao M: Controlling cell behavior electrically: current views and future potential. Physiol Rev 2005; **85:** 943.
13. Pullar CE, Baier BS, Kariya Y, Russell AJ, Horst BA, Marinkovich MP, and Isseroff RR: beta4 integrin and epidermal growth factor coordinately regulate electric field-mediated directional migration via Rac1. Mol Biol Cell 2006; **17:** 4925.
14. Fitzsimmons RJ, Gordon SL, Kronberg J, Ganey T, and Pilla AA: A pulsing electric field (PEF) increases human chondrocyte proliferation through a transduction pathway involving nitric oxide signaling. J Orthop Res 2008; **26:** 854.
15. Gordon GA: Designed electromagnetic pulsed therapy: clinical applications. J Cell Physiol 2007; **212:** 579.
16. Ramadan A, Elsaidy M, and Zyada R. Effect of low-intensity direct current on the healing of chronic wounds: a literature review. J Wound Care 2008; **17:** 292.
17. Kloth LC and Zhao M: Endogenous and exogenous electrical fields for wound healing. In: *Wound Healing: Evidence-Based Management*, 4th edition, edited by McCulloch L and Kloth LC. Brick: F.A. Davis, 2009.
18. Junger M, Arnold A, Zuder D, Stahl HW, and Heising S: Local therapy and treatment costs of chronic, venous leg ulcers with electrical stimulation (Dermapulse): a prospective, placebo controlled, double blind trial. Wound Repair Regen 2008; **16:** 480.
19. Brighton CT, Wang W, and Clark CC: The effect of electrical fields on gene and protein expression in human osteoarthritic cartilage explants. J Bone Joint Surg 2008; **90:** 833.
20. Mathew NT: Dynamic optimization of chronic migraine treatment: current and future options. Neurology 2009; **72(5 Suppl):** S14.
21. Reinold MM, Macrina LC, Wilk KE, Dugas JR, Cain EL, and Andrews JR: The effect of neuromuscular electrical stimulation of the infraspinatus on shoulder external rotation force production after rotator cuff repair surgery. Am J Sports Med 2008; **36:** 2317.
22. Griffin XL, Warner F, and Costa M: The role of electromagnetic stimulation in the management of established non-union of long bone fractures: what is the evidence? Injury 2008; **39:** 419.
23. Brem H and Tomic-Canic M: Cellular and molecular basis of wound healing in diabetes. J Clin Investig 2007; **117:** 1219.
24. Eaglstein WH and Falanga V: Chronic wounds. Surg Clin North Am 1997; **77:** 689.
25. Kantor J and Margolis DJ: Expected healing rates for chronic wounds. Wounds 2000; **12:** 155.
26. Du Bois-Reymond E: *Untersuchungen uber thierische Elektricitat, Zweiter Band, Zweite Abtheilung (Erste Lieferung).* Berlin: Georg Reimer.
27. Mukerjee EV, Isseroff RR, Nuccitelli R, Collins SD, and Smith RL: Microneedle array for measuring wound generated electric fields. Conf Proc IEEE Eng Med Biol Soc 2006; **1:** 4326.
28. Nuccitelli R, Nuccitelli P, Ramlatchan S, Sanger R, and Smith PJ: Imaging the electric field associated with mouse and human skin wounds. Wound Repair Regen 2008; **16:** 432.
29. Reid B, Nuccitelli R, and Zhao M: Non-invasive measurement of bioelectric currents with a vibrating probe. Nat Protoc 2007; **2:** 661.
30. Reid B, Song B, McCaig CD, and Zhao M: Wound healing in rat cornea: the role of electric currents. FASEB J 2005; **19:** 379.
31. Ramamurthi S, Rahman MQ, Dutton GN, and Ramaesh K: Pathogenesis, clinical features and management of recurrent corneal erosions. Eye 2006; **20:** 635.
32. Robinson KR: The responses of cells to electrical fields: a review. J Cell Biol 1985; **101:** 2023.
33. Nuccitelli R: A role for endogenous electric fields in wound healing. Curr Top Dev Biol 2003; **58:** 1.
34. Farahani RM: Biological mediators of wound healing: the importance of the big picture. Int Wound J 2008; **5:** 414.
35. Jaffe LF and Vanable JW Jr: Electric fields and wound healing. Clin Dermatol 1984; **2:** 34.
36. Zhao M, Dick A, Forrester JV, and McCaig CD: Electric field-directed cell motility involves upregulated expression and asymmetric redistribution of the epidermal growth factor receptors and is enhanced by fibronectin and laminin. Mol Biol Cell 1999; **10:** 1259.
37. Brown MJ and Loew LM: Electric field-directed fibroblast locomotion involves cell surface molecular reorganization and is calcium independent. J Cell Biol 1994; **127:** 117.
38. Fenteany G, Janmey PA, and Stossel TP: Signaling pathways and cell mechanics involved in wound closure by epithelial cell sheets. Curr Biol 2000; **10:** 831.
39. Zhao M, Bai H, Wang E, Forrester JV, and McCaig CD: Electrical stimulation directly induces preangiogenic responses in vascular endothelial cells by signaling through VEGF receptors. J Cell Sci 2004; **117(Pt 3):** 397.
40. Fernandez-Chimeno M, Houghton PE, Holey L. Electrical stimulation for chronic wounds [Protocol]. Cochrane Database of Systematic Reviews 2004, Issue 1. Art. No.: CD004550. DOI: 10.1002/14651858.CD004550
41. Fang KS, Ionides E, Oster G, Nuccitelli R, Isseroff RR: Epidermal growth factor receptor relocalization and kinase activity are necessary for directional migration of keratinocytes in DC electric fields. 1999; J Cell Sci 112 (Pt 12):1967.

WHS
Wound
Healing
Society

The Value of Wound Care Devices

Kris Kieswetter,[1,*] Gregory D. Kunst,[2] and Maggie McMahon[3]

[1]Concept Management, [2]Global Reimbursement, and [3]Global Health Economics, Kinetic Concepts, Inc., San Antonio, Texas.

Abbreviations and Acronyms

EBM = evidence-based medicine

LOS = length of stay

NPWT = negative pressure wound therapy

V.A.C.® = vacuum-assisted closure

*Correspondence: 8023 Vantage Drive, San Antonio, Texas 78230 (e-mail: kieswetk@kci1.com).

Background: The overall cost of wound-related healthcare expenses is expected to increase as a greater proportion of the population becomes older and more susceptible to disease.

The Clinical Problem: Large wounds, as well as those susceptible to deleterious conditions such as considerable bacterial exposure, an ischemic environment, or significant clinical pathology do not readily heal and require considerable attention to achieve final closure.

The Clinical Solution: Active, integrated wound care technologies are capable of promoting wound healing via their ability to reduce infectious material and edema, control exudate, establish perfusion to the wound bed, and stimulate granulation tissue formation.

Market—History, Current, and Prospects: Many technologies have been developed to aggressively treat wounds. These technologies, however, are generally best at augmenting a particular portion of the wound healing process and often do not have a significant evidence basis.

Business Challenges—Policies and Practices: The current climate of short-term payment incentives and fragmented care threaten the opportunity to maximize patient outcomes and health system efficiencies by focusing on cost versus value.

Public–Private Partnership—Strength, Weakness, Opportunity, and Threat (SWOT) Analysis: Practitioners, payers, manufacturers, governmental agencies, and academia must come together to not only capture but also deeply understand data related to costs and value. This information can be well utilized to drive further product development and therapy utilization.

Conclusions: Collaborations between stakeholders can be created that maximize healthcare value by recommending the appropriate use of techniques, therapies, and devices.

BACKGROUND

The total cost of wound care in 2007, including associated expenses such as extended hospital stays and increased clinician time, has been estimated to be greater than $15 billion in the United States.[1] These costs are expected to rise significantly over the next few years, particularly as an increasing proportion of the population becomes older and is more susceptible to diseases such as diabetes and obesity.

Traditionally, wound care has not been perceived as a practice of medicine that requires a high level of sophistication with respect to either treatment modalities or its therapeutic value. Persistence and patience were more commonly the norm rather than aggressive therapeutic intervention. Winter's elucidation of the tenets of moist wound healing[2] initiated a more modern, scientific approach to wound care and has led to the development of many of the

ADVANCES IN WOUND CARE, VOLUME 1

Printed in U.S.A.
DOI: 10.1089/awc.2009.0089

advanced dressings currently available in the marketplace. As knowledge of biological processes, in general, and wound healing, in particular, has expanded, other more sophisticated technologies have arisen to address difficult to heal wounds. Because of the complexities of the wound healing process, various technologies, such as those designed to decrease the level of infectious agents or to increase the body's own reparative capacity through mechanical modalities, application of cells, growth factors, or genetic information, have been developed to aid in this process. These technologies, however, while designed to aid in the entire wound healing process, are generally best at augmenting a particular phase of the process or treating a particular niche of the population.

While it can be argued that the use of these more advanced modalities may increase the cost of healthcare, efforts have only recently begun to address the value of utilizing aggressive methodologies to rapidly heal a patient to decrease the overall utilization of healthcare resources that occurs when an individual has an open wound and is susceptible to infections, requires pain management, and has decreased quality of life due to their inability to participate in their normal activities of daily living.

THE CLINICAL PROBLEM

Open wounds, in the broadest sense, are any violation of the structural integrity of the skin. Small, acute wounds in healthy individuals undergo an orderly progression through the phases of wound healing: inflammation, proliferation, maturation, and remodeling. These wounds are generally closed via primary or secondary intention.

Large wounds, as well as those susceptible to deleterious conditions such as considerable bacterial exposure, an ischemic environment, or significant clinical pathology, however, do not readily heal, and after a given, arbitrary period of recalcitrance are labeled as chronic. These wounds generally require considerable attention with respect to reducing bacterial bioburden and edema, controlling exudate, establishing perfusion to the wound bed, stimulating granulation tissue to fill in the defect, and finally obtaining closure, be it by epithelialization, delayed primary closure, or coverage with a skin graft or flap.

Worthwhile products such as Regranex and Apligraf have come to market by performing stringent clinical trials[3–5] that required use of these products, in conjunction with appropriate adjuncts such as debridement and offloading, until final closure. In large and complicated wounds, however, the end goal of rapid, aggressive re-establishment of the skin's integrity generally cannot be accomplished using a single treatment modality; it generally requires sequential application of therapies that have been developed to perform optimally during a particular phase of wound healing. Unfortunately, clear, widely recognized intermediate clinical endpoints for these phases do not exist and the clinical effectiveness of a particular product or intervention is assessed by how it impacts overall time to closure, rather than the specific biological process(es) it is intended to address.[6] In these situations, the cost of the therapy is readily captured, while the potential value of utilizing a given device or therapy can easily be de-emphasized or lost due to downstream treatment decisions. For instance, a product that creates robust granulation tissue, thereby allowing a clinician to shift his or her focus toward epithelialization earlier than otherwise, may not appear as impactful to the patient's ability to return to his or her normal activities depending on whether the clinician chooses to achieve closure by secondary intention or by a more aggressive method such as application of a split-thickness skin graft.

A CLINICAL SOLUTION (PRODUCT)

One of the key advances in wound care over the past 15 years has been the development of Vacuum-Assisted Closure (V.A.C.®) Therapy (Kinetic Concepts, Inc., San Antonio, TX). The therapy system administers negative (subatmospheric) pressure to the wound site through a proprietary reticulated open-cell polyurethane foam dressing (GranuFoam® Dressing) using a pressure-sensing control mechanism (Therapeutic Regulated Accurate Care® Technology). Briefly, the dressing is cut to size and placed into the wound. This construct is then covered with an adhesive drape that maintains a vacuum seal when the system is in operation. A hole is cut in the drape and covered with a pressure-sensing connective pad that connects to a canister in the therapy unit.

The system is indicated for use with patients in acute, extended, and home care settings who have chronic, acute, traumatic, subacute, and dehisced wounds; partial thickness burns; ulcers (diabetic or pressure); and flaps and grafts. This therapy, along with several of those that have received pre-market approval from the Food and Drug Administration (*i.e.*, Apligraf and Dermagraft), has a significant bases of evidence. Since the vast majority of the data and publications (more than 550 peer-reviewed articles and 16 published randomized clinical trials[7–20]) regarding negative pressure wound therapy (NPWT) are specific to a single system, the proprietary name associated with the studies is being used in this text. Considerable scientific work has been performed to describe how this product promotes wound healing by preparing the wound bed for closure,[8,9,11,12,16,20–24] reducing edema,[23,25,26] promoting granulation tissue formation[8,9,11–13,23,24] and perfusion,[12,15,27,28] and removing exudate and infectious materials. More recently, work has been published that the reticulated open-cell polyurethane foam manifold stimulates granulation tissue by interacting with the underlying tissue to stimulate cellular, protein, and genomic changes that elicit pro-wound healing responses.[29,30] Less robust responses are evident when other manifolding materials are utilized.[29,30]

The above benefits can be further leveraged by combining this technology with controlled delivery and removal of topical treatment solutions and suspensions to the wound bed as performed by the V.A.C. Instill® System (Kinetic Concepts, Inc., San Antonio, TX). The reported literature describes its use in a wide range of clinical conditions and with various solutions.[31,32]

MARKET—HISTORY, CURRENT, AND PROSPECTS

Since its introduction in 1997, V.A.C. Therapy has been utilized to treat over 1,650,000 patients. In addition to the benefits seen in promoting wound healing, the product has received attention for perceived issues such as wound complications, pain, and costs. The issues of pain and wound complications can be easily ameliorated with good clinical practice, and several publications have addressed how best to do so.[33–35] By minimizing the factors that contribute to direct and indirect wound care costs, V.A.C. Therapy has emerged as a cost-effective option for wound healing.[7,8,22,26,36–38] Several studies have demonstrated that use of V.A.C. Therapy can result in fewer adverse events, which results in fewer hospitalizations, fewer emergent care incidents, fewer complications, fewer amputations, fewer dressing changes, decreased personnel commitments, shorter hospitalization, and reduced treatment times.[7,8,22,26,36–38]

The use of this and other similarly well-studied technologies such as Apligraf and Regranex have been successful in driving changes in the practice of medicine. Given the economic times and sensitivity to healthcare expenditures, the issue of cost deserves further attention and has required considerable partnership with public sector organizations. For instance, in combat settings, high-energy traumatic wounds are notoriously susceptible to infections. In one study, retrospective analysis of 88 patients showed a decrease in hospital infections from an anecdotally reported value of 80% to a documented level of 0% with the use of V.A.C. Therapy.[39] The impact of reductions of infections in such dramatic terms resulted in cooperation with the military to perform airworthiness testing that allowed forward deployment of units so that wounded soldiers could receive therapy before, rather than after, transport to Germany. In a civilian setting, the ability to reduce healthcare utilization secondary to increased adoption of V.A.C. Therapy has also been illustrated. Parrett *et al.*[24] reported that after incorporation of V.A.C. Therapy into their organization's practice, there was a trend down the reconstructive ladder toward using fewer free flaps and more delayed closures and skin grafts.

BUSINESS CHALLENGES—POLICIES, PRACTICES, LEGAL, AND GEOGRAPHICAL

Wound management presents an enormous challenge to patients, clinicians, and healthcare systems alike. One of the key challenges in wound care is in the area of aligning product selection with the overall clinical and economic value derived from evidenced-based decision making. Specifically, value-driven healthcare can be defined as the alignment of clinical decision making on the direct interaction between clinical outcomes, quality, and cost. Wound care products that have high acquisition costs when compared to the standard of care but have demonstrated enhancements to clinical outcomes, economic outcomes, and the quality of care reduce the overall cost of care. As an example, V.A.C. Therapy, based on published clinical evidence, has been able to demonstrate an overall reduction in the cost of care by

- reducing time to wound closure,[7,8]
- reducing length of stay (LOS),[7,19,26,36,40]
- reducing relative risk of secondary amputation rates and other surgical procedures,[7,22,41]
- reducing emergency care or readmission rates,[22,36]
- increasing graft/flap take rates,[21] and
- increasing provider productivity[19,26,38,40,42]

With over 7,000 wound care products currently available, each of which can be used during one or more stages of wound healing, the need to standardize the application of wound care products is of paramount concern in moving wound care to a state of the art medical specialty. Additionally, a focus on aligning the specific goals of therapy, available evidentiary support, and product applicability is a critical step forward to developing wound care best practices.

PUBLIC–PRIVATE PARTNERSHIP—STRENGTH, WEAKNESS, OPPORTUNITY, AND THREAT (SWOT) ANALYSIS

The development of best practices and the integration of evidence-based medicine (EBM) in wound care cannot be done by any one stakeholder. Broad collaboration between providers, payers, manufacturers, academia, and governments is the only way to ensure that all incentives are aligned with the goal of improving clinical outcomes and reducing the cost of care (Fig. 1). This strength, weakness, opportunity, and threat (SWOT) analysis is intended to highlight the current situation and potential opportunities afforded in the field by public–private partnerships and should not be construed as focusing on an individual product. Any examples provided are illustrative.

Strengths

Global desire for EBM integration. The wound care sector has begun to see a renewed interest in the integration of EBM defined as, "the conscientious, explicit, and judicious use of current best evidence in making decisions about the care of individual patients."[43]

Weaknesses

Difficulties of treating wounds across the continuum of care. Wounds manifest themselves in all areas of the healthcare system from acute hospitals to long-term care facilities to the outpatient environment. Frequently, the payment incentives across these care settings are not well aligned. In many instances, initial diagnosis and treatment

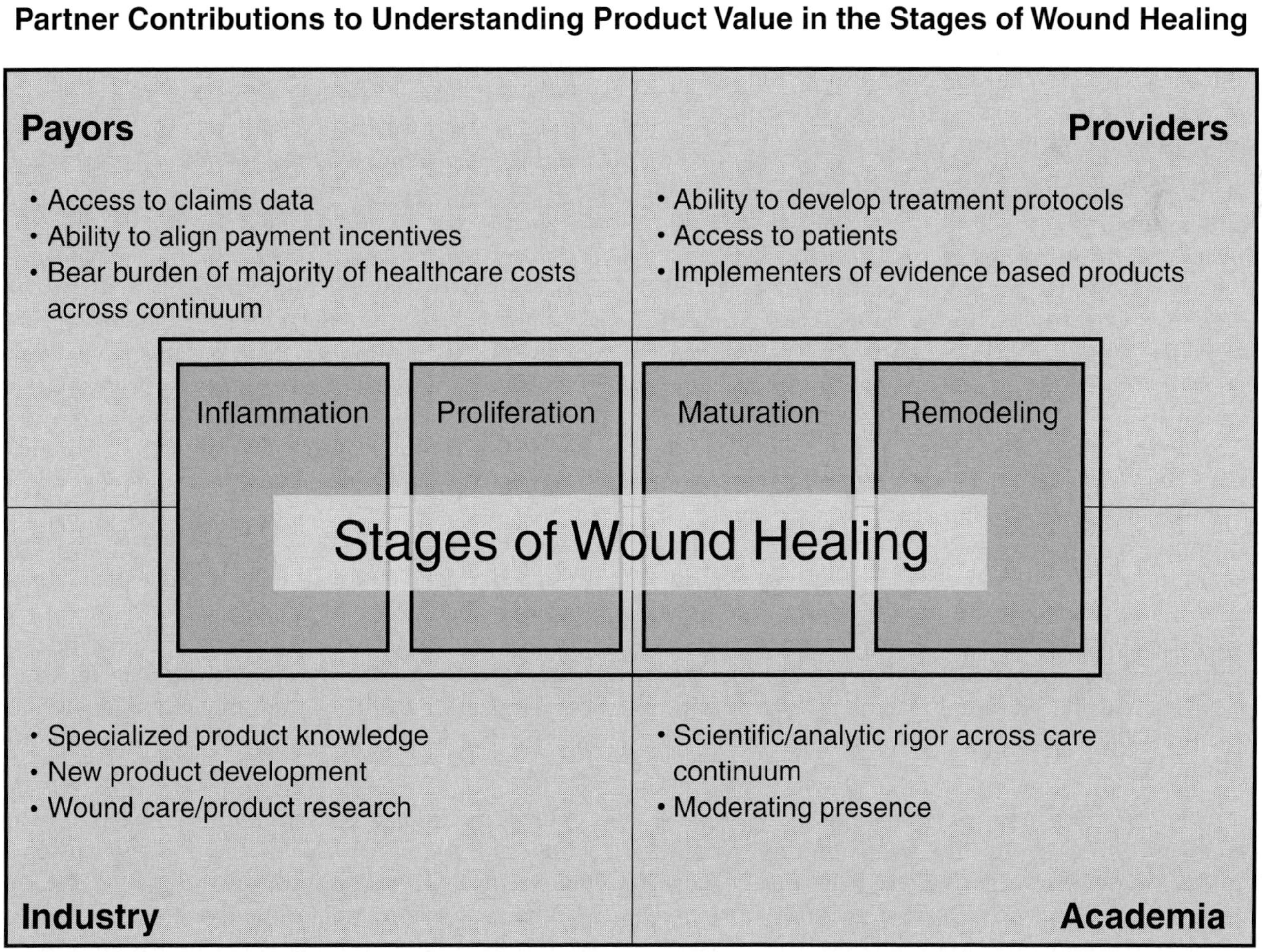

Figure 1. Development of devices and protocols that will deliver the best value requires that all interested parties contribute to understanding how therapies and products impact the various phases of wound healing.

plans are provided by multiple providers in multiple sites of service. Additionally, the initial provider and subsequent providers rarely see wound care patients through to wound closure, therefore minimizing the opportunity to develop best practices. Thus, this multidisciplinary approach to wound care leads to nonprotocolized care.

Weak evidentiary starting foundation. Many wound care products and procedures lack strong clinical evidence to support their use. Implementation of evidence-based decision making requires the development of time-consuming and costly clinical evidence and guidelines to support the standardization of care. This is particularly true when technologies may be used in tandem or sequentially.

Research funding dependent on industry. Where research is available, much of the clinical evidence supporting wound care products has been financed by wound care product manufacturers. There is a continued bias against using industry-financed clinical evidence if the evidence is to be used in evidenced-based decision making. Thus, collaboration between payers, providers, academia, and manufacturers is critical in the validation and expansion of clinical evidence to drive evidence-based decision making in wound care.

Opportunities

Improve understanding of clinical and cost-effective outcomes. Global opportunities exist for expanding Coverage with Evidence Development programs. For promising therapies, these programs should be designed to benefit patients, governments, and sponsoring institutions while data on clinical and cost outcomes are collected. In a current project with Kinetic Concepts, Inc., the German government and insurance companies are developing additional evidence to support outpatient reimbursement of V.A.C. Therapy while providing patient access and provider/manufacturer reimbursement. While the German project uses randomized clinical trials and a registry, retrospective review of electronic medical records and/or claims data also provides ongoing outcomes assessments.

Optimize product use for improved delivery system efficacy. Programs like the Complex Wound Management Program, Kinetic Concepts, Inc.'s pilot partnership with Bupa Australia, are designed to standardize wound treatment, assess outcomes, and demonstrate reduction in overall healthcare costs, inpatient LOS, and hospitalizations. Pilot programs, with meaningful data analysis, that demonstrate overall improved care delivery and cost reductions provide opportunities for better patient care, renewed collaboration between all healthcare stakeholders, and improved reimbursement for efficacious interventions.

Novel technology development partnerships. Enhancing public–private partnerships may also highlight new product development needs and make room for novel technology development partnerships. Robust data sharing and aligned outcome measures/payment incentives create opportunities to identify and then test the efficacy of new products. For example, the Combat Wound Initiative is a multidisciplinary collaborative effort chartered to "provide state-of-the-art wound care through targeted clinical and translation research incorporating advanced technology and treatment, informatics, tissue banking, and research."[44] The studies performed under this initiative utilize inputs from public institutions such as Walter Reed Army Medical Center and Naval Medical Research Center as well as its partners to develop and test novel technologies. One of the Combat Wound Initiative's ongoing efforts involves evaluating the effects of extracorporeal shockwave therapy on wound healing utilizing a device produced by Tissue Regeneration Technologies, Inc. (Atlanta, GA).

Threats

Short-term payment incentives and fragmented care. Globally, few payment structures allow care to be optimized in the most efficient and lowest cost care setting. In England, Primary Care Trusts and Hospitals struggle to manage the appropriate discharge of patients into the community due to discrepancies in incentives created by their separate budgets. The constrained, separate budgets do not create incentives to use products that minimize overall healthcare costs; similar disincentives exist in Canada and Australia. In the United States, hospitals are incented primarily to reduce LOS, inpatient costs, and readmissions, regardless of overall costs across the continuum. Continued fragmentation will threaten opportunities to maximize patient outcomes and health system efficiencies.

Distrust among stakeholders. Capitalizing on collaborative opportunities to efficiently deliver wound care will be difficult given historic distrust between stakeholders. Misalignment in global healthcare systems that results in anything other than payment for clinically and cost effective care has caused stakeholders to turn suspicious eyes toward each other. Realigning payment-based incentives for all players around the same outcome-based metrics may minimize this threat.

Potential destructive pressure on new product development. Severe pressures to minimize costs coupled with expensive and restrictive premarket outcomes data requirements may create destructive pressure on innovation, threatening advances in wound treatment. For example, as standards of care continue to improve, the challenges in demonstrating significant improvement become more and more difficult and may require a prohibitively large number of patients. Partnerships that seek to bring innovative products, aligned with the overall goals of improving clinical and cost outcomes, meet true clinical needs and measure impact, while funding portions of Research and Development activities can help to allay these problems, as well as contribute to improved efficiency and value in our global health systems.

CONCLUSIONS

The value, or balance offered by the aggregate of quality and cost effectiveness outcomes, provided by a given technology or device will continue to gain greater relevance in the upcoming years. The increased pressure on utilization of wound care resources by a greater proportion of the population underscores the importance of developing public–private partnerships whereby industry aligns along the quality and economic objectives of the provider community. By bringing these groups (healthcare practitioners, payers, manufacturers, governmental agencies, and academia) together to not only capture but also deeply understand data related to costs and value, practices can be created that maximize the appropriate use of techniques, therapies, and devices. This information can then be utilized to drive appropriate development of further advances in the wound care space.

The combination of the complexities of the wound healing process and the onerous premarket burdens of clinical proof required for reimbursement, however, may provide a very real disincentive toward future product development. The opportunity for new products to undergo a limited, well-defined period of broad clinical utilization to find their niche with respect toward effectiveness in augmenting a particular phase of the healing process or treating a particular niche of the population should be considered so that their value can be optimized.

CRITICAL REMARKS AND RECOMMENDATIONS

- Wound care technologies must be able to clearly demonstrate their economic as well as clinical benefit to meet widespread acceptance and reimbursement.
- Regulatory and reimbursement strategies should be developed in parallel during the development process.
- New technologies should be offered an opportunity to collect health economic data early in their product life cycle to clearly show their value.
- Health policy and payment decisions should be made in alignment with the best available comparative evidence supporting the use of a particular wound care product.

AUTHOR DISCLOSURE STATEMENT

All authors are employees of and hold stock options in Kinetic Concepts, Inc.

REFERENCES

1. U.S. Advanced Wound Management Markets: N46C-54. 9-5-2008. Palo Alto, CA: Frost & Sullivan.
2. Winter GD and Scales JT: Effect of air drying and dressings on the surface of a wound. Nature 1963; **197:** 91.
3. Wieman TJ: Clinical efficacy of becaplermin (rhPDGF-BB) gel. Becaplermin Gel Studies Group. Am J Surg 1998; **176(2A Suppl):** 74S.
4. Falanga V and Sabolinski M: A bilayered living skin construct (APLIGRAF) accelerates complete closure of hard-to-heal venous ulcers. Wound Repair Regen 1999; **7:** 201.
5. Veves A, Falanga V, Armstrong DG, Sabolinski ML, and Apligraf Diabetic Foot Ulcer Study: Graftskin, a human skin equivalent, is effective in the management of noninfected neuropathic diabetic foot ulcers: a prospective randomized multicenter clinical trial. Diabetes Care 2001; **24:** 290.
6. Steed DL, Hill DP, Woodske ME, Payne WG, and Robson MC: Wound-healing trajectories as outcome measures of venous stasis ulcer treatment. Int Wound J 2006; **3:** 40.
7. Blume PA, Walters J, Payne W, Ayala J, and Lantis J: Comparison of negative pressure wound therapy using vacuum-assisted closure with advanced moist wound therapy in the treatment of diabetic foot ulcers: a multicenter randomized controlled trial. Diabetes Care 2008; **31:** 631.
8. Armstrong DG, Lavery LA, and Diabetic Foot Study Consortium: Negative pressure wound therapy after partial diabetic foot amputation: a multicentre, randomised controlled trial. Lancet 2005; **366:** 1704.
9. Eginton MT, Brown KR, Seabrook GR, Towne JB, and Cambria RA: A prospective randomized evaluation of negative-pressure wound dressings for diabetic foot wounds. Ann Vasc Surg 2003; **17:** 645.
10. Wanner MB, Schwarzl F, Strub B, Zaech GA, and Pierer G: Vacuum-assisted wound closure for cheaper and more comfortable healing of pressure sores: a prospective study. Scand J Plast Reconstr Surg Hand Surg 2003; **37:** 28.

11. McCallon SK, Knight CA, Valiulus JP, Cunningham MW, McCulloch JM, and Farinas LP: Vacuum-assisted closure versus saline-moistened gauze in the healing of postoperative diabetic foot wounds. Ostomy Wound Manage 2000; **46:** 28.

12. Joseph E, Hamori CA, Bergman S, Roaf E, Swann NF, and Anastasi GW: A prospective, randomized trial of vacuum-assisted closure versus standard therapy of chronic nonhealing wounds. Wounds 2000; **12:** 60.

13. Moues CM, Vos MC, Van Den Bemd GJ, Stijnen T, and Hovius SE: Bacterial load in relation to vacuum-assisted closure wound therapy: a prospective randomized trial. Wound Repair Regen 2004; **12:** 11.

14. Braakenburg A, Obdeijn MC, Feitz R, van Rooij IA, van Griethuysen AJ, and Klinkenbijl JH: The clinical efficacy and cost effectiveness of the vacuum-assisted closure technique in the management of acute and chronic wounds: a randomized controlled trial. Plast Reconstr Surg 2006; **118:** 390.

15. Timmers MS, Le CS, Banwell P, and Jukema GN: The effects of varying degrees of pressure delivered by negative-pressure wound therapy on skin perfusion. Ann Plast Surg 2005; **55:** 665.

16. Moisidis E, Heath T, Boorer C, Ho K, and Deva AK: A prospective, blinded, randomized, controlled clinical trial of topical negative pressure use in skin grafting. Plast Reconstr Surg 2004; **114:** 917.

17. Wild T, Stremitzer S, budzanowski A, Hoelzenbein T, Ludwig C, and Ohrenberger G: Definition of efficiency in vacuum therapy—a randomized controlled trial comparing Redon drains with V.A.C.® Therapy. Int Wound J 2008; **5:** 641.

18. Stannard JP, Robinson JT, Anderson ER, McGwin G Jr., Volgas DA, and Alonso JE: Negative pressure wound therapy to treat hematomas and surgical incisions following high-energy trauma. J Trauma 2006; **60:** 1301.

19. Vuerstaek JD, Vainas T, Wuite J, Nelemans P, Neumann MH, and Veraart JC: State-of-the-art treatment of chronic leg ulcers: a randomized controlled trial comparing vacuum-assisted closure (V.A.C.) with modern wound dressings. J Vasc Surg 2006; **44:** 1029.

20. Jeschke MG, Rose C, Angele P, Fuchtmeier B, Nerlich MN, and Bolder U: Development of new reconstructive techniques: use of Integra in combination with fibrin glue and negative-pressure therapy for reconstruction of acute and chronic wounds. Plast Reconstr Surg 2004; **113:** 525.

21. Genecov DG, Schneider AM, Morykwas MJ, Parker D, White WL, and Argenta LC: A controlled subatmospheric pressure dressing increases the rate of skin graft donor site reepithelialization. Ann Plast Surg 1998; **40:** 219.

22. Page JC, Newswander B, Schwenke DC, Hansen M, and Ferguson J: Retrospective analysis of negative pressure wound therapy in open foot wounds with significant soft tissue defects. Adv Skin Wound Care 2004; **17:** 354.

23. DeFranzo AJ, Argenta LC, Marks MW, Molnar JA, David LR, Webb LX, Ward WG, and Teasdall RG: The use of vacuum-assisted closure therapy for the treatment of lower-extremity wounds with exposed bone. Plast Reconstr Surg 2001; **108:** 1184.

24. Parrett BM, Matros E, Pribaz JJ, and Orgill DP: Lower extremity trauma: trends in the management of soft-tissue reconstruction of open tibia-fibula fractures. Plast Reconstr Surg 2006; **117:** 1315.

25. Kamolz LP, Andel H, Haslik W, Winter W, Meissl G, and Frey M: Use of subatmospheric pressure therapy to prevent burn wound progression in human: first experiences. Burns 2004; **30:** 253.

26. Kaplan M: Negative pressure wound therapy in the management of abdominal compartment syndrome. Ostomy Wound Manage 2004; **50 (11A Suppl):** 20S.

27. Wackenfors A, Gustafsson R, Sjogren J, Algotsson L, Ingemansson R, and Malmsjo M: Blood flow responses in the peristernal thoracic wall during vacuum-assisted closure therapy. Ann Thorac Surg 2005; **79:** 1724.

28. Greene AK, Puder M, Roy R, Arsenault D, Kwei S, Moses MA, and Orgill DP: Microdeformational wound therapy: effects on angiogenesis and matrix metalloproteinases in chronic wounds of 3 debilitated patients. Ann Plast Surg 2006; **56:** 418.

29. Derrick KL, Norbury K, Kieswetter K, Skaf J, and McNulty AK: Comparative analysis of global gene expression profiles between diabetic rat wounds treated with vacuum-assisted closure therapy, moist wound healing or gauze under suction. Int Wound J 2008; **5:** 615.

30. McNulty AK, Schmidt M, Feeley T, and Kieswetter K: Effects of negative pressure wound therapy on fibroblast viability, chemotactic signaling, and proliferation in a provisional wound (fibrin) matrix. Wound Repair Regen 2007; **15:** 838.

31. Wolvos T: Wound instillation with negative pressure wound therapy. Ostomy Wound Manage 2005; **51(2A Suppl):** 21S.

32. Gabriel A, Shores J., Heinrich C, Baqai W, Kalina S, Sogioka N, and Gupta S: Negative pressure wound therapy with instillation: a pilot study describing a new method for treating infected wounds. Int Wound J 2008; **5:** 399.

33. Baharestani M, De Leon J, Mendez-Eastman S, Powell G, Weir D, Niezgoda J, Payne W, Nanney LB, Pelham F, and Gupta S: Consensus statement: a practical guide for managing pressure ulcers with negative pressure wound therapy utilizing vacuum-assisted closure—understanding the treatment algorithm. Adv Skin Wound Care 2008; **21(Suppl 1):** 1.

34. Orgill DP, Austen WG, Butler CE, Fine NA, Horvath KA, Mihaljevic T, Song DH, and Wolfe WG: Guidelines for treatment of complex chest wounds with negative pressure wound therapy. Wounds 2004; **16(SupplB):** 1.

35. Andros G, Armstrong DG, Attinger C, Boulton AJM, Frykberg RG, Joseph WS, Lavery LA, Morbach S, Niezgoda JA, and Toursarkissian B: Consensus statement on negative pressure wound therapy (V.A.C.® Therapy) for the management of diabetic foot wounds. Wounds 2006; **52(6-Suppl):** 1.

36. Schwien T, Gilbert J, and Lang C: Pressure ulcer prevalence and the role of negative pressure wound therapy in home health quality outcomes. Ostomy Wound Manage 2005; **51:** 47.

37. Frykberg RG and Williams DV: Negative-pressure wound therapy and diabetic foot amputations: a retrospective study of payer claims data. J Am Podiatr Med Assoc 2007; **97:** 351.

38. Niezgoda JA: The economic value of negative pressure wound therapy. Ostomy Wound Manage 2005; **51(2A Suppl):** 44S.

39. Leininger BE, Rasmussen TE, Smith DL, Jenkins DH, and Coppola C: Experience with wound VAC and delayed primary closure of contaminated soft tissue injuries in Iraq. J Trauma 2006; **61:** 1207.

40. Moues CM, Van Den Bemd GJ, Meerding WJ, and Hovius SE: An economic evaluation of the use of TNP on full-thickness wounds. J Wound Care 2005; **14:** 224.

41. Sjogren J, Gustafsson R, Nilsson J, Malmsjo M, and Ingemansson R: Clinical outcome after post-sternotomy mediastinitis: vacuum-assisted closure versus conventional treatment. Ann Thorac Surg 2005; **79:** 2049.

42. Lavery LA, Boulton AJ, Niezgoda JA, and Sheehan P: A comparison of diabetic foot ulcer outcomes using negative pressure wound therapy versus historical standard of care. Int Wound J 2007; **4:** 103.

43. Sackett DL, Rosenberg WM, Gray JA, Haynes RB, and Richardson WS: Evidence based medicine: what it is and what it isn't. Br Med J 1996; **312:** 71.

44. Elster EA, Davis JM, and Stojadinovic A: Combat Wound Initiative Summary. International Society for Musculoskeletal Shockwave Therapy 2007 Meeting, Toronto, Canada, 72, 2007.

Section 12

Public–private Partnership

Section Editors: Kris Kieswetter and Katy Rowland

PUBLIC–PRIVATE PARTNERSHIP

WHS Wound Healing Society

Wound Management Services and Academic Partnerships

Katy Rowland[1,*] and Peter Metcalfe[2]

[1]*Departments of Clinical Services and* [2]*Information Services, National Healing Corporation, Boca Raton, Florida.*

*Correspondence: Department of Clinical Services, National Healing Corporation, 4850 T-Rex Ave., Boca Raton, Florida 33431 (e-mail: krowland@nationalhealing.com).

Background: Building a partnership for research between wound management service companies and academia has the potential to create a model that facilitates translational research while developing physician scientists.

Clinical Problem: Building a partnership between academia and wound management services requires reaching a mutually agreed vision. There are multiple stakeholders and requirements in this partnership that can easily come into conflict and limit the effectiveness of the research program.

Clinical Solution: Ensuring that there are shared values, goals, and research priorities is critical to the development of a successful partnership. A research advisory board that represents the interests of both parties while advancing the goals of the partnership is essential.

Market—History, Current, and Prospects: Evaluating the effectiveness of such guidelines in practice will require access to large data sets that have already been shown to provide valuable prognostic information for the prediction of wound healing.

Business Challenges—Policies, Practices, Legal, and Geographical: As research is costly, and to mitigate such cost burdens, management companies need to ensure that the model is practical to implement and integrates reasonably into everyday practice. The academia needs to ensure that research protocols will be followed and that data quality and integrity are viewed as being of paramount importance.

Public–Private Partnership: Partnerships between wound management service companies and academic research centers can be a powerful research engine for improving the effectiveness of wound practices. The broad reach of such companies provides significant opportunities for a nationally relevant translational research model. Failure to align interests and maintain a balanced perspective on development in the industry while protecting each stakeholder's needs can undermine the sustainability of the entity.

BACKGROUND

THE CLINICAL RESEARCH infrastructure of the United States is currently at a critical crossroad. Fragmented, outdated, and ailing, it is rapidly emerging as a rate-limiting step in transferring novel basic research into improved patient care.[1]

As a discipline, wound management is particularly affected by this situation. The concept of organized wound management services, specifically in the outpatient setting, emerged in the United States in the mid-1990s. As organized entities, providers of these services should provide clinicians with the best available evidence in the form of tools and education that preprocesses the latest wound research.

Academic Medicine's traditional mission of education, research, and clinical care can serve as a catalyst to the development of these tools and to

Printed in U.S.A.
DOI: 10.1089/awc.2009.0107

the maturation of practicing wound specialists in multiple and diverse clinical settings. Conducting research is time consuming and costly. Researchers need access to large study populations to achieve an adequate sample size and the potential for rapid enrollment in their studies. Outpatient wound centers operated by these service companies have the potential to be a rich source of subjects for such researches. The services they provide currently represent a $4.2 billion market which is projected to grow by 10% per year.[2] It is estimated that over 500 hospitals are managed by a wound management company.

Building a partnership for research between wound management service companies and academia has the potential to create a model that facilitates translational research while developing physician scientists. However, creating such a partnership can be challenging and there is no good model for reference. A research advisory board is an essential component of such a partnership and in overcoming these challenges. Its fundamental role is to ensure a shared vision and to oversee the activities of the program and the needs of each partner to sustain a translational research program.

CLINICAL PROBLEM

Building a partnership between academia and wound management services requires reaching a mutually agreed vision. There are multiple stakeholders and requirements in this partnership that include the hospital and their desire to do research, management company leadership and their strategic objectives, university researchers and their research interests, investors in the management company and their targets for return on investment, physician principal investigators in the centers and their time commitments, and university objectives. The management company partners with the hospital to establish an outpatient wound service and with that certain quality and performance achievements are expected of the management company as a condition of maintaining the partnership. Research projects that deviate substantially from routine clinical practice can absorb additional resources and prevent hospital client's expectations from being met. This can be problematic for the sustenance of ongoing partnerships.

Hospital and community sizes vary, and although many hospitals desire to get involved in research, their experience in conducting research may be minimal. Experience and instruction in conducting such researches may be lacking for both the physicians and the center's staff.

Finally, academia may have needs to support their mission related to ownership of publication rights and authorship which may impose undesirable constraints to a project in which the management company might otherwise be desirable.

CLINICAL SOLUTION

Key challenges in building a partnership:

1. What are the needs of each partner?
2. How to access whether there are shared values, goals, and research priorities?
3. What are the limits of one's organization and competing demands?
4. How can the partnership help build capacity to conduct research?
5. What is the value added for each partner from involvement in research versus the risks inherent in participation?
6. How do the partners build effective relationships?
7. What does a balanced collaboration with equal power sharing entail?
8. How do the management company goals mirror academic goals?
9. How do the partners use a research advisory board effectively?[3]

Ensuring that there are shared values, goals, and research priorities is critical to the development of a successful partnership. In addition to the large number of wound patients they treat, wound management companies provide a single set of policies and documentation tools that are used across the centers managed by them. This provides for consistency in terminology and practices, such as how wounds are measured, along with a common set of data elements that can be aggregated and analyzed. In addition, hospital size and geography vary, thus contributing to the ability to generalize study findings and results.

There are three key steps to development of this model:

1. Creating a mutually agreed vision.
2. Developing a memorandum of understanding about the partnership and the needs of each party.
3. Establishing a research advisory board to oversee the program on behalf of all parties.

Duties of a research advisory board:

1. Responding to individual parent organizations is necessary to ensure continued authority and resources.
2. Targeting only those issues critical to the enterprise's success that require multiple stakeholders for a solution.
3. Overseeing and integrating.
4. Agreeing on standards, integrating them into workflow, and sustaining them over time.
5. Developing or ensuring that there is a good research training program.

MARKET—HISTORY, CURRENT, AND PROSPECTS

In addition to the cost of research and time involved for the sponsoring companies, there is also a need for good clinical data to establish best practice. The Wound Healing Society has published guidelines for diagnosing and treating the major types of chronic wounds. During the development of these guidelines, it was noted by Adrian Barbul, M.D., President of the Wound Healing Society, that despite many recent advances in wound care, the challenge of managing chronic wounds is compounded by the current lack of uniformly accepted diagnostic methods to evaluate the outcomes and consensus on clearly defined, comprehensive wound standards. (The Wound Care Guidelines were compiled by the Wound Healing Society in the December 2006 issue of *Wound Repair and Regeneration*.) Evaluating the effectiveness of such guidelines in practice will require access to large data sets that have already been shown to provide valuable prognostic information for the prediction of wound healing.[4]

BUSINESS CHALLENGES—POLICIES, PRACTICES, LEGAL, AND GEOGRAPHICAL

Research is very resource consuming. The drug companies spent $39.4 billion in research and development in 2005. DiMasi, Hansen, and Grabowski[5] (2003) estimated the cost of bringing a drug from phase I to market. Their work was based on data from the Tufts Center for the Study of Drug Development. The firms included in their survey represent 42% of all pharmaceutical R&D expenditures in the United States. The authors found that the time from the start of clinical testing to marketing approval was approximately 90.3 months. The final estimate was that it costs—including the expense of failed drugs—$802 million to take a drug from phase I trials to approval. Over 50% of this figure is the cost of capital needed to finance the R&D over such a long period.

To mitigate such cost burdens, management companies need to ensure that the model is practical to implement and integrates reasonably into everyday practice. The academia needs to ensure that research protocols will be followed and that data quality and integrity are viewed as being of paramount importance. All parties desire research that is conducted ethically, is scientifically sound, and satisfies prevailing regulatory requirements.[6] Unfortunately, because of such potentially conflicting requirements, many times the research conducted in these settings does not translate to a change in outcome for patients.

PUBLIC–PRIVATE PARTNERSHIP—SWOT ANALYSIS

Strengths

The need for good clinical research in wound care that results in changes in the way clinicians practice is central to achieve the best possible clinical outcomes for chronic wound patients. A partnership between academia and wound management services has the potential to combine the highest level of scientific rigor with a broad, multiregional influence in healthcare. Diffusion of the practice improvements that emerge from such a partnership can be accelerated in the wound management services environment. The structure of the wound management services provides an educational platform that trains physicians and nurses new to wound care in the most current protocols and science available. Their clinical policies and quality management processes provide an essential means of monitoring knowledge retention and practice adoption. Subsequently, the partnership also provides the essential conduits for broadcast (marketing) and dissemination (research publications) of advances translated from research and proven in practice. One such promising example is the development of a tissue bank of chronic wound biopsies, which holds the potential to identify genetic markers associated with delayed healing.[7]

Weaknesses

As mentioned earlier, failure to align values and goals of the partners can limit the potential and effectiveness of the partnership. Academic requirements such as publication rights, researcher interests, and overall university objectives may not be congruent with management services' objectives. Conflict of interest may arise in the area of ownership of intellectual property which may emerge from partnership research activities.

Unusual operational requirements for a specific research project may impose a burden or disruption to the efficient operation of the center, impacting productivity and return for both the company and the hospital. As private entities, management companies must meet shareholder expectations, both short and long term, which can compete with the timeline and focus of an academic setting.

Opportunities

Undoubtedly, public–private partnerships in this field can provide significant opportunities for improvements in care delivery and patient outcomes. Through such research and care delivery platforms, comparative new research products can be evaluated more effectively and brought to market more efficiently. These studies can provide funding agencies with good cost comparison data, which can maximize the resources available for wound care via a strategy that allocates resources based on better comparative research. Importantly, this type of platform can also fuel a commercialization strategy to sustain the partnership and further increase its influence and impact. Finally, data and new knowledge generated from this partnership can shape and mature evidence-based algorithms that are applied to multiple clinical practice settings.

Threats

Despite the proliferation of wound management service companies in the 1990s, today there are only a small number of organizations with the needed infrastructure and reach to effect such an effective partnership with major academic research institutions. As a result, the potential exists for such partnerships to evolve in a manner that does not provide an exposure to a broad scientific influence, which in turn can lead to an undesirable narrowing of perspective and focus.

CONCLUSION

Evidence in wound care is sparse. Research to advance best practice is needed but is very costly. Patient enrolment in clinical research is a key variable in the amount of time and resources it takes to complete a good clinical trial. A partnership between an academic setting and a management services company can provide an effective and compelling platform for conducting translational research that impacts the care in multiple geographic communities. This can result not only in the creation of new knowledge but also the adoption of that knowledge into real bedside practice. To build an effective and self-sustaining partnership, it is vital to establish a common vision, create a written document representing both parties' needs, and establish a research advisory committee to oversee the needs of each party while respecting and advancing the goals of the partnership. Developing and supporting physician scientists, which is part of this process, will advance the needs of the academic researchers, the effectiveness and success of the management company, and most importantly the quality of care given to the wound patients in communities across the United States.

CRITICAL REMARKS AND RECOMMENDATIONS

- Wound healing research is needed to advance the industry.
- Partnerships between wound management services and academic institutions can enhance wound research in both quality and quantity and support the development of physician scientists.
- This type of partnership can create an ideal platform for translational research, thereby improving direct care to patients in multiple communities.
- Sharing a clear vision is paramount for these partnerships to work effectively.

AUTHOR DISCLOSURE STATEMENT

No competing financial interests exist.

REFERENCES

1. Crowley WF, Sherwood L, Salber P, *et al.*: Clinical research in the United States at a crossroads: proposal for a novel public-private partnership to establish a National Clinical Research Enterprise. JAMA 2004; **291:** 1120.
2. The Advisory Board: *Considerations for Developing a Wound Care Center.* Washington, DC; The Advisory Board, April 11, 2007, No. 9.
3. Norris KC, Brusuelas R, *et al.*: Partnering with community-based organizations: an academic institution's evolving perspective. Ethn Dis 2007; **17(1 Suppl 1):** S27.
4. Margolis DJ, Gelfand JM, Hoffstad O, and Berlin JA: Surrogate end points for the treatment of diabetic neuropathic foot ulcers. Diabetes Care 2003; **26:** 1696.
5. DiMasi JA, Hansen RW, and Grabowski HG: The Price of innovation: new estimates of drug development costs. J of Health Economics 2003; **22:** 151.
6. Bozik M: He who pays the piper calls the tune: the role of the industry sponsor in acute stroke trials. Eur Neurol 2003; **49:** 128.
7. Roy S, Patel D, *et al.*: Transcriptome-wide analysis of blood vessels laser captured from human skin and chronic wound-edge tissue. Proc Natl Acad Sci USA 2007; **104:** 14472.

Time is Tissue—How Early and Accurate Assessment of Lower Extremity Peripheral Arterial Disease Leads to Favorable Outcomes

Paul L. Vaughn*

Chandler Wound Healing and Hyperbaric Oxygen Center, Chandler Regional Hospital, Chandler, Arizona.

Background: Lower extremity arterial disease can be a significant impediment to wound healing often resulting in delayed/nonhealing, especially in compromised patient populations. Peripheral arterial disease prevalence and influential comorbid rates remain on the rise with 50% of the patients having peripheral arterial disease being asymptomatic thereby further crippling their ability to heal effectively.
Clinical Problem: Complicating the landscape is a montage of technologies fraught with limitations, inaccuracies, or both, which are recommended as the standard of care for lower limb arterial patency and perfusion assessment.
Clinical Solution: Improve the "clinician tool box" by identifying noninvasive technologies that are timely, accurate, and convenient for the patient and end-user.
Market—History, Current, and Prospects: A variety of noninvasive test modalities (NITMs) have been established and include Ankle-Brachial Index, Toe-Brachial Index, segmental pressures, pulse volume recording, transcutaneous partial oxygen, and skin perfusion pressure measurements.
Business Challenges—Policies, Practices, Legal, and Geographical: Despite known limitations, certain preference-sensitive NITMs remain as standards regardless of clinical situation and/or economic need. The effective-care NITM is supported by evidence, provides relevant documentation, is multispecialty oriented and serves as a front-line, point-of-care reference. Combining skin perfusion pressure and pulse volume recording yields an effective tool for assessing tissue viability and directing therapy.
Public–Private Partnership—Strengths, Weaknesses, Opportunities, Threats (SWOT) Analysis: A cohesive relationship between industry and care providers is crucial to ensuring delivery of medically economic and accountable patient care.
Conclusion: Provision of and access to more efficient and clinically diagnostic tools can serve the clinician and patient well through improved coordination of care, uniformity of service, and timely direction of therapeutic intervention.

Abbreviations and Acronyms

CLI = critical limb ischemia
DM = diabetes mellitus
NITM = noninvasive test modality
NIVT = noninvasive vascular test or noninvasive vascular testing
PAD = peripheral arterial disease
SPP = skin perfusion pressure
SWOT = strengths, weaknesses, opportunities, threats

*Correspondence: Chandler Wound Healing and Hyperbaric Oxygen Center, Chandler Regional Hospital, 1875 West Frye Road, Chandler, Arizona 85224 (e-mail: plvmd@aol.com).

BACKGROUND

Lower extremity arterial disease can be a significant impediment to wound healing and often results in delayed or nonhealing, especially in compromised patient populations such as those with poorly managed heart failure, noncompliant peripheral vessels, diabetes mellitus (DM), and/or renal insufficiency. Impairment of regional and localized flow and the effects this has on endothelial health and the pliancy and/or patency of vessels can prevent sufficient nourishment from reaching the wound to effect tissue healing. With the increasing burden of a diabetic population that is projected to

Printed in U.S.A.
DOI: 10.1089/awc.2009.0045

escalate to 37.7 million by the year 2031,[1] a current obesity epidemic involving more than 72 million U.S. adults (one-third of the U.S. adult population)[2] and documented rates of peripheral arterial disease (PAD) affecting 12 million people in the United States alone,[3] the potential health resource utilization and financial impact to our national health and economic climate are undeniable.

From a patient's perspective, the effect of PAD is felt through diminished quality of life, claudication or rest pain, decreased mobility, need for revascularization, cardiovascular disease, foot ulcerations, nontraumatic amputations, and significant morbidity and mortality.[4] PAD serves to further complicate the lower extremity wound landscape as 50% to 70% of the patients with the disease are asymptomatic.[3,5–7] Without adequate evaluation and testing, the disease may go undetected until the severity increases to a symptomatic level, thereby further prolonging a patient's ability to heal effectively and/or leading to undesirable outcomes that include critical limb ischemia (CLI) and amputation. Early identification of PAD can influence and effectively help direct the appropriate treatment pathway whether it be aggressive risk factor modification and/or actual revascularization for the individual patient suffering its affect.

When evaluating the lower extremity wound environment, we must ensure our patient assessment informs us sufficiently through provision of high-level objective of data obtained in a timely manner, to comfortably and confidently determine an optimal treatment care plan for the circumstance. This cannot be achieved solely though physical examination but should incorporate systemic and local evaluation, pathogenic influence, cellular failure, and noninvasive testing as first-line defense mechanisms.

CLINICAL PROBLEM

While the ability to effect tissue healing is multivariant with one variable being the in-line arterial blood supply,[8] there are four common pathways to nonhealing wounds: infection, malperfusion, cellular failure, and unrelieved pressure/repetitive trauma.[9] It is imperative to assess for all four components both during the initial presentation and continually throughout the wound care phase; however, this review will focus on the commonality of the vascular element of supply and malperfusion.

The health provider is presented with multiple challenges in assessing patients presenting with lower extremity wounds. As an example, in the evaluation of PAD a clinician must choose the best modality that will provide the required information in a cost-effective[10] and timely manner. Ideally the modality will provide an upstream analysis of the large arterial vessels (regional macrovascular component) and a distal arterial vessel assessment (local capillaries, the microvascular component). To accurately gauge lower limb arterial patency and thus the adequacy for healing potential or the need for vascular intervention at the point of care, both assessments are necessary. Complicating the landscape, however, is a montage of technologies fraught with limitations, inaccuracies, or both, which are recommended as the standard of care for evaluation of lower limb arterial patency. Choice of these technologies is in large part preference driven versus algorithm driven, often luring the physician into ordering tests with speculative interpretations suggesting further and unnecessary additional testing.

CLINICAL SOLUTION

We can improve the "clinician tool box" by identifying NITM technologies that are timely, accurate, reproducible, and convenient for the patient and the end-user. However, in search of a solution to the NITM dilemma, a review of each technology's benefits and limitations is necessary.

Although the Ankle-Brachial Index is the front-line assessment tool for PAD detection as recommended by the American Heart Association/ American College of Cardiology Guidelines that cites its cost effectiveness, the same document warns that it is proven inaccurate in the following populations: patients with DM and/or renal compromise, those with calcified or noncompliant vessels, and the elderly.[11] When considering the current patient landscape with its ever-increasing diabetes rate and that we are quickly approaching the largest elderly population in the history of our nation,[12] identification of effective technologies to assess PAD becomes ever important. Toe-Brachial Indices are not affected by calcified vessels and are cost effective but have anatomic limitations and require careful technique to preserve accuracy.[11] Segmental pressures provide good anatomic localization of disease level but as with Ankle-Brachial Index, it is inaccurate in the presence of noncompressible arteries, DM, and advanced age.[11] Pulse volume waveforms are useful in the diagnosis and monitoring of PAD level and severity, CLI, and interventions. It is unaffected by noncompressible vessels; however, it is limited in that it is non-specific and a qualitative not quantitative tool.[11] Transcutaneous partial oxygen monitoring is not affected by vessel calcification but is time consuming, often problematic to perform,[13] has anatomical limitations, and is operator dependent. Skin perfusion pressure (SPP) requires little time to perform, is cost effective, user friendly, has few site limitations,[14] is a functional tool for regional mapping, correlates well with other more costly testing (multidetector-row computed tomography),[15] and is not hampered by noncompliant or calcified vessels,[16] issues previously discussed. By combining SPP and pulse volume recording, the clinician can readily and effectively assess the lower extremities for both local and regional health using the following parameters: local, a SPP value of <30 mmHg strongly correlates with CLI and nonhealing; regional, the presence and severity of arterial disease may be observed as a diminished pulse volume recording waveform evidenced in the loss of the dicrotic notch, a delay in the systolic upstroke and diastolic downstroke creating a wider pulse width, and a dampening or blunting of the peak.

MARKET—HISTORY, CURRENT, AND PROSPECTS

Although PAD incidence rates are inclining, the disease remains largely underdiagnosed and undertreated.[3] One method of impact is to implement appropriate diagnostic protocols that are user friendly and accurately reflect a patient's condition irrespective of their comorbidities. Accuracy is important since the unreliable referral of a patient for more invasive and expensive testing only serves to increase the financial burdens placed on payers. In addition, provision of an optimal tool for arterial status assessment that adequately detects lower extremity disease presence and level of severity at the point of care (*i.e.*, in the clinic or office setting) providing fast and easy access to critical limb perfusion data would help to rapidly triage patients into appropriate therapeutic algorithms (conservative specialty care such as a wound clinic, vascular intervention, and planned amputation) earlier in their disease process, thereby permitting implementation of focused therapies that have evidence-based success.

For many disciplines from cardiology to emergency medicine, the "golden hour" concept is well known and refers to early reperfusion to salvage tissue and the beneficial effect on outcomes and prognosis.[17] The same "time-is-tissue" principle can be readily applied to lower limb management. For example, early detection of PAD in advance of the manifestation of clinical symptomology can translate to earlier cardiovascular risk factor modification and revascularization before the limb becoming ischemic. This is important since first-motivation for a patient to seek treatment is frequently severe limb pain (nociceptive tissue injury that may be secondary to vascular compromise) or a foul smelling and draining chronic ulcer in the circumstance of patients with significantly decreased sensation secondary to diabetic neuropathy. Accurate and timely point-of-care testing can expedite the diagnosis and assist in the management of a targeted goal-focused treatment plan compared to a patient presenting with late-stage PAD as evidenced in the patient with mixed disease such as a DM neuropathic ulcer with malperfusion secondary to occlusive disease of the tibial artery. As with other disciplines,[18] rapid diagnosis and treatment can be a key factor in decreasing morbidity and mortality rates.

BUSINESS CHALLENGES—POLICIES, PRACTICES, LEGAL, AND GEOGRAPHICAL

There are numerous business challenges that face organizations and individuals who care for patients with comorbid disease. Improving quality and costs requires organization and accountability across multiple dimensions not to mention specialties. Care providers of this patient population are charged with ensuring appropriate policies and practices are in place with respect to staff training, mitigating potential patient risks, and ensuring medical–legal requirements are met in terms of documentation and recordkeeping. Beyond these, administrative elements are the crucial nuts-and-bolts of everyday patient care. As healthcare providers, we must make sure that certain appropriate patient treatment algorithms are evidenced and followed to an acceptable standard, and that the care we offer is of the highest quality. This directive applies to the lower extremity noninvasive vascular testing (NIVT) we order and/or perform. We want to foster organizational accountability across medical disciplines to provide the best management at the best price for the highly comorbid patient populations we serve. The role of point-of-care NIVT/NITM within this context is to provide the 5 R's: Rapid, Right Result (the first time), Reliability, Record of Result, and Repertoire (clinical/customer/payor need). In the case of lower extremity wounds and PAD, the ideal NIVT/NITM will provide sufficient documentation, serve as a front-line, point-of-care reference tool that supports decision making, supplies accurate, relevant, and current patient data, and is available without delay. The combination of SPP measurements and pulse volume waveforms may be a best fit for the ideal NIVT/NITM since they yield an effective tool for assessing tissue viability[19,20] and directing therapy including the monitoring of peripheral vascular interventions.[21–23] In this model, a requisite base of fundamental knowledge of the natural history of PAD is required by the physician providing point-of-care NIVT/NITM.

PUBLIC–PRIVATE PARTNERSHIP—SWOT ANALYSIS

Many considerations loom on the forefront of PAD management not the least of which is healthcare reform that focuses on this very high-cost disease. The underdiagnosis of PAD in the primary care setting may thwart effective secondary preventive strategies.[3,24] In consideration of disease prevalence, the coming storm of escalating comorbid rates (DM, hypertension, obesity, renal compromise, and tobacco use) and the underlying element of occult PAD, it becomes imperative that we both strengthen and broaden the relational supporting medical structure. Dr. Elliott S. Fisher[25] published the "Medical House" concept, referring to the coordination and delivery of healthcare to patients with chronic diseases through the creation and management of a continuous relationship between the patient and providers to optimally navigate the healthcare system. This concept is especially important to treating PAD resultant of its systemic polyvascular nature.

Recognizing that PAD is impacted by the above cited conditions, and that subclinical PAD is associated with numerous systemic conditions including atherosclerotic vascular disease, increased cardiovascular disease events, and even erectile dysfunction, a coordinated care model that is both medically and economically driven is needed. As an example, timely, objective, and precise patient data can influence the clinician to: (a) determine if more invasive testing is necessary, (b) initiate treatment, (c) refer the patient to another appropriate specialty, or (d) pursue vascular intervention. This scenario can be an effective medical–economic marker, but only if the level of information provided is accurate, not ambiguous. It can guide the physician to mitigate ordering potentially unnecessary and more expensive tests, affect initiation of treatment earlier in the treatment cycle, ensure that assessment/testing is performed initially at the point of care rather than prolonged secondary to patient noncompliance or transportation issues, and ultimately impact patient outcomes. However, at-risk patient populations often have limited access to PAD assessment by their primary care physician due to logistics, time, resources, or general awareness particularly in the case of occult PAD.

To effectively impact the observed influence and effect of PAD, it must be diagnosed early in the disease process, that is, ideally before the development of clinical symptomology. Hirsch *et al.* demonstrated through conduct of a large study that the under-utilization of early screening and diagnosis of PAD could be a barrier to preventing further cardiovascular risk.[3] Disease presence and severity can readily be detected through utilization of established technologies as screening and diagnostic tools. However, current practices that support screening assessments and standardize the current variations in treatment algorithms exercised throughout the care process remain unadopted. Professional organizations have ardently worked toward this end including the American Heart Association/American College of Cardiology, the American Diabetes Association, and the American College of Preventive Medicine. Their ongoing work is demonstrated in the establishment of the PAD treatment guidelines and diabetic guidelines and recommendations. Despite the undeniable and notable progress of professional organizations, additional alliances could be beneficial in this arena. As Dr. Fisher suggests, the medical home has great potential to improve the delivery of coordinated healthcare to patients, but that significant obstacles still exist.

As a care group treating patients we would be well suited to align patient care models with shared strategies across disciplines to attack the disease process early in the cycle through detection and effective treatment. At-risk and standard populations should have provisional access to screening procedures by knowledgeable providers, yet there are obstacles that remain even here (Fig. 1). In an already burdened healthcare system where reimbursement for "PAD screening" is in most instances not a provision, and medical clinics strive to provide the best quality care for the lowest cost, often NIVT for lower extremity assessment is not conducted. Unfortunately, the reality of this circumstance is that the disease process is actually observable and underway but for lack of appropriate training in recognizing its manifestations in other areas of the body, it is frequently first noticed only when the patient presents with symptoms including evidence of CLI or gangrenous wounds.

To truly effect change whether observed in a reduction of amputation rates through the adoption of advanced diagnostic and therapeutic

SWOT Analysis Summary Illustrating Relational Impact of Care Providers and Industry

Strengths

- Existence of effective tools for disease detection/severity determination and tissue viability
- Existence of diverse medical and health care networks
- Early detection of PAD translates to early treatment integration and potentially better outcomes

Weaknesses

- Lack of strategic alliances
- Lack of uniformity in conduct of NIVT across centers
- Lack of evidence-based, standardized treatment algorithms
- Efficient care coordination/referral networks
- Complications of the "polyvascular" umbrella

Opportunities

- Build upon stronger "medical house and community" concept
- Orchestration of disease care to include screening, monitoring, and treatment options
- Effective targeting of PAD identification and evaluation
- Reduce disease severity and resource utilization

Threats

- Increasing PAD prevalence and comorbid rates
- Limited access for at-risk patients to have PAD assessment by their PCP
- No change in amputation rates by not adopting advanced diagnostic and therapy technologies
- Lack of a multidisciplinary approach to treating patients with PAD/CLI

Figure 1. SWOT analysis summary illustrating relational impact of care providers and industry.

technologies, or by affecting a reduction in the long-term rates of PAD severity and associated complications, development of cohesive relationships between professional medical organizations, care providers, regulatory agencies, and industry is crucial to ensuring delivery of quality patient care.

CONCLUSION

PAD rates in the U.S. adult population are substantial, and inadequate recognition of the local, regional, and systemic effects of the disease may place many more patients at risk for complications. Through timely application of currently available technologies that are user friendly and provide accurate and objective individualized patient data, we have an opportunity to impact disease progression through early detection and standardization of treatment models. The author believes that provision of, and access to, better tools can serve the clinician and patient well through optimal and timely directed therapeutic pathways. Further, by bridging medical specialties for care coordination, implementation of cross-discipline treatment care plans, and broadening relational organization scopes, we have the potential to improve our ability to save time, save tissue, and ultimately, save lives.

CRITICAL REMARKS AND RECOMMENDATIONS

- Early assessment for tissue viability and disease presence may translate to overall improved outcomes through more timely intervention and goal-directed therapies.

- Formation of strategic alliances across disciplines, larger organizations, and industry may yield positive dividends in terms of patient care and overall lower limb outcomes regardless of whether the etiology is disease or wound based.
- Combining the technologies of SPP and pulse volume waveforms yield an optimal point-of-care tool for the clinician who provides prompt, accurate, objective, and meaningful individualized patient data to better direct treatment plans.

ACKNOWLEDGMENT

No financial support or compensation was received for manuscript development.

AUTHOR DISCLOSURE STATEMENT

No competing financial interests exist.

REFERENCES

1. Mainous AG, Baker R, Koopman RJ, Saxena S, Diaz VA, Everett CJ, and Majeed A: Impact of the population at risk of diabetes on projections of diabetes burden in the United States: an epidemic on the way. Diabetologia 2007; **50:** 934.
2. CDC publication: Obesity at a glance 2009 (CS123149). Centers for Disease Control and Prevention, National Center for Chronic Disease Prevention and Health Promotion, Atlanta, GA.
3. Hirsch AT, Criqui MH, Treat-Jacobson D, Regensteiner JG, Creager MA, Olin JW, *et al.*: Peripheral arterial disease detection, awareness, and treatment in primary care. JAMA 2001; **286:** 1317.
4. Norgren L, Hiatt WR, Dormandy JA, Nehler MR, Harris KA, Fowkes FG, *et al.*: Inter-society consensus for the management of peripheral arterial disease (TASC II). Eur J Vasc Endovasc Surg 2007; **33:** S1.
5. McDermott MM, Guralnik JM, Ferrucci L, Tian L, Liu K, Liao Y, *et al.*: Asymptomatic peripheral arterial disease is associated with more adverse lower extremity characteristics than intermittent claudication. Circulation 2008; **117:** 2484.
6. Kanjwal MK, Cooper C, and Bashir R: Peripheral arterial disease–the silent killer. JK Pract 2004; **11:** 225.
7. Dormandy JA and Rutherford RB: Management of peripheral arterial disease (PAD). TASC Working Group. TransAtlantic Inter-Society Concensus (TASC). J Vasc Surg 2000; **31(1Pt2):** S1.
8. Rose SC: Noninvasive vascular laboratory for evaluation of peripheral arterial occlusive disease: part II-clinical applications: chronic, usually atherosclerotic, lower extremity ischemia. JVIR 2000; **11:** 1257.
9. Warriner RA: Wound assessment. In: *Wound Care Practices*, 2nd edition, edited by Sheffield PJ and Fife CE. Flagstaff, AZ: Best Publishing Company, 2007, pp. 83–108.
10. de Vries, Ouwendijk R, Flobbe K, Nelemans PJ, Kessels AG, Schurink GH, *et al.*: Peripheral arterial disease: clinical and cost comparisons between duplex US and contrast-enhanced MR angiography—a multicenter randomized trial. Radiology 2006; **240:** 401.
11. Hirsch AT, Haskal ZJ, Hertzer NR, Bakal CW, Creager MA, Halpern JL, *et al.*: ACC/AHA guidelines for the management of patients with peripheral arterial disease (lower extremity, renal, mesenteric, and abdominal aortic): executive summary: a collaborative report for the American Association for Vascular Surgery/Society for Vascular Surgery, Society for Cardiovascular Angiography and Interventions, Society of Interventional Radiology, Society for Vascular Medicine and Biology, and the American College of Cardiology/American Heart Association Task Force on Practice Guidelines. JACC 2006; **47:** 1239.
12. Hobbs, Frank and Nichole Stoops, U.S. Census Bureau, Census 2000 Special Reports, Series CENSR-4, Demographic Trends in the 20th Century, U.S. Government Printing Office, Washington, DC, 2002.
13. Castronuovo JJ: The role of skin perfusion pressure and transcutaneous partial pressure oxygen measurements in chronic critical limb ischemia. In: *Vascular Diagnosis*, 1st edition, edited by Mansour MA and Labropoulos N. Philadelphia, PA: Elsevier Saunders, 2005, pp. 247–255.
14. Kondo Y, Muto A, Dardik A, Nishibe M, and Nishibe T: Laser Doppler skin perfusion pressure in the diagnosis of limb ischemia in patients with diabetes mellitus and/or hemodialysis. Int Angiol 2007; **26:** 258.
15. Okamoto K, Oka M, Maesato K, Ikee R, Mano T, Moriya H, *et al.*: Peripheral arterial occlusive disease is more prevalent in patients with hemodialysis: comparison with the findings of multidetector-row computed tomography. Am J Kidney Dis 2006; **48:** 269.
16. Yamada T, Ohta T, Ishibashi H, Sugimoto I, Iwata H, Takahashi M, and Kawanishi J: Clinical reliability and utility of skin perfusion pressure measurement in ischemic limbs-comparison with other noninvasive diagnostic methods. J Vasc Surg 2008; **47:** 318.
17. Yesil M: Management of arrhythmias during transportation in patients with acute myocardial infarction. Anatol J Cardiol 2007; **7 Suppl 1:** 85.
18. Sirlin CB, Brown MA, Deutsch R, Andrade-Barreto OA, Fortlage DA, Hoyt DB, and Casola G: Screening US for blunt abdominal trauma: objective predictors of false-negative findings and missed injuries. Radiology 2003; **229:** 766.
19. Dwars BJ, Van den Broek TA, Rauwerda JA, and Baaker FC: Criteria for reliable selection of the lowest level of amputation in peripheral vascular disease. J Vasc Surg 1992; **15:** 536.
20. Schechter RR and Bailey BB: Clinical utility evaluation of lower extremity wound assessment and healing potential. Wounds 2008; **20:** A32 (Abstract).
21. Iida O, Nanto S, Uematsu M, Morozumi T, Akahori H, and Negata S. Endovascular therapy for limb salvage in a case of critical lower limb ischemia resulting from fibromuscular dysplasia. J Vasc Surg 2007; **46:** 803.
22. Tsai Y, Hiroto T, Kitano I, Tahara S, and Sugiyama D: Importance of skin perfusion pressure in treatment of critical limb ischemia. Wounds 2008; **20:** 95.
23. Akahori H, Uematsu M, Morozumi T, Watanabe T, Awata M, Onishi T, *et al.*: Magnitude of the improvement in skin perfusion pressure is as important as skin perfusion pressure immediately following intervention for predicting limb salvage in critical limb ischemia. Abstract presented at American College of Cardiology 56th Annual Scientific Session, New Orleans, LA.
24. Gey DC, Lesho EP, and Manngold J: Management of peripheral arterial disease. Am Fam Physician 2004; **69:** 525.
25. Fisher ES: Building a medical neighborhood for the medical home. NEJM 2008; **359:** 1202.

WHS
Wound
Healing
Society

Developing a Gene-Activated Matrix Product for Chronic Wounds: A Biotech's Perspective

Barbara K. Sosnowski,[1,*] Robert Engler,[2,3] and Lois A. Chandler[1]

[1]*Tissue Repair Company, San Diego, California.*
[2]*Cardium Therapeutics, Inc., San Diego, California.*
[3]*Professor of Medicine Emeritus, Department of Medicine, Cardiovascular Division, University of California, San Diego, California.*

Background: The normal wound healing process is mediated by specific cells and cytokines, especially growth factors. In chronic wounds, there is often a deficiency of endogenous growth factors, which impairs healing.
The Clinical Problem: Administration of exogenous growth factor proteins has had limited success because of inefficient delivery, inadequate persistence, and poor patient compliance with daily treatment regimens for prolonged periods of time.
The Clinical Solution: If the gene encoding a growth factor could be transfected into cells in the tissue defect, prolonged production of growth factor could improve therapeutic efficacy. Formulating the DNA vector in a biocompatible matrix (Gene Activated Matrix) can further enhance the product potential. GAM501 (an adenovector encoding platelet-derived growth factor-B gene within 2.6% collagen matrix) has progressed to a phase 2b clinical trial.
Market—History, Current, and Prospects: Only recombinant human platelet-derived growth factor-B homodimer (becaplermin) has been approved by the U.S. Food and Drug Administration for the treatment of diabetic ulcers. There remains a compelling medical need for a more practical and effective therapy for nonhealing ulcers, which is a large and expanding market.
Business Challenges—Policies & Practices: An ideal wound healing product would promote faster healing, be more effective and easier to use, and be less expensive itself or require fewer associated medical resources than current products (*i.e.*, faster, better, and cheaper). A combination product must generally demonstrate that both components are required for efficacy, or that the combination is superior to the individual components.
Public–Private Partnership—SWOT (strength, weakness, opportunities, threat) Analysis: Developing a combination wound healing product requires collaboration with the U.S. Food and Drug Administration, and gene therapy trials must be reviewed by the Recombinant DNA Advisory Committee at National Institutes of Health.
Conclusion: Collaboration with regulatory agencies during all phases of clinical development and periodic reanalysis of trial design strategies and commercial plans is essential in developing combination products for wound healing.

Abbreviations and Acronyms

Ad5PDGF-B = adenovirus serotype 5, E1a/b deleted, encoding PDGF-B
FDA = U.S. Food and Drug Administration
GAM = gene-activated matrix
GAM501 = Ad5PDGF-B in 2.6% collagen
NIAMS = National Institute of Arthritis and Musculoskeletal and Skin Diseases
NIH = National Institutes of Health
PDGF-BB = platelet-derived growth factor-B homodimer
PMOA = primary mode of action
RAC = Recombinant DNA Advisory Committee
SOC = Standard of Care
SWOT = strength, weakness, opportunities, threat

*Correspondence: Tissue Repair Company, 12255 El Camino Real #250 San Diego, CA 92130 (e-mail: bsosnowski@t-r-co.com).

BACKGROUND

Wound healing of lower extremity ulcers in diabetic patients is significantly impaired relative to acute wound healing in healthy individuals. Diabetes-associated vascular insufficiency, neuropathy, and infection all contribute to impairment of wound healing. As a result, a significant percentage of diabetic ulcers do not heal and become chronic wounds that persist for months or years.

Printed in U.S.A.
DOI: 10.1089/awc.2009.0007

Nonhealing ulcers are susceptible to infections that can eventually lead to amputation. Individuals with lower-limb amputations are at risk for developing further medical complications and have a 50% mortality rate at 3 years.[1]

The current standard of care (SOC) for the treatment of diabetic foot ulcers consists of a combination of (i) sharp surgical debridement to remove necrotic soft tissue, bio-burden, debris, sinus tracts, and callus, (ii) daily dressing changes with saline-moistened gauze, and (iii) use of a weight off-loading device to remove pressure from the ulcer area. Even with regular treatment, only 31% of wounds treated with SOC will heal over a 20-week period.[2] Other approved treatment modalities include devices such as vacuum pumps for exudate removal, hyperbaric oxygen, living skin equivalents, and becaplermin (human platelet-derived growth factor-BB protein [PDGF-BB]; Regranex® Systagenix, North Yorkshire, UK). However, several of these products have demonstrated limited benefit over SOC, and their use requires frequent clinic visits or repeated treatments at home in a patient population in which compliance is often a major problem. A more ideal therapeutic for diabetic ulcers would have a higher degree of therapeutic efficacy, would require fewer clinic visits and applications (*e.g.*, application only once or at intervals of several weeks), and would be less dependent on patient compliance.

Gene therapy vectors formulated in biocompatible matrices represent a versatile combination product approach to tissue repair. The primary mode of action (PMOA) of these so-called gene-activated matrices (GAMs) is attributed to the DNA vector, and therefore primary regulatory oversight is provided through the Center for Biologics Evaluation and Research with a Center for Devices and Radiological Health consult.

THE CLINICAL PROBLEM

Clinical results have shown that approximately 24% of diabetic ulcers attain complete healing after 12 weeks with a standardized care regime, and approximately 31% of diabetic ulcers heal after 20 weeks[2]. While living skin equivalents such as Apligraf® (Organogenesis, Canton, MA) and Dermagraft® (Advanced Biohealing, Westport, CT) have been shown in clinical trials to be effective in accelerating wound repair (56% and 30% wound closures respectively after 12 weeks),[3,4] the current usage of these approved products has been limited by their relatively short shelf life (5–10 days), logistics with ordering product (which are manufactured on demand), and associated costs. Clinical studies have also suggested the need for up to 6–8 weekly applications to achieve wound closure; however, Medicare guidelines have restricted reimbursement for living skin equivalents to only one application under most circumstances.[5] Two devices in use (vacuum-assisted and hyperbaric oxygen) are also very expensive and time consuming, and require multiple clinic visits. Vacuum-assisted therapy has recently been shown to lead to a 43.2% wound closure compared to 28.9% SOC within the 16-week study period.[6] Becaplermin (PDGF-BB; Regranex), is the only growth factor protein that has been approved for use in diabetic ulcers. However, clinical studies have shown that the ulcer healing incidence compared to placebo was only 15% greater for becaplermin, which must be applied daily over an extended period of time (with a single course of treatment lasting up to 20 weeks).[7] Maintenance of the therapeutic protein at the wound site in sufficient quantities and for a sufficient period of time has been identified as the likely cause of this relatively low rate of efficacy and requirement for numerous reapplications over the treatment course. All existing therapeutic approaches in this patient population are further limited by the fact that they require repeated administrations in a patient population for whom compliance is frequently an important underlying problem. In view of these limitations, there remains a compelling medical need for a more practical, safe, and effective therapy for nonhealing diabetic ulcers of the lower extremities.

THE CLINICAL SOLUTION

In chronic wounds such as lower extremity neuropathic ulcers in diabetics, the wound healing process is impaired, in part owing to reduced levels of endogenous growth factors,[8,9] and becaplermin was developed to address this problem. Difficulty in maintaining therapeutic growth factors at the wound site in sufficient quantities and for a sufficient period of time likely contributes to the low rate of healing. An investigational combination product, GAM501, utilizes a technology in which a nonintegrating, replication incompetent adenoviral vector containing the human PDGF-B gene (Ad5PDGF-B, a biologic) is incorporated into a three-dimensional biocompatible matrix (2.6% collagen, a device) and applied topically once or twice to an ulcer site. The PMOA of GAM501 is attributed to expression of PDGF-BB by Ad5PDGF-B. The duration of PDGF-BB expression is transient and continues for approximately 2 weeks. GAM501 preclinical studies have shown that fibroblasts, endothelial cells, inflammatory cells, and other connective tissue cell types, which originate in viable tissue surrounding a wound site, migrate into and proliferate within the gene-containing matrix, where they are transfected and then secrete the encoded PDGF-BB growth factor locally where it is needed within wound site, and over an extended period of time. The matrix of GAM501 has at least two key beneficial functions: (i) it holds the Ad5PDGF-B vector in place at the wound site by electrostatic forces (positively charged collagen and negatively charged vector) until infiltrating wound-healing cells arrive, and (ii) it acts as a biocompatible scaffolding that promotes in-growth of cells that are responsible for accumulation of granulation tissue, a key part of the wound healing process. Once in the matrix, transfected cells act as local *in vivo* bioreactors that transiently produce PDGF-BB protein within the wound site on a sustained basis to stimulate wound repair. The protein is synthesized by wound repair cells only for as long as the gene is expressed, which is generally days to a couple of weeks for adenoviral vectors since they do not integrate into the genome of transfected cells, and gene expression is naturally turned off after those cells expressing the protein are either remodeled or resorbed. This duration of localized protein availability is substantially prolonged relative to topical protein therapy (which must be reapplied daily), and may more closely match the natural healing process in such wounds, which generally takes place over days to weeks. The sustained presence of the active therapeutic protein at the precise location where it is required is believed to lead to the acceleration and augmentation of a normal wound healing response.

MARKET—HISTORY, CURRENT, AND PROSPECTS

In the United States alone there are 1.2 million patients with diabetic neuropathic ulcers (the initial target population for GAM501), and the potential market size for wound healing products or devices is considered to be several billion dollars. The incidence of obesity and diabetes in the general population is projected to increase significantly, and so too will the market potential for wound healing products. Despite the recent development of guidelines for an SOC regimen[10] and the availability of advanced wound healing technologies, persistent low closure rates indicate a substantial need for improved therapeutic options. Practitioners express frustration with their lack of success in treating chronic wounds, the time-consuming nature of the treatment regimens, and the resultant patient noncompliance. Patients express anxiety over lack of improvements to their wound despite repeated treatments (because of the slow and inefficient healing process), as well as the need for frequent clinic or hospital visits and the fear of amputation.[11] A novel therapy that can address these problems might be regarded as fulfilling a significant unmet need by both physicians and patients. Factors that will help drive the successful development of a combination wound healing product include the product's superiority over SOC, safety profile, single application use, and an expanding market potential.

BUSINESS CHALLENGES—POLICIES & PRACTICES

The majority of the development work for GAM501 was completed utilizing three different avenues of support: venture capital funds, National Institutes of Health (NIH) Small Business Innovation Research grants (up to 2 million dollars), and academic collaborations. Venture capital funds enabled preclinical research in-house to first evaluate and select the optimum gene, and then to test GAM501 in five different animal models. This was supplemented with funds from the NIH through a Small Business Innovation Research grant. Lastly, when expertise or time was not available in-house, collaborative efforts with experts in the field contributed to the needed research. Manuscripts describing the preclinical results were published in peer-reviewed journals to disseminate important information and to stimulate a spirit of openness in the wound healing field.

Combination products such as GAM501 have special regulatory considerations. Each component is subject to the corresponding Current Good Laboratory Practices and Current Good Manufacturing Practices regulations; however, the center primarily responsible for the U.S. Food and Drug Administration (FDA) oversight of a combination product is determined based on the PMOA of the product. To streamline the review of combination products, FDA has established an Intercenter Consultative and Collaborative Review Process (www.fda.gov/oc/combination/consultative.html). In addition to FDA, all recombinant DNA product trials in humans must be reviewed by the Recombinant DNA Advisory Committee (RAC) at the NIH. RAC meets every 3 months, and RAC approval is required before Institutional Review Board for Human Subjects approval. The review and approval processes can be further streamlined if one of the components of a combination product has prior regulatory approval. For GAM501, Center for Biologics Evaluation and Research has primary regulatory jurisdiction, with consultation from Center for Devices and Radiological Health for the collagen component, which is already approved as a dermal filler.

PUBLIC–PRIVATE PARTNERSHIP—SWOT (STRENGTH, WEAKNESS, OPPORTUNITIES, THREAT) ANALYSIS

In the case of GAM501, since bovine collagen is an approved product that is routinely injected into human tissue and has more than 18 years of safety information, there were no significant safety concerns expected for that component of the combination product. When bovine collagen is injected in other approved applications, prior allergy testing is routinely required. However, since GAM501 is applied only topically within the wound site, and there was no evidence of allergy, induration, or erythema in preclinical testing or in the phase 1/2 trial, allergy testing was not required by FDA. Very extensive preclinical studies were used to show that Ad5PDGF-B alone (aqueous formulated) was not retained in wounds and was not effective at stimulating granulation tissue where it was needed most. Only when Ad5PDGF-B was formulated with collagen was robust granulation tissue generated in the wound bed. Thus, the control arm (vector alone) was not required to be evaluated in the clinic. The protein produced by GAM501 is already approved for use in the same clinical application, further raising confidence in expected safety. Extensive preclinical safety, allergy, and biodistribution studies further supported the trial design.[12] The extensive preclinical data, including five different wound models to demonstrate mechanism of action and testing of other growth factor genes for optimum growth factor selection, gave the company and FDA additional confidence in moving to phase 2. Several of these studies were carried out in collaboration with academic partners, thus reducing the need for internal costs and headcount. During such extensive preclinical studies it is important to keep patent life in mind and maintain a strategy of extending patent life through additional filings as new methods are discovered or improved. Deciding between optimizing the product in preclinical testing versus moving as fast as possible to and through the clinic requires careful balance and judgment.

After planning discussions with FDA it was decided to test SOC[10] and collagen alone in separate control arms in the randomized, double-blinded phase 2b trial. It was agreed, unless further warranted, that if GAM501 proved to be superior to SOC alone in phase 2b, then collagen alone could be the control arm in phase 3. The company presented its overall development plan to FDA and made modifications based on Agency comments.

Our approach to regulatory affairs has been to "go early and go often," but always with a carefully drawn proposed development plan. Agency comments on the plan can be very helpful in optimizing development and shortening the time to approval. We also consider the FDA to be an important partner in the process, since they often have extensive experience and knowledge of ongoing developments in the field and their overall guidance can therefore be extremely helpful.

Strengths of the GAM501 development program include the thorough understanding of mechanism of action and biology (see "Matrix Enabled Gene Delivery for Tissue Repair" chapter), extensive toxicology, selection of the optimum growth factor for this GAM application, extensive history of use of one of the two elements in this combination product (collagen) and the protein encoded by the other (PDGF-BB), the safety profile of both collagen and the adenovector, and the fact that the protein that the product produces, PDGF-BB, is already approved for human use. Further, the one- or two-time application will be much more efficient than other approved products, and the combination product seems to overcome the primary reason other growth factor protein products have failed. The market penetration opportunity is great as existing products are very expensive and cumbersome to use, there is an important clinical need, and there is a very large and growing patient population. The main difficulties or weaknesses have been raising funds to support development of a wound care product with the history of so many failures and the long duration of observation required in the clinical trials. The potential risks include the outcome of the phase 2b trial and the burden of 16% Gross Domestic Product health care costs to reimbursement of the product, although we believe that the costs of not effectively treating such wounds are far greater, both in dollars and in quality of life.

CONCLUSION

The development of GAM501 as a combination therapeutic holds great promise in overcoming the relatively mediocre results of growth factor proteins that have been developed or have failed in the wound healing market. Applying growth factor gene therapy to wound healing using GAM technology has the potential to take an effective but very difficult-to-apply treatment and transforming it into one that is effective, practical, and easy to use. Development of a combination product requires planned collaboration with regulatory agencies. Both elements of the GAM501 combination product have strong safety records independently, and the protein produced by GAM501 is already approved for clinical use. A thumbnail analysis of the product's development is shown in the table.

SUMMARY ILLUSTRATION

Strengths: Extensive preclinical testing Understanding primary mechanism of action Optimum growth factor selection Safety profile (collagen and PDGF-BB approved) One- or two-time application	**Weaknesses:** Wound care market history and fundraising Clinical trial duration
Opportunities: Wound care market expansion Product reimbursement Mediocre efficacy of existing products	**Risks:** Not yet known results of phase 2b trial Obtaining significant reimbursement codes

Figure 1. Chart showing the key aspects of GAM501 development.

CRITICAL REMARKS AND RECOMMENDATIONS

- The benefits of extensive mechanism of action and product selection preclinical studies must be balanced by time factors.
- Work in close collaboration with FDA, bring a full development plan, and listen carefully to their guidance.
- Select the best formulation and combination product, but the use of already-known safe and/or effective elements can shorten development time and facilitate regulatory interactions.
- GAM technology holds great promise for transforming protein growth factor therapy into a more efficient and effective therapeutic.

AUTHOR DISCLOSURE STATEMENT

L.A.C. and B.K.S. are employees of Tissue Repair Company and hold stock options in Cardium Therapeutics, Inc. R.E. is a consultant to and owns stock options in Cardium Therapeutics. The Phase 1/2 clinical study was partially supported by a grant from NIH/NIAMS (5R44 AR46154-03).

REFERENCES

1. Reiber GE, Vileikyte L, Boyko EJ, del Aguila M, Smith DG, Lavery LA, and Boulton AJ: Causal pathways for incident lower-extremity ulcers in patients with diabetes from two settings. Diabetes Care 1999; **22:** 157.
2. Margolis DJ, Kantor J, and Berlin JA: Healing of diabetic neuropathic foot ulcers receiving standard treatment. Diabetes Care 1999; **22:** 692.
3. Veves A, Falanga V, Armstrong DG, and Sabolinski ML: Graftskin, a human skin equivalent, is effective in the management of noninfected neuropathic diabetic foot ulcers. Diabetes Care 2001; **24:** 290.
4. Marston WA, Hanft J, Norwood P, and Pollak R: The efficacy and safety of Dermagraft in improving the healing of chronic diabetic foot ulcers. Diabetes Care 2003; **26:** 1701.
5. Eisenbud D, Huang NF, Luke BS, and Silberklang M: Skin substitutes and wound healing: current status and challenges. Wounds 2004; **16:** 2.
6. Blume PA, Walters J, Payne W, Ayala J, and Lantis J: Comparison of negative pressure wound therapy using vacuum-assisted closure with advanced moist wound therapy in the treatment of diabetic foot ulcers. Diabetes Care 2008; **31:** 631.
7. Smiell JM, Wieman TJ, Steed DL, Perry BH, Sampson AR, and Schwab BH: Efficacy and safety of becaplermin (recombinant human platelet-derived growth factor-BB) in patients with non-healing, lower extremity diabetic ulcers: a combined analysis of four randomized studies. Wound Repair Regen 1999; **7:** 335.
8. Cooper DM, Yu EZ, Hennessey P, Ko F, and Robson MC: Determination of endogenous cytokines in chronic wounds. Ann Surg 1994; **219:** 688.
9. Pierce GF, Tarpley JE, Tseng J, Bready J, Chang D, Kenney WC, Rudolph R, Robson MC, Vande Berg J, Reid P, Kaufman S, and Farrell CL: Detection of platelet-derived growth factor (PDGF)-AA in actively healing human wounds treated with recombinant PDGF-BB and absence of PDGF in chronic nonhealing wounds. J Clin Invest 1995; **96:** 1336.
10. Steed DL, Attinger C, Colaizzi T, Crossland M, Franz M, Harkless L, Johnson A, Moosa H, Robson M, Serena T, Sheehan P, Veves A, and Wiersma-Bryant L: Guidelines for the treatment of diabetic ulcers. Wound Repair Regen 2006; **14:** 680.
11. Searle A, Campbell R, Tallon D, Fitzgerald A, and Vedhara K: A qualitative approach to understanding the experience of ulcerations and healing in the diabetic foot: patient and podiatrist perspective. Wounds 2005; **17:** 16.
12. Gu DL, Nguyen T, Gonzalez AM, Printz MA, Pierce GF, Sosnowski BA, Phillips ML, and Chandler LA: Adenovirus encoding human platelet-derived growth factor-B delivered in collagen exhibits safety, biodistribution, and immunogenicity profiles favorable for clinical use. Mol Ther 2004; **9:** 699.

Ultrasound Therapy for Wound Healing, Evidence-Informed Treatment Decision Making

Malgorzata Plummer,[1] Patricio Meneses,[2] and William J. Ennis[3,*]

[1]Wound Healing and Tissue Repair, University of Illinois, Chicago, Illinois.
[2]Center for Comprehensive Wound and Disease Management, St. James Olympia Fields Hospital, Olympia Fields, Illinois.
[3]Section of Wound Healing and Tissue Repair, University of Illinois, Chicago, Illinois.

Abbreviation and Acronym

US = ultrasound

*Correspondence: Section of Wound Healing and Tissue Repair, University of Illinois, 840 S. Wood St., Mail Code 958, Suite 518, Chicago, Illinois 60612 (e-mail: wtc211@pol.net, shelliec@uic.edu).

Background: Wound care has advanced from moist wound healing to the use of gene therapy, stem cells, and proteomics within a 40-year time frame. Despite the advances, wound care clinicians are still confronted with a large number of nonhealing wound patients for whom there appears to be no clinical answer. The use of therapeutic modalities such as ultrasound (US) can reestablish healing in certain cases. Understanding the cellular and biochemical mechanism of action of US can help the clinician determine when to consider this therapeutic option.

The Problem: How does US impact healing? Are there predictive qualitative or quantitative indicators that help identify which patients would benefit from US therapy? This chapter will review the biophysical mechanisms by which US can reestablish a healing trajectory in a chronic, nonhealing wound.

Basic/Clinical Science Advances: For over 20 years, megahertz-based US therapy has been employed in clinical practice. The majority of wound-related indications have focused on treating peri-wound tissue. Recently, kilohertz-based US therapy has entered the mainstream with implications for wound healing, vascular disease, and bone stimulation.

Clinical Care Relevance: As a result of several clinical trials in wound healing, the use of kilohertz-based US therapy allows clinicians another option for the treatment and debridement of hard to heal wound care patients.

Conclusion: As wound care therapeutic options continue to evolve, it becomes important for the clinician to analyze the available literature, and combine that knowledge with their clinical experience to make to best evidence-informed treatment decisions for their patients. Therapeutic US may well represent an important tool in the treatment armamentarium. Comparative effectiveness studies will need to be conducted in the future to help clarify when US should be used, for how long, in what sequence, and if other treatments are synergistic or antagonistic.

BACKGROUND

The care of nonhealing wounds has developed into a multi-billion-dollar worldwide industry. Although the science has evolved, there are currently a myriad of treatment options with little comparative effectiveness data to support one over the other. The clinician is therefore left to practice evidence-informed clinical care with more emphasis on clinical experience. Recently, there have been peer-reviewed, evidenced-based guidelines that aid the clinician through diagnostic and treatment pathways for nonhealing wounds.[1] There is preclinical and clinical evidence that physical therapy–based

ADVANCES IN WOUND CARE, VOLUME 1

Printed in U.S.A.
DOI: 10.1089/awc.2009.0051

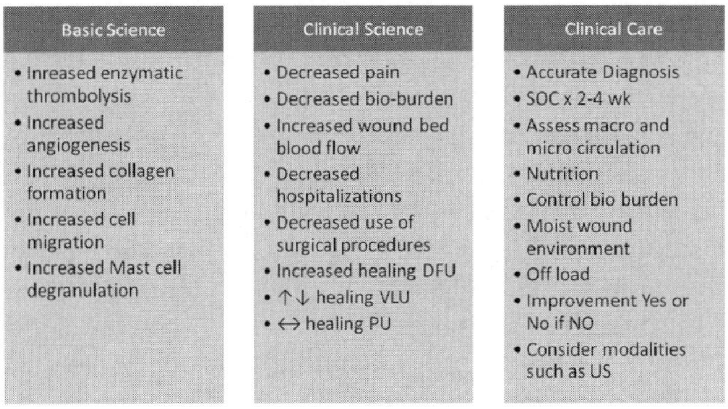

Figure 1. Basic and clinical science effects of US are used to make evidence-informed clinical care decisions. After an accurate diagnosis and 2–4 weeks of therapy, the clinician can consider using modalities such as US as a therapeutic option.

modalities can impact healing at a biochemical level and might be stimulated through calcium ion channels and the nitric oxide pathway.[2] Ultrasound (US), one of these energy-based treatments, is the subject of this brief review (Fig. 1).

CLINICAL PROBLEM ADDRESSED

The skin is the largest organ in the body and is our first line of defense. A wound puts a patient at higher risk for infection and loss of water/nutrients. The patient is subjected to painful dressing changes and multiple invasive treatments, and often has to deal with profuse drainage and wound odor. Taken together, there is a great impact on an individual's life, including work performance, family life, and the ability to enjoy leisure activities. Patients are also under financial strain as they have to buy dressings and travel for their medical appointments.

BASIC SCIENCE CONTEXT

A chronic wound is one that fails to heal within an expected time frame. Wounds can become chronic because of an imbalance in the molecular environment, increases in inflammatory cytokines and proteases, a nonfunctional extracellular matrix, and senescent cells that are unable to proliferate or produce an appropriate matrix.[3] US is a mechanical vibration transmitted at a frequency above the human limit of hearing (above 20 kHz).[2] US causes several bioeffects that are divided into thermal and nonthermal effects. Thermal effects are mainly used in rehabilitation medicine to improve joint and muscle mobility. Wound care applications mainly rely on nonthermal effects. Cavitation refers to the formation of micron-size bubbles within the extracellular fluid matrix.[4] Cavitation bubbles vibrate, compress, and expand within the ultrasonic field. US also causes a mechanical pressure wave that is responsible for the unidirectional movement of fluids along acoustic boundaries known as acoustic streaming.[4] Currently, two versions of therapeutic US are available to wound care professionals. Contact US and, more recently, noncontact US. Contact US is used mainly on periwound tissues through a coupling gel. Contact US can be used over the wound itself; however, the process is somewhat cumbersome and limited by infection control issues and wound tenderness. Contact US therapy mainly employs the use of 1–3-MHz devices. There are several kilohertz-based contact ultrasonic debriding tools now on the market. Noncontact US therapy was recently developed by Celleration, Inc. (MIST Therapy™, Eden Prairie, MN). This device provides low-intensity (0.1–0.5 W/cm^2), low-frequency (40 kHz) US via a saline mist with uniform droplet size (60 μm). This technique allows for treatment to the wound bed and peri-wound tissue. Kilohertz therapy provides a deeper tissue penetration and causes both increased cavitation and microstreaming.[4]

EXPERIMENTAL MODEL OR MATERIAL

The majority of US research has been performed *in vitro*, leading some authors to question the translational relevance of those preclinical studies.[5] Many studies have employed US therapy applied to cell cultures through a water bath. The use of various wavelengths and frequencies makes comparative analysis and meta-analysis difficult. Clinical trials have either been uncontrolled or not adequately defined standard of care in the control arm. Another complication has been the absence of a sham device in many clinical trials.

DISCUSSION OF FINDINGS AND RELEVANT LITERATURE

Dyson *et al.*, working with a rabbit ear model, reported that US may enhance tissue regeneration through the nonthermal mechanism of cavitation and microstreaming.[6] Further studies confirmed that US affects tissue healing at many levels, including increased blood flow through a nitric oxide pathway and angiogenesis.[7,8] US can also potentiate enzymatic thrombolysis.[9] During the inflammatory phase US has an effect on macrophages as evidenced by increased cytokine production and increased leukocyte adhesion and migration.[10,11] Mast cells have been shown to demonstrate increased degranulation as a result of US treatment.[12] Many cellular processes depend on intercellular communication and cellular adhesion to the extracellular matrix. US may influence these processes through bypassing usual signaling systems.[13] US may also promote increased collagen production, thereby improving the growth of the extracellular matrix.[14] US leads to morphological changes in fibroblasts, including a dilated endoplasmic reticulum as noted through an *in vitro* electron microscopy study by Lai.[15] Additional studies have proposed an increased expression of transforming growth factor-β, and subsequently collagen production, through gene upregulation.[16]

Clinical examples

Patients with diabetes are likely to develop a foot ulcer, which puts them at high risk of limb loss. A randomized, sham-controlled trial using noncontact kilohertz-based US (MIST therapy; Celleration, Inc.) was published by Ennis et al.[17] The study design was appropriate, but due to protocol violations, the intent to treat data failed to reach statistical significance. A sub-group evaluable for efficacy cohort, however, did achieve healing in 40.7% compared to 14.3% in sham-treated ulcers ($p = 0.0366$) after 12 weeks of treatment.[17] Time to healing was also shorter in active group with a mean of 9.12 weeks versus 11.74 weeks in the placebo group ($p = 0.0144$). The use of US for the treatment of venous ulcers has been studied more widely. An early study published by Dyson in 1976 demonstrated a reduction in ulcer size compared to controls after 4 weeks of three times per week therapy to periwound tissue.[18] Another study by Callam evaluated weekly applications of 1-MHz-pulsed US therapy for the periwound skin of patients with venous ulcers. Results revealed a statistically different cumulative percentage of cases healed in relation to time ($p = 0.03$) and decrease in ulcer area.[19] Other authors have not demonstrated improved healing rates for venous ulcers using US therapy.[20] Peschen *et al.* evaluated low-frequency US using a foot bath and 30-kHz continuous US three times per week.[21] Treatment consisted of 10 min of 30-kHz continuous US three times a week. The study was single-blinded and controlled with a sham US group. After 12 weeks, there was a statistically significant 55.4% decrease in wound size in the study group compared to a 16.5% decrease in the control group ($p < 0.0070$). Kavros *et al.* compared low-frequency US therapy plus standard of care to a group that received standard of care alone.[22] The study was a retrospective observational study, and the patients who received US had a larger number of healed wounds and a faster rate of healing compared to controls (53% vs. 32%, $p = 0.009$). The study evaluated patients with a variety of wounds, but a subgroup analysis of patients with venous ulcers demonstrated an even more impressive healing percentage when compared to controls (65% vs. 21%, $p = 0.02$).[22] The reestablishment of macro-vascular flow for ischemic ulcers is primary, but the establishment of an adequate microcirculation plays an integral role in the patient's ability to heal. The connection between the macro circulation and the micro circulation as it relates to wound healing has recently been elucidated.[23] Kavros *et al.* studied the influence of noncontact kilohertz US therapy for the treatment of ischemic wounds.[24] In a prospective, parallel group, standard of wound care alone was compared to standard of care plus US therapy three times per week. The author found a statistically significant difference in positive outcomes (>50% healing in 12 weeks) in the study group compared to controls (63% vs. 29%, $p < 0.001$). The mainstay of treatment for pressure ulcers is to offload the pressure, maximize the underlying medical condition of the patient, and provide appropriate local wound care. Recently, the *Journal of the American Medical Association* published a systematic review of pressure ulcer treatment options.[25] The authors concluded that there was no healing benefit

TAKE-HOME MESSAGE

Basic science advances

- US affects healing mainly through nonthermal actions.
- The mechanism of action includes cavitation and microstreaming.
- US results in increased blood flow through a nitric oxide pathway.
- Intracellular calcium ion levels temporarily rise after US treatment.

Clinical science advances

- US treatment results in increased wound healing and decreased pain.
- US treatment can alter the wound bioburden.

Relevance to clinical care

- US may improve healing for patients with nonhealing wounds of various etiologies.
- Diabetic foot ulcer healing improved in a sub-group of patients from a RCT trial.
- US can be used for wound debridement and cell stimulation.

through the use of modalities such as US. The study, however, limited the review of literature to randomized controlled trials, and therefore most of the published literature on US therapy was not included in the final analysis. US has also been used to treat a number of specific aspects of the healing process, for example, wound pain. Gehling *et al.* evaluated 15 patients receiving noncontact kilohertz US therapy.[26] Pain was reduced by approximately 80% from pretreatment scores (8.07 vs. 1.67, $p = 0.0003$). Patients with chronic wounds benefit from periodic wound debridement. One of the main side effects of this treatment is significant pain and bleeding. A study by Breuing *et al.* evaluated the usefulness of low-frequency US therapy for debridement and found it appealing for relatively painless, bloodless debridement.[27] The usefulness of US has to be further studied as there is no study available that compares the US device to any other debridement technique, sham device or to no debridement treatment.[28] In two separate studies by Ennis *et al.*, one on diabetic foot ulcers and the other focused on leg ulcers, they noted a reduction in wound drainage.[17,29] In a recent study, Serena *et al.* confirmed that US has the ability to destroy bacteria such as *Pseduomonas aeruginosa*, *Escherichia coli*, and *Enterococcus fecalis*; however, no influence was noted on strains of *Staphylococcus aureus*, including Methicillin-resistant *S. aureus*.[30] An *in vivo* component to this study demonstrated a reduction in overall bacterial quantity that was comparable with treatment using a topical silver impregnated dressing. In one study, the use of US therapy for nonhealing wounds resulted in a reduction in hospitalization and surgical procedures compared to historic controls.[29]

CAUTION, CRITICAL REMARKS, AND RECOMMENDATIONS

- As with many wound healing therapeutics in wound care, there are few randomized controlled trials to support efficacy. Clinicians therefore need to combine their experience with the best literature available to create informed decision making for their complicated wound care patients. Support for US therapy continues to grow in the literature, and further trials will help better identify the most appropriate patient populations.

FUTURE DEVELOPMENTS

Further work on US and other modalities will focus on identifying specific biochemical effects. It is likely that US will be combined with other modalities such as gene or cellular therapy to maximize the effectiveness of both. For example, the use of US alters the properties of the cell membrane that could theoretically increase viral plasmid transfection rates.

ACKNOWLEDGMENT

This work was not financially supported.

AUTHOR DISCLOSURE STATEMENT

M.P. has no financial disclosures.

W.J.E. received funds for clinical trials in the past from Celleration, Inc., and was a consultant for the company. At the time of this writing W.J.E. is neither a consultant nor a speaker for Celleration, Inc.

P.M. has no financial disclosures.

REFERENCES

1. Robson MC and Barbul A: Guidelines for the best care of chronic wounds. Wound Repair Regen 2006; **14:** 647.
2. Ennis WJ, Lee C, and Meneses P: A biochemical approach to wound healing through the use of modalities. Clin Dermatol 2007; **25:** 63.
3. Schultz G *et al.*: Wound healing and TIME; new concepts and scientific applications. Wound Repair Regen 2005; **13(4 Suppl):** S1.
4. Dalecki D: Mechanical bioeffects of ultrasound. Annu Rev Biomed Eng 2004; **6:** 229.
5. Baker KG, Robertson VJ, and Duck FA: A review of therapeutic ultrasound: biophysical effects. Phys Ther 2001; **81:** 1351.
6. Dyson M *et al.*: The stimulation of tissue regeneration by means of ultrasound. Clin Sci 1968; **35:** 273.
7. Young SR and Dyson M: The effect of therapeutic ultrasound on angiogenesis. Ultrasound Med Biol 1990; **16:** 261.
8. Suchkova VN *et al.*: Ultrasound improves tissue perfusion in ischemic tissue through a nitric oxide dependent mechanism. Thromb Haemost 2002; **88:** 865.
9. Suchkova VN, Baggs RB, and Francis CW: Effect of 40-kHz ultrasound on acute thrombotic ischemia in a rabbit femoral artery thrombosis model: enhancement of thrombolysis and improvement in capillary muscle perfusion. Circulation 2000; **101:** 2296.
10. Maxwell L *et al.*: The augmentation of leucocyte adhesion to endothelium by therapeutic ultrasound. Ultrasound Med Biol 1994; **20:** 383.
11. Young SR and Dyson M: Macrophage responsiveness to therapeutic ultrasound. Ultrasound Med Biol 1990; **16:** 809.
12. Fyfe MC and Chahl LA: Mast cell degranulation and increased vascular permeability induced by 'therapeutic' ultrasound in the rat ankle joint. Br J Exp Pathol 1984; **65:** 671.
13. Mahoney CM *et al.*: Therapeutic ultrasound bypasses canonical syndecan-4 signaling to activate Rac1. J Biol Chem 2009; **284:** 8898.
14. Doan N *et al.*: *In vitro* effects of therapeutic ultrasound on cell proliferation, protein synthesis, and cytokine production by human fibroblasts, osteoblasts, and monocytes. J Oral Maxillofac Surg 1999; **57:** 409; discussion 420.

15. Lai J and Pittelkow MR: Physiological effects of ultrasound mist on fibroblasts. Int J Dermatol 2007; **46:** 587.

16. Tsai WC *et al.*: Ultrasound stimulation of types I and III collagen expression of tendon cell and upregulation of transforming growth factor beta. J Orthop Res 2006; **24:** 1310.

17. Ennis WJ, Foreman P, Mozen N, Massey J, Conner-Kerr T, and Meneses P: Ultrasound therapy for recalcitrant diabetic foot ulcers: results of a randomized, double-blind, controlled, multicenter trial. Ostomy Wound Manage 2005; **51:** 24.

18. Dyson M, Franks C, and Suckling J: Stimulation of healing of varicose ulcers by ultrasound. Ultrasonics 1976; **14:** 232.

19. Callam MJ *et al.*: A controlled trial of weekly ultrasound therapy in chronic leg ulceration. Lancet 1987; **2:** 204.

20. Lundeberg T *et al.*: Pulsed ultrasound does not improve healing of venous ulcers. Scand J Rehabil Med 1990; **22:** 195.

21. Peschen M *et al.*: Low-frequency ultrasound treatment of chronic venous leg ulcers in an outpatient therapy. Acta Derm Venereol 1997; **77:** 311.

22. Kavros SJ *et al.*: Expedited wound healing with noncontact, low-frequency ultrasound therapy in chronic wounds: a retrospective analysis. Adv Skin Wound Care 2008; **21:** 416.

23. Ennis WJ, Meneses P, and Borhani M: Push-pull theory: using mechanotransduction to achieve tissue perfusion and wound healing in complex cases. Gynecol Oncol 2008; **111(2 Suppl):** S81.

24. Kavros SJ, Miller JL, and Hanna SW: Treatment of ischemic wounds with noncontact, low-frequency ultrasound: the Mayo clinic experience, 2004–2006. Adv Skin Wound Care 2007; **20:** 221.

25. Reddy M *et al.*: Treatment of pressure ulcers: a systematic review. JAMA 2008; **300:** 2647.

26. Gehling ML and Samies JH: The effect of noncontact, low-intensity, low-frequency therapeutic ultrasound on lower-extremity chronic wound pain: a retrospective chart review. Ostomy Wound Manage 2007; **53:** 44.

27. Breuing KH *et al.*: Early experience using low-frequency ultrasound in chronic wounds. Ann Plast Surg 2005; **55:** 183.

28. Ramundo J and Gray M: Is ultrasonic mist therapy effective for debriding chronic wounds? J Wound Ostomy Continence Nurs 2008; **35:** 579.

29. Ennis WJ *et al.*: Evaluation of clinical effectiveness of MIST ultrasound therapy for the healing of chronic wounds. Adv Skin Wound Care 2006; **19:** 437.

30. Serena T *et al.*: The impact of noncontact, nonthermal, low-frequency ultrasound on bacterial counts in experimental and chronic wounds. Ostomy Wound Manage 2009; **55:** 22–30.

WHS
Wound
Healing
Society

Microvascular Diagnostics in Wound Care

Jenny Ellen Freeman[1,*] and Anita Karcz[2]

[1]JEF Core, Inc., Weston, Massachusetts.
[2]Healthcare Opportunities Inc., Watertown, Massachusetts.

Background: While progress has been made in diagnosis and therapy of macrovascular disease in wound care, treatment of microvascular disease has lagged, often secondary to lack of appropriate diagnostics.
The Clinical Problem: Despite diagnostic/therapeutic advances, amputation rates remain constant. Focused management of the microcirculation may favorably impact wound healing and decrease amputations.
The Clinical Solution: Two methods for assessing microcirculation are (a) categorization as local, regional, and systemic and (b) evaluation of metabolic versus physiologic influences.
Market—History, Current, Prospects: Products delivering reliable quantitative information about wound microvasculature are needed, but have been historically unavailable. Ankle-brachial index lacks sufficient information to direct care. Transcutaneous oxygen is limited by anatomic constraints and implementation difficulties. Laser Doppler has not proven to be clinically useful. More recently, skin perfusion pressure has been developed and implemented alongside pulse volume recording to provide a combined assessment of regional macrocirculatory and microcirculatory status. Bioimpedance cardiac output can be used to report systemic blood flow and vascular resistance. Hyperspectral technology illustrates the adequacy of oxygen delivered to local tissue in an image format. A novel technology, sublingual CO_2 measurement, can rapidly and quantitatively demonstrate adequacy of the systemic circulation.
Business Challenges, Policies, and Practices: Bridging new modalities and concepts is challenging, as is diagnostic reimbursement. Shaping diagnosis and treatment of systemic microvascular compromise may be difficult, particularly because of cross-discipline care requirements.
Public–Private Partnership—SWOT Analysis: Increasing economic and public health impact of peripheral vascular disease places emphasis on collaborative approaches to public and professional education and applied research.
Strength: Potential for improving patient care, lowering healthcare costs.
Weakness: Implementation requires learning new concepts and methods.
Opportunity: Shifting focus from passive salvage to aggressive tissue preservation.
Threat: Multidisciplinary, coordinated care is required.
Conclusion: Careful evaluation of the microcirculation has the potential to substantially improve wound management and patient outcomes.

Abbreviations and Acronyms

APG = ambulatory patient groups
CMS = Center for Medicaid and Medicare Services
MHSI = medical hyperspectral imaging
NIH = National Institutes of Health
PAD = peripheral arterial disease
PVD = peripheral vascular disease
SPP = skin perfusion pressure

*Correspondence: JEF Core, Inc., 59 Ash St., Weston, Massachusetts 02493 (e-mail: jefreeman07@gmail.com).

BACKGROUND

While progress has been made over the last 30 years in the management of macrovascular disease in wound care patients, treatment of microvascular disease has lagged, in large part because of the lack of appropriate diagnostics. Local, regional, and

Printed in U.S.A.
DOI: 10.1089/awc.2009.0071

Table 1. *Noninvasive Vascular Diagnostic Tools*

Diagnostic tool	Benefits	Limitations
Regional measures	*Macrovascular*	
Ankle-Brachial indices[a]	Quick, inexpensive	Inaccurate in noncompressible arteries, diabetics, and elderly
Toe-Brachial indices[a]	Quick, inexpensive	Requires small cuffs and careful technique for accuracy
	Measures digital perfusion in PAD	
Segmental pressure[a]	Anatomic localization, diagnosis of PAD, and monitoring interventions	Inaccurate in noncompressible arteries, diabetics, or elderly
Pulse volume recording[a]	Diagnosis and monitoring of PAD level and severity, chronic critical limb ischemia, and interventions	Qualitative result
	Unaffected by noncompressible vessels	Nonspecific; abnormal with low cardiac stroke volume
Regional measures	*Microvascular*	
Transcutaneous oxygen	Oxygenation: unaffected by noncompressible vessels	Lengthy, expensive
		Anatomical limitations, operator dependent, ambiguous results
Skin perfusion pressure	Blood perfusion	Movement artifact in patients with tremors
	Quick, cost effective, and easy	
	Unaffected by noncompressible vessels	
Local measures	*Microvascular*	
Laser Doppler	Blood perfusion	Motion sensitive
	Scanning mode provides image format	Primarily research tool
Hyperspectral imaging	Quantified tissue oxygenation	Emerging technology
	Imaging format	Not yet in widespread use
	Anatomically relevant data	
Systemic measures	*Microvascular*	
Bioimpedance cardiac output	Perfusion, blood flow, and vascular resistance	Early generation devices were inaccurate
Sublingual carbon dioxide	Hypercarbia due to decrease in GI perfusion	Emerging technology
	Rapid, early metric of perfusion collapse	Validated in critical care setting
	Small, portable, cost effective, and user friendly	

[a]PAD, peripheral arterial disease.

systemic evaluation of microvascular disease has been largely confined to the nonspecific physical examination and limited diagnostic testing modalities. Newer technologies offer tremendous value in supporting clinical decision making, resulting in better clinical outcomes for many local, regional, and systemic pathophysiological conditions.

A variety of noninvasive diagnostic tools that have been developed to assess both macrovascular and microvascular disease are outlined in Table 1.

THE CLINICAL PROBLEM

Despite advances in diagnosis and therapy of macrovascular disease in patients with lower extremity ulcers, and other chronic wounds, amputation rates have remained relatively constant, with 105,309 lower extremity nontraumatic amputations performed annually in the United States.[1] Tissue perfusion and, ultimately, tissue viability require both macrocirculatory and microcirculatory adequacy.

Systemic factors including poor cardiac output, increased systemic vascular resistance, poor oxygenation, and anemia impact the clinical response of local microvasculature. Metabolic factors such as diabetes, sepsis, renal failure, nutritional impairment, steroid therapy, and growth factors also impair local tissue function and injury response. Vasoconstrictive effects of smoking, caffeine, or bronchodilators play important negative roles.[2] Regionally, microvascular disease compounds macrovascular obstruction. Locally, infection or trauma increases tissue metabolic demand and requirements for increased capillary perfusion.

Accurate assessment of systemic, regional, and local microcirculation in patients who present with lower extremity wounds can assist in guiding the patient into an optimal therapeutic pathway (Table 2). Ultimately, the evaluation and improvement of the microcirculation may favorably impact wound healing and decrease amputations.

THE CLINICAL SOLUTION

Emerging technologies have the potential to revolutionize diagnosis and treatment of impaired microvascular flow at local, regional, and systemic levels (Table 3). Improved outcomes and faster/

Table 2. *Microcirculatory Assessment Guides Optimal Therapy*

Anatomy	*Test result*	*Clinical result*
Local	Show tissue injured or at risk	Strategies to prevent ulceration Earlier indication for surgical/endovascular intervention Successful wound closure Optimal amputation level for healing and functional recovery
Regional	Quantitate result of intervention at the tissue level	Better design surgical/endovascular procedures Evaluate embolization prevention techniques
Systemic	Evaluate systemic tissue perfusion	Eliminate drugs/substances that decrease perfusion Maintain adequate hydration Improve cardiac performance Treat infection

better/cheaper are the value propositions driving this market.

Skin perfusion pressure (SPP) provides regional microvascular perfusion evaluation. SPP measures automatically the minimal external pressure above which cutaneous blood flow ceases using algorithm controlled cuff pressure. Values <30 mmHg are indicative of chronic critical limb ischemia. The current easy-to-use, point-of care system (Sensi-Lase®; Väsamed) combines SPP with pulse volume recording to provide timely, accurate, and objective data (in comparison to ankle-brachial index and transcutaneous oxygen) for evaluating critical limb ischemia,[3–5] predicting wound-healing potential[6,7] or detecting peripheral arterial disease in patients with noncompressible vessels.[8] It is well suited for use during endovascular procedures for assessing impact on tissue perfusion and potentially for assessing embolization.[9] Figure 1 demonstrates the use of SPP in the catheterization laboratory.

Medical hyperspectral imaging (MHSI) demonstrates microvascular oxygenation, visually depicting local tissue viability. MHSI systems have been used to quantitate oxy- and deoxy-hemoglobin pixel-by-pixel and display a tissue oxygenation image in a clinically relevant manner.[10] MHSI can evaluate the microcirculation in diabetics[11,12] and predict diabetic foot ulcer healing.[13,14] Preliminary data support its utility in defining tissue at risk for ulceration,[15] evaluating claudication,[16] determining the level of amputation and planning surgeries,[17] and assessing how revascularization procedures have impacted tissue around a wound.[18,19] Figure 2 contrasts the MHSI assessments in two patients with healing and nonhealing amputation sites. Additional screening applications exist based on the anatomic information provided by MHSI including screening inpatients on admission who are at risk for pressure ulcers to help identify deep tissue injury.

Sublingual CO_2 measurements are perfomed using a thermometer-like probe placed under the tongue. When systemic perfusion is inadequate, to preserve the heart and brain, blood flow is reduced to other organs, and of these, the gut is the first. Therefore, increased sublingual CO_2 is a very early indicator of blood flow inadequate to support the body's metabolism.[20] It has been used successfully in patients with sepsis[21,22] and hemorrhagic shock.[23] In wound evaluation, it has the potential to identify patients with early sepsis and those with suboptimal peripheral perfusion. It is well positioned to supplant other systemic indicators since it is portable, inexpensive, and provides measurement in less than a minute. Figure 3 demonstrates the device in use.

Table 3. *Noninvasive Diagnostic Indicators*

Anatomy	*Traditional diagnostics*	*Advanced microvascular diagnostics*
Local	Laser Doppler	Hyperspectral
Regional	Transcutaneous oxygen	Skin perfusion pressure
Systemic	Bioimpedance cardiac output	Sublingual CO_2

MARKET—HISTORY, CURRENT, AND PROSPECTS

Despite perennial budget concerns in health care, there is a demand for more efficient, accurate, rapid, and cost-effective diagnostics. Early diagnosis and therapy offer to not only reduce amputations and improve quality of life for patients with lower extremity wounds but also provide huge cost savings. In America, over $16 billion is spent annually to treat nearly 7 million people with problem wounds resulting from diabetes, pressure ulcers, vascular insufficiency, radiation injury, and other conditions (www.diversifiedclinicalservices.com/news/news_072707RF.php [July 27, 2007]). Annual U.S. costs of foot ulcer care and lower limb amputations

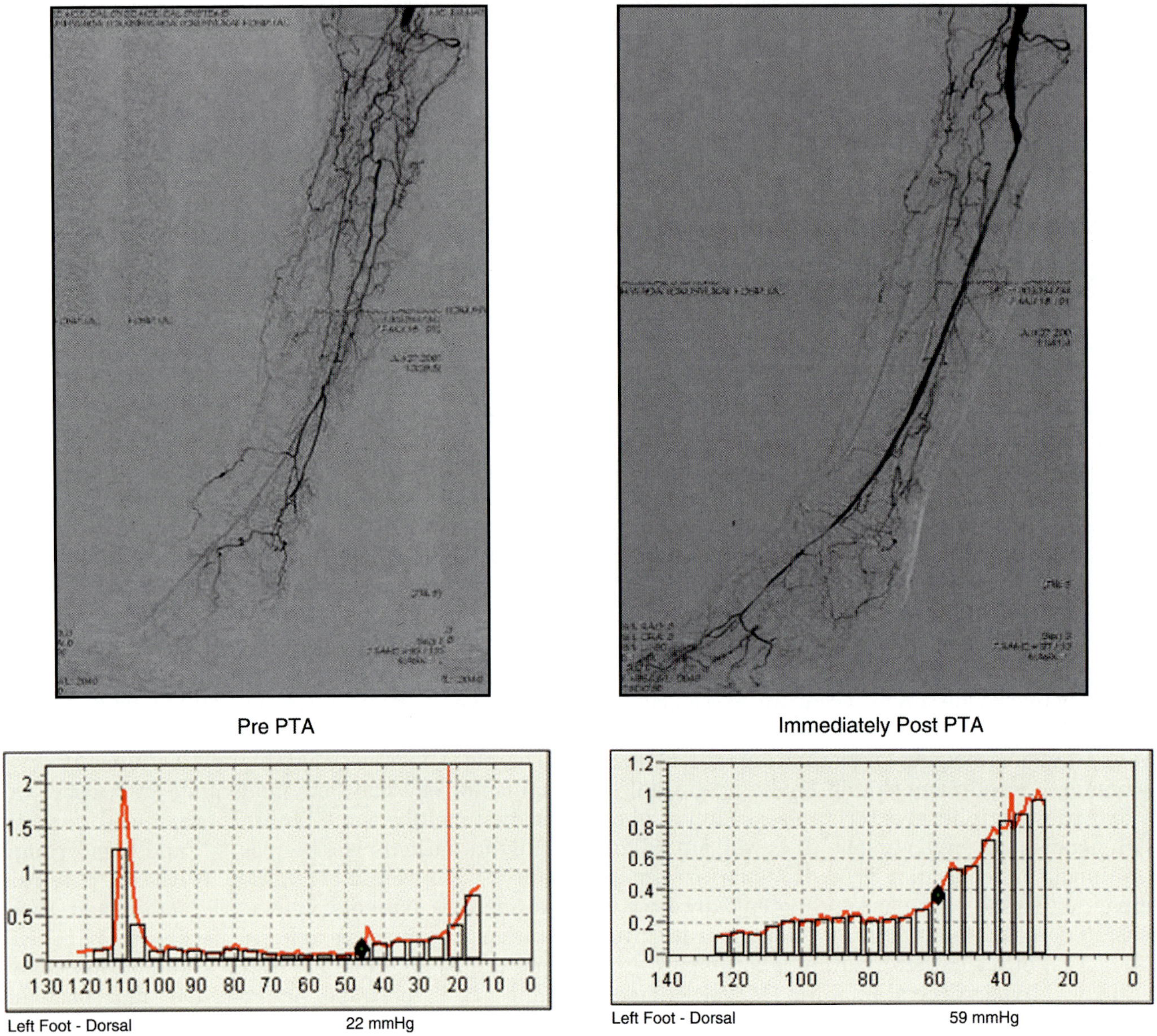

Figure 1. Skin perfusion pressure (SPP) measurements before and after posterior tibial angioplasty. Note that the SPP from the foot dorsum rose from 22 mmHg before to 59 mmHg after revascularization. The plantar SPP changed from 26 to 35 mmHg (courtesy of Dr. Osami Kawarada).

approach $13 billion.[24] Total costs for treating a diabetic foot ulcer range from $10,000 to $60,000.[25]

The majority of peripheral ulcer patients have diabetes. Twenty-four million Americans have diabetes and another 57 million have prediabetes. New cases jumped 40% in the last decade and with an increase in 2007 of over 3 million new patients in 2 years, the Center for Disease Control[26] predicts epidemic levels (www.cdc.gov/media/pressrel/2008/r080624.htm). A foot ulcer develops in 25% of these diabetics during their lifetime.[27]

Peripheral vascular disease (PVD) affects 12 million Americans, of which 2.1 million require pharmacologic management.[28] Annually, 315,450 patients undergo peripheral vascular procedures, bypass surgery (112,200), or angioplasty (203,250).[29] All are candidates for screening or pre- and postprocedure testing.

To serve these chronic wound populations, wound care centers are proliferating, resulting in an accessible and interested target market for new diagnostic testing modalities. There are over 500 free standing wound care centers, over 4,100 hospitals with wound care services, and over 4,700 home health agencies with wound care services (www.firstmark.com/fmkcat/woundcare.htm).

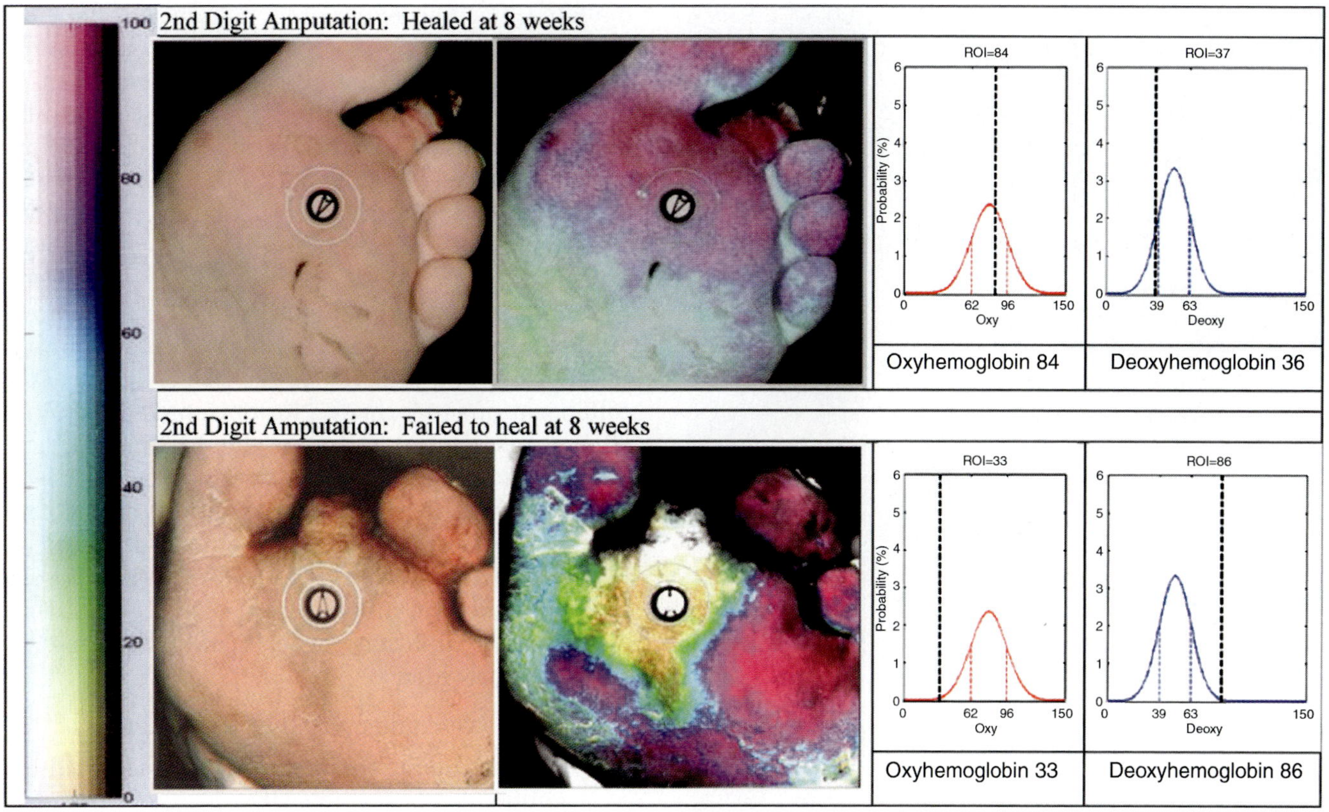

Figure 2. Medical hyperspectral imaging has been used to predict ulcer healing and to help plan amputations. At left a color scale depicts increasing oxyhemoglobin (yellow to purple) and a luminosity scale depicts increasing deoxyhemoglobin (faded to bright). Oxy- and deoxyhemoglobin values derived from the doughnut around the target are represented in arbitrary medical hyperspectral imaging units at right. The patient whose foot is demonstrated on the top row had a periwound oxyhemoglobin of 84 that is consistent with adequate tissue oxygenation for healing. He went on to heal his amputation in 8 weeks. The patient on the bottom row had a periwound oxyhemoglobin of 33 that has been demonstrated in foot ulcer studies to predict nonhealing. His amputation site had failed to heal 8 weeks after surgery (courtesy of Dr. Robert Frykberg).

Advanced diagnostics and earlier, more targeted therapy would benefit all the patient groups served by these wound centers.

BUSINESS CHALLENGES—POLICIES, PRACTICES, LEGAL, AND GEOGRAPHICAL

Obtaining adequate reimbursement for products and services is a challenge for medical device companies with emerging technologies. This has been recently exacerbated by budgetary cuts and focus on decreasing healthcare spending. Even if it provides a patient care advantage, a novel diagnostic will have little hope of wide acceptance without a clear and easy way for physicians and/or the hospital to be reimbursed. When appropriate, billing can be done under existing current procedural terminology or ambulatory patient group (APG) codes used for reimbursing other vascular assessments. It is occasionally possible to apply to the Center for Medicaid and Medicare Services (CMS) for a modification of an existing code to incorporate a new technology. Applying to CMS for a new reimbursement code can take many years and requires citation of articles in the published U.S. literature that documents the utility of the device. For private carriers in particular, cost–benefit documentation also may be required. While prevention of complications is the best way to both improve patient outcomes and decrease overall costs, screening tests are still generally not reimbursed. Hopefully, as the care burden of diabetes complications and chronic wounds from other causes becomes even greater, the focus will shift toward disease management and complication prevention, with more resources for early diagnostics.

PUBLIC–PRIVATE PARTNERSHIP—SWOT ANALYSIS

A public/private partnership or collaboration is an interaction between a government agency and one or more public or private sector organizations in which all parties work together to carry out

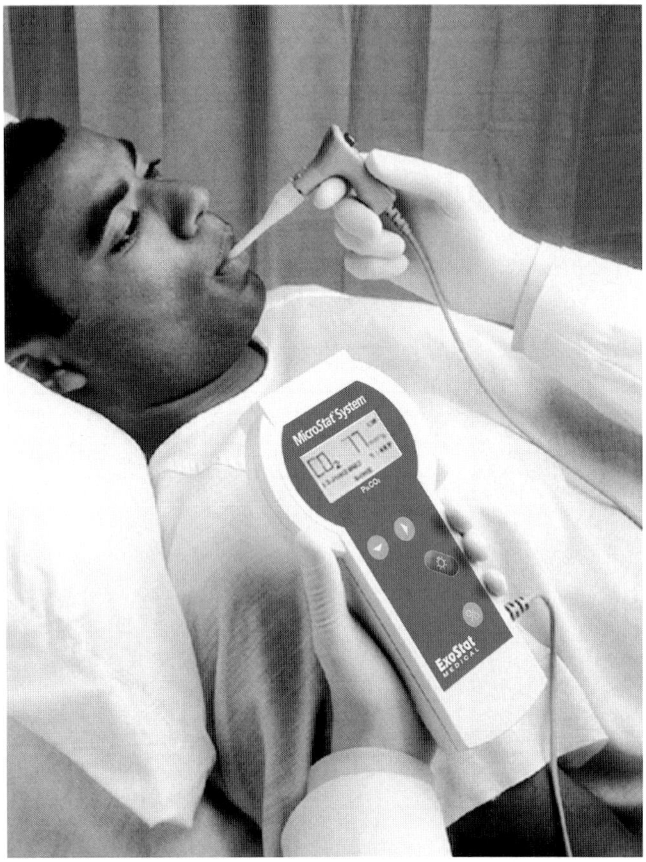

Figure 3. Sublingual CO_2 ($SLCO_2$) measurements (Microstat[R], ExoStat Medical, Inc., Eden Prairie, MN) can be performed in less than a minute at the point of care and deliver useful information about early sepsis and the adequacy of systemic perfusion.

a common mission. The interaction is voluntary, not based on statutory authority or other law. Collaborations may involve public education, professional education, and applied research or evaluation. Given the costs associated with PVD and diabetes and the expanding populations at risk, there is an increasing government interest in developing strong, nationally visible and effective public/private partnerships to promote community education about PVD and wounds and to promote advances in research and healthcare delivery to prevent and better treat both underlying disease states and complications. A SWOT analysis is presented in Fig. 4.

Promoting vascular health is a central component of improving overall health of the community. Given the rising prevalence of PVD, it is logical for collaborations to form and for national educational efforts to include vascular health messages.[30] Professional organizations are also increasingly active in their focus on education and applied research. For example, current combined American Heart Association/American College of Cardiology guidelines for the management of PVD state that diagnostic evaluation for critical limb ischemia should be provided:

1. Objective confirmation of the diagnosis
2. Localization of the responsible lesion(s) and a gauge of relative severity
3. Assessment of the hemodynamic requirements for successful revascularization (vis-à-vis proximal vs. multilevel revascularization)
4. Assessment of individual patient endovascular or operative risk.[2]

Such guidelines that promote the collection of objective diagnostic data will clearly provide performance metrics to assess the quality of care. If this can be paired with government funding agencies such as the National Institutes of Health (NIH) providing appropriate funds for development of

Strength:	Weakness:
• Enhanced credibility of a collaborative • Collaborative itself elevates visibility and priority of the problem	• Long dissemination cycle for new information to public and professionals • Delay: time spent making collaborative a working group
Opportunity:	**Threat:**
• Addressable gaps in public PVD knowledge • Addressable gaps in health care professionals' PVD knowledge • Greater access to research funding for private sector • Reduce dissemination cycle	• Multiple organizations move slowly • Lack of patience: will take years to see outcomes change • Different drivers for different partner participants

Figure 4. SWOT table of public/private partnership opportunities.

new technologies and for clinical trials to demonstrate benefit, and with assistance from CMS and third-party payors in providing appropriate reimbursement for methods and protocols that reduce overall cost, we can hope to see both improvement in outcomes and a decrease in healthcare spending.

CONCLUSION

Preventing wounds in high-risk populations and optimizing treatment of patients with wounds to speed recovery and deliver the best possible functional result are huge and growing challenges. Wound care centers and limb preservation programs have been developed to address these needs. Multidisciplinary care is now recognized as mandatory to deliver superior results. This provides the infrastructure for the emerging concept that diagnosis and treatment of the microcirculation can favorably impact outcomes in these patient populations.

Microcirculatory changes that impact wound healing can occur at the systemic, regional, or local levels. Regionally and locally emerging technologies such as SPP and hyperspectral imaging offer promise. Systemically, poor perfusion due to low cardiac output, high systemic resistance, dehydration, edema, or other factors can profoundly alter the blood flow to a lower extremity wound. Medications prescribed to address other medical problems such as congestive heart failure or hypertension may have a detrimental effect on a wound that is being treated by a different set of physicians and care givers. Understanding and monitoring the effects of medications such as β-blockers and diuretics should enable the wound care practitioner to improve wound outcomes. Understanding the needs related to extremity perfusion in the wound care patient should enable the cardiologist and primary care physician to help care for "the whole patient." Technologies such as bioimpedance cardiac output and sublingual carbon dioxide measurements should prove useful to identify and quantify the status of the microcirculation and help physicians optimize tissue perfusion to improve wound-healing outcomes.

Emerging technologies such as SPP and hyperspectral imaging can deliver otherwise unavailable information about the status of the microvasculature in the region or locale of a wound. This information about the regional and local microcirculation can assist decisions regarding likelihood of wound healing, necessity for revascularization, choice of specific revascularization procedure, and evaluation of the results of revascularization and can be useful in designing surgical procedures such as flap closures of wounds, elective reconstructions, or determining the necessity and level of amputation.

CRITICAL REMARKS AND RECOMMENDATIONS

- Wound healing requires adequate tissue perfusion and metabolism.
- Compromised tissue perfusion is the sum of macrovascular and microvascular insufficiencies.
- It is important to perform both microvascular and macrovascular assessments of patients with chronic wounds.
- Microvascular assessment may be performed at the local, regional, and systemic level.
- Physicians can utilize microvascular assessment tools to assist in choosing, altering, and monitoring therapies in wound care patients to optimize outcomes.
- Emerging technologies of SPP, hyperspectral imaging, and sublingual CO_2 measurement may provide clinically useful microvascular information.
- SPP can:
  - evaluate microvascular physiology and perfusion
  - complement macrovascular assessment (pulse volume recording)
  - determine level of amputation
  - evaluate results of revascularization during procedure
- Hyperspectral imaging can:
  - evaluate tissue oxygenation in an anatomically relevant fashion
  - predict which diabetic foot ulcers will heal
  - predict which areas of tissue are predisposed to breakdown
  - help determine level of amputation and plan surgical procedures
- Sublingual CO_2 measurement may be used to evaluate for:
  - adequacy of systemic circulation
  - early sepsis
  - dehydration/overhydration
  - detrimental effects on peripheral circulation of drugs such as β-blockers

AUTHOR DISCLOSURE STATEMENT

Jenny Freeman is a consultant to Exostat Medical, Inc.

REFERENCES

1. Reiber GE, Boyko EJ, and Smith DG: Lower extremity foot ulcers and amputations in diabetes, Chapter 18. In: *Diabetes in America*, 2nd edition. National Diabetes Data Group, National Institutes of Health, National Institute of Diabetes and Digestive and Kidney Diseases. Bethesda, MD: NIH Publication No. 95–1468, 1995, pp. 409–428. www.diabetes.niddk.nih.gov/dm/pubs/America/pdf/chapter18.pdf.

2. Hirsch AT, Haskal ZJ, Hertzer NR, Bakal CW, Creager MA, Halperin JL, Hiratzka LF, Murphy WR, Olin JW, Puschett JB, Rosenfield KA, Sacks D, Stanley JC, Taylor LM Jr., White CJ, White J, White RA, Antman EM, Smith SC Jr., Adams CD, Anderson JL, Faxon DP, Fuster V, Gibbons RJ, Hunt SA, Jacobs AK, Nishimura R, Ornato JP, Page RL, and Riegel B: American Association for Vascular Surgery; Society for Vascular Surgery; Society for Cardiovascular Angiography and Interventions; Society for Vascular Medicine and Biology; Society of Interventional Radiology; ACC/AHA Task Force on Practice Guidelines Writing Committee to Develop Guidelines for the Management of Patients With Peripheral Arterial Disease; American Association of Cardiovascular and Pulmonary Rehabilitation; National Heart, Lung, and Blood Institute; Society for Vascular Nursing; TransAtlantic Inter-Society Consensus; Vascular Disease Foundation: ACC/AHA 2005 Practice Guidelines for the management of patients with peripheral arterial disease (lower extremity, renal, mesenteric, and abdominal aortic): a collaborative report from the American Association for Vascular Surgery/Society for Vascular Surgery, Society for Cardiovascular Angiography and Interventions, Society for Vascular Medicine and Biology, Society of Interventional Radiology, and the ACC/AHA Task Force on Practice Guidelines (Writing Committee to Develop Guidelines for the Management of Patients with Peripheral Arterial Disease): endorsed by the American Association of Cardiovascular and Pulmonary Rehabilitation; National Heart, Lung, and Blood Institute; Society for Vascular Nursing; TransAtlantic Inter-Society Consensus; and Vascular Disease Foundation. www.circ.ahajournals.org/cgi/reprint/113/11/e463.

3. Iida O, Nanto S, Uematsu M, Morozumi T, Akahori H, and Nagata S: Endovascular therapy for limb salvage in a case of critical lower limb ischemia resulting from fibromuscular dysplasia. J Vasc Surg 2007; **46:** 803.

4. Castronuovo JJ, Adera HM, Smiell JM, and Price RM: Skin perfusion pressure measurement is valuable in the diagnosis of critical limb ischemia. J Vasc Surg 1997; **26:** 629.

5. Castronuovo JJ: The role of skin perfusion pressure and transcutaneous partial pressure oxygen measurements in chronic critical limb ischemia. In: *Vascular Diagnosis*, 1st edition, Chapter 23, edited by Mansour MA and Labropoulos N. Philadelphia, PA: Elsevier Saunders, 2005, pp. 247–255.

6. Yamada T, Ohta T, Ishibashi H, Sugimoto I, Iwata H, Takahashi M, and Kawanishi J: Clinical reliability and utility of skin perfusion pressure measurement in ischemic limbs—comparison with other noninvasive diagnostic methods. J Vasc Surg 2008; **47:** 318.

7. Schechter R and Bailey B: Paired non-invasive vascular testing modalities for clinical utility and arterial disease assessment. Diabetic Foot Conference, 2008 (Abstract/Poster Presentation). www.opsi.com/documents/DFCon2008PosterAbstracts.pdf.

8. Okamoto K, Oka M, Maesato K, Ikee R, Mano T, Moriya H, Ohtake T, and Kobayashi S: Peripheral arterial occlusive disease is more prevalent in patients with hemodialysis: comparison with the findings of multidetector-row computed tomography. Am J Kidney Dis 2006; **48:** 269.

9. Akahori H, Uematsu M, Morozumi T, Watanabe T, Awata M, Ohnishi T, Nanto S, Iida O, Ohshima F, Minamiguchi H, Yano M, Yasui H, and Nagata S: Magnitude of the improvement in skin perfusion pressure is as important as skin perfusion pressure immediately following intervention for predicting limb salvage in critical limb ischemia. J Am Coll Cardiol, March 6, 2007, p. 316A (Abstract). www.content.onlinejacc.org/cgi/reprint/49/9_Suppl_A/315A.pdf.

10. Kellicut DC, Weiswasser JM, Arora S, Freeman J, Lew RA, Shuman C, and Mansfield JM: Emerging technology: hyperspectral imaging. Perspect Vasc Surg Endovasc Ther 2004; **16:** 53.

11. Greenman RI, Panasyuk S, Wang X, Lyons TE, Dinh T, Longorio L, Giurini JM, Freeman J, Khaodhiar L, and Veves A: Early changes in the skin microcirculation and muscle metabolism of the diabetic foot. Lancet 2005; **366:** 1711.

12. Freeman J, Nouvong A, Mohler E, Davis B, Medenilla E, Tajaddini E, Cornejo M, Arriga W, Panasyuk, Schomacker K, and Veves A: Microcirculatory changes in diabetic subjects. Circulation 2007; **116:** II_837 (Abstract).

13. Khaodhiar L, Dinh T, Schomacker KT, Panasyuk SV, Freeman JE, Lew R, Vo T, Panasyuk AA, Lima C, Giurini JM, Lyons TE, and Veves A: The use of medical hyperspectral technology to evaluate microcirculatory changes in diabetic foot ulcers and to predict clinical outcomes. Diabetes Care 2007; **30:** 903.

14. Nouvong A, Davis B, Hoogwerf B, Tajadini A, Mohler E, and Medenilla E: Evaluation of diabetic foot ulcer healing with hyperspectral imaging of oxyhemoglobin and deoxyhemoglobin. Diabetes Care 2009; **32:** Number 11 2056–2061.

15. Keevey S, Davis V, Hoogwerf B, Mohler E, Medinilla E, Neverov M, Nouvong A, and Schomacker K: Hyperspectral imaging to assess and predict diabetic foot ulcers. Proceedings of 32nd Annual Conference of the American Society of Biomechanics, 2008 (Abstract). www.health.uottawa.ca/biomech/csb/Conference%20Proceedings/NACOB/Abstracts/284.pdf.

16. Sidawy A: Diabetic foot: lower extremity arterial disease and limb salvage, chapter 13. In: *Abnormalities of Microcirculation in Diabetes*. Philadelphia, PA: Lippincott Williams & Wilkins. p. 148.

17. Frykberg RG, Tierney E, and Tallis A: Applying hyperspectral imaging to limb preservation. Proceedings of 9th Annual New Cardiovascular Horizons, 2008. www.newcvhorizons.com/uploads/Abstract_751%5D.pdf.

18. Freeman JE, Schomacker KT, Panasyuk SV, Panasyuk AA, Lew RA, and Sidawy AN: The use of hyperspectral technology in a Cuff-Ischemia model. FASEB J 2007; **21:** 957. Svetlana V. Panasyuk1, Alexander A. Panasyuk1, Robert A. Lew2 and Anthony N. Sidawy3.

19. Johnson O, Slidell M, Kreishman P, Walcott R, Scanlon J, Arora S, Macsata R, and Sidawy A: Hyperspectral imaging: an emerging technology as a potential novel adjunct in assessing peripheral perfusion deficits and success of lower extremity revascularizations. J Am Coll Surg 2008; **207:** S114 (Abstract). www.journalacs.org/arti-article/S1072-7515(08)00883-1/pdf.

20. Sato Y, Weil M, and Tang W: Tissue hypercarbic acidosis as a marker of acute circulatory failure (shock). Chest 1998; **114:** 263.

21. Marik PE: Sublingual capnography: a clinical validation study. Chest 2001; **120:** 923.

22. Creteur J, De Backer D, Sakr Y, Koch M, and Vincent JL: Sublingual capnometry tracks microcirculatory changes in septic patients. Intensive Care Med 2006; **32:** 516. Epub 2006 Feb 17.

23. Jin X, Weil MH, Sun S, Tang W, Bisera J, and Mason, EJ: Decreases in organ blood flows associate with increases in sublingual PCO_2 during hemorrhagic shock. J Appl Physiol 1998; **85:** 2360.

24. Gordois A, Scuffham P, Sheerer A, Oglesby A, and Tobin J: The health care costs of diabetic peripheral neuropathy in the U.S. Diabetes Care 2003; **26:** 1790.

25. Sheehan P, Jones P, Caselli A, Giurini JM, and Veves A: Percent change in wound area of diabetic foot ulcers over a 4-week period is a robust predictor of complete healing in a 12-week prospective trial. Diabetes Care 2003; **26:** 1879.

26. Center for Disease Control: National Diabetes Fact Sheet, last modified: December 20, 2005. Content Source: National Center for Chronic Disease Prevention and Health Promotion, Division of Diabetes Translation. www.cdc.gov/diabetes/pubs/estimates.htm.

27. Singh N, Armstrong DG, and Lipsky BA: Preventing ulcers in patients with diabetes. JAMA 2005; **293:** 217.

28. Golomb BA, Dang TT, and Criqui MH: Peripheral arterial disease: morbidity and mortality implications. Circulation 2006; **114:** 688.

29. Mahoney EM, Wang K, Cohen DJ, Hirsch AT, Alberts MJ, Eagle K, Mosse M, Jackson JD, Steg G, and Bhatt DL on behalf of the REACH Registry Investigators: One-year costs in patients with a history of or at risk for atherothrombosis in the United States. Circ Cardiovasc Qual Outcomes 2008; **1:** 38.

30. NHLBI Workshop on Peripheral Arterial Disease (PAD): Developing a Public Awareness Campaign Meeting Summary, Bethesda Marriott Hotel, Bethesda, Maryland, January 15, 2003. U.S. Department of Health and Human Services, National Institutes of Health, National Heart, Lung, and Blood Institute. www.nhlbi.nih.gov/health/prof/heart/other/pad_sum.pdf.

INDEX